Skeletal Trauma of the Upper Extremity

Skeletal Trauma of the Upper Extremity

Edited by

Grant E. Garrigues, MD

Orthopaedic Surgeon
Associate Professor, Shoulder and Elbow Surgery
Rush University Medical Center
Chicago, Illinois

Marc J. Richard, MD

Associate Professor
Hand, Upper Extremity, and Microvascular Surgery
Department of Orthopaedic Surgery
Duke University Medical Center
Durham, North Carolina

Mark J. Gage, MD

Assistant Professor
Director of Orthopaedic Trauma
Duke University Hospital
Department of Orthopaedic Surgery
Duke University Medical Center
Durham, North Carolina

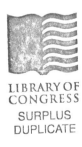

ELSEVIER

Elsevier
1600 John F. Kennedy Blvd.
Ste 1800
Philadelphia, PA 19103-2899

SKELETAL TRAUMA OF THE UPPER EXTREMITY   ISBN: 978-0-323-76180-2

Notice

Practitioners and researchers must always rely on their own experience and knowledge in evaluating and using any information, methods, compounds or experiments described herein. Because of rapid advances in the medical sciences, in particular, independent verification of diagnoses and drug dosages should be made. To the fullest extent of the law, no responsibility is assumed by Elsevier, authors, editors or contributors for any injury and/or damage to persons or property as a matter of products liability, negligence or otherwise, or from any use or operation of any methods, products, instructions, or ideas contained in the material herein.

Library of Congress Control Number: 2021940077

Cover Image: Francois Auguste Rene Rodin (1840-1917) sculpted *Le Penseur,* more commonly known as *The Thinker.* The juxtaposition of physical strength with intellect mirrors the complexities of the upper extremity and the various techniques used for its reconstruction. Just as Rodin hoped to demonstrate the beauty of the balance that exists between the physical and the intellectual, that same beauty and balance is reflected in these chapters outlining the treatment of upper limb disorders.

Content Strategist: Humayra Khan
Senior Content Development Manager: Kathryn DeFrancesco
Senior Content Development Specialist: Lisa M. Barnes
Publishing Services Manager: Shereen Jameel
Senior Project Manager: Manikandan Chandrasekaran
Illustration Buyer: Muthukumaran Thangaraj
Cover Design and Design Direction: Brian Salisbury

Printed in The United States of America.

Last digit is the print number: 9   8   7   6   5   4   3   2   1

Working together to grow libraries in developing countries

www.elsevier.com • www.bookaid.org

Contributors

Leonard Achenbach, MD
Department of Trauma Surgery
University Medical Centre Regensburg
Regensburg, Germany

Julie Adams, MD
Professor of Orthopaedic Surgery
University of Tennessee College of Medicine—Chattanooga
Chattanooga, Tennessee

Nicholas S. Adams, MD
Hand, Upper Extremity, and Microsurgery Fellow
Department of Orthopaedics
University of Arizona
Phoenix, Arizona

Julian McClees Aldridge III, MD, FAOA
Hand, Upper Extremity, and Microsurgery
Emerge Orthopaedics
Durham, North Carolina

Kyle M. Altman, MD
Resident Physician
Department of Orthopaedics
Prisma Health-Upstate
Greenville, South Carolina

Emilie J. Amaro, MD
Resident Physician
Department of Orthopaedic Surgery
Vanderbilt University
Nashville, Tennessee

Ivan Antosh, MD
Brooke Army Medical Center
San Antonio, Texas

Edward Arrington, MD
Madigan Army Medical Center
Tacoma, Washington

Francis J. Aversano, MD
Resident Physician
Department of Orthopaedic Surgery
Washington University School of Medicine
St. Louis, Missouri

Hassan J. Azimi, MD
Fellow
Department of Orthopaedic Surgery
Rush University Medical Center
Chicago, Illinois

Jonathan Barlow, MD
Assistant Professor
Department of Orthopaedic Surgery
Mayo Clinic
Rochester, Minnesota

Daniel P. Berthold, MD
Department of Orthopaedic Sports Medicine
Technical University of Munich
Munich, Germany;
Department of Orthopaedic Surgery
University of Connecticut
Farmington, Connecticut

Chelsea C. Boe, MD
The Doctors Clinic
Silverdale, Washington

Nicholas A. Bonazza, MD, MHA
Allegheny Health Network
Pittsburgh, Philadelphia

David M. Brogan, MD, MSc
Assistant Professor
Department of Orthopaedic Surgery
Washington University School of Medicine
St. Louis, Missouri

David F. Bruni, MD
Resident Physician
Department of Orthopaedic Surgery
University of Texas—Dell Medical School
Austin, Texas

Ryan P. Calfee, MD, MSc
Associate Professor
Department of Orthopaedic Surgery
Washington University School of Medicine
St. Louis, Missouri

Louis W. Catalano III, MD
Clinical Professor
Department of Orthopaedic Surgery
New York University Langone Medical Center
New York, New York

Brian Christie, MD, MPH
Assistant Professor of Surgery
Division of Plastic Surgery
Adjunct Assistant Professor of Orthopaedic Surgery
Indiana University School of Medicine
Indianapolis, Indiana

Zachary Christopherson, MD
Clinical Specialist
Department of Sports Physical Therapy;
Clinical Specialist
Orthopaedic Physical Therapy
Senior II Sports Physical Therapist
Duke University Athletics
Durham, North Carolina

Joseph B. Cohen, MD
Department of Orthopaedic Surgery
Loyola University Medical Center
Chicago, Illinois

Matthew R. Cohn, MD
Resident
Department of Orthopaedic Surgery
Rush University Medical Center
Chicago, Illinois

Brian J. Cole, MD, MBA
Professor
Department of Orthopaedic Surgery
Rush University Medical Center
Chicago, Illinois

Peter A. Cole, MD, FAOA
Division Medical Director
HealthPartners Trauma Network;
Orthopaedic Trauma Director
Regions Hospital;
Professor
University of Minnesota
St. Paul, Minnesota

Bert Cornelis, MD
Department of Orthopaedic and Traumatology
University Hospital Ghent
Ghent, Belgium

William M. Cregar, MD
Department of Orthopaedic Surgery
Rush University Medical Center
Chicago, Illinois

Gregory L. Cvetanovich, MD
Assistant Professor
Department of Clinical Orthopaedics
The Ohio State University Wexner Medical Center
Columbus, Ohio

Nicholas C. Danford, MD
Department of Orthopaedic Surgery
Columbia University Irving Medical Center/New York
    Presbyterian Hospital
New York, New York

Nicholas J. Dantzker, MD
Knoxville Orthopaedic Clinic
Knoxville, Tennessee

Malcolm R. DeBaun, MD
Department of Orthopaedic Surgery
Stanford University
Palo Alto, California

Lieven De Wilde, MD
Ghent University Hospital
Ghent, Belgium

Mihir J. Desai, MD
Associate Professor of Orthopaedic Surgery
Department of Orthopaedic Surgery
Vanderbilt University Medical Center
Nashville, Tennessee

Scott G. Edwards, MD
Professor or Orthopaedics Surgery
Director, Hand, Upper Extremity, and Microsurgery
    Fellowship
Department of Orthopaedics Surgery
University of Arizona College of Medicine
Phoenix, Arizona

Andy Eglseder Jr., MD
Professor of Orthopaedics
Department of Orthopaedics
University of Maryland School of Medicine
Baltimore, Maryland

Bryant P. Elrick, MD, MSc
Steadman Philippon Research Institute
Vail, Colorado;
Department of Orthopaedic Surgery
University of Colorado School of Medicine
Aurora, Colorado

Peter J. Evans, MD, PhD
Director, Upper Extremity Center
Department of Orthopaedic Surgery
Cleveland Clinic
Stuart, Florida

Gregory K. Faucher, MD
Assistant Professor
Department of Orthopaedic Surgery
Prisma Health University of South Carolina Greenville
Greenville, South Carolina

John J. Fernandez, MD
Midwest Orthopaedics at Rush
Rush University Medical Center
Chicago, Illinois

Zachary J. Finley, MD
Tulane Institute of Sports Medicine
Tulane University School of Medicine
New Orleans, Louisiana

Nathaniel Fogel, MD, MS
Resident Physician
Department of Orthopaedic Surgery
Stanford University School of Medicine
Redwood City, California

Antonio M. Foruria, MD, PhD
Shoulder and Elbow Reconstructive Surgery
Department of Orthopaedic Surgery
Fundación Jiménez Díaz
Associate Professor of Orthopaedics
Orthopaedic Surgery
Autonoma University
Madrid, Spain

Travis L. Frantz, MD
Resident
Department of Orthopaedics
The Ohio State University Wexner Medical Center
Columbus, Ohio

Michael C. Fu, MD
Midwest Orthopaedics at Rush University Medical Center
Chicago, Illinois

Michael J. Gardner, MD
Professor
Department of Orthopaedic Surgery
Stanford University
Palo Alto, California

R. Glenn Gaston, MD
Hand Fellowship Director
Department of Orthopaedics
OrthoCarolina Hand Center;
Chief of Hand Surgery
Atrium Musculoskeletal Institute
Charlotte, North Carolina

William B. Geissler, MD
Alan E. Freeland Chair of Hand Surgery,
Professor and Chief, Division of Hand and Upper Extremity
    Surgery,
Chief: Arthroscopic Surgery and Sports Medicine,
Department of Orthopaedic Surgery,
University of Mississippi Medical Center
Jackson, Mississippi

Ron Gilat, MD
Department of Orthopaedic Surgery
Rush University Medical Center
Chicago, Illinois

Robert J. Gillespie, MD
Michael and Grace Drusinsky Chair in Orthopaedic Surgery and
    Sports Medicine
Department of Orthopaedic Surgery;
Associate Professor
Department of Orthopaedic Surgery
Case Western Reserve University;
Orthopaedic Surgery Residency Program Director
Department of Orthopaedic Surgery
University Hospitals, Case Western Reserve University
Cleveland, Ohio

Joshua A. Gillis, MD
Assistant Professor
Department of Plastic Surgery
McFarlane Hand and Upper Limb Centre
London, Ontario, Canada

L. Henry Goodnough, MD, PhD
Department of Orthopaedic Surgery
Stanford University
Palo Alto, California

Jordan Grier, MD
Assistant Professor of Orthopaedic Surgery
Case Western Reserve University School of Medicine
Division of Hand & Upper Extremity Surgery
University Hospitals Cleveland Medical Center
Cleveland, Ohio

Warren C. Hammert, MD
Professor of Orthopaedic and Plastic Surgery
Department of Orthopaedic Surgery
University of Rochester Medical Center
Rochester, New York

Armodios M. Hatzidakis, MD
Western Orthopaedics P.C.
Medical Director, Rose Medical Center Shoulder Surgery Program
Fellowship Director, Western Orthopaedics and Rose Medical
    Center Shoulder and Elbow Fellowship
Denver, Colorado

Eric D. Haunschild, BS
Midwest Orthopaedics at Rush University Medical Center
Chicago, Illinois

Daniel E. Hess, MD
Clinical Assistant Professor
Department of Orthopaedic Surgery
Michigan State University College of Human Medicine
Spectrum Health Medical Group
Grand Rapids, Michigan

Bettina Hochreiter, MD
Resident
Department of Orthopaedics and Traumatology
Kantonsspital St. Gallen
St. Gallen, Switzerland

Rachel Honig, MD
Resident
Mayo Clinic
Rochester, Minnesota

Harry A. Hoyen, MD
Associate Professor
Department of Orthopaedic Surgery
Case Western Reserve University, MetroHealth Medical Center,
Cleveland, Ohio

Jerry I. Huang, MD
Associate Professor
Department of Orthopaedics and Sports Medicine
University of Washington Medical Center
Seattle, Washington

Thomas B. Hughes, MD
Associate Clinical Professor of Orthopaedic Surgery
Department of Orthopaedic Surgery
University of Pittsburgh School of Medicine
Pittsburgh, Pennsylvania

Jaclyn M. Jankowski, DO
Division of Orthopaedic Trauma
Department of Orthopaedic Surgery
Jersey City Medical Center—RWJBarnabas Health
Jersey City, New Jersey

Devon Jeffcoat, MD
Department of Orthopaedic Surgery
David Geffen School of Medicine at UCLA
Los Angeles, California

Pierce Johnson, MD
Department of Orthopaedic Surgery
University of Arizona College of Medicine—Phoenix
Phoenix, Arizona

Bernhard Jost, MD
Professor
Department of Orthopaedics and Traumatology
Kantonsspital St. Gallen
St. Gallen, Switzerland

Sanjeev Kakar, MD
Professor of Orthopaedics—College of Medicine
Department of Orthopaedic Surgery
Mayo Clinic
Rochester, Minnesota

Robin Kamal, MD
Assistant Professor, Chase Hand and Upper Limb Center
Department of Orthopaedic Surgery
Stanford University
Palo Alto, California

Robert A. Kaufmann, MD
Associate Professor
Department of Orthopaedic Surgery
University of Pittsburgh Medical Center
Pittsburgh, Pennsylvania

June Kennedy, PT, DPT
Physical Therapist
Duke Sports Medicine Physical Therapy
Duke University Health Systems;
Affiliate Clinical Faculty
Doctor of Physical Therapy Program
Duke University Medical Center
Durham, North Carolina

Thomas J. Kremen Jr., MD
Assistant Professor-in-Residence
Department of Orthopaedic Surgery
David Geffen School of Medicine at UCLA
Los Angeles, California

John E. Kuhn, MD, MS
Kenneth D. Schermerhorn Professor of Orthopaedics
Department of Orthopaedic Surgery
Vanderbilt University Medical Center
Nashville, Tennessee

Laurent Lafosse, MD
Chairman
Clinique Generale d'Annecy
Alps Surgical Institue
Annecy, France

Thibault Lafosse, MD
Clinique Générale d'Annecy
Alps Surgery Institute
Annecy, France

Chris Langhammer, MD, PhD
Assistant Professor
Department of Orthopaedic Trauma
University of Maryland
Baltimore, Maryland

Frank A. Liporace, MD
Chair of Orthopaedic Surgery
St. Barnabas Medical Center-RWJ Barnabas Health
Jersey City, New Jersey

Daniel A. London, MD, MS
Assistant Professor
Department of Orthopaedic Surgery
Missouri Orthopaedic Institute
University of Missouri
Columbia, Missouri

Bhargavi Maheshwer, BS
Research Fellow Division of Sports Medicine
Midwest Orthopaedics at Rush
Chicago, Illinois

Jed I. Maslow, MD
Assistant Professor
Department of Orthopaedic Surgery
Vanderbilt Orthopaedic Institute
Nashville, Tennessee

Nina Maziak, MD
Department of Shoulder and Elbow Surgery
Center for Musculoskeletal Surgery
Charite´–Universitaetsmedizin Berlin, Campus-Virchow
Berlin, Germany

Augustus D. Mazzocca, MS, MD
Professor and Director
The University of Connecticut Musculoskeletal Institute
Department of Orthopaedic Surgery
University of Connecticut
Farmington, Connecticut

Michael McKee, MD, FRCS(C)
Professor and Chairman, Department of Orthopaedic Surgery
University of Arizona College of Medicine—Phoenix
Phoenix, Arizona

Sunita Mengers, MD
Resident Physician
Department of Orthopaedic Surgery
University Hospitals, Case Western Reserve University
Cleveland, Ohio

Peter J. Millett, MD, MSc
Director of Shoulder Surgery
Shoulder, Knee, and Elbow Surgery and Sports Medicine
The Steadman Clinic
Chief Medical Officer
The Steadman Philippon Research Institute
Vail, Colorado

M. Christian Moody, MD
Hand and Upper Extremity Surgeon
Department of Orthopaedics
Prisma Health University of South Carolina School of Medicine
Greenville, South Carolina

Mark E. Morrey, MD, MSc
Associate Professor
Department of Orthopaedics;
Consultant
Department of Orthopaedics
Mayo Clinic
Rochester, Minnesota

Michael N. Nakashian, MD
Hand and Upper Extremity Surgeon
Brielle Orthopaedics
Brick, New Jersey

Andrew Neviaser, MD
Associate Professor of Orthopaedic Surgery
Ohio State University Wexner Medical Center
Columbus, Ohio

Gregory Nicholson, MD
Associate Professor
Sports Medicine and Shoulder & Elbow Surgery
Rush University Medical Center
Chicago, Illinois

Luke T. Nicholson, MD
Assistant Professor of Orthopaedic Surgery
Department of Orthopaedic Surgery
University of Southern California
Los Angeles, California

Philip C. Nolte, MD, MA
Steadman Philippon Research Institute
Vail, Colorado;
Department of Trauma and Orthopaedic Surgery
BG Trauma Center Ludwigshafen
Ludwigshafen, Germany

Michael J. O'Brien, MD
Associate Professor
Department of Orthopaedics
Tulane University School of Medicine
New Orleans, Louisiana

Marc J. O'Donnell, MD
Assistant Professor of Clinical Orthopaedics
Department of Orthopaedics
University of Rochester Medical Center
Rochester, New York

Reza Omid, MD
Associate Professor of Orthopaedic Surgery
Keck Medical Center of USC
Department of Orthopaedic Surgery
University of Southern California
Los Angeles, California

Jorge L. Orbay, MD
Medical Director
Department of Orthopaedic Surgery
The Miami Hand and Upper Extremity Institute
Miami, Florida

Maureen O'Shaughnessy, MD
Assistant Professor
Department of Orthopaedic Surgery
University of Kentucky
Lexington, Kentucky

A. Lee Osterman, MD
Professor
Department of Orthopaedics
Thomas Jefferson
Philadelphia, Pennsylvania

Belén Pardos Mayo, MD
Orthopaedic Surgeon
Department of Orthopaedic and Traumatology Surgery
Hospital Universitario Fundación Jiménez Díaz
Madrid, Spain

Christine C. Piper, BA, MD
Fellow, Shoulder & Elbow Division
Department of Orthopaedic Surgery
University of Pennsylvania
Philadelphia, Pennsylvania

Austin A. Pitcher, MD, PhD
Hand and Upper Extremity Surgeon Webster Orthopaedics
Oakland, California

David Potter, MD
Professor of Orthopaedics
Sanford Orthopaedics and Sports Medicine
Sanford USD Medical Center
Sioux Falls, South Dakota

Kevin Rasuli, MD, MEd, FRCSC
Department of Orthopaedic Surgery
Bassett Healthcare Network
Cooperstown, New York

Lee M. Reichel, MD
Associate Professor Orthopaedic Surgery
Department of Surgery and Perioperative Care
Dell Medical School
Austin, Texas

Jonathan C. Riboh, MD
OrthoCarolina
Charlotte, North Carolina
Atrium Health Musculoskeletal Institute
Charlotte, North Carolina

David Ring, MD, PhD
Associate Dean for Comprehensive Care
Department of Surgery and Perioperative Care
Dell Medical School—The University of Texas at Austin
Austin, Texas

Marco Rizzo, MD
Professor
Department of Orthopaedic Surgery
Mayo Clinic
Rochester, Minnesota

David Ruch, MD
Chief of Division of Hand Surgery
Department of Orthopaedic Surgery
Duke University Medical Center
Durham, North Carolina

Frank A. Russo, MD
Hand and Upper Extremity Surgery
Department of Orthopaedic Surgery
Providence Medical Institute
Los Angeles, California

Casey Sabbag, MS, MD
Hand Surgery Fellow
Department of Orthopaedic Surgery
OrthoCarolina Hand Center
Charlotte, North Carolina

Joaquin Sanchez-Sotelo, MD, PhD
Consultant and Professor of Orthopaedic Surgery
Chair, Division of Shoulder and Elbow Surgery
Mayo Clinic
Rochester, Minnesota

Felix H. Savoie, MD
Ray J. Haddad Professor and Chairman
Department of Orthopaedics
Tulane University School of Medicine
New Orleans, Louisiana

Markus Scheibel, MD
Professor
Department of Shoulder and Elbow Surgery
Center for Musculoskeletal Surgery
Charite´–Universitaetsmedizin Berlin, Campus-Virchow
Berlin, Germany;
Department of Shoulder and Elbow Surgery
Schulthess Clinic
Zurich, Switzerland

Lisa K. Schroder, BSME, MBA
Director, Geriatric and Orthopaedic Trauma Academic Programs
Department of Orthopaedic Surgery
University of Minnesota/Regions Hospital
St. Paul, Minnesota

Benjamin W. Sears, MD
Orthopaedic Surgeon
Department of Orthopaedics
Western Orthopaedics
Denver, Colorado

Anshu Singh, MD
Shoulder and Elbow Surgeon
Department of Orthopaedics
Kaiser Permanente;
Associate Professor
Department of Orthopaedic Surgery
University of California, San Diego
San Diego, California

Christian Spross, MD
Consultant
Department of Orthopaedics and Traumatology
Kantonsspital St. Gallen
St. Gallen, Switzerland

Ramesh C. Srinivasan, MD
Adjunct Clinical Professor
Department of Orthopaedic Surgery
University of Texas Health Science Center of San Antonio
The Hand Center of San Antonio
San Antonio, Texas

Scott Steinmann, MD
Emeritus Professor of Orthopaedic Surgery
Mayo Clinic
Rochester, Minnesota;
Professor and Chair of Orthopaedic Surgery
University of Tennessee College of Medicine
Chattanooga, Tennessee

Eloy Tabeayo, MD
Upper Extremity Surgeon
Assistant Professor of Orthopaedic Surgery
Department of Orthopaedic Surgery
Albert Einstein College of Medicine
Montefiore Medical Center
Bronx, New York

Ryan Tarr, DO
Hand Surgeon
Orthopaedic Specialists of North Carolina
Raleigh, North Carolina

Tracy Tauro, BS, BA
Researcher
Department of Orthopaedics
Rush University Medical Center
Chicago, Illinois

Paul A. Tavakolian, MD
Hand and Upper Extremity Surgeon
Department of Orthopaedic Surgery
University of Arizona—Phoenix
Phoenix, Arizona

John M. Tokish, MD
Professor
Orthopaedic Surgery;
Fellowship Director
Orthopaedic Sports Medicine
Mayo Clinic Arizona
Scottsdale, Arizona;
Team Orthopaedic Surgeon
Arizona Coyotes Hockey Club

Rick Tosti, MD
Assistant Professor
Orthopaedic Surgery
Thomas Jefferson University
Devon, Pennsylvania

Leigh-Anne Tu, MD
Orthopaedic Surgeon
Illinois Bone and Joint Institute
Morton Grove, Illinois

Colin L. Uyeki, BA
Clinical Research Assistant
Department of Orthopaedic Surgery
University of Connecticut Health Center
Farmington, Connecticut

Alexander Van Tongel, MD, PhD
Professor
Department of Orthopaedic and Traumatology
University Hospital Ghent
Ghent, Belgium

David R. Veltre, MD
Hand and Upper Extremity Surgeon
Department of Orthopaedic Surgery
Southwestern Vermont Medical Center
Bennington, Vermont

Nikhil N. Verma, MD
Orthopaedic Surgery
Division of Sports Medicine
Midwest Orthopaedics at Rush
Chicago, Illinois

J. Brock Walker, MD
Resident
Department of Orthopaedic Surgery
University of Arizona College of Medicine—Phoenix
Phoenix, Arizona

Adam C. Watts, MBBS, BSc, FRCS (Tr and Ortho)
Consultant Elbow Surgeon
Upper Limb Unit
Wrightington Hospital
Wigan, United Kingdom

Brady T. Williams, MD
Department of Orthopaedic Surgery
University of Colorado Medical Center
Aurora, Colorado

Joel C. Williams, MD
Department of Orthopaedic Surgery
Rush University Medical Center
Chicago, Illinois

David Wilson, MD, FAAOS
Chief
Hand & Elbow Surgery
Brooke Army Medical Center
San Antonio, Texas

Theodore S. Wolfson, MD
OrthoConnecticut
Danbury, Connecticut

Robert W. Wysocki, MD
Associate Professor
Department of Orthopaedic Surgery
Rush University Medical Center
Chicago, Illinois

Jeffrey Yao, MD
Professor
Department of Orthopaedic Surgery
Stanford University Medical Center
Palo Alto, California

Richard S. Yoon, MD
Director, Orthopaedic Research
Division of Orthopaedic Trauma and Adult Reconstruction
Department of Orthopaedic Surgery
Jersey City Medical Center—RWJBarnabas Health
Jersey City, New Jersey

Foreword

Dr. Frankle and I were asked to write a foreword for this text edited by Grant E. Garrigues, MD, Marc J. Richard, MD, and Mark J. Gage, MD; we are delighted to do so. The addition of new textbooks that provide information to aid in the treatment of patients with upper-extremity trauma become valuable as our understanding and experience improves. The description of the pathoanatomic classifications, treatment options, indications for surgery, different surgical approaches, and outcomes that are reasonably expected when applying these methods allows us to access lots of information in a single source. The illustrations and descriptions of surgical technique are clearly the highlight of this book. They provide clear instructions for applying the various surgical options in managing traumatic injuries to the upper extremities.

The editors have assembled a great combination of senior leaders in the field and young, gifted clinicians and educators to create this excellent text, *Skeletal Trauma of the Upper Extremity*. It is well referenced for readers who would like to delve deeper into the original articles and texts. The balance between in-depth discussion and surgical technique is excellent. This will be a durable reference text for those of us who take care of patients with upper-extremity trauma.

Dr. Frankle and I respect and are familiar with all three editors. A project like this requires a hardworking team, including the editors as well as the publisher's project managers and other key personnel. We have both worked closely with Dr. Garrigues on a number of projects; he exceeds expectations on a regular basis and has already achieved so much in his career. This text by his co-editors and him is just the next chapter. From my own personal perspective, I am always happy and proud to see one of my previous fellows excel. Grant was a superstar from his first day on the job. He will be a leader in our field for years to come and I am very proud of him. I applaud Grant, his co-editors, and the many authors of this superb text.

Gerald R. Williams, Jr., MD
Mark Frankle, MD

Introduction

Orthopaedic trauma of the upper extremity is common, diverse, and complex. This should not be surprising given the myriad roles of the upper limb—so diverse in function and requisitely complex in form. As humans, the upper extremity is the tool we use to interact with and manipulate the world around us. Our bipedal nature, opposable thumb, and extensive range of motion create an upper limb made for daily tasks such as grasping, pushing, and pulling. But this elegant anatomy also makes us capable of pitching a 100 mph fastball, playing concert violin, or knocking out an opponent in the ring. The torsional embryology that has led to this highly specialized anatomy of the upper limb means that neurovascular structures wrap around the extremity, complicating exposures. The diverse injuries and functions of the upper extremity mean that the surgeon must be comfortable with a wide variety of techniques, in order to provide the optimal treatment to their patients. Our aim with this textbook was to bring international experts and thought leaders in all the various disciplines that address upper extremity trauma under one title—shoulder and elbow surgeons, traumatologists, hand and upper-extremity surgeons, sports medicine surgeons, physical and occupational therapists. Our aim was to write the book you keep in your call room that gets you through the night!

As an example of the frequency, diversity, and complexity of these injures, consider the clavicle. The clavicle is a commonly fractured bone and, depending on the patient and the pathoanatomy, the ideal treatment can range from a simple sling to internal fixation of both fracture and associated ligamentous injury. To thoroughly master treatment of this "simple" bone, the surgeon may, at times, need to employ skills most frequently used by such an array of specialists from traumatologists to shoulder specialists to sports medicine arthroscopists to thoracic surgeons.

Other fractures of the upper limb—including distal radius and proximal humerus, routinely make the list of most commonly encountered fractures. The proximal humerus is another perfect example of a fracture that can be best treated with treatment ranging from a sling to open reduction and internal fixation (with plate or nail) to arthroplasty with reverse total shoulder arthroplasty. These diverse skill sets are not typically taught in the same fellowship and, as upper-limb surgery advances so quickly, even those who have training in these injuries will need frequent updates on best practices and the latest techniques.

The editors of this book come from a background of running an upper-limb trauma service at a large, academic, Level-I trauma center. They come with different fellowship training (Dr. Grant E. Garrigues—Shoulder and Elbow Surgery; Dr. Marc J. Richard—Hand and Upper Extremity; Dr. Mark J. Gage—Orthopaedic Trauma Surgery). The esteemed chapter authors are, likewise, a diverse group selected for their international expertise in upper extremity trauma treatment. This diversity of thought leadership is intended to allow you, the surgeon, to learn the fracture fixation skills of a traumatologist, the arthroplasty techniques of a shoulder surgeon, the arthroscopy skills of a sports medicine arthroscopist, and the hand surgery knowledge of a hand specialist. Any orthopaedic surgeon taking call will be faced with these common injuries, and with this textbook, will be well-prepared to care for the entirety of the upper limb.

The book is organized into two types of entries. The traditional chapter format has been updated with rich illustrations and also allows for an in-depth understanding of a topic—anatomy, fracture classification, results, and complications of various treatment options. *Technique spotlights* are a deep dive into treatment techniques from the thought leaders who made them possible. This section includes detailed surgical steps, indications, preoperative evaluation, as well as pearls and pitfalls.

Whether you are a resident, fellow, or attending orthopaedic surgeon, we hope you enjoy this textbook. May it help you get your patients from the sudden and unfortunate disability of an upper limb trauma, back to throwing a fastball, playing the violin, or throwing a punch in the ring.

Sincerely,
The Editors

Grant E. Garrigues, MD
Marc J. Richard, MD
Mark J. Gage MD

Contents

Video Contents

1

Sternoclavicular Joint Dislocations

NICHOLAS J. DANTZKER AND JOHN E. KUHN

Relevant Anatomy

The sternoclavicular joint (SCJ) is a saddle-shaped, diarthrodial synovial joint that provides the only bony articulation between the axial skeleton and upper extremity. It is an important fulcrum for the movement of the shoulder girdle, as translation and rotation of the clavicle through the SCJ and acromioclavicular joint (ACJ) dictate the position of scapula as it moves against the posterior chest wall.[1,2] The joint is formed by the articulation of the medial end of the clavicle, the clavicular notch of the sternum, and the cartilage of the first rib. Developmentally, the clavicle is the first bone to ossify in utero; however, the physis of the medial clavicle is the last to fuse in adulthood, doing so at a mean age of 23–25 years.[3] The medial clavicle articulates with both the reciprocal notch of the sternum and the superior surface of the first costal cartilage. The articulating surfaces of the clavicle and sternum are not fully congruent, with less than half of the medial clavicular surface articulating with the corresponding articular facet on the sternum. Due to this incongruent osseous geometry, the SCJ is inherently unstable and has been described as the least constrained joint in the human body (Fig. 1.1).[4] Functionally, however, the SCJ is remarkably stable, owing to the robust surrounding fibrocartilaginous, ligamentous, and muscular structures.

Positioned between the clavicle and the sternum is a well-developed fibrocartilaginous intra-articular disc, which is closely associated with the medial end of the clavicle and is analogous to the menisci of the knee or the intra-articular disc of the ACJ (Fig. 1.2). The SCJ disc has robust insertions on the posterosuperior aspect of the clavicle, with peripheral attachments to the anterior and posterior sternoclavicular ligaments and surrounding joint capsule.[5] The thickness of the disc tapers centrally, causing a central concavity on both the sternal and clavicular sides. This disc undergoes physiologic degenerative changes with aging and is often incomplete by the seventh decade of life.[6]

The stabilizing ligamentous structures of the SCJ include the costoclavicular ligament, anterior and posterior sternoclavicular ligaments, the interclavicular ligament, and the intra-articular disco-ligamentous complex[4,5,7–9] (Fig. 1.1). The costoclavicular ligament is a short, robust ligament connecting the first-rib costal cartilage to the medial end of the clavicle. It consists of an anterior and posterior fasciculus, separated by a bursa. From its origin on the first rib, the costoclavicular ligament extends from medial to lateral to insert on the anteroinferior aspect of the clavicle. The costoclavicular ligament

has the largest footprint of the SCJ-associated ligaments, with its insertion on the clavicle reported to average 182.8 mm.[2,5] Several anatomic studies have sought to establish the distance between the inferior articular surface of the medial clavicle and the most medial aspect of the clavicular insertion of the costoclavicular ligament, reporting average distances ranging from 1.0 to 1.3 cm.[5,7,8] The anterior sternoclavicular ligament is an oblique capsular thickening that courses from inferomedial to superolateral across the anterior aspect of the SCJ and serves as the anterior attachment of the intra-articular disc. The posterior sternoclavicular ligament is a diffuse thickening of the posterior joint capsule with broad attachments on both the posterosuperior sternum and posteroinferior clavicle. The interclavicular ligament is a discrete ligament that extends between the medial ends of the clavicle and is continuous with deep cervical fascia superiorly.[5,9]

The SCJ is enveloped by a closely applied muscular layer both anteriorly and posteriorly. Anteriorly, the sternal insertion of sternocleidomastoid muscle (SCM) is a tendinous extension of the muscle that covers the medial aspect of the SCJ (Fig. 1.3). The clavicular head of the SCM has a broad, linear insertion on the superior surface of the clavicle, with the most medial extent of the tendon reported to be an average of 9.9 mm lateral to the superior articular margin of the clavicle.[5] The subclavius originates on the inferomedial aspect of the clavicle and courses obliquely to insert on the lateral aspect of the first-rib costal cartilage. Posteriorly, the sternohyoid is a thin strap muscle that inserts onto the posterior aspect of the SCJ joint capsule and clavicle. The sternothyroid runs deep to the sternohyoid, with a more inferior insertion on the posterior aspect of the sternum and costal cartilage. A fascial attachment is present between the right and left muscle bellies of both strap muscles, with a midline raphe that inserts onto the posterior aspect of the sternum. No vascular structures are present anterior to this fascial layer.

Biomechanics

The SCJ is one of five articulations of the shoulder girdle and plays a critical role in maintaining normal glenohumeral and scapulothoracic motion. The normally functioning SCJ achieves 35 degrees of movement in both the horizontal and coronal planes, as well 45 degrees of rotation along its longitudinal axis.[10] The majority of scapulothoracic movement occurs through the SCJ and relies on both translation and rotation between the sternum and clavicle.

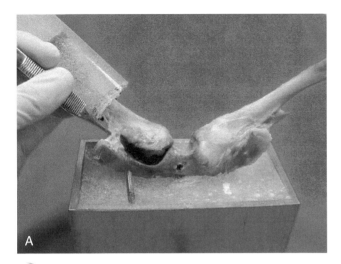

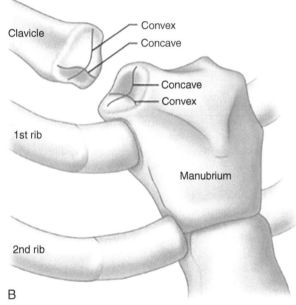

• **Fig. 1.1** Bony anatomy of the sternoclavicular joint. The sternal facet has less than half of the articulating surface of the medial clavicle, as such the sternoclavicular joint is highly unconstrained. (Illustration B from Warth RJ, Millett PJ. (2015) The Sternoclavicular Joint. In: Physical Examination of the Shoulder. Springer, New York, NY. https://doi.org/10.1007/978-1-4939-2593-3_8.)

In regard to stability, several authors have proposed the costoclavicular ligament to be the primary stabilizer of the SCJ.[7,8,11–13] Abbott and Lucas[12] reported that medial clavicle resections that included any portion of bone lateral to the costoclavicular ligament resulted in proximal displacement and instability of the remaining clavicle. These findings were further supported by an investigation of medial clavicle resections performed by Rockwood et al.,[13] in which they reported superior clinical outcomes in patients whose resection spared the costoclavicular ligament as compared with those in which the ligament was violated. A close review of this literature, however, provides little biomechanical evidence for the importance of the costoclavicular ligament in the normally functioning and intact SCJ joint.

The most rigorous biomechanical investigation of the SCJ ligamentous structures was performed by Spencer and Kuhn,[4] in which they established the contribution of each individual ligament to the translational stability of the joint. In their study, the anterior capsule, posterior capsule, costoclavicular ligament, and interclavicular ligament were singularly divided, and the resulting change

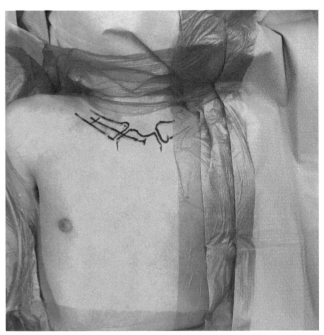

• **Fig. 1.2** Ligamentous support of the sternoclavicular joint. The posterior sternoclavicular joint capsule is the primary restraint to both posterior and anterior translation of the joint (Spencer et al., 2002). (Kuhn JE. Treatment. In: Arciero RA, Cordasco FA, Provencher MT, eds. *Shoulder and Elbow Injuries in Athletes*. Philadelphia, PA: Elsevier; 2018:362; Fig. 17.3.)

in anterior and posterior translation of the SCJ was recorded using a custom biomechanical testing fixture. The results of this study clearly showed the posterior capsule to be the most important stabilizing structure to both anterior and posterior translation of the SCJ. The anterior capsule was shown to be a significant, but less important stabilizer to anterior translation. Interestingly, neither the costoclavicular nor interclavicular ligaments were not found to be important primary stabilizers of the SCJ.

Pathoanatomy

Sternoclavicular injuries are rare, accounting for 1% of all dislocations and 3% of all shoulder girdle injuries.[14] Owing to the strong supporting ligamentous structures, traumatic dislocations of the SCJ generally only occur after a tremendous, high-energy force has been applied through the shoulder, such as those seen in collisions during contact sports or motor vehicle collisions.[3,9,15,16] Several epidemiological studies on traumatic SCJ dislocations have reported motor vehicle collisions to be the most common cause of injury (40%), while sports injuries are also common (25%). The remaining SCJ injuries resulted from a combination of falls and other miscellaneous low-energy traumatic mechanisms.[3,16,17]

Traumatic dislocations can result from a force applied directly to the SCJ or from an indirect compressive force applied to the lateral aspect of the shoulder, which is transmitted along the long axis of the clavicle. When an SCJ dislocation occurs, the direction is classified as either anterior or posterior based on the direction of displacement of the medial clavicle, with anterior dislocations occurring much more commonly than posterior.[3,16,18] The direction of displacement of the clavicle is dependent on the position of ipsilateral shoulder at the moment of impact. If the shoulder is rolled backward (i.e., the acromion is posterior to the sternum) during lateral compression, the force applied to the clavicle produces an anterior dislocation of the SCJ. When the shoulder is at rest and in a neutral anatomic orientation, the acromion is positioned posterior

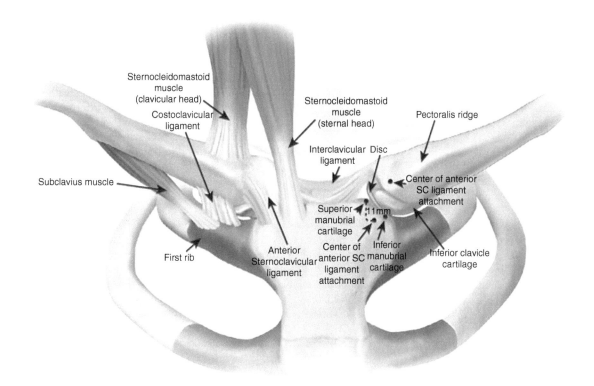

• **Fig. 1.3** Muscle attachments of the sternoclavicular *(SC)* joint. (From Lee JT, Campbell KJ, Michalski MP, et al. Surgical anatomy of the sternoclavicular joint: a qualitative and quantitative anatomical study. *J Bone Joint Surg Am*. 2014;96(19):e166.)

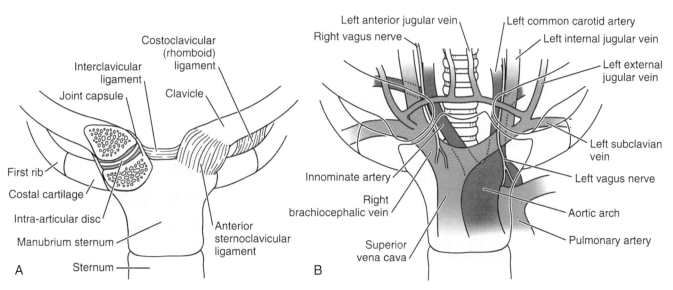

• **Fig. 1.4** Retrosternal vascular anatomy: (A) ligaments and (B) vasculature.

to the sternum. It is this spatial relationship, as well the fact that the posterior capsular ligaments are the strongest of the sternoclavicular ligaments, that likely explains why anterior dislocations are much more common.[3,4,15] Conversely, if the shoulder is rolled forward (i.e., the acromion is anterior to the sternum), a laterally applied compressive force will produce a posterior dislocation of the SCJ. Posterior dislocations can also result from a direct posterior force applied to the anteromedial aspect of the clavicle.[3,15]

Although posterior SCJ dislocations represent a small subset of a rare injury that only accounts for 1% of dislocations overall, the consequences of this injury can be devastating and life-threatening

due to the close proximity of the critical cardiopulmonary structures located in retrosternal mediastinal space.[19–27] The critical mediastinal structures include the great vessels of the neck, subclavian vessels, brachial plexus, brachiocephalic vein, trachea, and esophagus (Fig. 1.4). Serious sequelae of posterior SCJ dislocations reported in the literature include brachial plexus compression, pneumothorax, respiratory distress, dysphagia, vascular compromise, and death.[19–27] Worman and Leagus[19] performed a retrospective review of patients with posterior SCJ dislocations and reported that 16 of 60 patients (27%) had a serious injury of the trachea, esophagus, or great vessels. Other studies have reported compression of critical mediastinal structures in as many as 30% of posterior SCJ dislocations with a 3%–4% mortality rate.[17] Ponce et al.[28] investigated the proximity of critical mediastinal structures to the SCJ by reviewing computed tomography (CT) angiograms of the neck of 49 patients and reported that the nearest critical structure is, on average, only 6.6 mm deep to the posterior aspect of the SCJ. The closest structure in most patients was the brachiocephalic vein, but in >20% of patients the closest structure was an artery.

Clinical Presentation

Patients who have a traumatic injury to the SCJ will have pain and swelling over the joint. If involved in athletics, they may come off the field with the arm hanging at the side and an unwillingness to move the arm. Patients involved in motor vehicle accidents will have pain and swelling over the SCJ. If the dislocation is posterior, some patients will present with symptoms related to injury to the retrosternal structures, including thoracic outlet syndrome,[26] mediastinal compression,[29] subclavian artery compression,[25] innominate vein compression,[30] and compression of the brachial plexus.[31] Traumatic venous tearing has also been reported with acute posterior SCJ dislocations.[32,33]

Although severe pain and deformity are commonly present with traumatic SCJ dislocations, determining the direction of the dislocation by clinical examination can be surprisingly difficult due to significant swelling. Moreover, the medial physis of the clavicle does not fuse until 23–25 years of age, predisposing patients <25 years to physeal fractures with clavicular displacement rather than true SCJ dislocations.[3,34] The unique ossification of the medial clavicle can lead to further difficulty in clinically diagnosing traumatic SCJ instability in the young adult population, with some studies reporting clavicular physeal fractures as accounting for up to 16% of traumatic SCJ injuries in the adult population.[16] Proper imaging of the SCJ joint is thus critical to the accurate diagnosis of traumatic SCJ injuries and associated injuries of the critical surrounding structures.

Radiographic Evaluation

Unfortunately, routine radiographs of the chest are of limited utility in diagnosing SCJ disruption due to the overlap of the medial clavicle, sternum, ribs, and vertebrae. However, Rockwood[35] developed an oblique view of the SCJ, commonly called "the serendipity view," that captures both of SCJs and medial clavicles and allows for comparison of the injured and uninjured sides. The serendipity view is obtained by centering X-ray beam on the SCJ with the beam tilted 40 degrees cephalically. If the injured SCJ is dislocated posteriorly, the clavicle will appear to be displaced inferiorly when compared with the uninjured side. If the injured SCJ is dislocated anteriorly, the clavicle will appear to be displaced superiorly when compared with the uninjured side.

CT has become of the study of choice for the evaluation of traumatic SCJ injuries, as it can easily distinguish between medial clavicle or transphyseal fractures, sprains, and true dislocations. Moreover, a CT of the chest can identify injuries to the structures that surround the SCJ and provide a rapid diagnosis of potentially devastating complications.[3,34]

Classification

SCJ instability can be classified based on the direction of dislocation (anterior and posterior), etiology (traumatic and atraumatic), duration (acute and chronic), or severity (sprain, ligament rupture without dislocation, and ligament rupture with joint dislocation). The most commonly cited classification system for traumatic SCJ injuries was first proposed by Allman in 1967[36] and stratifies injuries based on the degree of joint subluxation and ligamentous damage. Grade I injuries are defined as sprains of the SCJ capsule without rupture of the supporting ligaments or joint laxity. Grade II injuries are defined by rupture of the sternoclavicular ligaments without injury to the costoclavicular ligament and only mild deformity. Grade III injuries are defined by rupture of the sternoclavicular and costoclavicular ligaments resulting in dislocation of the joint. This system, however, does not consider the direction of displacement or chronicity of the injury and thus has limited utility in guiding treatment or establishing operative indications. In response to these limitations, several authors have proposed more expansive and detailed classification systems with a focus on guiding treatment and providing indications for operative intervention of SCJ dislocations.[15,37] Jaggard et al.[15] described a five-tier classification system that incorporates direction of displacement, mode of displacement, and degree of displacement according to the Allman classification (Table 1.1). More recently, Sewell et al.[37] proposed utilizing the Stanmore triangle system, originally developed as an aid in classifying and managing patients with glenohumeral instability, to classify SCJ instability (Fig. 1.5).[38] In type I instability, there is a clear history of trauma. In type II, there is structural capsular pathology without a history of trauma. In type III instability, there is no structural abnormality, but a definite muscle-patterning component underlying the instability. This system allows for the presence of multiple concurrent pathologies and for these pathologies the change over time. Moreover, a patient's response to treatment can be monitored using the same system. Although a patient may present with SCJ instability caused by a certain initial pathology, they would likely migrate around the triangle, depending on the intervention and their subsequent healing and improvement.

Treatment Options

The types of injury and treatment approaches are detailed in Table 1.2. The appropriate treatment of a patient presenting with an SCJ dislocation is dependent on the acuity and severity of the injury, the direction of displacement of the medial clavicle, and the integrity of the ligamentous stabilizers of the SCJ.

TABLE 1.1 Classification of Sternoclavicular Joint Injury

Classification	Disruption	Treatment
Type I	Mild/moderate sprain	Immobilize and physiotherapy
Type II	Acute anterior traumatic dislocation	Reduce early and immobilize
Type III	Chronic anterior traumatic dislocation	Reduce early, immobilize, and physiotherapy. Operate if recurrent and symptomatic
Type IV	Chronic anterior atraumatic dislocation	Reduce, immobilize, and physiotherapy. Do not operate
Type V	Posterior dislocation	Reduce early, immobilize, and physiotherapy. Operate if reduction is chronic

From Jaggard MKJ, Gupte CM, Gulati V, Reilly P. A comprehensive review of trauma and disruption to the sternoclavicular joint with the proposal of a new classification system. *J Trauma.* 2009;66(2):576-584.

Atraumatic Sternoclavicular Joint Instability

Patients without a history of injury may present with instability of the SCJ. These patients are typically adolescent females with generalized ligamentous laxity.[39] They typically have anterior subluxation and can demonstrate this in the office. Historically, most authors have recommended avoiding surgery in these patients unless their symptoms are severe, as capsular plication may lead to failure. In such cases, anterior capsule reconstruction using allograft tendon may produce better outcomes.[40]

Capsular Sprain and Subluxation

In cases with a traumatic injury to the capsular and ligamentous structures of the SCJ, but without a true dislocation, conservative treatment is the standard of care. Treatment should consist of ice, analgesics, and immobilization of the ipsilateral upper extremity in a sling or clavicle strap for 3–6 weeks.[34,37,41] The recovery is similar to ACJ injuries, whereas mild injuries may be ready to play sports in approximately 4 weeks, with more severe injuries sometimes taking over 12 weeks to recover.

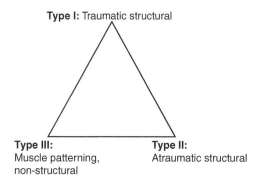

• **Fig. 1.5** The Sewell-Stanmore triangular classification for sternoclavicular joint instability. This conceptual way of classifying instability allows patients to move around the triangle as their pathology changes. For example, patients who originally had a traumatic dislocation then subsequently were able to demonstrate instability by muscle patterning would fit in this diagram. (From Sewell MD, Al-Hadithy N, Le Leu A, Lambert SM. Instability of the sternoclavicular joint: current concepts in classification, treatment and outcomes. *Bone Joint J*. 2013;95-B(6):721-731.)

Anterior Dislocation

Closed reduction of traumatic anterior dislocations is the current treatment of choice and should be attempted as soon as possible from the time of injury.[3,15,18,34,37] The time from injury has a significant impact on the likelihood of a successful closed reduction, with most authors advocating for closed reduction within 48–72 hours of the injury.[15,18,37,42] Closed reduction can be performed with the patient under conscious sedation in the emergency room setting or under general anesthesia in the operating room. The patient is placed supine on a table with a bolster placed between the scapulae. Traction is applied to the ipsilateral abducted arm and pressure on the medial clavicle is applied in the posterior direction. A towel clip on the clavicle with thumb pressure pushing the clavicle head back into place can help with the reduction (Fig. 1.6). After successful reduction, the patient should be immobilized in a plain sling that keeps the arm in front of the body and maintains scapular protraction for 4–6 weeks.

The treatment of acute anterior dislocations that exhibit recurrent symptomatic dislocations or instability after closed reduction is controversial. The redislocation rate after anterior dislocation is reported to be higher than 50%.[43] Historically, the literature has advocated for leaving these injuries in the dislocated position and treating patients symptomatically.[34,44] Like a Grade III ACJ separation, if the scar tissue that develops produces stability with little motion, patients may not have significant symptoms. If there is motion of the clavicle with translation across the manubrium, patients will be symptomatic. More recently, however, larger studies and systematic reviews have reported poor overall outcomes in patients with nonreduced anterior SCJ dislocations or symptomatic instability in those who are treated nonsurgically, and advocate for open reduction and stabilization in healthy active patients.[18,45–47] While most case series are small, between 38% and 42% of patients with unreduced anterior sternoclavicular joint dislocations will have pain with activity and decreased function.[18] In addition, some patients will develop posttraumatic arthritis and others will be unhappy with the appearance of the deformity.[18] These data have led some authors to recommend open reduction of a failed anterior dislocation.[18,45–47]

Posterior Dislocation

Management of traumatic posterior dislocations requires adequate imaging, a careful history, and a thorough physical examination. The presence of any signs or symptoms of mediastinal compression, such

TABLE 1.2	Types of Sternoclavicular Injuries, Findings, and Treatment	
Sternoclavicular Joint Injury	**Findings**	**Treatment**
Sprain	Tenderness at sternoclavicular joint. No displacement of joint on imaging	Symptomatic, symptoms resolve in a few weeks
Subluxation	Significantly more swelling, slight displacement of joint on imaging	Symptomatic, may require surgery if symptoms persist >3 months
Dislocation-clavicle head anterior	Significant pain, swelling, inability to move arm. Anterior displacement of clavicle on imaging	Closed reduction and immobilization. Many chronic anterior dislocations will scar and be symptom free (like Grade III acromioclavicular separation)
Dislocation-clavicle head posterior	Significant pain, swelling, inability to move arm. May have mediastinal compression symptoms (dyspnea, dysphagia, vascular compromise), posterior displacement of clavicle on imaging	Closed reduction. If fails, open reduction and repair/reconstruction of ligaments. Chronic posterior dislocation should under open reduction and reconstruction of ligaments

From Kuhn JE. Open management of traumatic disorders of the sternoclavicular joint. Indications, techniques, outcomes, and complications. In: Rockwood CA, Matsen FA, eds. *The Shoulder*. 6th ed. Philadelphia, PA: Elsevier; 2021.

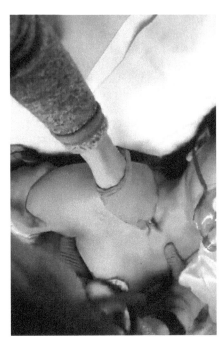

• **Fig. 1.6** Reduction of anterior sternoclavicular joint dislocation. The surgeon's thumb can be used to help push the clavicle lateral and posteriorly into place. In this case, the patient's dislocation was performed in the intensive care unit (ICU), and a towel clip provided lateral traction.

as dyspnea, choking, or hoarseness, should prompt an urgent consultation with a thoracic or cardiothoracic surgeon. As with anterior dislocations, closed reduction should be attempted in all posterior SCJ dislocations that present within 7–10 days of injury.[3,18,34,37,42] Beyond 10 days, open reduction is indicated, as these patients are at an increased risk of scarring and adhesion formation to posterior structures, which could tear during closed reduction. Closed reduction of posterior dislocations should be performed in the operating room under sedation or general anesthesia. Most authors recommend having a thoracic surgeon, thoracic instruments, and sternal saw available during closed reduction in the event of mediastinal involvement. Moreover, we recommend the same thoracic surgery backup if an open reduction is required, as there is the risk of operative injury to nearby structures.[3,34,37]

The patient is placed supine on the operating table with a bolster between the scapulae to extend the shoulders (Fig. 1.7A). The patient should be shifted on the table toward the injured side, such that the ipsilateral extremity is near the edge of the table to allow the arm to be extended and abducted. Gentle traction is applied to the abducted upper extremity, in line with the clavicle (Fig. 1.7B). An assistant stabilizes the patient's torso by providing counter-traction via a sheet wrapped around the patient's thoracic cage just distal to the ipsilateral axilla. Traction on the affected arm is slowly increased as the arm is brought into extension. If this initial technique is unsuccessful, traction can be applied with the arm in abduction while posterior pressure is applied to the shoulder with the goal of levering the clavicle over the first rib.[3,34] Should both traction techniques fail, the skin should be surgically prepped and a sterile towel clip can be used to percutaneously grasp the medial clavicle. The towel clip should be used to completely grasp around the medial clavicle rather than to penetrate the cortical bone. While traction is applied to the ipsilateral arm, the clavicle is lifted anteriorly using the towel clip (Fig. 1.7C). The overall success rate of closed reduction as the definitive treatment for posterior dislocations has been reported to be between 38% and 55%, with higher success rates in patients treated within 48 hours of injury.[42,48]

After closed reduction of a posterior dislocation, a figure-of-eight brace is used to keep the scapulae in retraction with very limited activity for 4–6 weeks. Sleeping on the affected side is to be avoided. After 6 weeks the patient can start to work on glenohumeral range of motion, avoiding crossed body adduction for 8 weeks. After 8 weeks any motion would be allowed and strengthening, particularly scapula control, can begin. Athletes could return to play after 12–16 weeks.

If closed reduction fails, open reduction is indicated, as unreduced posterior dislocations are associated with a variety of severe complications, including vascular compromise, thoracic outlet syndrome, and late erosion of visceral structures by the medial clavicle.[20,24,25]

Medial Clavicular Physeal Fracture

The medial clavicular physis does not begin to ossify until 18–20 years of age and does not fuse until 23–25 years of age, making it the last bone in the body to reach skeletal maturity. Due to this unique anatomy, a sternoclavicular injury in an adolescent patient may represent a medial clavicular physeal fracture with displacement, rather than a true SCJ dislocation.[49] The reported treatment of displaced SCJ injuries in adolescents is varied. Some authors have argued that closed reduction of medial clavicular physeal fractures is ineffective due to entrapment of the periosteum[50] and others have argued that good outcomes can be expected even if the fracture is nonreduced, given the healing and remodeling potential of physeal fractures.[3] Recent literature, however, has favored operative management to prevent recurrent instability.[51] In the largest systematic review of traumatic SCJ injuries in the adolescent population, Tepolt et al.[42] report that closed reduction and open reduction with internal fixation are utilized with equal frequency as the definitive treatment of these injuries. Just as in true SCJ dislocations, the success rate of closed reduction is greatly impacted by the time from injury. Successful closed reduction was reported in >50% of patients treated within 48 hours of injury, as compared with only 30% in patients treated >48 hours from their injury.

Indications for Surgical Treatment

There is a general consensus among authors that surgical stabilization of the SCJ is indicated in recurrent or irreducible posterior dislocations and chronic symptomatic anterior instability.[43] Opinions on the treatment of acute anterior dislocations in which a stable closed reduction cannot be achieved, however, are greatly varied. Historically, recommendations have favored conservative treatment of patients with recurrent anterior instability in the acute period, but there has been growing support in recent years for acute open reduction and stabilization of irreducible or unstable anterior dislocations in healthy active patients.[18,46,47] Like the Grade III ACJ separation, a period of time to determine if symptoms will develop may be entertained prior to recommending surgery for anterior dislocations that have not been reduced.

Surgical Approaches

Numerous techniques have been described for the treatment of SCJ instability. Whether addressing an acute traumatic dislocation or chronic instability resulting from remote trauma, five common categories of SCJ stabilization are reported in the published literature: open reduction and internal fixation,[45,52] medial clavicle resection with or without ligament transfer,[13,48,51] local soft tissue repair or augmentation with synthetic materials,[24,47,50,53–55] tendon transfer techniques,[25,51,56] and ligament reconstruction with allograft or autograft.[46,57–62] All five of these categories of SCJ stabilization

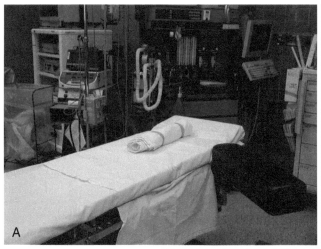
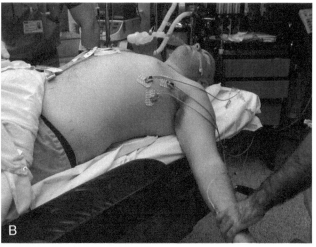
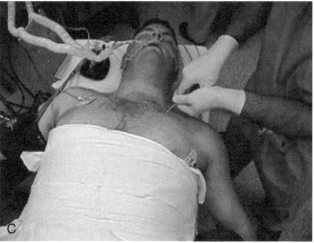

• **Fig. 1.7** Closed reduction of a posterior sternoclavicular joint dislocation. (A) Setup with bolster for placement behind the patient. (B) Attempt at reduction without towel clip. (C) A towel clip is placed around the clavicle and direct anterior and lateral traction is applied.

have been described for the treatment of both anterior and posterior dislocations and no specific surgical approach or technique of stabilization has been reported to be superior in regard to the direction of instability. Early case reports utilized wires or pins for stabilization of the SCJ, but due to reported lethal complications secondary to pin migration, this technique is no longer recommended.[63–66] Franck et al.[45] reported the use of a hooked Balser plate to provisionally fix the SCJ after acute dislocation to allow for healing of the capsule. Rockwood et al.[13] reported a case series in which the medial clavicle was resected and the stabilizing ligaments of the SCJ were reconstructed utilizing the joint capsule and disc, while preserving the periosteal attachments of the medial clavicle. Reconstruction with sutures either through drill holes or suture anchors has been performed, although robust biomechanical evaluation of this technique is lacking.[47,53,55] Armstrong and Dias[56] reported a technique in which they transferred the sternal head of sternocleidomastoid through a single drill hole in the medial clavicle.

More recently, reconstruction utilizing tendon grafts has become popular given its theoretically improved biomechanical properties. Figure-of-eight reconstructions utilizing gracilis,[57] semitendinosus,[57,58] palmaris longus, or occasionally sternocleidomastoid[59,60] tendon grafts have gained increasing support among recent authors. Although satisfactory clinical outcomes have been reported for each of these graft reconstruction techniques, these reports have been based on low-level case reports and series, making comparison of outcomes between techniques difficult.

Biomechanical testing has revealed the figure-of-eight reconstruction with tendon graft to be superior to other graft reconstruction techniques for both anterior and posterior SCJ instability. Spencer and Kuhn[67] compared the mechanical strength of three different reconstruction techniques, including semitendinosus figure-of-eight reconstruction, subclavius tendon reconstruction, and intramedullary ligament reconstruction. Their results demonstrated that the figure-of-eight reconstruction had significantly higher mechanical strength than the other two reconstruction techniques in both the anterior and posterior directions. Although subsequent modifications on this figure-of-eight technique have been described,[68] mechanical strength testing[69] has revealed the technique originally described by Spencer and Kuhn to be biomechanically superior. Because of its biomechanical advantages and satisfactory initial clinical outcomes, figure-of-eight reconstruction with semitendinosus graft is the senior author's preferred surgical technique (see Chapter 2).

Outcomes of Surgical Treatment

Traumatic injuries to the SCJ leading to dislocation or symptomatic instability are rare, resulting in a paucity of high-level prospective studies that are able to evaluate long-term outcomes of surgical treatment.[43,70,71] Review of the literature is limited by the preponderance

TABLE 1.3   Reported Outcomes After Surgical Treatment of Sternoclavicular Joint Instability Using Standard and Modified Figure-of-Eight Ligament Reconstructions

Author	N	Technique	Outcome	Failure Rate/Complications
Standard Figure-of-Eight Technique				
Bae et al.[62]	N = 15 4M, 11F 15 anterior and 9 treated with figure of eight	8 semitendinosus and 1 sternocleidomastoid in figure of eight	SST score improved to 11.4 out of 12	None
Gowd et al.[72]	N = 10 patients who had 12 surgeries	Figure of eight	ASES score improved 29.7 points VAS improved by 2.3 44.4% return to sport 50% could do push-ups 42.9% returned to work No heavy workers returned to heavy activities	
Singer et al.[57]	N = 5 3M and 3F 3 anterior, 2 posterior, and 1 combined	Hamstring autograft figure of eight	DASH score improved 25 points. All patients returned to full activity including contact sports	No recurrence One infection
Kusnezov et al.[46]	N = 14 13M, 1F 8 anterior and 6 posterior	Figure of eight, mixture of allograft and autograft	10/12 returned to full active military duty	21% osteoarthritis 14.3% persistent instability 14.3% reoperation
Petri et al.[73]	N = 21 10M, 9F	Figure of eight Hamstring tendon autograft	ASES score improved 30.6 points SANE score improved by 16.3–82.5	None
Modifications of Figure-of-Eight Technique				
Bak et al.[74]	N = 27 27 anterior	Suture anchor in sternum modification with palmaris autograft in 7, gracilis autograft in 25	WOSI score improved 31%	Two failures (7.4%), 68% had complaints with donor site, 40% had some discomfort at surgical site
Guan et al.[75]	N = 6 1M, 5F 6 anterior	Hamstring autograft	VAS score was no pain in 5 and mild pain in 1 All returned to preoperative activities including sports	One patient sustained failure at 4 years after surgery
Sabatini et al.[61]	N = 10 3M, 7F 9 anterior and 1 posterior	Figure-of-eight allograft tendon with two tenodesis screws	ASES improved 49 points. VAS improved from 7.0 to 1.2	One hematoma One superficial infection One patient with pain and osteoarthritis
Sanchez-Sotelo et al.[76]	N = 19 13 anterior, 3 posterior, and 3 arthritis resection	5–10 mm of medical clavicle excised, drill holes are unicortical anterior, with graft spanning joint space	VAS improved from 5.0 to 1.0	2 (10.5%) required revision surgery 1 (5%) continued to have symptoms of instability

ASES, American Shoulder and Elbow Surgeons; *DASH*, The Disability of the Arm, Shoulder and Hand; *SANE*, Single Assessment Numerical Evaluation; *SST*, Simple Shoulder Test; *VAS*, Visual Analog Scale; *WOSI*, Western Ontario Shoulder Instability.

From Kuhn JE. Open management of traumatic disorders of the sternoclavicular joint. Indications, techniques, outcomes, and complications. In: Rockwood CA, Matsen FA, eds. *The Shoulder*. 6th ed. Philadelphia, PA: Elsevier; 2021.

of reports on single cases or small series of patients and surgical technique papers that lack the adequate follow-up necessary to compare the efficacy of one technique with another. Moreover, these low-level studies often report outcomes on mixed patient populations representing both anterior and posterior instability, making any inference on differential outcomes between anterior and posterior dislocations unreliable.[13,45,46,53,55,57,61] Although a small subset of studies have reported outcomes of surgical stabilization for only anterior[47,56,58,59,62] or posterior[24,25,48,50–52,54,60,71] dislocations, no significant difference in outcomes between these groups has been established. Results from all of the techniques discussed in this chapter, regardless of the direction of instability of the SCJ, have indicated generally favorable outcomes. Validated patient-reported and objected outcomes, however,

are absent from many of these reports.[43,71] Results from open reduction and internal fixation reveal that in a majority of cases (80%), a second procedure from implant removal was required. Patient outcomes, however, demonstrate satisfactory outcomes at a mean follow-up of 9.1 months. Outcomes of medial clavicle resection with or without ligament transfer have also been successful, with the majority of patients reporting normal function or only slight restriction with overhead movements at a mean follow-up of 59 months. Techniques utilizing synthetic materials to augment or repair capsular and ligamentous tissue have proved successful with a very low overall complication rate (3%). Studies documenting tendon transfer techniques reported good to excellent results using either the subclavius or sternocleidomastoid tendons (Table 1.3). Ligament reconstruction using allograft or autograft have similarly documented satisfactory outcomes, with no reports of recurrent instability or limitations with return to activity, and the fewest reported complications among the five categories of techniques described in this chapter.

Relevant Complications

Given their close proximity to the SCJ, iatrogenic injury to the critical visceral and vascular structures within the mediastinum during posterior dissection or drilling of bone tunnels is considered the most serious potential operative complication by many authors. Due to this concern, numerous sources have made the recommendation to have a cardiothoracic or thoracic surgeon available during operative stabilization of the SCJ.[18] However, in a systematic review of 32 studies in which intraoperative complications were reported, Kendal et al.[71] found no documented cases of neurovascular injury or other forms of mediastinal injury. Moreover, a subsequent meta-analysis by Sernandez et al.[18] reported that there is not a single case documented anywhere in the literature in which the intervention of a cardiothoracic surgeon was required. Overall, intraoperative or postoperative complications have been reported to occur in approximately 16% of cases.[71] In cases where open reduction and internal fixation with hardware was performed, a second procedure to remove symptomatic hardware was required in 80% of patients. Among all reconstruction techniques, recurrent instability was the most common complication, occurring in 4% of patients. Additional complications that have been reported in single case reports or small case series include transient scapular winging and posttraumatic arthritis.[25,46]

Summary

SCJ instability is rare, but often described in the literature. Traumatic posterior dislocations can be associated with injury to retrosternal structures and deserve special concern. Acute dislocations should undergo reduction. If closed reduction fails for anterior dislocations, the dislocated medial clavicle may be left in the dislocated position for many, especially relatively elderly, patients with low demands. All acute and chronic posterior dislocations should be reduced. A variety of techniques have been described, but the figure-of-eight technique using tendon graft seems to have biomechanical properties that are superior, and as such, is often employed with good results.

References

1. Doody SG, Freedman L, Waterland JC. Shoulder movements during abduction in the scapular plane. *Arch Phys Med Rehabil.* 1970;51(10):595–604.
2. Teubner E, Gerstenberger F, Burgert R. [Kinematic consideration of the shoulder girdle and its consequences on common surgical methods]. *Unfallchirurg.* 1991;94(9):471–477.
3. Wirth MA, Rockwood Jr CA. Acute and chronic traumatic injuries of the sternoclavicular joint. *J Am Acad Orthop Surg.* 1996;4(5):268–278.
4. Spencer EE, Kuhn JE, Huston LJ, Carpenter JE, Hughes RE. Ligamentous restraints to anterior and posterior translation of the sternoclavicular joint. *J Shoulder Elbow Surg.* 2002;11(1):43–47.
5. Lee JT, Campbell KJ, Michalski MP, et al. Surgical anatomy of the sternoclavicular joint: a qualitative and quantitative anatomical study. *J Bone Joint Surg Am.* 2014;96(19):e166.
6. van Tongel A, MacDonald PM, Leiter J, Pouliart N, Peeler J. A cadaveric study of the structural anatomy of the sternoclavicular joint. *Clin Anat.* 2012;25(7):903–910.
7. Bisson LJ, Dauphin N, Marzo JM. A safe zone for resection of the medial end of the clavicle. *J Shoulder Elbow Surg.* 2003;12(6):592–594.
8. Carrera EF, Archetti Neto N, Carvalho RL, Souza MA, Santos JB, Faloppa F. Resection of the medial end of the clavicle: an anatomic study. *J Shoulder Elbow Surg.* 2007;16(1):112–114.
9. Dhawan R, Singh RA, Tins B, Hay SM. Sternoclavicular joint. *Shoulder Elbow.* 2018;10(4):296–305.
10. Philipson M, Wallwork N. Traumatic dislocations of the sternoclavicular joint. *Orthop Trauma.* 2012;26(6):380–384.
11. Bearn JG. Direct observations on the function of the capsule of the sternoclavicular joint in clavicular support. *J Anat.* 1967;101(Pt 1):159–170.
12. Abbott LC, Lucas DB. The function of the clavicle; its surgical significance. *Ann Surg.* 1954;140(4):583–599.
13. Rockwood Jr CA, Groh GI, Wirth MA, Grassi FA. Resection arthroplasty of the sternoclavicular joint. *J Bone Joint Surg Am.* 1997;79(3):387–393.
14. Cave EF. *Fractures and Other Injuries.* Chicago, IL: Year Book Publishers; 1958.
15. Jaggard MKJ, Gupte CM, Gulati V, Reilly P. A comprehensive review of trauma and disruption to the sternoclavicular joint with the proposal of a new classification system. *J Trauma.* 2009;66(2):576–584.
16. Boesmueller S, Wech M, Tiefenboeck TM, et al. Incidence, characteristics, and long-term follow-up of sternoclavicular injuries: an epidemiologic analysis of 92 cases. *J Trauma Acute Care Surg.* 2016;80(2):289–295.
17. Nettles JL, Linscheid RL. Sternoclavicular dislocations. *J Trauma.* 1968;8(2):158–164.
18. Sernandez H, Riehl J. Sternoclavicular joint dislocation: a systematic review and meta-analysis. *J Orthop Trauma.* 2019;33(7):e251–e255.
19. Worman LW, Leagus C. Intrathoracic injury following retrosternal dislocation of the clavicle. *J Trauma.* 1967;7(3):416–423.
20. Jain S, Monbaliu D, Thompson JF. Thoracic outlet syndrome caused by chronic retrosternal dislocation of the clavicle. Successful treatment by transaxillary resection of the first rib. *J Bone Joint Surg Br.* 2002;84(1):116–118.
21. Howard FM, Shafer SJ. Injuries to the clavicle with neurovascular complications. A study of fourteen cases. *J Bone Joint Surg Am.* 1965;47(7):1335–1346.
22. Nakayama E, Tanaka T, Noguchi T, Yasuda JI, Tereda Y. Tracheal stenosis caused by retrosternal dislocation of the right clavicle. *Ann Thorac Surg.* 2007;83(2):685–687.
23. Gardner MA, Bidstrup BP. Intrathoracic great vessel injury resulting from blunt chest trauma associated with posterior dislocation of the sternoclavicular joint. *Aust N Z J Surg.* 1983;53(5):427–430.
24. Mirza AH, Alam K, Ali A. Posterior sternoclavicular dislocation in a rugby player as a cause of silent vascular compromise: a case report. *Br J Sports Med.* 2005;39(5):e28.
25. Noda M, Shiraishi H, Mizuno K. Chronic posterior sternoclavicular dislocation causing compression of a subclavian artery. *J Shoulder Elbow Surg.* 1997;6(6):564–569.
26. Gangahar DM, Flogaites T. Retrosternal dislocation of the clavicle producing thoracic outlet syndrome. *J Trauma.* 1978;18(5):369–372.
27. O'Connor PA, Nolke L, O'Donnell A, Lingham KM. Retrosternal dislocation of the clavicle associated with a traumatic pneumothorax. *Interact Cardiovasc Thorac Surg.* 2003;2(1):9–11.
28. Ponce BA, Kundukulam JA, Pflugner R, et al. Sternoclavicular joint surgery: how far does danger lurk below? *J Shoulder Elbow Surg.* 2013;22(7):993–999.
29. Jougon JB, Lepront DJ, Dromer CE. Posterior dislocation of the sternoclavicular joint leading to mediastinal compression. *Ann Thorac Surg.* 1996;61(2):711–713.
30. Ono K, Inagawa H, Kiyota K, Terada T, Suzuki S, Maekawa K. Posterior dislocation of the sternoclavicular joint with obstruction of the innominate vein: case report. *J Trauma.* 1998;44(2):381–383.
31. Rayan GM. Compression brachial plexopathy caused by chronic posterior dislocation of the sternoclavicular joint. *J Okla State Med Assoc.* 1994;87(1):7–9.

32. di Mento L, Staletti L, Cavanna M, Mocchi M, Berlusconi M. Posterior sternoclavicular joint dislocation with brachiocephalic vein injury: a case report. *Injury.* 2015;46(suppl 7):S8–S10.

33. Southworth S, Merritt T. Asymptomatic innominate vein tamponade with retromanubrial clavicular dislocation. A case report. *Orthop Rev.* 1998;17(8).

34. Groh GI, Wirth MA. Management of traumatic sternoclavicular joint injuries. *J Am Acad Orthop Surg.* 2011;19(1):1–7.

35. Rockwood C, Wirth M. Disorders of the sternoclavicular joint. In: Rockwood C, et al., ed. *The Shoulder.* Philadelphia, PA: Saunders; 2009:527–560.

36. Allman Jr FL. Fractures and ligamentous injuries of the clavicle and its articulation. *J Bone Joint Surg Am.* 1967;49(4):774–784.

37. Sewell MD, Al-Hadithy N, Leu AL, Lambert SM. Instability of the sternoclavicular joint: current concepts in classification, treatment and outcomes. *Bone Joint Lett J.* 2013;95-b(6):721–731.

38. Lewis A, Kitamura T, Bayley J. The classification of shoulder instability: new light through old windows. *Curr Orthop.* 2004;18(2):97–109.

39. Rockwood CA, Odor JM. Spontaneous atraumatic anterior subluxation of the sternoclavicular joint. *J Bone Joint Surg Am.* 1989;71(9):1280–1288.

40. Lemos MJ, Tolo ET. Complications of the treatment of the acromioclavicular and sternoclavicular joint injuries, including instability. *Clin Sports Med.* 2003;22(2):371–385.

41. Deren ME, Behrens SB, Vopat BG, Blaine TA. Posterior sternoclavicular dislocations: a brief review and technique for closed management of a rare but serious injury. *Orthop Rev.* 2014;6(1):5245.

42. Tepolt F, Carry PM, Heyn PC, Miller NH. Posterior sternoclavicular joint injuries in the adolescent population: a meta-analysis. *Am J Sports Med.* 2014;42(10):2517–2524.

43. Thut D, Hergan D, Dukas A, Day M, Sherman OH. Sternoclavicular joint reconstruction—a systematic review. *Bull NYU Hosp Jt Dis.* 2011;69(2):128–135.

44. de Jong KP, Sukul DM. Anterior sternoclavicular dislocation: a long-term follow-up study. *J Orthop Trauma.* 1990;4(4):420–423.

45. Franck WM, Jannasch O, Siassi M, Hennig FF. Balser plate stabilization: an alternate therapy for traumatic sternoclavicular instability. *J Shoulder Elbow Surg.* 2003;12(3):276–281.

46. Kusnezov N, Dunn JC, DeLong JM, Waterman BR. Sternoclavicular reconstruction in the young active patient: risk factor analysis and clinical outcomes at short-term follow-up. *J Orthop Trauma.* 2016;30(4):e111–e117.

47. Tytherleigh-Strong G, Pecheva M, Titchener A. Treatment of first-time traumatic anterior dislocation of the sternoclavicular joint with surgical repair of the anterior capsule augmented with internal bracing. *Orthop J Sports Med.* 2018;6(7). 2325967118783717.

48. Groh GI, Wirth MA, Rockwood Jr CA. Treatment of traumatic posterior sternoclavicular dislocations. *J Shoulder Elbow Surg.* 2011;20(1):107–113.

49. Tepolt F, Carry PM, Taylor M, Hadley-Miller N. Posterior sternoclavicular joint injuries in skeletally immature patients. *Orthopedics.* 2014;37(2):e174–e181.

50. Laffosse JM, Espie A, Bonnevialle N. Posterior dislocation of the sternoclavicular joint and epiphyseal disruption of the medial clavicle with posterior displacement in sports participants. *J Bone Joint Surg Br.* 2010;92(1):103–109.

51. Ting BL, Bae DS, Waters PM. Chronic posterior sternoclavicular joint fracture dislocations in children and young adults: results of surgical management. *J Pediatr Orthop.* 2014;34(5):542–547.

52. Gerich T, Hoffmann A, Backes F, Duinslaeger AD, Seil R, Pape D. Anterior buttress plate is successful for treating posterior sterno-clavicular dislocation. *Knee Surg Sports Traumatol Arthrosc.* 2019;27(1):251–258.

53. Abiddin Z, Sinopidis C, Grocock CJ, Yin Q, Frostick SP. Suture anchors for treatment of sternoclavicular joint instability. *J Shoulder Elbow Surg.* 2006;15(3):315–318.

54. Quispe JC, Herbert B, Chadayammuri VP, et al. Transarticular plating for acute posterior sternoclavicular joint dislocations: a valid treatment option? *Int Orthop.* 2016;40(7):1503–1508.

55. Thomas DP, Williams PR, Hoddinott HC. A 'safe' surgical technique for stabilisation of the sternoclavicular joint: a cadaveric and clinical study. *Ann R Coll Surg Engl.* 2000;82(6):432–435.

56. Armstrong AL, Dias JJ. Reconstruction for instability of the sternoclavicular joint using the tendon of the sternocleidomastoid muscle. *J Bone Joint Surg Br.* 2008;90(5):610–613.

57. Singer G, Ferlic P, Kraus T, Eberl R. Reconstruction of the sternoclavicular joint in active patients with the figure-of-eight technique using hamstrings. *J Shoulder Elbow Surg.* 2013;22(1):64–69.

58. Guan JJ, Wolf BR. Reconstruction for anterior sternoclavicular joint dislocation and instability. *J Shoulder Elbow Surg.* 2013;22(6):775–781.

59. Uri O, Barmpagiannis K, Higgs D, Falworth M, Alexander S, Lambert SM. Clinical outcome after reconstruction for sternoclavicular joint instability using a sternocleidomastoid tendon graft. *J Bone Joint Surg Am.* 2014;96(5):417–422.

60. Widodo W, Fahrudin M, Kamal AF. Joint reconstruction using sternocleidomastoid tendon autograft as a treatment for traumatic posterior dislocation of sternoclavicular joint: a case report. *Trauma Case Rep.* 2018;18:8–16.

61. Sabatini JB, Shung JR, Clay B, Oladeji LO, Minnich DJ, Ponce BA. Outcomes of augmented allograft figure-of-eight sternoclavicular joint reconstruction. *J Shoulder Elbow Surg.* 2015;24(6):902–907.

62. Bae DS, Kocher MS, Waters PM, Micheli LM, Griffey M, Dichtel L. Chronic recurrent anterior sternoclavicular joint instability: results of surgical management. *J Pediatr Orthop.* 2006;26(1):71–74.

63. Clark RL, Milgram JW, Yawn DH. Fatal aortic perforation and cardiac tamponade due to a Kirschner wire migrating from the right sternoclavicular joint. *South Med J.* 1974;67(3):316–318.

64. Gerlach D, Wemhoner SR, Ogbuihi S. [2 cases of pericardial tamponade caused by migration of fracture wires from the sternoclavicular joint]. *Z Rechtsmed.* 1984;93(1):53–60.

65. Leonard JW, Gifford Jr RW. Migration of a Kirschner wire from the clavicle into the pulmonary artery. *Am J Cardiol.* 1965;16(4):598–600.

66. Lyons FA, Rockwood Jr CA. Migration of pins used in operations on the shoulder. *J Bone Joint Surg Am.* 1990;72(8):1262–1267.

67. Spencer Jr EE, Kuhn JE. Biomechanical analysis of reconstructions for sternoclavicular joint instability. *J Bone Joint Surg Am.* 2004;86(1):98–105.

68. Martetschläger F, Braun S, Lorenz S, Lenich A, Imhoff AB. Novel technique for sternoclavicular joint reconstruction using a gracilis tendon autograft. *Knee Surg Sports Traumatol Arthrosc.* 2016;24(7):2225–2230.

69. Martetschlager F, Reifenschneider F, Fischer N. Sternoclavicular joint reconstruction fracture risk is reduced with straight drill tunnels and optimized with tendon graft suture augmentation. *Orthop J Sports Med.* 2019;7(4). 2325967119838265.

70. Martetschlager F, Warth RJ, Millett PJ. Instability and degenerative arthritis of the sternoclavicular joint: a current concepts review. *Am J Sports Med.* 2014;42(4):999–1007.

71. Kendal JK, Thomas K, LO IKY, Bois A. Clinical outcomes and complications following surgical management of traumatic posterior sternoclavicular joint dislocations: a systematic review. *JBJS Rev.* 2018;6(11):e2.

72. Gowd AK, Liu JN, Garcia GH, et al. Figure of eight reconstruction of the sternoclavicular joint: outcomes of sport and work. *Orthopedics.* 2019;42(4):205–210.

73. Petri M, Greenspoon JA, Horan MP, Martetschläger F, Warth RJ, Millett PJ. Clinical outcomes after autograft reconstruction for sternoclavicular joint instability. *J Shoulder Elbow Surg.* 2016;25(3):435–441. https://doi.org/10.1016/j.jse.2015.08.004.

74. Bak K, Fogh K. Reconstruction of the chronic anterior unstable sternoclavicular joint using a tendon autograft: medium-term to long-term follow-up results. *J Shoulder Elbow Surg.* 2014;23:245–250.

75. Guan JJ, Wolf BR. Reconstruction for anterior sternoclavicular joint dislocation and instability. *J Shoulder Elbow Surg.* 2013;22:775–781.

76. Sanchez-Sotelo J, Baghdadi Y, Nguyen NTV. Sternoclavicular joint allograft reconstruction using the sternal docking technique. *JSES Open Access.* 2018;2(4):190–193. https://doi.org/10.1016/j.jses.2018.08.002.

2

Technique Spotlight: Allograft Stabilization of the Sternoclavicular Joint

NICHOLAS J. DANTZKER AND JOHN E. KUHN

Authors' Preferred Surgical Technique: Figure-of-Eight Sternoclavicular Joint Reconstruction Using Autograft Tendon

Rationale

As described in the previous chapter, a variety of techniques have been described to treat the unstable sternoclavicular joint (SCJ). The figure-of-eight technique was developed after biomechanical testing determined that the posterior capsule was the primary restraint to posterior translation of the SCJ and the posterior capsule and anterior capsule were restraints to anterior translation.[1] When compared with other techniques, the figure-of-eight reconstruction has superior biomechanical properties preventing anterior and posterior translation.[2] A number of case series in the literature demonstrate significant improvements in patient-reported outcomes using this technique (see Table 1.3 of Chapter 1).

Indications

This technique is recommended for chronic anterior or posterior dislocations of the SCJ. In addition, acute posterior dislocations that require open reduction and where the capsule is irreparable, is another indication for this technique.

Surgical Technique

The procedure is performed with the patient in the supine position under general anesthetic. The entire chest and neck are prepped and draped as complications during surgery may require a sternotomy (Fig. 2.1). A thoracic surgeon assisting is recommended as dissection behind the manubrium is required to perform this surgery. The ipsilateral arm is also draped free to allow for dynamic examination and manipulation of the SCJ throughout the operation and if the patient is small and a palmaris longus tendon is going to be used as the graft for the reconstruction. The ipsilateral leg is prepped and draped if a semitendinosus graft will be used for the reconstruction. In the senior author's experience, the semitendinosus is used in approximately 80% of cases.

A 6- to 8-cm curved skin incision from the medial clavicle over the SCJ and sternum is carried down through the skin and subcutaneous tissues following Langer's lines. The platysma is incised parallel to the skin incision and reflected superiorly and inferiorly (Fig. 2.2). This exposes the sternocleidomastoid insertions on the clavicle and manubrium—which should be preserved—and the capsule of the SCJ. The capsule is then opened with an incision on the ventral aspect of the joint from lateral to medial using electrocautery (Fig. 2.3). The periosteum of the medial clavicle is elevated with the use of electrocautery and a periosteal elevator until a thorough circumferential capsular release is completed, mobilizing the medial clavicle. If the joint is dislocated posteriorly, it is reduced by grasping the medial clavicle with a towel clamp, and pulling laterally and ventrally.

At this point, our thoracic surgeon will make an incision just superior to the sternal notch, and the underlying platysma is also incised in the same plane (Fig. 2.4). Blunt finger

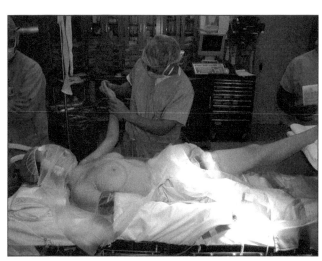

• **Fig. 2.1** Patient position and preparation. The entire chest and one leg are prepped and draped. (From Mansour AA, Kuhn JE. Sternoclavicular joint reconstruction using semitendinosus graft. In: Lee DH, Neviaser RJ, eds. *Operative Techniques. Shoulder and Elbow Surgery*. Philadelphia, PA: Elsevier Saunders; 2011:415, Fig. 5.)

dissection directly under the bony surface of the manubrium is carried out to create a space under the manubrium. When performing an SCJ reconstruction for an acute dislocation, the retromanubrial space can also be accessed by dissecting under the manubrial side of the SCJ if the posterior capsule has been avulsed or is significantly damaged. Placement of a broad ribbon retractor in this space is recommended when drilling the manubrium to prevent damage to the underlying retrosternal structures (Fig. 2.5).

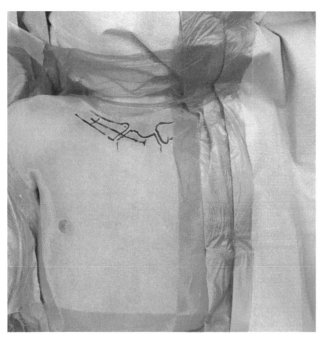

• **Fig. 2.2** Skin incision. The skin incision should follow Langer's lines and proceed to the midsternum. (From Kuhn JE. Treatment. In: Arciero RA, Cordasco FA, Provencher MT, eds. *Shoulder and Elbow Injuries in Athletes*. Philadelphia, PA: Elsevier; 2018:362, Fig. 17.3.)

Obtaining the Semitendinosus Graft

A skin incision is made over the pes anserinus. The overlying fascia is incised parallel to the course of the tendons. The semitendinosus is typically found deep and posterior to the gracilis and the sartorius tendon insertions. Once isolated, sutures are passed in the distal end of the semitendinosus, and the tendon is released from its insertion, and then sutured with #2 locking sutures. Fascial bands frequently tether the tendon to other structures and must be released. A long tendon stripper is then gently pushed up the leg until the tendon is released from its muscular attachments (Fig. 2.6). The residual muscle is dissected from the tendon, and the other end of the tendon is sutured with #2 locking sutures (Fig. 2.7). The diameter of the graft is measured prior to drilling bone tunnels to ensure the tunnels are of adequate diameter.

Preparing the Tunnels for the Graft

Two parallel drill holes are made in the clavicle a few millimeters lateral to the subchondral plate of the SCJ. Two drill holes in the manubrium are made a few millimeters to the subchondral plate of the SCJ. It is important to make all of these drill holes parallel, as deviations can produce torsion on the construct (Fig. 2.8). The size of the drill is usually determined by the graft thickness. Starting with a 4-mm bit is common, and the drill holes may be enlarged by using sequentially larger curettes. Parts of the graft may have to be trimmed to allow for passage into the tunnels. Suture loops are passed from each drill hole into the space above the sternal notch. These loops will be used to pass the graft through the tunnels in the appropriate order and direction (Fig. 2.9).

Graft Passage

At this point, the graft is passed through the tunnels in a figure-of-eight fashion. The sutures that have been woven into the smallest end of the graft are placed in the suture loop, then pulled through the drill hole. The graft is passed through sequential drill holes to create the figure-of-eight construct (Fig. 2.10).

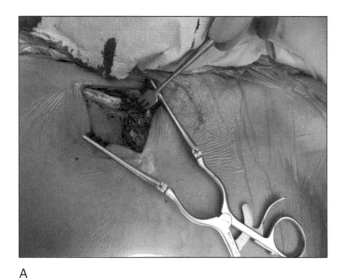

A

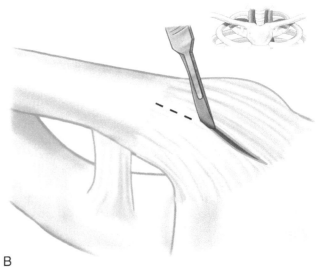

B

• **Fig. 2.3** Incision of the anterior capsule. (From Mansour AA, Kuhn JE. Sternoclavicular joint reconstruction using semitendinosus graft. In: Lee DH, Neviaser RJ, eds. *Operative Techniques. Shoulder and Elbow Surgery*. Philadelphia, PA: Elsevier Saunders; 2011:416, Fig. 6B.)

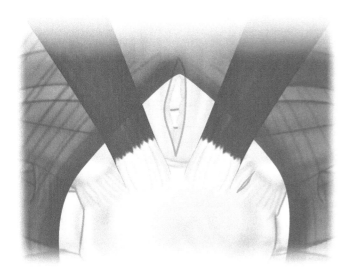

• **Fig. 2.4** Sternal notch incision. (From Mansour AA, Kuhn JE. Sternoclavicular joint reconstruction using semitendinosus graft. In: Lee DH, Neviaser RJ, eds. *Operative Techniques. Shoulder and Elbow Surgery*. Philadelphia, PA: Elsevier Saunders; 2011:418, Fig. 8.)

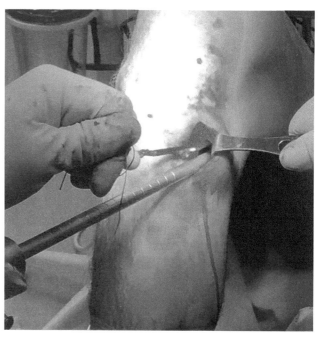

• **Fig. 2.6** Hamstring tendon harvest from right knee. (From Kuhn JE. Treatment. In: Arciero RA, Cordasco FA, Provencher MT, eds. *Shoulder and Elbow Injuries in Athletes*. Philadelphia, PA: Elsevier; 2018:361, Fig. 17.2.)

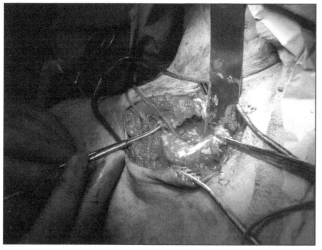

• **Fig. 2.5** Placement of the ribbon retractor before drilling the manubrium. (From Mansour AA, Kuhn JE. Sternoclavicular joint reconstruction using semitendinosus graft. In: Lee DH, Neviaser RJ, eds. *Operative Techniques. Shoulder and Elbow Surgery*. Philadelphia, PA: Elsevier Saunders; 2011:418, Fig. 9.)

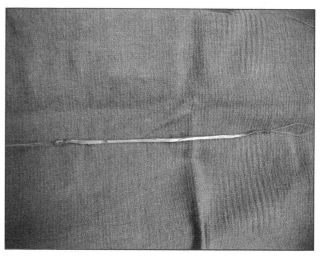

• **Fig. 2.7** Semitendinosus graft ready for passage. (From Mansour AA, Kuhn JE. Sternoclavicular joint reconstruction using semitendinosus graft. In: Lee DH, Neviaser RJ, eds. *Operative Techniques. Shoulder and Elbow Surgery*. Philadelphia, PA: Elsevier Saunders; 2011:417, Fig. 7.)

It is important to note that on one surface the graft will have parallel limbs, and on the other surface the graft will cross. In general, the parallel limbs are more secure than the crossed limbs, and as such the graft may be passed so that the parallel limbs are on the side of the instability (e.g., for a patient with posterior SCJ instability, the parallel limbs should be on the posterior side of the construct).

After the graft has been passed, it is gently tensioned. It is important to avoid overtensioning the graft which could produce tunnel failure. The free ends of the graft are tied to each other and secured with multiple figure-of-eight #2 permanent sutures. The free ends of the graft may be secured to residual capsule to reinforce the construct anteriorly (Fig. 2.11).

After the graft is secured, the wound is closed in layers. Any residual capsule may be repaired to itself of the graft to reinforce the construct. Look to be certain the sternocleidomastoid insertions have remained intact, and if not repair these. The platysma is closed with 2-0 absorbable sutures, and the skin is closed with 2-0 absorbable sutures in the deep layer and then a running 4-0 absorbable monofilament suture (Fig. 2.12). A sterile dressing is applied and the patient's arm is placed into a regular arm sling.

Postoperatively, it is important to avoid excessive motion early to allow the graft to heal into the tunnels. The author's postoperative rehabilitation protocol is provided in Table 2.1.

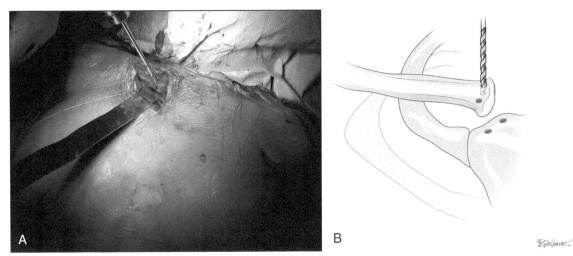

• **Fig. 2.8** Drill hole preparation. (From [A] Mansour AA, Kuhn JE. Sternoclavicular joint reconstruction using semitendinosus graft. In: Lee DH, Neviaser RJ, eds. *Operative Techniques. Shoulder and Elbow Surgery*. Philadelphia, PA: Elsevier Saunders; 2011:419, Fig. 10A; and [B] Kuhn JE. Treatment. In: Arciero RA, Cordasco FA, Provencher MT, eds. *Shoulder and Elbow Injuries in Athletes*. Philadelphia, PA: Elsevier; 2018:363, Fig. 17.5.)

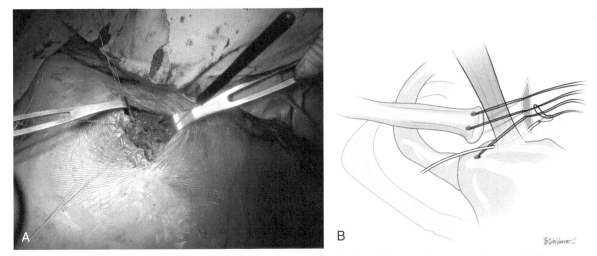

• **Fig. 2.9** Suture loops are passed. Suture loops are passed using a Hewson suture passer from each drill hole into the incision above the sternal notch. These suture loops will be used to pass the tendon graft. (From [A] Mansour AA, Kuhn JE. Sternoclavicular joint reconstruction using semitendinosus graft. In: Lee DH, Neviaser RJ, eds. *Operative Techniques. Shoulder and Elbow Surgery*. Philadelphia, PA: Elsevier Saunders; 2011:420, Fig. 11A; and [B] Kuhn JE. Treatment. In: Arciero RA, Cordasco FA, Provencher MT, eds. *Shoulder and Elbow Injuries in Athletes*. Philadelphia, PA: Elsevier; 2018:363, Fig. 17.6.)

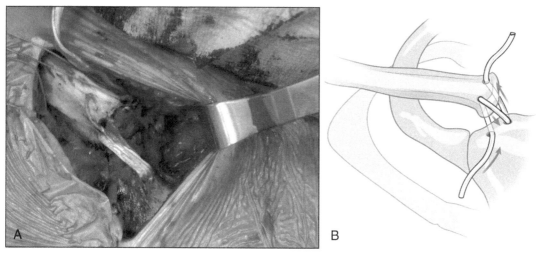

• **Fig. 2.10** Passing the graft to create a figure-of-eight construct. (From [A] Mansour AA, Kuhn JE. Sternoclavicular joint reconstruction using semitendinosus graft. In: Lee DH, Neviaser RJ, eds. *Operative Techniques. Shoulder and Elbow Surgery*. Philadelphia, PA: Elsevier Saunders; 2011:421, Fig. 12A; and [B] Kuhn JE. Treatment. In: Arciero RA, Cordasco FA, Provencher MT, eds. *Shoulder and Elbow Injuries in Athletes*. Philadelphia, PA: Elsevier; 2018:364, Fig. 17.7.)

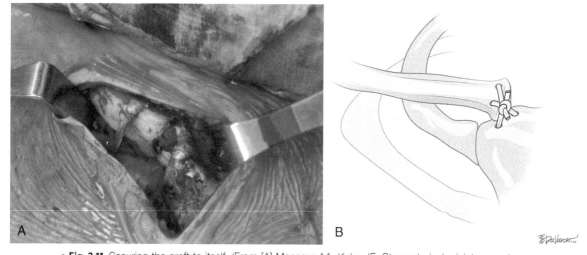

• **Fig. 2.11** Securing the graft to itself. (From [A] Mansour AA, Kuhn JE. Sternoclavicular joint reconstruction using semitendinosus graft. In: Lee DH, Neviaser RJ, eds. *Operative Techniques. Shoulder and Elbow Surgery*. Philadelphia, PA: Elsevier Saunders; 2011:422, Fig. 14A; and [B] Kuhn JE. Treatment. In: Arciero RA, Cordasco FA, Provencher MT, eds. *Shoulder and Elbow Injuries in Athletes*. Philadelphia, PA: Elsevier; 2018:363, Fig. 17.8.)

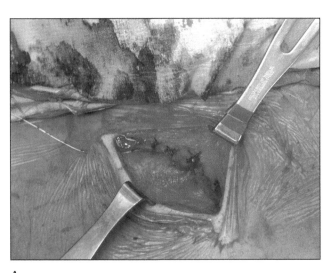

A

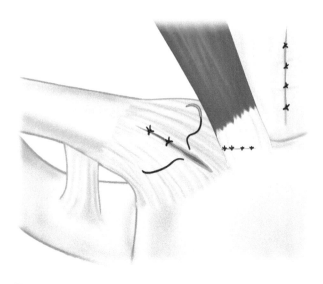

B

• **Fig. 2.12** Closing the wound. (From Mansour AA, Kuhn JE. Sternoclavicular joint reconstruction using semitendinosus graft. In: Lee DH, Neviaser RJ, eds. *Operative Techniques. Shoulder and Elbow Surgery.* Philadelphia, PA: Elsevier Saunders; 2011:423, Fig. 15A.)

TABLE 2.1 **Postoperative Rehabilitation Protocol for Figure-of-Eight Sternoclavicular Joint Reconstruction**

	Immobilization	Range of Motion	Strengthening	Return to Play	Comments
0–6 weeks	In brace that prevents scapula motion. For posterior instability, a sling that places arm in external rotation. For anterior instability, a sling that places arm in internal rotation.	None	None	None	
6–8 weeks		Passive range of motion begins at 6 weeks.	None	None	Early motion should avoid extremes of extension and crossed body adduction.
8–12 weeks	Sling is for comfort only.	Active range of motion begins at 8 weeks. Expect full shoulder motion at 12 weeks.	None	None	
12–16 weeks	None		Strengthening begins at 12 weeks and progresses as tolerated. Strengthening should include periscapular muscles, especially lower trapezius.		Expect full shoulder motion at 12 weeks.
16–20 weeks				Begin sport- or work-specific drills.	
20–24 weeks				Return to play.	

From Kuhn JE. Open management of traumatic disorders of the sternoclavicular joint. In: Rockwood CA, Matsen FA, eds. *The Shoulder.* 6th ed. Philadelphia, PA: Elsevier; in press.

References

1. Spencer EE, Kuhn JE, Huston LJ, Carpenter JE. Ligamentous restraints to anterior and posterior translation of the sternoclavicular joint. *J Shoulder Elbow Surg.* 2002;11(1):43–47.

2. Spencer Jr EE, Kuhn JE. Biomechanical analysis of reconstructions for sternoclavicular joint instability. *J Bone Joint Surg Am.* 2004;86(1):98–105.

3

Technique Spotlight: Sternal Docking Technique for Sternoclavicular Joint Instability

RACHEL HONIG, JONATHAN BARLOW, AND JOAQUIN SANCHEZ-SOTELO

Indications

Sternoclavicular joint dislocations occur secondary to trauma or develop spontaneously in patients with collagen disorders, such as Ehler-Danlos syndrome. They are anatomically classified as either anterior or posterior, and further classified as acute or chronic. Joint reconstruction is generally indicated for patients with acute posterior dislocations, which have failed closed reduction, and for patients with chronic instability who have failed nonoperative management. Occasionally, medial clavicle resection and ligament reconstruction is considered for primary osteoarthritis or inflammatory arthropathy.

The technique described here has some potential advantages or disadvantages compared with alternative procedures.[1,2] No graft needs to be passed behind or completely through the sternum, which increases the safety of the procedure. In addition, the graft is placed centrally in the coronal plane, which optimizes clavicle alignment with the sternum. However, resection of the medial end of the clavicle may be perceived as a disadvantage, since it has the potential to impact the strut function of the clavicle in a negative way if shortening is excessive.

Preoperative Evaluation/Imaging

Sternoclavicular joint pathology is difficult to assess on plain radiographs. Our advanced imaging modality of choice is computed tomography (CT) with three-dimensional volume rendering. Magnetic resonance imaging (MRI) may be useful when physeal injuries are suspected. CT arthrogram may help understand the location of adjacent vascular structures, and is particularly useful in posterior dislocations. Any patient with atraumatic instability should be evaluated for collagen disorder. We recommend a vascular or thoracic surgeon should be available at the time of surgery due to the close proximity to mediastinal neurovascular structures.

Positioning and Equipment

The sternal docking procedure is performed with the patient supine with the head of the bed raised 30 degrees from horizontal. A regular operating room (OR) table or a dedicated beach-chair table may be used. The entire ipsilateral upper extremity and both sternoclavicular joints are draped into the surgical field. We recommend prepping and draping to include the entire sternum distal to the xiphoid, and having the sternal saw and vascular tray available in case emergency access to the great vessels is necessary. The reconstruction procedure itself will require a tendon allograft, a microsagittal saw, a high-speed 4.0-mm bur, a small angled curette, free needles, and heavy nonabsorbable suture. Our allograft of choice is semitendinous tendon.

Technique Description

An incision is made on the anterior aspect of the sternoclavicular joint centered across the inferior portion of the joint. The medial end of the clavicle is exposed and the intra-articular disc between the sternum and the clavicle is visualized and resected. A microsagittal saw is used to perform an osteotomy of the medial end of the clavicle to remove a minimal amount of bone (typically 5–10 mm). The osteotomy is performed approximately perpendicular to the medial end of the clavicle. A 4.0-mm bur is used to open the medial end of clavicular endosteal canal. The same bur is then used to create two anterior cortical perforations, one anterior and superior and one anterior and inferior, approximately 10–15 mm from the resected end of the clavicle. The small angled curette is then inserted in the medial end of the clavicle to clear cancellous bone between the end of the canal and the cortical perforations.

Attention is then turned to the anterior sternum. The sternal facet of the sternoclavicular joint is identified and an oblong perforation into this facet is created with the 4.0-mm bur. This perforation is centered at the articular facet, oblong in a superior to

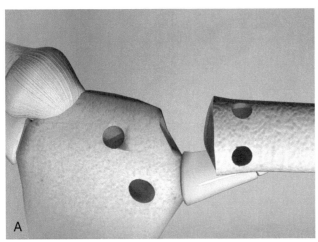
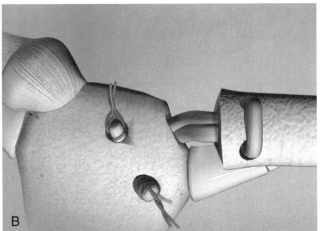
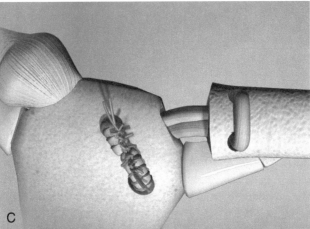

• **Fig. 3.1** (A) illustrates the bone tunnels needed for the procedure. (B) illustrates the graft being threaded into the medullary canal and through the bone tunnels in the sternum. (C) illustrates how the two ends of the graft should be sutured together to create a flush well-tensioned reconstruction.

inferior direction, and approximately 8–10 mm deep. Two additional 4.0-mm perforations are then created in the anterior cortex of the sternum, one proximal and one distal. The small angled curette is then used to clear cancellous bone such that the anterior cortical sternal perforations connect with the oblong tunnel made in the sternal articular facet.

The tendon allograft is then prepared in the back table with a running, locking stitch of heavy, nonabsorbable suture on one end of the graft. The heavy stitches are then used to thread the graft into the medullary canal of the clavicle (Fig. 3.1). The graft is first inserted through the anterior inferior cortical perforation in the clavicle, then reinserted through the anterior superior perforation so that now both ends of the graft are exiting the clavicle intramedullary canal. The two ends of the heavy suture are then inserted into the perforation at the sternal articular facet and retrieved through the anterior cortical holes of the sternum. The allograft is tensioned and the estimated length is measured so that the two ends of the allograft will exit through both holes in the front of the sternum with just the right length. Then, a second heavy nonabsorbable suture is placed on the second limb of the graft in a locking stitch configuration and the rest of the graft is resected and discarded. The sutures from each end of the graft are then tied over the anterior cortex of the sternum. This reconstruction can then be reinforced with multiple interrupted sutures if needed (Fig. 3.2).

Postoperative Management

Postoperatively, patients are recommended to use a shoulder immobilizer for 6 weeks. Active assisted and active range-of-motion exercises and scapular isometric exercises are initiated at 6 weeks. Between 10 and 12 weeks patients can initiate shoulder strengthening with elastic bands. Return to sports and other strenuous activities are allowed at 6 months.

PEARLS

- CT scan with three-dimensional volume rendering is the most useful advanced imaging modality to assess sternoclavicular joint pathology.
- Due to proximity to mediastinal neurovascular structures, vascular surgery availability is imperative.
- Minimize the amount of medial clavicle resected.
- Beware of patients with small clavicles or osteopenia to avoid intraoperative fracture of the tunnels.
- Carefully tension the graft to provide the exact length required to reestablish stability.

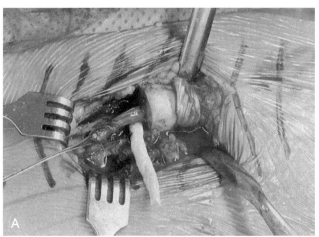
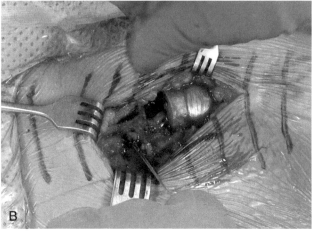
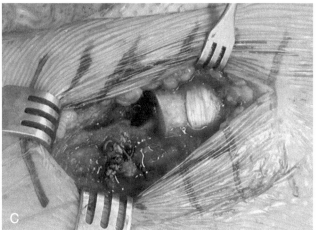

• **Fig. 3.2** (A–C) intraoperative images from graft passage during the sternal docking procedure.

References

1. Sanchez-Sotelo J. In: *Mayo Clinic Principles of Shoulder Surgery.* 1st ed. Rochester, MN: Mayo Clinic Scientific Press; 2018.

2. Sanchez-Sotelo J, Baghdadi Y, Nguyen NTV. Sternoclavicular joint allograft reconstruction using the sternal docking technique. *JSES Open Access.* 2018;2(4):190–193. https://doi.org/10.1016/j.jses.2018.08.002. eCollection 2018 Dec.

4

Medial Clavicle Fractures

ALEXANDER VAN TONGEL, BERT CORNELIS, AND LIEVEN DE WILDE

Relevant Anatomy

The clavicle is the first long bone to ossify. However, the epiphysis at the medial end of the clavicle is the last of the long bones to appear and is the last epiphysis to close. It does not ossify until 18–20 years of age. The epiphysis does not fuse with the shaft of the clavicle until age 23–25 years.[1] Until then, the growth plate remains the weakest point and more likely to sustain a displaced physeal fracture than a true dislocation.

The medial part of the S-shaped clavicle articulates with the sternum through a saddle-shaped joint with little intrinsic bony stability. Concerning the osseous anatomy, in both the anteroposterior and superoinferior directions, the clavicle is thickest at its medial part and looks more like a square (on average 25 mm on a side).

The clavicle is stabilized to the sternum via the sternoclavicular joint capsule and the anterior and posterior sternoclavicular ligaments. The posterior sternoclavicular ligament is particularly thick and stout. Further stability is provided by the costoclavicular ligament at the inferior border connecting with the first rib and the interclavicular ligament at the superior border connecting with the contralateral medial clavicle.[2]

Only the anteroinferior surface of the sternal end of the clavicle is covered by cartilage[3] (Fig. 4.1) and the clavicular articular surface is much larger than the sternal articular surface. There is also an intra-articular disc. Probably, as for meniscus in the knee, the function of the disc is to work as a shock absorber. Degenerative tears of the disc are commonly seen with aging and most of the time are asymptomatic in contrast to uncommon traumatic disc tears.[3,4]

Several muscles originate or insert on the medial clavicle. These include the clavicular part of the pectoralis major muscle, the sternocleidomastoid muscle, and the subclavius muscle.

In the case of a medial clavicle fracture, depending on the location of the fracture, any of these can act as deforming forces to displace the fracture and impede reduction. Typically, the lateral fragment is displaced anteriorly and inferiorly due to the pull of the pectoralis major muscle and the force of gravity on the upper limb while the sternocleidomastoid pulls the medial fragment superiorly.

Evaluation

A medial clavicle fracture is a rare injury, accounting for <5% of all clavicle fractures.[5–7] They commonly occur in middle-aged men as a result of auto or motorcycle accidents. The high incidence of segmental fractures (9%) and chest trauma (49%) implies an association with high-energy trauma.[8] These injuries, especially if nondisplaced or minimally displaced, are frequently missed during general clinical examination of the polytrauma patient, especially as more severe head, chest, and cervical injuries often coexist and can distract from the diagnosis. Furthermore, even if a standard trauma screening chest radiograph is taken, the overlapping shadows around the sternoclavicular joint and the medial clavicular metaphyseal cortices make diagnosis somewhat challenging even on standard radiographs. In the case of a hematoma, there should be a high suspicion of fracture. Even if displacement is visualized in the acute setting, it can be hard to distinguish between an anterior sternoclavicular dislocation and a medial clavicular fracture. When there is a suspicion of medial clavicle fracture, we recommend computed tomography (CT) scan for evaluation.

In children and young adults, fractures at the medial end of the clavicle are most commonly physeal separation. In contrast to adults, in which the lateral fragment displaces anteriorly, in this population, the lateral fragment can also displace anteriorly but much more commonly displaces posteriorly[9] (Fig. 4.2). When the lateral fragment is displaced posteriorly, this can cause dysphagia and/or dyspnea. Symptoms of mediastinal compression are a clear operative indication. Because the medial clavicular epiphysis is the latest bone to ossify, in patients under the age of 20, magnetic resonance imaging (MRI) or ultrasound can be helpful to distinguish between a physeal separation or a real dislocation.[10–12] In younger patients without symptoms, physeal injuries may remodel but closer to skeletal maturity, even physeal injuries with significant displacement may benefit from treatment.

Classification

Several classification systems have been described. According to the classification system of Allman, a medial clavicle fracture is localized in the medial one-third of the clavicle.[6] The Edinburgh classification describes a different segmentation of the clavicle with Type 1 medial fractures located within the one-fifth of clavicle bone lying medial to a vertical line drawn upward from the center of the first rib. Also, subclassifications A and B describe the aspect of displacement. Displacement is defined as >100% translation of the major fragments. Finally, Type 1A and Type 1B fractures are further subdivided into extra- or intra-articular[5] (Fig. 4.3). In 2007 Throckmorton and Kuhn described a new classification system in two ways, one system based on the fracture pattern and another based on the fracture displacement.[13] Fractures were classified as transverse, oblique intra-articular, oblique extra-articular,

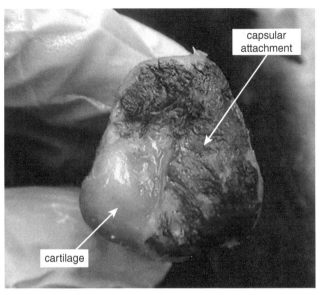

• **Fig. 4.1** Articular surface medial clavicle.

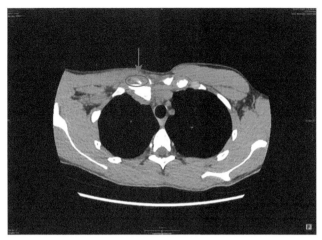

• **Fig. 4.2** Displaced Salter-Harris I fracture.

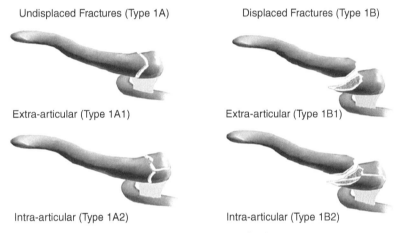

• **Fig. 4.3** Edinburgh classification.

comminuted, or avulsion. Fractures were classified as minimally, moderately, or severely displaced. In 2018 we described a new classification system based on the location of the fracture line and its relationship with the costoclavicular ligament[14] (Fig. 4.4). We described that the most common fracture line originates medial to the costoclavicular ligament. This fracture line starts just anteriorly at the limit of the articular surface but includes a larger piece of bone posteriorly. As we have described anatomically, there is a thick posterior sternoclavicular ligament/capsule that is attached to the superior and posterior two-thirds of the area of the medial surface of the clavicle and the posterior surface of the clavicle.[3] It seems that in this type of fracture pattern, the posterior piece of bone is still attached to the posterior sternoclavicular capsule. If there is no or minimal displacement, it seems the costoclavicular ligaments are still attached to the lateral fragment (Type 1A). In the case of rupture of the costoclavicular ligaments, the clavicular head of the pectoralis major can pull the lateral fragment of the clavicle anteriorly (Type 1B) (Fig 4.5). A much less common pattern is a Type 2 fracture. In this type, the fracture line is lateral to the costoclavicular ligament. In contrast to the oblique pattern in Type 1, the fracture line is transverse. In the case of displacement, shortening is probably caused by scapular protraction and loss of the strut effect normally provided by the clavicle.[15]

In medial physeal clavicle fractures, the Salter-Harris classification together with the direction of displacement of the lateral fragment is used to describe the fracture pattern.

Treatment Options

Nonoperative Treatment of Medial Clavicle Fractures

Similar to midshaft clavicle fractures, a nonoperative approach is preferred for the treatment of nondisplaced medial clavicle fractures. In our study, the healing rate was 100% for nondisplaced fractures (Type 1A and Type 1B). But even when significantly displaced, a nonoperative approach is traditionally preferred.[14] This is due to concerns about intraoperative complications and anticipated high union rates with nonoperative treatment.[16,17] A sling or a figure-of-eight bandage can be proposed for comfort but is not obligatory and will not have an influence on the long-term outcome, even in displaced fractures. However, several studies have shown symptomatic nonunion in up to 50% of all patients with displaced medial clavicle fractures.[13,18] In our study, 4 out of 19 patients (21%) with Type IB fractures developed a symptomatic nonunion.

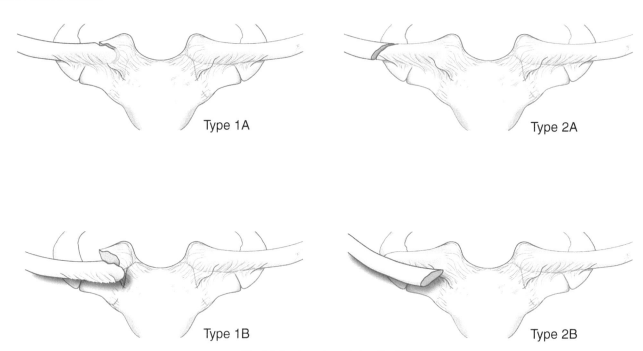

• **Fig. 4.4** Anatomy-based classification.

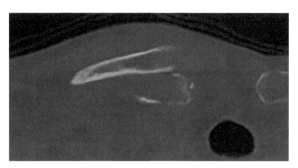

• **Fig. 4.5** Type 1B medial clavicle fracture.

Operative Treatment of Medial Clavicle Fractures

Because there seems to be a higher risk of symptomatic nonunion, primary operative treatment of displaced medial clavicle fractures has gained importance in recent literature.

As no specific implant for medial clavicle fractures or nonunion is available, multiple internal fixation methods have been utilized (Table 4.1). In a study by Frima et al., 14 patients received surgery for a primary displaced medial-end clavicle fracture. Three types of plates were used: six patients were treated with a radial (VA)-LCP Distal Humerus Plate, one patient with a standard 3.5 LCP Plate, and eight patients with an inverted LCP Superior Anterior Clavicle Plate with lateral extension. A mean QuickDASH and Subjective Shoulder Value (SSV) of 0.81 and 96, respectively, were found after a mean follow-up period of 39 months (range: 9–79), both indicating a good functional outcome. Seven of the 14 patients (50%), however, had their implant removed due to implant irritation after a mean period of 16 months.[17] Sidhu et al. investigated 24 patients undergoing primary operative fixation for a displaced medial clavicle fracture. In their study various fixation methods were used: 8 patients were treated with transosseous sutures and 16 patients with plate and screw. Plate and screw fixation included Medical and Optical 2.3-mm distal clavicle plate, a 3.5-mm Synthes distal clavicle plate, an ASDM distal clavicle

plate, distal radius plates, and standard locking compression plates. In this study, 17 patients (71%) reported mild symptoms of plate irritation. A median DASH (The Disabilities of the Arm, Shoulder and Hand) score of 0.4 was reported at 12 months postoperatively.[19] Oe et al. conducted a similar study. In their paper, 10 patients with a displaced medial-end clavicle fracture were included and treated primarily with various locking and nonlocking plates. Good functional results were reported in seven patients (70%). Two patients (20%) had their plate removed early due to local irritation and wound infection.[20] Similar results were found in a study by Low et al. on five patients.[21] Less implant and wound irritation were reported in a study by Titchener, possibly due to a more distant incision.[22]

At our institution, we use a hook plate developed for lateral clavicle fractures and acromioclavicular joint separations in the treatment of both acute and symptomatic nonunion medial clavicle fractures of Type 1B. In this fracture type, the medial fragment is too small for three bicortical screws. Furthermore, the hook placed posterior to the manubrium offsets the displacement force of the clavicular head of the pectoralis major. When evaluating all these arrays of surgical options, implant-related complications are very common (up to 70%).[17,19,23–25] The most common complication is hardware irritation. In our technique, we recommend standard removal of the hook plate after 3–6 months. Numerous dramatic cases of K-wires migrating dangerously in this region have been reported and we recommend avoiding this technique in this region. In the case of large fragments, tension band sutures seem to be less preferable. Despite the high complication rate, a good functional outcome was reported in most cases, and in the case of plate fixation (hook plate, plate and screw) no vascular complications have been described.

Nonoperative Treatment of Medial Physeal Fractures

Nondisplaced fractures can be treated nonoperatively. Literature is scarce on nondisplaced physeal fractures because most of the

TABLE 4.1 Various Studies of Internal Fixation Methods

Author	Number of Patients	Time of Fixation	Fixation Technique(s)	Outcome	Complications
Al-Yassari et al.[25]	3	After nonunion	Tension band wiring with mid clavicle osteotomy, plate, and screws with 4-month interval	Union in 3/3 Mean DASH 14.96, Constant score 75	Nil
Bartonicek et al.[24]	3	Primary fixation	Cerclage wires	Union in 3/3 Mean DASH 25.97	Nil
Der Tavitian et al.[23]	1	After nonunion	Lag screw	Union in 1/1 Severe pain at 32 months	Nil
Frima et al.[17]	14	Primary fixation	Plate and screws	Union in 14/14 Mean DASH 0.81, SSV 96	Implant irritation (8/14) Implant failure (1/14) Deep infection (1/14)
Low et al.[21]	5	Primary fixation (4/5) and after nonunion (1/5)	Plate and screws (4/5) and screw and sutures (1/5)	Union in 5/5 Mean DASH 9.0	Nil
Oe et al.[20]	10	Primary fixation	Plate and screws	Union in 9/10 Mean DASH 13.54	Implant irritation (2/10) Plate loosening (1/10)
Salipas et al.[16]	2	After nonunion	Plate and screws	Union in 2/2 Mean ASES 83, SSV 70	Intraoperative vascular complication (1/2)
Sidhu et al.[19]	27	Primary fixation (24/27) and after nonunion (3/27)	Plate and screws (19/27) and transosseous sutures (8/27)	Union in 27/27 Mean DASH 0.4	Implant irritation (17/27)
Titchener et al.[22]	8	Primary fixation	Plate and screws	Union in 8/8 Mean DASH 0.6	Nil

ASES, American Shoulder and Elbow Surgeons; *DASH*, The Disabilities of the Arm, Shoulder and Hand; *SSV*, Subjective Shoulder Value.

time they are probably not diagnosed correctly (diagnosed as a contusion).

In case of nonoperative treatment of displaced physeal fractures, activity-related pain can occur but also more serious complications like vascular compression, brachial plexopathy, exertional dyspnea, tracheal stenosis, sepsis, and even death from a tracheoesophageal fistula have been described.[26]

Operative Treatment of Medial Physeal Fractures

In the case of posteriorly displaced physeal fracture, a closed reduction can be attempted initially. This should preferentially be performed under general anesthesia. First, both shoulder blades are brought in retraction with a bump between the scapula, and the lateral fragment is pulled anteriorly with the use of a towel clip. Closed reduction is successful in >50% of the cases if attempted during the first 48 hours after the trauma. After 48 hours, the success rate drops to one-third. In case of failed closed reduction, an open reduction is the next step. After the reduction, if the fracture is unstable, several fixation techniques have been described in case reports. Because of several case fatalities or near fatalities, fixation with metallic pin fixation is contraindicated. Currently, the most common technique is suturing the epiphysis to the metaphysis with heavy sutures.[9,27] Open reduction and internal fixation in symptomatic chronic posterior sternoclavicular joint

fracture-dislocations in children and young adults is not possible. In these situations, a medial clavicle resection with stabilization has been described with acceptable results.[26]

References

1. Webb PA, Suchey JM. Epiphyseal union of the anterior iliac crest and medial clavicle in a modern multiracial sample of American males and females. *Am J Phys Anthropol*. 1985;68(4):457–466.
2. Cave AJ. The nature and morphology of the costoclavicular ligament. *J Anat*. 1961;95:170–179.
3. Van Tongel A, Macdonald P, Leiter J, Pouliart N, Peeler J. A cadaveric study of the structural anatomy of the sternoclavicular joint. *Clin Anat*. 2012;25(7):903–910.
4. Tytherleigh-Strong GM, Getgood AJ, Griffiths DE. Arthroscopic intra-articular disk excision of the sternoclavicular joint. *Am J Sports Med*. 2012;40(5):1172–1175.
5. Robinson CM. Fractures of the clavicle in the adult. Epidemiology and classification. *J Bone Joint Surg Br*. 1998;80(3):476–484.
6. Allman Jr FL. Fractures and ligamentous injuries of the clavicle and its articulation. *J Bone Joint Surg Am*. 1967;49(4):774–784.
7. Postacchini F, Gumina S, De Santis P, Albo F. Epidemiology of clavicle fractures. *J Shoulder Elbow Surg*. 2002;11(5):452–456.
8. Asadollahi S, Bucknill A. Acute medial clavicle fracture in adults: a systematic review of demographics, clinical features and treatment outcomes in 220 patients. *J Orthop Traumatol*. 2019;20(1):20–24.

9. Kasse AN, Limam SO, Diao S, Sane JC, Thiam B, Sy MH. [Fracture-separation of the medial clavicular epiphysis: about 6 cases and review of the literature]. *The Pan African Medical Journal.* 2016;25:19.

10. Baessler AM, Wessel RP, Caltoum CB, Wanner MR. Ultrasound diagnosis of medial clavicular epiphysis avulsion fracture in a neonate. *Pediatr Radiol.* 2020;50(4):587–590.

11. Sferopoulos NK. Fracture separation of the medial clavicular epiphysis: ultrasonography findings. *Arch Orthop Trauma Surg.* 2003;123(7):367–369.

12. Benitez CL, Mintz DN, Potter HG. MR imaging of the sternoclavicular joint following trauma. *Clin Imaging.* 2004;28(1):59–63.

13. Throckmorton T, Kuhn JE. Fractures of the medial end of the clavicle. *J Shoulder Elbow Surg.* 2007;16(1):49–54.

14. Van Tongel A, Toussaint A, Herregods S, Van Damme S, Marrannes J, De Wilde L. Anatomically based classification of medial clavicle fractures. *Acta Orthop Belg.* 2018;84(1):62–67.

15. Van Tongel A, De Wilde L. To the editor. *J Orthop Trauma.* 2015;29(9):e347–e348.

16. Salipas A, Kimmel LA, Edwards ER, Rakhra S, Moaveni AK. Natural history of medial clavicle fractures. *Injury.* 2016;47(10):2235–2239.

17. Frima H, Houwert RM, Sommer C. Displaced medial clavicle fractures: operative treatment with locking compression plate fixation. *Eur J Trauma Emerg Surg.* 2018(ePub).

18. Robinson CM, Court-Brown CM, McQueen MM, Wakefield AE. Estimating the risk of nonunion following nonoperative treatment of a clavicular fracture. *J Bone Joint Surg Am.* 2004;86-a(7):1359–1365.

19. Sidhu VS, Hermans D, Duckworth DG. The operative outcomes of displaced medial-end clavicle fractures. *J Shoulder Elbow Surg.* 2015;24(11):1728–1734.

20. Oe K, Gaul L, Hierholzer C, et al. Operative management of periarticular medial clavicle fractures-report of 10 cases. *J Trauma Acute Care Surg.* 2012;72(2):e1–e7.

21. Low AK, Duckworth DG, Bokor DJ. Operative outcome of displaced medial-end clavicle fractures in adults. *J Shoulder Elbow Surg.* 2008;17(5):751–754.

22. Titchener A, See A, Van Rensburg L, Tytherleigh-Strong G. Displaced medial end clavicular fractures treated with an inverted distal clavicle plate contoured through 90 degrees. *J Shoulder Elbow Surg.* 2019;28(4):e97–e103.

23. Der Tavitian J, Davison JN, Dias JJ. Clavicular fracture non-union surgical outcome and complications. *Injury.* 2002;33(2):135–143.

24. Bartonicek J, Fric V, Pacovsky V. Displaced fractures of the medial end of the clavicle: report of five cases. *J Orthop Trauma.* 2010;24(4):e31–35.

25. Al-Yassari G, Hetzenauer M, Tauber M, Resch H. Novel method to treat sterno-clavicular joint instability and medial clavicle fracture symptomatic nonunion. *J Shoulder Elbow Surg.* 2009;18(4):553–555.

26. Ting BL, Bae DS, Waters PM. Chronic posterior sternoclavicular joint fracture dislocations in children and young adults: results of surgical management. *J Pediatr Orthop.* 2014;34(5):542–547.

27. Goldfarb CA, Bassett GS, Sullivan S, Gordon JE. Retrosternal displacement after physeal fracture of the medial clavicle in children treatment by open reduction and internal fixation. *J Bone Joint Surg Br.* 2001;83(8):1168–1172.

5

Technique Spotlight: Medial Hook Plate

ALEXANDER VAN TONGEL AND LIEVEN DE WILDE

Indications

The authors prefer this technique for symptomatic medial clavicular nonunions type 1 or acute displaced fractures (relative indication) (type 1B) (see Chapter 4, Fig. 4.4).[1] For this fracture morphology, the hook plate provides resistance to the anterior deforming forces of the clavicular head of the pectoralis major even though the amount of bone on the medial aspect of the fracture is insufficient to obtain adequate bony purchase.

Preoperative Evaluation

A medial clavicle fracture is a rare injury, accounting for less than 5% of all clavicle fractures.[2–4] They commonly occur in middle-aged men as a result of auto or motorcycle accidents. These injuries are frequently missed during the general clinical examination of the polytrauma patient. In the acute setting, it can be hard to distinguish between an anterior sternoclavicular dislocation and a medial clavicular fracture (Fig. 5.1). Computed tomography (CT) scan is preferred for both diagnosis and evaluation of fracture type (Fig. 5.2). CT angiogram can be helpful in cases where great vessel injury is suspected.

Timing for Surgery

If performed in the acute setting, we ideally operate within 10 days after the injury as fracture mobility is simplified without extensive mobilization and dissection required. If there is symptomatic delayed union (minimum 3 months after trauma), a modified version of this same technique can be used, but the fracture mobilization and scar tissue make the procedure more difficult and potentially more prone to complications.

Positioning and Equipment

The patient is placed in a low beachchair position (20 degrees elevation). Care is taken not to create a plexopathy, but some degree of cervical rotation and extension is needed to allow access to the medial clavicle without hindrance from the chin. When draping, make sure the thorax is free to perform a sternotomy if necessary. The contralateral arm should be draped free so it can be mobilized during surgery.

Depending on surgeon comfort, it may be helpful to have a thoracic surgeon nearby and aware of the case, as well as having

the sternal saw and vascular tray in the room should great vessel injury occur.

Detailed Technique Description

Make a curved incision extending over the sternoclavicular joint and laterally along the anterior aspect of the clavicle (Fig. 5.3). Divide the overlying fascia and retract the fascia covering the sternocleidomastoid cranially, the clavicle in the middle and the pectoralis major caudally. Identify the sternal insertion of the sternocleidomastoid and retract medially.

Localize the sternoclavicular joint line. Open the anterior periosteal sleeve and expose the fracture edges (Fig. 5.4), afterwards the displaced lateral fragment needs to be reduced to the nondisplaced medial fragment. The clavicular part of the pectoralis major is partially released from the proximal clavicle and the costochondral junction for the first rib is visualized.

Carefully dissecting on bone between the medial fragment and the first rib and with the help of a periosteal elevator, soft-tissue is released from the posterior part of the sternum to create a space between the sternum anteriorly and the sternal muscles (sternothyroid and sternohyoid muscle) posteriorly (Fig. 5.5). Next, the hook of a hook plate (3.5 mm, Synthes) is inserted in the prepared area, posterior to the sternum with the hook portion caudad to the sternoclavicular joint (i.e., a left hook plate is used for a left proximal clavicular fracture; Fig. 5.6). The thickness of the hook plate is based on the preoperative CT evaluation of the thickness of the sternum. We measure the thickness of the sternum and until now we always used the 18-mm offset. This fits with the findings of Murty who described that the average thickness of the sternum was 16 mm.[5]

Next, the shaft portion of the hook plate is used as a reduction tool to lever the shaft fragment into place and minimal three bicortical screws are used in the lateral fragment (Fig. 5.7). If feasible, a lag screw through the plate is inserted to secure the avulsed segment to the rest of the clavicle. The direction based on the standard fracture plane is most commonly aiming 45 degrees medially. Care is taken not to plunge posteriorly beyond the posterior cortex with the drill bit.

The wound is closed in a layered fashion, first repairing the fascia between the pectoralis major and sternocleidomastoid and then the platysma layer if this is sufficiently thick for a separate, identifiable layer. The skin is closed in the standard fashion. We typically use a running subcuticular suture given the propensity

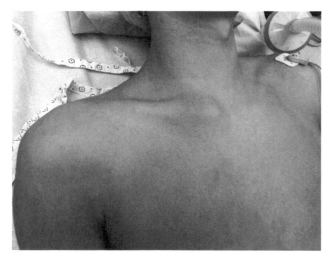

• **Fig. 5.1** Anteriorly displaced medial clavicle fracture.

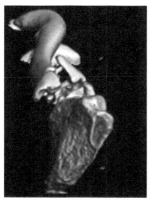

• **Fig. 5.2** Three-dimensional computed tomography (3D-CT) reconstruction of medial clavicle fracture type 1B. We routinely order a CT scan with 3D volume rendering reformats on medial clavicle fractures as we feel it provides the best appreciation for the fracture type and assists with surgical reduction.

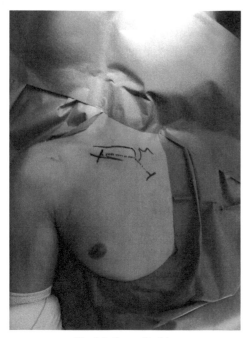

• **Fig. 5.3** Curved incision.

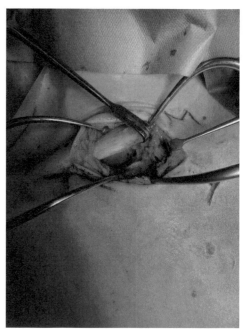

• **Fig. 5.4** Exposure of the fracture fragments.

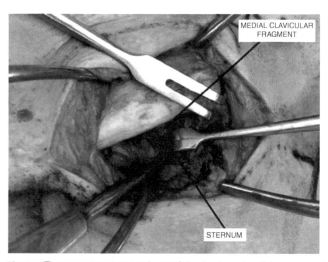

MEDIAL CLAVICULAR FRAGMENT

STERNUM

• **Fig. 5.5** The retrosternal space is carefully developed until large enough for the hook to enter.

of this area to form keloid scars and the goal for an optimal cosmetic result.

The patient is given a sling for comfort. We allow light activities with arms in front of the body (i.e., eating, computer work). Lifting, pushing, or pulling more significant weight and overhead activities are not allowed during the first 6 weeks. In our practice, a postoperative CT scan is routinely used to evaluate the correct position of the plate behind the sternum (Fig. 5.8).

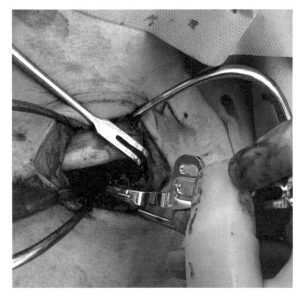

• **Fig. 5.6** Positioning hook retrosternal.

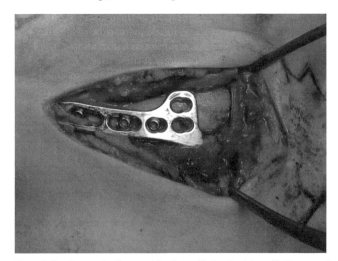

• **Fig. 5.7** Fracture reduction and fixation with hook plate with three cortical screws.

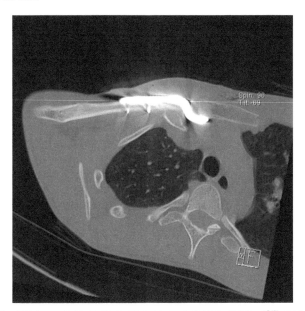

• **Fig. 5.8** Immediate postoperative computed tomography (CT) evaluation. Note the proper retrosternal positioning of the hook and the reduction of the clavicle.

PEARLS AND PITFALLS

- Although no literature currently exists describing neurovascular injuries after plate fixation of medial clavicle fracture, it is very important to know the anatomy of the mediastinal region and, depending on training and comfort level, have a thoracic surgeon available or even assist during the surgery.
- Although not proposed, the hook can also be positioned intraosseous within the sternum because a hole is created in the sternum and not behind the sternum. The disadvantage of this is the potential for a sternal cyst and the weaker resistance to anterior translation given a single cortex only. The advantage is that no hardware or instrumentation is required behind the sternum which theoretically could be safer with respect to great vessel injury (Fig. 5.9).

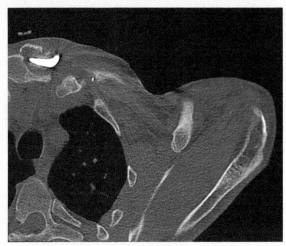

• **Fig. 5.9** Sternal cyst secondary to intraosseous placement of the hook within the manubrium and hardware left in place for 3 months. Again, we recommend routine hardware removal between 3 and 6 months and placement extraosseously posterior to the manubrium.

- While we do recommend routine hardware removal between 3 and 6 months after the surgery, this second surgery is straightforward, has minimal downtime for rehabilitation, and eliminates the possibility of residual discomfort from retained hardware.

References

1. Van Tongel A, Toussaint A, Herregods S, Van Damme S, Marrannes J, De Wilde L. Anatomically based classification of medial clavicle fractures. *Acta Orthop Belg.* 2018;84(1):62–67.
2. Robinson CM. Fractures of the clavicle in the adult. Epidemiology and classification. *J Bone Joint Surg Br.* 1998;80(3):476–484.
3. Allman Jr FL. Fractures and ligamentous injuries of the clavicle and its articulation. *J Bone Joint Surg Am.* 1967;49(4):774–784.
4. Postacchini F, Gumina S, De Santis P, Albo F. Epidemiology of clavicle fractures. *J Shoulder Elbow Surg.* 2002;11(5):452–456.
5. Murty O. Variability in thickness of skull bones and sternum. *Journal of Forensic Medicine and Toxicology ISSN.* 2009:0971–1929.

6

Midshaft Clavicle Fractures

PIERCE JOHNSON AND MICHAEL McKEE

Introduction

Clavicle fractures are among the most common bony injuries in the body, representing 2.5%–10% of all adult fractures and over 40% of shoulder girdle fractures.[1,2] Common injury mechanisms include skiing, mountain biking, American football, soccer/European football, as well as higher energy mechanisms like motor vehicle accidents. Due to the small bone diameter and limited soft tissue attachments, approximately 70%–80% of clavicle fractures occur in the middle one-third shaft.[2] In the past nearly all clavicle fractures were treated nonoperatively. This was likely due to the low nonunion rates reported in several studies. In 1960 Neer et al. published an analysis of 2000 patients with midshaft clavicle fractures reporting a nonunion rate of 0.13%.[3] Following this in 1968 Rowe subsequently published a nonunion rate of 0.8% in 566 midshaft clavicular fractures.[4] In addition to the extremely low nonunion rates reported, malunion was essentially not considered to be a real clinical entity as function and satisfaction were believed to be excellent no matter the orientation, alignment, or morphology of the healed fracture.[3,4] Today, nonoperative management remains the predominant treatment for most clavicle fractures but there has been a significant increase in surgical fixation. This shift in management is largely driven by investigations with an emphasis on patient outcomes that showed malunion to be a clear clinical entity, careful reporting of outcomes that has shown a significantly higher nonunion rate with certain fracture patterns, as well as multiple modern randomized trials that have shown benefit to fixation in certain types of clavicle fractures.[1,5–9]

Relevant Anatomy

The clavicle acts as a bony strut maintaining the distance between the lateral glenohumeral joint and medial axial skeleton at the sternoclavicular joint. It also serves a shoulder suspensory function maintaining the position of the shoulder girdle via coracoclavicular (CC) ligamentous attachment. The clavicle is a thin tubular S-shaped bone on average 12–15 cm in length with medial sternoclavicular and lateral acromioclavicular articulations.[10,11] The medial and lateral segments form widened flairs leaving the middle third with the smallest diameter. Because of this, the middle-third clavicle is the most susceptible and thus the most commonly fractured portion of the bone. The clavicle has a characteristic coronal plane S-shape with convex curvature medially and concave curvature involving middle and lateral portions of the bone.

The clavicle forms ligamentous attachments at the acromioclavicular joint, sternoclavicular joint, and coracoid. The acromioclavicular joint is a synovial joint that is stabilized by both superior and inferior acromioclavicular ligaments in addition to the CC ligaments. The conoid ligament medially and trapezoid ligament laterally make up the CC ligaments. The two ligaments come together to attach to the posterosuperior aspect of the coracoid base. Superiorly they separate and are often divided by a bursa at their superior attachment on the inferior aspect of the clavicle.[11,12] These ligaments provide stabilization of the clavicle mainly in the coronal plane. Injury to these ligaments can be associated with concomitant injuries to the acromioclavicular and/or sternoclavicular joints leading to dislocations at these sites.

The muscular attachments also play an important role in stabilization as well as creating the typical midshaft deformity often seen in clavicle fractures (Fig. 6.1). Medially, the pectoralis major attaches to the inferior aspect of the clavicle with the sternocleidomastoid (SCM) attaching to the superomedial aspect of the bone. The unopposed pull of the SCM results in the commonly observed superior displacement of the medial fragment. Laterally, the anterior attachments include both the deltoid and the pectoralis origins. The superolateral attachments are comprised of a combination of deltoid and trapezius fibers. The classic deformity of the lateral fragment is that of inferior and medial (shortening) caused by a combination of deltoid and pectoralis pull inferiorly and medially, respectively.

The relative proximity of major neurovascular structures including subclavian artery/vein, thoracoacromial vessels, supraclavicular nerves, and brachial plexus requires significant anatomic knowledge and surgical awareness in order to avoid injury when performing clavicle fixation. Multiple studies have described the anatomic relationship of these structures to the clavicle.[10,13,14] The mean distance from the subclavian and axillary vessels to the nearest surface of the clavicle has been reported to be 17–26 mm for the arteries and 3–12 mm for the veins. However, the artery can be as close as 5 mm, and in rare situations the vein may be directly opposed to the undersurface of the clavicle.[13] This is most commonly observed in revision situations where the vessels are distorted by scar tissue.

Robinson et al. performed a separate cadaveric study to evaluate these anatomic relationships and found the subclavian vein and artery were most closely associated with the clavicle medially (4.8 and 18.6 mm, respectively). The brachial plexus, however, was most closely associated with the clavicle (15.2 mm) in the middle third of the clavicle. In the lateral third of the clavicle, the subclavian vein was consistently identified as the closest structure and was never found to be within 2 cm of the clavicular cortex.[10] In an attempt to determine "safe zones" for fracture fixation, Steinmetz et al. performed a computed tomography (CT) angiogram-based study in which they evaluated the location of the major vascular structures around the clavicle and again determined that the subclavian vein is most closely located to the clavicle averaging

<10 mm to the clavicular cortex in the medial half of the bone.[15] These studies highlight the importance of anatomic awareness and the surgeon's ability to refrain from "plunging" during drill or screw placement, leading to possible neurovascular injury. Although often debated, the surgical approach and plate placement do not appear to significantly affect the proximity of neurovascular structures. Hussey et al. compared the distance of

hardware to neurovascular structures between anterior and superior plating. They found no significant difference in the distance to the subclavian vein/artery and brachial plexus in the superior plate position (9.2 ± 4.6, 12.2 ± 5.8, and 9.8 ± 5.2 mm, respectively) compared with the anterior plate position (8.3 ± 3.5, 12.2 ± 6.5, and 9.7 ± 5.3 mm, respectively).[16]

Another structure in relative proximity and thus at-risk during clavicle fixation is the pleural space. A recent CT-based study by Mulder et al. reported the average distance of 15.4 mm between the inferior aspect of the clavicle and the pleural space at the closest location which was medial. The average distances of 22 and 44 mm were also reported from the middle and lateral clavicle, respectively.[17] Due to the close proximity of the pleural space to the clavicle, iatrogenic pneumothorax is a potential complication of aberrant drilling during fixation.

The supraclavicular nerve is a superficial sensory nerve that originates from the C3 and C4 nerve roots of the superficial cervical plexus. This nerve ramifies proximally to provide sensation over the clavicle, anteromedial shoulder, and proximal chest and has three major branches (anterior, middle, posterior). These branches often cross the surgical field in the subcutaneous tissue during clavicle fracture fixation. Although high-level studies are lacking on this subject, some surgeons recommend identifying and preserving these cutaneous branches during approach while others do not. In either scenario, it is recommended to discuss with the patient the possibility of some numbness inferior to the clavicle postoperatively.

Pathoanatomy

Clavicle fractures are common injuries frequently resulting from a direct blow to the shoulder. Although previously thought to be caused by falls on the outstretched hand, current data suggest a direct blow to the shoulder is the more commonly observed mechanism.[18] A force directed inferomedially is applied to the shoulder or lateral aspect of the clavicle (Fig. 6.2). This places a compressive stress on the clavicle often leading to resultant injuries which can affect either

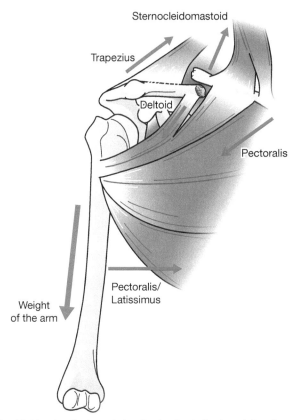

• **Fig. 6.1** Muscle attachments leading to classic fracture deformity.

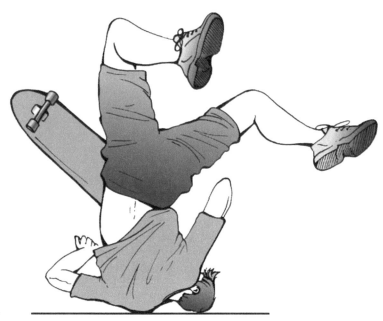

• **Fig. 6.2** Common mechanism of injury resulting in clavicle fracture with downward force applied to distal clavicle/shoulder. (From Court-Brown, Charles M. Rockwood and Green's Fractures in Adults, 8. Lippincott Williams and Wilkins; 2014.)

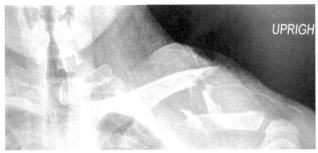

• **Fig. 6.3** Upright clavicle X-ray showing displaced midshaft clavicle fracture with classic deformity including proximal superior and distal anteroinferior displacement.

the laterally positioned acromioclavicular joint, the clavicle itself, or more infrequently resulting in a medial injury at the sternoclavicular joint injury. A common deformity seen after midshaft clavicle fracture is one in which the distal fragment is translated or rotated anteriorly, medialized (shortened), and inferiorly translated compared with the medial fragment (Fig. 6.3). As previously mentioned, this common deformity is due to a combination of force vector, bone morphology, gravity, and the deforming forces from muscle attachments.

Classification

An ideal classification system provides some direction towards treatment while describing the type of injury with high intra- and interobserver reliability. There are several proposed clavicle fracture classification systems. The original system developed by Allman placed fractures into one of three groups based on location with group I occurring proximally, group II mid-clavicle, and group III in the distal third.[19] However, because this system lacked important descriptive qualities such as displacement, comminution, or shortening, other systems emerged in order to address these important characteristics. The Edinburgh classification subclassifies type II (midshaft) fractures based on the degree of comminution. Simple or wedge-type fracture patterns make up subgroup 1, and comminuted or segmental fracture patterns represent subgroup 2.[20]

Treatment Options

Historically the vast majority of clavicle fractures were managed conservatively. Today many continue to be successfully managed in this fashion, although there has been a significant increase in rates of surgical fixation due to multiple recent high-level studies suggesting a lower rate of nonunion and symptomatic malunion with primary operative fixation.[5,7–9]

Nonoperative Management

Nonoperative management generally consists of placement of a sling for comfort for 7–10 days followed by an early gradual increase in shoulder motion as the patient is able to tolerate. Historically, figure-of-eight braces were also commonly used which have since largely fallen out of favor mainly due to patient discomfort and lack of data suggesting benefit for fracture healing.[21] Also of historical interest only, reduction of displaced clavicle fractures, achieved by lying the patient supine with a bump between the scapulae, was practiced since at least the days of the Edwin Smith Papyrus in 3500 BCE. Unfortunately, by the days of Hippocrates in 400 BCE, this was already known to be ineffective as gravity

and the deforming muscle forces soon returned the fracture to its prereduction alignment.[22]

Indications for Surgical Treatment

The majority of data available on completely displaced and/or shortened midshaft clavicle fractures involve only patients over the age of 16.[5,7–9] With the exclusion of adolescent and pediatric patients, it is difficult to completely generalize these results to include this population. As one would expect, due to improved healing and remodeling abilities of younger pediatric patients, the nonunion rates remain relatively low in this population. However, pediatric patients can still develop nonunions or symptomatic malunions affecting upper extremity function and thus surgeons may consider all treatment options in this age group. Vander Have et al. performed a retrospective study on 43 adolescent patients with a mean age of 15.4 years with displaced midshaft clavicle fractures. Seventeen underwent surgical fixation, and 25 were treated nonoperatively. They showed decreased time to union and return to function in the operative group. Five patients in the nonoperative group went on to develop symptomatic malunions whereas all surgically treated patients went on to complete fracture union.[23] This study suggests that even in this adolescent population, some displaced midshaft clavicle fractures go on to have suboptimal results following nonoperative management.

Indications for midshaft clavicle fracture fixation in the adult population have been further elucidated by the previously mentioned recent prospective studies.[5,7–9] These indications include injury characteristics such as open fractures or those with skin tenting, significant displacement >2 cm or 100%, shortening >2 cm, clinical deformity, segmental fractures, floating shoulder injuries, and those with significant comminution. They also include patient factors such as patient activity status, motivation to rapidly return to sport or work, or polytrauma injuries with the need for early upper extremity weight-bearing (Table 6.1).[5,6,9] In patients with concomitant lower extremity injuries, we do allow platform weight-bearing after clavicle fixation. As with any other surgery, patient lifestyle, comorbidities, and medical stability must also be taken into account. Although a patient's smoking status may negatively affect fracture healing, we do not routinely use this as a contraindication for surgery.

The classic clinical deformity often seen in patients with displaced clavicle fractures includes both medially displaced and anteriorly rotated shoulder girdles. In addition, there may be scapular winging and/or protraction noted in some patients posteriorly. The combination of these altered shoulder kinematics leading to symptomatic malunions if left to heal in a shortened position. Clinically, this often presents as a noticed reduction in strength and endurance due to altered muscle mechanics. Overhead positioning of the arm can result in neurological symptoms due to narrowing of the dimensions of the thoracic outlet. Physical examination often reveals clavicular asymmetry, an anteriorly rotated shoulder girdle, and scapular prominence with protraction. McKee et al. reported results from a recent meta-analysis of six randomized clinical trials including a total of 212 cases of operative versus nonoperative management for displaced midshaft clavicle fractures that showed 3/212 cases (1.4%) in the operative group versus 46/200 cases (23%) in the nonoperative group going on to either nonunion or symptomatic malunion.[5] A multicenter randomized trial was conducted by the Canadian Orthopaedic Trauma association that compared operative versus nonoperative outcomes and reported significant improvements in shoulder

TABLE 6.1 Indications for Clavicle Fracture Fixation

Fracture Specific	Associated Injuries	Other Factors
>2 cm displacement	Vascular injury requiring repair	Polytrauma/need for early UE weight-bearing
>2 cm shortening	Progressive neurological deficit	Patient motivation (elite athlete or self-employed professional)
Significant comminution	Ipsilateral UE/rib fractures	
Segmental fractures	Bilateral clavicle fractures	
Open fractures	Floating shoulder	
Impending open fractures		
Clinical deformity		

UE, Upper extremity.

Data from McKee RC, Whelan DB, Schemitsch EH, McKee MD. Operative versus nonoperative care of displaced midshaft clavicular fractures: a meta-analysis of randomized clinical trials. *J Bone Jt Surg-Am.* 2012;94(8):675-684; and Canadian Orthopaedic Trauma Society. Nonoperative treatment compared with plate fixation of displaced midshaft clavicular fractures. A multicenter, randomized clinical trial. *J Bone Joint Surg Am.* 2007;89(1):1-10.

and DASH (The Disabilities of the Arm, Shoulder and Hand) scores, improved time to healing (16.4 vs. 28.4 weeks), lower rate of nonunion (2%) and symptomatic malunion (<1%), and higher patient-reported shoulder outcomes in the operative group.[9]

Based on current available data, many midshaft clavicle fractures may still be managed nonoperatively with the majority of fractures going on to union. However, the aforementioned studies among others have shown decreased rates of nonunions and symptomatic malunions with surgical fixation of completely displaced (>100%) and shortened (>2 cm) clavicle fractures. It is for these fractures that the current data suggest surgical intervention is beneficial.

Techniques

Intramedullary Fixation

Another option for clavicle fracture fixation is the use of intramedullary fixation devices. There are several intramedullary implant devices today specifically designed for clavicle fracture fixation. Proposed benefits of this technique include minimal soft tissue disruption, potentially lower rates of hardware prominence, fewer cortical holes left in the clavicle as future stress risers, and a smaller incision/scar with a lower risk of residual paresthesias from cutaneous nerve injury. Complications such as nail migration, prominence, and continued shortening have often been cited especially with comminuted fractures. The nail may be inserted in an antegrade or retrograde fashion depending on the device. Some involve entering the nail at the fracture site which often requires an open approach. Fuglesang et al. performed a randomized controlled trial (RCT) evaluating outcomes for open reduction plate fixation versus intramedullary nail in displaced midshaft clavicle fractures at both 1- and 5-year postoperative intervals. They found no difference in nonunion rates between the two groups at both 1- and 5-year marks. They also reported no significant difference in DASH scores at 1 year (2.0 for nail vs. 1.4 for plate) but did report higher patient cosmetic satisfaction scores in the intramedullary group (8.6 vs. 7.7).[24] Of note, due to higher complication rates when 2.0-mm nails were placed, the authors recommend using plate fixation in smaller diameter clavicles (<2.5 mm). In another

study looking at implant irritation, Hulsman et al. found a significant difference in patient-reported irritation with comminuted and laterally localized fractures.[25] They recommend considering plate fixation for these types of fractures. In general, most intramedullary implant studies report good outcomes when used in simple, noncomminuted midshaft clavicle fractures. However, it is generally accepted that due to the risk of continued shortening and implant migration, these devices should be avoided in fractures with significant comminution. Also, due to limited fixation, these implants should be avoided in laterally based fractures.

Plate Fixation

The gold standard for clavicle fixation remains open reduction and fixation with plate and screw construct. Multiple studies have produced excellent and reproducible results regarding fracture healing with plate fixation, yet controversy still exists regarding the best type and location of plate fixation with options being anteroinferior versus superior, 3.5 mm versus small fragment dual plating, locking versus nonlocking, reconstruction versus nonrecon plates, and precontoured versus straight plates. Studies comparing different plate fixation methods vary widely in outcomes; however, multiple studies have shown increased failure rates with reconstruction plates when compared with compression plates.[26,27] Ashman et al. compared operative outcomes of 143 midshaft clavicular fractures treated with 51 compression plates and 92 reconstruction plates and reported implant failure rates of 1.4% for compression group, which was significantly lower than that of reconstruction plates which had a failure rate of 8.5%.[26] Multiple studies have reproduced these results as well, reporting failure of reconstruction plates between 7% and 12.5%.[7,28,29]

Precontoured plates have become increasingly popular due to improved fit in relation to the clavicle, which theoretically may avoid the complication of hardware prominence which can necessitate a second surgery for implant removal. Several studies have shown excellent fracture healing rates with these plates. Two multicenter RCTs reported implant failure rates as low as 1.1% and 0.6% with the use of precontoured locking compression plates (LCP).[1,30] A recent study showed significantly decreased rates of patient-reported hardware irritation and removal surgeries with the use of precontoured plates when compared with straight plates.[31] These plates have both locking and nonlocking options. Locking holes are often helpful in osteoporotic bone or with distal fractures in which there is minimal lateral bone for screw purchase. Some argue the use of locked plates allows for unicortical fixation minimizing the risk of iatrogenic neurovascular injury caused by bicortical drilling and screw placement. However, biomechanical studies have shown conflicting results regarding the strength of fixation of unicortical locking screws with load and stress testing.[32,33] We recommend the use of bicortical screws when able with the decision to use locking versus nonlocking screws based on bone quality and available bone for purchase. Typically, the cortical thickness of the midshaft clavicle is sufficient for cortical screws while fractures with more lateral and medial extension where the clavicular cortices are thinner may benefit from locking screw fixation.

Regarding plate placement, the two main techniques commonly used are anteroinferior and superior plating. Anterior plating was initially proposed to have drilling/screw trajectories farther from neurovascular structures, but, as discussed in the "Relevant Anatomy" section, this is not the case.[16] Anterior plating also has the theoretical benefit of allowing the thicker "width" of the plate resisting the bending moment imparted by gravity upon the upper limb versus the thinner plate thickness for a superiorly placed plate. One potential disadvantage is the theoretically increased need for plate bending given that the clavicle is essentially straight when viewed from anterior, allowing a superiorly based plate to simply be rotated slightly to fit a variety of anatomies, but has a variable "S-shaped" curvature when viewed from superior. Furthermore, with anterior plating the origin of the clavicular head of the pectoralis major and anterior deltoid must be released and repaired to allow access to the anterior clavicle. All told, much controversy still exists regarding which technique results in better outcomes and fewer complications as multiple biomechanical and clinical studies report conflicting results. Wilkerson et al. showed improved strength with anterior plates in cadaveric models. They reported superiorly plated specimens failed after significantly fewer cycles and with lower force than the anteriorly plated specimens.[34] Conversely, Toogood et al. performed a similar study but evaluated different force vectors acting on the clavicle and found increased stiffness with axial compression and torsion with a superior plate, whereas increased stiffness was observed with cantilever bending with an anterior plate. Given the unknown clinical relevance of various loading conditions, they stated that absolute recommendations for either superior or anterior plates cannot be made based solely off of biomechanical data.[35]

Studies evaluating rates of hardware irritation for anteroinferior versus superior plating again report varying results. A 2016 retrospective review comparing these techniques reported no difference in rates of patient-reported hardware irritation or implant removal.[25] A separate meta-analysis by Nourian et al. showed similar operative outcomes with respect to union, nonunion, malunion, and implant failure, as well as similar functional outcomes scores, but did show that superior plates were associated with significantly higher rates of symptomatic hardware and implant removal.[36] A meta-analysis by Ai et al. including four RCTs and eight observational studies showed no difference between the two methods regarding Constant score, and the rate of infection, nonunion, and complications. They did, however, report a shorter time to union, decreased operative time, and blood loss in the anteroinferior group compared with the superior group.[37] Thus due to the conflicting results of multiple studies, the present

literature has not shown any definitive significance whether superior or anterior plating produces better biomechanical or clinical outcomes.

Regardless of the approach, hardware irritation is the most common reason for subsequent surgeries following clavicle fixation with reported rates of hardware removal as high as 45% with a wide range of reported rates (5.6%–45%).[38–40] It has become clear that a technique that would provide sufficient stability while decreasing the rate of hardware irritation would be of great interest. In order to address this problem, a dual plating technique was developed that has become increasingly popular in recent years. This technique consists of low-profile dual minifragment plates applied to the anteroinferior and superior surfaces of the clavicle. The idea is that the two, smaller, lower profile plates will be less prominent thus causing less irritation with the same fracture stability than more traditional thicker plates. Multiple studies have been published regarding this technique including a recent biomechanical study that compared low-profile dual plating technique with either traditional 3.5-mm anterior or superior plates. They found no difference in stiffness or load to failure in the dual plate group.[41] A retrospective clinical study compared a single 2.7-mm plate versus a 3.5-mm plate and found no difference in time to union, nonunion rates, or outcome scores at 1 year. They did report a significant improvement in patient-reported cosmetic outcome (95% vs. 50%) with a trend towards decreased reoperation rates when compared with the 3.5-mm plate (0% vs. 17%).[29] There have been several studies reporting relatively low rates of reoperation using minifragment dual plating technique; however, none of them to date include comparative control groups and are subjected to significant possible biases. A relative contraindication to this technique is a fracture pattern with significant comminution. To date, there are limited data regarding clinical outcomes of low-profile dual plating. It is currently unknown whether or not this technique offers lower rates of hardware irritation and subsequent removal. Further clinical trials including comparative, prospective trials with objective criteria for reintervention are needed to further investigate.

Relevant Complications

The two most likely complications with nonoperative treatment are symptomatic malunion and nonunion. Malunion, discussed briefly in the "Indications for Surgical Treatment" section, is the healing of a fracture in a nonanatomic position. Several risk factors for symptomatic clavicle malunion can be seen in Table 6.1. In most clavicle fracture malunions, this includes shortening (>2 cm) and residual angulation. This can often lead to alterations of shoulder girdle mechanics, which in turn result in weakness and patient dissatisfaction. This has been shown in recent studies reporting objective shoulder strength loss of 18%–33%, poor early function, and up to 42% of patients with residual sequelae 6 months after injury.[6,42]

We define nonunion as a failure of fracture healing determined by radiographs or fragment motion on physical examination after a minimum of 9 months since the injury.[43] As discussed, the rate of nonunion was initially felt to be quite low with nonoperative management, but more recent trials have shown this rate to be closer to 15%–20%[42] in the subset of midshaft clavicle fracture displaced >100%. Surgical management can reduce this rate to approximately 1%[5,9] but carries its own risks such as infection, neurovascular injury, and soft tissue irritation requiring additional surgery for hardware removal. The ultimate goal of surgical fixation is to obliviate the risk of symptomatic malunion and nonunion, and it has been shown to be extremely successful in doing so.

Although relatively rare, complications such as surgical site infections (SSIs), wound dehiscence, neurovascular injury, and iatrogenic pneumothorax are possible. Reported infection rates after clavicle fixation range from 0.4%–7.8%.[44–46] Liu et al. reported an infection rate of 4.9% (7 out of 142) that had undergone clavicle fixation. All of their patients were treated with 24 hours of intravenous (IV) antibiotics prior to discharge. In all cases, the infections were noted to communicate with the hardware and all plates were eventually removed at an average of 21 days (range: 6–42) after surgery. All fractures eventually healed in appropriate position except one that went on to form a symptomatic malunion.[44] In a 2005 study Duncan discussed the significance of deep infection with regard to fracture healing. They found that four out of the six identified cases of deep infection went on to persistent nonunion with functional limitations.[47] This highlights the importance of ruling out deep infection in patients with continued functional limitations and/or radiographic evidence of nonunion following clavicle fixation. In the case of suspected deep infection, we will generally perform a formal irrigation and debridement down to the hardware and evaluate the plate and screw stability. If the hardware appears loose, we will remove it. However, if stable, we will usually leave the hardware in place after performing a thorough irrigation and debridement of the plate and surrounding tissues. Limited data exist regarding specific length of postoperative antibiotic use in this situation. We routinely leave a gram of powdered antibiotic (such as vancomycin) in the wound prior to closure when performing irrigation debridement for infected cases. The most commonly used regimens are between 2 and 6 weeks of oral or IV antibiotics based on culture and susceptibility profiles. Another important aspect of clavicle fixation SSI is in regard to the soft tissue closure at the time of surgery. Proponents of anterior plating argue this as one of the benefits of the technique. That is, that there is more available soft tissue to protect from hardware irritation as well as deep infection. There are no available studies showing significant differences in infection rates between anteroinferior and superior plating.

Fortunately, iatrogenic neurovascular complications during clavicle fracture fixation are very rare. Wijdicks et al. performed a meta-analysis of 582 cases of clavicle fixation and did not report a single vascular complication suggesting the relative rarity of these injuries.[48] However, the proximity of the subclavian vessels and brachial plexus to the clavicle requires detailed anatomic knowledge, as well as substantial intraoperative care by the operating surgeon as injuries to these structures may be devastating.

The incidence of brachial plexus injury is much higher in the surgical fixation of chronic nonunion/malunion cases. This is especially true in situations where the clavicle has healed or scarred down in a shortened position. During attempted reduction and fixation to an elongated position, an increased traction stress is placed on the surrounding neurovascular structures which can lead to neuropraxic injury. Jeyaseelan et al. reported a series of 21 cases of brachial plexus injury all following delayed fixation of a displaced clavicle fracture.[49] They postulated that the passing brachial plexus structures become adherent to the deep surface of the clavicle near the fracture site making them susceptible to traction injury. Thus care must be taken during late fixation to avoid overdistraction resulting in neurovascular stretch injuries.

Vascular injury is another serious complication of clavicle fixation. Although rare, these injuries are serious and if not immediately recognized and addressed can lead to significant complications such as loss of limb. This may be either due to acute vascular perforation by a drill or screw or more commonly due to more chronic injury caused by prominent screw placement. In a 2014 study Clitherow et al. evaluated reports of arterial injury caused by prominent screw placement and found four cases of arterial pseudoaneurysm and one case of subclavian arteriovenous (AV) fistula. All were associated with prominent screws, that is, overpenetrated past the far (inferior) cortex. There were no reported fatalities from arterial injury due to clavicle fixation.[50] There have been two reports of fatal air emboli caused by drilling and perforating the subclavian vein during placement of the medial screws.[51] One must take great care to be aware and protect the neurovascular structures during clavicle fixation, keeping in mind the anatomic relationship of the vessels and the clavicle. Medially, the vessels are normally situated posterior to the clavicle whereas laterally they are in a more inferior position and the vein is almost always closer to the clavicle than the artery.

Due to the relative proximity of the pleural space, pneumothorax is another potential complication of clavicle fixation. Although the actual rate of iatrogenic pneumothorax during clavicle fixation has not been reported, several case reports have been published. In a 2019 retrospective study, 89 patients without preoperative pneumothorax were evaluated for intraoperative iatrogenic pneumothorax by obtaining postoperative chest X-ray.[52] They reported zero cases of intraoperative iatrogenic pneumothorax thus recommending against the routine use of postoperative chest X-ray. However, if the patient has a known preoperative pneumothorax, a postoperative X-ray should be obtained to evaluate for any change in size, which is commonly seen after mechanical ventilation. Should there be any indication during surgery that the lung parenchyma has been penetrated such as excessive plunging during drilling, bleeding indicating vascular injury, or observed bubbling during lung inflation, a chest X-ray should be obtained. If bubbling is observed after drilling, the anesthesiologist should be notified and made aware of the possibility of iatrogenic injury. If a chest X-ray shows evidence of pneumothorax, chest tube placement may be warranted based on size and respiratory status. In the rare event of a tension pneumothorax, immediate chest tube insertion is indicated.

Review of Treatment Outcomes

A number of high-quality prospective, randomized studies are now available to better determine the role of primary operative fixation for midshaft clavicle fractures. While the majority of clavicle fractures heal with nonoperative management, there is a subset of fractures that benefit from operative fixation. Poor prognostic signs include significant fracture displacement, shortening, and comminution, especially if associated with scapular malposition or winging. Several meta-analyses of randomized clinical trials comparing operative versus nonoperative treatment for displaced midshaft fractures of the clavicle have produced some consistent findings.[5–9] We now know that plate fixation is a reliable technique with an extremely low nonunion rate of <2%.[5,8] Nonoperative treatment of displaced midshaft fractures results in a reported nonunion rate of 15%–25%[5,6,9,36] and symptomatic malunion continues to affect some patients treated conservatively. Finally, primary fixation results in modest patient-reported improvement in the operative group compared with the nonoperative group.[5,9,36]

Plate fixation remains the gold standard although other fixation methods are available. Anteroinferior plate placement has some theoretical advantages over superior plate positioning with respect to soft tissue irritation, but this has not yet been proven conclusively. Both techniques have been shown to produce >95% success rates regarding fracture healing. Low-profile dual plating is a relatively new technique of interest due to the proposed benefit of less hardware irritation; however, additional prospective studies are needed to better elucidate this. Intramedullary fixation also has several theoretical advantages and a high rate of success in skilled hands, although results in the literature remain inconsistent regarding indications, outcomes, and complications. Finally, although the difference is small, primary plate fixation provides significantly improved results in terms of strength and shoulder scores compared with delayed reconstruction.[5,8,9,36] Future randomized prospective studies are needed to refine the indications for primary operative repair and determine the ideal method of fixation.

References

1. Robinson CM, Goudie EB, Murray IR, et al. Open reduction and plate fixation versus nonoperative treatment for displaced midshaft clavicular fractures. *J Bone Jt Surg-Am.* 2013;95(17):1576–1584. https://doi.org/10.2106/jbjs.l.00307.

2. Postacchini F, Gumina S, De Santis P, Albo F. Epidemiology of clavicle fractures. *J Shoulder Elbow Surg.* 2002;11(5):452–456. https://doi.org/10.1067/mse.2002.126613.

3. Neer CS. Nonunion of the clavicle. *J Am Med Assoc.* 1960;172(10):1006–1011. https://doi.org/10.1001/jama.1960.03020100014003.

4. Rowe CR. An atlas of anatomy and treatment of midclavicular fractures. *Clin Orthop.* 1968;58:29–42.

5. McKee RC, Whelan DB, Schemitsch EH, McKee MD. Operative versus nonoperative care of displaced midshaft clavicular fractures: a meta-analysis of randomized clinical trials. *J Bone Jt Surg-Am.* 2012;94(8):675–684. https://doi.org/10.2106/jbjs.j.01364.

6. McKee MD. Deficits following nonoperative treatment of displaced midshaft clavicular fractures. *J Bone Jt Surg Am.* 2006;88(1):35–40. https://doi.org/10.2106/jbjs.d.02795.

7. Woltz S, Krijnen P, Schipper IB. Plate fixation versus nonoperative treatment for displaced midshaft clavicular fractures. *J Bone Jt Surg.* 2017;99(12):1051–1057. https://doi.org/10.2106/jbjs.16.01068.

8. Xu J, Xu L, Xu W, Gu Y, Xu J. Operative versus nonoperative treatment in the management of midshaft clavicular fractures: a meta-analysis of randomized controlled trials. *J Shoulder Elbow Surg.* 2014;23(2):173–181. https://doi.org/10.1016/j.jse.2013.06.025.

9. Canadian Orthopaedic Trauma Society. Nonoperative treatment compared with plate fixation of displaced midshaft clavicular fractures. A multicenter, randomized clinical trial. *J Bone Joint Surg Am.* 2007;89(1):1–10. https://doi.org/10.2106/JBJS.F.00020.

10. Robinson L, Persico F, Lorenz E, Seligson D. Clavicular caution: an anatomic study of neurovascular structures. *Injury.* 2014;45(12):1867–1869. https://doi.org/10.1016/j.injury.2014.08.031.

11. Hyland S, Varacallo M. *Anatomy, shoulder and upper limb, clavicle. StatPearls.* Treasure Island, FL: StatPearls Publishing; 2020. http://www.ncbi.nlm.nih.gov/books/NBK525990/.

12. Marchese RM, Bordoni B. *Anatomy, shoulder and upper limb, coracoclavicular joint (coracoclavicular ligament). StatPearls.* Treasure Island, FL: StatPearls Publishing; 2020. http://www.ncbi.nlm.nih.gov/books/NBK545221/.

13. Sinha A, Edwin J, Sreeharsha B, Bhalaik V, Brownson P. A radiological study to define safe zones for drilling during plating of clavicle fractures. *J Bone Joint Surg Br.* 2011;93-B(9):1247–1252. https://doi.org/10.1302/0301-620x.93b9.25739.

14. Jeon A, Seo CM, Lee J-H, Han S-H. The distributed pattern of the neurovascular structures around clavicle to minimize structural injury in clinical field: anatomical study. *Surg Radiol Anat.* 2018;40(11):1–5. https://doi.org/10.1007/s00276-018-2091-4.

15. Steinmetz G, Conant S, Bowlin B, et al. The anatomy of the clavicle and its in vivo relationship to the vascular structures. *J Orthop Trauma.* 2020;34(1):14–19. https://doi.org/10.1097/bot.0000000000001633.

16. Hussey MM, Chen Y, Fajardo RA, Dutta AK. Analysis of neurovascular safety between superior and anterior plating techniques of clavicle fractures. *J Orthop Trauma.* 2013;27(11):627–632. https://doi.org/10.1097/bot.0b013e31828c1e37.

17. Mulder FJ, Mellema JJ, Ring D. Proximity of vital structures to the clavicle: comparison of fractured and non-fractured side. *Arch Bone Jt Surg.* 2016;4(4):318–322.

18. Stanley D, Trowbridge E, Norris S. The mechanism of clavicular fracture. A clinical and biomechanical analysis. *J Bone Joint Surg Br.* 1988;70-B(3):461–464. https://doi.org/10.1302/0301-620x.70b3.3372571.

19. Allman FL. Fractures and ligamentous injuries of the clavicle and its articulation. *J Bone Jt Surg.* 1967;49(4):774–784. https://doi.org/10.2106/00004623-196749040-00024.

20. Robinson CM. Fractures of the clavicle in the adult. Epidemiology and classification. *J Bone Joint Surg Br.* 1998;80(3):476–484. https://doi.org/10.1302/0301-620x.80b3.8079.

21. Waldmann S, Benninger E, Meier C. Nonoperative treatment of midshaft clavicle fractures in adults. *Open Orthop J.* 2018;12:1–6. https://doi.org/10.2174/1874325001812010001.

22. Blomstedt P. Orthopedic surgery in ancient Egypt. *Acta Orthop.* 2014;85(6):670–676. https://doi.org/10.3109/17453674.2014.950468.

23. Vander Have KL, Perdue AM, Caird MS, Farley FA. Operative versus nonoperative treatment of midshaft clavicle fractures in adolescents. *J Pediatr Orthop.* 2010;30(4):774–784. https://doi.org/10.1097/bpo.0b013e3181db3227.

24. Fuglesang HFS, Flugsrud GB, Randsborg PH, Oord P, Benth JŠ, Utvåg SE. Plate fixation versus intramedullary nailing of completely displaced midshaft fractures of the clavicle. *Bone Jt J.* 2017;99-B(8):774–784. https://doi.org/10.1302/0301-620x.99b8.bjj-2016-1318.r1.

25. Hulsmans MHJ, van Heijl M, Houwert RM, et al. High irritation and removal rates after plate or nail fixation in patients with displaced midshaft clavicle fractures. *Clin Orthop Relat Res.* 2016;475(2):523–529. https://doi.org/10.1007/s11999-016-5113-8.

26. Ashman BD, Slobogean GP, Stone TB, et al. Reoperation following open reduction and plate fixation of displaced mid-shaft clavicle fractures. *Injury.* 2014;45(10):1549–1553. https://doi.org/10.1016/j.injury.2014.04.032.

27. Chiu Y-C, Huang K-C, Shih C-M, Lee K-T, Chen K-H, Hsu C-E. Comparison of implant failure rates of different plates for midshaft clavicular fractures based on fracture classifications. *J Orthop Surg.* 2019;14(1):1–7. https://doi.org/10.1186/s13018-019-1259-x.

28. Özkul B, Saygılı MS, Dinçel YM, Bayhan IA, Akbulut D, Demir B. Comparative results of external fixation, plating, or nonoperative management for diaphyseal clavicle fractures. *Med Princ Pract.* 2017;26(5):458–463. https://doi.org/10.1159/000481865.

29. Galdi B, Yoon RS, Choung EW, et al. Anteroinferior 2.7-mm versus 3.5-mm plating for AO/OTA type B clavicle fractures. *J Orthop Trauma.* 2013;27(3):121–125. https://doi.org/10.1097/bot.0b013e3182693f32.

30. Ahrens PM, Garlick NI, Barber J, Tims EM. The clavicle trial. *J Bone Jt Surg.* 2017;99(16):1345–1354. https://doi.org/10.2106/jbjs.16.01112.

31. VanBeek C, Boselli KJ, Cadet ER, Ahmad CS, Levine WN. Precontoured plating of clavicle fractures: decreased hardware-related complications? *Clin Orthop Relat Res.* 2011;469(12):3337–3343. https://doi.org/10.1007/s11999-011-1868-0.

32. Little KJ, Riches PE, Fazzi UG. Biomechanical analysis of locked and non-locked plate fixation of the clavicle. *Injury.* 2012;43(6):921–925. https://doi.org/10.1016/j.injury.2012.02.007.

33. Khan LAK, Bradnock TJ, Scott C, Robinson CM. Fractures of the clavicle. *J Bone Jt Surg-Am.* 2009;91(2):447–460. https://doi.org/10.2106/jbjs.h.00034.

34. Wilkerson J, Paryavi E, Kim H, Murthi A, Pensy RA. Biomechanical comparison of superior versus anterior plate position for fixation of distal clavicular fractures. *J Orthop Trauma*. 2017;31(1):13–17. https://doi.org/10.1097/bot.0000000000000707.

35. Toogood P, Coughlin D, Rodriguez D, Lotz J, Feeley B. A biomechanical comparison of superior and anterior positioning of precontoured plates for midshaft clavicle fractures. *Am J Orthop Belle Mead NJ*. 2014;43(10):E226–E231.

36. Nourian A, Dhaliwal S, Vangala S, Vezeridis PS. Midshaft fractures of the clavicle: a meta-analysis comparing surgical fixation using anteroinferior plating versus superior plating. *J Orthop Trauma*. 2017;31(9):461–467. https://doi.org/10.1097/BOT.0000000000000936.

37. Ai J, Kan S-L, Li H-L, et al. Anterior inferior plating versus superior plating for clavicle fracture: a meta-analysis. *BMC Musculoskelet Disord*. 2017;18(1):1–9. https://doi.org/10.1186/s12891-017-1517-1.

38. Mok D, Wang J, Chidambaram R. Is removal of clavicle plate after fracture union necessary? *Int J Shoulder Surg*. 2011;5(4):85–89. https://doi.org/10.4103/0973-6042.90998.

39. Baltes TPA, Donders JCE, Kloen P. What is the hardware removal rate after anteroinferior plating of the clavicle? A retrospective cohort study. *J Shoulder Elbow Surg*. 2017;26(10):1838–1843. https://doi.org/10.1016/j.jse.2017.03.011.

40. Granlund AS, Troelsen A, Ban I. Indications and complications in relation to removal of clavicle implants. *Dan Med J*. 2017;64(12):1–4.

41. Ziegler CG, Aman ZS, Storaci HW, et al. Low-profile dual small plate fixation is biomechanically similar to larger superior or anteroinferior single plate fixation of midshaft clavicle fractures. *Am J Sports Med*. 2019;47(11):2678–2685. https://doi.org/10.1177/0363546519865251.

42. Hill JM, McGuire MH, Crosby LA. Closed treatment of displaced middle-third fractures of the clavicle gives poor results. *J Bone Joint Surg Br*. 1997;79(4):537–539. https://doi.org/10.1302/0301-620x.79b4.7529.

43. Calori GM, Mazza EL, Mazzola S, et al. Non-unions. *Clin Cases Miner Bone Metab Off J Ital Soc Osteoporos Miner Metab Skelet Dis*. 2017;14(2):186–188. https://doi.org/10.11138/ccmbm/2017.14.1.186.

44. Liu P-C, Hsieh C-H, Chen J-C, Lu C-C, Chuo C-Y, Chien S-H. Infection after surgical reconstruction of a clavicle fracture using a reconstruction plate: a report of seven cases. *Kaohsiung J Med Sci*. 2008;24(1):45–48. https://doi.org/10.1016/s1607-551x(08)70073-1.

45. Bostman O, Manninen M, Pihlajamaki H. Complications of plate fixation in fresh displaced midclavicular fractures. *J Trauma Inj Infect Crit Care*. 1997;43(5):778–783. https://doi.org/10.1097/00005373-199711000-00008.

46. Shen W-J, Liu T-J, Shen Y-S. Plate fixation of fresh displaced midshaft clavicle fractures. *Injury*. 1999;30(7):497–500. https://doi.org/10.1016/s0020-1383(99)00140-0.

47. Duncan SFM, Sperling JW, Steinmann S. Infection after clavicle fractures. *Clin Orthop*. 2005;439:74–78. https://doi.org/10.1097/01.blo.0000183088.60639.05.

48. Wijdicks F-JG, Van der Meijden OAJ, Millett PJ, Verleisdonk EJMM, Houwert RM. Systematic review of the complications of plate fixation of clavicle fractures. *Arch Orthop Trauma Surg*. 2012;132(5):617–625. https://doi.org/10.1007/s00402-011-1456-5.

49. Jeyaseelan L, Singh VK, Ghosh S, Sinisi M, Fox M. Iatropathic brachial plexus injury. *Bone Jt J*. 2013;95-B(1):106–110. https://doi.org/10.1302/0301-620x.95b1.29625.

50. Clitherow HD, Bain GI. Major neurovascular complications of clavicle fracture surgery. *Shoulder Elb*. 2014;7(1):3–12. https://doi.org/10.1177/1758573214546058.

51. Bain GI, Eng K, Zumstein MA. Fatal air embolus during internal fixation of the clavicle. *JBJS Case Connect*. 2013;3(1):e24. https://doi.org/10.2106/jbjs.cc.l.00194.

52. Shubert DJ, Shepet KH, Kerns AF, Bramer MA. Postoperative chest radiograph after open reduction internal fixation of clavicle fractures: a necessary practice? *J Shoulder Elbow Surg*. 2019;28(5):e131–e136. https://doi.org/10.1016/j.jse.2018.09.016.

7

Technique Spotlight: ORIF Midshaft Clavicle Fracture with Plate and Screws

PIERCE JOHNSON AND MICHAEL McKEE

Indications

Indications for clavicle fixation include open fractures, skin tenting or soft tissue compromise, significant displacement >2 cm, shortening >2 cm, clinical deformity, significantly associated scapular winging from malrotation, segmental fractures, "floating shoulder" injuries and those with significant comminution. Patient factors are also important considerations including patient activity status and motivation to rapidly return to sport or work or polytrauma injuries with the need for early upper extremity weight-bearing. We generally allow modified weight-bearing postoperatively including platform weight-bearing in patients with concomitant lower extremity injuries. Contraindications include patients who are medically unstable to undergo surgery, patients with substance abuse disorders, and those unlikely to benefit from surgery.

Technique

Preoperative Planning and Patient Positioning

Preoperative planning including evaluating X-rays and consideration of the type and size of plate, and the possibility of lag screw placement is completed prior to incision. Care is taken to scour the radiographs for nondisplaced fracture lines which may affect the surgical tactic.

We generally request an interscalene block to be performed by our anesthesia colleagues prior to incision. Because of this we do not routinely use local anesthetic. We prefer the patient in either semi-sitting or beach chair position under general anesthesia. The patient must be positioned high and lateral on the bed to allow unencumbered radiographs of the affected clavicle. The endotracheal tube should be secured toward the opposite shoulder and care is taken for a neutral head position; kyphotic, flexed, or rotated cervical posture can place the head and jaw in the way of the drill, especially for superior plating of fractures on the medial half of the clavicle. X-ray is set up to approach from the contralateral side allowing for anteroposterior (AP) and inlet views of the clavicle (Fig. 7.1).

The skin is then prepped and draped leaving the entire clavicle exposed including the sternoclavicular joint. Some surgeons prep and drape the entire ipsilateral upper extremity; however, we do not include typically the arm in the surgical field for isolated clavicular injuries.

Surgical Approach

A straight or oblique incision in line with the clavicle is carried out over the fracture site identified by either preoperative imaging or intraoperative fluoroscopy (Fig. 7.2). The incision is made through the skin and subcutaneous tissue identifying both the platysma muscle and deltotrapezial fascial layers (Fig. 7.3). While some surgeons prefer to identify and protect the supraclavicular nerves, we do not routinely identify these nerves during the approach except for large branches seen with primary, simple fracture fixation (the patient is cautioned preoperatively that there may be some numbness inferior to the incision). Following the skin incision, the deltotrapezial fascial layer is identified, and electrocautery is used to incise one continuous myofascial layer allowing a two-layer closure (myofascial, skin/subcutaneous tissue). Identification and dissection of the layers during the approach is an important step in that it allows a layered closure that acts as a barrier to infection and may decrease hardware prominence and irritation.

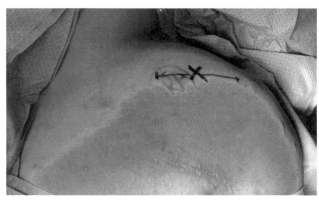

• **Fig. 7.1** Marking showing straight incision directly over the fracture site.

36

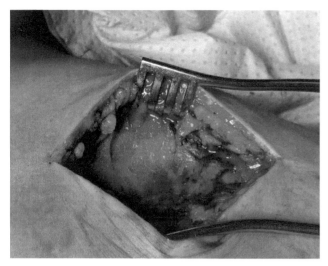

• **Fig. 7.2** Incision is carried down through the skin to clavipectoral fascia.

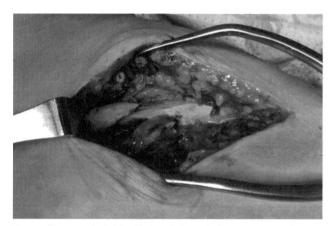

• **Fig. 7.3** Fracture site is identified and cleared of hematoma and intervening tissue.

Fracture Reduction and Provisional Fixation

The clavicle and fracture site are then identified and the fragments are mobilized keeping the most soft tissue attachments intact as possible but still allowing adequate mobilization for reduction (Fig. 7.4). Hematoma and soft tissue interposed at the fracture site are then debrided and irrigated. Reduction is performed with the use of reduction clamps, one on each end of the fracture site. Simple fractures are often able to be reduced with minimal traction and rotation (see Video 7.1). Segmental or butterfly fragments can be reduced and provisionally fixed with a pointed reduction clamp or K-wire (Fig. 7.5). If amenable to lag screw fixation, this should be performed with appropriately sized screw (2.7 or 3.5 mm) for the corresponding fragment size prior to plate placement (Fig. 7.6). For small butterfly fragments not amenable to lag screw fixation, high tensile cerclage sutures can be placed carefully around the fragment, plate, and clavicle at the end of the procedure and secured with a racking half hitch. For significantly comminuted fractures, the same principles apply with the primary goal of restoring length, alignment, and rotation. After sufficient reduction is obtained, provisional fixation may be obtained again with either pointed reduction clamps or K-wires. If K-wires are used, care must be taken to avoid deep penetration past the far cortex risking neurovascular injury.

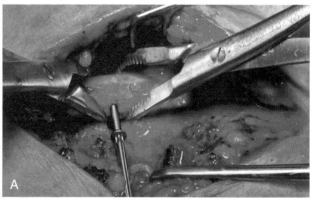

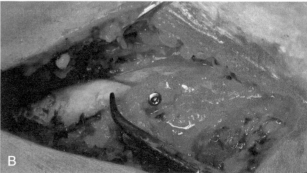

• **Fig. 7.4** Intraoperative photos showing segmental piece (A) before and (B) after reduction and provisional fixation with reduction clamp.

• **Fig. 7.5** (A and B) Placement of 2.7-mm lag screw securing segmental fragment.

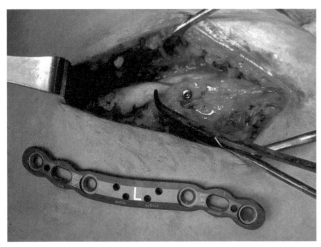

• **Fig. 7.6** Appropriately sized precontoured plate is chosen.

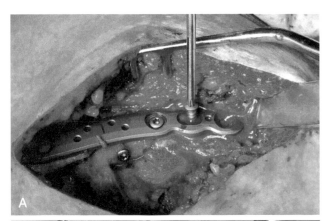

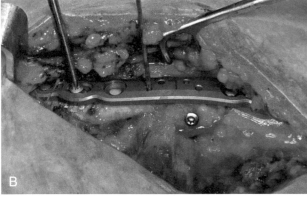

• **Fig. 7.7** (A) A screw is placed lateral to the fracture site in a static fashion. (B) Then an eccentrically placed screw is placed medial to the fracture site to provide compression. Note the K-wire being used to hold plate position during screw placement.

Internal Fixation

Once the fracture is provisionally fixed, the correct size and shape plate is chosen and applied (Fig. 7.7). We prefer 3.5-mm precontoured titanium plates placed on the superior aspect of the bone. Although the literature has not definitively shown that plate placement matters in regard to clinical outcomes, we prefer superior plate placement due to ease of plate application and what we feel requires less soft tissue dissection and deltoid release. For relatively simple fracture patterns with minimal comminution, a static screw is placed laterally followed by an eccentric screw

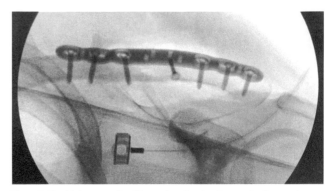

• **Fig. 7.8** Final intraoperative X-ray showing fracture reduction and proper plate/screw placement.

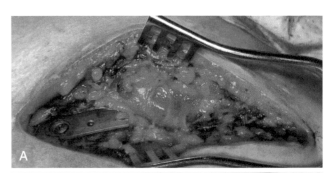

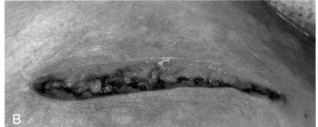

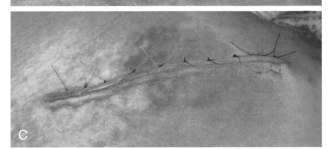

• **Fig. 7.9** Wound closure includes (A, B) fascial coverage followed by (C) skin closure.

placed medial to the fracture site to apply compression (Fig. 7.8). This step is not done in significantly comminuted fractures where the plate is acting in bridging mode and may lead to overshortening if overcompressed. After the plate is secured to both sides of the fracture, an intraoperative X-ray image is obtained to evaluate the position of the plate. If acceptable, screws are placed in the remaining holes with the goal of three screws (six cortices) on each side of the fracture.

Closure and Aftercare

At this point, a final X-ray (Fig. 7.9) should be obtained prior to wound closure to ensure accurate fracture reduction and screw

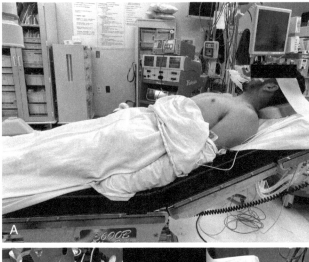
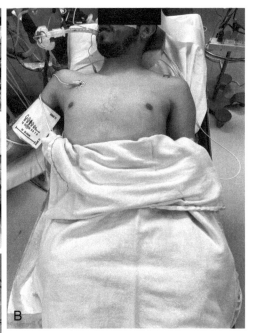
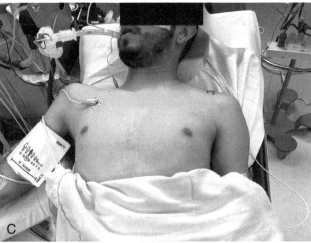

• **Fig. 7.10** Preoperative patient positioning in a semi-sitting position with the ipsilateral arm tucked. Note the C-arm approaching from the contralateral side allowing for appropriate radiographic views. Also note the head and endotracheal tube positioning away from the surgical site.

position/length. After thorough irrigation, a two-layered closure should be performed including the fascial layer followed by skin closure (Fig. 7.10). We do not routinely use local anesthetic prior to or after the case because patients usually receive an interscalene block prior to incision. Sterile dressings and sling are then applied. The patient is seen in the clinic 10 to 14 days after surgery for a wound check. At this time the sling is discontinued, sutures are removed and unrestricted range of motion (ROM) is allowed. We generally initiate partial weight-bearing 2 weeks after surgery for isolated injuries. However, for polytrauma patients with concomitant lower extremity injuries we do allow platform weight-bearing immediately after surgery. Following confirmation of fracture healing at 6 weeks, strengthening and resisted exercises are initiated. Return to contact sports is allowed at 8 to 12 weeks postsurgery provided a full ROM and protective strength have been restored.

PEARLS AND PITFALLS

- Select patients for clavicle fracture fixation carefully: it is a finesse operation with a narrow risk-benefit ratio. Healthy individuals with completely displaced fractures who are motivated for a rapid return of function are ideal candidates.
- In order to reduce the risk of infection, preserve two distinct layers during dissection including the superficial skin and subcutaneous layer as well as the deeper myofascial layer. These should be closed separately at the end of the case.
- Minimize rates of nonunion formation by handling the soft tissue with care. Avoid significant disruption of soft tissue attachments to the large fracture fragments during approach and reduction.
- Hardware irritation (and subsequent removal) can be minimized by using a precontoured plate to better fit the native clavicle. This can be applied either superiorly or in the anteroinferior position.
- Reconstruction plates should be avoided, especially in larger individuals due to the increased risk of plate breakage.
- To avoid loss of reduction, plates with appropriate size and strength should be used. A minimum of six cortices should be used on each side of the fracture. A lag screw improves fixation strength and can help maintain reduction prior to plate placement in fractures that are amenable.
- Intramedullary devices should be avoided in fractures with significant comminution in order to avoid shortening.

8

Technique Spotlight: Intramedullary Fixation of Clavicle Fractures

IVAN ANTOSH, EDWARD ARRINGTON, AND DAVID WILSON

Introduction

Recent literature recommends consideration of surgical treatment for completely displaced and/or significantly shortened middle-third clavicle fractures.[1–3] In certain fracture patterns, intramedullary clavicle fracture fixation has been shown to be an effective option for treatment while offering the potential advantages of reduced soft tissue irritation and a relative paucity of potentially bone-weakening screw holes when compared with traditional plate constructs.[2–4] While plate constructs are widely used with reliably high union rates and functional outcomes, hardware removal due to symptomatic prominence is often required.[5,6] Intramedullary fixation offers a lower profile solution, which can be performed through a smaller incision(s).

Indications

Displaced, midshaft clavicle fractures may be amenable to intramedullary fixation. Transverse and short oblique fracture patterns are ideal as these offer the option for interfragmentary compression. Some intramedullary implants (pins, screws, and flexible rods) have little intrinsic rotational or length stability. These should be avoided for transverse or highly comminuted fractures, though in an adolescent population these can still be effective given the robust biologic response. Intramedullary fixation can yield primary or secondary bone healing, based on the stability of the construct. Key technique considerations include anatomic reduction and obtaining endosteal canal purchase, which maximize fracture and construct stability.

Preoperative Evaluation

The determination of intramedullary versus plate fixation is made based on both fracture morphology and patient factors. Simple fracture patterns such as transverse and short oblique represent ideal indications for intramedullary fixation (Fig. 8.1).

Comminuted or segmental patterns may be more reliably treated with traditional plate constructs, though a small butterfly fragment in an otherwise length-stable fracture pattern is often easily addressed using racking half hitches with a heavy, braided suture. Consideration should be given to concomitant injuries (specifically shoulder girdle injuries), acute or chronic cervical spine pathology, and body habitus. These factors impact the surgeon's ability to gain adequate fluoroscopic visualization of the fracture reduction and landmarks for intramedullary fixation.

Lifestyle and work activities may increase intolerance of prominent hardware. Intramedullary fixation is very popular for military populations. In particular, this approach has a long history with airborne troops and infantry where the need to wear a parachute or ruck-sack may make plate prominence intolerable. In addition, cyclists have a high rate of clavicle fractures and repeat clavicle fractures. Intramedullary fixation can avoid the stress risers of multiple bicortical screw holes and leave only one cortical disruption—lateral to the conoid tubercle where the clavicle sees little force given the forces borne by the coracoclavicular ligaments. In cyclists, we frequently advocate removal of the device 4 months after union given the high rate of recurrent fractures leading to a desire to not leave any hardware which may complicate future management. Lastly, adolescent patients with significant shortening (>2 cm) and a simple fracture pattern are excellent candidates

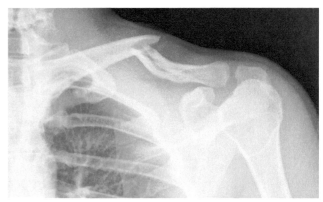

• **Fig. 8.1** Anteroposterior (AP) radiograph of short oblique, middle-third clavicle shaft fracture indicated for intramedullary fixation.

for intramedullary fixation as the biology for healing is excellent and the fracture fragments simply need to be held in suitable alignment.

Lastly, morphometric analysis of the clavicle demonstrates isthmic diameter and curvature variations associated with age, gender, and height.[7] For rigid, straight intramedullary devices, a "curvy" clavicle may be a relative contraindication.

Positioning and Equipment

Intramedullary clavicle fixation may be performed in numerous positions. The authors' preferred technique is a modified "lazy" beach chair position using a radiolucent backed table. The arm can be kept at the side out of the sterile field or draped in using an articulated arm holder or padded mayo. At a minimum, the surgical field should extend medially from the sternoclavicular joint to lateral to the acromioclavicular joint, with adequate superior exposure to allow posterolateral access to the conoid tubercle (Fig. 8.2).

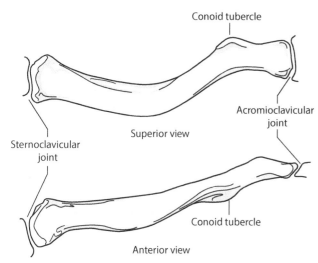

• **Fig. 8.2** Illustration demonstrating sigmoidal shape of clavicle when viewed from superior *(top)* and anterior *(bottom)*. Note the positioning of conoid tubercle which is the starting point when using a retrograde isthmic access technique.

A large C-arm fluoroscope is typically used. A 9-inch image intensifier can be easier to maneuver than the standard 12-inch version. The C-arm is brought in from the head on the operative side, and the beam is oriented from posterior to anterior (Fig. 8.3). After positioning, but prior to draping, radiographs are taken to confirm adequate fluoroscopic visualization as many commercially available positioning systems include metallic attachments (side posts, hinges, etc.) that may prevent adequate fracture and hardware visualization.

The C-arm receiver is "rolled over" the shoulder in a semi-reclined position to allow frontal plane imaging, and "rolled back" to allow a "top-down" view which more accurately visualizes the sigmoidal curvature of the bone (Fig. 8.4).

This latter view is key to visualizing the posterior-lateral start point for isthmic access when using a device that requires a lateral-to-medial trajectory. The combination of these views allows orthogonal plane confirmation of anatomic reduction and hardware position.

Technique Description

The authors' preferred technique is a two-incision technique for intramedullary fixation. The first incision is placed at the level of the fracture and can be oriented vertically or horizontally. In both cases, the incision is centered over the fracture. A vertical incision facilitates access and reduction of superiorly displaced medial fragments while minimizing the incision length. The correct site for a vertically oriented incision is best identified under fluoroscopic guidance. The horizontal incision is more extensile and may be considered when addressing widely displaced or more complex fracture patterns. A horizontal incision also allows versatility to convert to a traditional plate construct should intramedullary fixation be aborted intraoperatively.

The fracture is exposed through an anterior window with subperiosteal dissection limited to what is required for fracture fragment identification and anatomic reduction. Care should be taken to avoid devascularization of fracture fragments. Manual maintenance of the reduction (i.e., with two "lobster claw" serrated clamps) is often required to prevent displacement during isthmic access, canal preparation, and hardware implantation. The canal can be accessed from medial or lateral. The authors' preferred technique for most middle-third fracture patterns is to access the canal in a retrograde fashion. The conoid tubercle is the landmark for retrograde isthmic access. The conoid tubercle is a posterior

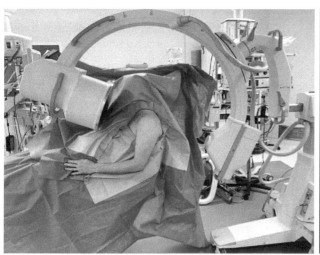
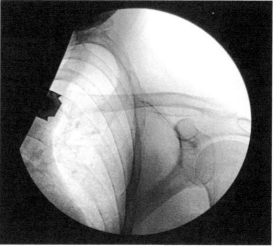

• **Fig. 8.3** Intraoperative large C-arm positioning in "rolled over" configuration to allow frontal plane imaging *(left)* and correlating fluoroscopic view *(right)*.

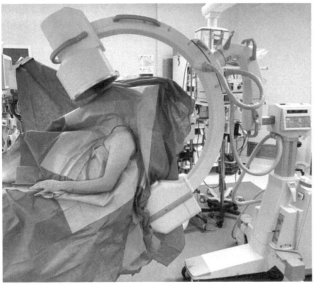
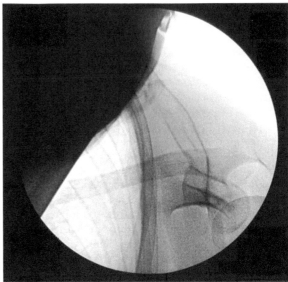

• **Fig. 8.4** Intraoperative large C-arm positioning in "rolled back" configuration to allow top-down imaging *(left)* and correlating fluoroscopic view *(right)*.

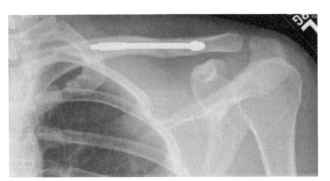

• **Fig. 8.5** Hagie pin (Smith & Nephew, Memphis, TN). An implant placed in a retrograde fashion. Note medial fragment screw threads completely across fracture site to allow intrafragmentary compression.

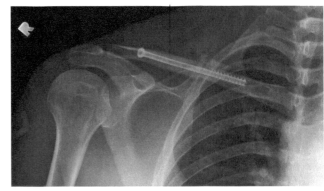

• **Fig. 8.7** Partially threaded cancellous screw of 4.0 mm (Depuy Synthes, West Chester, PA). An implant placed in a retrograde fashion.

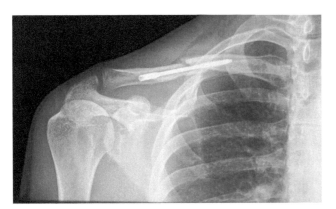

• **Fig. 8.6** Dual-Trak clavicle screw (Accumed, Hillsboro, OR). An implant placed in a retrograde fashion.

and lateral structure, the site of attachment of the conoid ligament, and the most medial of the two coracoclavicular ligaments. Isthmic access immediately lateral to this bony prominence allows a linear entry trajectory into the clavicular midshaft.

Typical isthmic access follows a cannulated technique, with a guide pin, followed by a cannulated drill or reamer. This can be accomplished using a hand or battery-powered technique. Proprietary entry awls can be helpful to place the device path in a best-fit-corridor based on the chosen implant's design. Cannulated screws have a limited ability to adjust to the sigmoidal curvature of the clavicle (Fig. 8.5).

Based on the fracture morphology, these may best be inserted from medial or lateral to maximize far-end-implant purchase, which is important for construct stability. When a threaded implant is used for compression, all screw threads should be within the far fracture fragment to maximize purchase. Figs. 8.6–8.9 demonstrate various implant options for intramedullary clavicle fixation.

Rehabilitation and postoperative restrictions are highly dependent on implant design, fracture morphology, and surgeon preference. In the majority of cases, we recommend early active range of shoulder motion with lifting/pushing/pulling up to 5 pounds of weight below the horizontal plane for the first 6 weeks. Given the significant rotational forces with an elevation beyond 90 degrees and the fact that glenohumeral stiffness is uncommon with this extra-articular injury, we delay active and passive range of motion until reassuring radiographs are visualized—typically at 6 weeks. When bridging callus is visualized, active motion and increased weight-bearing are gradually instituted. We typically recommend adding 5 pounds per week after week 6.

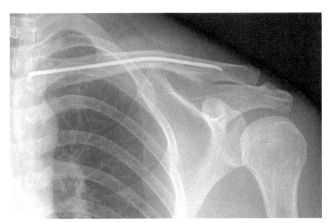

• **Fig. 8.8** Flexible intramedullary nail (Depuy Synthes, West Chester, PA). An implant placed in an antegrade fashion. This technique will not allow for intrafragmentary compression and may be predisposed to hardware migration.

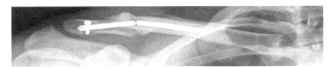

• **Fig. 8.9** Hardware failure reported by the authors in 2013.[11]

PEARLS AND PITFALLS

• Determine whether intramedullary fixation is a viable option. Key determinants include the following: bony morphology, fracture characteristics, and implant design. The clavicle has a sigmoidal shape with an apex posterolateral curve and an apex anteromedial curve (Fig. 8.5). Both of these morphological characteristics vary slightly between males and females.[7] Careful attention should be given to the medial radius of curvature and isthmic width within the clavicular midshaft. Intramedullary implant rigidity can affect trajectory within a constrained tortuous isthmic corridor. Fracture patterns that force intramedullary implants to negotiate a tight radii of curvature or rely on inadequate medial and/or lateral isthmic purchase may be best suited for flexibly inserted implant options. There is some evidence that in comminuted patterns, early patient satisfaction, function, and time to healing are improved with plate fixation.[8,9] We recommend always having a plate/screw system on backup to reliably adapt to anatomy or fracture morphology that is not well suited for intramedullary fixation. A horizontal incision is more extensile and facilitates adaptability of the surgical plan.

• Once intramedullary fixation is chosen, patient positioning and adequate fluoroscopic imaging are confirmed. Prior to a sterile prep and drape, the authors recommend establishing adequate orthogonal plane fluoroscopic visualization. Keeping the patient high and lateral in the beach chair minimizes bed interference with imaging. During the actual prepping and draping, care must be taken to preserve a surgical field from the sternoclavicular joint to the acromioclavicular joint.

• An intramedullary implant should be chosen that maximizes axial and rotational stability. Proprietary designs carry recommended minimum purchase lengths, in an effort to maximize stability. Adequate endosteal purchase on both sides of the fracture is a key factor involved in mechanical strength. Various systems allow for compression through the construct at the fracture site. Stable compression of an anatomically reduced fracture facilitates healing and construct stability.

• Finally, care must be taken when counseling and progressing motion in the postoperative setting. The middle one-third of the clavicular shaft experiences torsional and axial compressive forces transferred from the upper extremity.[10,11] Early mobilization of the upper extremity results in compressive and torsional loading of clavicular hardware which can result in early hardware failure.[10] Early hardware failure can also be seen in constructs with inadequate stability[11,12] (Fig. 8.9). Early active range of motion can be achieved in certain settings when the length and rotational stability are restored; however, gradual progression for active overhead motion is sometimes needed. One should consider hardware removal after adequate fracture healing in patients at high risk of re-fracture.

References

1. Wiesel B, Nagda S, Mehta S, Churchill R. Management of midshaft clavicle fractures in adults. *J Am Acad Orthop Surg.* 2018;26(2):e468–e476. PMID: 30180095.

2. Eichinger JK, Balog TP, Grassbaugh JA. Intramedullary fixation of clavicle fractures: anatomy, indications, advantages, and disadvantages. *J Am Acad Orthop Surg.* 2016;24:455–464. PMID: 27227985.

3. King PR, Ikram A, Eken MM, Lamberts RP. The effectiveness of a flexible locked intramedullary nail and an anatomically contoured locked plate to treat clavicular shaft fractures. *J Bone Joint Surg Am.* 2019;101:628–634. PMID: 30946197.

4. Ricci WM. In Completely displaced midshaft fractures of the clavicle, plate fixation and elastic stable intramedullary nailing did not differ in function at one year. *J Bone Joint Surg Am.* 2018;100(10):883. PMID: 29762287.

5. Woltz S, Krijnen P, Schipper IB. Mid-term patient satisfaction and residual symptoms after plate fixation or nonoperative treatment for displaced midshaft clavicular fractures. *J Orthop Trauma.* 2018 Nov; 32(11):e435–e439.

6. Nourian A, Dhaliwal S, Vangala S, Vezeridis PS. Midshaft fractures of the clavicle: a meta-analysis comparing surgical fixation using anteroinferior plating versus superior plating. *J Orthop Trauma.* 2017 Sep;31(9):461–467.

7. Aira JR, Simon P, Gutierrez S, Santoni BG, Frankle MA. Morphometry of the human clavicle and intramedullary canal: a 3D, geometry-based quantification. *J Orthop Res.* 2017;35(10):2191–2202. PMID: 28150886.

8. Hulsmans MHJ, Van Heijl M, Frima H, Van Der Meijden OAJ, Van Den Berg HR, et al. Predicting suitability of intramedullary fixation for displaced midshaft clavicle fractures. *Eur J Trauma Emerg Surg.* 2018;44(4):581–587. PMID: 28993839.

9. Fuglesang HFS, Flugsrud GB, Randsborg PH, Oord P, Benth JS, Utvag SE. Plate fixation vs. intramedullary nailing of completely displaced midshaft fractures of the clavicle: a prospective randomised controlled trial. *Bone Joint Lett J.* 2017;99-B(8):1095–1101. PMID: 28768788.

10. Wilson DJ, Scully WF, Min KS, Harmon TA, Eichinger JK, Arrington ED. Biomechanical analysis of intramedullary vs. superior plate fixation of transverse midshaft clavicle fractures. *J Shoulder Elbow Surg.* 2016;25(6):949–953. PMID: 26775744.

11. Wilson DJ, Weaver DL, Balog TP, Arrington ED. Early postoperative failures of a new intramedullary fixation device for midshaft clavicle fractures. *Orthopedics.* 2013;36(11):e1450–e1453. PMID: 24200452.

12. Wang SH, Lin HJ, Shen HC, Pan RY, Yang JJ. Biomechanical comparison between solid and cannulated intramedullary devices for midshaft clavicle fixation. *BMC Musculokelet Disord.* 2019;20(1):178. PMID 31027505.

9

Distal Clavicle Fractures

CHRISTINE C. PIPER AND ANDREW NEVIASER

Introduction

Distal clavicle fractures, also known as lateral clavicle fractures, account for approximately 25% of all clavicle fractures, the second most common subset after midshaft fractures.[1] This fracture is unique because of its high potential for nonunion, potential effects on scapulothoracic motion, and cosmetic deformity. Distal clavicle fractures have a predilection for elderly and middle-aged individuals, due to an overall decrease in bone mineral density.[1] The outcome for nonoperative treatment of distal clavicle fractures is largely dependent on the location of the fracture and the integrity of the coracoclavicular (CC) ligaments. These two factors are the primary determinants of displacement, stability, and operative versus nonoperative treatment.

Relevant Anatomy/Pathoanatomy

The cross-sectional area of the clavicle enlarges laterally, as the bone transitions from the thick cortices of the middle third to the thinner cortices with cancellous bone in the lateral third.[2] Bone mineral density is greater in the medial aspect of the distal clavicle (at the conoid tubercle and intertubercle space) as compared with the more lateral aspect.[3] These factors make the lateral region more prone to fracture, especially in an osteoporotic population. The subclavian artery and vein, which lie posteroinferiorly to the clavicle, are, on average, 63 and 76 mm from the distal clavicle, respectively.[4]

The surrounding ligamentous and capsular anatomy is of paramount importance in influencing displacement of these fractures. The four acromioclavicular (AC) ligaments, confluent with the joint capsule itself, act primarily to prevent anterior-posterior instability of the distal clavicle. The superior AC ligament has been shown to provide rotational stability of the distal clavicle.[5] The CC ligaments prevent vertical displacement of the distal clavicle. The posteromedial, conoid ligament thickens at its clavicular end, attaching 4.6 cm from the AC joint.[6–8] The trapezoid ligament attaches anterolaterally on the undersurface of the distal clavicle, 2.5 cm from the AC joint.[6,7] One can evaluate for injury to the CC ligaments radiographically by measuring the CC interspace; a measurement exceeding 1.3 cm indicates injury.[9]

Both muscular forces and gravity exacerbate fracture displacement. The pectoralis major, trapezius, anterior deltoid, and sternocleidomastoid (SCM) muscles all originate from the clavicle. The SCM and trapezius displace the proximal fragment superiorly and posteriorly, while the weight of the arm displaces the lateral fragment inferiorly and medially.[10]

Classification

Neer was the first to propose a classification system specific to distal clavicle fractures (Fig. 9.1).[10] Type I fractures occur lateral to intact CC ligaments and spare the AC joint. Type III fractures occur lateral to the intact CC ligaments; however, they extend into the AC joint. Type II fractures are inherently unstable and occur medial to one of both of the CC ligaments. This fracture type was further subdivided by Craig, into Types IIA and IIB.[11] In Type IIA, both CC ligaments remain intact, and the fracture lies medial to the conoid ligament (Fig. 9.2). In Type IIB, one or both of the CC ligaments are torn, rendering it an even more unstable injury (Fig. 9.3). A Type IV injury is a physeal fracture seen exclusively in the pediatric population. Because the distal clavicle physis does not fuse until early in the second decade, this fracture can occur later in life than most physeal injuries.[12] These injuries heal reliably well without surgical intervention, as the CC ligaments prevent significant displacement through their attachment to the robust periosteal sleeve. A Type V injury is a comminuted distal clavicle fracture where the CC ligaments, while intact, are attached to a comminuted free-floating bone fragment from the inferior aspect of the clavicle. In this regard, Type II and Type V injuries present with similar deformities and treatment challenges.

The Robinson classification for clavicle fractures, also referred to as the Edinburgh classification, was proposed in 1998.[13] Based on data gathered from over 1000 patients, it subdivides distal clavicle fractures according to the degree of displacement and joint involvement. More recently, Cho et al. created a new classification system for distal clavicle fractures based on fracture stability and fragment size, two factors previously identified as influential for guiding treatment strategy.[14,15] Despite the fact that both classification systems report superior intra- and interobserver reliability scores compared with Neer's, neither has been successful in superseding his classification system in terms of widespread use and popularity.

Treatment: Nonoperative

Nonoperative management is widely accepted for minimally displaced, stable distal clavicle fractures. These injuries, which typically include Neer Type I, III, and IV fractures, have an acceptably low nonunion rate of 5%.[16] The continuity of the coracoid, CC ligaments, and medial 2/3 of the clavicle make these stable injuries. Treatment consists of a short period of immobilization in a sling, with initiation of shoulder mobilization when acute pain

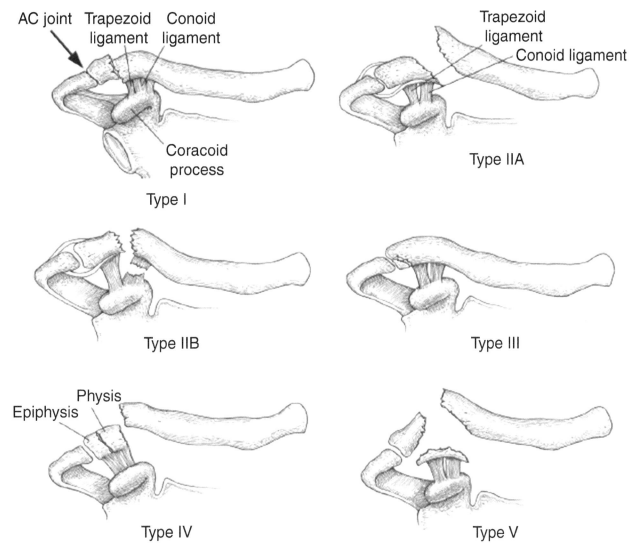

• **Fig. 9.1** Neer classification for distal clavicle fractures. *AC joint*, acromioclavicular joint. (From Banerjee R, Waterman B, Padalecki J, Robertson W. Management of distal clavicle fractures. *J Am Acad Orthop Surg.* 2011;19(7):392-401.)

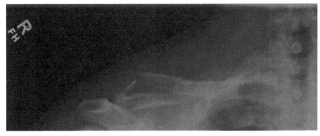

• **Fig. 9.2** Neer Type IIA distal clavicle fracture.

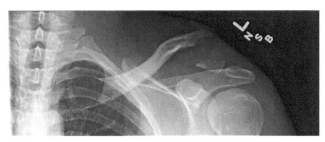

• **Fig. 9.3** Neer Type IIB distal clavicle fracture.

subsides. Routine radiographs are advised to monitor fracture healing.

Conservative treatment for displaced distal clavicle fractures is a more controversial topic, with reported nonunion rates ranging from 11.5% to 44%.[1,16–20] The greatest risk factors for nonunion are degree of fracture displacement and advanced age (Table 9.1).[17] Interestingly, the vast majority of nonunions are asymptomatic or minimally symptomatic.[17–20] Robinson et al. examined 101 patients treated conservatively for a displaced distal clavicle fracture and found no significant differences in functional outcome scores between those patients who had healed and those with asymptomatic nonunions.[1] The 14% of patients with symptomatic nonunions did require delayed surgical intervention, yet their ultimate Constant and SF-36 scores did not differ significantly from the other two patient cohorts. Rokito et al. performed a retrospective study to evaluate outcomes following operative and nonoperative treatment for displaced distal clavicle fractures in 30 patients.[18] They reported an almost 50% nonunion rate for the nonoperative group (average age 47), yet their functional scores (UCLA, Constant, ASES [American Shoulder and Elbow Surgeons]) did not differ from those patients with healed fractures.

TABLE 9.1	Probability of Distal Clavicle Nonunion Based on Age and Displacement	
	PROBABILITY OF A NONUNION	
Age (Years)	**Not Displaced (%)**	**Displaced (%)**
20	1	16
30	3	21
40	5	27
50	6	37
60	10	44
70	17	52

(Reproduced with permission from Khan, LK, Bradnock, TJ. Fractures of the Clavicle. *JBJS.* 2009;91(2):447-460.)

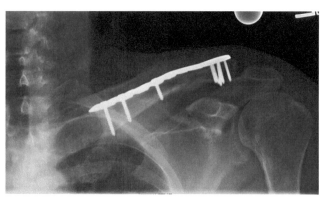

• **Fig. 9.4** Precontoured locking plate used for distal clavicle fracture fixation.

They also found no differences between the two patient groups with regard to range of motion or strength.

Poor outcomes following nonoperative management for distal clavicle fractures are due to one or more of the following: persistent pain, cosmetic deformity, decreased strength or range of motion, and symptomatic nonunion. Additionally, Neer observed that Type III fractures are susceptible to AC joint arthrosis if articular incongruity is present.[10] The finding was later refuted by Nordqvist, who reported on the natural history of distal clavicle fractures with a 15-year follow-up.[16] Regardless, AC joint arthritis can be addressed with a distal clavicle resection if symptoms should warrant it. Excluding nonunion, the complication rate for nonoperative treatment is low at 6.7%.[16]

Treatment: Operative

Absolute indications for surgery include open fracture, skin tenting with potential compromise, and certain polytrauma patients dependent on the upper extremities for mobilization. Outside of these circumstances, surgery may be considered for unstable type II and V distal clavicle fractures, as well as symptomatic nonunions. In brief, any fracture subtype where the coracoid is not functionally connected to the medial two-thirds of the clavicle may require surgery. Bishop et al. determined fracture stability to be the most important factor in a surgeon's decision to operate, while the size of the fragment was most influential in determining the choice of fixation.[15] Modern surgical techniques involve distal clavicle fracture fixation, CC stabilization, or a combination of the two.

There are many described techniques for surgical fixation of distal clavicle fractures. Originally described by Neer, transacromial K-wiring lost favor after unacceptably high complication and nonunion rates were published.[21] Cautionary case reports of wire migration to the mediastinum made this technique entirely obsolete.[22] The intramedullary Knowles pin, originally described by Neviaser for use in midshaft clavicle fractures, can be used transacromially or extra-articularly, as described by Jou.[23,24] Both Fann and Jou published case series with 100% union rates using the Knowles pin to treat distal clavicle fractures, yet complications of painful hardware and AC joint arthrosis were also reported.[24,25] Similar hardware-related complications were seen with cerclage and tension-band wiring techniques.[26]

CC screw fixation was originally described by Bosworth for treatment of AC separations, and later adapted by Ballmer for use in distal clavicle fracture.[27,28] This surgery, while technically demanding, is favored by some because it does not violate the AC joint or devitalize the distal clavicle of its soft tissue. Fazal and Macheras both reported a 100% union rate for their respective case series, although screw backout and AC joint ossification were observed in some cases.[29,30] Jin et al. later introduced a cannulated screw technique, which made it possible to perform the procedure under fluoroscopic guidance alone.[31] To allow for full shoulder range of motion, screw removal is recommended when callus is visible radiographically.

Plate osteosynthesis is widely employed for surgical treatment of distal clavicle fractures. Because these implants do not cross the AC joint, they do not require removal. Locking plate technology is generally preferred in the distal clavicle, where the cancellous bone makes screw pullout more likely. The surgical approach is straightforward due to the clavicle's subcutaneous location. An incision is made in line with the distal clavicle to the level of the AC joint. Once through the platysma and at the level of bone, periosteal flaps are created for later repair. Far lateral fractures can be challenging, as there is often insufficient bone for adequate distal fragment fixation. Kalamaras et al. introduced the use of the distal radius locking plate for distal clavicle fractures to address this problem.[32] The plate's inherent angular stability, low profile design, and multiple distal locking holes make it an appealing fixation option. Their small case series reported a 100% union rate and excellent Constant scores.

Precontoured locking plates provide yet another option for distal clavicle internal fixation, with a variety of divergent locking holes in the distal segment to increase pullout strength and options for fixation (Fig. 9.4).[33–35] In cases of complete CC ligament disruption, surgeons can choose to augment this construct with a form of CC stabilization. Theoretically, healing of the CC ligaments *or* the fracture is all that is required for a stable shoulder, but multiple studies show improved stability and functional outcomes in patients who have been treated with both techniques simultaneously.[36–38] Beirer et al. reported significantly lower Taft scores, a parameter for grading AC joint stability, in patients with Neer Type IIB fractures treated with a locking plate alone compared with all other distal clavicle fracture types.[39] These results suggest that this fracture type would benefit from additional CC stabilization. Two biomechanical studies further supported this theory; cadaveric specimens with type IIB fractures that were fixed with both a locking plate and CC fixation had a higher load to failure than those fixed with a plate alone.[40,41] By contrast, Shin et al. showed bony union and satisfactory functional outcome scores for patients treated with a precontoured plate

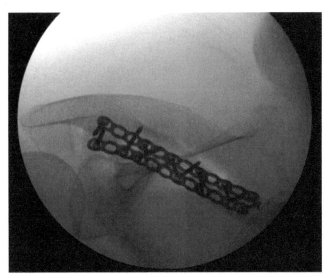

• **Fig. 9.5** Intraoperative fluoroscopy of a distal clavicle fracture fixed using the dual plating technique.

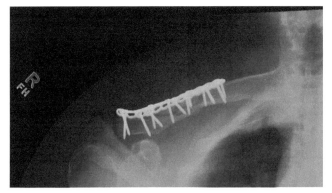

• **Fig. 9.6** Postoperative films of a distal clavicle fracture fixed using the dual plating technique.

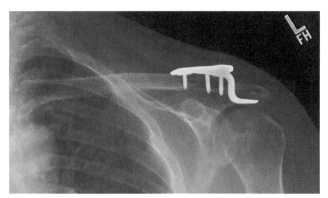

• **Fig. 9.7** Radiograph showing hook plate fixation.

alone, including those patients found to have an increased CC distance radiographically.[42] Data extracted from seven contemporary studies evaluating contoured plates in distal clavicle fractures reveal a 97% union rate.[43] Ten percent of patients complained of hardware irritation, necessitating a second surgery for hardware removal in 9 of 11 cases.

A double-plating technique was proposed by Kaipel, wherein two manually contoured 2.4-mm locking plates are placed superiorly and anteriorly in the distal clavicle (Figs. 9.5 and 9.6).[44] In addition to being cost-effective, low profile, and technically facile, this fixation construct was deemed stable enough to allow for immediate active postoperative mobilization. Interestingly, a recent biomechanical study comparing double-plate fixation to precontoured single plating found that the two techniques had comparable failure loads.[45]

Originally described for use following AC separations, the hook plate is typically reserved for those fractures that are too distal or too comminuted to accommodate adequate screw fixation in the lateral fragment(s). The distal aspect of the plate hooks under the acromion, counteracting the deforming forces on the proximal clavicle (Fig. 9.7). This feature of the plate makes hardware removal a necessity to avoid acromial osteolysis, subacromial bursitis, and/or rotator cuff tear. With a 97% union rate, this is

a widely accepted treatment option that is less technically challenging than most others described.[43] While most patients exhibit good to excellent functional outcome scores, the overall complication rate (minor and major) for this procedure is 41%.[46] Stegeman et al. corroborated these findings, reporting an 11-fold increased risk of major complications using the hook plate compared with intramedullary fixation, and a 24-fold increased risk when compared with CC fixation.[47] The most common complications are subacromial osteolysis, AC arthrosis, and periprosthetic fracture.[48]

CC stabilization procedures can be used in the treatment of distal clavicle fractures either alone or in combination with one of the previously mentioned fixation techniques. There are a variety of described techniques, including CC screw fixation (previously discussed), a sling or loop technique, and CC ligament reconstruction. The latter two options offer nonrigid suspensory fixation, which more closely mimics the biomechanics of an intact CC ligament complex. Regardless of the technique chosen, this open procedure requires a vertically based incision made from the posterior aspect of the clavicle to the coracoid base. If drilling the coracoid, proper identification of its center and base is critical in avoiding iatrogenic fracture.[49,50] Using smaller diameter drill holes in both the clavicle and coracoid also aids in reducing the incidence of fracture.

In the sling technique, cable or nonabsorbable suture material is looped under the coracoid and either tied around the clavicle or passed through it by way of a drill hole. Goldberg et al. pioneered this technique, and all nine patients in their initial prospective study achieved union, with no reported complications.[51] Webber and Soliman both advocate sling techniques that loop graft or suture material without the use of drill hole, as this creates a stress riser and can result in iatrogenic fracture.[45,52,53] Soliman reported a mean Constant score of 96 for his cohort of 14 patients, and 1 asymptomatic nonunion.[53] However, there have been results in the non–peer-reviewed literature of the heavy, nonresorbable suture material looped around the coracoid "gigli sawing" through the bone over time.[54]

CC ligament reconstruction, originally indicated for AC separations, is another treatment option for distal clavicle fractures requiring CC stabilization. Graft options include autograft, allograft, or synthetic material such as a suture button (Fig. 9.8). The graft is either looped under or passed through a drill hole in the coracoid and each end, after proper tensioning, is affixed in drill holes through the clavicle by way of interference screws.[55] There are many variations for both placement and number of drill holes. Milewski reported a significantly lower complication rate after CC reconstruction when the graft was looped

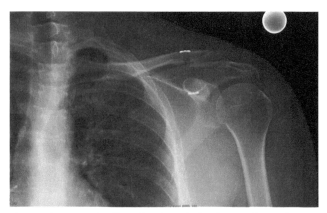

• **Fig. 9.8** Postoperative films of a distal clavicle fracture fixed using cora-coclavicular stabilization with a suture button technique.

under the coracoid as opposed to drilling through it.[49] Yagnik recommended the use of both allograft and cortical button fixation when treating unstable distal clavicle fractures, to strengthen the repair while recreating the anatomic soft tissue attachments between the clavicle and coracoid.[56] A recent biomechanical study comparing cortical button, suture anchor, and sling techniques found no significant differences in construct strength or displacement after cyclic loading.[57]

Arthroscopy made possible the minimally invasive techniques that have emerged more recently for CC stabilization.[58–60] It carries with it, however, a higher complication rate, as it is a more technically demanding operation with a steeper learning curve. Identification of the coracoid base is a more challenging task when performed arthroscopically and is critical in avoiding coracoid fracture, button migration, and damage to surrounding structures.[45,58] Among the studies performed to evaluate nonarthroscopic suspension fixation, there is a 98% union rate and 6% complication rate. A sampling of studies from the same time frame (2011 to present) which use arthroscopic methods to achieve CC fixation reveals a 94% union rate and a 15% complication rate.[45] The most common complication for arthroscopic procedures was nonunion, while for the open procedures it was wound infection.

Outcomes

While the data from Robinson and Rokito seem to support nonoperative treatment for displaced distal clavicle fractures, these data should be interpreted with caution. The majority of the patients in these studies were middle-aged or elderly; this group may better tolerate a nonunion due to lower functional demand compared with a younger cohort of patients. In fact, the group of patients in Robinson's study that required delayed surgery for a symptomatic nonunion were, on average, 10 years younger than the rest of the patients. While a younger patient is at a lower risk of nonunion overall, the data suggest that they are more likely to be symptomatic should they have one (Table 9.1). Delayed surgery (>4 weeks from injury) may also carry additional risk of complication.[61] In Klein's retrospective cohort study of 38 patients treated surgically for a distal clavicle fracture, there was a 36% complication rate in the delayed surgery group compared with a 7% complication rate for those patients treated acutely.

Meta-analysis and systematic review are useful for comparing surgical outcomes for varying distal clavicle fracture fixation methods. Oh et al. showed there was no significant difference in

nonunion rates among the following techniques: CC stabilization, hook plate, intramedullary fixation, interfragmentary fixation, and K-wire plus tension-band wiring.[18] There was, however, a notable difference in the complication rate. Compared with other described treatment modalities, hook plating and K-wire plus tension-band wiring had far higher complication rates at 40% and 20%, respectively. The most recent systematic review and meta-analysis to date, performed by Boonard et al., compared postoperative shoulder function and complications for a variety of fixation methods: the hook plate, locking plate, tension-band wiring, transacromial pinning, and CC stabilization.[62] Superior locking plates and CC fixation demonstrated the highest functional outcome scores (Constant Murley and UCLA). Locking plates had the lowest complication rate of any method studied, while transacromial pinning had the highest. A cost-effectiveness analysis by Fox et al. revealed that, when compared with hook and locking plates, the CC suture button technique was the least expensive and most effective treatment modality.[63] While no one surgical technique has proven to be superior, it is prudent to take these outcomes data into consideration.

Summary

Distal clavicle fractures are the second most common type of clavicle fracture. The exact location of the fracture and the integrity of the CC ligaments are two key factors in determining stability. Outcomes for conservative treatment of stable distal clavicle fractures are reliably good, whereas optimal management of a displaced distal clavicle fracture is controversial. While conservative treatment has a high nonunion rate and a low complication rate, surgical management has a low nonunion rate but a high complication rate. There has been no proven gold standard in operative care for a displaced distal clavicle fracture, and there are many variations of fixation that work equally well. Given that distal clavicle nonunions are often asymptomatic, it is important to consider not only the personality of the fracture but also the characteristics of the patient in making the decision whether or not to operate.

References

1. Robinson CM, Cairns DA. Primary nonoperative treatment of displaced lateral fractures of the clavicle. *JBJS*. 2004;86(4):778–782.
2. Tornetta III P, Ricci W, McQueen MM. *Rockwood and Green's Fractures in Adults*. Philadelphia: Lippincott Williams & Wilkins; 2019.
3. Chen RE, Soin SP, El-Shaar R, et al. What regions of the distal clavicle have the greatest bone mineral density and cortical thickness? A cadaveric study. *Clin Orthop Relat Res*. 2019;477(12):2726–2732.
4. Sinha A, Edwin J, Sreeharsha B, Bhalaik V, Brownson P. A radiological study to define safe zones for drilling during plating of clavicle fractures. *The Journal of Bone and Joint Surgery. British Volume*. 2011;93(9):1247–1252.
5. Branch TP, Burdette HL, Shahriari AS, Carter FM, Hutton WC. The role of the acromioclavicular ligaments and the effect of distal clavicle resection. *Am J Sports Med*. 1996;24(3):293–297.
6. Renfree KJ, Riley MK, Wheeler D, Hentz JG, Wright TW. Ligamentous anatomy of the distal clavicle. *J Shoulder Elbow Surg*. 2003;12(4):355–359.
7. Saccomanno MF, De Ieso C, Milano G. Acromioclavicular joint instability: anatomy, biomechanics and evaluation. *Joints*. 2014;2(02):87–92.
8. Harris RI, Vu DH, Sonnabend DH, Goldberg JA, Walsh WR. Anatomic variance of the coracoclavicular ligaments. *J Shoulder Elbow Surg*. 2001;10(6):585–588.

9. Bosworth BM. Complete acromioclavicular dislocation. *N Engl J Med.* 1949;241(6):221–225.

10. Neer CS. Fractures of the distal third of the clavicle. *Clin Orthop.* 1968;58:43e50.

11. Craig EV. Fractures of the clavicle. In: Rockwood Jr CA, Green DP, Bucholz RW, Heckman JD, eds. *Rockwood and Green's Fractures in Adults.* 4th ed. Philadelphia: Lippincott-Raven; 1996:1109–1193.

12. Bishop JY, Flatow EL. Pediatric shoulder trauma. *Clin Orthop Relat Res.* 2005;432:41–48.

13. Robinson CM. Fractures of the clavicle in the adult: epidemiology and classification. *The Journal of Bone and Joint Surgery. British Volume.* 1998;80(3):476–484.

14. Cho C-H, Kim BS, Kim DH, Choi CH, Dan J, Lee H. Distal clavicle fractures: a new classification system. *J Orthop Traumatol: Surgery & Research.* 2018;104(8):1231–1235.

15. Bishop JY, Jones GL, Lewis B, Pedroza A, MOON Shoulder Group. Intra-and interobserver agreement in the classification and treatment of distal third clavicle fractures. *Am J Sports Med.* 2015;43(4):979–984.

16. Nordqvist A, Petersson C, Redlund-Johnell I. The natural course of lateral clavicle fracture: 15 (11–21) year follow-up of 110 cases. *Acta Orthop Scand.* 1993;64(1):87–91.

17. Robinson CM, McQueen MM, Wakefield AE. Estimating the risk of nonunion following nonoperative treatment of a clavicular fracture. *JBJS.* 2004;86(7):1359–1365.

18. Rokito AS, Zuckerman JD, Shaari JM, Eisenberg DP, Cuomo F, Gallagher MA. A comparison of nonoperative and operative treatment of type II distal clavicle fractures. *Bulletin-Hospital for Joint Diseases.* 2002;61(1–2):32–39.

19. Oh JH, Kim SH, Lee JH, Shin SH, Gong HS. Treatment of distal clavicle fracture: a systematic review of treatment modalities in 425 fractures. *Arch Orthop Trauma Surg.* 2011;131(4):525–533.

20. Edwards DJ, Kavanagh TG, Flannery MC. Fractures of the distal clavicle: a case for fixation. *Injury.* 1992;23(1):44–46.

21. Kona J, Bosse MJ, Staeheli JW, Rosseau RL. Type II distal clavicle fractures: a retrospective review of surgical treatment. *J Orthop Trauma.* 1990;4(2):115–120.

22. Lyons FA, Rockwood Jr CA. Migration of pins used in operations on the shoulder. *JBJS.* 1990;72(8):1262–1267.

23. Neviaser RJ, Neviaser JS, Neviaser TJ. A simple technique for internal fixation of the clavicle. A long term evaluation. *Clin Orthop Relat Res.* 1975;109:103–107.

24. Jou IM, Chiang EP, Lin CJ, Lin CL, Wang PH, Su WR. Treatment of unstable distal clavicle fractures with Knowles pin. *J Shoulder Elbow Surg.* 2011;20(3):414–419.

25. Fann CY, Chiu FY, Chuang TY, Chen CM, Chen TH. Transacromial Knowles pin in the treatment of Neer type 2 distal clavicle fractures. A prospective evaluation of 32 cases. *Journal of Trauma and Acute Care Surgery.* 2004;56(5):1102–1106.

26. Wu K, Chang CH, Yang RS. Comparing hook plates and Kirschner tension band wiring for unstable lateral clavicle fractures. *Orthopedics.* 2011;34(11):e718–e723.

27. Bosworth BM. Acromioclavicular separation new method of repair. *Surgery, Gynecology and Obstetrics.* 1941;73:866–871.

28. Ballmer FT, Gerber C. Coracoclavicular screw fixation for unstable fractures of the distal clavicle. A report of five cases. *The Journal of Bone and Joint Surgery. British Volume.* 1991;73(2):291–294.

29. Fazal MA, Saksena J, Haddad FS. Temporary coracoclavicular screw fixation for displaced distal clavicle fractures. *J Orthop Surg.* 2007;15(1):9–11.

30. Macheras G, Kateros KT, Savvidou OD, Sofianos J, Papagelopoulos PJ, Fawzy EA. Coracoclavicular screw fixation for unstable distal clavicle fractures. *Orthopedics.* 2005;28(7):693–696.

31. Jin CZ, Kim HK, Min BH. Surgical treatment for distal clavicle fracture associated with coracoclavicular ligament rupture using a cannulated screw fixation technique. *Journal of Trauma and Acute Care Surgery.* 2006;60(6):1358–1361.

32. Kalamaras M, Cutbush K, Robinson M. A method for internal fixation of unstable distal clavicle fractures: early observations using a new technique. *J Shoulder Elbow Surg.* 2008;17(1):60–62.

33. Andersen JR, Willis MP, Nelson R, Mighell MA. Precontoured superior locked plating of distal clavicle fractures: a new strategy. *Clin Orthop Relat Res.* 2011;469(12):3344–3350.

34. Lee SK, Lee JW, Song DG, Choy WS. Precontoured locking plate fixation for displaced lateral clavicle fractures. *Orthopedics.* 2013;36(6):801–807.

35. Fleming MA, Dachs R, Maqungo S, du Plessis JP, Vrettos BC, Roche SJ. Angular stable fixation of displaced distal-third clavicle fractures with superior precontoured locking plates. *J Shoulder Elbow Surg.* 2015;24(5):700–704.

36. Schliemann B, Roßlenbroich SB, Schneider KN, Petersen W, Raschke MJ, Weimann A. Surgical treatment of vertically unstable lateral clavicle fractures (Neer 2b) with locked plate fixation and coracoclavicular ligament reconstruction. *Arch Orthop Trauma Surg.* 2013;133(7):935–939.

37. Johnston PS, Sears BW, Lazarus MR, Frieman BG. Fixation of unstable type II clavicle fractures with distal clavicle plate and suture button. *J Orthop Trauma.* 2014;28(11):e269–272.

38. Fan J, Zhang Y, Huang Q, Jiang X, He L. Comparison of treatment of acute unstable distal clavicle fractures using anatomical locking plates with versus without additional suture anchor fixation. *Med Sci Mon Int Med J Exp Clin Res: International Medical Journal of Experimental and Clinical Research.* 2017;23:5455.

39. Beirer M, Siebenlist S, Crönlein M, et al. Clinical and radiological outcome following treatment of displaced lateral clavicle fractures using a locking compression plate with lateral extension: a prospective study. *BMC Muscoskel Disord.* 2014;15(1):380.

40. Madsen W, Yaseen Z, LaFrance R, et al. Addition of a suture anchor for coracoclavicular fixation to a superior locking plate improves stability of type IIB distal clavicle fractures. *Arthrosc J Arthrosc Relat Surg.* 2013;29(6):998–1004.

41. Rieser GR, Edwards K, Gould GC, Markert RJ, Goswami T, Rubino LJ. Distal-third clavicle fracture fixation: a biomechanical evaluation of fixation. *J Shoulder Elbow Surg.* 2013;22(6):848–855.

42. Shin SJ, Ko YW, Lee J, Park MG. Use of plate fixation without coracoclavicular ligament augmentation for unstable distal clavicle fractures. *J Shoulder Elbow Surg.* 2016;25(6):942–948.

43. Hohmann E, Tetsworth K, Glatt V. Operative treatment of Neer Type-II distal clavicular fractures: an overview of contemporary techniques. *JBJS Reviews.* 2019;7(5):e5.

44. Kaipel M, Majewski M, Regazzoni P. Double-plate fixation in lateral clavicle fractures—a new strategy. *Journal of Trauma and Acute Care Surgery.* 2010;69(4):896–900.

45. Suter C, von Rohr M, Majewski M, et al. A biomechanical comparison of two plating techniques in lateral clavicle fractures. *Clin BioMech.* 2019;67:78–84.

46. Sambandam B, Gupta R, Kumar S, Maini L. Fracture of distal end clavicle: a review. *Journal of Clinical Orthopaedics and Trauma.* 2014;5(2):65–73.

47. Stegeman SA, Nacak H, Huvenaars KH, Stijnen T, Krijnen P, Schipper IB. Surgical treatment of Neer type-II fractures of the distal clavicle: a meta-analysis. *Acta Orthop.* 2013;84(2):184–190.

48. Asadollahi S, Bucknill A. Hook plate fixation for acute unstable distal clavicle fracture: a systematic review and meta-analysis. *J Orthop Trauma.* 2019;33(8):417–422.

49. Milewski MD, Tompkins M, Giugale JM, Carson EW, Miller MD, Diduch DR. Complications related to anatomic reconstruction of the coracoclavicular ligaments. *Am J Sports Med.* 2012;40(7):1628–1634.

50. Zheng YR, Lu YC, Liu CT. Treatment of unstable distal-third clavicle fractures using minimal invasive closed-loop double endobutton technique. *J Orthop Surg Res.* 2019;14(1):37.

51. Goldberg JA, Bruce WJ, Sonnabend DH, Walsh WR. Type 2 fractures of the distal clavicle: a new surgical technique. *J Shoulder Elbow Surg.* 1997;6(4):380–382.

52. Webber MC, Haines JF. The treatment of lateral clavicle fractures. *Injury*. 2000;31(3):175–179.

53. Soliman O, Koptan W, Zarad A. Under-coracoid-around-clavicle (UCAC) loop in type II distal clavicle fractures. *The Bone & Joint Journal*. 2013;95(7):983–987.

54. Reider B, Terry M, Provencher M. In: *Operative Techniques: Sports Medicine Surgery*. 1st ed. Philadelphia: Saunders Elsevier; 2009:50.

55. Carofino BC, Mazzocca AD. The anatomic coracoclavicular ligament reconstruction: surgical technique and indications. *J Shoulder Elbow Surg*. 2010;19(2):37–46.

56. Yagnik GP, Jordan CJ, Narvel RR, Hassan RJ, Porter DA. Distal clavicle fracture repair: clinical outcomes of a surgical technique utilizing a combination of cortical button fixation and coracoclavicular ligament reconstruction. *Orthopaedic Journal of Sports Medicine*. 2019;7(9). 2325967119867920.

57. Alaee F, Apostolakos J, Singh H, et al. Lateral clavicle fracture with coracoclavicular ligament injury: a biomechanical study of 4 different repair techniques. *Knee Surg Sports Traumatol Arthrosc*. 2017;25(7):2013–2019.

58. Pujol N, Philippeau JM, Richou J, Lespagnol F, Graveleau N, Hardy P. Arthroscopic treatment of distal clavicle fractures: a technical note. *Knee Surg Sports Traumatol Arthrosc*. 2008;16(9):884–886.

59. Checchia SL, Doneux PS, Miyazaki AN, Fregoneze M, Silva LA. Treatment of distal clavicle fractures using an arthroscopic technique. *J Shoulder Elbow Surg*. 2008;17(3):395–398.

60. Nourissat G, Kakuda C, Dumontier C, Sautet A, Doursounian L. Arthroscopic stabilization of Neer type 2 fracture of the distal part of the clavicle. *Arthrosc J Arthrosc Relat Surg*. 2007;23(6): 674–e1.

61. Klein SM, Badman BL, Keating CJ, Devinney DS, Frankle MA, Mighell MA. Results of surgical treatment for unstable distal clavicular fractures. *J Shoulder Elbow Surg*. 2010;19(7):1049–1055.

62. Boonard M, Sumanont S, Arirachakaran A, et al. Fixation method for treatment of unstable distal clavicle fracture: systematic review and network meta-analysis. *Eur J Orthop Surg Traumatol*. 2018;28(6):1065–1078.

63. Fox HM, Ramsey DC, Thompson AR, Hoekstra CJ, Mirarchi AJ, Nazir OF. Neer Type-II distal clavicle fractures: a cost-effectiveness analysis of fixation techniques. *JBJS*. 2020;102(3):254–261.

10

Technique Spotlight: Hook Plate Fixation Technique for Displaced Distal Clavicle Fractures

THOMAS J. KREMEN Jr. AND DEVON JEFFCOAT

Indications

The most common indications for use of the hook plate are for cases of displaced distal clavicle fractures in which the coracoclavicular (CC) ligaments (trapezoid and conoid) provide insufficient connection between the coracoid and the clavicle, thus allowing the medial clavicle to elevate and the weight of the arm to displace the distal fragment(s) inferiorly (Fig. 10.1).[1] Distal clavicle fractures, as characterized by Neer, include type I injuries (lateral to the CC ligaments), type IIA injuries (medial to the CC ligaments), type IIB injuries (between the CC ligaments with torn conoid), type III injuries (extending into the acromioclavicular [AC] joint), type IV injuries (physeal fractures), and type V injuries (unstable comminuted fractures with intact CC ligaments and medial clavicle displacement).[1] Injuries with significant fracture displacement and widening of the CC interspace on upright views to indicate disruption of these ligaments are amenable to this technique.

Although recently some authors have shown that different fixation constructs, such as dual plating or suture augmented superior plating, can result in similar biomechanical properties to hook plate constructs,[2] the versatility of hook plate constructs and their predictable and easily manageable associated complications make the hook plate implants quite appealing. Hook plate constructs function to reduce the distal clavicle with sufficient fixation regardless of the degree of comminution at the distal clavicle or injury to the coracoid. This is not always the case when dual plating is attempted or suture augmented superior plating is performed with cortical buttons at the inferior coracoid. Despite attempts to minimize the degree of hardware removal, every construct carries the potential for this secondary procedure and when cortical buttons inferior to the coracoid do fail, the complications can be difficult to manage including coracoid fracture, a potentially technically challenging surgical dissection, or a risk of hardware migration adjacent to important neurovascular structures. Whereas with hook plate fixation constructs, the risk of acromial osteolysis and even acromial fracture is foreseeable and rarely requires treatment beyond removal of hardware. Preplanned hardware removal at approximately 4 months after the index procedure (the norm for the authors of this chapter) can be perceived as more of an inconvenience rather than a true complication, and preoperative counseling of patients is important to set expectations. Finally, hook plate constructs can also be used to treat chronically displaced AC injuries including the treatment of these injuries with biologic fixation (soft tissue grafts) placed deep to the plate. If used for a fracture (clavicle or coracoid), it is best treated early to minimize the need for mobilization of the fragments. If treatment is delayed (>3 weeks after injury) for a displaced purely ligamentous injury (AC separations), there may be a need for augmentation of fixation with a heavy braided nonabsorbable implant as well as a soft tissue allograft or autograft placed deep to the hook plate device. Placing these implants deep to the plate ensures retention after planned removal of the hook plate itself.

While there are many techniques for treating distal clavicle instability, the hook plate is the only implant that uses the leverage point under the acromion and the hook to resist the relevant deforming forces. This strength is also its weakness in that it is occupying the subacromial space, exerting force onto the undersurface of the acromion and therefore must be removed to minimize any potential for injury to the rotator cuff and the undersurface of the acromion.

Positioning and Equipment

Equipment

Preoperative planning should include thought regarding operating table choice, operating room orientation including C-arm

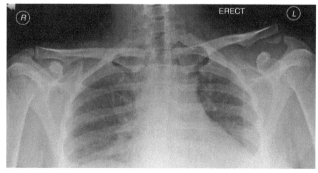

• **Fig. 10.1** Displaced distal clavicle fracture with coracoclavicular ligament disruption.

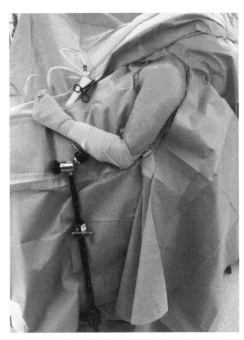

• **Fig. 10.2** Beach chair positioning with McConnell arm holding device.

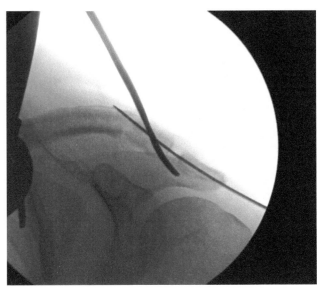

• **Fig. 10.3** Periosteal elevator passed inferior to the posterior acromion, posterior to the acromioclavicular joint.

positioning, and proper implant availability. Hook plate implants are manufactured by several different companies and these various vendors can be contacted to ensure the availability of implants. Many of these implants come sterile packed or in a specialized tray with various size options. The use of regional anesthetic blocks is institution dependent but can provide significant pain relief if performed appropriately.

Positioning

Generally, these fractures can be fixed with the patient in either supine or beach chair position. Proponents of supine position-ing enjoy the quick setup, but may struggle with access to the operative field while the opposite is true for beach chair. The authors prefer a gentle beach chair with ~60 degrees of eleva-tion at the head of the bead with the head secured into a head holder. It is essential to ensure that appropriate fluoroscopic images can be obtained prior to prepping the patient. Given the tendency for the lateral fragment to drop with the weight of the upper extremity, an arm holder can help neutralize these forces and help facilitate fracture reduction. An adjustable arm hold-ing device such as a Spider (Smith and Nephew, Andover, MA), Trimano (Arthrex Inc., Naples, FL), or McConnell (McConnell Orthopaedic Manufacturing, Greenville, TX) is recommended, particularly if no assistant is available. Alternatively resting the forearm on a padded mayo will suffice. The patient's head can be tilted and rotated axially slightly away from the operative field to allow the surgeon to more easily achieve appropriate screw trajectories (Fig. 10.2). A series of U-shaped drapes can help match the contours of the neck, axilla, and shoulder to allow for a large field and good adhesion to the skin. Placing drapes such that the medial border of the operating field is located at the medial clavicle is ideal. To minimize exposure to axillary skin flora, after sterile prep, the authors prefer to capture the opera-tive field with a sterile Ioban "sandwich" covering the entire sur-gical field and wrapping circumferentially around the brachium and axilla.

Technique Description

The skin incision is typically oriented from the anterosuperior aspect of the middle portion of the clavicle (depending on desired plate length) to 1 cm distal to the AC joint, crossing the postero-lateral aspect AC joint. This will make placing the hook under the acromion easier and with less need for lateral soft tissue dissection and skin retraction. Full-thickness skin flaps are created to allow a mobile skin window and a layered closure. The platysma and deltotrapezial fascia are then divided in a layered fashion and the fracture and planned plate area are exposed. This typically requires elevating some of the trapezius insertion with the deltotrapezial fascia. This allows exposure of the bone with minimal soft tissue detachment, subsequent imbrication and repair of the stretched/injured deltotrapezial fascia, and soft tissue closure over the plate to minimize plate irritation. There is generally no need to violate the AC joint. We have found that after dissection of the major fracture fragments, a small incision (~1–2 cm) along the medial border of the acromion posterior to the AC joint followed by the placement of a small periosteal elevator under the acromion (Fig. 10.3) and sweeping it from anterior to posterior will create an adequate potential space to accommodate the hook portion of the implant. A curved Crego Periosteal Elevator can be especially helpful for this step.

Reduction and Fixation

Reduction begins with reducing the deforming forces on the frac-ture. In this case, that is the force of gravity on the upper limb. Thus using the arm holder or an assistant to lift up on the arm can help with the reduction. Occasionally the fracture is a simple pattern that is conducive to clamp reduction and temporary wire fixation. Often these are transverse or short oblique and can be provisionally reduced using bone reduction forceps followed by a K-wire to resist vertical translation. The K-wire is placed from lateral to medial in-line with the long axis of the clavicle via percu-taneous puncture anterolateral to the incision (Fig. 10.4).

More often, the distal fragment is comminuted or the fracture is complex enough to make the use of K-wires not feasible. In this

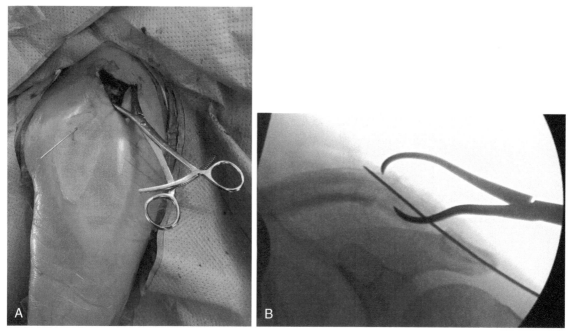

• **Fig. 10.4** (A) Clinical image and (B) fluoroscopic image demonstrating capture of the fracture fragments (provisional reduction) using bone reduction forceps and a K-wire.

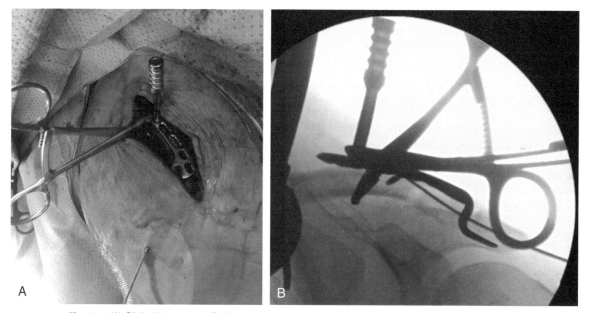

• **Fig. 10.5** (A) Clinical image and (B) fluoroscopic image demonstrating the passage of the hook posterior to the acromioclavicular (AC) joint and inferior to the acromion (posterior to the AC joint) followed by clamping of the medial aspect of the plate to correct the main deformity. A locking drill guide sleeve has been threaded into the medial aspect of the plate to aid in positioning and reduction.

case, the passage of the hook posterior to the AC joint and inferior to the acromion followed by clamping of the medial aspect of the plate to the clavicle can correct the main deformity as the hook plate itself acts as a powerful reduction tool (Fig. 10.5).

There are several options for the magnitude of hook offset (e.g., 12, 15, 18 mm). A 15-mm offset device will suffice in the vast majority of cases unless there is a significant acromion morphologic abnormality, and the authors typically do not employ the templates. The editors, however, *do* use the templates and find that a radiograph of the template with the hook under the acromion

and a clamp to hold the template to the clavicle medially can be very helpful (Fig. 10.6). This view should be assessed to ensure that the CC interspace is reduced, or even slightly over-reduced (Fig. 10.7), such that there is less than one clavicle width between the underside of the clavicle and the superior aspect of the coracoid. In addition, the inferior aspect of the clavicle should align with the inferior aspect of the acromion. If these alignments are not correct, this can indicate that the offset is too great and the displacement is under-reduced. The superior-inferior portion of the hook should be assessed to ensure that it is up against the

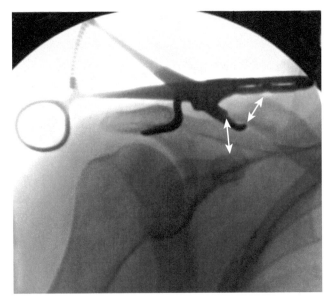

• **Fig. 10.6** Provisional reduction of hook plate construct with proposed 15-mm offset. Note the increased coracoclavicular distance *(double-headed white arrow)* relative to the distal clavicle height *(double-headed yellow arrow)* indicating inadequate reduction. Other clues to inadequate reduction include the inferior cortex of the distal clavicle not aligned with the undersurface of the acromion, the medial portion of the plate not being reduced to bone, and the angulation of the hook plate shim relative to the inferior acromion. Note the alignment of the inferior distal clavicle, medial portion of the hook plate at the shaft of the clavicle and alignment of the hook plate shim under the acromion in Fig. 10.7 for comparison.

medial aspect of the acromion. This will appear as coincident with the AC joint when the device is, in reality, directly behind the joint. Lastly the medial-to-lateral shim portion of the hook should sit flat and parallel to the underside of the acromion—if it sits at an angle (Fig. 10.6) this indicates that the offset does not appropriately match the patient's anatomy or your plate is not adequately reduced medially. Often this mismatch is too little offset in this scenario.

An implant with five screw holes is typically used and provides appropriate fixation, though fracture patterns with functional CC ligament disruption and more medial extension may require longer plates. Passage of the hook under the acromion and reduction of the medial portion of the plate to the medial clavicle can be aided by threading a locking drill guide sleeve into one of the medial screw holes of the plate to act as both a handle and a fulcrum for the medially placed bone reduction clamp (e.g., lobster claw). By tightening this medially placed clamp, apposition of the plate to bone and lateralization of the plate can be achieved. Appropriate lateralization of the plate ensures that the hook component adequately engages the inferior acromion and minimizes the risk of escape postoperatively. Fluoroscopy can be used to assess adequate alignment (Fig. 10.6) by evaluating the same parameters if

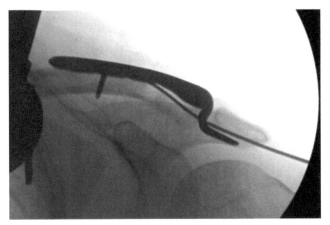

• **Fig. 10.7** Fluoroscopic image obtained after initial fixation with a single medial cortical screw. Note the bent provisional K- wire.

a template is used. Fixation is initiated by placing a single cortical screw at the medial portion of the plate. This effectively reduces the distal clavicle fracture. Note, this may lead to bending of the provisional fixation K-wire (Fig. 10.7). Attention is then paid to ensure the distal portion of the plate is well centered within the distal clavicle in the anterior-posterior plane. There is often an anterior-posterior mismatch between the plate and the distal fracture fragment. A clamp from the superior aspect of the plate can correct this prior to further screw placement. Once the position of the plate in all planes is adequate, the remaining screws are then placed into the plate definitively capturing and reducing the clavicle fracture fragments. At times, hook plate positioning can result in the distal holes of the plate being positioned directly over the AC joint. In this scenario these holes should not be utilized. It should be noted that the cortical bone of the distal clavicle is very thin. If the screw trajectory will not penetrate the AC joint, then locking screws are recommended in the lateral holes in order to achieve adequate fixation in this region.

The CC ligaments are never exposed or repaired. The indirect reduction of the torn ligaments and the maintenance of this reduction with the hook plate allow them to heal.

Closure and Rehabilitation

The closure is multilayered with care taken to close the deep fascia and platysma as separate layers. A simple arm sling is used and patients are encouraged to remove it as soon as pain allows them to start active range-of-motion exercises. Aside from any restriction from pain, no specific range of motion restrictions are given. No lifting or weight-bearing is recommended for the first 6 weeks until healing is observed on radiographs. Plate removal is performed routinely at 4 months postoperatively as the plate can lead to subacromial bursitis, rotator cuff irritation, acromial osteolysis, and even fracture of the acromion if left implanted for a prolonged time period.

PEARLS AND PITFALLS

- The most common error is to under-reduce. If you are using the 18-mm largest offset plate, unless there is unusual acromial anatomy, you are likely making a mistake.
- The vast majority of the time a five-hole implant with a 15-mm hook offset is the appropriate implant.
- Place the plate as lateral as possible in order to prevent escape of the hook from under the acromion. This is more important to the strength of the construct than ensuring that the lateral-most screw holes are medial to the AC joint.
- If distal clavicle bone quality is poor, place three or four screws in the medial fragment: avoiding distal clavicle fixation is often of little

consequence, whereas AC joint penetration can lead to symptomatic AC arthrosis in the future.
- It is recommended that the hook plate implant be removed by ~4 months after implantation. While the plate can be retained longer without significant symptoms, severe osteolysis or complete acromial erosion is a problem, which is difficult to reconstruct and is preventable with hardware removal. Although acromial osteolysis is apparent on the image in Fig. 10.8, this patient had minimal symptoms at the site of the hook plate at 1.5 years after implantation.
- CC ligaments do "heal" even without direct repair, particularly when fixed acutely. While not performed routinely, the reconstituted ligaments can be visualized on follow-up magnetic resonance imaging.

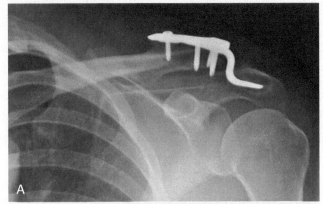

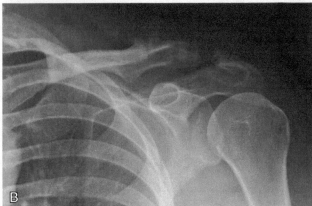

• **Fig. 10.8** (A) Hook plate at 1.5 years after implantation. Note the acromion osteolysis due to the hook portion of the implant. Also of note, this noncompliant patient had hardware migration at 2 weeks postoperatively; however, no further hardware migration was observed even at 1.5 years' follow-up. (B) X-ray images after hardware removal in this same patient at 1.5 years after implantation. The patient had no pain and full function after hardware removal.

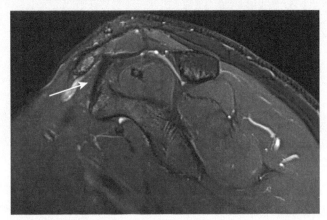

• **Fig. 10.9** Reconstituted coracoclavicular ligament visualized on follow-up magnetic resonance imaging (MRI) at 2 years after hook plate removal (MRI) after hardware removal. The low signal intensity structure connecting the coracoid to the distal clavicle as indicated by the *yellow arrow* on this sagittal T2 MRI image demonstrates the reconstituted coracoclavicular ligaments which are still intact 2 years after hook plate removal in a patient treated previously with a hook plate for an acute type 5 AC joint injury.

References

1. Neer 2nd, CS. Fracture of the distal clavicle with detachment of the coracoclavicular ligaments in adults. *J Trauma*. 1963;3:99–110.

2. Garlich J, Little M, Nelson TJ, et al. A comparison of three fixation strategies in the treatment of Neer type IIb distal clavicle fractures. *J Orthop Trauma*. 2020.

11

Technique Spotlight: Arthoscopic-Assisted Reduction and Internal Fixation of Distal Clavicle Fractures

TRAVIS L. FRANTZ, ANDREW NEVIASER, AND GREGORY L. CVETANOVICH

Indications

Clavicle fractures account for 2.6%–4% of all adult fractures, with 10%–30% of these occurring in the distal third of the clavicle.[1–3] The stability and displacement of the fracture determine whether surgery is indicated as the coracoclavicular (CC) ligaments (conoid and trapezoid) can be affected in these injuries.[1,4–8] Essentially, fractures of the lateral third of the clavicle in adult patients where the coracoid no longer has structural continuity to the clavicle are considered for operative treatment. The Neer classification for distal clavicle fractures is most commonly used, with displaced type IIA, type IIB, and type V commonly considered relative indications for surgical intervention due to the functional disruption of the ligaments leading to an unstable fracture pattern with high nonunion rates.[4,5] For acute fractures that are unstable and/or displaced, multiple surgical options exist including dynamic compression plating, hook plating, acromioclavicular (AC) joint spanning fixation, transacromial fixation, tension band techniques, intramedullary screw fixation, CC screw, and CC ligament repair or reconstruction.[9–14] Surgery is associated with both faster time to and higher rates of union with improved functional outcomes and less pain, particularly with overhead activities. However, it does come with the risk of symptomatic hardware, increased need for future procedures, and wound complication/infection.[4,9–17] The incidence of hardware removal can be as high as 100% for devices where this is routinely recommended (hook plate and AC spanning fixation) but even for devices where hardware removal is not routinely recommended and removal rates can be as high as 30%, and thus alternative surgical techniques have been sought.[3,15,16,18–20]

Fracture stability, disruption of the CC ligaments, and pattern according to the Neer classification are considered. An unstable fracture is a relative indication for surgical treatment. For lower-demand patients, nonoperative treatment can be considered and certain patients may be willing to accept the risk of and even tolerate a nonunion. Many studies combine all Neer classification types, thus making interpretation of the results for unstable patterns more difficult.[2,21,22] For unstable fractures with disruption of the CC ligaments and insufficient distal bone for locking plate fixation screws, hook plates have traditionally been used, but with relatively high complication rates and recommendations for routine removal with a second procedure.[3,16,21,23–25] In these cases, the authors prefer arthroscopic-assisted reduction and CC fixation to allow fracture reduction to near anatomic alignment and relative fracture stability for fracture healing in the acute setting (<2 weeks from time of injury). Treatment of these fractures in a subacute or delayed fashion has generated mixed outcomes due to the CC ligaments' poor ability to heal and the need to provide autograft or allograft collagen to supplement this deficiency. The arthroscopic-assisted technique is minimally invasive, facilitates treatment of associated pathology, maintains fracture site biology, and typically avoids complications seen with plating or more bulky hardware including secondary hardware removal.

Preoperative Evaluation

Standard preoperative evaluation should begin with a pertinent history and physical examination. Distal clavicle fractures are most commonly the result of a fall or trauma. The hand dominance, activity level, relevant employment or sport demands, and necessity of overhead activity should all be documented. Physical examination should assess for any gross deformity. The presence of tenting of the skin or any abnormal neurovascular examination finding may impact surgical decision-making. Standard shoulder radiographs of the affected shoulder should be obtained. Dedicated clavicle or Zanca views may help better determine the true extent of displacement (Fig. 11.1). Gravity is the major deforming force for distal clavicle fractures and thus given that the assessment of the connection between the medial portion of the clavicle and

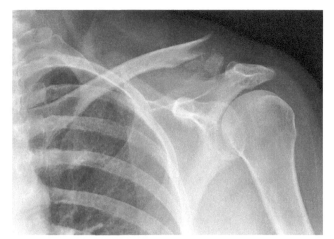

• **Fig. 11.1** Left shoulder X-ray demonstrating comminuted distal-third clavicle fracture.

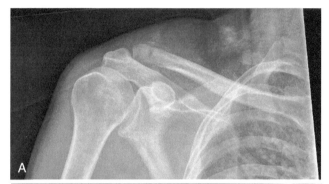

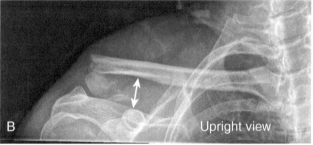

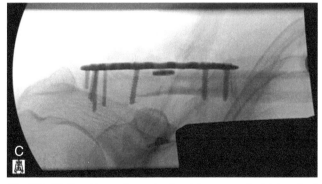

• **Fig. 11.2** (A) Shoulder radiograph of polytrauma patient taken in the supine position suggesting minimal displacement of a distal clavicle fracture. (B) Upright view (in this case seated due to patient's severe lower extremity injuries) reveal widening of the coracoclavicular (CC) distance *(arrow)* indicating incompetence of the CC ligaments—an unstable fracture pattern. (C) In this case, arthroscopic-assisted placement of a CC button was supplemented with a plate. Note the two metallic ends of the CC fixation above the clavicle and under the coracoid as well as the reduction of the CC distance. (Images courtesy Grant E. Garrigues, MD.)

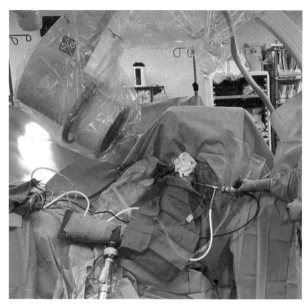

• **Fig. 11.3** Operating room set-up demonstrating beach chair positioning with the arthroscope currently placed through the posterior portal of the left shoulder, and C-arm coming over the top of the patient's head to obtain necessary shoulder and clavicle fluoroscopic images.

the coracoid is so critical, upright views are mandatory to allow assessment of widening of the CC distance (Fig. 11.2). On a case-by-case basis, the use of a computerized tomography (CT) scan can further help to evaluate displacement, shortening, comminution, and intra-articular involvement, but is rarely necessary when assessing distal-third clavicle fractures unless there is some concern that the coracoid base/scapula may also be involved.

For operative distal clavicle fractures, arthroscopic-assisted reduction and CC fixation can be considered when there is an intact coracoid and when the clavicular bone will allow a drill hole and cortical support for metal button fixation around 3–4.5 cm from the AC joint, which is the normal clavicular attachment site for the CC ligaments. If there is fracture extension into this area, significant comminution, or if the coracoid is compromised, we recommend choosing a different surgical tactic. If the clavicle fracture compromises the clavicular location of the button, supplementary plate fixation with a button superior to the plate can be used (Fig 11.2C). If the coracoid is compromised, fixation with a hook plate is typically chosen as it does not rely on the coracoid for fixation. Once the decision has been made to proceed with surgery, the patient is placed into a sling with limited shoulder range of motion (ROM) until the day of the procedure.

Positioning and Equipment

The patient is brought to the operating room and placed into the standard beach chair position used for shoulder arthroscopy with an arm holder (Trimano; Arthrex, Naples, FL, USA). The bed is then turned 90 degrees to allow full access to the shoulder for arthroscopy anteriorly and posteriorly as well as for positioning of the C-arm fluoroscopy. The operative shoulder is prepped and draped including the clavicle to enable conversion to an open approach if needed. The C-arm is then brought in from the head of the patient and parallel to the patient's body (Fig. 11.3). The C-arm can then be canted over the top in order to obtain the necessary shoulder and clavicle intraoperative fluoroscopy X-rays. Be sure to allow enough room at the head of the bed for the C-arm to

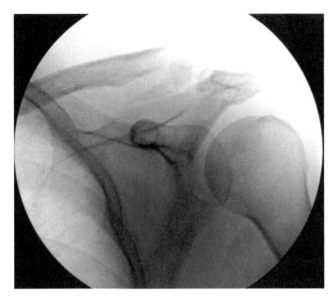

• **Fig. 11.4** Initial fluoroscopic C-arm view demonstrating fracture displacement.

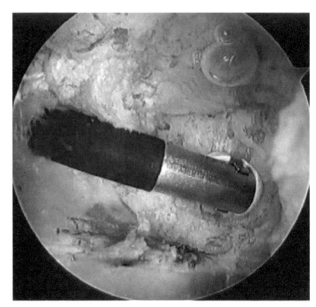

• **Fig. 11.5** Arthroscopic imaging demonstrating adequate visualization of the coracoid.

be maneuvered without difficulty. Also, make sure your arthroscopy set-up (arthroscope, cords, instruments, extra Mayo stand, etc.) are placed more toward the foot of the patient as to not block the C-arm. We use a large C-arm to enable room for instrumentation anteriorly and arthroscopic viewing posteriorly.

Technique

We begin with imaging to confirm fracture pattern (Fig. 11.4). Using a combination of upward pressure on the arm and downward pressure on the clavicle medial to the fracture site, we confirm that the fracture can be appropriately reduced without opening. If we are unable to achieve a closed reduction or for chronic fractures or nonunion, we would then perform a limited open reduction of the fracture site to confirm fracture reduction before proceeding with arthroscopy. In nonunions, we often supplement with allograft bone at the fracture site and semitendinosus allograft to reconstruct the chronically deficient CC ligaments in addition to the suture fixation. If closed reduction is successful, a 1.5- to 2-cm incision can be made outside the fracture site in the location of planned CC fixation to accommodate the titanium button down to the bone. Perhaps surprisingly, this incision can be smaller than that used for the similar technique applied to AC joint separation. In the latter technique, the AC joint capsule and deltotrapezial fascia are imbricated and repaired, where that is often unnecessary depending on the pathoanatomy of the fracture pattern. In a medial-lateral dimension, the button should be directly superior to the coracoid base, as visualized by the coracoid cortical ring sign, and in the midportion of the clavicle in an anteroposterior dimension.[26] Once fracture reduction is confirmed, the draped C-arm can be moved medially across the patient's body to be out of the way during arthroscopy until necessary later in the case for reduction and fixation.

Standard shoulder arthroscopy is initiated, beginning with the introduction of a 30-degree arthroscope into the posterior portal of the glenohumeral joint. The joint should be examined to rule out any additional pathology. A low anterior rotator interval portal is created using a standard spinal needle localization technique just above the subscapularis. With the use of a shaver and electrocautery device, we open the rotator interval and dissect down to the coracoid from an inferolateral direction. The inferior aspect of the coracoid is skeletonized working toward the base and once the

30-degree arthroscope can no longer view around the corner to see the posteriormost aspect of the base, we switch to a 70-degree scope viewing from posteriorly and continue the dissection of the coracoid with electrocautery until the base is visualized. The coracoid base blends with the scapular body and thus when the curved shape of the underside of the coracoid begins to curve almost vertically, then sufficient posterior exposure of the coracoid base has been achieved. The common error is not to expose far enough posterior or medial, leading to fixation that does not recreate the centroid of the CC ligaments and can break out of the weaker bone of the lateral coracoid tip. Care should be taken to expose the coracoid along the entire base and clearly palpate the medial and lateral edges of the coracoid (Fig. 11.5). Be mindful that the suprascapular nerve travels through the suprascapular notch just medial to the coracoid base and thus while the medial edge should be identified, exposing into the soft tissues farther medially is unnecessary and unwise. A 70-degree scope through the posterior portal is typically sufficient for this, but alternatively changing view to an accessory anterosuperolateral portal with a 30-degree scope can allow appropriate visualization. After dissection is complete, we insert a large flexible anterior cannula into the anterior portal to enable instrumentation and suture passage (10 mm PassPort Button Cannula; Arthrex).

There are multiple devices that use tensioned sutures between two buttons for fixation that accurately recreates the properties of a ligament to resist displacement but allow rotation and motion in other planes. We typically use the Arthrex Dog Bone and the steps here will follow that technique. However, similar devices from multiple manufacturing companies exist and can be utilized using similar principles. Next, the guide for the CC drill is brought in along with the C-arm. The fracture is reduced by an assistant and the guide is secured in the desired position. The specialized drill guide (Arthrex) inserted through the flexible anterior cannula seats a paddle on the bottom of the coracoid base and a sleeve secures the guide to the superior cortex of the clavicle through the previously made incision (Figs. 11.6 and 11.7). Proper placement of the fixation in the coracoid is critical (Fig. 11.8). Avoid placement too lateral or in the coracoid tip. The exit should be centered in the medial-lateral dimension and in the coracoid base. Practically, this will mean posterior to the upper border of the subscapularis where the inferior aspect of the coracoid base is curving inferiorly.

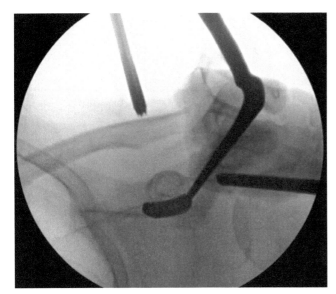

• **Fig. 11.6** Drill guide placed through low anterior working portal and into appropriate position to aid with drilling of the tunnel through the clavicle and coracoid.

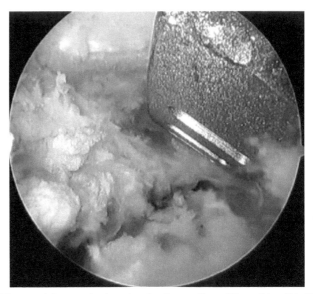

• **Fig. 11.7** Arthroscopic view showing the position of the guide within the shoulder.

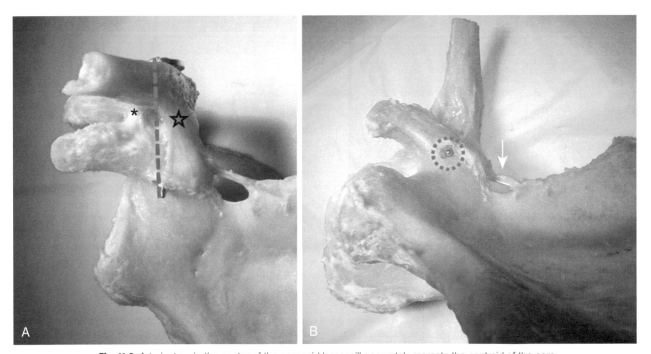

• **Fig. 11.8** A trajectory in the center of the coracoid base will accurately recreate the centroid of the coracoclavicular ligaments. This example shows a coracoclavicular screw (Bosworth screw) but the principles are identical. (A) and (B) Proper trajectory *(red dotted line)* in the coracoid base will travel between the posteromedial conoid ligament *(star)* and the anterolateral trapezoid ligament *(asterisk)*. (B) Fixation exiting centered on the coracoid base *(red dotted circle)*. Note the proximity of the suprascapular notch *(yellow arrow)*. (Images courtesy Grant E. Garrigues MD and adapted from Garrigues GE, Marchant MH Jr, Lewis GC, Gupta AK, Richard MJ, Basamania CJ. The cortical ring sign: a reliable radiographic landmark for percutaneous coracoclavicular fixation. *J Shoulder Elbow Surg.* 2010;19:121-129.)

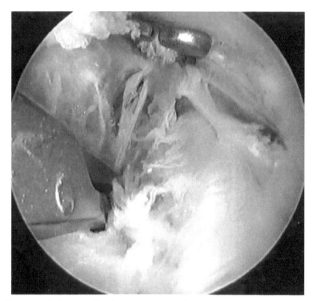

• **Fig. 11.9** Arthroscopic view demonstrating the position of the button flush against the coracoid surface.

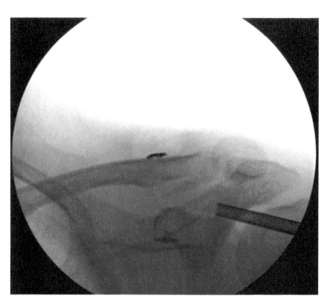

• **Fig. 11.10** Final fluoroscopic C-arm images demonstrating final titanium button and suture tape construct.

While the fracture and CC space are held reduced, C-arm imaging is used to confirm appropriate guide positioning of the sleeve on the mid clavicle about 3–4 cm from the AC joint and of the paddle on the coracoid base. A second assistant is extremely helpful at this portion of the case as the primary surgeon typically holds the arthroscope and the aiming guide, while one assistant and the arm holder hold the fracture and the CC space reduced, and a third assistant prepares to drill. After achieving the desired position, a 3.0-mm drill tunnel is created through the guide, drilling four cortices through the clavicle and coracoid base. Direct arthroscopic visualization will confirm the drill bit exiting the midportion of the coracoid base at the center of the guide paddle. The guide is removed and C-arm imaging is used to confirm the appropriate location and trajectory. Next, a nitinol suture is inserted through the cannulated drill through the clavicle and coracoid and retrieved from the anterior working portal. The drill is then removed and the assistant can relax on maintaining the fracture reduction.

Because the nitinol can break during suture shuttling, a high tensile shuttle suture is then shuttled with the nitinol through the

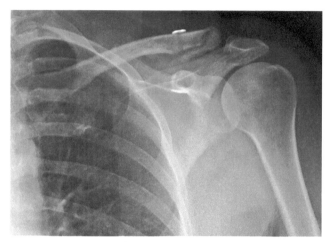

• **Fig. 11.11** Six-week postoperative X-ray.

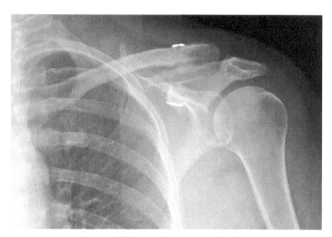

• **Fig. 11.12** Six-month postoperative X-ray.

coracoid and clavicle. Sutures are secured on either end with hemostat. Next, two high-tensile suture tapes are loaded into the first titanium button. With the sutures of each now tight and flush against the button, the tails of the sutures are shuttled into the shoulder via the shuttle suture through the anterior portal, coracoid tunnel, and out the top of the clavicular tunnel. Suture tails are again snapped with a hemostat and tension on the sutures brings the button through the anterior cannula down to the undersurface of the coracoid base under arthroscopic visualization. The button should now seat flush against the inferior cortex of the coracoid base (Fig. 11.9).

The suture tapes existing through the clavicle are loaded into the second titanium button. The button is slid down until it is seated flush against the superior surface of the clavicle. Again using fluoroscopy, the fracture is held reduced, or preferably slightly over reduced, through upward pressure on the arm and downward pressure on the medial clavicle. Reduction is confirmed fluoroscopically. The two suture tapes are then sequentially tied and cut. Alternatively, some devices utilize knotless tensioning. Advantages to this are the ease of tensioning and holding the tension without losing reduction during the tying step. The disadvantage is they typically require a larger hole in the coracoid with a smaller button and smaller sutures as opposed to the stronger tapes. Reduction of the fracture, appropriate hardware positioning, and alignment are all confirmed fluoroscopically (Fig. 11.10). The skin and portals are closed in a standard fashion.

The patient is placed into a sling postoperatively to support the weight of the arm that pulls on the CC fixation. The patient should be seen back at standard postoperative time intervals with repeat X-ray imaging (Figs. 11.11 and 11.12). Patients are maintained in a sling for 6 weeks. They can perform gentle shoulder passive- and active-assisted ROM with physical therapy to avoid stiffness as well as elbow, wrist, and hand motion. We typically avoid flexion beyond 90 degrees for the first 6 weeks given the rotational forces imparted by this action. In addition, we do emphasize passive external rotation as the dissection around the coracoid base coupled with the internal rotation position of sling immobilization can lead to rotational contracture. After 6 weeks, motion is advanced with physical therapy. Strengthening begins at 12 weeks according to fracture healing and return to sports at 3–6 months after fracture union and return of full strength and ROM.

PEARLS AND PITFALLS

- Preoperatively, ensure that the coracoid is intact and the clavicle fracture pattern will allow a drill hole and cortical support for metal button fixation around 3–4.5 cm from the AC joint.
- When setting up the room, make sure to allow enough room at the head of the bed for the C-arm to be maneuvered without difficulty, and make sure your arthroscopy set-up (arthroscope, cords, instruments, extra Mayo stand, etc.) are placed more toward the foot of the patient.
- After patient positioning, ensure that adequate fluoroscopic views can be obtained and that the fracture can be appropriately reduced; if it cannot, the fracture site may need to be reduced through open means.
- When not in use, move the C-arm medially over the patient's head and nonoperative shoulder rather than taking it in and out.
- Use of the 70-degree scope will facilitate better visualization of the coracoid if viewing from a posterior portal.
- When drilling the clavicle and coracoid, typically the camera and guide are held by the surgeon while an assistant drills the four cortices.
- Use of a robust suture or passer is needed to facilitate suture tape passage through the coracoid and clavicle.
- Ensure the reduction is maintained when tensioning the suture tapes. We recommend a slight over reduction.

References

1. Banerjee R, Waterman B, Padalecki J, Robertson W. Management of distal clavicle fractures. *J Am Acad Orthop Surg*. 2011;19:392–401.
2. Robinson CM, Cairns DA. Primary nonoperative treatment of displaced lateral fractures of the clavicle. *J Bone Jt Surg - Ser A*. 2004;86:778–782.
3. Oh JH, Kim SH, Lee JH, Shin SH, Gong HS. Treatment of distal clavicle fracture: a systematic review of treatment modalities in 425 fractures. *Arch Orthop Trauma Surg*. 2011;131:525–533.
4. Neer CS. Fracture of the distal clavicle with detachment of the coracoclavicular ligaments in adults. *J Trauma-Inj Infect Crit Care*. 1963;3:99–110.
5. Neer CS. Fractures of the distal third of the clavicle. *Clin Orthop Relat Res*. 1968;58:43–50.
6. Herrmann S, Schmidmaier G, Greiner S. Stabilisation of vertical unstable distal clavicular fractures (Neer 2b) using locking T-plates and suture anchors. *Injury*. 2009;40:236–239.
7. Moverley R, Little N, Gulihar A, Singh B. Current concepts in the management of clavicle fractures. *J Clin Orthop Trauma*. 2019;11:S25–S30.
8. Webber MCB, Haines JF. The treatment of lateral clavicle fractures. *Injury*. 2000;31:175–179.
9. Andersen JR, Willis MP, Nelson R, Mighell MA. Precontoured superior locked plating of distal clavicle fractures: a new strategy. *Clin Orthop Relat Res*. 2011;469:3344–3350 (Springer New York LLC, 2011).
10. Badhe SP, Lawrence TM, Clark DI. Tension band suturing for the treatment of displaced type 2 lateral end clavicle fractures. *Arch Orthop Trauma Surg*. 2007;127:25–28.
11. Hessmann M, Kirchner R, Baumgaertel F, Gehling H, Gotzen L. Treatment of unstable distal clavicular fractures with and without lesions of the acromioclavicular joint. *Injury*. 1996;27:47–52.
12. Kalamaras M, Cutbush K, Robinson M. A method for internal fixation of unstable distal clavicle fractures: early observations using a new technique. *J Shoulder Elbow Surg*. 2008;17:60–62.
13. Nourissat G, Kakuda C, Dumontier C, Sautet A, Doursounian L. Arthroscopic stabilization of Neer type 2 fracture of the distal part of the clavicle. *Arthroscopy*. 2007;23:674.e1–674.e4.
14. van der Meijden OA, Gaskill TR, Millett PJ. Treatment of clavicle fractures: current concepts review. *J Should Elb Surg*. 2012;21:423–429.
15. Carofino BC, Mazzocca AD. The anatomic coracoclavicular ligament reconstruction: surgical technique and indications. *J Should Elb Surg*. 2010;19:37–46.
16. Flinkkilä T, Ristiniemi J, Hyvönen P, Hämäläinen M. Surgical treatment of unstable fractures of the distal clavicle: a comparative study of Kirschner wire and clavicular hook plate fixation. *Acta Orthop Scand*. 2002;73:50–53.
17. Kashii M, Inui H, Yamamoto K. Surgical treatment of distal clavicle fractures using the clavicular hook plate. *Clin Orthop Rel Res*. 2006;447:158–164. https://doi.org/10.1097/01.blo.0000203469.66055.6a.
18. Suter C, von Rohr M, Majewski M, et al. A biomechanical comparison of two plating techniques in lateral clavicle fractures. *Clin Biomech*. 2019;67:78–84.
19. Suter C, Majewski M, Nowakowski AM. Comparison of 2 plating techniques for lateral clavicle fractures, using a new standardized biomechanical testing setup. *J Appl Biomater Funct Mater*. 2018;16:107–112.
20. Bishop JY, Roesch M, Lewis B, Jones GL, Litsky AS. A biomechanical comparison of distal clavicle fracture reconstructive techniques. *Am J Orthop (Belle Mead. NJ)*. 2013;42:114–118.
21. Klein SM, Badman BL, Keating CJ, Devinney DS, Frankle MA, Mighell MA. Results of surgical treatment for unstable distal clavicular fractures. *J Shoulder Elbow Surg*. 2010;19:1049–1055.
22. Meda PVK, Machani B, Sinopidis C, Braithwaite I, Brownson P, Frostick SP. Clavicular hook plate for lateral end fractures - a prospective study. *Injury*. 2006;37:277–283.
23. Vaishya R, Vijay V, Khanna V. Outcome of distal end clavicle fractures treated with locking plates. *Chinese J Traumatol - English Ed*. 2017;20:45–48.
24. Good DW, Lui DF, Leonard M, Morris S, McElwain JP. Clavicle hook plate fixation for displaced lateral-third clavicle fractures (Neer type II): a functional outcome study. *J Shoulder Elbow Surg*. 2012;21:1045–1048.
25. Charity RM, Haidar SG, Ghosh S, Tillu AB. Fixation failure of the clavicular hook plate: a report of three cases. *J Orthop Surg (Hong Kong)*. 2006;14:333–335.
26. Garrigues GE, Marchant Jr MH, Lewis GC, Gupta AK, Richard MJ, Basamania CJ. The cortical ring sign: a reliable radiographic landmark for percutaneous coracoclavicular fixation. *J Shoulder Elbow Surg*. 2010;19:121–129.

12

The Acromioclavicular Joint: Anatomy, Injury, Pathoanatomy, and Treatment Options

GREGORY NICHOLSON AND KEVIN RASULI

The clavicle functions as an anterior strut supporting the upper limb. The distal aspect of the clavicle articulates with the acromion, thus forming the acromioclavicular (AC) joint, via a posterolaterally oriented facet. The acromion has a reciprocal facet, which is oriented anteromedially.[1] The AC joint is a diarthrodial joint and includes a capsule, articular cartilage, and synovium (Fig. 12.1). An intra-articular disc is typically present, but its size and shape vary significantly.[1] This intra-articular disc begins deteriorating in the second decade of life, and the joint itself undergoes an age-related degeneration.[2]

The AC joint capsule is thin, but has regions that are thickened and are thought of as distinct ligaments: the superior, inferior, anterior, and posterior AC ligaments. The superior and posterior portions of the AC joint capsule are the thickest. They insert 2.8 mm laterally onto the acromial surface and extend onto the distal clavicle an average of 16 mm from the joint line.[3] The AC ligament complex, of which the superior and posterior portions are the thickest and strongest, is the primary stabilizer of the AC joint in the horizontal plane.[1,4,5] Vertical stability of the AC joint is maintained by the coracoclavicular (CC) ligament complex, which consists of the trapezoid and conoid ligaments (Fig. 12.2).[1,5] Specifically, the conoid ligament is the greatest contributor to AC joint stability in the vertical plane.[5] The conoid ligament is the more medial ligament and attaches to the clavicle at the conoid tubercle (a readily visible radiographic landmark on the inferior clavicle). Distally, it attaches to the posterior-most aspect of the dorsum of the coracoid and extends to the posterior coracoid precipice (the vertical component of the posterior coracoid as it blends with the supraspinatus fossa).[6] The trapezoid ligament is the more lateral of the CC ligaments and attaches to the undersurface of the clavicle along the trapezoid line (an oblique ridge that runs from the conoid tubercle anterolateral towards the anterior aspect of the AC joint) and to the coracoid base anterior and lateral to the conoid ligament. Familiarity with the attachments of the CC ligament complex is essential for successful reconstruction of the AC joint. The trapezoid and conoid ligaments originate 2.5 and 4.6 cm from the lateral edge of the clavicle, respectively. Alternatively, this represents a constant ratio of 17% and 31% from the lateral edge of the clavicle, respectively, which is consistent regardless of race or sex.[7,8]

The deltotrapezial fascia (DTF) may also play a role in AC joint stability. As fibers of the superior AC ligament weave into the DTF, it may act as a static and/or dynamic stabilizer of the AC joint.[9] Although some authors have suggested that additional injury to the DTF may be responsible for the increased displacement observed between Rockwood Type III and V injuries, strong biomechanical and clinical studies supporting this hypothesis are lacking. In a recent cadaveric study, Pastor et al. found a relatively small but statistically significant increase in translation and rotation following sectioning of the AC ligaments and the DTF, compared with isolated sectioning of the AC ligaments.[10]

Pathoanatomy

AC joint injuries typically occur as a result of direct trauma to the shoulder girdle with the arm adducted at the side.[11] An inferiorly directed force is applied to the acromion and scapula. This drives the entire scapula anteriorly, medially, and frequently inferiorly, causing variable injury to the AC and CC ligament complexes. Indirect trauma, such as a fall on an outstretched hand, may also lead to AC joint injury by driving the humeral head superiorly into the undersurface of the acromion, also resulting in injury to the AC and CC ligament complexes.[12]

AC joint injuries can be thought of as a continuum of injury severity, with sequential failure of the AC and CC ligaments. Low-grade injuries typically only involve the failure of the, comparatively less stout, AC ligament complex and lead to instability of the AC joint in the horizontal plane, but do not lead to significant instability in the vertical plane if the CC ligament complex remains intact.[5] The vertically oriented CC ligament complex is capable of partially compensating for AC ligament complex insufficiency with some resistance to force in the horizontal plane. In this injured scenario, the conoid ligament becomes the primary stabilizer to anteriorly directed forces, while the trapezoid ligament becomes the primary stabilizer to posteriorly directed forces.[5] Higher grade AC joint injuries lead to both failure of the AC ligaments and partial or complete failure of the CC ligaments with resultant instability in the horizontal and vertical planes. Ultimately, failure of the AC and/or the CC ligaments leads to abnormal AC joint kinematics and load transmission, which may

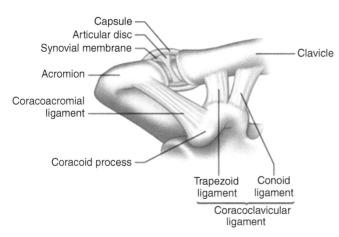

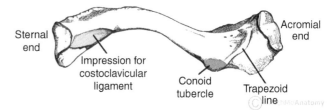

• **Fig. 12.2** Illustration highlighting the clavicular attachment sites of the trapezoid ligament *(trapezoid line)* and conoid ligament *(conoid tubercle)*. The trapezoid and conoid ligaments originate 2.5 and 4.6 cm from the lateral edge of the clavicle, respectively.

• **Fig. 12.1** Illustration highlighting the intra-articular structure of the acromioclavicular joint. The intra-articular disc typically adheres to the acromial side of the joint. (From https://musculoskeletalkey.com/the-acromioclavicular-joint/#CR24.)

result in pain, instability, and accelerated joint degeneration.[13] Additionally, as the clavicle functions as an anterior strut to support the scapula, AC joint instability may contribute to the development of scapular dyskinesis.[14–16]

Classification

The Rockwood classification remains the most widely used system guiding management of AC joint injuries.[17] First published in 1984, it expanded on the previous work of Cadenat, Tossy, and Allman.[18–21] It is a radiographic classification system that focuses on direction and extent of displacement at the level of the AC joint. The extent of vertical displacement is determined by measuring the CC distance of the injured extremity and comparing it with the presumably normal CC distance of the contralateral extremity. It is imperative that the assessed films be taken with the patient in the upright position as the extent of the ligamentous injury is inferred from the displacement induced by gravity upon the shoulder girdle.

Rockwood's six-part classification system can be thought of as a continuum of increasing injury severity (Fig. 12.3). A Type I injury involves a sprain of the AC joint without a complete tear of either the AC or CC ligament complexes; anteroposterior (AP) shoulder or Zanca view radiographs reveal no increase in CC distance. A Type II injury involves a complete tear of the AC ligament complex, but the CC ligament complex remains intact; radiographs reveal an increase in CC distance <25%. A Type III injury involves a complete tear of both the AC and CC ligament complexes; radiographs reveal an increase in CC distance between 25% and 100%. A Type IV injury involves posterior displacement of the lateral aspect of the clavicle. Radiographs may look relatively normal in the AP plane, but an axillary view will reveal posterior displacement of the lateral aspect of the clavicle in relation to the acromion. A Type V injury also involves a complete tear of both the AC and CC ligament complexes, but is significantly more displaced than a Type III injury. The distal clavicle is typically incarcerated in the DTF. Radiographs reveal an increase in CC distance in excess of 100%. A Type VI injury involves a complete tear of both the AC and CC ligament complexes accompanied by displacement of the lateral aspect of the clavicle inferior to the coracoid or acromion. This is an exceedingly rare injury.

Despite its widespread use, the Rockwood classification does have certain limitations; it has been criticized for being a purely

radiographic system attempting to infer and stratify a soft tissue injury.[17] In particular, the optimal management of Type III injuries remains a source of significant controversy.[11,17,22] In a recent consensus statement, The International Society of Arthroscopy, Knee Surgery and Orthopaedic Sports Medicine (ISAKOS) proposed subdividing Type III injuries into Type IIIA (stable) and Type IIIB (unstable) injuries. Type IIIB injuries are differentiated from Type IIIA injuries on the basis of functional criteria such as persistent pain, rotator cuff weakness, decreased flexion and abduction, scapular dyskinesis, and a positive cross-body adduction view (Basamania view).[17,23] They argue that this modified Rockwood classification may help with early identification of the subset of patients with Type III injuries who would benefit from early surgical management.

Clinical Evaluation

AC joint injuries are common and account for up to 9% of shoulder injuries.[24,25] Forty-four percent of these injuries occur in the third decade of life, and they are five times more common in men than in women.[24] Athletes are at increased risk compared with the general population, especially those participating in contact sports such as hockey, wrestling, rugby, and American football.[26,27] Falls onto the shoulder from cycling, skateboarding, skiing, and snowboarding are also common etiologies. Most acute injuries will be accompanied by pain, tenderness, and swelling of the AC joint. Patients typically present with the arm adducted and supported to alleviate the pain. They should be examined in a standing or sitting position as the weight of the extremity will allow full appreciation of the deformity (Fig. 12.4). High-grade injuries may be associated with significant deformity and skin tenting over the distal clavicle. Pain and tenderness along the trapezius muscle may also be observed in high-grade injuries due to soft-tissue injury and stripping of the DTF. Pain to palpation over the AC joint is typical. Cross-body abduction of the arm, which loads the AC joint, can create pain or instability of the distal clavicle.[28] A shrug test has also been described, which may help differentiate a Type III injury from a Type V injury.[1] If the patient is capable of reducing their AC joint with a shoulder shrug, this indicates an intact DTF and suggests a Type III injury. The scapulothoracic function should also be assessed when pain permits. Scapular dyskinesis may be observed in patients presenting with Type II–VI injuries and is often associated with ipsilateral prominence of the medial scapular border due to scapular internal rotation and/or anterior tilt.[17]

A thorough examination, including a neurovascular assessment, of the appendicular and axial skeleton should be performed to rule out associated injuries. In recent years, there has been increased awareness of concomitant intra-articular glenohumeral injuries.[29,30] These injuries occur in 15%–53% of patients presenting with high-grade (Types III–VI) AC joint injuries. Superior

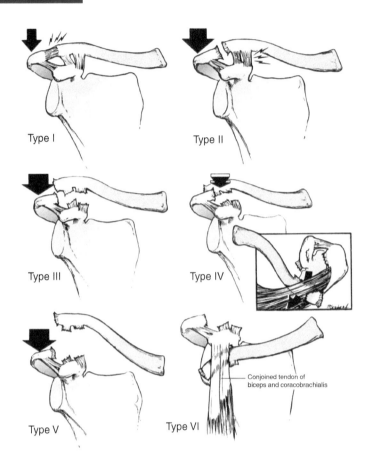

- **Type I**
  - minor sprain of the fibers of the AC ligaments

- **Type II**
  - distal end of the clavicle is unstable in the horizontal plane
  - widening of the AC joint. There may be a slight, relative upward displacement of the distal end of the clavicle

- **Type III**
  - 25% to 100% increase in the coracoclavicular space

- **Type IV**
  - clavicle is posteriorly displaced into or through the trapezius muscle

- **Type V**
  - coracoclavicular space is increased greater than 100%

- **Type VI**
  - Inferior dislocation of the distal clavicle

• **Fig. 12.3** Rockwood's classification system of acromioclavicular (AC) joint injuries.

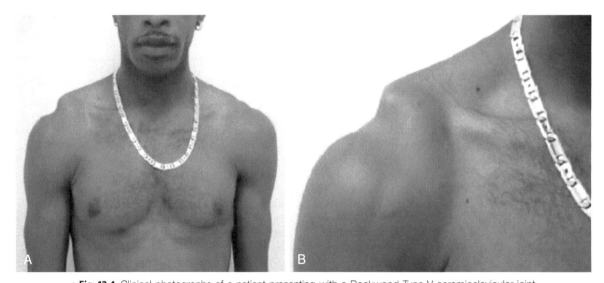

• **Fig. 12.4** Clinical photographs of a patient presenting with a Rockwood Type V acromioclavicular joint injury. (From Provencher MT, Leclere LE, Romeo A, Mazzocca A. Avoiding and managing complications of surgery of the acromioclavicular joint. In: Meislin RJ, Halbrecht J, eds. *Complications in Knee and Shoulder Surgery, Management and Treatment Options for the Sports Medicine Orthopedist.* Heidelberg, Germany: Springer Science + Business Media, LLC; 2009:245-264. https://doi.org/10.1007/978-1-84882-203-0_14.)

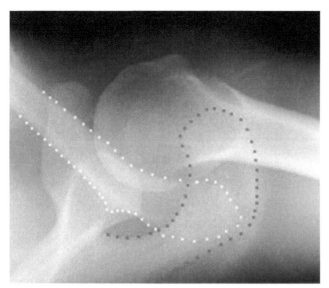

• **Fig. 12.5** Axillary radiograph of a left shoulder in a patient presenting with a Rockwood Type IV acromioclavicular joint injury. The lateral aspect of the clavicle *(white)* is displaced posteriorly in relation to the acromial facet of the acromioclavicular joint.

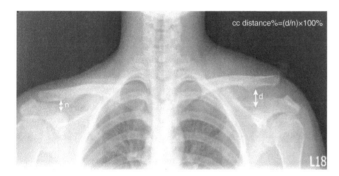

cc distance%=(d/n)×100%

• **Fig. 12.6** Measurement of coracoclavicular (*CC*) distance on a bilateral Zanca view in a patient presenting with a Rockwood Type V injury.

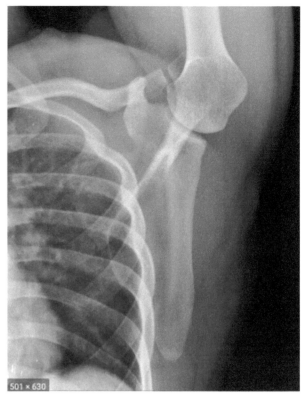

• **Fig. 12.7** The Stryker notch view provides an excellent view of the coracoid and may be considered to diagnose a coracoid fracture in the setting of a normal coracoclavicular distance despite a complete acromioclavicular joint dislocation.

labrum from anterior to posterior (SLAP) tears and rotator cuff tears were among the most commonly identified lesions.[30–32] While SLAP tears and rotator cuff tears are common findings in an asymptomatic population and the exact connection to the AC joint injury remains unclear, at least one group, Jensen et al., felt that 12% of their patients had concomitant glenohumeral pathology requiring surgical intervention. Factors that increase the likelihood of concomitant glenohumeral pathology include advanced age, chronicity, and high-grade injury (especially Type V).[30,32]

Radiographic Evaluation

Radiographs are the initial imaging modality of choice and should include a standard shoulder series (AP, scapula Y, axillary). Particular attention should be paid to the axillary view to rule out posterior displacement of the clavicle (Type IV injury) (Fig. 12.5). A Zanca view should also be obtained as it provides the most accurate radiographic assessment of the AC joint. The X-ray beam is directed with a 10- to 15-degree cephalic tilt and penetration strength is decreased by half compared with a standard AP shoulder radiograph to avoid overexposure of the AC joint.[33] A bilateral Zanca view allows visualization of both AC joints on a single X-ray cassette. Displacement is assessed by measuring the ipsilateral CC distance and comparing it with the CC distance on the uninjured contralateral side on upright films (Fig.

12.6). A side-to-side difference >25% signifies a complete disruption of both the AC and CC ligament complexes.[34] For reference, the normal CC distance ranges from 1.1 to 1.3 cm.[35] The Stryker notch view is taken with the patient supine and the X-ray cassette beneath the affected shoulder (Fig. 12.7).[36] The palm of the affected arm is placed on the superior aspect of the head, with forward flexion of the shoulder just beyond 90 degrees and slight internal rotation. The X-ray tube is tilted 10 degrees cranially and centered over the coracoid process. The Stryker notch view provides an excellent view of the coracoid and may be considered to diagnose a coracoid fracture in the setting of a normal CC distance despite a complete AC joint dislocation.[17]

Two additional views, the Alexander view and the Basamania view, characterize overlap of the distal clavicle in relation to the acromion in cross-body adduction and scapula internal rotation. Identification of overlap on these stress views suggests clinically relevant instability of the AC joint. The Alexander view is taken with the patient standing. The affected shoulder is shrugged forward, and the arm is adducted across the chest with the hand placed in the contralateral axilla. The affected shoulder is pressed against the X-ray cassette, with the uninjured shoulder creating an angle of 30–35 degrees with the cassette. The X-ray tube is angled 15 degrees caudad and the beam is directed at the coracoid.[37,38] A similar view, known as the cross-body adduction (Basamania) view, described by Garrigues et al., is an AP view of the AC joint obtained with the patient standing against the X-ray cassette. The arm is adducted across the chest, with the shoulder flexed to 90 degrees.[23] In a recent consensus statement, the ISAKOS has recommended obtaining a cross-body adduction (Basamania or Alexander) stress view to differentiate between stable (Type IIIA) and unstable (Type IIIB) injuries; instability is confirmed if the clavicle overlaps the acromion on this projection (Fig. 12.8).[17]

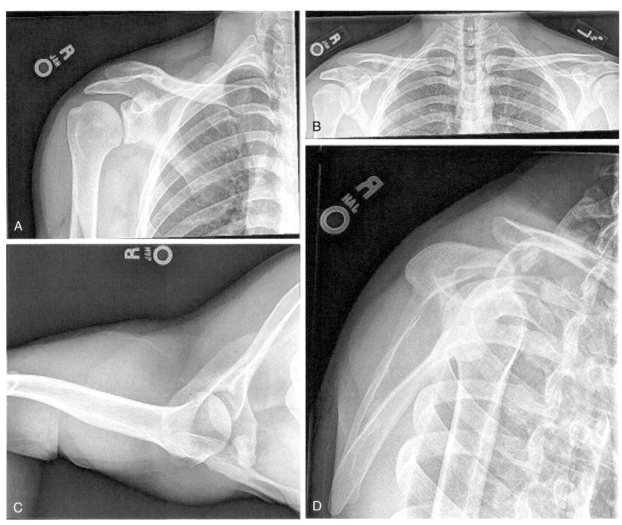

• **Fig. 12.8** The four projections recommended by the International Society of Arthroscopy, Knee Surgery and Orthopaedic Sports Medicine (ISAKOS) Upper Extremity Committee in a patient presenting with a chronic modified Rockwood Type IIIB injury: (A) true anteroposterior, (B) Zanca, (C) axillary, and (D) cross-body adduction (Basamania) views. (From Garrigues GE, Lewis, GC, Gupta AK, et al. The cortical ring sign: clinical results of percutaneous coracoclavicular fixation. *Shoulder and Elbow.* 2011;3(2):88-94.)

The cortical ring sign, described by Garrigues et al., is a useful view that can be obtained intraoperatively to assist in targeting the base of the coracoid for devices that include fixation into the coracoid base including the Bosworth screw, suture anchors, or as an augment to arthroscopically assisted "button" devices such as the TightRope (Arthrex, Naples, FL, USA) or ENDOBUTTON (Smith & Nephew, Memphis, TN, USA).[23,39] The fluoroscopic C-arm is arched over the shoulder and centered on the coracoid in a slight anterolateral to posteromedial direction until the coracoid base is visualized as a ring, which represents the cortical ring sign (Fig. 12.9). Specifically, the X-ray beam should be perpendicular to the medial border of the scapula in the parasagittal plane and approximately 45 degrees off the axis of the scapular spine in the axial plane. While a superiorly directed force is applied to the arm by an assistant to reduce the AC joint, the primary surgeon can confidently drill the fixation trajectory into the center of the cortical ring under fluoroscopic guidance, thus maximizing fixation within the coracoid base, using a uniplanar view.

Weighted stress radiographs have previously been described in the literature, but they are not routinely performed in the acute setting as they are painful and rarely influence management.[11,40] The role of magnetic resonance imaging (MRI) in the management of acute AC joint injuries remains undefined at this time. However, given the high incidence of concomitant intra-articular glenohumeral pathology associated with high-grade injuries, some authors have proposed that obtaining a preoperative MRI may assist in preoperative planning.[31,32]

Management of Acute Acromioclavicular Joint Injuries

Low-Grade Injuries (Rockwood Types I–II)

The management of acute AC joint injuries remains a topic of intense debate within the orthopedic community.[11,22,41] However, most authors agree that acute low-grade (Rockwood Types I–II) injuries should be treated nonoperatively.[11,22,24,42,43] In a study of 134 patients with Types I–II injuries, Park et al. noted that symptoms typically resolved within 6 weeks.[44] Although nonoperative treatment remains the standard of care for Types I–II injuries, Mikek reported that approximately half of the patients still experience some degree of pain and dysfunction at a mean of 10 years following the injury.[45] Similarly, Mouhsine et al. determined

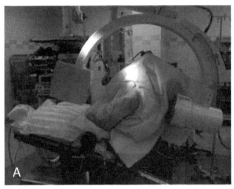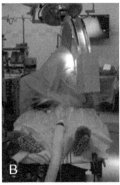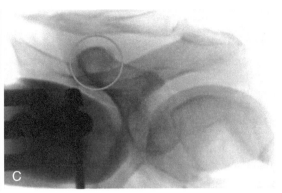

• **Fig. 12.9** Cortical ring sign: The C-arm is arched over the shoulder and centered on the coracoid in a slight anterolateral to posteromedial direction (A and B) until the coracoid base is fluoroscopically visualized as a ring (*circled*) (C). (From Garrigues GE, Marchant Jr MH, Lewis GC, Gupta AK, Richard MJ, Basamania CJ. The cortical ring sign: a reliable radiographic landmark for percutaneous coracoclavicular fixation. *J Shoulder Elbow Surg.* 2010;19(1):121-129.)

that one-third of patients with low-grade injuries treated nonoperatively complain of persistent pain and instability at long-term follow-up.[46] The severity of symptoms does not correlate with the degree of radiographic displacement.[45] Thus the long-term disability associated with Types I–II injuries may be underappreciated at this time.

High-Grade Injuries (Rockwood Types III–VI)

Acute high-grade injuries, particularly Type III injuries, have been the focus of the ongoing debate due to a lack of high-level evidence guiding management of Types III–VI injuries.[17,41,47,48] A recent Cochrane Review by Tamaoki et al. concluded that there was insufficient evidence to determine the relative effects of operative versus nonoperative treatment of high-grade AC joint injuries.[41] Only three studies, published between 1975 and 1989, met the authors' inclusion criteria. Furthermore, these studies included surgical techniques such as CC screw and K-wire fixation that are no longer commonly performed today due to their high complication rates.[41] Numerous recent systematic reviews and meta-analyses have echoed the Cochrane Review's findings.[11,22,49]

In comparison, the randomized controlled trial published in 2015 by the Canadian Orthopaedic Trauma Society (COTS), which was not included in the Cochrane Review, has been much more impactful. They reported no clinically significant differences between nonoperative and operative management of acute (<4 weeks) high-grade (Types III, IV, and V) AC joint injuries at 2-year follow-up.[48] All patients randomized to operative management were treated using hook plate fixation. Return to work was quicker and outcome scores were greater at 6 weeks, 3 months, and 6 months in the nonoperative group. However, the superiority of nonoperative treatment was not sustained beyond this time point, with no difference identified at the 1- and 2-year follow-up. Although the COTS trial supports initial nonoperative management of Type III–V injuries, the authors' failure to report the percentage of Type III, IV, and V injuries included in the study significantly affects our ability to interpret the results. Including a disproportionate number of Type III injuries within the study, which may be more amenable to nonoperative treatment, could potentially skew the results and lead to a Type II error.

Nevertheless, the results of the COTS trial are supported by a randomized controlled trial published by Larsen et al. in 1986.[50] They concluded that nonoperative treatment of acute high-grade AC joint injuries resulted in faster rehabilitation than operative

treatment (K-wire fixation), but that clinical outcomes were equivalent at 13 months.

Murray et al. recently published the results of the ACORN trial, a prospective randomized controlled trial comparing operative versus nonoperative treatment of acute (<2 weeks) Type III and IV injuries in young patients (16–35 years old).[51] Patients randomized to operative management were treated with loop suspensory fixation (LSF) using a double TightRope (Arthrex) technique. The results of their study also mirror those of the COTS trial; they found no significant difference in outcomes between operative and nonoperative treatment after a minimum 1-year follow-up, despite a faster initial recovery in the nonoperative group. Five patients from the nonoperative group required operative intervention due to persistent disability or cosmetic concerns, but the authors were unable to identify patient or injury-related factors that predicted a poor outcome with nonoperative treatment.

A prospective randomized controlled trial by Joukainen et al. informs on the long-term outcomes of AC joint injuries.[52] They reported no difference in clinical outcome scores between operative and nonoperative treatment of Type III and V injuries at long-term follow-up of 18–20 years. Although they noted increased deformity and instability in the nonoperative group, there was no difference in the prevalence of AC joint degeneration at long-term follow-up. Results of this study should be interpreted with caution considering that operative treatment involved direct ligamentous repair and temporary transarticular K-wire fixation, which is a technique that has largely been abandoned due to a high complication rate.

Although the literature seems to support nonoperative treatment of most high-grade AC joint injuries, a subset of patients with these injuries will fail nonoperative treatment and require surgical intervention. This is of particular concern as delayed AC joint reconstruction following a failed trial of nonoperative treatment yields inferior results compared with acute AC joint reconstruction.[53–55] However, nonoperative treatment of AC joint injuries provides good-to-excellent outcomes in most cases, and these studies should not be interpreted as a justification to pursue widespread operative management.[56,57] Thus the challenge is to identify the subset of patients who may benefit from early operative treatment.

Rockwood Type III Injuries

The optimal management of Rockwood Type III remains a source of controversy. Results following nonoperative treatment of these injuries have been mixed, with some authors reporting good or excellent outcomes, while others report persistent disability.[43,53,56–62] Schlegel et al. prospectively studied the natural history of Type III injuries.[60] At 1 year, 4 of 20 patients judged their outcome as suboptimal, although only 1 patient felt their current functional status warranted surgical management. Objective assessment revealed no significant difference in range of motion, military press, or rotational shoulder strength compared to the contralateral extremity. However, the authors did note a significant decrease (17%) in bench press strength. The authors concluded that initial nonoperative management of Type III injuries is appropriate for most patients, but that competitive weightlifters and manual laborers may benefit from early surgical management. Similarly, Dias et al. reported good or excellent outcomes following nonoperative management of Type III injuries in 43 of 44 patients at 5-year follow-up.[63] However, 55% of patients reported mild persistent AC joint symptoms. Overall, the literature suggests that most patients presenting with a Type III injury can be successfully treated with nonoperative management, but that a minority of patients will experience suboptimal outcomes. As a result, numerous authors have explored the role of surgical management in the setting of Type III injuries in an attempt to determine which patients may benefit from early surgical management.

A small retrospective study published by Gstettner et al. is one of the few studies that both include a control group and support operative management of Type III injuries.[64] They reported significantly improved Constant scores (90.4 vs. 80.7) following surgical treatment of acute Rockwood Type III using hook plate fixation compared with nonoperative treatment. However, there was no significant difference between groups in the Oxford or Simple shoulder scores. Based on the improvement in Constant scores, the authors recommended operative treatment of acute Rockwood Type III injuries, especially in young and active patients.

In contrast to the findings above reported by Gstettner et al., a preponderance of evidence within the literature supports initial nonoperative management of Type III injuries.[11,22,41,48–52,57–60,65–74] In a systematic review specifically comparing operative versus nonoperative management of Type III injuries, Smith et al. identified no significant difference in postintervention strength, pain, throwing ability, or incidence of AC joint arthritis.[72] Although operative management was associated with a better cosmetic outcome, it also resulted in a slower return to work. In another recent systematic review, Beitzel et al. also recommended initial nonoperative management for all Type III injuries.[73]

Despite the evidence supporting initial nonoperative management of Type III injuries, some authors have proposed early surgical management for overhead throwing athletes and young patients with higher functional demands, although these recommendations are often based on anecdotal experience.[43,63,64,75–77] In contrast, McFarland et al. surveyed Major League Baseball team physicians and found that 69% of respondents favored initial nonoperative management of Type III injuries.[71] They reported that 16 of 20 professional pitchers were successfully treated nonoperatively and displayed normal pain-free function. In comparison, 11 of 12 professional pitchers displayed normal pain-free function following early operative management. Similarly, Schlegel et al. reported acceptable outcomes following nonoperative management of Type III injuries in a small retrospective study of 15 NFL quarterbacks.[78] In light of these findings, Trainer et al. recommended initial nonoperative treatment of all Type III injuries, including overhead throwing athletes and those with higher functional demands.[74] However, they did recognize that additional factors may influence treatment decisions, including timing of the injury relative to the athletic season. In their opinion, early operative management may

be considered for Type III injuries occurring near the end of the athletic season or the beginning of the off-season, which provides additional time to recover from surgical treatment.

Despite the ongoing controversy regarding Type III injuries, the lack of high-level evidence clearly supporting early operative treatment of these injuries appears to be influencing community practice. In 2007 Nissen and Chatterjee reported that 81% of surgeons associated with the American Orthopaedic Society for Sports Medicine preferred nonoperative treatment for acute Type III injuries.[69]

Rockwood Type IV Injuries

Type IV injuries are relatively rare and management of these injuries has been guided by small case series or case reports.[11,79–82] Posterior displacement of the clavicle may lead to incarceration of the distal clavicle in the DTF, which often requires open reduction. Most authors have recommended early surgical management based on the available level IV and V evidence.[11,22,83]

Rockwood Type V Injuries

Type V injuries are typically treated with early surgical management, although little evidence exists to support this practice.[22] Several recent studies evaluating high-grade AC joint injuries (including Type V injuries) have consistently reported no significant difference in outcomes between operative and nonoperative treatment of these injuries.[41,48,52] However, the results of these studies must be interpreted with caution as they group Type III injuries, which may be more amenable to nonoperative treatment, along with Type V injuries. In one of the few studies assessing the effectiveness of nonsurgical management exclusively in Type V injuries, Dunphy et al. described their experience in a recent retrospective review of 22 patients.[84] At a mean of 34 months post injury, very few patients were found to have a normal DASH (Disability of the Arm, Shoulder and Hand) score (23%) or ASES (American Shoulder and Elbow Surgeons) score (9%). However, age <40 years at the time of injury was predictive of better functional outcomes with nonoperative treatment. The authors were unable to make a recommendation for or against nonoperative treatment of Type V injuries based on the results of their study. Thus the optimal management of Type V injuries has also become increasingly controversial with some authors calling for an initial trial of nonoperative treatment, while others continue to recommend early surgical management.[11,22,83]

Rockwood Type VI Injuries

Type VI injuries are exceedingly rare. Accordingly, management of these injuries has been guided by case reports and expert opinion.[85–90] Type VI injuries are often associated with high-energy trauma and may present with concomitant acromion, clavicle, scapula, and/or rib fractures.[86,88] Neurologic injury, including brachial plexus injury, has been reported in the literature, but these injuries are typically transient and resolve following reduction of the AC joint.[86,90] Based on the available evidence and expert opinion, early operative treatment is typically recommended for Type VI injuries.

Recommendations: High-Grade (Types III–VI) Injuries

Despite the lack of high-level evidence guiding management, Li et al. recommend an initial trial of nonoperative treatment for Type III injuries of 3–4 months, and early operative intervention for Type IV–VI injuries.[11] Relative indications for surgical management of Type III injuries include persistent pain despite a trial of nonoperative treatment, significant AC deformity, tenting of the skin, and high-demand patients.[11] Alternatively, Cook et al. recommend a 3- to 6-month trial of nonoperative treatment for Type III injuries, as well as Type V injuries with < 2 cm of displacement and a negative Basamania view.[22] They recommend early surgical intervention for open injuries, Type IV injuries, Type VI injuries, and Type V injuries with >2 cm of displacement or a positive Basamania view in a high-demand patient.

In summary, the indications for surgical intervention of high-grade AC joint injuries remain a highly controversial topic and well-designed randomized controlled trials are required to provide further guidance.

Management of Chronic Acromioclavicular Joint Injuries

Chronic AC joint injuries are typically associated with delayed presentation or a failed trial of nonoperative management. The definition of a chronic AC joint injury varies within the literature, with most authors differentiating a chronic injury from an acute injury after 3–6 weeks.[29,53,91,92] Historically, there has been a fundamental difference in the approach toward acute versus chronic injuries. In the acute setting, surgical techniques aim to maintain reduction of the AC joint to promote healing of the native AC and CC ligaments. In the chronic setting, the native AC and CC ligaments are presumed to lack this healing potential, and most surgical techniques aim to provide biological or synthetic augmentation in addition to maintenance of reduction.[93]

Borbas et al. performed a systematic review including 590 patients with high-grade (Rockwood III–VI) injuries undergoing chronic AC joint reconstruction (>6 weeks).[94] Interestingly, they found no significant difference in secondary loss of reduction or overall complication rate between nonbiologic fixation, biologic reconstruction of the CC ligaments using allograft or autograft, or ligament/tendon transfer techniques.[94]

Despite the heterogeneity of surgical techniques, satisfactory outcomes following operative management of chronic AC joint injuries have been reported in 76%–93% of patients.[54,95,96] However, compared with acute injuries, several studies suggest inferior outcomes in the chronic setting.[53,54,97] Specifically, secondary loss of reduction remains significantly higher in chronic AC joint reconstruction.[94] Of note, chronic AC joint injuries are also more likely to present with concomitant intra-articular glenohumeral pathology and scapular dyskinesis compared with acute injuries, which may negatively affect reported outcomes.[30,98]

Distal clavicle excision, also known as the Mumford procedure, may also be considered as an alternative to AC joint reconstruction for symptomatic, low-grade, chronic AC joint injuries.[93] This procedure is typically reserved for patients presenting with chronic Type I and II injuries, as they are more likely to develop posttraumatic degeneration of the AC joint compared with patients with high-grade injuries. In addition, the concern for destabilizing a previously injured AC joint is minimal as the CC ligaments are intact in these low-grade injuries. Good outcomes have been reported in 100% of patients following distal clavicle excision, with 75% of patients reporting excellent results.[99] A maximum resection of 8–10 mm is recommended to prevent disruption of a significant portion of the trapezoid ligament.[93] Ultimately, further research is required to clarify optimal management of chronic AC joint injuries as the current literature is dominated by level IV evidence.

Treatment Options

Nonoperative Treatment

Although numerous approaches to nonoperative treatment have been proposed, this typically involves a brief period (3–7 days) of immobilization, ice, analgesia, and anti-inflammatory medication followed by physical therapy to oversee the recovery of strength and range of motion.[11,41] High-grade injuries may require a longer duration of immobilization, often approaching 3–4 weeks.[83] Contact sports should be avoided until the patient has symmetric strength and range of motion; return to full activity may take up to 3 months.

Numerous methods of immobilization have been proposed in the literature including adhesive strapping, slings, bandages, braces, traction, pressure dressings, and plaster casts.[43,50,100,101] Notably, although the figure-of-eight brace may promote scapular retraction, it has recently fallen out of favor due to its association with higher pain scores and poor patient tolerance compared to a simple sling in the setting of clavicle fracture.[42,102] Transient brachial plexus injury has also been described as a result of incorrect application of the figure-of-eight brace.[103] The Kenny Howard brace combines a sling with an additional strap over the distal clavicle that provides a downward force in an attempt to maintain reduction of the AC joint. Due to poor patient tolerance and the risk of skin breakdown beneath the strap, the Kenny Howard brace has also fallen out of favor and become mostly of historical interest.[104] In contrast, immobilization with a simple sling has become the standard of care for nonoperative treatment of AC joint injuries due to its comfort and ease of use.

Operative Treatment

Over 60 different surgical techniques have been described to treat AC joint injuries, some have said more than any other orthopedic malady, but none has been identified as clearly superior.[83] In the acute setting, both reparative and reconstructive techniques have been described. The goal of reparative techniques is to maintain reduction of the AC joint to promote healing of the native AC and CC ligaments. Reconstructive techniques, however, aim to provide biological or synthetic augmentation as well as maintain reduction of the AC joint. Reconstructive techniques do not depend on successful healing of the native AC and CC ligaments.[93]

Acromioclavicular Joint Reduction and Internal Fixation

The goal of AC joint reduction and internal fixation is to obtain and maintain anatomic reduction of the AC joint to promote healing of the native AC and CC ligaments. These techniques are typically reserved for acute AC joint injuries, as the native AC and CC ligaments are presumed to lack this healing potential in the chronic setting—perhaps as soon as 2–3 weeks out from injury.[93] Historically, fixation methods have included primary transarticular fixation of the AC joint using smooth or threaded K-wires. K-wire fixation has been abandoned due to the rare, but catastrophic complications associated with wire migration; case reports have described pin migration to the spinal canal, heart, lungs, and great vessels.[105,106] Transarticular fixation has also been shown to increase the rate of posttraumatic AC joint arthrosis.[107]

CC screw fixation was first described by Bosworth in 1941 (Fig. 12.10).[108] This procedure was initially described as an

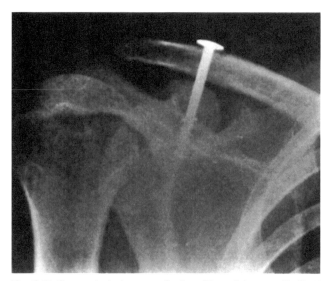

• **Fig. 12.10** Coracoclavicular screw fixation. (From Johansen JA, Grutter PW, McFarland, EG, Petersen SA. Acromioclavicular joint injuries: indications for treatment and treatment options. *J Shoulder Elbow Surg.* 2011; 20(2): S70-S82.)

inpatient procedure performed in the operating theater, but was subsequently modified to an outpatient procedure performed under local anesthesia. With the patient in a seated position, the surgeon positioned himself behind the patient to drill and insert the screw through a minimally invasive or percutaneous approach. The medial and lateral borders of the coracoid were palpated with the drill bit to determine the path to the coracoid base, but given the risk of fracture, no attempt was made to drill the coracoid prior to screw insertion. Bosworth recommended a screw with a wide-flanged thread of minimal pitch and a broad, flat head.[109] In most patients, a 1.5-inch screw was of appropriate length to obtain bicortical fixation within the coracoid and maintain AC joint reduction. Despite fluoroscopic guidance, accurately targeting the base of the coracoid proved to be challenging due to the shape of the coracoid, which curves in two planes, and likely contributed to failure rates as high as 32%.[110] However, the use of the cortical ring sign, as previously described, significantly improves accurate fluoroscopic targeting of the coracoid base and may lead to improved outcomes. Regardless, the high failure rates reported in the literature and obligatory screw removal decreased the popularity of this technique.[110,111] The screw and washer devices used for this procedure were pulled from the market due to low sales and this technique has now become of historical interest.

Hook plate fixation (DePuy-Synthes, Warsaw, IN, USA) has become a popular adjunct in the treatment of AC joint injuries as the architecture of the plate makes it a powerful reduction tool and provides a rigid construct to maintain reduction (Fig. 12.11). This technique involves open reduction of the AC joint and subsequent fixation using a uniquely designed plate. The hook-shaped lateral aspect of the plate is inserted directly posterior to the AC joint into the subacromial space and the medial aspect of the plate is affixed to the superior aspect of the distal clavicle with screws to maintain reduction of the AC joint. Of note, hook plates are available with varying hook depths to match patient anatomy. A detailed description of their use for AC joint injuries is presented in Chapter 10.

One of the major disadvantages of hook plate fixation remains the need to perform a secondary procedure for implant removal; this is typically performed between 2 and 6 months postoperatively. Timely removal of the implant is important, as Lin et al. identified the development of subacromial impingement syndrome in 37.5% of patients and acromial erosion in 50% at 2 months postoperatively.[112] Complications specifically associated with hook plate fixation include plate pull-off from the lateral aspect of the clavicle and acromial erosion. These complications are typically a result of over-reduction of the AC joint, often due to incorrect subacromial insertion of the hook or inappropriate hook depth of the implant.[48] Specifically, selecting a hook plate with insufficient hook depth will lead to over-reduction of the AC joint. Over-reduction is a technical error and is the most common cause of mechanical failure.[48] Obtaining an intraoperative radiograph to confirm satisfactory reduction may help prevent this complication.[48]

Recent biomechanical studies support the use of hook plate fixation as it closely replicates native AC joint stability.[113] Clinical studies have reported reliably good outcomes, but with sobering complication rates.[64,97] In their landmark study, the COTS reported a 35% complication rate within the operative group randomized to acute hook plate fixation.[48] Major complications included plate loosening, acromial erosion, clavicle fracture, frozen shoulder, and deep infection. Minor complications included superficial wound infection and peri-incisional numbness. However, the mean time to plate removal was 8.2 months, and 21% of patients did not undergo plate removal during the study period, which may have contributed to the high complication rate.

First described by Struhl in 2007, LSF techniques were developed in an effort to address the previously described shortcomings of hook plate fixation.[114] Since then, various LSF techniques have been described including coracoid loop, single-bundle, and double-bundle techniques (Fig. 12.12).[115–118] Double-bundle techniques attempt to recreate the anatomic relationships of the conoid and trapezoid ligaments and have been shown to most closely replicate native stiffness compared with single-bundle and coracoid loops techniques.[119] Although most LSF techniques are capable of restoring vertical stability, double-bundle techniques provide improved rotational and horizontal stability compared with single-bundle and coracoid loop techniques due to an increased number of fixation points.[119–122] Commonly used LSF devices include the TightRope (Arthrex) and the ENDOBUTTON (Smith & Nephew, Andover, MA, USA).

LSF techniques have been shown to be safe and provide a predictably good outcome.[123] Loss of reduction is the most common complication following these techniques and ranges from 16.6% to 50%.[124–126] Other complications of LSF include suspensory button pull-out, as well as coracoid and clavicle fracture.[124,126,127] Meticulous surgical technique may decrease the risk of these complications as they are frequently secondary to tunnel malposition.[128] Additionally, one-third of patients report hardware irritation following LSF techniques, but unlike hook plate fixation, a secondary procedure for hardware removal is rarely required.[123] A recent meta-analysis comparing LSF with hook plate fixation suggests that LSF may improve shoulder function and decrease postoperative pain scores, but is associated with a higher complication rate.[129] LSF techniques can be performed via an open approach, or more commonly, via an arthroscopic-assisted approach. Notably, arthroscopic techniques facilitate the diagnosis and management of concomitant glenohumeral pathology.[130]

In 2011 Scheibel et al. described an arthroscopically-assisted double TightRope technique.[116] However, they noted persistent posterior instability of the AC joint in nearly half of patients, which significantly affected outcomes. Subsequently, they modified their technique to

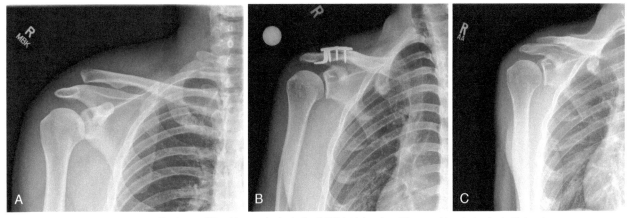

• **Fig. 12.11** Acute Rockwood Type V acromioclavicular (AC) joint injury in a 29-year-old male treated with hook plate fixation. (A) Preoperative anteroposterior view revealing >100% displacement of the AC joint. (B) Immediate postoperative Grashey view demonstrating hook plate fixation with satisfactory reduction of the AC joint. (C) Grashey view demonstrating plate removal at 4 months with mild loss of reduction of the AC joint.

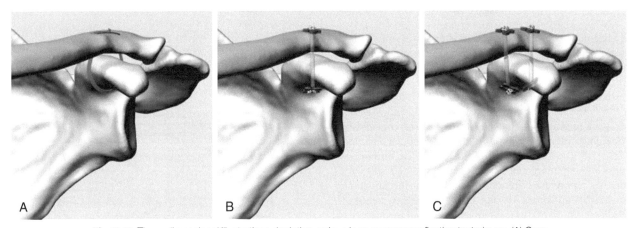

• **Fig. 12.12** Three-dimensional illustrations depicting various loop suspensory fixation techniques. (A) Coracoid loop, (B) single bundle, and (C) double bundle.

include a nonabsorbable AC cerclage tape to provide horizontal stability to their construct.[131] In their series of 34 patients, they reported good-to-excellent outcomes and a significantly decreased incidence of posterior instability compared with their original technique. They reported a revision rate of 11.7% due to hardware irritation, recurrent instability, and surgical site infection. A detailed description of their use for AC joint injuries is presented in Chapter 13.

Acromioclavicular Joint Reconstruction

AC joint reconstruction is an appropriate treatment for both acute and chronic high-grade AC joint injuries. AC joint reconstruction techniques can be classified as anatomic versus nonanatomic. Nonanatomic techniques do not seek to recreate native AC and CC ligament anatomy, but simply seek to provide biologic or synthetic augmentation and maintenance of reduction.

Nonanatomic Reconstruction

Described in 1972, the Weaver-Dunn procedure is a classic non-anatomic technique that involves distal clavicle excision and transposition of the coracoacromial (CA) ligament off the acromion into the intramedullary canal of the distal clavicle.[132] The native ligament still originates from the coracoid. However, the resulting

construct has been shown to be biomechanically inferior to the native CC ligament complex, and failure rates as high as 30% have been reported in the literature.[54,133] Therefore several modifications to the Weaver-Dunn procedure have been published over the years, all of which have the common goal of enhancing primary stability of the construct until ligamentous healing has been achieved. Modifications include enhanced CC fixation using subcoracoid suture loops, suture anchors, and tendon grafts.[134,135] These augmented CA ligament transfer techniques have shown biomechanical superiority over the original Weaver-Dunn procedure.

In 2019 Boileau et al. reported their short-term results of an all-arthroscopic modified Weaver-Dunn technique (Fig. 12.13).[29] In their series of 57 patients with chronic high-grade (Rockwood Types III–V) AC joint injuries, they noted a 95% satisfaction rate and a secondary loss of reduction in 12% of patients. The authors highlighted the ability to diagnose and treat concomitant intra-articular pathology as an advantage of their arthroscopic technique over previous open techniques.

Anatomic Reconstruction

There has been increased interest in anatomic reconstruction techniques in recent years as numerous biomechanical studies have demonstrated initial stability comparable to that of the native AC

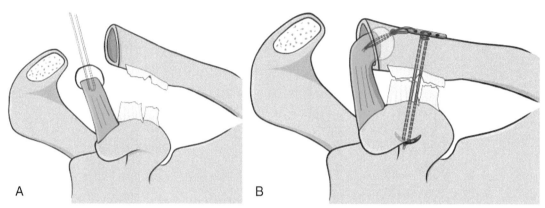

• **Fig. 12.13** All-arthroscopic modified Weaver-Dunn procedure described by Boileau et al. (A) The cora-coacromial ligament is harvested with the tip of the acromion and rerouted in the distal end of the clavicle after its distal resection and cavitation. (B) The coracoclavicular reduction is maintained with the help of two cortical buttons connected with four strands of tape to protect the transferred ligament for the period of bone healing; the lateral suture, attached to the clavicular button, is used to fix the tip of the acromion and coracoacromial ligament inside the clavicular socket.

and CC ligament complexes as well as superiority over nonana-tomic techniques.[136–139] Several open and arthroscopic techniques have been proposed in the literature; although they differ based on graft type, configuration, and fixation method, they all attempt to recreate the native functions of the AC and CC ligament com-plexes.[140–146] The technique described by Carofino and Mazzocca, which loops a semitendinosus allograft around the coracoid in a figure-of-eight fashion, remains one of the most popular techniques (Fig. 12.14).[141] The graft is docked into the clavicle through two bone tunnels using interference screw fixation. In their series of 17 patients, they reported a significant improvement in radiographic and functional outcomes despite three treatment failures.[141] A detailed description of this technique is presented in Chapter 14.

Malposition of clavicular and/or coracoid bone tunnels follow-ing anatomic reconstruction techniques can lead to early failure. Martetschlager et al. reported coracoid or clavicular fractures in up to 20% of cases following anatomic AC joint reconstruction, which significantly affected postoperative outcomes.[126] Numerous recommendations have been proposed to reduce this risk includ-ing preoperative templating, adequate spacing between bony tunnels, avoiding excessively lateral clavicular tunnels, and sub-stituting bony tunnels with loop fixation around the clavicle or coracoid.[22,126,147,148] Additionally, arthroscopic techniques may decrease the risk of coracoid and clavicular fracture compared with open techniques.[149]

Yoo et al. described an arthroscopically assisted technique using semitendinosus autograft, which attempts to replicate the native anatomy of the CC ligament complex.[142] The graft is passed through a coracoid bone tunnel and the ends are docked into two clavicular tunnels using interference screw fixation. In their series of 13 patients, they reported significant postoperative improve-ment in functional outcomes despite persistent displacement of the AC joint in all patients at final follow-up.

Tauber et al. also described an arthroscopically assisted recon-struction technique. Their triple-bundle technique involves recon-struction of the conoid, trapezoid, and superior AC ligament using a semitendinosus autograft and interference screw fixation.[150] Nonabsorbable suture tape fixation provides additional protection to the construct during the early postoperative period. In their series of 12 patients, they reported a significantly decreased (8% vs. 21%) rate of recurrent instability compared with single-bundle

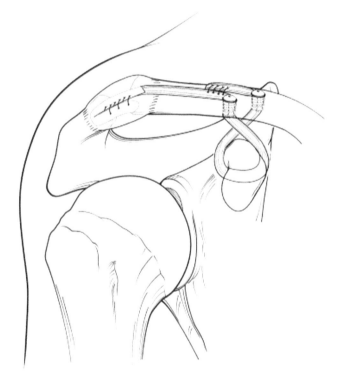

• **Fig. 12.14** Anatomic acromioclavicular (AC) joint reconstruction tech-nique described by Carofino and Mazzocca. The semitendinosus allograft is secured in bone tunnels with PEEK anchors, and the AC ligaments have been reconstructed with the remaining graft exiting the trapezoid tunnel.

reconstruction using the AC GraftRope (Arthrex) with a gracilis tendon. They reported no revisions, fractures, or infections.

Complications

Complications may occur following both operative and nonop-erative management of AC joint injuries, although nonoperative management is associated with a lower risk and severity of com-plications. Nonoperative treatment can be complicated by post-traumatic AC joint arthrosis, persistent pain and instability, and distal clavicle osteolysis.[24,151] Cosmetic deformity is also the norm following nonoperative treatment of high-grade AC joint injuries. Operative treatment carries additional surgical risks such as infection, neurovascular injury, clavicle and coracoid fractures, as well as the unique complication profile associated with the chosen surgical technique. The risk of secondary loss of reduction is also relatively high, regardless of the surgical technique.[22,123]

A recent systematic review by Woodmass et al. reported a superficial infection rate of 3.8% following arthroscopic AC joint reconstruction techniques, and no deep infections.[123] In comparison, open procedures such as hook plate fixation are associated with a total infection rate of 5%, which increases to 8% with the use of semitendinosus autograft.[47,152] The incidence of coracoid or clavicular fracture following arthroscopic techniques is 5.3%, with coracoid fracture being much more common than clavicular fracture.[123] Fracture was more commonly associated with techniques utilizing bony tunnels, although this complication can still occur following loop fixation techniques. The risk of fracture is comparable between open and arthroscopic techniques utilizing bony tunnels.[123]

Author's Preferred Approach

Although optimal management remains controversial, we believe that the highest level of evidence supports initial nonoperative treatment of the vast majority of AC joint injuries—including high-grade injuries. Routine imaging includes a standard shoulder series (AP, scapula Y, axillary) as well as a Zanca view. We do not obtain a cross-body adduction (Basamania) stress view as it does not alter initial management based on our current treatment algorithm. We do not routinely obtain a preoperative MRI unless we identify specific signs or symptoms suggestive of concomitant intra-articular pathology.

Relative indications for early surgical treatment include posteriorly displaced (Type IV) injuries, in which mechanical abutment of the distal clavicle against the scapular spine and acromion occurs with elevation. This causes pain and poor motion, which seldom improves with physical therapy. Type V injuries associated with significantly painful motion at the clavicle after 6 weeks of nonoperative treatment may be considered for operative intervention. Manual laborers with jobs that require significant overhead motion or strength are also considered for early intervention.

Nonoperative treatment consists of sling immobilization for 4–6 weeks. This allows the soft tissue envelope to become stable around the AC complex. Patients who remain significantly symptomatic at 3–6 months are deemed to have failed a trial of nonoperative treatment and are offered surgical treatment.

Our preferred surgical technique is a modification of the Weaver-Dunn-Chuinard technique.[153] The Weaver-Dunn-Chuinard procedure involves resecting the distal clavicle and transferring the CA ligament, along with a bone block from the anterior acromion, to the medullary canal of the distal clavicle. This results in bone-to-bone healing of the transferred ligament and may decrease the risk of ligament pull-out compared with the original Weaver-Dunn procedure, in which the ligament is transferred without a bony block. Our modification of the Weaver-Dunn-Chuinard technique involves synthetic augmentation with heavy nonabsorbable suture. Sutures are passed around the base of the coracoid and passed through a bicortical drill hole in the distal clavicle. This stabilizes the distal clavicle in the vertical and horizontal planes and protects the CA ligament transfer construct during the early postoperative period.

The operation is performed through an incision in Langer's lines just lateral to the AC joint. The DTF is split with needle-tip cautery down to the surface of the distal clavicle, across the injured AC joint, and onto the superior surface of the acromion. The deltoid is carefully elevated off the distal clavicle and CA ligament. An acromioplasty with an osteotome is performed to harvest the ligament. The bone typically needs to be debulked to fit into the distal clavicle's medullary canal. The CA ligament is exposed down to its origin off the coracoid. Heavy #2 nonabsorbable suture is run along both edges of the CA ligament in Krackow fashion, with the suture limbs exiting proximally.

The coracoid is identified and the interval tissue is released off the coracoid base. A curved vascular (Satinsky) clamp is passed around the coracoid to pass two #5 braided nylon sutures. A distal clavicle resection is performed removing 8–10 mm of bone and the intramedullary canal is opened.

A bicortical drill hole is placed through the clavicle approximately 1.5–2 cm from the edge of the resected distal clavicle. It should be at the midpoint of the bone from anterior to posterior. This allows maintenance of reduction in the horizontal and vertical planes. The lateral limbs of the augmentation (subcoracoid) sutures are brought up through the clavicular drill hole and tied sequentially while holding the clavicle reduced with an awl. Once these are tied, two drill holes are placed on the superior surface of the distal clavicle. The CA ligament sutures are passed through the intramedullary canal and up through the drill holes, reducing the CA ligament transfer into the clavicle. Once again, the distal clavicle is reduced with an awl, and the CA ligament sutures are tied over the superior clavicle surface with appropriate tension. The DTF, including the released portion of the anterior deltoid, and AC capsular remnant should be meticulously closed.

Postoperatively a sling is worn for 4 weeks. Pendulums are allowed at 2–3 weeks, but active motion is not instituted until 6 weeks. This technique is versatile for all types of distal clavicle instability patterns and for acute and chronic pathology.

Summary

AC joint injuries occur along a continuum of injury severity due to sequential failure of the AC and CC ligaments, which is reflected by Rockwood's classification system. A thorough physical examination should be performed at the time of presentation followed by appropriate radiographic imaging. MRI may also be considered to rule out concomitant intra-articular glenohumeral joint pathology for preoperative planning. The management of AC joint injuries remains a highly controversial topic. We recommend an initial trial of nonoperative treatment regardless of injury severity. However, individualized decision-making is essential as some patients may benefit from acute surgical management. Both reparative and reconstructive techniques have been described in the treatment of acute AC joint injuries. The goal of reparative techniques is to maintain reduction of the AC joint to promote healing of the native AC and CC ligaments. Reconstructive techniques aim to provide biological or synthetic augmentation as well as maintain reduction of the AC joint. In the chronic setting, reconstructive techniques are favored due to a presumed lack of healing potential of the native AC and CC ligaments. Numerous techniques have been proposed in the literature, most of which report satisfactory outcomes. However, no particular technique has been identified as clearly superior. Further research is required to determine the optimal management of acute and chronic AC joint injuries.

References

1. Saccomanno MF, De Ieso C, Milano G. Acromioclavicular joint instability: anatomy, biomechanics and evaluation. *Joints*. 2014;2(2):87–92.
2. DePalma AF, Callery G, Bennett GA. Variational anatomy and degenerative lesions of the shoulder joint. *AAOS Instructional Course Lectures*. 1949;6:255–281.
3. Stine IA, Vangsness Jr CT. Analysis of the capsule and ligament insertions about the acromioclavicular joint: a cadaveric study. *Arthroscopy*. 2009;25(9):968–974.
4. Salter Jr EG, Nasca RJ, Shelley BS. Anatomical observations on the acromioclavicular joint and supporting ligaments. *Am J Sports Med*. 1987;15(3):199–206.
5. Debski RE, Parsons IM, Woo SL-Y, Fu FH. Effect of capsular injury on acromioclavicular joint mechanics. *J Bone Joint Surg Am*. 2001;83(9):1344–1351.
6. Harris RI, Vu DH, Sonnabend DH, Goldberg JA, Walsh WR. Anatomic variance of the coracoclavicular ligaments. *J Shoulder Elbow Surg*. 2001;10(6):585–588.
7. Rios CG, Arciero RA, Mazzocca AD. Anatomy of the clavicle and coracoid process for reconstruction of the coracoclavicular ligaments. *Am J Sports Med*. 2007;35(5):811–817.
8. Salzmann GM, Paul J, Sandmann GH, Imhoff AB, Schottle PB. The coracoidal insertion of the coracoclavicular ligaments: an anatomic study. *Am J Sports Med*. 2008;36(12):2392–2397.
9. Sellards R. Anatomy and biomechanics of the acromioclavicular joint. *Oper Tech Sports Med*. 2004;12(1):2–5.
10. Pastor MF, Averbeck AK, Welke B, Smith T, Claassen L, Wellmann M. The biomechanical influence of the deltotrapezoid fascia on horizontal and vertical acromioclavicular joint stability. *Arch Orthop Trauma Surg*. 2016;136(4):513–519.
11. Li X, Ma R, Bedi A, Dines DM, Altchek DW, Dines JS. Management of acromioclavicular joint injuries. *J Bone Joint Surg Am*. 2014;96(1):73–84.
12. Bontempo NA, Mazzocca AD. Biomechanics and treatment of acromioclavicular and sternoclavicular joint injuries. *Br J Sports Med*. 2010;44(5):361–369.
13. Flatow EL. The biomechanics of the acromioclavicular, sternoclavicular, and scapulothoracic joints. *Instr Course Lect*. 1993;42:237–245.
14. Seo YJ, Yoo YS, Noh KC, et al. Dynamic function of coracoclavicular ligament at different shoulder abduction angles: a study using a 3-dimensional finite element model. *Arthroscopy*. 2012;28(6):778–787.
15. Izadpanah K, Weitzel E, Honal M, et al. In vivo analysis of coracoclavicular ligament kinematics during shoulder abduction. *Am J Sports Med*. 2012;40(1):185–192.
16. Ludewig PM, Phadke V, Braman JP, Hassett DR, Cieminski CJ, LaPrade RF. Motion of the shoulder complex during multiplanar humeral elevation. *J Bone Joint Surg Am*. 2009;91(2):378–389.
17. Beitzel K, Mazzocca AD, Bak K, et al. ISAKOS upper extremity committee consensus statement on the need for diversification of the Rockwood classification for acromioclavicular joint injuries. *Arthroscopy*. 2014;30(2):271–278.
18. Cadenat F. The treatment of dislocations and fractures of the outer end of the clavicle. *Int Clin*. 1917;1:145–169.
19. Tossy JD, Mead NC, Sigmond HM. Acromioclavicular separations: useful and practical classification for treatment. *Clin Orthop Relat Res*. 1963;28:111–119.
20. Rockwood CAJ. Injuries to the acromioclavicular joint: subluxations and dislocations about the shoulder. In: Rockwood CAJ, Green DP, eds. *Fractures in Adults*. Philadelphia: JB Lippincott; 1984:860–910.
21. Allman Jr FL. Fractures and ligamentous injuries of the clavicle and its articulation. *J Bone Joint Surg Am*. 1967;49(4):774–784.
22. Cook JB, Krul KP. Challenges in treating acromioclavicular separations: current concepts. *J Am Acad Orthop Surg*. 2018;26(19):669–677.
23. Garrigues GE, Lewis GC, Gupta AK, et al. The cortical ring sign: clinical results of percutaneous coracoclavicular fixation. *Shoulder Elbow*. 2011;3(2):88–94.
24. Mazzocca AD, Arciero RA, Bicos J. Evaluation and treatment of acromioclavicular joint injuries. *Am J Sports Med*. 2007;35(2):316–329.
25. Chillemi C, Franceschini V, Dei Giudici L, et al. Epidemiology of isolated acromioclavicular joint dislocation. *Emerg Med Int*. 2013;2013:171609.
26. Gorbaty JD, Hsu JE, Gee AO. Classifications in brief: Rockwood classification of acromioclavicular joint separations. *Clin Orthop Relat Res*. 2017;475(1):283–287.
27. Pallis M, Cameron KL, Svoboda SJ, Owens BD. Epidemiology of acromioclavicular joint injury in young athletes. *Am J Sports Med*. 2012;40(9):2072–2077.
28. Chronopoulos E, Kim TK, Park HB, Ashenbrenner D, McFarland EG. Diagnostic value of physical tests for isolated chronic acromioclavicular lesions. *Am J Sports Med*. 2004;32(3):655–661.
29. Boileau P, Gastaud O, Wilson A, Trojani C, Bronsard N. All-arthroscopic reconstruction of severe chronic acromioclavicular joint dislocations. *Arthroscopy*. 2019;35(5):1324–1335.
30. Jensen G, Millett PJ, Tahal DS, Al Ibadi M, Lill H, Katthagen JC. Concomitant glenohumeral pathologies associated with acute and chronic grade III and grade V acromioclavicular joint injuries. *Int Orthop*. 2017;41(8):1633–1640.
31. Tischer T, Salzmann GM, El-Azab H, Vogt S, Imhoff AB. Incidence of associated injuries with acute acromioclavicular joint dislocations types III through V. *Am J Sports Med*. 2009;37(1):136–139.
32. Pauly S, Gerhardt C, Haas NP, Scheibel M. Prevalence of concomitant intraarticular lesions in patients treated operatively for high-grade acromioclavicular joint separations. *Knee Surg Sports Traumatol Arthrosc*. 2009;17(5):513–517.
33. Zanca P. Shoulder pain: involvement of the acromioclavicular joint. (Analysis of 1,000 cases). *Am J Roentgenol Radium Ther Nucl Med*. 1971;112(3):493–506.
34. Rockwood CA, Young DC. Disorders of the acromioclavicular joint. In: Rockwood CA, Matsen FA, eds. *The Shoulder*. Philadelphia: WB Saunders; 1990:413–476.
35. Bearden JM, Hughston JC, Whatley GS. Acromioclavicular dislocation: method of treatment. *J Sports Med*. 1973;1(4):5–17.
36. Hall RH, Isaac F, Booth CR. Dislocations of the shoulder with special reference to accompanying small fractures. *J Bone Joint Surg Am*. 1959;41-A(3):489–494.
37. Alexander OM. Radiography of the acromioclavicular articulation. *Med Radiogr Photogr*. 1954;30(2):34–39.
38. Waldrop JI, Norwood LA, Alvarez RG. Lateral roentgenographic projections of the acromioclavicular joint. *Am J Sports Med*. 1981;9(5):337–341.
39. Garrigues GE, Marchant Jr MH, Lewis GC, Gupta AK, Richard MJ, Basamania CJ. The cortical ring sign: a reliable radiographic landmark for percutaneous coracoclavicular fixation. *J Shoulder Elbow Surg*. 2010;19(1):121–129.
40. Melenevsky Y, Yablon CM, Ramappa A, Hochman MG. Clavicle and acromioclavicular joint injuries: a review of imaging, treatment, and complications. *Skeletal Radiol*. 2011;40(7):831–842.
41. Tamaoki MJ, Lenza M, Matsunaga FT, Belloti JC, Matsumoto MH, Faloppa F. Surgical versus conservative interventions for treating acromioclavicular dislocation of the shoulder in adults. *Cochrane Database Syst Rev*. 2019;10:CD007429.
42. Cote MP, Wojcik KE, Gomlinski G, Mazzocca AD. Rehabilitation of acromioclavicular joint separations: operative and nonoperative considerations. *Clin Sports Med*. 2010;29(2):213–228 (vii).
43. Bannister GC, Wallace WA, Stableforth PG, Hutson MA. The management of acute acromioclavicular dislocation. A randomised prospective controlled trial. *J Bone Joint Surg Br*. 1989;71(5):848–850.

44. Park JP, Arnold JA, Coker TP, Harris WD, Becker DA. Treatment of acromioclavicular separations. A retrospective study. *Am J Sports Med.* 1980;8(4):251–256.

45. Mikek M. Long-term shoulder function after type I and II acromioclavicular joint disruption. *Am J Sports Med.* 2008;36(11):2147–2150.

46. Mouhsine E, Garofalo R, Crevoisier X, Farron A. Grade I and II acromioclavicular dislocations: results of conservative treatment. *J Shoulder Elbow Surg.* 2003;12(6):599–602.

47. Modi CS, Beazley J, Zywiel MG, Lawrence TM, Veillette CJ. Controversies relating to the management of acromioclavicular joint dislocations. *Bone Joint Lett J.* 2013;95-B(12):1595–1602.

48. Canadian Orthopaedic Trauma Society. Multicenter randomized clinical trial of nonoperative versus operative treatment of acute acromio-clavicular joint dislocation. *J Orthop Trauma.* 2015;29(11):479–487.

49. Chang N, Furey A, Kurdin A. Operative versus nonoperative management of acute high-grade acromioclavicular dislocations: a systematic review and meta-analysis. *J Orthop Trauma.* 2018;32(1):1–9.

50. Larsen E, Bjerg-Nielsen A, Christensen P. Conservative or surgical treatment of acromioclavicular dislocation. A prospective, controlled, randomized study. *J Bone Joint Surg Am.* 1986;68(4):552–555.

51. Murray IR, Robinson PG, Goudie EB, Duckworth AD, Clark K, Robinson CM. Open reduction and tunneled suspensory device fixation compared with nonoperative treatment for type-III and type-IV acromioclavicular joint dislocations: the ACORN prospective, randomized controlled trial. *J Bone Joint Surg Am.* 2018;100(22):1912–1918.

52. Joukainen A, Kroger H, Niemitukia L, Makela EA, Vaatainen U. Results of operative and nonoperative treatment of Rockwood types III and V acromioclavicular joint dislocation: a prospective, randomized trial with an 18- to 20-year follow-up. *Orthop J Sports Med.* 2014;2(12):1–9. https://doi.org/10.1177/2325967114560130.

53. Rolf O, Hann von Weyhern A, Ewers A, Boehm TD, Gohlke F. Acromioclavicular dislocation Rockwood III-V: results of early versus delayed surgical treatment. *Arch Orthop Trauma Surg.* 2008;128(10):1153–1157.

54. Weinstein DM, McCann PD, McIlveen SJ, Flatow EL, LU B. Surgical treatment of complete acromioclavicular dislocations. *Am J Sports Med.* 1995;23(3):324–331.

55. Liu HH, Chou YJ, Chen CH, Chia WT, Wong CY. Surgical treatment of acute acromioclavicular joint injuries using a modified Weaver-Dunn procedure and clavicular hook plate. *Orthopedics.* 2010;33(8).

56. Bjerneld H, Hovelius L, Thorling J. Acromio-clavicular separations treated conservatively. A 5-year follow-up study. *Acta Orthop Scand.* 1983;54(5):743–745.

57. Spencer Jr EE. Treatment of grade III acromioclavicular joint injuries: a systematic review. *Clin Orthop Relat Res.* 2007;455:38–44.

58. Taft TN, Wilson FC, Oglesby JW. Dislocation of the acromioclavicular joint. An end-result study. *J Bone Joint Surg Am.* 1987;69(7):1045–1051.

59. Calvo E, Lopez-Franco M, Arribas IM. Clinical and radiologic outcomes of surgical and conservative treatment of type III acromioclavicular joint injury. *J Shoulder Elbow Surg.* 2006;15(3):300–305.

60. Schlegel TF, Burks RT, Marcus RL, Dunn HK. A prospective evaluation of untreated acute grade III acromioclavicular separations. *Am J Sports Med.* 2001;29(6):699–703.

61. Hootman JM. Acromioclavicular dislocation: conservative or surgical therapy. *J Athl Train.* 2004;39(1):10–11.

62. Wojtys EM, Nelson G. Conservative treatment of Grade III acromioclavicular dislocations. *Clin Orthop Relat Res.* 1991;(268):112–119.

63. Dias JJ, Steingold RF, Richardson RA, Tesfayohannes B, Gregg PJ. The conservative treatment of acromioclavicular dislocation. Review after five years. *J Bone Joint Surg Br.* 1987;69(5):719–722.

64. Gstettner C, Tauber M, Hitzl W, Resch H. Rockwood type III acromioclavicular dislocation: surgical versus conservative treatment. *J Shoulder Elbow Surg.* 2008;17(2):220–225.

65. Galpin RD, Hawkins RJ, Grainger RW. A comparative analysis of operative versus nonoperative treatment of grade III acromioclavicular separations. *Clin Orthop Relat Res.* 1985;193:150–155.

66. Press J, Zuckerman JD, Gallagher M, Cuomo F. Treatment of grade III acromioclavicular separations. Operative versus nonoperative management. *Bull Hosp Jt Dis.* 1997;56(2):77–83.

67. Powers JA, Bach PJ. Acromioclavicular separations. Closed or open treatment? *Clin Orthop Relat Res.* 1974;104:213–223.

68. MacDonald PB, Alexander MJ, Frejuk J, Johnson GE. Comprehensive functional analysis of shoulders following complete acromioclavicular separation. *Am J Sports Med.* 1988;16(5):475–480.

69. Nissen CW, Chatterjee A. Type III acromioclavicular separation: results of a recent survey on its management. *Am J Orthop (Belle Mead NJ).* 2007;36(2):89–93.

70. Phillips AM, Smart C, Groom AF. Acromioclavicular dislocation. Conservative or surgical therapy. *Clin Orthop Relat Res.* 1998;353:10–17.

71. McFarland EG, Blivin SJ, Doehring CB, Curl LA, Silberstein C. Treatment of grade III acromioclavicular separations in professional throwing athletes: results of a survey. *Am J Orthop (Belle Mead NJ).* 1997;26(11):771–774.

72. Smith TO, Chester R, Pearse EO, Hing CB. Operative versus operative management following Rockwood grade III acromioclavicular separation: a meta-analysis of the current evidence base. *J Orthop Traumatol.* 2011;12(1):19–27.

73. Beitzel K, Cote MP, Apostolakos J, et al. Current concepts in the treatment of acromioclavicular joint dislocations. *Arthroscopy.* 2013;29(2):387–397.

74. Trainer G, Arciero RA, Mazzocca AD. Practical management of grade III acromioclavicular separations. *Clin J Sport Med.* 2008;18(2):162–166.

75. Ryhanen J, Niemela E, Kaarela O, Raatikainen T. Stabilization of acute, complete acromioclavicular joint dislocations with a new C hook implant. *J Shoulder Elbow Surg.* 2003;12(5):442–445.

76. Leidel BA, Braunstein V, Kirchhoff C, Pilotto S, Mutschler W, Biberthaler P. Consistency of long-term outcome of acute Rockwood grade III acromioclavicular joint separations after K-wire transfixation. *J Trauma.* 2009;66(6):1666–1671.

77. Lizaur A, Sanz-Reig J, Gonzalez-Parreno S. Long-term results of the surgical treatment of type III acromioclavicular dislocations: an update of a previous report. *J Bone Joint Surg Br.* 2011;93(8):1088–1092.

78. Schlegel TF, Boublik M, Hawkins RJ. Grade III acromioclavicular separations in NFL quarterbacks. In: *Paper Presented at: American Orthopaedic Society of Sports Medicine Annual Meeting; July.* Keystone, CO; 2005:14–17.

79. Malcapi C, Grassi G, Oretti D. Posterior dislocation of the acromio-clavicular joint: a rare or an easily overlooked lesion? *Ital J Orthop Traumatol.* 1978;4(1):79–83.

80. Hastings DE, Horne JG. Anterior dislocation of the acromioclavicular joint. *Injury.* 1979;10(4):285–288.

81. Nieminen S, Aho AJ. Anterior dislocation of the acromioclavicular joint. *Ann Chir Gynaecol.* 1984;73(1):21–24.

82. Sondergard-Petersen P, Mikkelsen P. Posterior acromioclavicular dislocation. *J Bone Joint Surg Br.* 1982;64(1):52–53.

83. Frank RM, Cotter EJ, Leroux TS, Romeo AA. Acromioclavicular joint injuries: evidence-based treatment. *J Am Acad Orthop Surg.* 2019;27(17):e775–e788.

84. Dunphy TR, Damodar D, Heckmann ND, Sivasundaram L, Omid R, Hatch 3rd GF. Functional outcomes of type V acromioclavicular injuries with nonsurgical treatment. *J Am Acad Orthop Surg.* 2016;24(10):728–734.

85. Patterson WR. Inferior dislocation of the distal end of the clavicle. A case report. *J Bone Joint Surg Am.* 1967;49(6):1184–1186.

86. McPhee IB. Inferior dislocation of the outer end of the clavicle. *J Trauma.* 1980;20(8):709–710.

87. Torrens C, Mestre C, Perez P, Marin M. Subcoracoid dislocation of the distal end of the clavicle. A case report. *Clin Orthop Relat Res.* 1998;348:121–123.

88. Grossi EA, Macedo RA. Acromioclavicular dislocation type VI associated with diaphyseal fracture of the clavicle. *Rev Bras Ortop.* 2013;48(1):108–110.

89. Schwarz N, Kuderna H. Inferior acromioclavicular separation. Report of an unusual case. *Clin Orthop Relat Res.* 1988;234: 28–30.

90. Gerber C, Rockwood Jr CA. Subcoracoid dislocation of the lateral end of the clavicle. A report of three cases. *J Bone Joint Surg Am.* 1987;69(6):924–927.

91. Mazzocca AD, Spang JT, Rodriguez RR, et al. Biomechanical and radiographic analysis of partial coracoclavicular ligament injuries. *Am J Sports Med.* 2008;36(7):1397–1402.

92. Phadke A, Bakti N, Bawale R, Singh B. Current concepts in management of ACJ injuries. *J Clin Orthop Trauma.* 2019;10(3): 480–485.

93. Cisneros LN, Reiriz JS. Management of chronic unstable acromioclavicular joint injuries. *J Orthop Traumatol.* 2017;18(4): 305–318.

94. Borbas P, Churchill J, Ek ET. Surgical management of chronic high-grade acromioclavicular joint dislocations: a systematic review. *J Shoulder Elbow Surg.* 2019;28(10):2031–2038.

95. Mignani G, Rotini R, Olmi R, Marchiodi L, Veronesi CA. The surgical treatment of Rockwood grade III acromioclavicular dislocations. *Chir Organi Mov.* 2002;87(3):153–161.

96. Dumontier C, Sautet A, Man M, Apoil A. Acromioclavicular dislocations: treatment by coracoacromial ligamentoplasty. *J Shoulder Elbow Surg.* 1995;4(2):130–134.

97. von Heideken J, Bostrom Windhamre H, Une-Larsson V, Ekelund A. Acute surgical treatment of acromioclavicular dislocation type V with a hook plate: superiority to late reconstruction. *J Shoulder Elbow Surg.* 2013;22(1):9–17.

98. Gumina S, Carbone S, Postacchini F. Scapular dyskinesis and SICK scapula syndrome in patients with chronic type III acromioclavicular dislocation. *Arthroscopy.* 2009;25(1):40–45.

99. Lancaster S, Horowitz M, Alonso J. Complete acromioclavicular separations. A comparison of operative methods. *Clin Orthop Relat Res.* 1987;(216):80–88.

100. Imatani RJ, Hanlon JJ, Cady GW. Acute, complete acromioclavicular separation. *J Bone Joint Surg Am.* 1975;57(3):328–332.

101. Galatz LM, Hollis Jr RF, Williams Jr GR. Acromioclavicular joint injuries. In: Bucholz RW, Heckman JD, Court-Brown CM, Tornetta P, eds. *Rockwood and Green's Fractures in Adults.* Vol. 1. Philadelphia, PA: Lippincott Williams & Wilkins; 2010:1210–1242.

102. Lenza M, Belloti JC, Andriolo RB, Faloppa F. Conservative interventions for treating middle third clavicle fractures in adolescents and adults. *Cochrane Database Syst Rev.* 2014;(5):CD007121.

103. McKee M. Clavicle fractures. In: Bucholz RW, Court-Brown CM, Heckman JD, Tornetta III P, eds. *Rockwood and Green's Fractures in Adults.* 7th ed. Philadelphia, PA: Lippincott Williams & Wilkins; 2010:1106–1143.

104. Nuber GW, Lafosse, L. Disorders of the acromioclavicular joint: pathophysiology, diagnosis, and management. In: Iannotti JP, Williams Jr GR, eds. Disorders of the Shoulder: Diagnosis & Management. Vol. 2, 2nd ed.. Philadelphia, PA: Lippincott Williams & Wilkins; 2006:979-1006.

105. Sethi GK, Scott SM. Subclavian artery laceration due to migration of a Hagie pin. *Surgery.* 1976;80(5):644–646.

106. Norrell Jr H, Llewellyn RC. Migration of a threaded Steinmann pin from an acromioclavicular joint into the spinal canal. A case report. *J Bone Joint Surg Am.* 1965;47:1024–1026.

107. Pavlik A, Csepai D, Hidas P. Surgical treatment of chronic acromioclavicular joint dislocation by modified Weaver-Dunn procedure. *Knee Surg Sports Traumatol Arthrosc.* 2001;9(5):307–312.

108. Bosworth BM. Acromioclavicular separation: new method of repair. *Surg Gynecol Obstet.* 1941;73:866–871.

109. Bosworth BM. Acromioclavicular dislocation: end-results of screw suspension treatment. *Ann Surg.* 1948;127(1):98–111.

110. Tsou PM. Percutaneous cannulated screw coracoclavicular fixation for acute acromioclavicular dislocations. *Clin Orthop Relat Res.* 1989;243:112–121.

111. Lee S, Bedi A. Shoulder acromioclavicular joint reconstruction options and outcomes. *Curr Rev Musculoskelet Med.* 2016;9(4):368–377.

112. Lin HY, Wong PK, Ho WP, Chuang TY, Liao YS, Wong CC. Clavicular hook plate may induce subacromial shoulder impingement and rotator cuff lesion—dynamic sonographic evaluation. *J Orthop Surg Res.* 2014;9:6.

113. McConnell AJ, Yoo DJ, Zdero R, Schemitsch EH, McKee MD. Methods of operative fixation of the acromio-clavicular joint: a biomechanical comparison. *J Orthop Trauma.* 2007;21(4):248–253.

114. Struhl S. Double Endobutton technique for repair of complete acromioclavicular joint dislocations. *Tech Shoulder Elbow Surg.* 2007;8(4):175–179.

115. Ladermann A, Grosclaude M, Lubbeke A, et al. Acromioclavicular and coracoclavicular cerclage reconstruction for acute acromioclavicular joint dislocations. *J Shoulder Elbow Surg.* 2011;20(3):401–408.

116. Scheibel M, Droschel S, Gerhardt C, Kraus N. Arthroscopically assisted stabilization of acute high-grade acromioclavicular joint separations. *Am J Sports Med.* 2011;39(7):1507–1516.

117. Venjakob AJ, Salzmann GM, Gabel F, et al. Arthroscopically assisted 2-bundle anatomic reduction of acute acromioclavicular joint separations: 58-month findings. *Am J Sports Med.* 2013;41(3):615–621.

118. Shin SJ, Kim NK. Complications after arthroscopic coracoclavicular reconstruction using a single adjustable-loop-length suspensory fixation device in acute acromioclavicular joint dislocation. *Arthroscopy.* 2015;31(5):816–824.

119. Celik H, Chauhan A, Flores-Hernandez C, et al. Vertical and rotational stiffness of coracoclavicular ligament reconstruction: a biomechanical study of 3 different techniques. *Arthroscopy.* 2020;36(5):1264–1270.

120. Park I, Itami Y, Hedayati B, et al. Biomechanical analysis of single-, double-, and triple-bundle configurations for coracoclavicular ligament reconstruction using cortical fixation buttons with suture tapes: a cadaveric study. *Arthroscopy.* 2018;34(11):2983–2991.

121. Beitzel K, Obopilwe E, Chowaniec DM, et al. Biomechanical comparison of arthroscopic repairs for acromioclavicular joint instability: suture button systems without biological augmentation. *Am J Sports Med.* 2011;39(10):2218–2225.

122. Abat F, Sarasquete J, Natera LG, et al. Biomechanical analysis of acromioclavicular joint dislocation repair using coracoclavicular suspension devices in two different configurations. *J Orthop Traumatol.* 2015;16(3):215–219.

123. Woodmass JM, Esposito JG, Ono Y, et al. Complications following arthroscopic fixation of acromioclavicular separations: a systematic review of the literature. *Open Access J Sports Med.* 2015;6:97–107.

124. Thiel E, Mutnal A, Gilot GJ. Surgical outcome following arthroscopic fixation of acromioclavicular joint disruption with the tightrope device. *Orthopedics.* 2011;34(7):e267–274.

125. Lim YW, Sood A, van Riet R, Bain G. Acromioclavicular joint reduction, repair and reconstruction using metallic buttons-early results and complications. *Tech Shoulder Elbow Surg.* 2007;8:213–221.

126. Martetschlager F, Horan MP, Warth RJ, Millett PJ. Complications after anatomic fixation and reconstruction of the coracoclavicular ligaments. *Am J Sports Med.* 2013;41(12):2896–2903.

127. El Sallakh SA. Evaluation of arthroscopic stabilization of acute acromioclavicular joint dislocation using the TightRope system. *Orthopedics.* 2012;35(1):e18–22.

128. Shin JJ, Popchak AJ, Musahl V, Irrgang JJ, Lin A. Complications after arthroscopic shoulder surgery: a review of the American Board of Orthopaedic Surgery database. *J Am Acad Orthop Surg Glob Res Rev.* 2018;2(12):e093.

129. Arirachakaran A, Boonard M, Piyapittayanun P, et al. Post-operative outcomes and complications of suspensory loop fixation device versus hook plate in acute unstable acromioclavicular joint dislocation: a systematic review and meta-analysis. *J Orthop Traumatol.* 2017;18(4):293–304.

130. Jensen G, Katthagen JC, Alvarado LE, Lill H, Voigt C. Has the arthroscopically assisted reduction of acute AC joint separations with the double tight-rope technique advantages over the clavicular hook plate fixation? *Knee Surg Sports Traumatol Arthrosc.* 2014;22(2):422–430.

131. Hann C, Kraus N, Minkus M, Maziak N, Scheibel M. Combined arthroscopically assisted coraco- and acromioclavicular stabilization of acute high-grade acromioclavicular joint separations. *Knee Surg Sports Traumatol Arthrosc.* 2018;26(1):212–220.

132. Weaver JK, Dunn HK. Treatment of acromioclavicular injuries, especially complete acromioclavicular separation. *J Bone Joint Surg Am.* 1972;54(6):1187–1194.

133. Mazzocca AD, Santangelo SA, Johnson ST, Rios CG, Dumonski ML, Arciero RA. A biomechanical evaluation of an anatomical coracoclavicular ligament reconstruction. *Am J Sports Med.* 2006;34(2):236–246.

134. Bostrom Windhamre HA, von Heideken JP, Une-Larsson VE, Ekelund AL. Surgical treatment of chronic acromioclavicular dislocations: a comparative study of Weaver-Dunn augmented with PDS-braid or hook plate. *J Shoulder Elbow Surg.* 2010;19(7):1040–1048.

135. Shin SJ, Yun YH, Yoo JD. Coracoclavicular ligament reconstruction for acromioclavicular dislocation using 2 suture anchors and coracoacromial ligament transfer. *Am J Sports Med.* 2009;37(2):346–351.

136. Michlitsch MG, Adamson GJ, Pink M, Estess A, Shankwiler JA, Lee TQ. Biomechanical comparison of a modified Weaver-Dunn and a free-tissue graft reconstruction of the acromioclavicular joint complex. *Am J Sports Med.* 2010;38(6):1196–1203.

137. Lee SJ, Nicholas SJ, Akizuki KH, McHugh MP, Kremenic IJ, Ben-Avi S. Reconstruction of the coracoclavicular ligaments with tendon grafts: a comparative biomechanical study. *Am J Sports Med.* 2003;31(5):648–655.

138. Lee SJ, Keefer EP, McHugh MP, et al. Cyclical loading of coracoclavicular ligament reconstructions: a comparative biomechanical study. *Am J Sports Med.* 2008;36(10):1990–1997.

139. Grutter PW, Petersen SA. Anatomical acromioclavicular ligament reconstruction: a biomechanical comparison of reconstructive techniques of the acromioclavicular joint. *Am J Sports Med.* 2005;33(11):1723–1728.

140. Banffy MB, van Eck CF, Stanton M, ElAttrache NS. A single-tunnel technique for coracoclavicular and acromioclavicular ligament reconstruction. *Arthrosc Tech.* 2017;6(3):e769–e775.

141. Carofino BC, Mazzocca AD. The anatomic coracoclavicular ligament reconstruction: surgical technique and indications. *J Shoulder Elbow Surg.* 2010;19(2 Suppl):37–46.

142. Yoo YS, Seo YJ, Noh KC, Patro BP, Kim DY. Arthroscopically assisted anatomical coracoclavicular ligament reconstruction using tendon graft. *Int Orthop.* 2011;35(7):1025–1030.

143. Kibler WB, Sciascia AD, Morris BJ, Dome DC. Treatment of symptomatic acromioclavicular joint instability by a docking technique: clinical indications, surgical technique, and outcomes. *Arthroscopy.* 2017;33(4):696–708. e692.

144. Haber DB, Golijanin P, Stone GL, et al. Primary acromio-clavicular-coracoclavicular reconstruction using 2 allografts, TightRope, and stabilization to the acromion. *Arthrosc Tech.* 2019;8(2):e147–e152.

145. Frank RM, Bernardoni ED, Cotter EJ, Verma NN. Anatomic acromioclavicular joint reconstruction with semitendinosus allograft: surgical technique. *Arthrosc Tech.* 2017;6(5):e1721–e1726.

146. Natera L, Sarasquete Reiriz J, Abat F. Anatomic reconstruction of chronic coracoclavicular ligament tears: arthroscopic-assisted approach with nonrigid mechanical fixation and graft augmentation. *Arthrosc Tech.* 2014;3(5):e583–588.

147. Cook JB, Shaha JS, Rowles DJ, Bottoni CR, Shaha SH, Tokish JM. Clavicular bone tunnel malposition leads to early failures in coracoclavicular ligament reconstructions. *Am J Sports Med.* 2013;41(1):142–148.

148. Eisenstein ED, Lanzi JT, Waterman BR, Bader JM, Pallis MP. Medialized clavicular bone tunnel position predicts failure after anatomic coracoclavicular ligament reconstruction in young, active male patients. *Am J Sports Med.* 2016;44(10):2682–2689.

149. Milewski MD, Tompkins M, Giugale JM, Carson EW, Miller MD, Diduch DR. Complications related to anatomic reconstruction of the coracoclavicular ligaments. *Am J Sports Med.* 2012;40(7):1628–1634.

150. Tauber M, Valler D, Lichtenberg S, Magosch P, Moroder P, Habermeyer P. Arthroscopic stabilization of chronic acromioclavicular joint dislocations: triple- versus single-bundle reconstruction. *Am J Sports Med.* 2016;44(2):482–489.

151. Simovitch R, Sanders B, Ozbaydar M, Lavery K, Warner JJ. Acromioclavicular joint injuries: diagnosis and management. *J Am Acad Orthop Surg.* 2009;17(4):207–219.

152. Tauber M, Gordon K, Koller H, Fox M, Resch H. Semitendinosus tendon graft versus a modified Weaver-Dunn procedure for acromioclavicular joint reconstruction in chronic cases: a prospective comparative study. *Am J Sports Med.* 2009;37(1):181–190.

153. Shoji H, Roth C, Chuinard R. Bone block transfer of coracoacromial ligament in acromioclavicular injury. *Clin Orthop Relat Res.* 1986;208:272–277.

13

Technique Spotlight: Arthroscopically Assisted Stabilization for Acute and Chronic High-Grade Acromioclavicular Joint Dislocations

MARKUS SCHEIBEL AND NINA MAZIAK

Indications

Combined coraco- and acromioclavicular stabilization using a low-profile single TightRope (Arthrex, Naples, FL, USA) device and an additional FiberTape (Arthrex) cerclage is indicated in acute high-grade bidirectional acromioclavicular (AC) joint instabilities (Rockwood type IV–VI dislocations), and depending on the patient's functional requirements, for select type IIIb separations. Chronic lesions, on the other hand, should initially be addressed conservatively and surgery should be reserved for patients in whom conservative measures have failed. If nonoperative treatment fails, combined coraco- and acromioclavicular stabilization with the aid of a free hamstring tendon autograft or allograft supported with a low-profile TightRope is our surgical procedure of choice for these patients.

The low-profile device used for the techniques described in this chapter was designed to reduce the risks of irritation from the knot stack and hardware as well as tunnel widening.[1,2]

Preoperative Evaluation

The diagnosis of an AC joint dislocation should always be based on the patient's history, clinical examination, and imaging.[2,3] It is important to evaluate the date of injury, to determine acute versus chronic, as well as possible pretreatments. Although the terms "acute" and "chronic" regarding the timing of surgery post injury are still not well defined, we, as most authors, consider AC joint separations as acute within 3 weeks after trauma.[4] A deformity, with the clavicle appearing elevated, can often be observed on physical examination. Reducing the clavicle manually (piano key sign) confirms the injury. Horizontal stability also needs to be examined and is likewise tested manually. For detection of possible concomitant lesions, a full physical examination of both shoulders should, furthermore, be performed in all cases. For

radiographic evaluation, bilateral anteroposterior stress views with 10 kg of axial load are recommended (Fig. 13.1). The amount of vertical dislocation can be determined on these by measuring the coracoclavicular difference. Additionally, bilateral Alexander or axillary views should be obtained for assessment of potential additional dynamic posterior translation (Fig. 13.1).

Arthroscopically Assisted Low-Profile Stabilization for Acute AC Joint Dislocations

Positioning and Equipment

Under general anesthesia, the patient is placed in a beach chair position with the affected shoulder prepped and draped in a sterile fashion. The patient's head should be slightly tilted to the contralateral side to enable enough space for establishment of the coracoclavicular tunnel. A standard posterior, lateral, and an anteroinferior portal are required for this minimally invasive technique (Fig. 13.2). Additionally, a 2- to 3-cm sagittal incision on the top of the clavicle is necessary.[1]

Surgical Technique

In the first step, a diagnostic arthroscopy is performed via the standard posterior portal. Concomitant glenohumeral lesions can thus be detected and addressed if required. The anteroinferior portal is then established using an outside-in technique. In a similar fashion, the lateral transtendinous portal is created through the supraspinatus tendon. To minimize the access-related trauma, the incision of this portal should be made parallel to the fibers of the tendon. Next, the arthroscope is introduced to the lateral portal. A

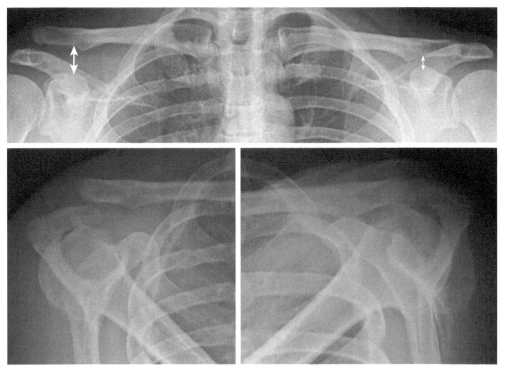

• **Fig. 13.1** Bilateral anteroposterior stress views (coracoclavicular distance marked with *arrows*) and Alexander views of a patient with a high-grade bidirectional acromioclavicular joint dislocation (type V according to Rockwood). (From Scheibel M, Maziak N. Arthroscopic and arthroscopic-assisted management of traumatic disorders of the ACJ: indications, techniques and outcomes. In: Matsen F, Cordasco FA, Sperling J, Lippitt S, eds. *Rockwood and Matsen's The Shoulder*. 6th ed. Philadelphia: Elsevier; 2021.)

shaver is inserted via the anteroinferior portal and the subcoracoid bursa and base of the coracoid are dissected to achieve sufficient visualization of the undersurface of the coracoid process. The sagittal incision over the clavicle, 2 to 3 cm long and approximately 3 cm medial to the AC joint, is subsequently created.

Next, the coracoclavicular tunnel, required for reduction of the AC joint, should be established. This step is performed with a combination of image intensifier control and visualization (through the incision and arthroscopically) and with the aid of a specially designed drill guide. The marking hook of this drill guide is first introduced through the anteroinferior portal and placed under the coracoid process (Fig. 13.3A). The drill sleeve is placed on the midpoint of the clavicle approximately 3 cm medial from the AC joint (Fig. 13.3A). With the aid of a drill bit with an internal K-wire, a 3-mm transclavicular and transcoracoidal drill hole is then created between the former coracoclavicular ligaments (Fig. 13.3B–C). The clavicle is then unicortically overdrilled using a 5.1-mm drill bit (Fig. 13.3D–E). The K-wire is subsequently removed and a nitinol suture passing wire is inserted via the drill bit. The nitinol wire is retrieved anteroinferiorly and the drill bit can be removed (Fig. 13.3F).

Transclavicular and transacromial tunnels for horizontal stabilization are then created with the marking hook of the drill guide positioned behind the clavicle, while the drill sleeve is introduced via the anteroinferior portal. A 1.25-mm K-wire can then be inserted in the clavicle from anterior to posterior (Fig. 13.4A–B). This K-wire should be placed approximately 1 cm lateral to the coracoclavicular drill hole. It is overdrilled using a 2.7-mm cannulated drill bit (Fig. 13.4C–D). The K-wire is removed next and a nitinol wire inserted into the drill bit and retrieved over the clavicular incision. In a similar fashion, the transacromial drill hole is established approximately at the midpoint of the acromion

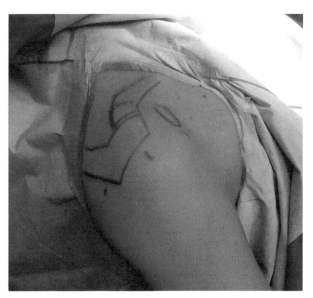

• **Fig. 13.2** Anatomic landmarks and marked portals.

from lateral-inferior to medial-superior via the lateral portal (Fig. 13.5A–B). A nitinol wire is again inserted via the drill bit and retrieved through the clavicular incision (Fig. 13.5C–D).

A low-profile TightRope (Arthrex) for joint reduction and coracoclavicular stabilization is then inserted (Fig. 13.6A). The inferior sutures of the device are therefore attached to the proximal eyelet of the coracoclavicular nitinol wire and shuttled through the clavicular and coracoidal tunnel and pulled out via the anteroinferior portal (Fig. 13.6B–C). Finally, a Dog Bone button (Arthrex)

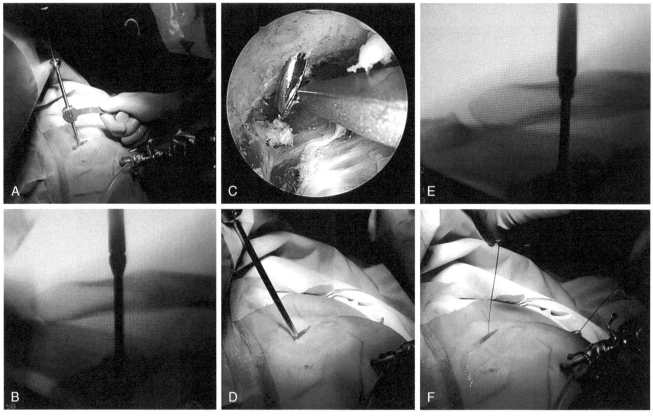

• **Fig. 13.3** (A–F) Establishment of the coracoclavicular tunnel.[1]

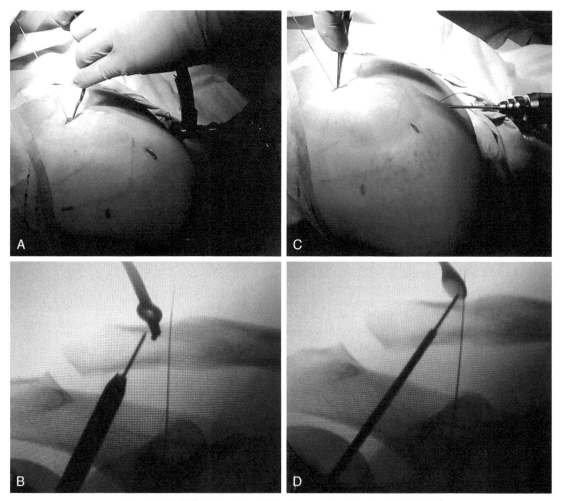

• **Fig. 13.4** (A–D) Transclavicular drilling for acromioclavicular stabilization.[1]

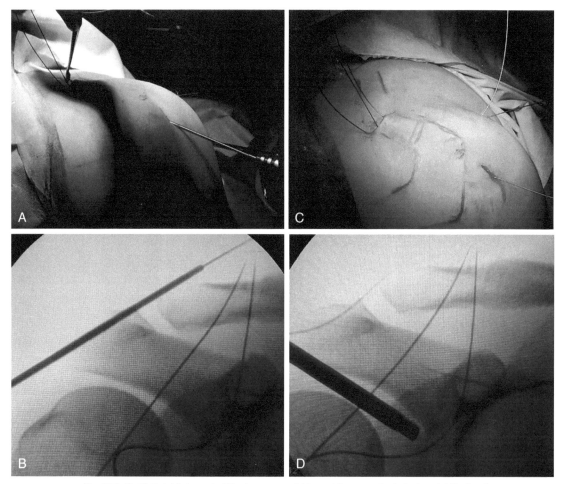

• **Fig. 13.5** (A–D) Establishment of the transacromial tunnel for acromioclavicular stabilization.[1]

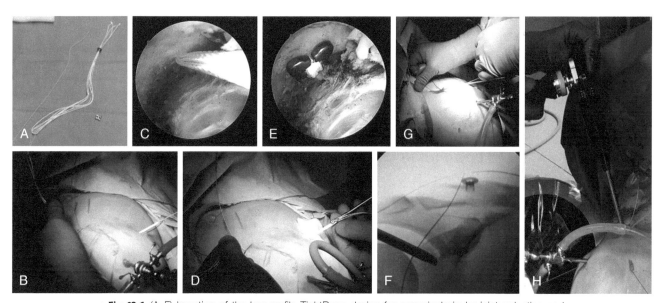

• **Fig. 13.6** (A–F) Insertion of the low-profile TightRope device for acromioclavicular joint reduction and coracoclavicular stabilization.[1]

is attached to the inferior sutures (Fig. 13.6D). Under arthroscopic visualization, it is positioned under the coracoid arch (Fig. 13.6E). The sutures of the TightRope (Arthrex) are then pulled in an alternating, "marionette" fashion, until the construct begins to become tight (Fig. 13.6F–G). A suture tensioner (Arthrex) is subsequently

used to tension the sutures (Fig. 13.6H). Approximately 80–100 N is applied to achieve a slight over-reduction of the AC joint (~3 mm). It is important to perform this step under image intensifier control to achieve sufficient reduction. We aim for slight over-reduction. Once reduction is obtained, the sutures are secured

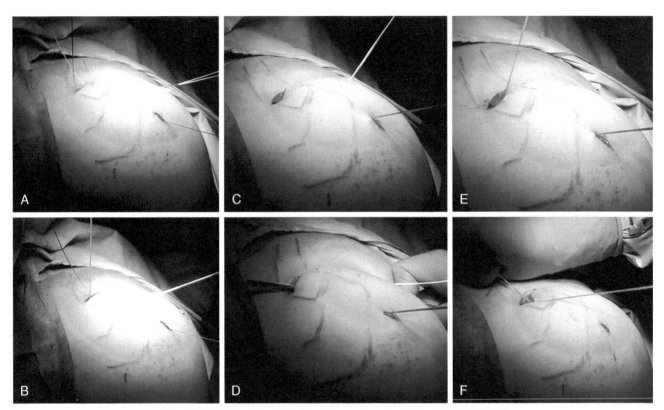

• **Fig. 13.7** (A–F) Insertion of the FiberWire cerclage for horizontal stabilization.[1]

with six knots (three per suture) which are countersunk in the top hat button of the low-profile TightRope device (Arthrex). At this point, the AC joint has been stabilized in a vertical dimension.

Now a FiberTape (Arthrex) is inserted for horizontal stabilization. It is first shuttled through the transclavicular tunnel via the respective nitinol suture passer (Fig. 13.7A). Then it is inserted into the transacromial tunnel by using the remaining nitinol wire and retrieved via the lateral portal (Fig. 13.7B). Both ends of the FiberTape are then shuttled back subcutaneously to be retrieved via the clavicular incision (Fig. 13.7D–E) and tightened and tied with knots (Fig. 13.7F). All portals and the clavicular incision are then closed in a standard fashion (Fig. 13.8).[1]

Arthroscopically Assisted Low-Profile Stabilization for Chronic AC Joint Dislocations

Positioning and Equipment

The same positioning, portals, and supraclavicular incision are required for this procedure as described above for acute cases.[2] For this technique, hamstring allograft is used to reconstruct the functions of the chronically ruptured ligaments.

Surgical Technique

After a diagnostic arthroscopy is performed, the coracoclavicular tunnel for the low-profile TightRope device (Arthrex) is established in the same way as described for stabilization of acute AC dislocations. The next step involves preparation for the hamstring tendon graft passage. While viewing through the transtendinous

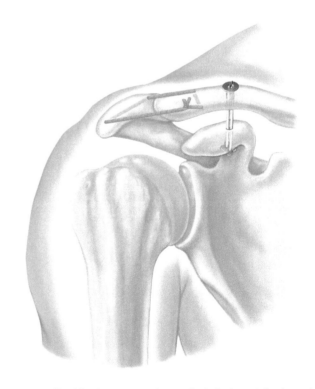

• **Fig. 13.8** Combined coraco- and acromioclavicular stabilization using a low-profile TightRope and acromioclavicular FiberTape cerclage.[3]

portal, the blunt end of a 2.0-mm K-wire is introduced through the superior incision, posterior to the clavicle, and close to the medial part of the coracoid process into the subcoracoid space. Without spinning, a 4-mm drill bit is placed over this K-wire. The K-wire is then exchanged for a nitinol suture passing wire. The free-end of the passing wire is retrieved through the anteroinferior portal and the drill bit is removed. With a similar maneuver, another nitinol suture passing wire is placed anterior to the clavicle and lateral to the coracoid process. The AC joint is subsequently reduced with the aid of a low-profile TightRope (Arthrex) as described above for stabilization of acute ACJ dislocations.

Once two nitinol passing loops have been passed on either side of the coracoid and clavicle, or concurrently if a surgical assistant is available, the hamstring allograft must be prepared. The graft should have an approximate length of at least 24 cm. Its diameter should be approximately 3 to 5 mm. Number 2 FiberWire (Arthrex) is then "baseball-stitched" in a running, locked fashion at both ends of the tendon to reinforce it. The previously passed nitinol suture passing wires are then used to pass the hamstring allograft. First, one limb of the graft is shuttled in through the superior incision, medial to the coracoid and retroclavicular exiting through the anteroinferior portal. The opposite limb is similarly shuttled with the nitinol passing loop in through the anteroinferior portal, lateral to the coracoid, anterior to the clavicle, and out through the superior incision.

For AC stabilization, a 1.25-mm K-wire is placed transacromially from lateral-inferior to medial-superior. The K-wire is then overdrilled using a 3.5-mm cannulated drill bit and subsequently removed. Another nitinol suture passing wire is inserted via the drill bit and retrieved via the clavicular incision. The retroclavicular end of the tendon graft can then be shuttled subcutaneously, superior to the AC joint capsule, and then through the transacromial drill hole. Finally, it is shuttled back subcutaneously, superior to the acromion, to the clavicular incision, where both FiberWire (Arthrex) ends of the tendon graft are knotted to each other (Fig. 13.9). The crossed ends of the tendon allograft are additionally sewed together using a Vicryl suture. The deltotrapezial fascia as well as all portals can now be closed in a standard fashion.[2]

Aftercare

We instruct patients after stabilization of acute injuries to wear an orthosis in neutral position (UltraSling Quadrant; DJO Global Inc., Dallas, TX, USA) for 6 weeks postoperatively. Only passive range-of-motion exercises are allowed during this time. Flexion and abduction, however, should be limited to 45 degrees, external rotation up to 30 degrees, and internal rotation to the belly of the patients in the first 3 weeks. Flexion and abduction up to 90 degrees, external rotation up to 60 degrees, and internal rotation to the belly are allowed in the following 3 weeks. After week 7, unrestricted passive range-of-motion exercises in all planes are allowed and an active-assisted to active range-of-motion progression is initiated. Muscle-strengthening exercises are allowed from week 13 on.

Patients after reconstruction of chronic AC joint separations are also instructed to wear an orthosis for 6 weeks postoperatively. Only elbow, wrist, and hand mobilization, however, is allowed during the first 2 weeks postsurgery. Passive range-of-motion exercises for the shoulder are allowed from the third week on, whereby flexion and abduction should be limited to 45 degrees, external rotation to 30 degrees, and internal rotation to the belly of the patient for 2 weeks and up to 90 degrees in the following 2 weeks.

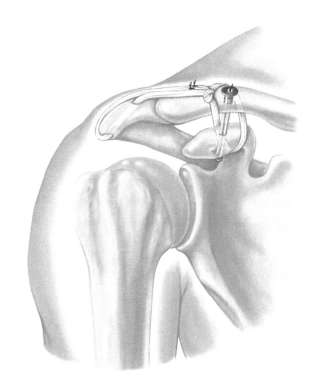

• **Fig. 13.9** Combined coraco- and acromioclavicular stabilization with the aid of a free hamstring tendon allograft augmented by a low-profile Tight-Rope.[3]

In weeks 7 and 8, active-assisted abduction up to 90 degrees, external rotation up to 60 degrees, and internal rotation to the belly are allowed. After week 9, unrestricted passive range-of-motion exercises in all planes are allowed and active range-of-motion progression is initiated. Free passive and each active range-of-motion exercises are allowed from week 9 on. Muscle-strengthening exercises start gradually after 12 weeks.

PEARLS AND PITFALLS

- Drill holes should always be created with the aid of a drill guide and under image intensifier control.
- We use a low-profile TightRope device to minimize the risk of suture irritations due to knot stacks.
- Loss of reduction may occur if the sutures of the TightRope device are not fully tensioned before they are knotted. A suture tensioner should therefore be used to achieve sufficient reduction and remove any slack in the construct. And it is crucial to perform this step under image intensifier control to assess the amount of reduction intraoperatively.
- Neurovascular structures medial to the coracoid include the suprascapular nerve, musculocutaneous nerve, and the brachial plexus. When passing the K-wire and drill bit, care must be taken to avoid plunging medially and/or distally. Staying just medial to the coracoid is ideal.
- The typical error for fixation placement in the coracoid is to be too lateral and not far enough back into the base. The tunnel should be centered in a medial-lateral dimension and located where the coracoid base begins to dive down into the scapular body.

References

1. Minkus M, Maziak N, Moroder P, Scheibel M. Arthroscopic low-profile reconstruction for acute acromioclavicular joint instability. *Obere Extremität.* 2019;14(1):60–65. https://doi.org/10.1007/s11678-019-0506-4.
2. Dittrich M, Wirth B, Freislederer F, Bellmann F, Scheibel M. Arthroscopically assisted stabilization of chronic bidirectional acromioclavicular joint instability using a low-profile implant and a free tendon graft. *Obere Extremität.* 2020;15,118–121.
3. Scheibel M, Maziak N. Arthroscopic and arthroscopic-assisted management of traumatic disorders of the ACJ: indications, techniques and outcomes. In: Matsen F, Cordasco FA, Sperling J, Lippitt S, eds. *Rockwood and Matsen's the Shoulder.* 6th ed. Philadelphia: Elsevier; 2021.
4. Flint JH, Wade AM, Giuliani J, Rue JP. Defining the terms acute and chronic in orthopaedic sports injuries: a systematic review. *Am J Sports Med.* 2014;42(1):235–241. PMID: 23749341.

14

Technique Spotlight: Anatomic Coracoclavicular Ligament Reconstruction

DANIEL P. BERTHOLD, COLIN L. UYEKI, AND AUGUSTUS D. MAZZOCCA

Indications

High-grade acromioclavicular (AC) joint injuries (Rockwood types IV, V, and VI)[1] are usually treated operatively due to considerable morbidity associated with a persistently dislocated AC joint and severe soft tissue disruption.[2,3] In some type IV–VI injuries, primary conservative treatment may be considered; however, if the patient remains chronically symptomatic, surgical intervention to improve range of motion (ROM), strength, and pain control is recommended.[2,3] Additionally, surgery is recommended in chronic AC joint instability (including type III) with previously failed conservative treatment and/or persistent horizontal instability, limited ROM, and scapular dyskinesia—especially if these symptoms occur in high-demand athletes or manual laborers.[2–9]

Contraindications

Lack of pain or dysfunction, advanced osteoarthritis, severe neurological pathology, and ongoing local or systemic infection are considered contraindications for AC joint reconstruction. Furthermore, all patients must be willing and able to undergo and comply with the proper postoperative rehabilitation and restrictions. Thus patients with alcoholism, end-stage Alzheimer's disease, severe psychiatric comorbidity, or other conditions which may affect postoperative adherence to the rehabilitation protocol are not good candidates for this procedure.

Preoperative Evaluation

A detailed clinical evaluation including a complete physical examination of the glenohumeral joint, sternoclavicular joint, cervical spine, and ipsilateral upper extremity along with a complete neurovascular exam is key for correct classification of the injury and to rule out any concomitant pathology.[3] Coexisting pathology is frequent, with lesions of the long head of the biceps tendon or SLAP (superior labral anterior-posterior) lesions reported in up to 18% of high-grade AC joint dislocations.[10]

Ecchymosis over the AC joint and a possible deformity (depending on the severity of injury) can be revealed by inspection.

Tenderness to direct palpation over the AC joint and pain with crossed body adduction confirms AC joint injury.[3,4,11,12] A less common way of confirming the diagnosis, but still helpful is relief of pain after injection of local anesthetic into the AC joint.

Subsequently, the physician should focus on evaluating vertical displacement, horizontal and rotational instability. Horizontal and rotational stability of the AC joint can be assessed by moving the clavicle in an anterior to posterior direction while stabilizing the acromion. Physical examination should detect if present horizontal or rotational instability may result in pain or scapula dysfunction.[13] Painful "scissoring" of the lateral clavicle over the acromion with cross-body adduction has been shown to be indicative of poor tolerance of a type III injury.[14]

Assessing the scapulothoracic rhythm is critical, as clavicle normally functions as a strut, working in tandem with the periscapular muscles to create a mobile platform for the glenohumeral joint. However, in AC joint injuries, especially those poorly compensated with weak and/or uncoordinated periscapular musculature, there is frequently scapular dyskinesia with excessive scapular internal rotation and anterior tilt.[3]

Imaging

In addition to a thorough clinical examination, a detailed radiological evaluation is required. Both vertical and horizontal instability have to be detected using feasible and precise methods. Numerous radiographic techniques have been described in the literature including the bilateral Zanca view, bilateral panoramic view, (dynamic) axillary view, and stress imaging. To date, a widely accepted standardized radiographic protocol does not exist.[15] Vertical instability can be diagnosed with high inter- and intraobserver reliability in a bilateral panoramic view by measuring the coracoclavicular (CC) distance, thus allowing for direct correlation of the CC distance to the uninjured contralateral AC joint.[16,17]

At the authors' institution, standard radiographs include an anteroposterior (AP) view, supraspinatus outlet view, axillary views, and bilateral Zanca views. By using the Zanca view, the source-to-image distance is increased to 72 inches in combination with increasing the tube voltage to 73–80 kV (Figs. 14.1–14.4).

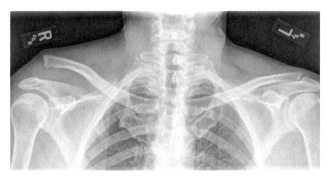

• **Fig. 14.1** Preoperative (panoramic) Zanca view.

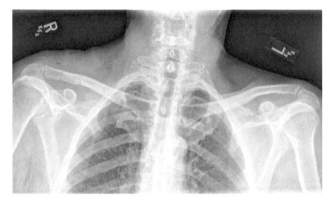

• **Fig. 14.2** Postoperative (panoramic) Zanca view.

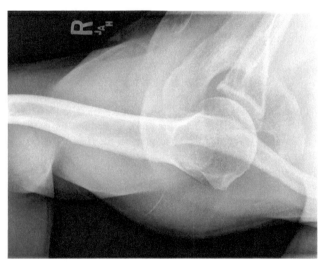

• **Fig. 14.3** Preoperative axial view.

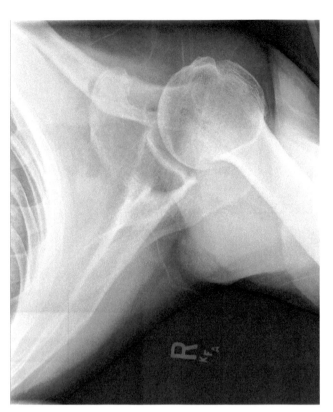

• **Fig. 14.4** Postoperative axial view.

Complete CC ligament disruption can be detected by an increase in the CC distance (usually 1.1–1.3 cm) of 25%–50% over the normal side. If a patient presents with a complete dislocation of the AC joint and a normal CC interspace (average 1.1–1.3 cm), this may indicate a fracture of the coracoid base. Thus AC joint dislocation (or CC interspace) may be better diagnosed with a Stryker notch view. To evaluate the coracoid base and to assist in differentiating a type III from a type IV AC joint injury, we recommend an axillary view of the shoulder.

Assessment of horizontal and rotational instability is considered as one of the most important steps in AC joint treatment recommendations. A correct and reliable diagnosis is often difficult with heterogeneous inter- and intraobserver reliability being reported in the current literature.[15] Bilateral modified Y-views with the arm in adduction (e.g., Alexander view) can be used to detect horizontal instability by quantifying posterior translation and "scissoring" over the acromion.[18,19] However, to date, there remains a lack of evidence regarding the advantage of this radiographic view.[15]

Magnetic resonance imaging (MRI) of the shoulder may be useful for detecting concomitant injuries of the glenohumeral joint. These often include SLAP lesions or rotator cuff tears.[10] In rare, chronic, or revision cases, computed tomography (CT) scans may be needed for detailed visualization of osseous structures or technical failures including insufficient fixation, bone tunnel widening or position, and clavicular and/or coracoid fractures.

Positioning and Equipment

After induction of anesthesia, the patient is positioned in a beach chair position and if necessary, with additional draping of the ipsilateral knee joint for harvest and preparation of the hamstring tendon graft. Allografts (such as semitendinosus, peroneus longus, tibialis anterior) can be used. The arm can either be placed in a movable arm holding device or be rested on the abdomen (surgeon's preference).

A standard table provides posterior support and stabilization of the scapula. Additionally, a small bump can be placed beneath the medial border of the scapula for stabilization and to improve operative access to the clavicle. Draping is performed to expose the sternoclavicular joint and posterior clavicle for complete visualization of the shoulder girdle. Besides, the arm is free draped to allow easy manipulation during reduction of the AC joint.

Surgical Technique

See Video 14.1 for the senior author's preferred surgical technique described in this section. Surgery starts with a skin incision centered 3.5 cm medial to the AC joint starting at the posterior clavicle in a curvilinear fashion toward the coracoid process along Langer's lines of skin tension. To guarantee full visualization of the AC joint laterally and the coracoid process medially, the incision can be placed obliquely (Fig. 14.1). Superficial skin bleeders are controlled down to the deep fascia with a needle-tip electrocautery. Full-thickness cutaneous flaps should be elevated to define the underlying deltotrapezial fascia attachment onto the clavicle and acromion. The deltoid has two attachments on to the clavicle, which is complex and must be preserved. The superior attachment is easily seen and can be carefully peeled off the superior and anterior aspect of the clavicle. The second attachment is on the inferior cortex of the clavicle. Because of its position, it is not easily seen but critical to also peel off. Once it is released, it is an easy "trip" inferior to the base of the coracoid. The surgeon then must "travel" anterior on the base of the coracoid to get to its tip. Dissection at the base runs the risk of damaging the suprascapular nerve, which is directly medial to the base of the coracoid in the suprascapular fossa (Fig. 14.2). Subsequently, using an electrocautery device, full-thickness fascioperiosteal flaps are elevated posteriorly and anteriorly to skeletonize the clavicle (Fig. 14.3). The raphe between the deltoid and trapezius attachments at the clavicle and acromion serves as an avascular plane for dissection. Then, tagging sutures are placed on the edges of the deltotrapezial fascia (Fig. 14.4). Continuous traction is then placed on the tagging sutures to retract the fascia. Alternatively,

a Gelpi retractor placed under the flaps can be used for improved visualization.

Once visualization is guaranteed, a trial reduction is attempted involving an upward displacement of the scapulohumeral complex combined with the use of a large, pointed reduction forceps placed on the undersurface of the coracoid process and the posterosuperior border of the clavicle. Thus the distal-most end of the clavicle should be freed from trapezius muscle, hypertrophic scar tissue, or any capsular remnant. Especially in chronic separations, interposition of soft tissue and scar inferior to the clavicle will prevent an anatomic reduction.

Graft Preparation

For graft preparation, an allograft (semitendinosus or peroneus longus) or autograft (semitendinosus) can be used for this procedure (Fig. 14.5). Both tendon ends are "bulleted" to facilitate future passage through bone tunnels. A whipstitch or grasping suture is placed in the two free ends of the tendon for graft passage through bone tunnels. The tendon is sized using standard tendon sizers, usually 5 or 6 mm.

Coracoid Preparation and Graft Fixation to Coracoid

As previously mentioned, the graft can be fixed to the coracoid by either looping the graft around the coracoid base in our "loop technique" or by performing a tenodesis of the graft into the coracoid base using an interference screw, the so-called tenodesis technique. The author's preferred technique is the "loop technique" to avoid potential fracture to the coracoid.

Soft tissue dissection is performed to expose the coracoid process from the base to the tip, including dissection of the medial and lateral margins of the coracoid. The pectoralis minor is released but the conjoint tendon is left intact. To this, the CA ligament is also kept intact, as there is no need to resect as its attachment to the acromion is anterior, inferior, and lateral.[20] Care is taken not to injure the suprascapular nerve as it traverses immediately medial to the coracoid base through the suprascapular notch.

An additional suture can be looped around the base of the coracoid process using an aortic cross-clamp (Satinsky clamp) or a suture-passing device (Fig. 14.6). A loop is created at one end of

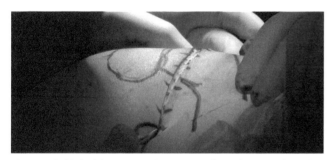

• **Fig. 14.5** A skin incision centered 3.5 cm medial to the acromioclavicular (AC) joint starting at the posterior clavicle in a curvilinear fashion toward the coracoid process along the Langer lines is placed. To guarantee full visualization of the AC joint laterally and the coracoid process medially, the incision can be placed obliquely.

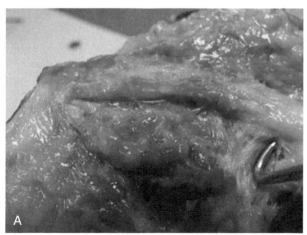
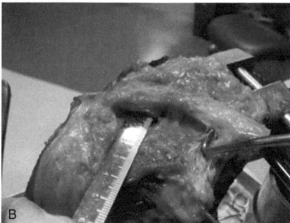

• **Fig. 14.6** (A) The superior attachment is easily seen and can be carefully peeled off the superior and anterior aspect of the clavicle. (B) The second attachment is on the inferior cortex of the clavicle. Because of its position, it is not easily seen but critical to also peel off. Once it is released, it is an easy "trip" inferior to the base of the coracoid. The surgeon then must "travel" anterior on the base of the coracoid to get to its tip.

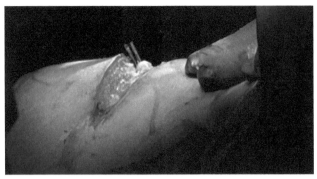

• **Fig. 14.7** Using an electrothermic device, full-thickness fascioperiosteal flaps are elevated from the midline of the clavicle both posteriorly and anteriorly to skeletonize the clavicle.

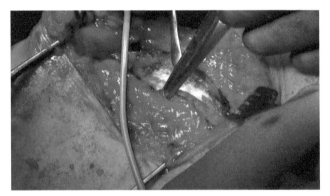

• **Fig. 14.8** Tagging sutures are placed on the edges of the deltotrapezial fascia.

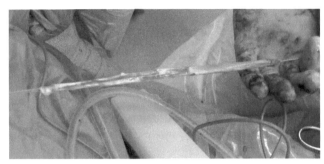

• **Fig. 14.9** For graft preparation, an allograft (semitendinosus or peroneus longus) or autograft (semitendinosus) can be used. Both tendon ends are bulleted for future passage through bone tunnels.

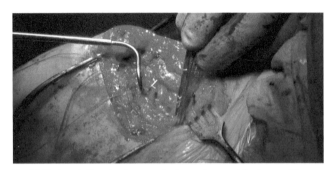

• **Fig. 14.10** An additional suture can be looped around the base of the coracoid process using a suture-passing device (Arthrex, Inc., Naples, FL, USA).

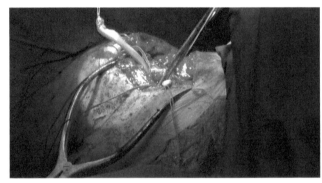

• **Fig. 14.11** A loop is created at one end of this suture and is used to shuttle the graft and collagen-coated No. 2 FiberWire (Arthrex, Inc., Naples, FL, USA) beneath the coracoid.

this suture and is used to shuttle the graft and collagen-coated No. 2 FiberWire (Arthrex, Inc., Naples, FL, USA) beneath the coracoid (Fig. 14.7). The advantage of this technique is that the graft provides a biologic form of fixation and collagen-coated No. 2 FiberWire provides the nonbiologic augment of fixation across the CC space.

Clavicle Preparation

For clavicle preparation, both bone tunnels are drilled in the clavicle to anatomically reconstruct the conoid and trapezoid ligaments. To recreate the conoid ligament, a cannulated guide pin is placed approximately 45–50 mm medial from the distal end of the clavicle at the conoid tubercle and the posterior aspect of the clavicle (Fig. 14.8). Alternatively, the conoid tubercle on the inferior surface of the lateral third of the clavicle can also be used as an anatomic landmark for this guide pin placement. The drill hole should be drilled as posterior as possible. Care has to be taken to avoid a "blow out" of the posterior cortical rim during subsequent reaming. Then, a 5-mm cannulated reamer is used to create the tunnel (Figs. 14.9 and 14.10). Again, we recommend starting with the smallest reamer and if necessary, the surgeon can ream sequentially to larger sizes. The goal is to select the smallest possible size, and therefore the tightest inference fit that can still allow graft passage. The bone tunnels are reamed in under power. After passing through the inferior cortex, the power driver is disconnected and the reamer can be pulled out manually to ensure that the tunnel is a perfect cylinder and not widened by uneven reaming on the way out.

The depth of the tunnel is measured for appropriate screw length placement. The same steps should be repeated for the trapezoid ligament, which is anatomically located more anteriorly

and laterally than the conoid ligament. The bone tunnel for the trapezoid ligament should be centered on the clavicle in an AP dimension, approximately 15–20 mm lateral to the center of the previous tunnel, but definitely 25–30 mm medial to the AC joint. Biomechanically, Geaney et al. showed that the bone mineral density in the lateral third of the clavicle progressively increases from lateral to medial.[21] The optimal bone density was found in the anatomic insertion area of the CC ligaments between 20 and 50 mm medially from the lateral end of the clavicle. The distance from the AC joint line demonstrated a positive correlation to the pullout strength of the graft in cadaveric clavicles.[21]

Graft Fixation to the Clavicle and Reconstruction of CC Space and AC Joint Anatomy

Subsequently, one limb of the biologic graft is placed through the posterior bone tunnel (representing the conoid ligament) with the other limb being passed through the anterior bone tunnel in the same fashion (representing the trapezoid ligament; Fig. 14.11). The graft is not crossed. Then, the No. 2 collagen-coated Fiber-Wire looped around the coracoid is passed through the tunnels for providing a nonbiologic augmentation of the repair. Additionally, a reduction maneuver for the AC joint is performed involving an upward-directed force on the scapulohumeral complex combined with the use of a large, pointed reduction forceps placed on the undersurface of the coracoid process and on the posterosuperior border of the clavicle to reduce the AC joint (Fig. 14.12). Fluoroscopy is used to confirm the adequate reduction of the AC joint. The next step is critical to ensure that no migration or movement occurs after fixation: the graft has to be tensioned cyclically multiple times and passed through the tunnels back and forth to reduce any displacement that might occur after fixation. The graft is then positioned such that the graft limb representing the conoid ligament is left 2 cm proud from the superior margin of the clavicle. The long limb of the graft exits the trapezoid tunnel and is later used to augment the AC joint capsule. Next, a screw of appropriate size and length is placed in the posteromedial tunnel, anterior to the conoid ligament graft, with the graft under traction to ensure tautness. The size varies depending on graft size, but typically we prefer a 5.5 mm × 8 mm PEEK screw (Arthrex, Inc., Naples, FL, USA) (Fig. 14.13).

Again, the graft is cyclically loaded multiple times. While holding reduction and tension on the ligament, a second nonabsorbable screw (5.5 mm × 8 mm PEEK screw) is placed in the lateral tunnel anterior to the graft. We prefer a 5.5 mm × 8 mm PEEK screw for this as well. Finally, with both grafts being secured, the No. 2 collagen-coated FiberWire is tied over the top of the clavicle, to further augment the construct stability.

Now, the entire superior complex of the AC capsule can be augmented by using the limb of the graft used for the CC ligament reconstruction. Our preferred approach is to perform a repair of the AC joint capsule (capsule reconstruction), as recent studies have shown that its integrity ensures physiological centering of the AC joint under rotational loading and supports the synergistic effect of CC ligaments and AC capsule for maintaining joint stability.[22,23] The short limb of the graft exiting the medial tunnel is folded laterally and sewn to the base of the graft exiting the trapezoid tunnel in series. The long limb exiting the lateral (trapezoid) tunnel is routed laterally and looped on top of the AC joint as an augmentation of the AC joint capsule repair. The posterior graft is sewn into the acromion. The authors try to avoid bone anchors due to obvious issues with motion.

Finally, the deltotrapezial fascia, a critical stabilizer of the AC joint, is meticulously closed using interrupted nonabsorbable sutures, taking care to leave the knots on the posterior aspect of the trapezius. A Barrel stitch can be used to bury the knot if it is prominent (Fig. 14.14). The suture goes from the outside first on the deltoid, then crosses to the trapezius outside to in. The needle is then reversed to go inside to out and then cross back and go inside to out ("out, out, in, in") (Figs. 14.15–14.19).

Postoperative Care

The aim of postoperative rehabilitation should be to reinforce AC joint stability through strength training of the supporting muscles of the shoulder girdle and restore pain-free movement of the shoulder. We recommend using postoperative support with a Lerman Shoulder Orthosis (DJO Inc., Vista,

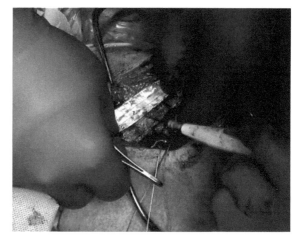

• **Fig. 14.12** To recreate the conoid ligament, a cannulated guide pin is placed approximately 45–50 mm medial from the distal end of the clavicle at the conoid tubercle and the posterior aspect of the clavicle.

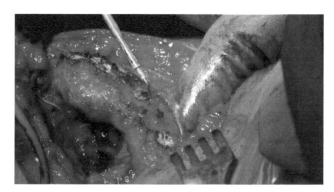

• **Fig. 14.13** The bone tunnel for the trapezoid ligament should be centered on the clavicle, approximately 15–20 mm lateral to the center portion of the previous tunnel, but definitely 25–30 mm medial to the acromioclavicular joint.

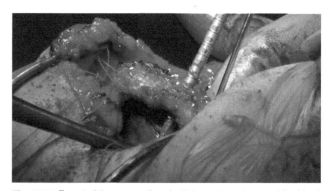

• **Fig. 14.14** For clavicle preparation, both bone tunnels are drilled in the clavicle to anatomically reconstruct the conoid and trapezoid ligaments. To recreate the conoid ligament, a cannulated guide pin is placed approximately 45–50 mm medial from the distal end of the clavicle at the conoid tubercle and the posterior inferior aspect of the clavicle. Alternatively, the conoid tubercle on the inferior surface of the lateral third of the clavicle can also be used as an anatomic landmark for this guide pin placement. The drill hole should be drilled as posterior as possible. Care has to be taken to avoid a "blow out" of the posterior cortical rim during subsequent reaming.

CA, USA) or a Gunslinger Shoulder Orthosis (Hanger Prosthetics & Orthotics Inc., Bethesda, MD, USA) for 6–8 weeks. These braces counter the downward pulling forces (gravity-dependent weight of the arm) on the CC and AC capsular repair. It is of great importance to educate the patient about

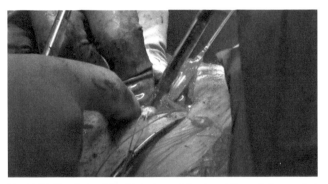

• **Fig. 14.15** One limb of the biologic graft is placed through the posterior bone tunnel (representing the conoid ligament) with the other limb being passed through the anterior bone tunnel in the same fashion (representing the trapezoid ligament).

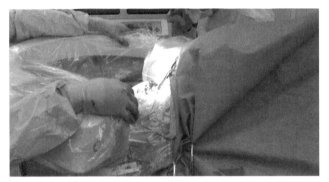

• **Fig. 14.16** A reduction maneuver for the acromioclavicular (AC) joint is performed involving an upward-directed force on the scapulohumeral complex combined with the use of a large, pointed reduction forceps placed on the undersurface of the coracoid process and on the postero-superior border of the clavicle to reduce the AC joint. Fluoroscopy is used to confirm the adequate reduction of the AC joint.

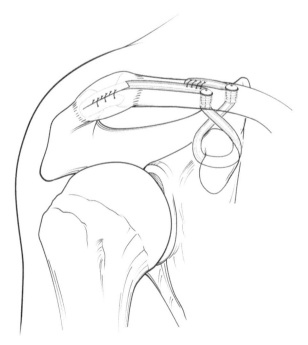

• **Fig. 14.17** The graft is positioned such that the graft limb representing the conoid ligament is left 2 cm proud from the superior margin of the clavicle. The long limb of the graft exits the trapezoid tunnel and is later used to augment the acromioclavicular joint capsule. Next, a screw of appropriate size and length is placed in the posteromedial tunnel, anterior to the conoid ligament graft, with the graft under traction to ensure tautness.

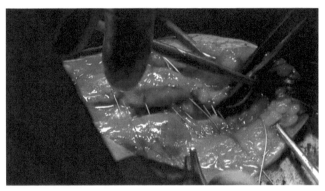

• **Fig. 14.18** The deltotrapezial fascia is meticulously closed using interrupted nonabsorbable sutures, taking care to leave the knots on the posterior aspect of the trapezius. A Barrel stitch can be used to bury the knot if it is prominent.

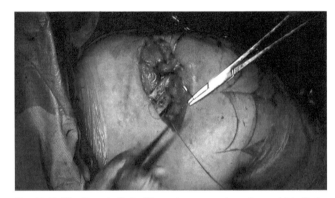

• **Fig. 14.19** The Barrel stitch: The suture goes from the outside first on the deltoid, then crosses to the trapezius outside to in. The needle is then reversed to go inside to out and then cross back and go inside to out ("out, out, in, in").

the importance of immobilization and protection of repair in the brace during the first 6 weeks, as it is critical in preventing early postoperative failure. Initial rehabilitative intervention is directed toward reducing pain and inflammation to allow for initiation of strength-based exercise as soon as possible. For the first 6–8 weeks, the brace may be removed for grooming and supine gentle passive ROM only. Active-assisted and active ROM exercises are progressively introduced starting at 6 weeks after surgery. If a painless ROM is obtained, strength training is started at 12 weeks. Full activity can be resumed after 24 weeks.

Complications

Complications include loss of reduction and recurrence of deformity, infection, stiff shoulder, graft failure, coracoid fracture, clavicle fracture, (distal) clavicle or coracoid osteolysis, tunnel osteolysis, hypertrophic distal clavicle, brachial plexopathy, implant-related complications (broken hardware, symptomatic hardware), and osteoarthritis of AC joint.[7,26]

PEARLS AND PITFALLS

Surgery-related risks include nerve (plexus brachialis) or vascular (Arteria subclavia) injuries, pneumothorax, hemothorax, fractures of the clavicle, coracoid or acromion, loss of reduction, material or hardware failure, required change to an open approach, revision or donor side morbidity due to graft harvest (lesion to N. saphenous).[24,25]

Positioning and approach	• The patient's head should be repositioned to the side, allowing access for conoid tunnel drilling. • A large bump is placed under the scapula to improve access and visualization. • Positioning can be checked by a mini C-arm. • An alternative is to displace the clavicle anteriorly with a towel clip to allow access for conoid tunnel drilling. • The deltoid and trapezius fascia should be tagged to ensure good repair.
Graft management	• Graft ends are bulleted to allow for easy passage through clavicle tunnels. • Graft and sutures should be shuttled under the coracoid from medial to lateral. • By exposing the medial coracoid base, shuttling the graft from lateral to medial can be facilitated. Additionally, by inserting a Darrach retractor on the medial base, the passing device can be caught.
Tunnel preparation and graft fixation	• The surgeon should ream in under full power. When the power driver is disconnected, the surgeon should pull the reamer out manually to ensure that the tunnel is a perfect circle and not widened by uneven reaming on the way out. • We recommend starting with the smallest reamer possible. The surgeon can ream up at half-millimeter increments if the graft is too large. • The bone tunnels should be tapped to 5.5 mm. • The tenodesis screw should be inserted anteriorly to the graft to equally recreate posterior CC ligaments.

CC, Coracoclavicular.

References

1. Rockwood C. Disorders of the acromioclavicular joint. In: Rockwood CA, Matsen FA, eds. *The Shoulder.* Vol. 1. Philadelphia: WB Saunders; 1998.
2. Beitzel K, Cote MP, Apostolakos J, et al. Current concepts in the treatment of acromioclavicular joint dislocations. *Arthroscopy.* 2013;29(2):387–397.
3. Beitzel K, Mazzocca AD, Bak K, et al. ISAKOS upper extremity committee consensus statement on the need for diversification of the Rockwood classification for acromioclavicular joint injuries. *Arthroscopy.* 2014;30(2):271–278.
4. Aliberti GM, Kraeutler MJ, Trojan JD, Mulcahey MK. Horizontal instability of the acromioclavicular joint: a systematic review. *Am J Sports Med.* 2020;48(2):504-510. doi:10.1177/0363546519831013. [Epub 2019 Apr 23.].
5. Braun S, Beitzel K, Buchmann S, Imhoff AB. Arthroscopically assisted treatment of acute dislocations of the acromioclavicular joint. *Arthrosc Tech.* 2015;4(6):e681–e685.
6. Dyrna F, Berthold DP, Feucht MJ, et al. The importance of biomechanical properties in revision acromioclavicular joint stabilization: a scoping review. *Knee Surg Sports Traumatol Arthrosc.* 2019;27(12):3844–3855.

7. Moatshe G, Kruckeberg BM, Chahla J, et al. Acromioclavicular and coracoclavicular ligament reconstruction for acromioclavicular joint instability: a systematic review of clinical and radiographic outcomes. *Arthroscopy.* 2018;34(6):1979–1995. e1978.
8. Muench LN, Kia C, Jerliu A, et al. Functional and radiographic outcomes after anatomic coracoclavicular ligament reconstruction for type III/V acromioclavicular joint injuries. *Orthop J Sports Med.* 2019;7(11). 2325967119884539.
9. Rabalais RD, McCarty E. Surgical treatment of symptomatic acromioclavicular joint problems: a systematic review. *Clin Orthop Relat Res.* 2007;455:30–37.
10. Tischer T, Salzmann GM, El-Azab H, Vogt S, Imhoff AB. Incidence of associated injuries with acute acromioclavicular joint dislocations types III through V. *Am J Sports Med.* 2009;37(1):136–139.
11. Braun S, Martetschläger F, Imhoff AB. *Acromioclavicular Joint Injuries and Reconstruction. Sports Injuries: Prevention, Diagnosis, Treatment and Rehabilitation*; 2015:1–12.
12. Martetschläger F, Kraus N, Scheibel M, Streich J, Venjakob A, Maier D. The diagnosis and treatment of acute dislocation of the acromioclavicular joint. *Dtsch Arztebl Int.* 2019;116(6):89–95.
13. Scheibel M, Dröschel S, Gerhardt C, Kraus N. Arthroscopically assisted stabilization of acute high-grade acromioclavicular joint separations. *Am J Sports Med.* 2011;39(7):1507–1516.
14. Garrigues G, Endres N, Singh A, et al. Clinical results of percutaneous acromioclavicular screw placement. *Shoulder Elbow.* 2011;3:88–94.
15. Pogorzelski J, Beitzel K, Ranuccio F, et al. The acutely injured acromioclavicular joint–which imaging modalities should be used for accurate diagnosis? A systematic review. *BMC Musculoskelet Disord.* 2017;18(1):515.
16. Gastaud O, Raynier JL, Duparc F, et al. Reliability of radiographic measurements for acromioclavicular joint separations. *Orthop Traumatol Surg Res.* 2015;101(8 Suppl):S291–S295.
17. Schneider MM, Balke M, Koenen P, et al. Inter- and intraobserver reliability of the Rockwood classification in acute acromioclavicular joint dislocations. *Knee Surg Sports Traumatol Arthrosc.* 2016;24(7):2192–2196.
18. Alexander OM. Dislocation of the acromioclavicular joint. *Radiography.* 1949;15(179):260 (illust).
19. Berthold D, Dyrna F, Imhoff A, Martetschlaeger F. Innovations for treatment of acromioclavicular joint instability. *Arthroskopie.* 2019;32(1):11–14.
20. Chahla J, Marchetti DC, Moatshe G, et al. Quantitative assessment of the coracoacromial and the coracoclavicular ligaments with 3-dimensional mapping of the coracoid process anatomy: a cadaveric study of surgically relevant structures. *Arthroscopy.* 2018;34(5):1403–1411.
21. Geaney LE, Beitzel K, Chowaniec DM, et al. Graft fixation is highest with anatomic tunnel positioning in acromioclavicular reconstruction. *Arthroscopy.* 2013;29(3):434–439.
22. Dyrna FGE, Imhoff FB, Voss A, et al. The integrity of the acromioclavicular capsule ensures physiological centering of the acromioclavicular joint under rotational loading. *Am J Sports Med.* 2018;46(6):1432–1440.
23. Morikawa D, Dyrna F, Cote MP, et al. Repair of the entire superior acromioclavicular ligament complex best restores posterior translation and rotational stability. *Knee Surg Sports Traumatol Arthrosc.* 2019;27: 3764–3770. https://doi.org/10.1007/s00167-018-5205-y.
24. Berthold DP, Muench LN, Dyrna F, et al. Komplikationsmanagement in der Versorgung von Verletzungen des Akromioklavikulargelenks. *Arthroskopie* 2020;33:171–175. https://doi.org/10.1007/s00142-020-00361-7.
25. Berthold DP, Muench LN, Dyrna F, et al. Radiographic alterations in clavicular bone tunnel width following anatomic coracoclavicular ligament reconstruction (ACCR) for chronic acromioclavicular joint injuries. *Knee Surg Sports Traumatol Arthrosc.* 2020. https://doi.org/10.1007/s00167-020-05980-z. [Epub ahead of print].
26. Carofino BC, Mazzocca AD. The anatomic coracoclavicular ligament reconstruction: surgical technique and indications. *J Shoulder Elbow Surg.* 2010;19(2 Suppl):37–46.

15

The Scapula—Body, Glenoid and Process Fractures

LISA K. SCHRODER AND PETER A. COLE

Introduction

Scapula fractures are receiving unprecedented attention in the orthopedic community, as illustrated by a simple PubMed search for "scapula fracture." Search results provide only 82 publications in the 150 years from 1818 to 1967, followed by the 30-year span from 1968 until 1999, a period dubbed as the dark ages of scapula fracture care when these injuries were largely treated with benign neglect, and new publications appeared at a rate of fewer than 15 per year. In the 20 years since the start of the new millennium, more than twice as many publications have emerged ($n = 983$) at a rate tripling the previous three decades, of 49 per year. In the last 2 years alone, 212 new publications regarding scapula fractures have been listed on PubMed. Presumably, this rapidly increasing interest is spawned by an awakening among orthopedic traumatologists and shoulder surgeons alike, to understand the nuances of scapula fractures in a way that aligns the diagnosis and treatment with that of other fractures. This phenomenon could also be related to the recognition that with significant malunion deformity of scapula comes substantial dysfunction, thus supporting the well-known AO (Arbeitsgemeinschaft für Osteosynthesefragen) axiom that musculoskeletal function follows skeletal form. As with other fractures surgically treated with open reduction and internal fixation (ORIF), rendering stability to the unstable and displaced "shoulder blade" fracture expedites pain relief and functional recovery.

Important early descriptions of scapula fractures were published in 1723 by Jean-Louis Petit, whose extraordinary work distinguished fractures of the body, neck, and processes.[1] These fractures were first documented radiographically by Grune in 1911,[2] nearly 200 years later. Albin Lambotte[3] published the first report of a scapular fracture treated with ORIF in 1910. In the United States, Longabaugh[4] reported successful operative fixation of a scapular body fracture of the distal angle, followed by a series from Reggio[5] and then Fischer.[6]

Despite larger surgical series emerging from Judet[7] and others,[8,9] a subsequent period of nonoperative management was widely embraced among orthopedists as appropriate for almost all scapula fractures.[10,11] Expectant management was supported by the premise that nearly all scapula fractures heal, and the shoulder has a capacity to compensate for morbidity due to its "global motion." This rationale was applied broadly to scapula fracture patients, except for the most significantly displaced intra-articular glenoid fractures, where there was general acceptance of the need to restore articular congruency.

Shoulder Anatomy and Biomechanics

The glenohumeral joint is a diarthrodial, multiaxial joint, and together with the smaller articulations of the sternoclavicular, acromioclavicular, and scapulothoracic joints ranks as the most mobile joint of the human body.[12,13] The proximal forequarter's extraordinary mobility is also attributed to the shallow glenoid fossa in which most of the stability is maintained by the compressive loading of opposing shoulder muscles and the labrum. The shoulder capsule provides the remainder of the restraint. The dynamic relationship of the humeral head to the glenoid, with all the muscles acting across this joint, has been likened to the balance of a ball on the nose of a seal with all the adjustments necessary to maintain equilibrium.[14] Correct muscle vectors and forces of the parascapular muscles are imperative for glenohumeral joint stability and pain-free full range of motion and shoulder strength.[15–18] Scapulohumeral rhythm, first described by Codman in the 1930s, describes the interplay between the scapulothoracic joint and the glenohumeral joint with a ratio of approximately 1:2, such that for every approximately 2 degrees of glenohumeral joint motion, the scapulothoracic joint will move 1 degree.[19] Thus the scapula acts as a mobile platform—a foundation that allows the glenoid to be oriented in a way that will resist subluxation forces and allow maximal range of motion.

Importantly, Goss[20] first described the concept of the superior shoulder suspensory complex (SSSC) to characterize the osseoligamentous ring that includes the glenoid, coracoid, clavicle, and acromion process along with the connecting soft tissues between these

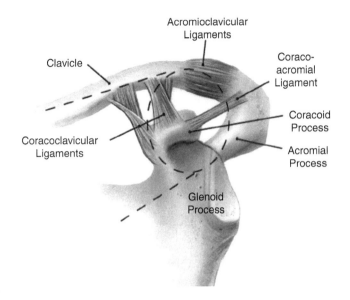

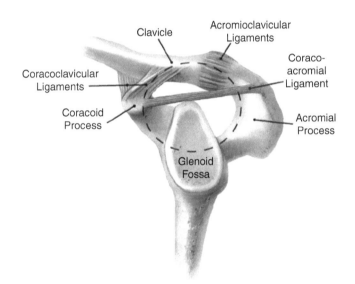

• **Fig. 15.1** The superior shoulder suspensory complex described by Goss characterizes the osseoligamentous ring that includes the glenoid, coracoid, clavicle, and acromion process along with the connecting soft tissues between these structures (i.e., coracoclavicular ligament and acromioclavicular joint capsule). (Reproduced with permission from Goss TP. Double disruptions of the superior shoulder suspensory complex. J Orthop Trauma. 1993;7(2):99-106. https://doi.org/10.1097/00005131-199304000-00001. PMID: 8459301.)

structures (i.e., coracoclavicular ligament and acromioclavicular joint capsule). Goss taught that an interruption of two or more structures within this ring resulted in a disruption of the suspension system between the axial and appendicular skeleton[20] (Fig. 15.1).

Our own recent work has also focused on the important aspects of the scapulothoracic joint allowing for gliding motion of the scapula across the chest wall. Chest wall injury, which commonly occurs concomitantly with scapula fracture, can result in abhorrent shoulder motion, impeding the patient's full recovery from high-energy injury[21] (Fig. 15.2).

Finally, within the orthopedic arena today, a discussion of shoulder biomechanics would not be complete without consideration for the introduction of modified biomechanics and bony

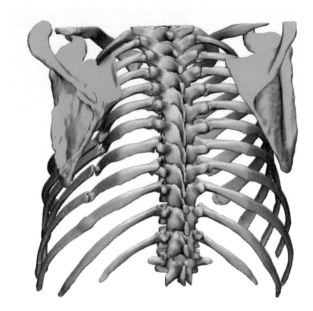

• **Fig. 15.2** A three-dimensional computed tomography reconstruction several years following successful open reduction and internal fixation of the patient's left scapula, illustrating the persistent deformity of the thoracic cage with malunions of ribs 3 through 7 and nonunions of ribs 8 and 9. The outlines of medial and lateral border plates on the healed scapula are visible. This patient has ongoing functional limitation and pain due to the underlying deformity of the scapulothoracic joint on which the scapula attempts to glide during range of motion of the left upper extremity. Retraction and protraction of the scapula are most symptomatic.

structures following joint replacement. Hemiarthroplasty of the shoulder (HSA), as well as total shoulder replacement (TSA) and reverse total shoulder arthroplasty (rTSA), may all be encountered in the setting of scapula fracture and the dilemmas presented to the orthopedic traumatologists. This has become especially true in regard to the growing awareness of acromion stress fractures in the presence of rTSA[22,23] (Fig. 15.3).

Mechanism of Injury, Concomitant Injuries, and Pathomechanics

Scapula fractures have been thought to occur at a rate of <1% of all fractures.[24] Though in epidemiological reports, they appear to occur at a rate similar to distal humerus fractures, midfoot and distal femur fractures.[24] A recent analysis from the National Trauma Data Bank (NTDB) included a review of 106,119 patients having scapula fractures occurring within the decade of 2002–12.[25] This study revealed a two-fold increase in the rate of diagnosis and reporting of scapula fractures coincidentally with an increase in the utilization of spiral computed tomography (CT) in most trauma patients. Other notable findings included a decrease in the proportion of scapula fractures occurring in motor vehicle accidents, with an increase in the number of fall-related injuries and an increasing proportion of these injuries occurring in the 60- to 79-year-old patient population (Fig. 15.4). Similar results to these were also found in a Finnish study covering the same general time period.[26]

Diagnosis of a scapula fracture remains a marker of high-energy trauma in the majority of patients and is associated with concomitant injury rates of 80%–95% in operative scapula series.[27–31] The

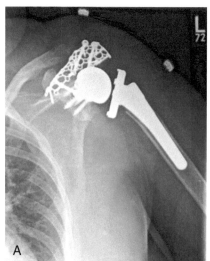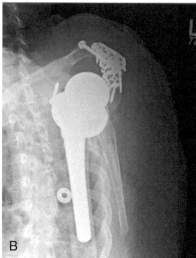

• **Fig. 15.3** (A) Anteroposterior and (B) scapular-Y radiographs of the left shoulder following reconstruction of an acromial stress fracture nonunion. A variable angle mesh plate was shaped intraoperatively and applied with 2.4/2.7 locking screws and (2) 2.7-mm lag screws were used across the fracture to gain compression.

most frequent combination of musculoskeletal injuries encountered includes concomitant rib fractures in >50%,[25,32] clavicle fracture (25%–39%), humeral fracture (11%–15%), and multiple disruptions to the SSSC.[32–34] More recently, periprosthetic fractures have also been reported, and there is evidence that the incidence in fragility fractures of the shoulder blade is increasing.[25,35]

Biomechanical and clinical studies of scapula fractures and forequarter injury have shown that severe displacement of scapula fractures can result in functional alterations and unsatisfactory outcomes if treated nonoperatively.[36–40] An understanding of the common fracture lines where the largest amount of fracture displacement has been found to occur will give the treating physician an understanding of both deforming muscular forces acting upon the fractured scapula and the likely dysfunction which may result if the scapula is left to heal with substantial displacement, malrotation, and angulation. Armitage and Cole mapped fracture patterns resulting in displaced common patterns, which can inform the reader and assist in clinical decision-making (Fig. 15.5).[41]

These patterns of highly displaced scapula fractures are, therefore, relevant to the work elucidating scapula neck malunions resulting in a loss of strength and altered muscle activation specifically during abduction shown in biomechanical models.[37] As the glenoid medializes or rotates inferiorly relative to the body and lateral border of the scapula, the rotator cuff shortens taking tension off these muscles which have essential upper extremity function, including the proper loading (vector and force) of the glenoid fossa. Compressive muscular forces change to shear forces as a function of this aberrancy. Gauger et al. documented by quantitative three-dimensional (3D) shoulder motion analysis, the altered motion in a scapular malunion patient, which was shown to be normalized following surgical reconstruction of the scapula and clavicle.[42] A series presented by the senior author at the 2017 OTA (Orthopaedic Trauma Association) described 26 patients with 34 malunions and/or nonunions of the scapula inclusive of neck, body, and process, which demonstrated statistically significant improved motion, strength, and functional outcome following scapula malunion reconstruction.[43] In a more recent investigation accepted for publication, the treatment of process malunions

and nonunions of the coracoid and acromion also reveals a morbid and dysfunctional baseline nearly completely reversible after reconstruction using a principled approach to restoring anatomy and bony union.[44] Unfortunately, it remains unknown how much displacement resulting in malunion is tolerable to retain adequate upper extremity functionality.

Evaluation

Due to the high-energy mechanisms causing most scapula fractures, it is vital to perform a thorough evaluation of any patient presenting with a scapula fracture because of the high associated injury rate.[30,31,45] Prioritization of injuries in terms of treatment follows full trauma resuscitation of patients. From several operative series which represent the severe end of the energy spectrum, we know a keen workup will yield positive findings for associated upper extremity fractures in up to 50% of patients, brachial plexus and peripheral nerve lesions in about 10%, significant chest injury in over 80%, as well as both cervical spine and traumatic brain injury in 15%. A thorough physical examination with a critical secondary survey alongside three X-ray views of the shoulder and a chest radiograph should provide the necessary information for clinical decision-making. We have seen a rapid adoption of spiral CT in the trauma patient over the past 10–15 years, which makes access to 3D CT reconstructions of the injured thorax and forequarter possible in most emergency centers.

Examination

In the immediate acute injury phase, an awake and cooperative patient can direct the physical examination by indicating the location of pain. Shoulder asymmetry with a slumped or depressed shoulder (so-called shoulder ptosis), if not medialized, is commonly observed.[46] This deformity becomes more apparent in some patients, particularly those who are upright and ambulatory post injury (Fig. 15.6). The skin should be inspected for abrasions and scabs, particularly over the prominent acromion (Fig. 15.7). This finding should affect surgical timing.

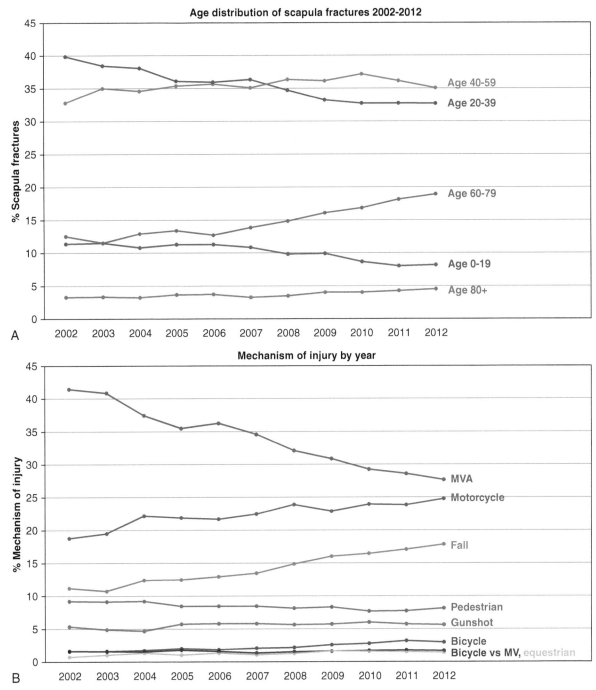

Fig. 15.4 From a study of the National Trauma Data Bank 2002 and 2012 registry data, changing demographics of scapula fractures can be understood. (A) Scapula fractures occurring due to motor vehicle accidents *(MVA)* are steadily declining, while motorcycle collision and fall-related injuries have increased during the same time period. (B) In the same time period, the percentage of fractures in the younger age group has declined (age 20–39), while the older age groups (age 60–79 and 80+) have increased. This increase indicates a rise in fall-related fragility fractures. (Reprinted with permission from Tatro JM, Schroder LK, Molitor BA, Parker ED, Cole PA. Injury mechanism, epidemiology, and hospital trends of scapula fractures: a 10-year retrospective study of the National Trauma Data Bank. *Injury.* 2019;50(2):376-381. https://doi.org/10.1016/j.injury.2019.01.017.)

Every bone and joint should be palpated and inspected to assess for swelling, crepitance, instability, and pain. The neck should be assessed for tenderness, and deep palpation of the clavicle and thorax should be performed to direct further radiographic assessment for the common ipsilateral rib and clavicle fractures. It should be assumed that the shoulder will hurt with motion, but active forward elevation should be attempted to delineate minimally displaced variants not requiring surgery from those variants in which shoulder motion of any magnitude is extremely painful. Specifically palpate the acromioclavicular and sternoclavicular joints, sites of sometimes subtle but relevant findings. Take the wrist and elbow through a full active and passive range-of-motion

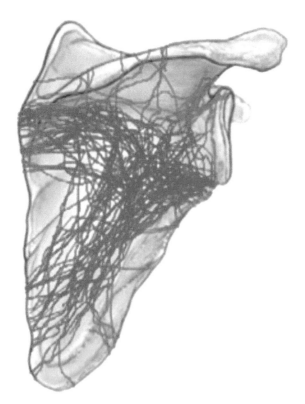

• **Fig. 15.5** From the work of Armitage et al., a cohort of 90 operative scapula fractures including all extra-articular fractures that entered (exited) the lateral border inferior to the glenoid were overlaid to create a fracture heat map. (Reproduced with permission from Armitage BM, Wijdicks CA, Tarkin IS, et al. Mapping of scapular fractures with three-dimensional computed tomography. *J Bone Joint Surg Am.* 2009;91(9):2222-2228.)

Area

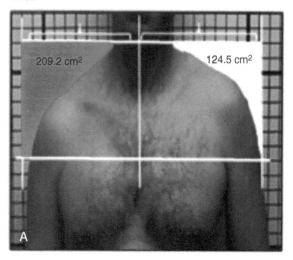

Angle

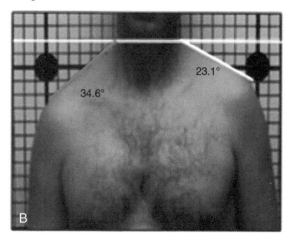

Shoulder Height

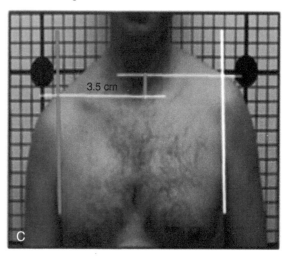

• **Fig. 15.6** Clinical examination of the upright patient with a scapula fracture can reveal marked shoulder deformity. In this illustration, using a posture grid behind the patient, the difference in area, angulation, and shoulder height can be quantified between the injured *(red)* and noninjured *(yellow)* shoulders.[46] (Reprinted with permission from Tatro JM, Anderson JP, McCreary DL, Schroder LK, Cole PA. Radiographic correlation of clinical shoulder deformity and patient perception following scapula fracture. *Injury.* 2020;51(7):1584-1591. https://doi.org/10.1016/j.injury.2020.04.017.)

examination. Next, pulses at the wrist and a detailed neurologic examination of C5-T1 should be documented.

Concomitant nerve lesions are particularly common, yet may only be detected by sensory examination because of the inability for active motion of the patient's shoulder. A high index of suspicion for axillary and suprascapular nerve lesions should be considered with particular attention to the fracture pattern which extends through the suprascapular notch and/or scapula neck areas. Due to most patients' inability to externally rotate because of pain, these findings often manifest later in treatment.

In the intubated or obtunded patient, palpation and motion to detect crepitation is important, including subcutaneous crepitation along the thorax and neck region, which will be positive in many patients with pneumothoraces. This finding may direct the placement of a chest tube unless already performed by the trauma service.

Imaging

Upon presentation to the emergency room, a chest X-ray and CT scan will often be the first opportunity to identify a scapula fracture. Tatro et al. recently found that the routine use of spiral CT in the emergency setting resulted in a two-fold increase in the diagnosis of scapula fracture among NTDB-reported patients.[25] Blunt chest trauma associated with shoulder pain, deformity, or the radiographic presence of other ipsilateral injuries warrants dedicated shoulder imaging. Three plain X-ray views should be evaluated: anteroposterior (AP) Grashey, scapula Y, and axillary

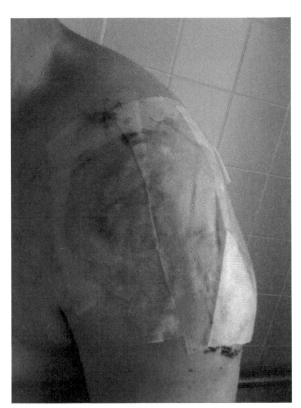

• **Fig. 15.7** A clinical image of commonly seen skin abrasions in a patient with a scapula fracture. The patient is shown with an ADAPTIC dressing applied. Reepithelialization is recommended prior to surgical intervention.

views (Figs. 15.8–15.10). It is not uncommon to be misled by displacement and fracture patterns seen on conventional shoulder X-rays.[47] CT scans with 3D reconstructions (Fig. 15.9) have proven to be a gold standard for evaluation of fracture displacement and ultimate treatment decisions. Measurement of lateral border offset (LBO), angulation, glenopolar angle (GPA), and translation of the scapula have become accepted methods forming a common language to quantitatively describe fracture displacement and deformity.[48]

Certain extra-articular injury patterns may be prone to progressive deformity in the early postinjury period.[49] Therefore it is recommended that serial radiographs be obtained on a weekly basis for up to 3 weeks post injury. Upright standing or seated films, when possible, help accentuate ligamentous injuries (e.g., AC separation) as the force of gravity becomes evident. Articular displacement and measurement of step-offs and gaps are best visualized on two-dimensional (2D) CT. Critical assessment of each scapula process and the articulations at each end of the clavicle is also important.

Diagnosis and Classification

Historical classifications for scapula fractures include those of Hardegger,[50] Ada-Miller,[36] as well as progressive iterations of AO/OTA.[51] Both Ada-Miller and Hardegger have been classically beneficial in that their subclassifications reflect patterns commonly encountered in practice. The 2018 AO/OTA Fracture and Dislocation Classification Compendium continues to refine its scapula classification, dividing the scapula into three basic segments: processes, body, and glenoid fossa.[51] The glenoid fossa fractures are further subdivided based on the quadrant and number of

fracture lines involved (Fig. 15.10). Focused classifications have also existed for the glenoid, acromion, and coracoid. Mayo et al.[45] expanded the Ideberg classification for intra-articular fractures, but some authors are finding improved reliability in the use of the AO/OTA classification for intra-articular glenoid fractures, as well (Fig. 15.11).[52]

3D reconstructions have been used to create a comprehensive scapula fracture map[40] (Fig. 15.12), though even this likely does not create the most accurate reconstruction of the complex anatomy of scapula fractures[53] (Fig. 15.13). Work still remains to be accomplished to form the basis of a comprehensive classification scheme with actual fracture patterns found clinically.

Ogawa's classification system is specific to the acromion and coracoid.[54,55] Coracoid fractures were classified based on whether the fracture line ran anterior or posterior to the coracoclavicular ligaments, while the acromion fractures were classified based on the fracture proximity to the spinoglenoid notch. Anavian et al. mapped fractures of 26 operatively treated process fractures.[56] There was a higher prevalence of coracoid base fractures that extended into the glenoid with the fracture line running posterior to the coracoclavicular ligaments (an Ogawa Type I fracture) and acromion fractures that extended into the region of the spinoglenoid notch, or included the entire scapular spine (Ogawa Type II fracture). Notably, this specific series only included fractures displaced >1 cm, which was the surgical indication for the senior author.

In the setting of rTSA, Levy et al.[57] followed a similar description to Ogawa in categorizing the acromion stress fractures as Type I, II, or III when occurring as a complication to these procedures. In some series, these are the most common complication after rTSA occurring up to 4% of the time. The mechanism for acromial stress fractures appears to be that the deltoid recruitment and increased activity afforded by the rTSA leads to increased forces through the acromion. This can be worsened by underlying osteoporosis or osteopenia, an excessively tight articulation, reverse baseplate screws into the scapular spine that may act as a stress riser, or an acromion compromised by acetabularization and the abrasive effects of long-standing cuff tear arthropathy.

Management

Emergent Treatment

High-energy scapula fractures serve as harbingers of associated life-threatening injuries that do warrant emergent treatment. Scapula fractures in and of themselves generally do not pose emergent threats, or conditions that warrant immediate surgical treatment, other than the occasional open fracture. Open fractures usually occur at the level of the acromion due to the superficial osseous structure, when the mechanism of injury is a direct superior blow. This condition should be treated using the principles of open fracture management and ideally stabilized with internal fixation, if the treating surgeon on call is familiar with techniques to fix the acromion.[58] Careful review of the chest X-ray and/or CT should also be accomplished in the emergent setting, as concomitant rib fractures are associated with >50% of scapula fractures, and a pneumothorax may require chest tube placement. The orthopedic team should work closely with the general surgery trauma team in the management of such patients, and timing of the scapula surgery with or without rib ORIF should be accomplished in a collaborative fashion.

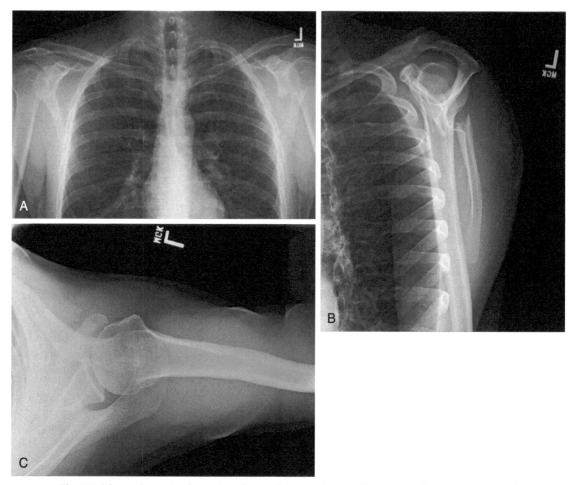

• **Fig. 15.8** Injury radiographs of an extra-articular left scapula fracture. (A) Anteroposterior view, (B) scapula Y view, and (C) axillary view of the left scapula.

Indications for Definitive Care

Specific radiographic measurements of scapula fracture displacement have begun to form a consistent basis for clinical decision-making and discussion in contemporary peer-reviewed literature including clinical reports and outcomes assessment. Though no Level 1 data exist, and operative indications remain relative and based upon expert opinion, there is a growing body of evidence to suggest that outcomes are good or excellent and risks of surgery are low.

Explicitly defined measurements of scapula fracture characteristics as described by Anavian et al. in 2011 have formed the basis of a common language in understanding the severity of scapula fracture injuries.[48] 3D CT reconstructions are now considered the gold standard in the severely displaced variants in which surgery is being considered. If operative indications are suspected based upon the 2D radiographic images, by obtaining 3D-CT reconstructions, a full and accurate assessment of LBO, angular deformity, and glenopolar angular deformity can be quantitatively measured. These measurements, best obtained from an appropriately oriented 3D CT reconstruction, include LBO, angulation, and GPA (Fig 15.9). This measurement technique has been shown to be valid in inter- and intrareader reliability.

Authors such as Hardegger et al.,[50] Ada and Miller,[36] Nordqvist and Petersson,[38] and Romero et al.[59] clearly influence and inform the surgical indications which have evolved. Findings from

these authors indicated a clear relationship in patients with the most severe injuries resulting in persistent shoulder disability and residual deformity, seen radiographically. These patients have been shown to be most likely to have functional complaints and pain following nonsurgical treatment.[36]

For extra-articular scapular fractures with or without concomitant ipsilateral shoulder girdle fractures, four articles, beginning with Ada and Miller in 1991,[36] have proposed medial displacement or LBO of >1 to >2.5 cm as one indication for surgery.[60–62] These same authors state that angular deformity of >25 to >45 degrees would also be an indication for operative treatment, as well as combined injuries with intra-articular involvement, or multiple disruptions of the SSSC. The senior author's preferred guidelines for surgical indications are summarized in Table 15.1. Although nondisplaced or minimally displaced, stable fractures are generally treated nonoperatively. The patient's functional demands and overall health status will, of course, guide care considerations in shared decision-making.

Nonoperative Treatment Outcomes

As with principles of fracture treatment in most other areas of the anatomy, minimally to moderately displaced, stable extra-articular fractures should be treated nonoperatively with a sling for 2–3 weeks, until fracture consolidation and pain subsidence occur. In

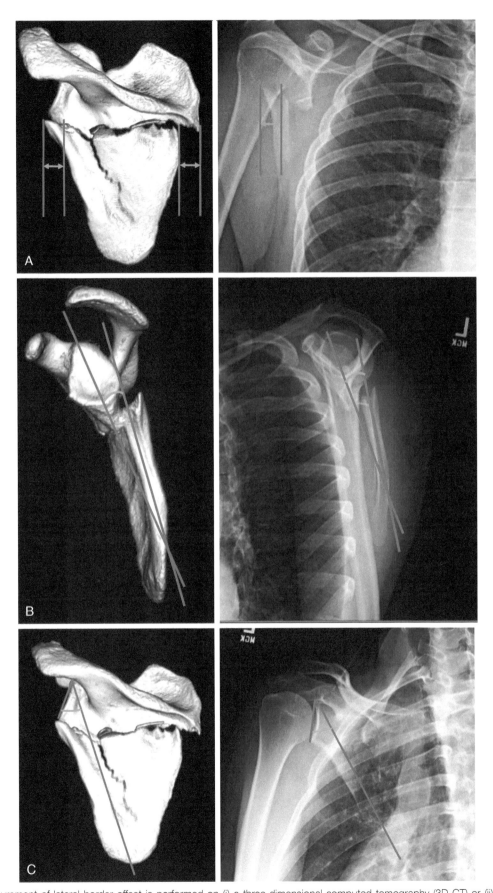

• **Fig. 15.9** (A) Measurement of lateral border offset is performed on (i) a three-dimensional computed tomography (3D CT) or (ii) scapular radiograph oriented in the posteroanterior view. Lateral border offset is measured by drawing a line from the lateral-most extent of the inferior fragment and another perpendicular line from the lateral-most aspect of the superior fragment. (B) Angulation deformity is measured on (i) a 3D CT image of a scapula in the trans-scapular Y orientation and (ii) a scapula Y radiograph. The angle is formed by the intersection of a line running parallel to the proximal fragment and a line running parallel to the distal fragment. Note that even though the inferior teardrop forms a concave surface over the rib cage, it is the more proximal straight portion of the intramedullary canal that is used for the measurement. (C) Measurement of glenopolar angle is performed on (i) a 3D CT oriented in the posteroanterior view and (ii) scapula Y radiographs. The glenopolar angle measurement is made by drawing a line from the inferior to the superior pole of the glenoid fossa and another line from the superior pole to the apex of the scapula body's inferior angle.

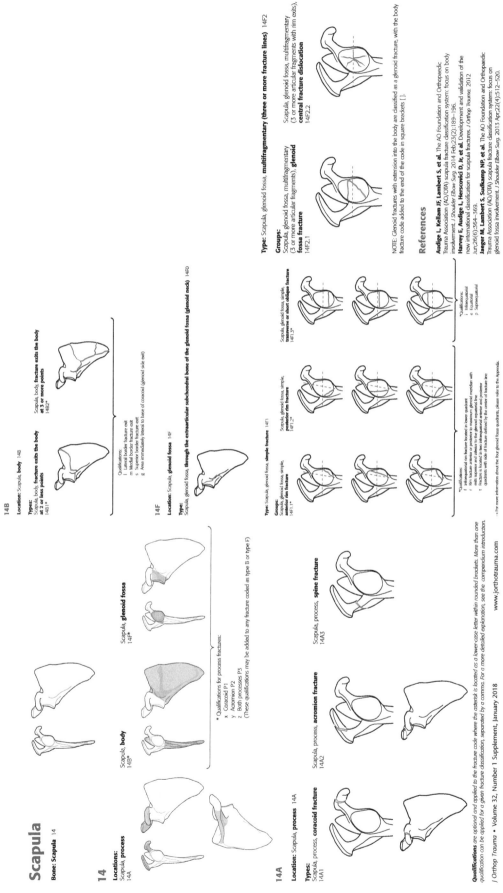

• **Fig. 15.10** The 2018 Arbeitsgemeinschaft für Osteosynthesefragen/Orthopaedic Trauma Association (AO/OTA or OTA/AO) Fracture and Dislocation Classification Compendium. This is the second and most recent revision of the compendium. (From Meinberg E, Agel J, Roberts C, et al. Fracture and dislocation classification compendium. *J Orthop Trauma.* 2018;32:[1]. With permission.)

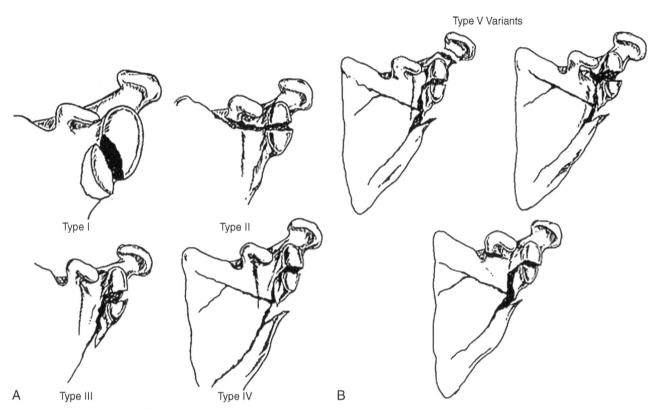

• **Fig. 15.11** Diagram of the modified Ideberg classification of glenoid fractures. (From Mayo KA, Benirschke SK, Mast JW. Displaced fractures of the glenoid fossa. Results of open reduction and internal fixation. *Clin Orthop Relat Res.* 1998;347:122–130, Fig. 1-A–B, p 125. With permission.)

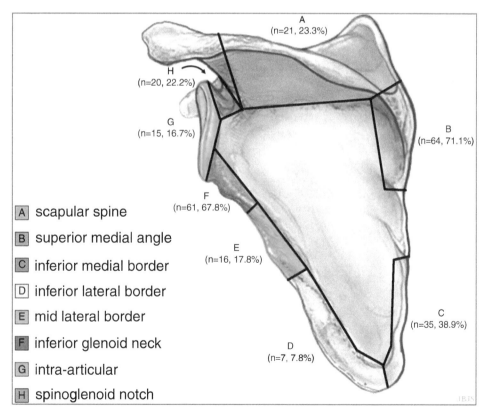

A scapular spine

B superior medial angle

C inferior medial border

D inferior lateral border

E mid lateral border

F inferior glenoid neck

G intra-articular

H spinoglenoid notch

• **Fig. 15.12** A code map demonstrating the frequency (totals and percentages) of involvement of different parts of the scapula by the fractures in the ninety subjects in this series. (From Armitage BM, Wijdicks CA, Tarkin IS, et al. Mapping of scapular fractures with three-dimensional computed tomography, *J Bone Joint Surg Am.* 2009;91[9]:2222–2228. With permission.)

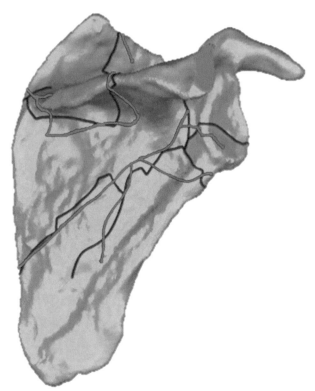

• **Fig. 15.13** Utilizing a proprietary 3D graphics software, Dugarte et al. traced fracture lines following re-orientation of the fracture fragments and tracing in 3D vs 2D. The *(red) lines* are from the 2D overlay process, the *(black) lines* are fracture line tracing in 3D for the same patients. (From Dugarte AJ, Tkany L, Schroder LK, Petersik A, Cole PA. Comparison of 2 versus 3 dimensional fracture mapping strategies for 3 dimensional computerized tomography reconstructions of scapula neck and body fractures: THREE-DIMENSIONAL SCAPULAR FRACTURE DATABASE. *Journal of Orthopaedic Research*. Published online June 2, 2017. https://doi.org/10.1002/jor.23603)

TABLE 15.1	Guidelines and Surgical Indications
Injury	**Displacement**
Lateral border offset	20 mm (sometimes called medialization measured on anteroposterior scapula)
Glenopolar angle	<22 degrees (sometimes called glenopolar angle)
Angulation	>45 degrees (measured on scapula Y view)
Articular step-off	> 4 mm (>20% required for instability)
Double lesions of superior shoulder suspensory complex (SSSC)	(each lesion should be displaced >1 cm)
Triple and quadruple lesions of the SSSC	(acromioclavicular dislocation, clavicle, coracoid + neck)
Coracoid fracture	>10 mm
Acromion fracture	>5 mm
Reverse total shoulder arthroplasty painful stress fracture	>1 mm (after conservative management failure)
Nonunion-malunion scapula	Pain dysfunction (commonly in fractures which would have been indicated)
Translation and anteversion	Undefined

These displacements are not commonly used for indications, but likely have important influence on outcome and should be studied.

our experience, approximately 10% of patients presenting through the emergency department meet established operative criteria due to fracture displacement.[63] Due to the lack of Level 1 evidence in the literature on this topic, there are conflicting opinions and only Level IV evidence of therapeutic outcomes to advise surgical indications. **In our center, nonoperative treatment is reserved for those patients with <20 mm of LBO (or medialization) or <45 degrees of angular deformity of the scapular body or neck on a scapula Y view.** In the presence of clinical healing and pain subsidence, management with a sling and progressive physical therapy generally provides good results in these patients.

During the early stages of healing, patients may experience pseudo paralysis and report altered or lack of function of the injured shoulder. Progressive displacement in the early post injury period has been reported and certain injury patterns may be more prone to this occurring.[49,64] In a recent review by Steinmetz et al.,[64] transverse scapular body fractures were found to be an independent risk factor for displacement, when compared with nontransverse fractures (relative risk [RR]: 6.5, 95% confidence interval [CI]: 1.96–21.6, *P* =.0023). Serial radiographs should be obtained on a weekly basis for up to 3 weeks post injury. The possibility for increasing deformity likely occurs through fracture instability, muscular spasm, the weight of the body in the supine position, and gravitational forces when patients are upright and mobile. Scapular fractures associated with multiple consecutive

rib fractures, or double lesions of the SSSC, may be more vulnerable, due to the compromised thoracic and appendicular skeletal support, though this hypothesis has not been tested.

In 2020, two reports have been published describing nonoperative care in displaced extra-articular scapula fractures, as well as one scientific presentation from 2016, unpublished as of this writing.[65–67] Zlowodzki et al.[68] completed a systematic review for the treatment of scapular fractures. The results of the analysis showed that 70% (*n* = 325) of the scapular fractures were treated nonoperatively and 30% (*n* = 140) operatively. At that time, 99% (135/137) of isolated body fractures were treated nonoperatively with excellent to good results achieved in 86% of these cases. Dienstknecht and colleagues[69] performed a meta-analysis of operative versus nonoperative treatment in scapular neck fractures. This study encompassed 463 cases from 22 case series. There were 249 isolated neck fractures and 7 neck fractures were combined with coracoid, acromion, body, spine, or glenoid fractures. Though the results of the analysis could not detect any statistically relevant difference in restrictions of day-to-day activities or the Constant score (*P* = .16 and *P* = .62, respectively), they did find that a greater number of patients were pain-free during day-to-day activities in the surgical group (*P* < .00001). Newly published systematic reviews continue to conclude that no clear evidence exists to definitively guide surgical indications.[70–72] In addition, variability in reporting of outcomes from clinical series and case reports further limits the ability of these authors to perform meta-analyses with the published data.

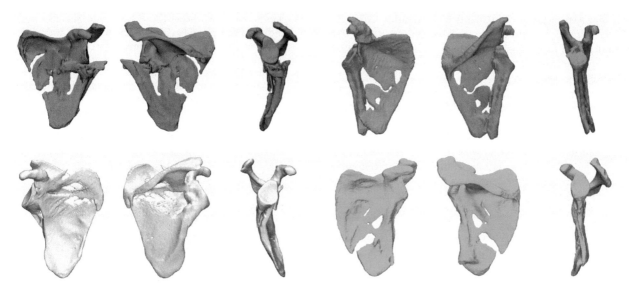

• **Fig. 15.14** 3D-CT reconstructions rotated to three views: Anteroposterior, Posterioanterior, and Scapula Y. Four patients with scapula malunions following nonoperative treatment of their injuries. All four had pain and dysfunction and sought reconstructive care.

There are reports of satisfactory outcomes for nonoperatively treated scapular fractures in the literature. Though some authors used only subjective surgeon assessments for the determination of "good" outcomes,[73] others made conclusions based upon the scoring systems of Rowe[10] or Constant and Murley.[74] It is impossible to discern from these reports the severity of injury since no discrete radiographic measures indicating degree of displacement are utilized.

Complications

Missed or Delayed Diagnosis

The anatomic position and morphology of the scapula, aligned off the coronal plane of the thorax by 30 degrees, may contribute to missed diagnoses of scapula fracture. In addition, associated injuries occur in up to 90% of scapula fractures, and therefore medical attention can be distracted from suspicion of scapular injury. Approximately 15% of scapular fracture patients have sustained a traumatic brain injury, further confounding the physical examination process. Missed or delayed diagnosis of scapula fractures can also occur when the clinician is unfamiliar with the anatomy or when expert care is not available at the treating center.[62,75,76]

Deformity and Malunion

Malunions of scapular fractures are likely more common than previously thought.[40,42] It stands to reason that nonoperatively treated fractures, which are displaced, predictably heal with poor alignment. Muscular deforming forces and the effect of gravity on the upper limb will influence this result, leading to pain, weakness, and glenohumeral imbalance.[37–39,59,77] Such forces acting on the shoulder girdle have been shown to continue to increase deformity in the early postinjury period in some patients, requiring certain unstable fracture patterns to be closely monitored radiographically.[49] Our center has become a referral center for these injuries, with patients presenting in a delayed fashion,[62] as well as several years post injury with ongoing pain, dysfunction, and dissatisfaction driving the patient to seek multiple opinions in their care. This can be true for both extra-articular neck and body fractures, and fractures of the acromion and coracoid processes[43,44] (Fig. 15.14).

Pain

In multiple case series reporting on nonoperative treatment of scapular fractures, pain is commonly described in association with healed scapular fractures. Pain is suspected to arise from deformity, scapulothoracic crepitus, rotator cuff dysfunction, and scarring.[38,39,59,77] Muscular imbalance leads to fatigue with sustained activities. Certainly, painful glenohumeral arthrosis results from ignored, displaced glenoid fractures as well.

Nonunion

The scapula is surrounded by a robust muscular envelope and rich vascular supply, leading to the rapid formation of callus, therefore making the nonunion of nonoperatively treated scapular body fractures an unexpected result.[78] Current controversy specifically exists in the care of acromial stress fractures following rTSA. While many centers are reporting acceptance of suboptimal outcomes in the presence of nonunion, other authors are applying principles of nonunion reconstruction with successful outcomes.[44,79,80]

Outcomes

Isolated Extra-Articular Fracture

Regardless of operative or nonoperative treatment in scapular fractures, nearly all reportedly heal. The circumstances of a well-protected muscular envelope with a rich blood supply contribute to rapid healing. This fact, combined with the shoulder's capability for compensatory motion, creates the basis of the continued controversy over operative indications.[65–67]

Studies stratifying outcomes by degree of initial deformity are lacking but necessary in the literature. One such study by Bozkurt et al.[39] in 18 patients with extra-articular fractures treated nonoperatively illustrates a positive correlation between the resulting deformity of decreased GPA and poorer shoulder Constant scores ($P < .05$). In the same way, Romero et al.[59] demonstrated that patients who healed with a GPA <20 degrees experienced significantly poorer outcomes ($P < .05$). Alternatively, Kim et al.[81]

showed improved outcomes in patients with resulting GPA >30 degrees versus patients with resulting GPA <30 degrees (P <.05). These studies form the basis of contemporary standards for one of the operative indications for displaced extra-articular fractures, an injury GPA ≤22 degrees.

Not all patients treated nonoperatively do well; not all scapular malunions are asymptomatic. Ada and Miller[35] first illustrated this in an evaluation of 24 nonoperatively treated scapular fractures, resulting in decreased range of motion (in 20%), residual pain (in 50%), and pain and weakness with exertion (in 40%) of the patients studied. The authors recommended operative treatment in patients with medial displacement or LBO >1 cm or angular deformity of >40 degrees.

Conclusions

Though the surgical treatment of scapula fractures was described one century ago, the past 15 years have provided a surge of scientific publications, which have aided in our current understanding of the importance of deformity and function after operative and nonoperative treatment. The goals of surgery for the scapula are now better aligned with those of other fractures throughout the body, and that is to render an anatomic reduction of the articular glenoid, establish length, alignment, and rotation of the neck and body to promote proper function, and provide stability to allow for effective rehabilitation, most often immediate passive and early active range of motion. These goals have borne out in multiple studies and expert observations of patients with malunions. In Chapter 16, we will discuss the complex decision-making involved in choosing approaches and describe the surgical options for ORIF of common fracture patterns.

References

1. Petit J. Traité des maladies des os. Tome second. Paris: Charles-Etienne Hochereau; 1723:122–138.
2. Grune O. Zur diagnose der frakturen im bereiche des collum scapulae. *Z Orthop Chir*. 1911;29:83–95.
3. Lambotte A. *Chirurgie opératoire des fractures*. Paris: Masson; 1913.
4. Longabaugh R. Surgical notes: fracture simple, right scapula. *United States Naval Medical Bulletin*. 1924;21:341.
5. Reggio A. Fracture of the shoulder girdle. In: Wilson P, ed. *Experience in the Management of Fractures and Dislocations, Based on an Analysis of 4,390 Cases*. Philadelphia: Lippincott; 1930:370–374.
6. Fischer WR. Fracture of the scapula requiring open reduction. *J Bone Joint Surg*. 1939;11(2):459–461.
7. Judet R. Traitement chirurgical des fractures de omoplate. *Acta Orthop Belg*. 1964;30:673–678.
8. Decoulx P, LeMerle MP. Fractures of the scapula. *Lille Chir*. 1956;11(4):215–227.
9. Tondeur G. [Recent shoulder fractures]. *Acta Orthop Belg*. 1964;30:1–144.
10. Rowe C. Fractures of the scapula. *Surg Clin North Am*. 1963;43:1565–1571.
11. Schnepp J, Comtet J, Cetre J, Ray A. Valeur du traitement non sanglant des fractures de l'omoplate [Value of nonsurgical treatment of omoplata fractures]. *Lyon Med*. 1968;220(40):809–813.
12. Howell S, Galinat B, Renzi A, Marone P. Normal and abnormal mechanics of the glenohumeral joint in the horizontal plane. *J Bone Joint Surg*. 1988;70(2):227–232.
13. De Palma A. *Surgery of the Shoulder*. 3rd ed. Philadelphia: Lippincott; 1983.
14. Hackney RG. Advances in the understanding of throwing injuries of the shoulder. *Br J Sports Med*. 1996;30(4):282–288. https://doi.org/10.1136/bjsm.30.4.282.
15. McClure PW, Michener LA, Karduna AR. Shoulder function and 3-dimensional scapular kinematics in people with and without shoulder impingement syndrome. *Phys Ther*. 2006;86(8):1075–1090.
16. Warner JJP, Micheli L, Arslanian LE, Kennedy J, Kennedy R. Scapulothoracic motion in normal shoulders and shoulders with glenohumeral instability and impingement syndrome. *Clin Orthop Relat Res*. 1992;285:191–199.
17. Myers JB, Riemann BL, Ju Y-Y, Hwang J-H, McMahon PJ, Lephart SM. Shoulder muscle reflex latencies under various levels of muscle contraction. *Clin Orthop Relat Res*. 2003;407:92–101. https://doi.org/10.1097/00003086-200302000-00017.
18. Latimer HA, Tibone JE, Pink MM, Mohr KJ, Perry J. Shoulder reaction time and muscle-firing patterns in response to an anterior translation force. *J Shoulder Elbow Surg*. 1998;7(6):610–615. https://doi.org/10.1016/S1058-2746(98)90009-X.
19. Codman EA. *The Shoulder*. Boston: Geo Miller & Co; 1934.
20. Goss TP. Double disruptions of the superior shoulder suspensory complex. *J Orthop Trauma*. 1993;7(2):99–106.
21. Ogunleye T, Carlson D, Schroder L, Cole P. Operative reconstruction of symptomatic rib nonunions and outcomes. In: *Chest Wall Injury Society Annual Summit*; 2020.
22. Patterson DC, Chi D, Parsons BO, Cagle PJ. Acromial spine fracture after reverse total shoulder arthroplasty: a systematic review. *J Shoulder Elbow Surg*. 2019;28(4):792–801. https://doi.org/10.1016/j.jse.2018.08.033.
23. Zmistowski B, Gutman M, Horvath Y, Abboud JA, Williams GR, Namdari S. Acromial stress fracture following reverse total shoulder arthroplasty: incidence and predictors. *J Shoulder Elbow Surg*. 2020;29(4):799–806. https://doi.org/10.1016/j.jse.2019.08.004.
24. Court-Brown CM, Caesar B. Epidemiology of adult fractures: a review. *Injury*. 2006;37(8):691–697. https://doi.org/10.1016/j.injury.2006.04.130.
25. Tatro JM, Schroder LK, Molitor BA, Parker ED, Cole PA. Injury mechanism, epidemiology, and hospital trends of scapula fractures: a 10-year retrospective study of the National Trauma Data Bank. *Injury*. 2019;50(2):376–381. https://doi.org/10.1016/j.injury.2019.01.017.
26. Launonen AP, Laitinen MK, Sumrein BO, Niemi ST, Kannus P, Mattila VM. Trends in scapular fractures: a nationwide 17-year study in Finland. *JSES Int*. 2020;4(1):59–62. https://doi.org/10.1016/j.jses.2019.10.111.
27. Imatani RJ. Fractures of the scapula: a review of 53 fractures. *J Trauma*. 1975;15(6):473–478.
28. McGahan JP, Rab GT, Dublin A. Fractures of the scapula. *J Trauma*. 1980;20(10):880–883.
29. Ideberg R, Grevsten S, Larsson S. Epidemiology of scapular fractures. Incidence and classification of 338 fractures. *Acta Orthop Scand*. 1995;66(5):395–397. https://doi.org/10.3109/17453679508995571.
30. Anavian J, Gauger EM, Schroder LK, Wijdicks CA, Cole PA. Surgical and functional outcomes after operative management of complex and displaced intra-articular glenoid fractures. *J Bone Joint Surg Am*. 2012;94(7):645–653. https://doi.org/10.2106/JBJS.J.00896.
31. Cole PA, Gauger EM, Herrera DA, Anavian J, Tarkin IS. Radiographic follow-up of 84 operatively treated scapula neck and body fractures. *Injury*. 2012;43(3):327–333. https://doi.org/10.1016/j.injury.2011.09.029.
32. Baldwin KD, Ohman-Strickland P, Mehta S, Hume E. Scapula fractures: a marker for concomitant injury? A retrospective review of data in the National Trauma Database. *J Trauma Inj Infect Crit Care*. 2008;65(2):430–435. https://doi.org/10.1097/TA.0b013e31817fd928.
33. Veysi VT, Mittal R, Agarwal S, Dosani A, Giannoudis PV. Multiple trauma and scapula fractures: so what? *J Trauma Inj Infect Crit Care*. 2003;55(6):1145–1147. https://doi.org/10.1097/01.TA.0000044499.76736.9D.

34. Mulawka B, Jacobson AR, Schroder LK, Cole PA. Triple and quadruple disruptions of the superior shoulder suspensory complex. *J Orthop Trauma*. 2015;29(6):264–270. https://doi.org/10.1097/BOT.0000000000000275.

35. Cole PA, Gilbertson JA, Cole PA. Functional outcomes of operative management of scapula fractures in a geriatric cohort. *J Orthop Trauma*. 2017;31(1):e1–e8. https://doi.org/10.1097/BOT.0000000000000710.

36. Ada JR, Miller ME. Scapular fractures: analysis of 113 cases. *Clin Orthop Relat Res*. 1991;(269):174–180. https://doi.org/10.1097/00003086-199108000-00025.

37. Chadwick EKJ, van Noort A, van der Helm FCT. Biomechanical analysis of scapular neck malunion—a simulation study. *Clin BioMech*. 2004;19(9):906–912. https://doi.org/10.1016/j.clinbiomech.2004.06.013.

38. Nordqvist A, Petersson C. Fracture of the body, neck, or spine of the scapula a long-term follow-up study. *Clin Orthop Relat Res*. 1992;(283):139–144. https://doi.org/10.1097/00003086-199210000-00019.

39. Bozkurt M, Can F, Kırdemir V, Erden Z, Demirkale İ, Başbozkurt M. Conservative treatment of scapular neck fracture: the effect of stability and glenopolar angle on clinical outcome. *Injury*. 2005;36(10):1176–1181. https://doi.org/10.1016/j.injury.2004.09.013.

40. Cole PA, Talbot M, Schroder LK, Anavian J. Extra-articular malunions of the scapula: a comparison of functional outcome before and after reconstruction. *J Orthop Trauma*. 2011;25(11):649–656. https://doi.org/10.1097/BOT.0b013e31820af67f.

41. Armitage BM, Wijdicks CA, Tarkin IS, et al. Mapping of scapular fractures with three-dimensional computed tomography. *J Bone Joint Surg Am*. 2009;91(9):2222–2228. https://doi.org/10.2106/JBJS.H.00881.

42. Gauger EM, Ludewig PM, Cole PA. Pre- and postoperative function after scapula malunion reconstruction: a novel kinematic technique. *J Orthop Trauma*. 2013;27(8):6.

43. Schirmers J, Gilbertson J, Schroder LK, Joscelyn T, Cole PA. AM17 Paper 121: extra-articular malunions and nonunions of the scapula: a comparison of functional outcome before and after reconstruction Orthopaedic Trauma Association (OTA). *AM17: Polytrauma and Post Traumatic Reconstruction*. OTA; 2017. https://ota.org/education/meetings-and-courses/abstracts/am17-paper-121-extra-articular-malunions-and-nonunions.

44. Ogunleye T, Schirmers J, Gilbertson JA, Schroder LK, Cole PA. Malunions and nonunions of the acromion and coracoid process: a comparison of functional outcome before and after reconstruction. *J Orthop Trauma*. 2020;34(12):669–674. https://doi.org/10.1097/BOT.0000000000001840.

45. Mayo KA, Benirschke SK, Mast JW. Displaced fractures of the glenoid fossa. *Clin Orthop Relat Res*. 1998;347:122–130.

46. Tatro JM, Anderson JP, McCreary DL, Schroder LK, Cole PA. Radiographic correlation of clinical shoulder deformity and patient perception following scapula fracture. *Injury*. 2020;51(7):1584–1591. https://doi.org/10.1016/j.injury.2020.04.017.

47. Wijdicks CA, Anavian J, Hill BW, Armitage BM, Vang S, Cole PA. The assessment of scapular radiographs: analysis of anteroposterior radiographs of the shoulder and the effect of rotational offset on the glenopolar angle. *Bone Joint J*. 2013;95-B(8):1114–1120. https://doi.org/10.1302/0301-620X.95B8.30631.

48. Anavian J, Conflitti JM, Khanna G, Guthrie ST, Cole PA. A reliable radiographic measurement technique for extra-articular scapular fractures. *Clin Orthop Relat Res*. 2011;469(12):3371–3378. https://doi.org/10.1007/s11999-011-1820-3.

49. Anavian J, Khanna G, Plocher EK, Wijdicks CA, Cole PA. Progressive displacement of scapula fractures. *J Trauma Inj Infect Crit Care*. 2010;69(1):156–161. https://doi.org/10.1097/TA.0b013e3181b40393.

50. Hardegger FH, Simpson LA, Weber BG. The operative treatment of scapula fractrures. *Bone Joint J*. 1984;66-B(5):725–731.

51. Meinberg EG, Agel J, Roberts CS, Karam MD, Kellam JF. Scapula. *J Orthop Trauma*. 2018;32:S101. https://doi.org/10.1097/BOT.0000000000001070.

52. Gilbert F, Eden L, Meffert R, et al. Intra- and interobserver reliability of glenoid fracture classifications by Ideberg, Euler and AO. *BMC Musculoskelet Disord*. 2018;19(1):89. https://doi.org/10.1186/s12891-018-2016-8. PMID: 29580228; PMCID: PMC5870213.

53. Dugarte AJ, Tkany L, Schroder LK, Petersik A, Cole PA. Comparison of 2 versus 3 dimensional fracture mapping strategies for 3 dimensional computerized tomography reconstructions of scapula neck and body fractures: three-dimensional scapular fracture database. *J Orthop Res*. 2018;36(1):265-271. https://doi.org/10.1002/jor.23603.

54. Ogawa K, Naniwa T. Fractures of the acromion and the lateral scapular spine. *J Shoulder Elbow Surg*. 1997;6(6):544–548. https://doi.org/10.1016/S1058-2746(97)90087-2.

55. Ogawa K, Yoshida A, Takahashi M, Ul M. Fractures of the coracoid process. *Bone Joint J*. 1997;79(1):17–19.

56. Anavian J, Wijdicks CA, Schroder LK, Vang S, Cole PA. Surgery for scapula process fractures: good outcome in 26 patients. *Acta Orthop*. 2009;80(3):344–350. https://doi.org/10.3109/17453670903025394.

57. Levy JC, Anderson C, Samson A. Classification of postoperative acromial fractures following reverse shoulder arthroplasty. *J Bone Joint Surg Am*. 2013;95(15):e104. https://doi.org/10.2106/JBJS.K.01516.

58. Hill BW, Anavian J, Jacobson AR. Surgical management of isolated acromion fractures: technical tricks and clinical experience. *J Orthop Trauma*. 2014;28(5):7.

59. Romero J, Schai P, Imhoff AB. Scapular neck fracture - the influence of permanent malalignment of the glenoid neck on clinical outcome. *Arch Orthop Trauma Surg*. 2001;121(6):313–316. https://doi.org/10.1007/s004020000224.

60. Jones CB, Cornelius JP, Sietsema DL, Ringler JR, Endres TJ. Modified Judet approach and minifragment fixation of scapular body and glenoid neck fractures. *J Orthop Trauma*. 2009;23(8):558–564. https://doi.org/10.1097/BOT.0b013e3181a18216.

61. Khallaf F, Mikami A, Al-Akkad M. The use of surgery in displaced scapular neck fractures. *Med Princ Pract*. 2006;15(6):443–448. https://doi.org/10.1159/000095491.

62. Herrera DA, Anavian J, Tarkin IS, Armitage BA, Schroder LK, Cole PA. Delayed operative management of fractures of the scapula. *J Bone Joint Surg*. 2009;91(5):8.

63. Schroder LK, Gauger EM, Gilbertson JA, Cole PA. Functional outcomes after operative management of extra-articular glenoid neck and scapular body fractures. *J Bone Joint Surg*. 2016;98(19):1623–1630. https://doi.org/10.2106/JBJS.15.01224.

64. Steinmetz RG, Maupin JJ, Johnson EB, et al. Are routine follow-up radiographs necessary for extra-articular scapula body fractures managed conservatively? *J Am Acad Orthop Surg*. 2020;28(23):990–995. https://doi.org/10.5435/JAAOS-D-19-00553.

65. Sharma J, Maenza C, Myers A, et al. Clinical outcomes and shoulder kinematics for the "gray zone" extra-articular scapula fracture in 5 patients. *Int J Orthop*. 2020;3(1):1017. Epub 2020 Feb 7. PMID: 32346675; PMCID: PMC7188186.

66. Rajfer RA, Salopek T, Mosier BA, Miller MC, Altman GT. Long-term functional outcomes of nonoperatively treated highly displaced scapular body and neck fractures. *Orthopedics*. 2020;43(3):e177–e181. https://doi.org/10.3928/01477447-20200314-05.

67. Jones CB, Sietsema DL, Ringler JR, Endres TJ. OTA AM16 Paper #97: should displaced scapular body fractures be operatively treated? A randomized controlled trial. In: *Podium Presentation Presented at the Orthopaedic Trauma Association Annual Meeting*. National Harbor, MD; 2016. https://ota.org/education/meetings-and-courses/meeting-archive/2016.

68. Zlowodzki M, Bhandari M, Zelle BA, Kregor PJ, Cole PA. Treatment of scapula fractures: systematic review of 520 fractures in 22 case series. *J Orthop Trauma*. 2006;20(3):230–233. https://doi.org/10.1097/00005131-200603000-00013.

69. Dienstknecht T, Horst K, Pishnamaz M, Sellei RM, Kobbe P, Berner A. A meta-analysis of operative versus nonoperative treatment in 463 scapular neck fractures. *Scand J Surg*. 2013;102(2):69–76. https://doi.org/10.1177/1457496913482251.

70. Bi AS, Kane LT, Butler BA, Stover MD. Outcomes following extra-articular fractures of the scapula: a systematic review. *Injury*. 2020;51(3):602–610. https://doi.org/10.1016/j.injury.2020.01.036.

71. Kannan S, Singh HP, Pandey R. A systematic review of management of scapular fractures. *Acta Orthop Belg*. 2018;84(4):497–508.

72. Dombrowsky AR, Boudreau S, Quade J, Brabston EW, Ponce BA, Momaya AM. Clinical outcomes following conservative and surgical management of floating shoulder injuries: a systematic review. *J Shoulder Elbow Surg*. 2020;29(3):634–642. https://doi.org/10.1016/j.jse.2019.09.029.

73. McGinnis M, Denton JR. Fractures of the scapula: a retrospective study of 40 fractured scapulae. *J Trauma*. 1989;29(11):1488–1493.

74. Constant CR, Murley AHG. A clinical method of functional assessment of the shoulder. *Clin Orthop Relat Res*. 1987;214:160–164.

75. Tadros AMA, Lunsjo K, Czechowski J, Abu-Zidan FM. Causes of delayed diagnosis of scapular fractures. *Injury*. 2008;39(3):314–318. https://doi.org/10.1016/j.injury.2007.10.014.

76. Stevens NM, Tejwani N. Commonly missed injuries in the patient with polytrauma and the orthopaedist's role in the tertiary survey. *JBJS Reviews*. 2018;6(12):e2. https://doi.org/10.2106/JBJS.RVW.18.00014.

77. Pace AM, Stuart R, Brownlow H. Outcome of glenoid neck fractures. *J Shoulder Elbow Surg*. 2005;14(6):585–590. https://doi.org/10.1016/j.jse.2005.03.004.

78. Marek DJ, Sechriest VF, Swiontkowski MF, Cole PA. Case report: reconstruction of a recalcitrant scapular neck nonunion and literature review. *Clin Orthop Relat Res*. 2009;467(5):1370–1376. https://doi.org/10.1007/s11999-008-0651-3.

79. Toft F, Moro F. Does ORIF of rare scapular spine fractures sustained after reverse shoulder arthroplasty benefit elderly patients? A case-series appraisal. *Orthop Traumatol Surg Res*. 2019;105(8):1521–1528. https://doi.org/10.1016/j.otsr.2019.07.023.

80. Kicinski M, Puskas GJ, Zdravkovic V, Jost B. Osteosynthesis of type III acromial fractures with locking compression plate, lateral clavicular plate, and reconstruction plate: a biomechanical analysis of load to failure and strain distribution. *J Shoulder Elbow Surg*. 2018;27(11):2093–2098. https://doi.org/10.1016/j.jse.2018.05.031.

81. Kim K-C, Rhee K-J, Shin H-D, Yang J-Y. Can the glenopolar angle be used to predict outcome and treatment of the floating shoulder? *J Trauma Inj Infect Crit Care*. 2008;64(1):174–178. https://doi.org/10.1097/01.ta.0000240982.99842.b9.

16

Technique Spotlight: ORIF Scapula

PETER A. COLE AND LISA K. SCHRODER

Introduction

This chapter builds on a new perspective of operative intervention in cases of marked displacement of scapular fractures, based on surgical indications covered in the last chapter (Table 16.1). These surgical indications should be assessed with measurements obtained on three-dimensional computed tomography (3D CT) scans for accurate reading, and of course applied to the patient's context including age and comorbidities, baseline and desired function, as well as concomitant injuries. As discussed, these surgical indications have been tested with application to many patient populations, which have yielded good or excellent results in early, midterm, and long-term well-documented outcome studies. These results are summarized in the last chapter, which should yield a reasonable approach to choosing surgical candidates.

The purpose of this chapter is to help the surgeon choose from a variety of surgical options and to execute the chosen operative approach while optimizing access and minimizing risk to the patient. Additionally, fracture reduction methods will be elucidated and placed into the context of common deforming forces on the typical fracture fragments. Common associated injuries, as well as potential complications of surgery to recognize and consider for intervention, will be discussed. Lastly, a protocol for rehabilitation after scapula open reduction internal fixation (ORIF) with a track record for success will be presented and will be applicable to the majority of patients.

Preoperative Evaluation

Choosing the Surgical Approach

It is important to select the best approach to most effectively accomplish open reduction and internal fixation with the least amount of trauma to the soft tissues. These principles will promote the quickest and most complete recovery (Table 16.2).

Generally, all scapular neck and body fractures, fractures of the acromion, inferior angle or posterior scapular spine, as well as the posterior glenoid, should be approached from posterior. Only anterior glenoid and coracoid fractures should be approached from anterior. It is rare that combined approaches are necessary and only applies to approximately 5% of cases overall. Additionally, other lesions that commonly occur must be considered for incorporation into the operative plan, inclusive of clavicle fractures and acromioclavicular (AC) dislocation. Clavicle fractures

occur in approximately 30% of operatively indicated scapular fractures. More uncommon are sternoclavicular lesions and proximal humerus fractures; however, the ipsilateral injury rate is approximately 50%.

Decision-Making on Anterior Approach

If the anterior glenoid fracture is small enough to treat arthroscopically, such as for the bony Bankart lesion more common to sports-related shoulder dislocation mechanisms, then management with suture anchors would be most appropriate. This scenario could apply to fractures that make up <10% of the articular surface (Fig. 16.1A–B). While it has been described for larger fragments, the surgeon should determine the best strategy in his or her hands to obtain an anatomic and stable reduction.

Sometimes glenoid fractures are more inferiorly located, and the surgeon must determine whether an anterior or posterior approach offers the best access. A 3D CT reconstruction can help to visualize where the apex of the fracture is in order to make this decision (Fig. 16.2). The inferior glenoid fracture is challenging to buttress from anterior due to inferior access through a deltopectoral interval, whereas it is entirely feasible through the interval of the teres minor and infraspinatus posteriorly.

An isolated coracoid fracture can be accessed through a 4- to 6-cm incision centered over the coracoid itself. There is a common superior glenoid fracture variant (Ideberg Type III Scapula or Eyers Type V Coracoid) (Fig. 16.3). This fracture often extends just inferior to the coracoid and is best accessed through a deltopectoral approach if the surgeon desires to visualize the articular surface or clean out the fracture which can only be performed through this glenoid vantage point. The need for an arthrotomy in this fracture variant is particularly relevant to delayed fractures in which the medially displaced superior glenoid with a typical caudal tilt is filled with callus after 10–14 days.

For the commonly associated AC dislocation or clavicle fracture, the incision is modified and extended as necessary to accommodate fixation of this pathology when present. The surgical tactic should involve reducing a distal clavicle fracture or AC dislocation prior to coracoid fixation because of the deforming forces which are more challenging to manage for the coracoid reduction and fixation.

Decision-Making on Posterior Approach

The variations of the posterior approach for scapular neck and body fractures depend on the fracture pattern, chronicity of the

TABLE 16.1 Indications for Surgery[a]

Lateral border offset	20 mm (sometimes called medialization measured on AP scapula)
Glenopolar angle	<22 degrees (sometimes called GPA)
Angulation	>45 degrees (measured on scapula Y view)
Articular Step-off	>4 mm (>20% required for instability)
Double lesions of superior shoulder suspensory complex	(each lesion should be displaced >1 cm)
Triple and quadruple lesions of the SSSC	(acromioclavicular dislocation, clavicle, coracoid + neck)
Coracoid fracture	>10 mm
Acromion fracture	>5 mm
Reverse total shoulder arthroplasty painful stress fracture	>1 mm (after conservative management failure)
Nonunion-malunion scapula	Pain-dysfunction (commonly in fractures which would have been indicated)
Translation and anteversion	Undefined

[a](See Chapter 15 for how to measure.)

These displacements are not commonly used for indications, but likely have important influence on outcome and should be studied.

TABLE 16.2 Approach and Position Based on Fracture Anatomy

Anterior (Beach Chair Position)

- Anterior, superior, and inferior articular glenoid

- Coracoid

Posterior (Lateral Decubitus Forward Leaning)

- Posterior articular glenoid

- Scapula body, neck, spine

Other Considerations

- The **associated acromion fracture** depends on the morphology of the fracture and may include a lateral decubitus approach or a beach chair with a medial scapular bump to allow acromial access.

- The **associated clavicle fracture** can be performed in a staged fashion, alternating positions as well as prep and drape, but can also be accomplished in the floppy lateral position before or after the posterior approach to the scapula.

- The **associated acromioclavicular dislocation** should be addressed independently after the ORIF of the scapular fracture. It is not wise to fix an acromioclavicular dislocation first because the scapular acromion position is not reduced with respect to the clavicle.

fracture, and experience of the surgeon. In general, it is a good idea in a surgeon's experience to begin with more open and invasive approaches until better knowledge of critical neurovascular anatomy, common deformities, and muscular planes is gained. It is far easier to obtain and maintain a reduction, and apply implants with an open and visual assessment of the posterior scapula, than it is to do the same through small surgical windows of exposure. As long as soft tissue handling is respectful, and proper anatomical and internervous intervals are used with good reattachment, open approaches have a favorable track record. With more experience will come less detachment of muscular origins and more tactical incisions and dissection.

At this juncture, the operative approach depends upon whether the surgeon desires limited or complete exposure to the posterior scapula. Intermuscular "windows" can be used to access specific portions of the fracture involving the scapular borders. An extensile approach can be executed to expose the entire posterior scapula. The extensile approach still respects the entire subscapularis muscular attachment on the anterior surface, and the elevated flap respects the neurovascular pedicle of the suprascapular nerve and artery (Table 16.3).

Decision-Making for Anterior and Posterior Combined

In severe associated scapular fractures, combined anterior and posterior approaches are necessary, such as when there is an associated body and/or neck fracture, with extensive comminution of the glenoid and/or a coracoid fracture. The surgical tactic in these cases should start with the posterior approach to restore the proper rotation and relationship of the body and neck and posterior glenoid surface, as well as to provide a foundation for fixation via the deltopectoral approach to restore stability to the coracoid or anterior glenoid (Fig. 16.9).

Surgical Anatomy. The scapula is a relatively flat and triangular bone, with a thin body surrounded by a well-developed perimeter and three unique processes, which are the key opportunities for plate and screw fixation. Deforming forces from muscle insertions determine the vector of fragment displacement (Fig. 16.10). The typical cephalad, glenoid-containing fragment often medializes with respect to the scapular body, and it tends to tilt caudal due to gravity and the pull of levator scapula and coracoid-based muscles (Fig. 16.11). The inferior body lateralizes often from the dominant pull of the triceps long head.

The scapular spine divides the anterior supraspinatus from the posterior infraspinatus fossa, the platform origin for their supraspinatus and infraspinatus muscles, respectively. The concave anterior body surface of the scapula serves as the origin for the subscapularis muscle providing a rich blood supply to the scapular body, along with the serratus anterior. The suprascapular, dorsal scapular, and circumflex scapular arteries provide a rich anastomosis and blood supply to this anatomy.

The acromion is the prominent, lateral most structure at the distal end of the scapular spine. The acromion and clavicle serve as the origin for the deltoid muscle and make up key links in the chain between the axial and appendicular skeleton. The trapezius originates on the acromion and scapular spine anteriorly. The anterior medial border of the scapula is the site of attachment of the serratus anterior, the main scapula protractor, and the rhomboid muscles inserting posterior medial, which function as scapula retractors.

The lateral border of the scapula forms a thick condensation of bone that ends at the base of the glenoid and forms the stable axis around which the glenohumeral joint provides rotation. The lateral border is the site of origin of the teres major and minor muscles,

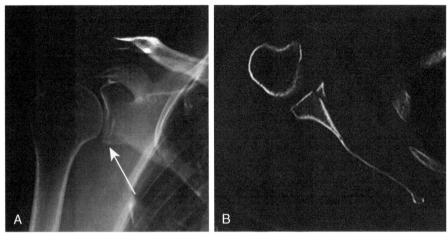

• **Fig. 16.1** (A) A Grashey view of the right scapula after a reduced glenohumeral dislocation. The articular lesion denoted by the *arrow* is recognized as a double opacity adjacent to the articular surface, which represents a displaced glenoid fracture which is further defined in the (B) axial computed tomography cut shown. It is approximately 10% of the articular surface. These lesions are amenable to arthroscopic reduction and stabilization.

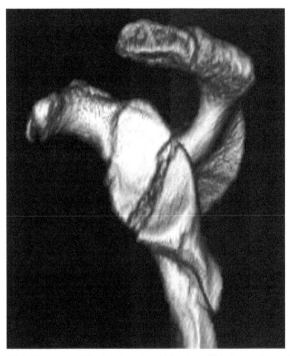

• **Fig. 16.2** The apex of the inferior glenoid fracture. This three-dimensional computed tomography image is imminently helpful in determining whether an anterior or posterior approach is more helpful for reduction and fixation of the glenoid articular fracture itself. In this case, a posterior approach was chosen.

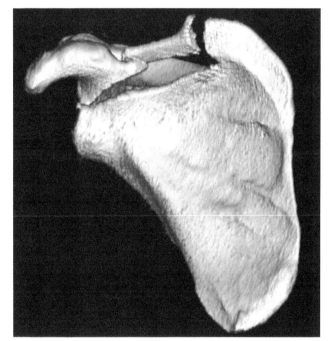

• **Fig. 16.3** A three-dimensional computed tomography from the anterior scapula shows a coracoid fracture pattern that exits into the glenoid cavity. Often these fractures exit medially through the suprascapular notch putting the suprascapular nerve at risk. These fractures can occur in isolation or in combination with scapular body or neck fractures.

as well as the insertion for the long head of the triceps inferior to the glenoid where it forms a thickening due to the tension forces imparted by this muscle. The latissimus dorsi inserts in part at the inferior angle and its contractile forces are responsible for this more formidable region of the scapular body in addition to teres major.

The coracoid process is a curved, osseous proboscis medial to the anterior neck of the scapula serving as the origin for the coracoacromial and coracoclavicular ligaments as well as for the coracobrachialis, short head of the biceps, and pectoralis minor muscles. Just medial to the coracoid process on the superior margin of the scapula is the scapular notch or incisura across which spans the transverse scapular ligament, above which runs the suprascapular artery and below which lies the suprascapular nerve.

The glenoid fossa has a fibrocartilaginous peripheral labrum that is confluent with the long head of the biceps tendon at the supraglenoid tubercle. The labrum increases the depth of the pear-shaped glenoid fossa which is approximately 4 cm in a superior-inferior direction and 3 cm in an anterior-posterior direction in its lower half.

There are 18 muscular origins and insertions on the scapula in total, each with its own contribution to deforming force on

TABLE 16.3	Posterior Approach Options From Most to Least Invasive

Extensile Judet (Fig. 16.4)

- Complex fracture patterns involving multiple exit points

- Delay to surgery >10 days or malunions

- Limited intra-articular access

- Consider for less experienced surgeon

Modified Judet Deltoid Detaching (Fig. 16.5)

- Best access for anatomic neck, complex glenoid patterns

- Greater need for longer protected rehabilitation

Modified Judet Deltoid Sparing (Fig. 16.6)

- The work-horse for more experienced surgeon

- 10%–15%< exposure than detaching deltoid

Mini-Modified Judet (Fig. 16.7A–B)

- Isolated lateral (glenoid and neck) fractures exiting spine

Minimally Invasive Osteosynthesis (Fig. 16.8A–B)

- Best for simple patterns in acute setting <7 days

- Requires more help to maintain surgical window for access

- More experienced surgeon

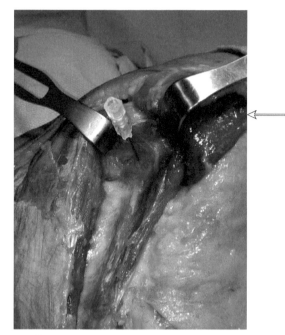

• **Fig. 16.5** This posterior shoulder dissection shows the exposure to the posterior glenoid and scapular neck through a modified deltoid detaching Judet approach. The IV needle is penetrating the glenohumeral joint and the arm would be to the right side of the picture. The infraspinatus is being retracted medially to the left, and the teres minor and detached deltoid *(yellow arrow)* is being retracted superiorly and to the right. There is easier access to the posterior glenoid and for intra-articular assessment with the deltoid detached.

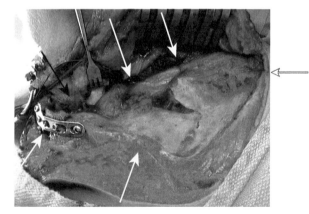

• **Fig. 16.4** This is an intraoperative image of an extensile Judet approach, in which the infraspinatus, teres minor, and deltoid are mobilized off of the posterior scapular body. This provides maximal visualization, and the flap is elevated on the neurovascular (nv) pedicle. The *black arrow* is pointing to the suprascapular nv bundle which exits the spinoglenoid notch at the base of the acromion. The acromion, in this case, has already been fixed. This approach was chosen because of the complexity of the fracture pattern with multiple exit points around the perimeter *(yellow arrows)*. Furthermore, it was 2 weeks from the time of injury and callus formation was inevitable. An arthrotomy has been made through which the humeral head can be visualized. This was done because the patient had a comminuted glenoid fracture and required an anterior approach subsequent to this posterior approach.

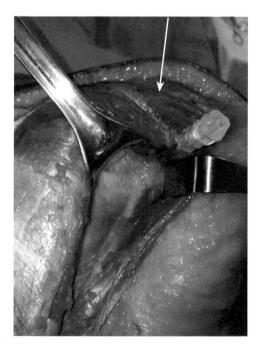

• **Fig. 16.6** This posterior shoulder dissection shows the exposure to the posterior glenoid and scapular neck through a modified deltoid sparing Judet approach. The IV needle is penetrating the glenohumeral joint and the arm would be to the right side of the picture. The infraspinatus is being retracted medially to the left, and the teres minor is being retracted laterally to the right. The deltoid is intact and sweeping across the cephalad part of the surgical field *(yellow arrow)*.

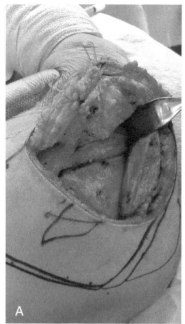
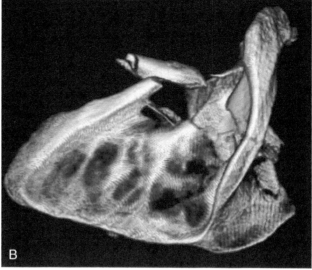

• **Fig. 16.7** (A) The purpose of this posterior shoulder image is to show the different size of the skin incision, which helps to limit exposure to the lateral scapula for certain fracture patterns that do not exit the vertebral border. The deltoid muscle is being retracted cephalad, exposing the interval between teres minor and infraspinatus. (B) This three-dimensional computed tomography image is an example of a scapular fracture pattern, which would be amenable to such an approach.

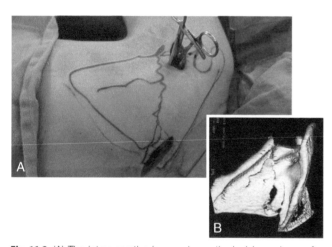

• **Fig. 16.8** (A) The intraoperative image shows the incisions chosen for a minimally invasive approach which yields windows down to the displaced fracture line. (B) A corresponding simple body fracture on a three-dimensional computed tomography scan, revealing a lot of lateral border offset. The surgeon will approach the two displaced ends of the scapula, medial and lateral, to reduce and fix this pattern.

fractured segments. It is helpful to understand both pathophysiology and surgical reduction maneuvers in the context of this rich myofibril endowment.

Surgical Techniques

Anterior Approach

Anterior Approach Positioning (Fig. 16.12)

The patient is placed in a beach chair position with an arm board attached to support the extremity. Place the arm board sufficiently

distal so as to be out of the way of shoulder fluoroscopy, and a table with a shoulder "cut-out" is very useful to facilitate imaging as well. An X-ray plate may be positioned prior to draping posterior to the shoulder for an intraoperative film, but it is helpful in complex glenoid fracture variants to have the use of intraoperative C-arm during the procedure to evaluate fracture reduction and ensure there is no intra-articular penetration by hardware.

Anterior Approach Surgical Technique

The coracoid and acromion are first palpated and marked on the skin. An incision is made from the coracoid toward the deltoid humeral insertion, lateral to the axillary fold (Fig. 16.13). The incision is taken down through the deltopectoral interval. The cephalic vein is the marker for this interval and should be protected and retracted medially. The incision can be extended distally to the deltoid insertion and proximally to the clavicle and may be extended as necessary to approach a clavicle fracture, or an AC dislocation.

After the cephalic vein is identified and protected, the dissection continues down to the clavipectoral fascia, which covers the pectoralis minor, coracobrachialis, and subscapularis tendons. The humerus can be rotated to appreciate tension on the subscapularis tendon and its insertion onto the lesser tuberosity. At the inferior margin of the subscapularis tendon lays the transversely running anterior humeral circumflex vessels, which can be ligated or cauterized if necessary, but the axillary nerve immediately inferior is at risk. No inferior dissection should be performed beyond the crossing vessels. The subscapularis tendon should be incised vertically approximately half a centimeter medial to its insertion on the lesser tuberosity for repair at the completion of the surgery. Some prefer a tuberosity osteotomy which can be fixed after glenoid fixation and capsulorrhaphy. It is preferable to identify the subscapularis tendon distinct from the capsule for capsulotomy,

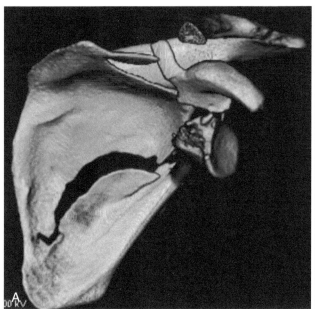 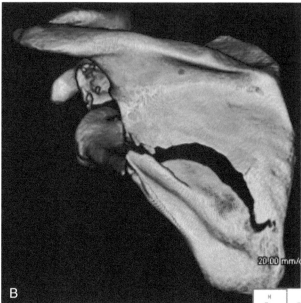

• **Fig. 16.9** The (A) anterior and (B) posterior three-dimensional computed tomography views demonstrate the need for an anterior approach and a posterior approach to address the pathology. The surgical tactic begins with the posterior approach to restore the lateral pillar and scapular neck. The anterior approach is then required to address the coracoid and glenoid. The surgeon must ensure that no screws from posterior interfere with the reduction and fixation of the coracoglenoid complex.

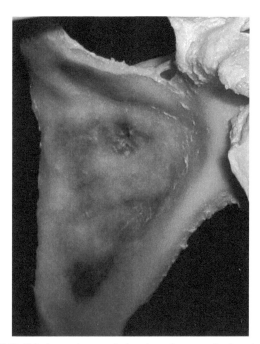

• **Fig. 16.10** This image is an anterior view of a scapula denuded of its musculature, revealing the bony opportunities for fixation. The vertebral medial border is only approximately 8-mm thick, while the lateral border provides about 14 mm. The glenoid yields approximately 30 mm at the subchondral bone but transitions quickly through the scapular neck to the translucent body.

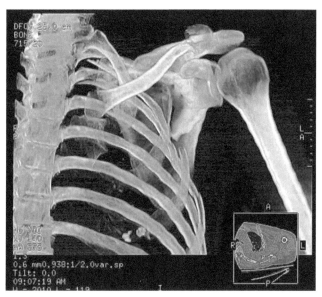

• **Fig. 16.11** This three-dimensional computed tomography of the left shoulder and thorax helps to reveal a medialized and anteverted glenoid with respect to the caudal body of the scapula. Less obvious is the inferior tilt of the glenoid; however, this deformity can be appreciated by noting the shallow glenopolar angle and understanding what would happen to the face of the glenoid were the lateral border reduced.

and each layer can be tagged; however, these layers can be quite adherent and can be handled with a single incision and repair (Fig. 16.13). To avoid taking down the subscapularis, it can be split rather than detached which allows adequate exposure for most Bankart lesions, albeit with more restricted access.

To allow intra-articular inspection, an arthrotomy can be performed by dividing the capsule vertically (with or without subscapularis tendon), just medial to the palpable glenoid rim. Alternatively, the surgeon can work through the fracture to wash out the joint and then obtain an indirect articular reduction by reducing the fragment from the neck for an indirect articular reduction which is possible in a simple anterior glenoid fracture pattern. If there is articular comminution, then capsulotomy is

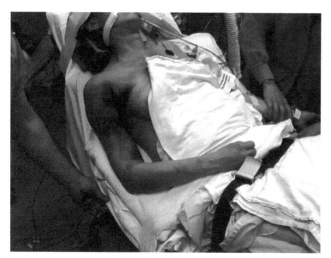

• **Fig. 16.12** This patient is set up in the beach chair position for an anterior deltopectoral approach, with the head carefully secured and the arm board positioned distal to allow for intraoperative C-arm imaging.

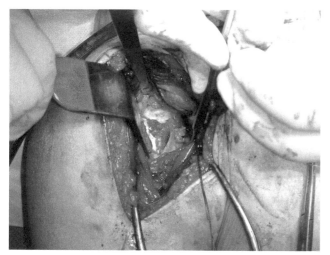

• **Fig. 16.13** This is an intraoperative image of a deltopectoral approach, after subscapularis tenotomy and capsulotomy with a red-handled Fukuda retractor levering off the intact posterior glenoid to retract the humeral head to allow for articular access. The glenoid is fractured into three dominant pieces with the inferior fragment pointed out by the dental pick in the surgeon's hand.

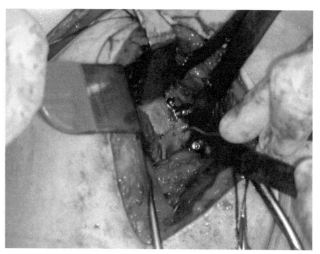

• **Fig. 16.14** This intraoperative photo shows the anterior glenoid minifragment plate and screw fixation of the anterior fragment, and a 2.7-mm lag screw through the inferior fragment. Although the Fukuda retractor has been relaxed, the anterior articular surface can now be appreciated to be reduced and stable.

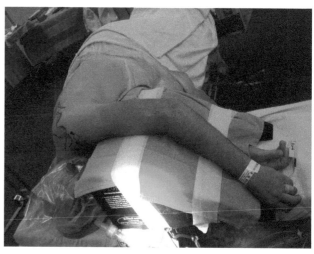

• **Fig. 16.15** This image is of a patient in the right lateral decubitus position, floppy lateral before prepping the left forequarter. Bony landmarks on the scapula have been marked with a marking pen.

important, and the surgeon must work on either side of the capsulolabral complex. For optimal joint inspection and access, the surgeon should place a Darrah or Fukuda retractor in the joint, on the posterior edge of the glenoid, to lever the humeral head away from the articular surface (Fig. 16.13).

Reduction is accomplished with a dental pick or shoulder hook, and provisional fixation obtained with K-wires. Direct inspection eliminates the need for arthroscopy. Depending on the size of the fragment or the degree of comminution, screw choices may range in size from 2.0 to 3.5 mm. A minifragment buttress plate can be applied on the anteroinferior edge of the glenoid, particularly if there is comminution or small fragment difficult to capture with screws (Fig. 16.14). In small bony Bankart fractures or labral tears, suture anchors are preferable to repair the capsulolabral junction. Suture anchors at the articular margin are preferable rather than outside the labrum to promote glenohumeral stability.

Closure of the capsule and subscapularis may be performed with a heavy, braided, nonabsorbable suture. The deltopectoral interval can be approximated with a running absorbable stitch.

Posterior Approach

Posterior Approach Positioning

The patient is placed in the lateral decubitus position, falling slightly forward for access to the posterior shoulder. An axillary roll is positioned to protect the brachial plexus, and positioning bumps (BoneFoam Inc., Cocran, MN) are optimal to support the extremity in 90 degrees of forward flexion and abduction. The entire upper extremity and forequarter should be prepped and draped to allow for manipulation of the arm and shoulder (Fig. 16.15). Shucking the shoulder is helpful to palpate landmarks before the incision is made; additionally, in delayed cases, manipulation of the shoulder pre- and postfixation is helpful in

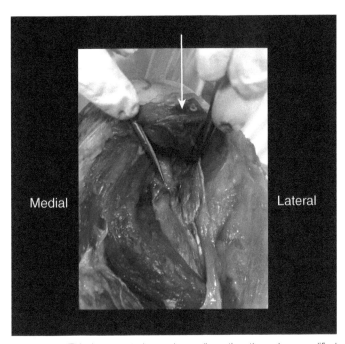

Medial

Lateral

• **Fig. 16.16** This is a posterior cadaver dissection through a modified deltoid detaching Judet approach. The deltoid muscle which has been detached from the spine of the scapula is retracted off the posterior surface exposing the interval between the infraspinatus and teres minor muscles. The deltoid is distinguished by the *yellow arrow*, the teres minor fascia is being held at the right of the image by the surgeon's forceps, while the medial circumflex scapular artery (pointed by the tenotomy scissors) crosses from the lateral border to the posterior scapula where it anastomoses with the suprascapular artery.

releasing and stretching the extrinsic contractures which occur during the delay to surgery. The prep should be wide, including the lower neck superiorly and the vertebral column medially, and the thorax. After the prep, the axilla is isolated with a towel and an impervious dressing to isolate the axilla and its flora.

Posterior Approach Surgical Technique

As aforementioned, depending on the fracture pattern, chronicity of the fracture, and the surgeon's experience, a multitude of approaches can be performed from posterior. The Judet approaches all begin with an incision from the posterior lateral acromion along the spine of the scapula, to the vertebral angle where it curves inferior along this medial scapula. For the classic extensile approach, the entire deltoid and infraspinatus is detached from their origins and elevated medial to lateral protecting the neurovascular pedicle from traction or direct injury as these exit the spinoglenoid notch. In the modified approaches, the subcutaneous flap is elevated off the posterior fascia overlying deltoid and infraspinatus.

Modified Judet Deltoid Detaching Approach (Case 1 [Fig. 16.16]). To operate through more limited intermuscular windows, the muscle plane entered at the spine of the scapula is between the trapezius, originating at the superior margin, and the deltoid at the inferior margin, which is elevated. The deltoid can then be dissected off the scapular spine and separated from the infraspinatus fascia, and tagged for reattachment later. It is retracted laterally to maximize exposure and access to the posterior glenoid.

Modified Judet Deltoid Sparing Approach (Case 2 [Fig. 16.17]). Recently, we have spared the deltoid origin based on cadaveric studies in the lab, which, we postulate, allows for improved rehabilitation.

At the vertebral border of the scapula, the intramuscular plane is between the infraspinatus, which is elevated, and the rhomboids, which are left attached. The most important window is between the infraspinatus and teres minor for access to the lateral border of the scapula and the posterior glenoid rim. Access to the glenohumeral joint is possible through this window. Either a stripe of fatty tissue defines the interval between these two muscles or dissection of the fascia on its posterior surface can take the surgeon right down to the lateral border. The course of these two muscular fibers varies slightly. Once this important interval is developed, the lateral border of the scapula can be accessed, and this is the typical location for the lateral primary fracture line. Direct visualization for the assessment of anteversion of the glenoid and medialization of the superior fragment is accomplished. Through this interval, the lateral border is reduced, the glenoid neck retracted laterally, and the inferior lateral border retracted medially. Overcoming these forces can be challenging, but the reduction of this lateral pillar is the most important maneuver of the case. If the articular glenoid must be assessed, a vertical capsulotomy is made in such a way as to leave a reparable cuff of tissue just distal to the labral attachment.

Extensile Judet Approach (Case 3 [Figs. 16.18 and 16.19]). For full-on exposure of the posterior scapula, the incision is taken down through subcutaneous tissue onto the bony ridge of the scapular spine around to the medial angle at the vertebral border and then caudad.

Palpation of the bony landmarks of the acromion, scapular spine, and vertebral border provides key landmarks for the surgical incisions. Marking out these structures, in addition to the assumed fracture lines of the scapula helps to locate incisions accurately. Manually protracting and retracting the scapula by grabbing the shoulder and "shucking" it medially and laterally helps to locate key landmarks.

The incision should be as generous as necessary to allow for flap retraction to expose the lateral scapular border and neck, and without traction on the suprascapular neurovascular bundle. The fascia along the incision at the acromial spine and medial border should be sutured back to its bony origin at the end of the procedure.

It is important at the end of the case, in patients who are delayed, days to weeks, to the operating room, to perform a manipulation of the extremity prior to awaking the patient. This ensures that all extrinsic adhesions and stiffness are eliminated prior to awaking the patient.

All devitalized muscle should be debrided prior to closure to decrease the opportunity for infection. A drain is placed under the muscular flap on the posterior surface of the scapula to prevent the accumulation of hematoma under the rotator cuff flap supplied by the vulnerable neurovascular bundle exiting the spinoglenoid notch.

For repair of the flap, three small drill holes are made along the scapular spine and three more on the vertebral border to repair the fascia back to its bony origin. The rest of the interval is closed with a figure-of-eight braided suture. The rest of the subcutaneous interval is approximated with braided absorbable suture and the skin closed with an absorbable subcuticular stitch.

Straight Posterior Approach (Case 4 [Fig. 16.20]). If the fracture is isolated to the true anatomic neck of the scapula or the posterior glenoid, a direct posterior approach through a straight incision over the glenoid neck is performed. The dissection is taken down to the deltoid fascia and more inferiorly the rotator cuff fascia.

The deltoid fascia is incised, and subdeltoid access becomes possible to place a retractor drawing the deltoid superiorly. This

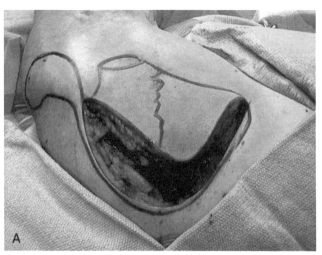

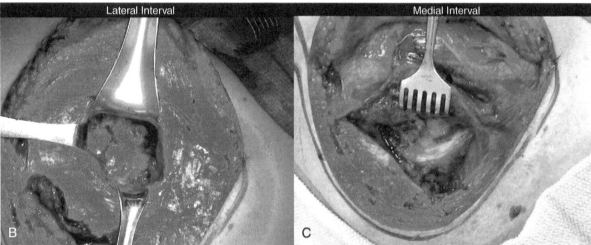

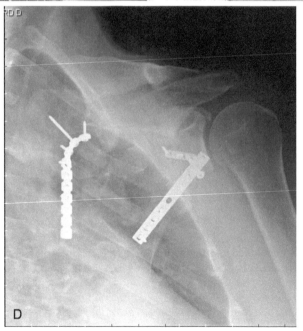

• **Fig. 16.17** (A) An image of the shoulder after the Judet incision and the development of a subcutaneous flap off the posterior deltoid and infraspinatus fascia. The next image will show retraction of this subcutaneous flap. (B) and (C) show the windows to the lateral and medial fractured borders, respectively. The lateral border is shown with the deltoid retracted with the left-side retractor, the teres minor with the superior retractor, and the inferior side with the appendiceal retractor on the infraspinatus. The rake in (C) is retracting the deltoid and infraspinatus detached from the scapular spine and vertebral border. The displacement of the fracture at the base of the spine of the scapula is quite significant. (D) A postoperative image showing the fixation typically utilized through the two surgical intervals of the modified deltoid sparing Judet approach.

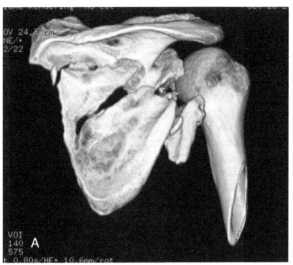 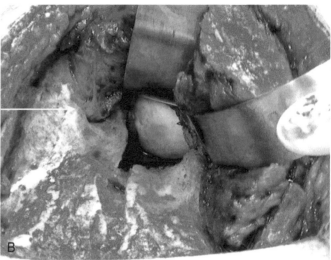

• **Fig. 16.18** (A) A posterior three-dimensional computed tomography view of a patient with a complex glenoid and scapular neck and body fracture. The intraoperative image in (B) is the corresponding extensile Judet approach showing the posterior surface of the scapular neck and acromion with the humeral head dislocated into the surgical field. The suprascapular neurovascular bundle is marked with *yellow arrow* as it exits the spinoglenoid notch at the base of the acromion.

exposes the rotator cuff fascia which is incised vertically to expose the infraspinatus and teres minor. This approach yields excellent access to the posterior glenoid and scapular neck.

Mini-Modified Approach (Case 5 [Fig. 16.21]). Instead of a large boomerang incision, a small boomerang cut is made to correspond with a far lateral fracture which exits up through the acromial spine. This yields the necessary exposure to the deltoid and rotator cuff, but also to the spine of the scapula which can be used to gain a reduction of a fracture line which exits here. The point of this shortened Judet incision is that there is no need to access the base of the spine or the vertebral border where most scapular body and neck fractures exit.

Minimally Invasive Approach (Case 6 [Fig. 16.22]). A minimally invasive approach can be used to limit detachment of muscular origins. Corresponding incisions at the level of the skin are dictated by the fracture pattern, so incisions are typically placed laterally over the glenoid neck, and medially where the fracture exits at the spine or medial border.

It is more challenging to operate through a window, so excellent retraction is paramount. The dissection is taken down to the deltoid fascia, which is then retracted cephalad to expose the fascia overlying infraspinatus and teres minor. The interval between these two muscles is then developed exposing the fracture site as it exits the lateral scapular border typically inferior to the glenoid. It is important that the surgeon remains aware of the axillary nerve and posterior circumflex humeral artery passing through the quadrilateral space, thus the skin incision should not be placed too lateral. Furthermore, once down to the lateral border at the level of the neck, the circumflex scapular artery is encountered and can bleed profusely. It may be cauterized.

The medial incision corresponds with the fracture exit point, usually at the base of the scapular spine. The dissection is taken down to the fascia and then to the periosteum and extending along the vertebral border distally as needed. These lateral and medial windows are usually adequate for reduction and plate application at the two most common sites of displacement at the periphery. This approach is best suited for simple fracture patterns treated within 2 weeks of injury. Fixation with this approach is similar to the other posterior approaches, though because of the small windows and limited incisions, shorter locking plates are used maximizing strength against failure.

Reduction Tools (Fig. 16.23)

Tools
    Schanz pin + T-handled chuck
    Jungbluth clamp
    Small distractor
    Lamina spreader
    Shoulder hook
    Pointed bone reduction clamps—small ×2

Reduction Techniques

The reduction techniques are nearly the same for each posterior approach because fracture patterns and deforming forces are common. After mobilizing the key fragments with a lamina spreader, and breaking up and clearing out posterior callus formation which is often well formed 10 days after injury, attention can be directed to obtaining and maintaining a reduction. Although this is a skill that is developed over time and to which one can apply many tricks, I have found certain maneuvers very helpful. It is useful to have the patient paralyzed anesthetically to facilitate reduction.

The cephalad fragment must be moved lateral and derotated from its anteverted position. A 5-mm Schanz pin in the glenoid neck with a T-handled chuck can be used to accomplish this most often.

Simultaneously, a shoulder hook (Bankart shoulder awl) can be placed into a 2.5-mm pilot hole in the lateral caudal border. This gives the surgeon a joystick for the left hand and right. The left hand draws the caudal fragment medial, while the right hand draws the cephalad fragment lateral and posterior. The goal is to line up the lateral border and most often the fracture ends can hitch up and be stable, or at least held with a pointed bone reduction forceps.

Once the lateral border is reduced, the medial border can be visualized and clamped with a small pointed bone reduction forceps. It is helpful to keep this tenaculum on the periphery to make way for the plate placement inside the scapular border.

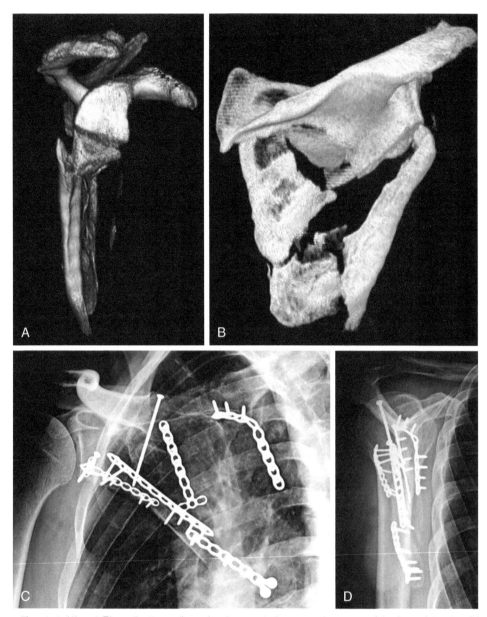

• **Fig. 16.19** (A) and (B) are the three-dimensional computed tomography scans, of the face of the glenoid (scapula Y) and the posterior scapula. In addition to a displaced glenoid fracture, there are three other exit points in the cortical perimeter which make an extensile approach the logical choice to reduce and fix each of these fracture points. (C) and (D) are the anteroposterior and scapula Y X-ray views after ORIF of the fracture shown in (A) and (B). An extensile Judet approach with 2.4- and 2.7-mm plates and screw fixation was used in addition to a 3.5-mm lag screw extending from the scapular spine into the lateral pillar.

It is the delayed and highly deformed cases, including malunions, when strong reduction aids are necessary, particularly on the lateral borders of the caudal and cephalad segments. It is for these cases where a small or medium distractor over two Schanz pins or a Jungbluth clamp over two 3.5 screws can be used to power the reduction.

Common Implants for Fixation

Lateral border	2.7-mm plate
Medial border	2.7- or 2.4-mm reconstruction plate
Inferior angle	2.7 plate + 3.5 T plate
Posterior glenoid	2.0-mm buttress plate or 2.0-mm T plate
Anterior glenoid	2.0-mm buttress plate or 2.0-mm T plate
Acromion	3.5-mm lag screws + 2.7-mm neutralization plate
	2.7 or 3.5 superior tension band
Coracoid	3.5-mm screws
Malunions	3.5-mm dynamic compression plate lateral

Special Considerations

Acromion Fractures (Case 7 [Figs. 16.24–16.27]). The fractured acromion can occur at the periphery in the body of the acromion, at its base, or extend up into the spine of the scapula. The most common pattern is across its base which is challenging

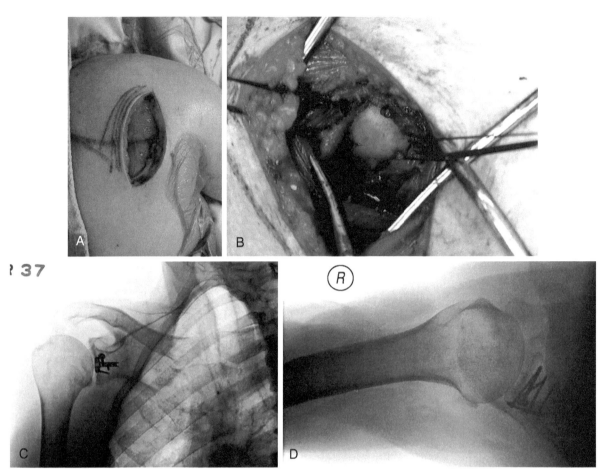

• **Fig. 16.20** (A) A straight incision is made over the scapular neck, and taken down to the deltoid fascia which is incised exposing the deltoid running horizontally from the scapular spine to the proximal humerus. Just anterior to the deltoid is the infraspinatus muscle shown here after the fascia is incised. With the deltoid retracted cephalad, the interval between infraspinatus and teres minor is developed exposing the posterior glenoid. (B) In posterior glenoid fractures, the humeral head subluxes into the field. (C) and (D) show the postoperative radiographs, Grashey view and axillary view, demonstrating the articular reduction and fixation with minifragment screws.

to treat. This scenario is like attempting to fix a diving board at its base and expecting it to withstand the forces imparted by a bouncing diver—very challenging.

Lag screw fixation across the fracture which must be anatomically reduced and compressed is paramount. However, even in good bone, this must be neutralized with a plate along the superior or posterior surface. The superior plate provides a tension band effect which may be of some value.

In comminuted variants or nonunions, the variable angled Mesh Plate (Depuy-Synthes, Paoli, PA) can be used to provide multiplanar stability with variable angled locking screws for maximizing fixation during the period of healing. It must be cut and contoured to match the acromion carefully, and soft tissue reattachment of the trapezius and deltoid is critical.

rTSA Stress Fractures of the Acromion (Case 8 [Figs. 16.28 and 16.29]). It is beyond the scope of this chapter to discuss the etiology of this common fracture pattern which occurs after approximately 5% of reverse total shoulder arthroplasties. This condition is gaining greater attention, because it manifests in a chronic painful shoulder with resultant severe disability.

Certain principles for fixation of these fractures should be applied if healing is to be expected. Many surgeons believe there

is no good treatment, but healing after stable fixation can be accomplished and pain abolished. These principles extend from the treatment of acromion fractures but in the setting of severe osteoporosis and disuse osteopenia. The principles are as follows:

1. lag screw fixation across the nonunion
2. dual or multiplane plates
3. long working length
4. tension band plate over the superior surface of the acromion
5. fixed angled screws

Coracoid (Case 9 [Figs. 16.30 and 16.31]). Isolated coracoid fractures involving the tip, shaft, and base (Ogawa Types I and II and Eyers Types I, II, and III, respectively) can be addressed using an anterior approach. The patient is placed in the beach chair position. A small towel roll is placed under the ipsilateral shoulder to help thrust the shoulder. The entire forequarter should be prepped including the entire extremity for intraoperative elbow flexion which can remove excess traction force on the coracoid during reduction.

An incision is centered directly over the coracoid in Langer's lines which is cosmetic and allows for extension to a formal deltopectoral approach for associated lesions of the anterior glenoid. The incision is taken down through the subcutaneous tissue to the clavipectoral fascia. The coracoid is palpated and

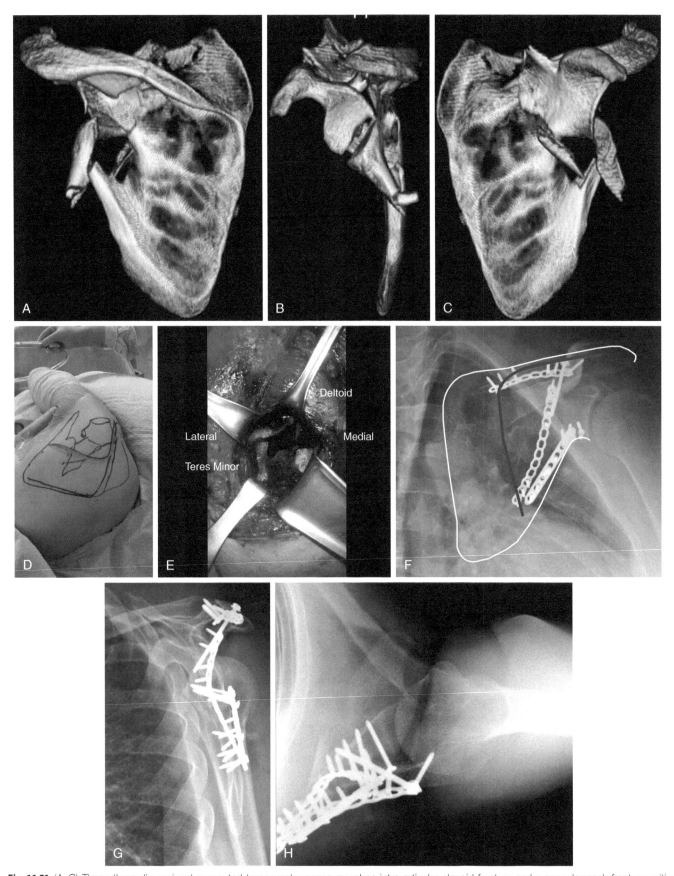

• **Fig. 16.21** (A–C) These three-dimensional computed tomography scans reveal an intra-articular glenoid fracture and a scapular neck fracture exiting through the scapular spine posteriorly and suprascapular notch anteriorly. There is no propagation of the fracture to the medial border or base of the spine of the scapula, so a full Judet incision and exposure would not be necessary. The fracture is all in the lateral scapular complex. (D) and (E) This surgical interval through a mini-modified Judet approach allows the surgeon to get down to the scapular neck without a large Judet incision, without taking down the deltoid or infraspinatus or teres minor, and with good exposure of the fracture. (F–H) This fracture was approached through a mini-modified Judet incision *(blue line)*, because the whole incision as indicated by the *yellow line* in the Grashey view image to the left would not be necessary. The fixation of the lateral fracture of the scapular neck and glenoid is shown in these three X-ray views: Grashey, scapula Y *(top right)*, and axillary view *(bottom right)*.

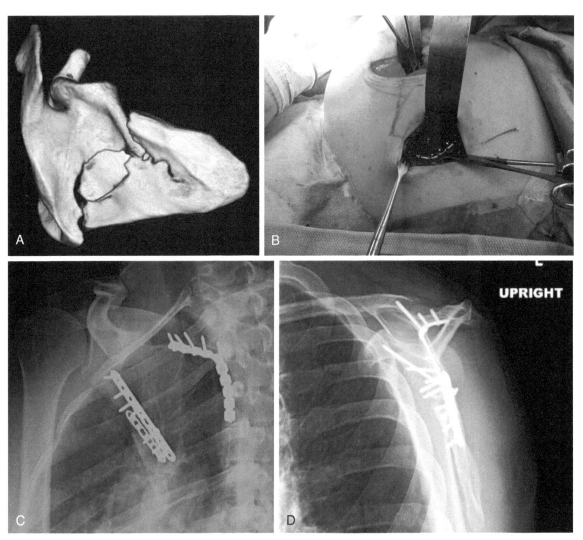

• **Fig. 16.22** (A) Three-dimensional computed tomography scan of a simple scapular body fracture, displaced and medialized with a decreased glenopolar angle. (B) The surgical approach applied to get down to the displaced medial and lateral border. (C) A Grashey view of the scapula and (D) a scapula Y X-ray view, respectively, showing the final fixation for the fracture shown in (A). With short plate fixation because of the limited approach, a parallel plate for the scapular border placed through the same surgical window can render more stable fixation without having to extend the incision.

the fascia is incised directly over it. The incision is extended cephalad from the coracoid to the clavicle through the pectoralis minor muscle. Blunt dissection is then executed with a Cobb elevator from the tip of the coracoid down its cephalad slope. Depending on the fracture pattern, this dissection can lead right to the base at the coracoclavicular ligament complex including the conoid (medial) and trapezoid (lateral) ligaments. The surgeon should appreciate the soft tissue structures attached to the coracoid including the coracoacromial ligament, conjoint tendon, and the coracoclavicular ligaments. The coracoid has a hooked shape which cannot usually be appreciated visually due to the enveloping structures, meaning a screw cannot be successfully placed through the tip of the coracoid and capture the base.

A small pointed bone tenaculum can be used to grasp the coracoid to manipulate it into a reduced position, and a 4.0-mm Schanz pin through the distal coracoid is a helpful adjunctive reduction aid. After reduction, provisional fixation can be obtained using a K-wire. If the fracture occurs through the base, then a 3.5-mm lag screw is often all that is needed for adequate stability, but our preference is to place a 3.5-mm neutralization screw as well to prevent rotational deformity.

One of the challenging aspects of surgery is the screw trajectory, which must be inferiorly directed and with a 20-degree lateral vector to capture the bone stock of the glenoid neck. A common mistake is to direct the screw to posterior and medial where there is little bone stock.

With regard to fractures through the base of the coracoid, the suprascapular nerve is at risk for injury secondary to displaced fractures traversing the suprascapular notch. The notch is located just medial and adjacent to the base of the coracoid so retractors and reduction aids should respect this zone.

A one-quarter tubular plate along the cephalad slope to fix a fracture through the neck of the coracoid is useful and may be added to supplement a single screw enhancing fixation against traction forces of the upper extremity.

In cases where a coracoid base fracture extends laterally and enters the superior glenoid fossa or if there is a concomitant

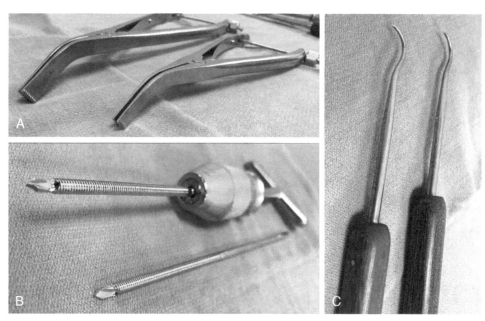

• **Fig. 16.23** (A) At *the top* is a large and a medium-sized lamina spreader used to stretch fragments apart and release extrinsic contractures, and to break apart early formed fracture callus. (B) To the *bottom left* is a Shanz pin with a universal T-handled chuck which is used for manipulating the cephalad fragment. The Shanz pin is placed into the scapular neck. (C) Two Bankart awls also known as shoulder hooks. One of these is placed into the lateral border through a pilot hole allowing the surgeon to joystick the caudal fragment.

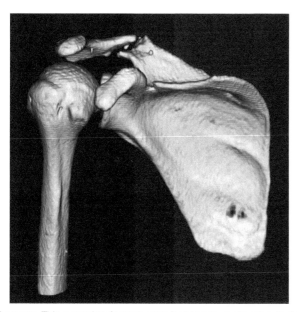

• **Fig. 16.24** This acromion fracture near its base is challenging to treat, particularly if comminuted. There is a tremendous moment arm across the fracture.

anterior glenoid fracture being addressed, fixation of the coracoid can be achieved by extending the incision distally to a formal deltopectoral approach. These cases benefit from an anatomic joint reduction with restoration of the arc of the glenoid, and a superior to inferior lag screw capturing the inferior glenoid. A cannulated screw can be used for this purpose in order to be able to image the screw just adjacent to the glenoid surface for maximal compression.

Postoperative Care and Rehabilitation

Immediately postoperative, the patient is given a sling for comfort and told to discontinue use once they find it a nuisance. The surgical drain is removed once drainage resolves, usually on postoperative day 1 or 2. They are immediately encouraged to move their fingers, wrist, and elbow to mitigate swelling. Patient follow-up is scheduled at 2, 6, and 12 weeks postoperatively for wound assessment, and mainly to encourage an aggressive plan of rehabilitation and ensure progression of motion.

One of the basic goals of surgery is a well-fixed and stable scapula, which means that the shoulder should be able to tolerate a physiologic range of motion. The patients will "autoprotect" sufficiently to advance their rehabilitation with this simple instruction. They should be told, no lifting, pushing, pulling, or carrying anything for 1 month, as a guideline. Note that for the minimally invasive approach in which essentially no muscles have been detached, immediate motion and resistance as tolerated can be allowed. This approach should be clear to patients and therapists. It is imperative that patients and their therapists understand this.

Codman's exercise, passive stretching, and active motion with a broomstick or wall assistance are appropriate activities with goals of achieving near full range of motion by the time the patient returns for the 6-week follow-up. Patients with extra-articular fractures should have an almost normal motion by 6 weeks after surgery, whereas intra-articular fractures require a little more patience until they are generally normal by 3 months postoperative. In patients who have had a deltopectoral approach, only passive- and active-assisted external rotation should be limited for the first 6 weeks to 30 degrees of external rotation.

On rare occasions, a patient may be stiff at 6 weeks and show evidence of failure to progress. Such stiffness occurs more commonly in patients with cognitive impairment or anxiety problems. Other patients with brachial plexus injury, or complex associated

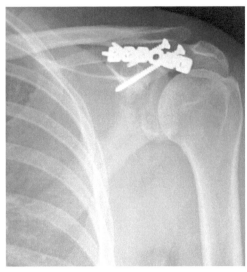
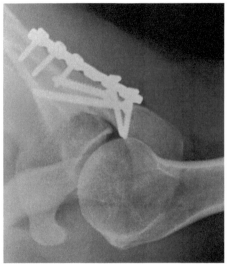

• **Fig. 16.25** An anteroposterior view of the shoulder and an axillary view post fixation showing lag screw fixation augmented by a posterior-based neutralization plate. In this case, there was no superior tension band plate used as the fracture was compressed and stable.

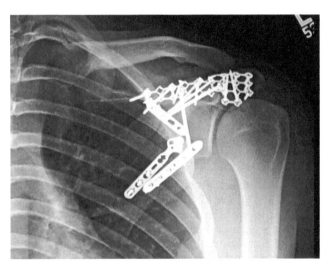

• **Fig. 16.26** This Grashey X-ray view of the shoulder shows a scapular body fracture and acromion fracture status post fixation. The acromion fracture was fixed with a variable angled locking mesh plate (Depuy-Synthes, Paoli, PA) in addition to two lag screws. This construct allows for multiplanar locked screws maximizing fixation in the distal segment.

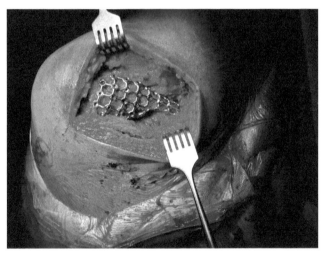

• **Fig. 16.27** The mesh plate technique provides multiplanar stability and should be considered in nonunions or comminuted fractures of the acromion. The surgeon should attempt to maximize the working length to decrease the plate strain in these variants. It is imperative that the deltoid and trapezius be securely repaired after fixation is complete, and the rehabilitation should respect the need for these muscle origins to heal.

ipsilateral injuries, and patients with a halo-vest for spine fractures are also at risk. In such instances, a manipulation under anesthesia (MUA) should be planned prior to 3 months postoperative. If such a patient has an intra-articular fracture, an intraoperative steroid injection should be performed to help prevent recurrence of intra-articular adhesions. Almost always, these interventions progress the patients in a far less painful context than the original injury.

At the 2- and 6-week postoperative visit, an anteroposterior (AP), scapula Y, and axillary radiograph is assessed. At all other follow-up visits, a single AP view of the shoulder is all that is required mainly to check for progression of glenohumeral arthrosis in

glenoid fractures or failure of fixation, though both are extremely rare in the stably and anatomically fixed scapula.

Strength training with 3–5-lb weights or Thera band should begin 4 weeks postoperative, and advanced as tolerated, with an emphasis on endurance training from 8 to 12 weeks and beyond. Therapeutic activities that help proprioception and scapular stabilization (wall wash, ball circles, scapular retraction/protraction) can also be initiated at this time. Restrictions are lifted after 12 weeks including impact sports and heavy labor. Generally, it is the patients with neurologic sequelae of their injuries who require work modifications and further therapy for work hardening or re-entry into other less demanding occupations.

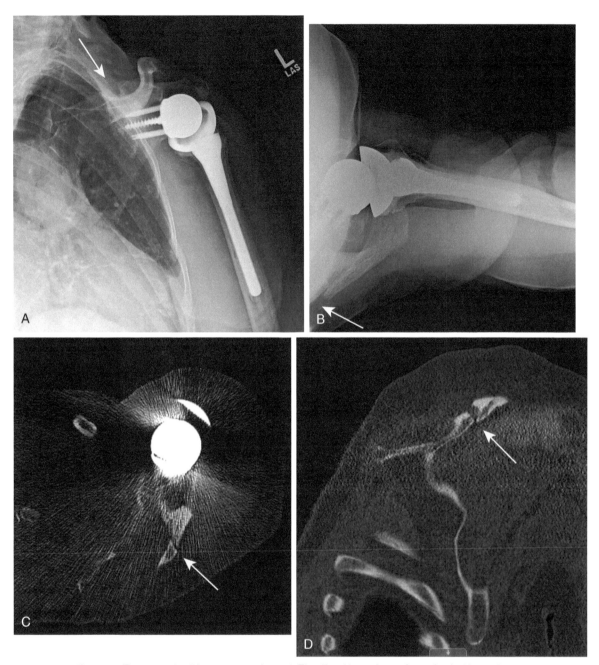

• **Fig. 16.28** These are the (A) anteroposterior and (B) axillary X-ray views of a patient's 12-month status post reverse total shoulder arthroplasty. The patient presented with a history of a spontaneous crack in the shoulder and severe debilitating pain which has been managed nonoperatively for 3 months with no resolution. The *yellow arrows* point to the acromion stress fracture which is displaced. The (C) axial and (D) coronal computed tomography cuts defining and confirming an atrophic nonunion. The *arrows* denote the united site.

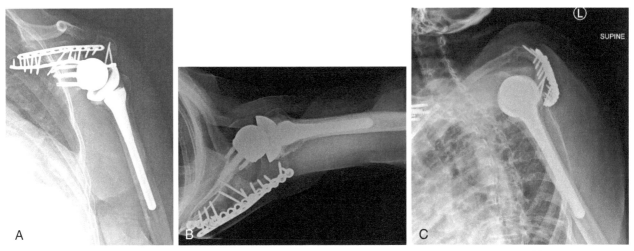

A

B

C

• **Fig. 16.29** These are the (A) anteroposterior, (B) axillary, and (C) scapula Y views of the patient from Fig. 16.28, 6 weeks after surgery. At this time the patient was pain free, but with limited motion, and had been followed up for 24 months and remained pain free.

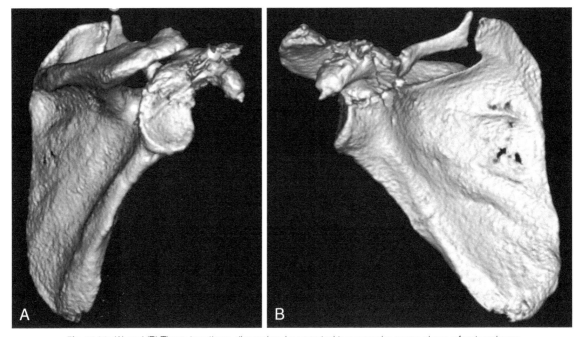

A

B

• **Fig. 16.30** (A) and (B) These two three-dimensional computed tomography scans show a fractured coracoid from two different angles. There is comminution at the base of the coracoid, and the process is displaced inferior and lateral because of the deforming force of the coracobrachialis and short head of biceps.

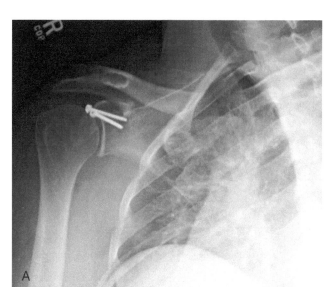
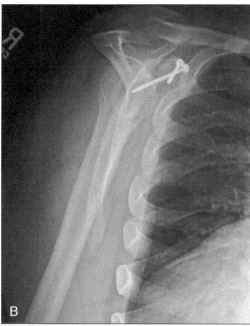

• **Fig. 16.31** This is an (A) anteroposterior and (B) scapula Y X-ray view taken 1 month postoperative of the patient whose fracture was depicted in Fig. 16.30A–B. The coracoid was reduced with a 4-mm Shanz pin and then lagged with a 3.5-mm screw. One more screw was placed to neutralize rotation.

17

The Superior Shoulder Suspensory Complex, Floating Shoulder Injuries, and Other Segmental Injuries to the Shoulder Girdle

CHRIS LANGHAMMER AND NICHOLAS C. DANFORD

Introduction

Segmental injury patterns about the shoulder have earned the name "floating shoulder" and "double disruptions" of the shoulder suspensory complex because they frequently consist of two radiographically distinct skeletal and/or ligamentous injuries about the shoulder girdle. The cumulative instability from two colocalized injuries has made this injury pattern difficult to conceptualize, and its clinical significance and optimal treatment remain controversial. The goal of this chapter is to provide a basis for understanding (1) the pathoanatomy and injury stratification of this injury pattern, (2) the rationale for available treatment options, and (3) the outcomes scoring systems used most frequently in the relevant primary literature. The surgical techniques for management of the various injuries at the clavicle and scapula that comprise the individual aspects of these double disruptions are described elsewhere in this book, and so have been excluded from this chapter in favor of an increased focus on pathoanatomy, indications, and outcomes when these multiple injuries simultaneously befall the same shoulder.

The term "floating" in orthopedic surgery is used to describe segmental injury patterns where skeletal injury has occurred above and below a joint. It is a commonly held belief that the loss of bony stability both above and below an articulation generates a *cumulative instability* that is more clinically disabling than the maximum instability caused by either of its component injury patterns as considered in isolation. In these cases, a risk-benefit assessment of surgical intervention at each individual injury may not justify surgical fixation, but the combination of the two injuries may. Many orthopedic surgeons advocate for partial or complete surgical stabilization of such injuries as a result of this cumulative instability.[1]

The concept of the superior shoulder suspensory complex (SSSC) was first described by Ganz and Noesberger in 1975 in their work *Treatment of Scapular Fractures*,[2] but did not gain the formal title of "floating shoulder" until discussed by Herscovici and coauthors in 1992.[3] The idea ties together the interconnected ring of bony and ligamentous structures about the glenohumeral joint and is perhaps articulated best by Goss shortly following its formal identification.[4] The bony structures of the coracoid, distal clavicle, acromion, and superior aspect of the glenoid are connected into a bony-ligamentous ring by the coracoclavicular (CC), coracoacromial (CA), and acromioclavicular (AC) ligaments which help create a stable platform for the glenohumeral joint This platform is supported away from the chest wall by the clavicular shaft (superior strut) and the scapular body/glenoid neck (inferior strut). In the context of glenoid neck fractures, the ligamentous interconnections of the CC, CA, and AC ligaments generate *redundant stability* around the glenoid platform, in which the stabilizing structures must be fully dissociated from all aspects of the superior struts (including both the anterior strut of the clavicle and the posterior strut of the acromion and spine) before clinically significant instability occurs,[4] as depicted in Fig. 17.1.

At the time of the writing of this chapter, there is insufficient evidence to indicate that any constellation of bony injuries about the shoulder girdle will benefit from surgical management if no single component of that constellation warrants surgical correction when considered in isolation. In other words, double disruptions of the SSSC (of which "floating shoulder" injuries are a subset) are not necessarily greater than the sum of their parts. Similarly, no specific fixation tactic can currently be recommended as superior to any other based on limited outcomes data, such as

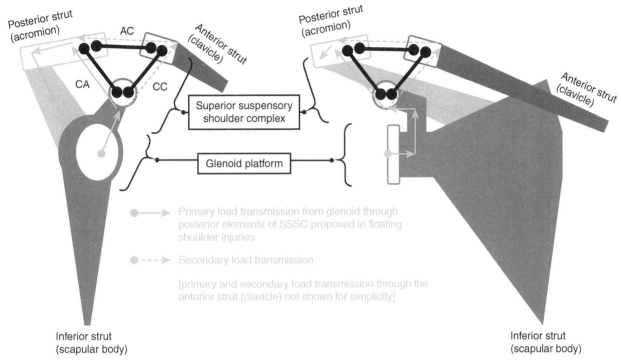

• **Fig. 17.1** Schematic of the superior shoulder suspensory complex *(SSSC)*. Ligamentous connectivity between the coracoid, clavicle *(dark gray)*, and acromion *(light gray)* provide redundant stability to the glenoid platform (acromioclavicular *[AC]*, coracoacromial *[CA]*, coracoclavicular *[CC]* ligaments illustrated in *black*). Load transmission through the posterior acromial strut is illustrated in *green arrows*. Load transmission through the anterior clavicular strut (not shown for simplicity) would be the mirror image.

fixation of the clavicle, scapula, or both. There is, however, growing consensus that treatment options should be considered with a goal of restoring scapular anatomy to within debated acceptable limits, with specific attention to glenopolar angle (GPA), as it is likely that this parameter correlates with shoulder function after injury.[5–7] An understanding of the redundant stability provided by the SSSC will help tailor fixation and rehabilitation strategies to each individual patients' injury. An example of this is the indirect reduction and stabilization of scapular neck fractures which may be achievable using only fixation of associated clavicle fractures.

Anatomy and Pathoanatomy—Historical Evolution of an Injury Definition

The purpose of this section is to define floating shoulder injuries and characterize which fracture patterns may experience redundant stability from the SSSC.

The term "floating shoulder" was originally used to describe the combination of a scapular neck and ipsilateral midshaft clavicle fracture.[3] These authors asserted that isolated fractures of the clavicle OR scapula both do well when treated conservatively, but that fractures of both the clavicle AND scapula do not, due to an assumed inherent instability. Their choice of "floating shoulder" as the name for this injury constellation is confusing, as the term "shoulder" usually refers to the glenohumeral joint. One would imagine that the term floating shoulder would refer to a floating glenohumeral joint, and other authors have noted this term is a misnomer and should best be applied to a glenoid neck fracture with ipsilateral humeral neck fracture.[8] In the case of floating shoulder as described initially and in the vast majority of the published literature, however, there

is no injury distal to the glenohumeral articulation, and so with this in mind it may be easier to conceptualize the idea of cumulative glenoid instability as being caused by a floating AC joint.

The original description was followed shortly by a theoretical description of the SSSC by Goss et al. in 1993.[4] The work was not focused on the concept of the floating shoulder specifically, but instead proposed a theoretical, conceptual framework for shoulder stability meant to facilitate understanding and treatment of complex and segmental injuries in the shoulder. Most importantly, it proposed how the shoulder architecture, when conceptualized as an osseoligamentous superior ring held by superior and inferior struts, may help guide treatment. For example, the redundancy of the superior and inferior struts means that if either the clavicle or scapular body/glenoid neck is disrupted in isolation, theoretically the other strut can provide stability. Similarly, as a ring structure, it is proposed that if a single aspect of the SSSC is disrupted, the remainder of the ring can impart stability (see Fig. 17.1).

In 2001 Williams et al. provided biomechanical evidence supporting the concept of the SSSC's redundant stability.[9] This cadaver-based biomechanical study involving serial sectioning of components of the SSSC showed that in the context of a glenoid neck fracture, gross instability occurred only after complete dissociation of the coracoid from its surrounding stabilizers, including all ligamentous attachments to the acromion and clavicle. It was only after indirect dissociation of the glenoid from the acromion, which is acting as a superior/posterior strut, through combinatorial ligamentous sectioning of the AC, CA, and CC ligaments (in addition to the superior and inferior struts through simulated fracture), that true instability was achieved (see Fig. 17.2). These and other authors make special note that ligamentous injury, while not directly visualized on plain films, can be inferred based on

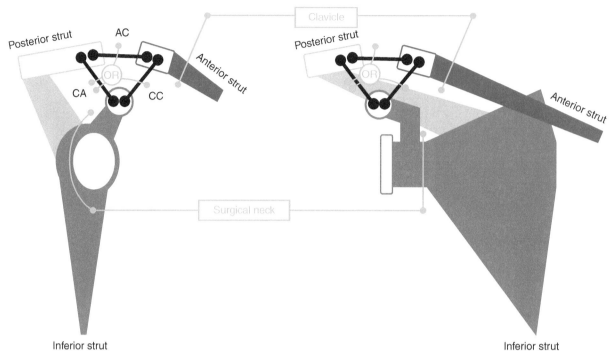

• **Fig. 17.2** Floating shoulder injuries—surgical neck and associated clavicle and ligamentous injury. Floating shoulder injuries as described by Williams and colleagues in their 2001 biomechanical study.[9] Surgical neck fractures were not unstable until the glenoid platform was fully separated from the superior supporting structures through either (1) clavicle fracture with sectioning of coracoacromial *(CA)* and acromioclavicular *(AC)* ligaments both or (2) sectioning of CA and coracoclavicular *(CC)* ligaments. Either of the two disruption sequences above fully dissociates load transmission as shown in Fig. 17.1.

displacement on plain films.[9,10] This biomechanical work implies the existence of a third, redundant, posterior strut: the acromion, although the authors do not specifically define it as such. Additional studies have speculated about the role acromial fracture may play in destabilizing this third strut, and if this should therefore be included in the concept of "floating shoulder."[11]

Based on these studies we are left with a model for shoulder stability in the context of segmental disruption as appears in Fig. 17.1. Due to the redundant stability of the SSSC, glenoid fractures at the surgical neck with *intact* ligamentous connections between the coracoid and acromion or clavicle are stable even in the context of a clavicle fracture as the glenoid platform is suspended from the acromial posterior strut (Fig. 17.2). Conversely, glenoid fractures at the surgical neck with *ruptured* connections between the coracoid and the acromion/clavicle complex will be unstable regardless of a fracture at either one. In general, large displacements (including medialization[12–14]) have been interpreted as markers for ligamentous instability, though this is unproven at this point as no studies cataloging magnetic resonance imaging (MRI) findings in floating shoulder injuries have been performed.[15]

Floating shoulder injuries are a subset of double disruptions of the SSSC in which a scapular neck fracture is one site of disruption. The second disruption can be at a number of locations, including fracture of the clavicle, acromion, or rupture of the AC, CA, or CC ligaments. It is important to note that the two concepts of cumulative instability (floating shoulder) and redundant stabilization (SSSC) overlap most importantly in the case of scapular neck fractures with a superior exit point MEDIAL to the coracoid process[16] (also called "surgical neck" fractures[17]). In these cases, the SSSC may impart stability to the glenoid through the coracoid process and its ligamentous association with the clavicle and acromion (Figs. 17.1 and 17.2).

Special attention must be paid to the character of the surgical neck fracture, because there are a variety of scapular fracture patterns that are frequently included under the heading of floating shoulder injuries, but which are expected to behave differently based on redundant stabilization through the SSSC (see Fig. 17.3). For example, fractures of the anatomic glenoid neck (with superior exit points LATERAL to the coracoid process) maintain no ligamentous connection to the SSSC and therefore do not benefit from its redundant stabilization. Similarly, fractures extending into the articular surface may cause loss of humeral containment or may have significant articular incongruence. The outcomes for these fractures are likely to be driven by different factors than scapular neck–associated floating shoulders and therefore will have distinct operative indications outside those associated with floating shoulder. The idea that there is an interaction between the SSSC and floating shoulder injuries that may direct treatment modalities and affect outcomes, however, requires one to limit this interpretation to surgical neck fractures only.

Quantifying Injury Severity and Outcomes in Floating Shoulder Injuries

Classification Systems and Injury Stratification

Isolated fractures of the scapular articular surface, glenoid anatomic neck, coracoid process, and body have all been discussed separately in this book and in multiple other resources.[18] A variety of different classification systems exist for describing the nature and severity of scapular injuries.[18,19] The term "floating shoulder" was first used by Herscovici et al. in 1992, defined as a

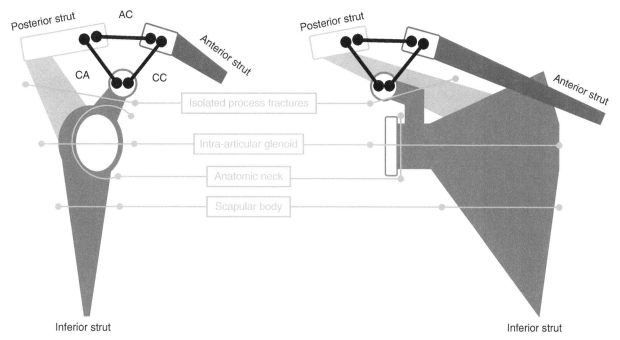

Posterior strut · AC · Anterior strut · CA · CC · Isolated process fractures · Intra-articular glenoid · Anatomic neck · Scapular body · Inferior strut

Posterior strut · Anterior strut · Inferior strut

• **Fig. 17.3** Scapular fractures unlikely to benefit from redundant stabilization by the superior shoulder suspensory complex (SSSC). Examples of scapular fractures frequently included in studies on floating shoulder injuries, but which are unlikely to benefit from the redundant stabilization of the SSSC. In isolated process fractures, load transmission is intact through the inferior strut. In intra-articular glenoid fractures, operative indications are dictated by step-off and concentricity. In anatomic neck fractures, the glenoid is dissociated from all stabilizing structures regardless of additional sites of injury. In scapular body fractures, there is residual communication of the neck to portions of the scapular body. *AC*, Acromioclavicular; *CA*, coracoacromial; *CC*, coracoclavicular.

scapular neck and ipsilateral midshaft clavicle fracture.[3] In much of the current literature, however, the term has come to be more loosely interpreted within the context of the term "floating" and now includes a variety of segmental skeletal disruptions around the shoulder girdle[1] (Fig. 17.4A). There is no widely used classification system for these combined injuries, however. Recent literature has attempted to develop a system based on displacement and stability (as determined by radiographic findings),[15] but has not been widely adopted in subsequent reports.

Concurrent Injuries (Multisystem Injury and Ipsilateral Limb Injury)

Recently, the clinical significance of the floating shoulder as defined by a clavicle fracture in conjunction with a nondisplaced scapular body or neck fracture has been called into question, since the later injury is found with increasing frequency following the addition of the "pan-scan" (computed tomography [CT] head, cervical spine, chest, abdomen, and pelvis) to the algorithmic workup of high-energy blunt trauma at level-1 trauma centers.[20] Clinically irrelevant scapular injuries are now identified with greater frequency, but there is little indication that fractures identifiable only on CT contribute to instability or disability. However, prior to the advent of the pan-scan, these injuries were considered rare and may represent an even higher energy variant of scapular neck fractures.

Floating shoulder injuries are high-energy events and coexist with severe injuries to multiple organ systems—complicating both treatment choice and collection of outcomes measures. Studies have indicated pneumothorax (45%), head injury (41%), lower extremity injury (28%), spine fracture (23%), and brachial plexus injury (23%) may occur at higher rates than with scapular fractures alone, as well as very high rates of ipsilateral limb injury.[10] The Injury Severity Score (ISS) and a thorough cataloging of associated extremity injuries (specifically brachial plexus injuries and ipsilateral limb injuries) will help identify if the appropriate outcome measures are being recorded, and how these injuries and global health status of the patient may drive both outcome and treatment choice (Fig. 17.4B).

Glenopolar Angle

The most frequently studied metric for displacement of glenoid neck fractures is the GPA. The GPA has been studied with regard to scapular neck fractures both in isolation and in association with clavicle fractures, showing that reduced GPA is a predictor of poor outcomes.[21] Further, GPA has shown a "dose-dependent" effect on shoulder function scores in a population of mixed scapular neck and floating shoulder patients.[22]

In the context of floating shoulder injuries specifically, decreased GPA (described initially as "caudal dislocation"[10] and later clarified in subsequent editorial letters[23]) was noted to correlate negatively with function following either conservative management or clavicular stabilization. In other words, patients treated by either modality did worse when their residual deformity as measured by GPA was greater.[10] Additionally, the correlation of GPA on outcomes following both conservatively and operatively treated floating shoulder injuries demonstrates dose dependence in retrospective studies[24,25] and meta-analyses.[7] Finally, the limited prospective literature in this field indicates surgical stabilization may be an effective tool at restoring normal GPA,[26,27] and that the effect on clinical outcome is similarly dose dependent.[26]

There are only two studies in which GPA has been studied and found NOT to be predictive of clinical outcome.[14,27] One

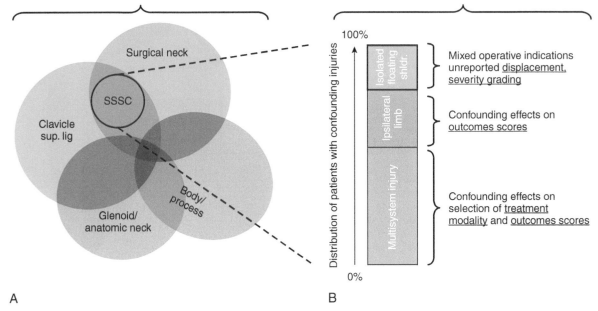

Local injury pattern - possible double disruptions of the SSSC

Global injury pattern - sources of variability in case series

• **Fig. 17.4** Schematic of local and global injury characteristics contributing to heterogeneity in study design. (A) Both local injury patterns based on the specifics of the segmental injury to the shoulder girdle and (B) global injury patterns based on the additional injuries sustained by the patient will have effects on the treatment modalities selected and the outcomes observed. When reading the primary literature, the location of each patient population in the above schematic should be noted as a means of helping generalize the conclusions to a larger population. Floating shoulder injuries as classically described appearing as isolated injuries (the ideal study population, and an obvious minority of total reported cases) are emphasized in *red*. *SSSC*, Superior shoulder suspensory complex.

of these used a single scoring scale only (the Herscovici scale), which has never been validated as an accurate patient-reported outcome measure, and used a threshold of correlation rather than a calculated *P* value to determine "significance." The authors likely meant simply that the correlation is shallow. A reexamination of their data, as available in the manuscript, looking at correlation between final GPA and outcome score for the whole population (rather than operative and nonoperative subpopulations), demonstrates that there *is* a correlation and that it only narrowly misses statistical significance. The second study finds that while reduced GPA is not associated with poor outcome, medialization of the glenoid neck is,[14] and their data are not available for review.

Due to its increasing popularity, the response characteristics of GPA measurement have been studied directly. GPA, as measured on plain radiography, has a high degree of accuracy when compared to 3D CT.[28] Measurement of GPA on plain film anteroposterior (AP) projections of the scapula can be expected to be within approximately 5 degrees of that measured with 3D CT and are expected to be reasonably accurate and reproducible to within approximately 20-degree deviation from an AP view in any plane before large measurement error is encountered.[29]

Given its reliability, reproducibility, and the increasing body of work demonstrating a correlation with outcomes, the GPA may be one of the best metrics to predict outcomes after floating shoulder injuries. In the absence of GPA, other quantitative measures of displacement, including medialization, should be noted.

Outcomes Scoring

The goal of this section is to provide an overview of the challenges in assessing outcomes after floating shoulder injuries, and the

history and characteristics of the scales used most frequently in the relevant literature.

The purpose of a scoring system is to facilitate comparison of results between populations, interventions, and across time by creating a reproducible and specific vocabulary with which to describe outcomes. A review of shoulder scoring scales emphasizes the importance of appropriately selecting instruments for a given clinical indication, and that instruments developed before modern validation techniques may not have appropriate response characteristics to capture the effect of interest. This creates confusion in the interpretation of both positive and negative results.[30] Additionally, the application of instruments that are not shoulder-specific should be interpreted with caution in a multiply-injured patient population, as global functional outcomes can be driven by disability occurring outside of the zone of interest. The importance of this cannot be overstated, as the injury pattern of interest is so frequently attached to patients with multiple extremities and organ systems affected by their trauma. Multiple studies, even within the context of floating shoulder injuries, have identified other injury, notably ipsilateral limb injury or injury to the central or peripheral nervous system, to be the primary driver of global outcome[3,22] (Fig. 17.4B).

A recent systematic review of floating shoulder injuries identified the multiple scoring systems used most frequently to assess clinical outcomes from this injury pattern.[5] Of the modern shoulder/upper limb–specific instruments used in more than one recent high-quality study, the most popular were the Constant score (nine studies), the DASH ([Disability of the Arm, Shoulder and Hand]; three studies), Rowe (three studies), UCLA rating scale (two studies), and the ASES (American Shoulder and Elbow Surgeons) score (two studies). Additional scores used which assess global patient status and lack validation or were used infrequently included the Herscovici score, the Short Form-36/12 (SF-36/12), and the Oxford Shoulder Score. These scales have been reviewed expertly.[31–33]

Treatment Options

The goal of this section is to provide an overview of the treatment options for floating shoulder injuries, accompanied by a nonexhaustive survey of the evidence and opinions supporting each option.

Proponents for surgical stabilization of floating shoulder injuries have traditionally advocated for either fixation of the clavicle only or fixation of both the clavicle and scapular neck. The few studies advocating for surgical fixation of the scapular neck in isolation are based on the recommendations of the authors rather than on clinical outcomes data.[6,15] They do an excellent job of enumerating their reasons this approach may be indicated, but are not mentioned further because they are based on author opinion rather than clinical outcome studies.

Nonoperative Treatment

While early authors suggested that combined neck and clavicle fractures were by definition unstable, little in the literature has demonstrated progressive deformity in the context of floating shoulder injuries. Progressive displacement of scapular fractures has been described in a single study.[34] In this report on 49 consecutive scapular ORIF (open reduction internal fixation) procedures, 8 were indicated for secondary displacement (interestingly, only 3 of which were classified as double disruptions of the SSSC). However, all cases had a very specific transverse body pattern, which is neither a common pattern within the floating shoulder literature nor a pattern that would be expected to benefit from the redundant stability of the SSSC (Fig. 17.3). The progressive deformity in GPA reported by the authors was accompanied by lateral translation of the inferior pole rather than a true angular deformity of the neck relative to the superior shoulder structures. This study demonstrates that progressive deformity may occur in some scapular fracture patterns. It should be interpreted with caution, however, as not all measures of displacement are likely to be relevant to all injury patterns, and there is little additional evidence to indicate a high rate of progressive displacement in scapular fractures.

Progressive displacement of a scapular neck fracture in the context of high-quality studies specifically reporting on floating shoulder injuries has been described in only two patients (one each in two separate series[10,14]). Late surgery for clavicle malunion and nonunion commensurate with isolated clavicle literature has been described in the context of floating shoulder injuries, but these patients have not been assessed for the purposes of subgroup analysis.

Overall, excellent results can be expected from nonoperative treatment when patients are selected appropriately. There is now consensus that appropriately selected minimally displaced fractures can be considered stable and can be treated successfully without surgical intervention due to the low rate of observed progressive deformity and the good clinical outcomes achieved with nonoperative treatment.

The success of nonoperative treatment should be considered cautiously, however, as it may not generalize to all patients. Due to the nonrandom assortment of patients to different treatment arms in retrospective case-series, studies examining nonoperative treatment frequently do not include patients who would benefit from surgical stabilization. An early study advocating for nonoperative treatment includes no mention of the displacement of

the injuries and uses only a single unvalidated outcomes tool.[35] A later study of 20 patients includes only 6 who would have arguably met modern indications for procedural intervention.[36] In patient series demonstrating no difference in operative treatment versus nonoperative treatment, the retrospective and nonrandomized application of treatment protocols prohibits interpretation. When an indication for surgery is "preference of the treating physician" or otherwise nondisclosed parameters, the most that can be taken from a study demonstrating equivalent outcomes is that the patients were assigned to treatment arms in an appropriate fashion, not that the effects of the treatment arms are equivalent.

Clavicle-Only Fixation

Many studies demonstrate good outcomes following clavicle-only stabilization of floating shoulder injuries. Proponents for clavicle-only fixation claim this technique provides adequate secondary stabilization of the glenoid, assuming there are intact ligamentous connections between the coracoid process and acromion or distal clavicle. Even before the accumulation of evidence regarding the efficacy of this technique, early authors suggested that "surgical management of one site (preferably the one that is easier to address) often reduces and stabilizes the other site secondarily."[4] Proponents additionally claim the technique reduces the surgical morbidity associated with a traditional Judet approach to the scapula, including muscle weakness, prolonged operative time, increased blood loss, and the possibility of neurologic injury.

These claims were eventually well supported, as authors have found that clavicle fixation using intramedullary fixation or plates has generally good outcomes and is not generally associated with late displacement of the unfixed scapular neck fracture.[25,37,38] In further support of clavicle-only fixation, there is evidence that reduction and fixation of the clavicle fracture may even reduce the glenoid indirectly[27,39] in patients where the ligamentous connectivity of the SSSC is preserved.

These results should be interpreted with caution, however, as many papers demonstrating good outcomes with isolated clavicle fixation frequently include only nondisplaced fractures of the neck, even going so far as to exclude patients with neck fractures so displaced they warranted independent fixation.[24] One would not expect these fractures to displace, regardless of whether the clavicle is stabilized. Additionally, the finding that scapular reduction is possible by manipulating the clavicle is not consistent between studies. A different, well-designed study demonstrated that while some correction of GPA is possible, it is not enough to correct GPA to the point that patients avoid the negative clinical impact of residual deformity.[26]

Combined Fixation

Despite the generally good results with nonoperative management and fixation of the clavicle alone reported in many case-series, many authors still advocate for fixation of the scapular neck directly. These authors endorse the belief that treatment should be dedicated to restoring glenoid reduction, and that clavicle-only fixation may be inadequate to achieve this in certain instances due to nonobvious ligamentous injury.[10]

The topic is fraught with conflicting reports due again in large degree to lack of randomization in treatment assignment. In general, patients with worse injuries to the shoulder (as described by displacement, comminution, or intra-articular involvement) receive operative fixation, whereas patients with less severe injuries to the shoulder are funneled selectively to the nonoperative or less invasive groups. There is an additional confounding factor that severe systemic injuries, ipsilateral limb injuries, and brachial plexus injury (all of which have a large effect on outcomes scores) frequently coexist with floating shoulder injuries.[12] Whether a study is biased in favor of surgical fixation or nonoperative treatment will be unpredictably determined by their inclusion and treatment criteria (Fig. 17.4). One frequently quoted study that did not find a difference between operative and nonoperative management used mixed inclusion criteria and the authors admit that it was profoundly affected by nonrandomization (patients with minimal displacement or too unstable for operative intervention received nonoperative treatment, the others received treatment for the most displaced injury).[14] Another study with similar findings which did not show a difference in the outcome between clavicle-only and combined fixation disproportionately includes non-neck scapular fractures in the clavicle-only group. Given these study designs, their results cannot be easily generalized to all "floating shoulder" injuries.[40]

While nonrandomized case-series demonstrate mixed and difficult to interpret results, one of the only prospective studies examining floating shoulder injuries provides excellent support for fixation of both injuries.[26] The authors show that fixation of both the clavicle and scapular neck provides superior correction of GPA relative to clavicular fixation alone, and that final deformity as measured by GPA correlates with poor outcomes in a dose-dependent fashion as measured by validated and translatable outcomes scores. The exclusion criteria effectively isolate the treatment effect to the shoulder injury and to floating shoulder injuries with preserved ligamentous complexes (which may theoretically benefit from clavicular fixation alone). This study demonstrated that while there was no secondary displacement in the "nonoperative" and "clavicle-only fixation" groups, that correction of the GPA was not achieved with clavicular fixation only.

The recommendation to perform open reduction should be interpreted carefully, however, as the procedure obviously comes with surgical risks that may outweigh any incremental benefit. One author reported equivalent outcomes with a more serious complication profile in the operative group, including iatrogenic nerve injury.[41] The loss of strength following combined fixation relative to nonoperative and clavicular fixation is a constant theme between multiple reports,[12,37,41,42] which many speculate is a consequence of separation of the infraspinatus from its scapular origin. Another author describes a four-fold increase in operative time and a six-fold increase in blood loss between clavicle-only and combined fixation, demonstrating the relative increase in surgical complexity and risk between these two fixation tactics.[40] While multiple techniques have been described to minimize operative complications, including the classic Judet approach, modified Judet approach, and minimally invasive approaches,[43–46] there is little evidence-based guidance regarding superiority of any one approach over another.

Treatment Algorithms

In the absence of definitive evidence of superiority of any one treatment modality, and in the context of conflicting studies of varied design, several durable themes can be qualitatively inferred from the literature. There is growing consensus regarding the following points:

1. Minimally displaced floating shoulder injuries are typically stable, and it is likely they can be treated nonoperatively with success.
2. Clinical outcomes appear to be correlated with glenoid reduction as measured by GPA, therefore surgical treatment of displaced floating shoulder injuries should be aimed at restoring the anatomic relationships of the glenoid.

3. Fixation of the clavicle alone is relatively straightforward and may indirectly assist with reduction of the glenoid in cases where there has not been additional disruption of the CC, AC, or CA ligaments.
4. In cases where there is still significant glenoid displacement despite reduction and stabilization of the clavicle, ORIF of the scapular neck may be considered to further restore normal anatomic parameters (although this procedure is more technically demanding and may result in muscle weakness and other sequelae).

Given the points above, many authors are now recommending variations on a treatment algorithm consisting of fixation of the clavicle first with the patient supine or in the beach chair position, followed by repeat radiographic examination of the scapular neck. If there is persistent unacceptable deformity, then proceed with fixation of the scapular neck after repositioning the patient as necessary.[6,10,13,47]

Systematic Reviews and Primary Literature Table

Provided is a tabulated list of the most widely cited high-quality primary studies of floating shoulder injuries.

Synthesizing treatment recommendations from the varied spectrum of literature regarding floating shoulder injuries is a challenge. This is a rare injury that occurs in medically complex patients, in which treatment preferences vary widely based on treating center and physician. As such, research on the topic is dominated by retrospective reviews which are overwhelmingly nonrandomized, predisposing them to powerful selection bias. These studies are best characterized by their heterogeneity on injury reporting, inclusion and exclusion criteria, treatment modality, and outcomes reporting.

In addition, because there is no widely accepted classification system or outcome reporting for this injury pattern, injury severity cannot be controlled for and outcome cannot be reproducibly reported in such a way to facilitate comparison between studies. With no ability to control for injury severity, it is impossible to tell if similar outcomes between treated and untreated groups mean that there is no beneficial effect of treatment, or if similar outcomes simply mean we are already doing a very good job of separating patients who would benefit from surgical intervention from patients who would not.

Several recent reviews have done an excellent job of consolidating the available primary literature and attempting to combine studies in a variety of ways to derive statistical significance from this body of work.[5–7] They have all found insufficient evidence to make specific treatment recommendations.

We (the authors) encourage you (the readers) to read each paper on your own, keeping in mind the points covered in this chapter regarding injury pathoanatomy and stratification (Figs. 17.1–17.3), selection bias in treatment modality, and outcome reporting. As a means of assessing the validity of each paper's conclusions, compare the inclusion criteria to the injury schematics in Figs. 17.1–17.3 and consider how treatment assignment and outcomes scoring will be affected by local (Fig. 17.4A) and global (Fig. 17.4B) injury severity (Table 17.1).

We believe the overwhelming majority of "floating shoulder" injuries are stable and will do well without fixation. The topic remains relevant, however, as a thorough understanding of the anatomic basis of the SSSC will assist with the clinical decision-making and management of the rare injuries that will benefit from surgical intervention.

TABLE 17.1   Primary Studies of Floating Shoulder Injuries

Ref. #	Design	N	Injury Description/Indication	No.	Clavicle	Scapula	Combo	Outcomes	Follow-up
Herscovici et al. (1992)[3]	Retrospective; Single center	7	Midshaft clavicle + scapular neck (presumed anatomic neck)	—	7	—	—	Noncomparable scales	Avg. ~4 years
Leung and Lam (1993)[42]	Retrospective; Single center	15	Displaced scapular fracture; Contains mix of anatomic neck/other	—	—	—	15	Noncomparable scales; 50% had subjective loss of strength	Avg. ~2 years
Ramos et al. (1997)[35]	Retrospective; Single center	16	Ipsilateral clavicle + scapula; No measure of displacement; Includes severely injured patients and ipsilateral injury	16	—	—	—	Herscovici—avg. 15	Avg. ~7 years
Edwards et al. (2000)[36]	Retrospective; Single center	20	3 operative based on SN; 5 operative based on clavicle; Majority clavicle shaft + neck; Exclude TBI and ipsilateral injury	20	—	—	—	Constant—96; Rowe—95; Herscovici—17 excellent/3 good; Symmetric strength	Avg. ~2 years
Egol et al. (2001)[41]	Retrospective; Single center	19	OTA classification; No clear description of indication or displacement; Includes intra-articular fractures in the operative group	12	—	—	7	DASH—52 vs. 46 (not significant); ASES—80 vs. 88 (not significant); ROM—20 degrees > in the operative group; Strength—NO > operative group; SF-36—no difference	Avg. ~4 years
van Noort et al. (2001)[10]	Retrospective; Multicenter	35	Anatomic/surgical neck + clavicle; Displacement (not defined); Nonunion/malunion of clavicle; GPA	28	7	—	—	Constant—76 vs. 71; (42 if displaced, 85 if nondisplaced)	Avg. ~3 years
Oh et al. (2002)[13]	Retrospective; Single center	3	Clavicle or AC + neck (± body); No neurovascular injury; Includes severe polytrauma in nonoperative group	3	5	—	5	Rowe—77 vs. 88; Medialization correlated with worse outcome	Avg. 20 months
Hashiguchi and Ito (2003)[37]	Retrospective; Single center	5	Anatomic neck + midshaft clavicle; Neck displacement not specified	—	5 (K-wires)	—	—	UCLA—34; Strength—no difference to contra	Avg. ~5 years
Labler et al. (2004)[12]	Retrospective; Single center	17	Displacement clavicle and scapula; GPA <30 degrees; Scapular fixation only if wide scapular displacement; Includes clavicle fixation for pulmonary function	8	7	—	2	Constant—no difference; SF-36—worse in the nonoperative group (driven by other injuries); Weakness noted in the operative group	Avg. ~6 years

Study	Design	Center	N	Indications/Notes					Outcomes	Follow-up
Kim et al. (2008)[24]	Retrospective	Single center	16	Displaced clavicle fractures; Excludes scapular neck fractures fixed directly	7	9	—	—	Constant—65 vs. 74; Dose-dependent effect of GPA on outcome	Avg. ~5 years
Izadpanah et al. (2012)[25]	Retrospective	Single center	16	Displaced clavicle + nondisplaced neck; Includes GPA	—	16	—	—	Constant—approximately 85; ASES—approximately 82	Avg. 3 years
Pailhes et al. (2013)[14]	Retrospective	Single center	40	Includes isolated body and intra-articular glenoid; Nonrandomized mixed fixation	24	10	3	3	Constant—84; DASH—15; Simple Shoulder Test—11; Oxford Shoulder Score—14; SANE—81%; SF-12—50 and 60; No difference in operative vs. nonoperative; Medialization correlated with poor outcome	Avg. 12 years
Yadav et al. (2013)[27]	Prospective randomized	Single center	25	Displaced clavicle and scapula; Excludes neurovascular and polytrauma	13	12	—	—	Herscovici—13 vs. 15; ROM improved in the operative group; GPA improved in the operative group	Avg. 2 years
Gilde et al. (2015)[38]	Retrospective	Single center	13	Clavicular displacement; No GPA <20	—	13	—	—	Herscovici—13; VAS—unreportable; All returned to employment	Avg. 16 months
Lin et al. (2015)[26]	Prospective	Stratified random	39	GPA <30 or clavicle displacement; Excludes ipsilateral UE injury and neurovascular injury	13	13	—	13	Constant—75 vs. 65; DASH—2 vs. 16; Dose-dependent effect of GPA on outcome; Superiority of combined fixation over clavicle-only fixation	Avg. 24 months
Zhou et al. (2017)[40]	Retrospective	Single center	56	Mixed indications	12	29	—	9	Constant—74 vs. 85; Herscovici—9 vs. 13; No difference in clavicle-only and combined fixation	Avg. 17 months
Samy and Darwish (2017)[39]	Retrospective	Single center	13	Displaced clavicle with GPA <30; +Intraoperative assessment of coracoclavicular ligaments	—	13	—	—	UCLA—32; Improvement noted in GPA following clavicle-only fixation	Avg. 24 months

AC, acromioclavicular; ASES, American Shoulder and Elbow Surgeons; DASH, The Disabilities of the Arm, Shoulder and Hand; GPA, glenopolar angle; OTA, Orthopaedic Trauma Association; ROM, range of motion; SANE, single assessment numeric evaluation; SF-36, Short Form-36; SN, scapular neck; TBI, traumatic brain injury; UE, upper extremity; UCLA, The University of California—Los Angeles; VAS, visual analog scale.

References

1. Mohamed SO, Ju W, Qin Y, Qi B. The term "floating" used in traumatic orthopedics. *Medicine (Baltim)*. 2019;98(7). e14497.
2. Ganz R, Noesberger B. [Treatment of scapular fractures]. *Hefte Unfallheilkd*. 1975;(126):59–62.
3. Herscovici Jr D, Fiennes AG, Allgöwer M, Rüedi TP. The floating shoulder: ipsilateral clavicle and scapular neck fractures. *J Bone Joint Surg Br*. 1992;74(3):362–364.
4. Goss TP. Double disruptions of the superior shoulder suspensory complex. *J Orthop Trauma*. 1993;7(2):99–106.
5. Dombrowsky AR, Boudreau S, Quade J, et al. Clinical outcomes following conservative and surgical management of floating shoulder injuries: a systematic review. *J Shoulder Elbow Surg*. 2019;29(3):634–642.
6. Hess F, Zettl R, Smolen D, et al. Decision-making for complex scapula and ipsilateral clavicle fractures: a review. *Eur J Trauma Emerg Surg*. 2019;45(2):221–230.
7. Morey VM, Chua KHZ, Ng ZD, et al. Management of the floating shoulder: does the glenopolar angle influence outcomes? A systematic review. *Orthop Traumatol Surg Res*. 2018;104(1):53–58.
8. Berkes MB, Little MTM, Pardee NC, et al. Outcomes of proximal humerus fracture open reduction internal fixation with concomitant ipsilateral shoulder girdle injuries: a case control study. *HSS J*. 2016;12(2):105–110.
9. Williams Jr GR, Naranja J, Klimkiewicz J, et al. The floating shoulder: a biomechanical basis for classification and management. *J Bone Joint Surg Am*. 2001;83(8):1182–1187.
10. van Noort A, te Slaa RL, van der Werken C, et al. The floating shoulder. A multicentre study. *J Bone Joint Surg Br*. 2001;83(6):795–798.
11. Lyons RP. Open reduction and internal fixation of os acromion fracture-separation as a component of a floating shoulder injury: a case report. *J Shoulder Elbow Surg*. 2010;19(7). e18-21.
12. Labler L, Platz A, Weishaupt D, et al. Clinical and functional results after floating shoulder injuries. *J Trauma*. 2004;57(3):595–602.
13. Oh W, et al. The treatment of double disruption of the superior shoulder suspensory complex. *Int Orthop*. 2002;26(3):145–149.
14. Pailhes RG, Pailhes RG, Bonnevialle N, et al. Floating shoulders: clinical and radiographic analysis at a mean follow-up of 11 years. *Int J Shoulder Surg*. 2013;7(2):59–64.
15. Friederichs J, Morgenstern M, Buhren V. Scapula fractures in complex shoulder injuries and floating shoulders: a classification based on displacement and instability. *J Trauma Manag Outcomes*. 2014;8:16.
16. Arts V, Louette L. Scapular neck fractures; an update of the concept of floating shoulder. *Injury*. 1999;30(2):146–148.
17. Hardegger FH, Simpson LA, Weber BG. The operative treatment of scapular fractures. *J Bone Joint Surg Br*. 1984;66(5):725–731.
18. Browner BD, Jupiter J, Cole PA. *Skeletal Trauma: Basic Science, Management, and Reconstruction*. 6th ed. St. Louis: Elsevier; 2019.
19. Ropp AM, Davis DL. Scapular fractures: what radiologists need to know. *AJR Am J Roentgenol*. 2015;205(3):491–501.
20. Brown C, Elmobdy K, Raja AS, et al. Scapular fractures in the pan-scan era. *Acad Emerg Med*. 2018;25(7):738–743.
21. Romero J, Schai P, Imhoff AB. Scapular neck fracture—the influence of permanent malalignment of the glenoid neck on clinical outcome. *Arch Orthop Trauma Surg*. 2001;121(6):313–316.
22. Bozkurt M, Can F, Kirdemir V, et al. Conservative treatment of scapular neck fracture: the effect of stability and glenopolar angle on clinical outcome. *Injury*. 2005;36(10):1176–1181.
23. Gerber C. The floating shoulder: a multicentre study. *J Bone Joint Surg Br*. 2002;84(5):776. author reply 776.
24. Kim KC, Rhee KJ, Shin HD, et al. Can the glenopolar angle be used to predict outcome and treatment of the floating shoulder? *J Trauma*. 2008;64(1):174–178.
25. Izadpanah K, Jaeger M, Maier D, et al. The floating shoulder—clinical and radiological results after intramedullary stabilization of the clavicle in cases with minor displacement of the scapular neck fracture. *J Trauma Acute Care Surg*. 2012;72(2). E8-13.
26. Lin TL, Li YF, Hsu CJ, et al. Clinical outcome and radiographic change of ipsilateral scapular neck and clavicular shaft fracture: comparison of operation and conservative treatment. *J Orthop Surg Res*. 2015;10:9.
27. Yadav V, Khare GN, Singh S, et al. A prospective study comparing conservative with operative treatment in patients with a 'floating shoulder' including assessment of the prognostic value of the glenopolar angle. *Bone Joint Lett J*. 2013;95-B(6):815–819.
28. Kejriwal R, Ahuja T, Hong T. Is radiograph glenopolar angle accurate for extraarticular scapular neck fractures? *Injury*. 2016;47(12):2772–2776.
29. Suter T, Henninger HB, Zhang Y, et al. Comparison of measurements of the glenopolar angle in 3D CT reconstructions of the scapula and 2D plain radiographic views. *Bone Joint Lett J*. 2016;98-B(11):1510–1516.
30. Kirkley A, Griffin S, Dainty K. Scoring systems for the functional assessment of the shoulder. *Arthroscopy*. 2003;19(10):1109–1120.
31. Wylie JD, Beckmann JT, Granger E, et al. Functional outcomes assessment in shoulder surgery. *World J Orthop*. 2014;5(5):623–633.
32. Wright RW, Baumgarten KM. Shoulder outcomes measures. *J Am Acad Orthop Surg*. 2010;18(7):436–444.
33. van de Water AT, Shields N, Taylor NF. Outcome measures in the management of proximal humeral fractures: a systematic review of their use and psychometric properties. *J Shoulder Elbow Surg*. 2011;20(2):333–343.
34. Anavian J, Khanna G, Plocher EK, et al. Progressive displacement of scapula fractures. *J Trauma*. 2010;69(1):156–161.
35. Ramos L, Mencía R, Alonso A, et al. Conservative treatment of ipsilateral fractures of the scapula and clavicle. *J Trauma*. 1997;42(2):239–242.
36. Edwards SG, Whittle AP, Wood 2nd GW. Nonoperative treatment of ipsilateral fractures of the scapula and clavicle. *J Bone Joint Surg Am*. 2000;82(6):774–780.
37. Hashiguchi H, Ito H. Clinical outcome of the treatment of floating shoulder by osteosynthesis for clavicular fracture alone. *J Shoulder Elbow Surg*. 2003;12(6):589–591.
38. Gilde AK, Hoffmann MF, Sietsema DL, et al. Functional outcomes of operative fixation of clavicle fractures in patients with floating shoulder girdle injuries. *J Orthop Traumatol*. 2015;16(3):221–227.
39. Samy MA, Darwish AE. Fixation of clavicle alone in floating shoulder injury: functional and radiological outcome. *Acta Orthop Belg*. 2017;83(2):292–296.
40. Zhou Q, Chen B, Zhou Y, et al. Comparisons of shoulder function after treatment of floating shoulder injuries with different methods. *Biomedical Research*. 2017;28(5):2320–2326.
41. Egol KA, Connor PM, Karunakar MA, et al. The floating shoulder: clinical and functional results. *J Bone Joint Surg Am*. 2001;83(8):1188–1194.
42. Leung KS, Lam TP. Open reduction and internal fixation of ipsilateral fractures of the scapular neck and clavicle. *J Bone Joint Surg Am*. 1993;75(7):1015–1018.
43. Cole PA, Dubin JR, Freeman G. Operative techniques in the management of scapular fractures. *Orthop Clin North Am*. 2013;44(3):331–343 (viii).
44. Gauger EM, Cole PA. Surgical technique: a minimally invasive approach to scapula neck and body fractures. *Clin Orthop Relat Res*. 2011;469(12):3390–3399.
45. Harmer LS, Phelps KD, Crickard CV, et al. A comparison of exposure between the classic and modified Judet approaches to the scapula. *J Orthop Trauma*. 2016;30(5):235–239.
46. Obremskey WT, Lyman JR. A modified Judet approach to the scapula. *J Orthop Trauma*. 2004;18(10):696–699.
47. Coleridge S, Ricketts D. The floating shoulder: a multicentre study. *J Bone Joint Surg Br*. 2003;85(2):308. author reply 308-309.

18

Scapulothoracic Dissociation

JACLYN M. JANKOWSKI, FRANK A. LIPORACE, AND RICHARD S. YOON

Introduction

Scapulothoracic dissociation is a rare and devastating injury of the shoulder girdle. Originally described by Oreck et al. in 1984, the injury was defined as a complete separation of the acromioclavicular (AC) joint with lateral displacement of the scapula and disruption of the brachial plexus and subclavian vessels with intact skin.[1] It is most often the result of high-energy trauma to the shoulder girdle with a subsequent massive traction force applied to the affected upper extremity. In 1987 Ebraheim et al. expanded the definition to include the addition of either a distracted clavicle fracture or sternoclavicular (SC) joint separation.[2] Currently, scapulothoracic dissociation is considered to be a spectrum of injury that includes AC joint separation (25%), clavicle fractures (55%), and/or SC joint separation (20%); vascular injury to subclavian or axillary vessels (64%); partial or complete disruption of the brachial plexus (40% have incomplete neurologic deficit, 36% with brachial plexus avulsions); severe soft-tissue swelling; and extensive disruption of the musculature surrounding the shoulder girdle (Fig. 18.1).[3,4] This constellation of injuries is considered to be analogous to a closed forequarter amputation.[5] It was originally reported that the mortality rate of scapulothoracic dissociation was 11%, but in reality, it is likely higher, due to many patients dying from associated injuries in the field prior to making it to the emergency room.[2]

Relevant Anatomy

The relevant osseous anatomy of this injury pattern includes the scapula and the clavicle. The scapula itself has no direct osseous attachment to the axial skeleton. Instead, it has indirect attachments via the AC and SC joints. Additionally, the scapula has an indirect relationship with the thorax via infraserratus and supraserratus bursae.[6]

Three muscle groups can be affected in this spectrum of injury: scapulothoracic, rotator cuff, and scapulohumeral. The scapulothoracic muscles include trapezius, serratus anterior, levator scapulae, rhomboid major, and pectoralis minor. The rotator cuff muscles include supraspinatus, infraspinatus, teres minor, and subscapularis. The scapulohumeral muscles include deltoid, latissimus dorsi, and triceps.[7]

The vasculature of the upper limb is redundant, with extensive collateral flow. The subclavian artery arises from the innominate artery on the right and directly off of the aortic arch on the left. The subclavian artery has five main branches: the internal mammary artery, the vertebral arteries, the high thoracic artery, and the thyrocervical trunk. At the level of the first rib, the subclavian artery ends and becomes the axillary artery.[8] The axillary artery has six main branches: the superior thoracic artery, the lateral thoracic artery, the thoracoacromial trunk, the subscapular artery, and the anterior and posterior circumflex humeral arteries.[9] The axillary then becomes the brachial artery once it courses over the anterior shaft of the humerus at the inferior margin of teres major (Fig. 18.2).

The nerve supply to the upper extremity originates from the C5-T1 nerve roots and is supplied mostly via the terminal branches of the brachial plexus (Fig. 18.3). Scapulothoracic dissociation can present with preganglionic nerve root injuries, meaning they occur proximal to the dorsal root ganglion, or postganglionic nerve root injuries, meaning they occur distal to the dorsal root ganglion. The dorsal root ganglion contains sensory neurons that relay information from thermoreceptors, nociceptors, proprioceptors, and chemoreceptors to the central nervous system.[10]

Pathoanatomy

Scapulothoracic dissociation, now understood to be a spectrum of injury, includes AC, clavicle, and/or SC injuries; damage to the subclavian or axillary vessels; brachial plexus injury/avulsion; as well as disruption of the musculature surrounding the shoulder, typically resulting from a high-energy traction mechanism. Traction injuries to the vasculature of the upper extremity can cause extensive internal bleeding and limb-threatening ischemia if not addressed in a timely manner. As noted above, there is extensive collateral vascular flow such that patients may have a perfused limb or even a palpable pulse even in the setting of a complete transection or thrombosis from intimal occlusion of the subclavian artery. Brachial plexus avulsions, while not necessary to treat emergently, dictate the long-term outcomes of this constellation of injuries.

With regard to the spectrum of osseous injury in scapulothoracic dissociation, it can be thought of within the framework of the superior shoulder suspensory complex (SSSC) originally described by Goss in 1993 and described in this text in Chapter 17.[11]

- **Fig. 18.1** Scapulothoracic dissociation is a spectrum of injury that includes acromioclavicular, clavicle, and/or sternoclavicular injuries. (A) Disruption of the musculature surrounding the shoulder and (B) damage to the subclavian or axillary vessels, and brachial plexus injury/avulsion. (From Flanigan BA, Leslie MP. Scapulothoracic dissociation. *Orthop Clin N Am.* 2013;44:1-7.)

The SSSC is a bone and soft tissue ring that comprises the glenoid, distal clavicle, acromion, AC joint, and coracoclavicular ligaments. This ring is held in place by two struts, which impart an element of redundancy: the superior strut is composed of the clavicle shaft and AC joint while the inferior strut is composed of the acromion, scapular spine, and lateral scapula. The SSSC concept posits that "double disruptions," when the ring fails in two locations, lead to a degree of instability that has decreased potential to heal without surgical intervention. Additionally, this increased degree of instability can lead to further neurovascular compromise in a patient where some degree of vascular compromise or brachial plexus disruption likely already exists.

Initial radiographic evaluation should begin with a well-centered chest X-ray to look for lateral displacement of the scapula (a finding that is considered pathognomonic for scapulothoracic dissociation). Lateral displacement of the scapula is quantified by the scapular index. This is obtained by measuring the distance from the medial border of the scapula to the thoracic spinous process, then obtaining the ratio between the measurement of the injured side compared with that of the uninjured side. A ratio of ≥1.29 on chest X-ray without rotation is consistent with scapulothoracic dissociation.[12] Rotation can be assessed by observing how the thoracic spinous processes line up with the sternum. Diagnosis is generally confirmed with dedicated radiographs of the scapula as well as computed tomography (CT) of the injured extremity (Fig. 18.4).

On physical examination, this injury typically presents as severe swelling about the shoulder due to the hematoma formation that results from the significant soft tissue damage that is characteristic of this injury. Inspection of the shoulder girdle should be followed by a thorough vascular examination to assess perfusion of the limb. Initial assessment of perfusion should begin with palpation, Doppler evaluation, and brachial-brachial indices, followed by angiography to evaluate for injury to the subclavian, axillary, or brachial vessels.[13]

Once determined that the patient is hemodynamically stabilized, a very thorough neurologic examination must be performed to determine the presence of incomplete or complete brachial plexus injury. As mentioned earlier, the vascular injury is a life- and limb-threatening event that often required emergent exploration and surgical treatment, but the severity of brachial plexus injury determines the long-term disability. Preganglionic neurologic injuries can present with weakness of the serratus anterior, rhomboids, and levator scapula, as well as with potential Horner's syndrome (miosis, ptosis, and anhidrosis).[5] Magnetic resonance imaging (MRI) or CT myelogram can be performed to evaluate for nerve root avulsion.[14]

Classification

In 1997, Damschen et al. initially classified scapulothoracic dissociation into three types.[4] Type 1 was musculoskeletal injury alone. Type 2A was musculoskeletal injury with associated vascular disruption. Type 2B was musculoskeletal injury with associated incomplete neurological impairment of the upper extremity. Type 3 was a musculoskeletal injury with both a vascular compromise and incomplete neurological injury. More recently, in 2004 Zelle et al. demonstrated that the initial classification system described by Damschen was not indicative of long-term patient outcomes.[15] In their series, patients classified as having type 3 injuries did not have significantly worse outcomes than those with type 1 or 2 injuries. Soberingly, all patients with complete brachial plexus avulsion either reported poor shoulder function or had an amputation by the time of follow-up. As such, they proposed the addition of a fourth type. Type 4 being a musculoskeletal injury with complete brachial plexus avulsion (Table 18.1).

Treatment Options

Scapulothoracic dissociation remains a rare injury pattern that has a wide variety of presentations, and as such, there is not a universally accepted treatment algorithm. In general, if the patient is hemodynamically unstable, vascular exploration and management of vascular injury should be completed first, with possible intraoperative angiography at the discretion of the vascular surgeon. If the patient is stable, CT angiography should be performed prior to surgical assessment of vascular injury. With regard to osseous fixation, some believe it should be performed as an adjunct to vascular repair as a means of providing the stabilization necessary to protect the repair. This most commonly means open reduction internal fixation of associated clavicle fractures with plate and screw fixation. If the patient does not require emergent surgical intervention for vascular injury, many feel that osseous fixation can be performed in a delayed manner.

Choo, Schottel, and Burgess, on the other hand, advocate that all clavicle fractures, AC and SC joint injuries be surgically stabilized regardless of the need for vascular repair. It is their belief that at least one point of osseous fixation is necessary to restore length of the limb, prevent worsening traction injuries to the already damaged surrounding soft tissue, and create a stable base to support an eventual prosthesis. Their preferred methods of fixation include orthogonal plating of midshaft clavicle fractures, the combination of a hook plate with a coracoclavicular screw,

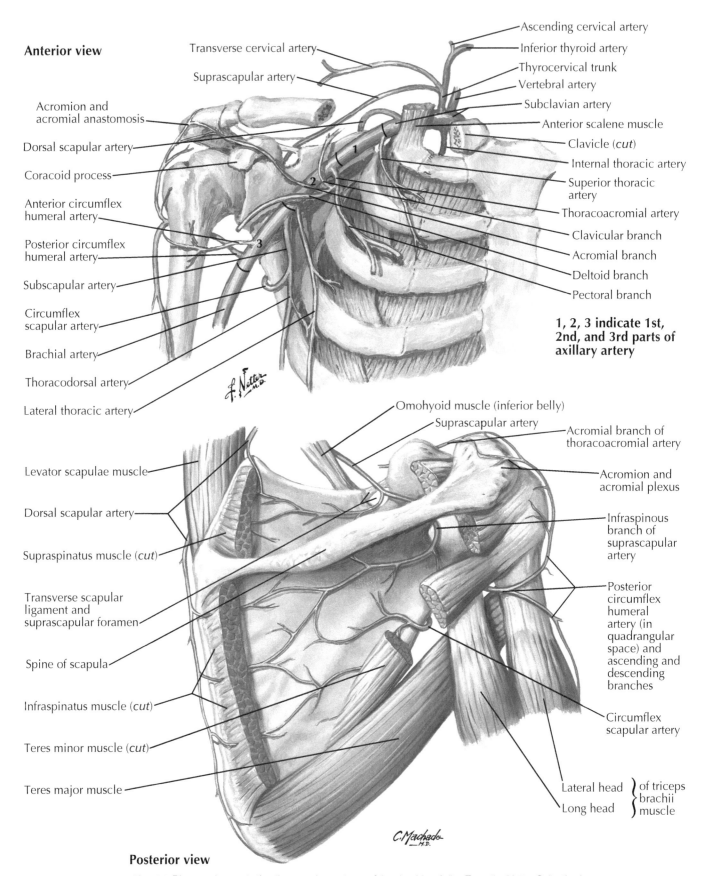

Anterior view

Transverse cervical artery

Suprascapular artery

Acromion and acromial anastomosis

Dorsal scapular artery

Coracoid process

Anterior circumflex humeral artery

Posterior circumflex humeral artery

Subscapular artery

Circumflex scapular artery

Brachial artery

Thoracodorsal artery

Lateral thoracic artery

Ascending cervical artery

Inferior thyroid artery

Thyrocervical trunk

Vertebral artery

Subclavian artery

Anterior scalene muscle

Clavicle (*cut*)

Internal thoracic artery

Superior thoracic artery

Thoracoacromial artery

Clavicular branch

Acromial branch

Deltoid branch

Pectoral branch

1, 2, 3 indicate 1st, 2nd, and 3rd parts of axillary artery

Levator scapulae muscle

Dorsal scapular artery

Supraspinatus muscle (*cut*)

Transverse scapular ligament and suprascapular foramen

Spine of scapula

Infraspinatus muscle (*cut*)

Teres minor muscle (*cut*)

Teres major muscle

Omohyoid muscle (inferior belly)

Suprascapular artery

Acromial branch of thoracoacromial artery

Acromion and acromial plexus

Infraspinous branch of suprascapular artery

Posterior circumflex humeral artery (in quadrangular space) and ascending and descending branches

Circumflex scapular artery

Lateral head } of triceps brachii muscle

Long head }

Posterior view

• **Fig. 18.2** Diagram demonstrating the vascular anatomy of the shoulder girdle. (From the Netter Collection.)

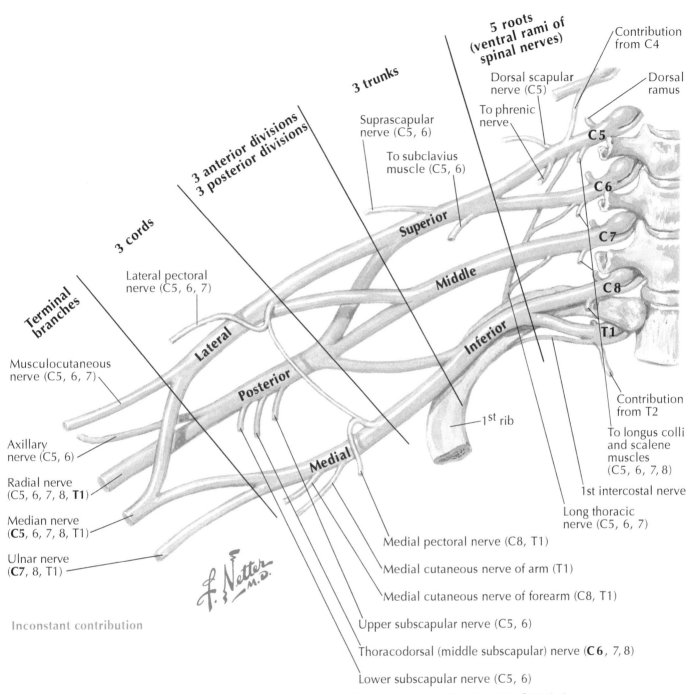

5 roots (ventral rami of spinal nerves)

3 trunks

3 anterior divisions
3 posterior divisions

3 cords

Terminal branches

Contribution from C4

Dorsal scapular nerve (C5)

Dorsal ramus

To phrenic nerve

Suprascapular nerve (C5, 6)

To subclavius muscle (C5, 6)

Lateral pectoral nerve (C5, 6, 7)

Superior

Middle

Lateral

Inferior

Posterior

Musculocutaneous nerve (C5, 6, 7)

Axillary nerve (C5, 6)

Radial nerve (C5, 6, 7, 8, **T1**)

Median nerve (**C5**, 6, 7, 8, T1)

Medial

Ulnar nerve (**C7**, 8, T1)

f. Netter M.D.

Inconstant contribution

C5

C6

C7

C8

T1

Contribution from T2

To longus colli and scalene muscles (C5, 6, 7, 8)

1st rib

1st intercostal nerve

Long thoracic nerve (C5, 6, 7)

Medial pectoral nerve (C8, T1)

Medial cutaneous nerve of arm (T1)

Medial cutaneous nerve of forearm (C8, T1)

Upper subscapular nerve (C5, 6)

Thoracodorsal (middle subscapular) nerve (**C6**, 7, 8)

Lower subscapular nerve (C5, 6)

• **Fig. 18.3** Diagram demonstrating the anatomy of the brachial plexus. (From the Netter Collection)

and anterior spanning plate for AC joint separations, and graft reconstruction of SC joint separations.[6]

Management of nervous injury is not generally performed emergently, but is recommended to be addressed within 6 months of injury to prevent atrophy and motor end-plate fibrosis. In the patient diagnosed with complete pan-brachial plexus avulsions, primary above-elbow amputation has been advocated due to its poor prognosis and likely resultant painful, functionless upper extremity.[16]

Nonoperative management has been advocated in patients without limb-threatening ischemia (due to the collateral flow to the upper extremity) and without complete brachial plexus avulsion. Sampson et al. performed a retrospective review of

11 patients and found that all had pale cool limbs with absent radial pulses; however, only one was found to have limb-threatening ischemia, which they defined by cold temperature and mottled blue skin. Five patients in this study group did not receive vascular reconstruction and were not found to have developed ischemia during long-term follow up. Six patients underwent revascularization (one of which subsequently became ischemic post repair). Regardless of whether patients received repair or not, all of them ended up with insensate flail limbs, thus leading us to believe that neurologic injury is the key predictive factor for long-term functional outcomes.[17] In cases where neurologic injury is not present or is incomplete, there is a chance for functional recovery that would not require surgical intervention.

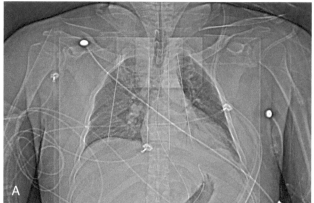

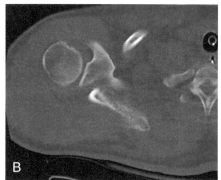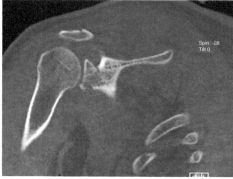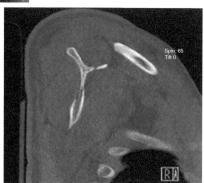

• **Fig. 18.4** (A) Portable anteroposterior chest X-ray of a 42-year-old male obtained in the trauma bay after the patient suffered a motorcycle accident showing lateral displacement of the right scapula. (B) Axial, coronal, and sagittal cuts of the patient's right upper extremity showing fractures of the glenoid, scapular neck, scapular body, and acromion.

TABLE 18.1	Damschen Classification of Scapulothoracic Dissociation With Zelle Modification
Type	**Definition**
1	Musculoskeletal injury alone
2A	Musculoskeletal injury and vascular disruption
2B	Musculoskeletal injury and incomplete neurological injury
3	Musculoskeletal injury with vascular disruption and incomplete neurological injury
4	Musculoskeletal injury with complete brachial plexus avulsion

Indications for Surgical Treatment

Ebraheim et al. devised a three-phase treatment protocol for patients with diagnosed scapulothoracic dissociation.[2] Phase 1 occurs within the first 24 hours after injury. The patient is primarily resuscitated and stabilized, after which angiography is performed to identify the level/location of vascular injury. Once identified, surgical exploration and vascular repair are performed. It is advocated to perform bony fixation while performing any necessary vascular repair in order to establish a stable setting that would be protective for the newly repaired vasculature. This is especially true in the setting of a double disruption to the SSSC. Even if it is later determined that above-elbow amputation is required, performing early osseous fixation can allow for early rehabilitation. Additionally, at the

time of vascular repair, the brachial plexus may be explored and possibly grafted if deemed appropriate.

Phase 2 encompasses the first 2 weeks following the injury where primary above-elbow amputation or glenohumeral arthrodesis is considered. Amputation is dictated by the presence of complete brachial plexus avulsion or extensive/irreparable skin defects.

Phase 3 is beyond 2 weeks from the initial injury and is considered the "chronic period" of the injury. During this phase, prosthetic fitting can occur, and, after 6 weeks from injury, baseline electromyography (EMG) can be established. Definitive nerve injury can be addressed via necessary tendon transfers or nerve transfers. Additional EMGs and further nerve grafting or neurolysis can also be performed in conjunction with the necessary physical and occupational therapy to improve long-term function.

Surgical Approaches

There are a variety of surgical approaches that may be utilized for the management of scapulothoracic dissociation based on the specific injury incurred. Initial approach is dictated by the presence and location of vascular injury. If there is damage to the proximal vasculature (e.g., within the subclavian artery), then a median sternotomy may be utilized. If there is damage to the more distal vasculature (e.g., within the axillary artery), then a high lateral thoracotomy may be utilized.[18]

The type of nerve reconstruction/grafting and potential muscle transfers are dictated by the location and degree of brachial plexus injury. Masmejean et al. advocated CT myelography as early as 3 weeks post injury in the cases of apparent complete brachial plexus avulsion, in order to confirm complete root avulsion, determine

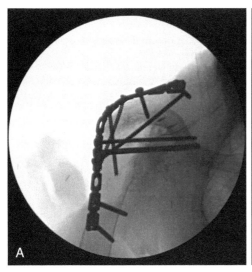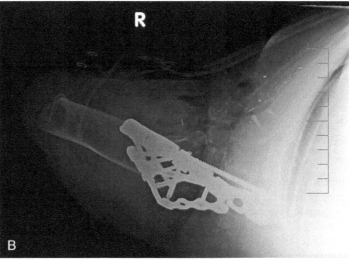

• **Fig. 18.5** Postoperative anteroposterior and axillary views of a patient 3 years' status posttraumatic scapulothoracic dissociation with associated brachial plexus injury and multiple cervical nerve root avulsions. The patient developed a flail limb with arthrofibrosis. Multiple nerve transfers were attempted at an outside institution, which were ultimately unsuccessful. The patient was then indicated for above-elbow amputation and shoulder arthrodesis.

the exact level of injury, and as a means of determining the feasibility of successful nerve grafting.[19] They advocate MRI for evaluation of incomplete brachial plexus avulsion.

Maldonado et al. reviewed the procedures that they have found give the best outcomes in the setting of traumatic brachial plexus injuries. Ulnar nerve fascicle transfer to biceps motor branch in the setting of upper trunk injuries was shown to provide excellent elbow flexion with minimal ulnar nerve deficits. Triceps nerve fascicle transfer to axillary motor branch in upper trunk injuries provides restoration of shoulder abduction and external rotation, which are the next most important planes of motion after elbow flexion. With regard to posterior cord injuries, they find inconsistent results with radial nerve grafting and rather advocate for radial nerve tendon transfers (pronator teres to extensor carpi radialis brevis, flexor carpi radialis to extensor digitorum communis, and palmaris longus to extensor pollicis longus for restoration of hand function).[20]

In cases of traumatic total brachial plexus palsy, double free-muscle transfers can be performed to restore combined elbow and finger function. This has been outlined by Dodakundi et al. as a four-step process.[21] Stage 1 being surgical exploration of the brachial plexus with nerve repair for restoration of shoulder function (if performed within 5 months of the injury). Stage 2 is the first free-muscle transfer, using the contralateral gracilis to restore elbow flexion and finger extension. Stage 3 consists of utilizing the ipsilateral gracilis for restoration of finger flexion. Stage 4 includes any necessary supplemental procedures to aid in finger function (tenolysis, wrist fusion, finger joint stabilization).[22] Satbhai et al. compared outcomes of double free-muscle transfer with those of single free-muscle transfer or nerve graft only and found that the double muscle transfer group showed the greatest improvement in motor function and DASH (The Disabilities of the Arm, Shoulder and Hand) scores.[23]

If development of flail extremity appears to be the likely end-result, management usually consists of above-elbow amputation alone, or above-elbow amputation with shoulder arthrodesis. The goals of amputation and arthrodesis are pain relief and to create a stable construct for prosthesis function. The ideal position of

fusion has also been debated in the literature, though deeper analysis shows that this is likely a result of variations in reference points and imprecise orientation aids when making measurements. Lerch et al. state that the most agreed upon positions of fusion are 20 degrees of abduction, 30 degrees of anteversion, and 40 degrees of internal rotation relative to the thorax in order to obtain a functional position for prosthesis use (Fig. 18.5).[24,25]

Following amputation and arthrodesis, early functional prosthesis fitting is encouraged for improved long-term outcomes. Goals of prostheses are to provide elbow flexion. New myoelectric prostheses provide elbow flexion and extension via the contralateral pectoralis major, pronation and supination via the contralateral latissimus, and pincer function via the ipsilateral trapezius.[26] These prostheses function by utilizing electromyographic signals from residual musculature. While technological advances are promising, those with upper limb prostheses function at <50% the level of those with intact anatomy.[27]

Relevant Complications

The complications/long-term sequelae of scapulothoracic dissociation can be devastating, and, as has been previously outlined, are most related to the degree of neurologic compromise occurring with the initial injury.[28] As Zelle et al. reported, those with a complete brachial avulsion had significantly lower Subjective Shoulder Rating System scores and significantly lower SF-36 scores than those with incomplete brachial plexus avulsions.[15] Patients with persistent pain 6 months after injury are less likely to see full return of neurologic function. Those with complete brachial plexus injuries are often left with insensate, flail limbs, and persistent pain.[24] Once this occurs, there are few options for treatment, mainly above-elbow amputation with or without shoulder arthrodesis.

Review of Current Treatment Outcomes

It is postulated that, due to improvements in the emergency field management of trauma patients in general, there has been an increase in the incidence of scapulothoracic dissociation managed in the emergency room as more patients with this injury survive long enough to present to medical care.[2,15] Despite this alleged increase in incidence, there is still a paucity of studies looking at long-term outcomes of those treated for scapulothoracic dissociation. In a recent review by Branca, Vergana, and Monesi, in those who did survive the initial trauma after >24 hours in the hospital, 50% were reported to have a flail limb and 20% required eventual above-elbow amputation.[29]

Damschen and Zelle reported an amputation rate ranging from 21% to 24%, but Riess et al. report an amputation rate of as low as 9%.[4,15,30] Riess and colleagues believe that they have lower rates of amputation due to a more aggressive approach to timely vascular repair. However, Brucker et al. report that, while aggressive timely vascular repair is obviously important for the hemodynamic stability of the patient, it does not necessarily have as great an impact on the long-term clinical outcomes.[16] Long-term functional outcomes and amputation rates are dictated by degree of brachial plexus injury.[31] In those where functional recovery is unlikely, early amputation with immediate prosthetic fitting is advocated due to improved functional outcomes.[15,26] With regard to bony fixation, it seems the most important and most reliable approach is orthogonal plating of the clavicle. This is largely due to the fact that the displaced midshaft clavicle fractures are at extreme high risk of nonunion due to the lateralization of the entire limb in this injury pattern. Therefore results are improved with surgical stabilization.[29]

In summary, scapulothoracic dissociation is still a rare and potentially devastating injury. Initial management of patients with scapulothoracic dissociation should be centered around resuscitation and evaluation for vascular injuries that would require emergent surgical intervention. Long-term outcomes are dictated by degree of neurologic injury, and those who have a low likelihood of recovering from their neurologic injury will have improved functional outcomes with early amputation and prosthesis fitting.

References

1. Oreck SL, Burgess A, Levine AM. Traumatic lateral displacement of the scapula: a radiographic sign of neurovascular disruption. *J Bone Joint Surg Am.* 1984;66:758–763.
2. Ebraheim NA, Pearlstein SR, Savolaine ER, et al. Scapulothoracic dissociation (closed avulsion of the scapula, subclavian artery, and brachial plexus): a newly recognized variant, a new classification, and a review of the literature and treatment options. *J Orthop Trauma.* 1987;1:18–23.
3. Merk BR, Minihane KP, Shah NA. Scapulothoracic dissociation with acromioclavicular separation: a case report of a novel fixation method. *J Orthop Trauma.* 2008;22(8):572–575.
4. Damschen DD, Cogbill TH, Siegel MJ. Scapulothoracic dissociation caused by blunt trauma. *J Trauma.* 1997;42:537–540.
5. Flanigan BA, Leslie MP. Scapulothoracic dissociation. *Orthop Clin N Am.* 2013;44:1–7.
6. Choo AM, Schottel PC, Burgess AR. Scapulothoracic dissociation: evaluation and management. *J Am Acad Orthop Surg.* 2017;25(5):339–347.
7. Conduah AH, Baker III CL, Baker CL. Clinical management of scapulothoracic bursitis and the snapping scapula. *Sports Health.* 2010;2(2):147–155.
8. Wu J, Bordoni B. Anatomy, shoulder and upper limb, scapulohumeral muscle. In: *StatPearls. Treasure Island (FL).* StatPearls Publishing; 2019.
9. Bajzer CT. Arterial supply to the upper extremities. In: Bhatt DL, ed. *Guide to Peripheral and Cerebrovascular Intervention.* London:

10. Thiel R, Daly DT. Anatomy, shoulder and upper limb, axillary artery. In: *StatPearls. Treasure Island (FL).* StatPearls Publishing; 2018. Available from: https://www.ncbi.nlm.nih.gov/books/NBK482174/.
11. Ahimsadasan N, Kumar A. Neuroanatomy, dorsal root ganglion. In: *StatPearls. Treasure Island (FL).* StatPearls Publishing; 2018. Available from: https://www.ncbi.nlm.nih.gov/books/NBK532291/.
12. Goss TP. Double disruptions of the superior shoulder suspensory complex. *J Orthop Trauma.* 1993;7(2):99–106.
13. Naunheim RS. Scapulothoracic dissociation. *Emergency Med.* 2013;3(3):1–2.
14. Maria SW, Sapuan J, Abdullah S. The flail and pulseless upper limb: an extreme case of traumatic scapulothoracic dissociation. *Malaysian Orthop J.* 2015;9(2):54–56.
15. Zelle BA, Pape HC, Gerich TG, Garapati R, Ceylan B, Krettek C. Functional outcome following scapulothoracic dissociation. *J Bone Joint Surg.* 2004;86A(1):2–8.
16. Brucker P, Gruen G, Kaufmann R. Scapulothoracic dissociation: evaluation and management. *Injury.* 2005;36:1147–1155.
17. Sampson LN, Britton JC, Eldrup-Jorgensen J, Clark DE, Rosenberg JM, Bredenberg CE. The neurovascular outcome of scapulothoracic dissociation. *J Vasc Surg.* 1993;17(6):1083–1089.
18. Katsamouris AN, Kafetzakis A, Kostas T, Tsetis D, Katonis P. The initial management of scapulothoracic dissociation: a challenging task for the vascular surgeon. *Eur J Vasc Endovasc Surg.* 2002;24(6):547–549.
19. Masmejean EH, Asfazadourian H, Alnot JY. Brachial plexus injuries in scapulothoracic dissociation. *J Hand Surg.* 2000;25(4):336–340.
20. Maldonado AA, Bishop AT, Spinner RJ, Shin AY. Five operations that give the best results after brachial plexus injury. *Plast Reconstr Surg.* 2017;140(3):545–556.
21. Dodakundi C, Doi K, Hattori Y, et al. Outcome of surgical reconstruction after traumatic total brachial plexus palsy. *J Bone Jt Surg Am Vol.* 2013;95(16):1505–1512.
22. Bedi A, Miller B, Jebson PJL. Combined glenohumeral arthrodesis and above-elbow amputation for the flail limb following a complete posttraumatic brachial plexus injury. *Tech Hand Up Extrem Surg.* 2005;9(2):113–119.
23. Satbhai NG, Doi K, Hattori Y, Sakamoto S. Functional outcome and quality of life after traumatic total brachial plexus injury treated by nerve transfer or single/double free muscle transfers. *The Bone & Joint Journal.* 2016;98-B(2):209–217.
24. Rorabeck CH, Harris WR. Factors affecting the prognosis of brachial plexus injuries. *JBJS(Br).* 1981;63-B3:404–407.
25. Lerch S, Berndt T, Ruhmann O, et al. Schraubenarthrodese der schulter. *Oper Orthop Truamatol.* 2011;23:215–226.
26. Burdette TE, Long SA, Ho O, Demas C, Bell JE, Rosen JM. Early delayed amputation: a paradigm shift in the limb-salvage time-line for patient with major upper-limb injury. *J Rehab Research Develop.* 2009;46(3):385–394.
27. Chadwell A, Kenney L, Thies S, Galpin A, Head J. The reality of myoelectric prostheses: understanding what makes these devices difficult for some users to control. *Front Neurorobot.* 2016;10:7.
28. Doi K, Otsuka K, Okamoto Y, et al. Cervical nerve root avulsion in brachial plexus injuries: magnetic resonance imaging classification and comparison with myelography and computerized tomography myelography. *J Neurosurg.* 2002;96:277–284.
29. Branca Vergano L, Monesi M. Scapulothoracic dissociation: a devastating "floating shoulder" injury. *Acta Biomed.* 2018;90(1-S):150–153.
30. Riess KP, Cogbill TH, Patel NY, Lambert PJ, Mathiason MA. Brachial plexus injury: long-term functional outcome is determined by associated scapulothoracic dissociation. *J Trauma Inj Infect Crit Care.* 2007;63(5):1021–1025.
31. Lavelle WF, Uhl R. Scapulothoracic dissociation. *Orthopedics.* 2010;33(6):417–421.

Remedica; 2004:4–6. Available from: https://www.ncbi.nlm.nih.gov/books/NBK27339/.

19

Anterior Glenohumeral Instability: Evaluation and Decision-Making

NICHOLAS A. BONAZZA, ZACHARY CHRISTOPHERSON, AND JONATHAN C. RIBOH

Introduction

Anterior instability represents over 70% of glenohumeral instability with a yearly incidence approaching 3% in high-risk populations.[1,2] Males sustain 70%–80% of instability episodes with subluxations being more common than frank dislocations.[1,2] About half (47%) of all dislocations occur in individuals between 15 and 29 years of age.[3] A fall represents the most common cause (59%) of a dislocation with half (48%) occurring during sport or recreation.[3]

Recurrent instability has short- and long-term consequences for the patient. In addition to immediate symptoms, recurrent instability results in an increased risk of glenoid and humeral bone loss as well as an increased risk of long-term arthropathy.[4–6] Within anterior instability, there is growing evidence that surgical management yields better clinical results, but a thorough evaluation of the patient must be coupled with an understanding of individual goals to come to a shared decision for management of each patient.

Pathophysiology

A clear understanding of anatomy and, especially, the patient's specific pathology are crucial to appropriate treatment of anterior instability. The limited bony stability of the glenohumeral joint allows significant motion which relies heavily on soft tissue stability. The dynamic stability provided by the concavity compression of the rotator cuff is the most important aspect, but critical stabilization is also provided by the passive effects of the capsuloligamentous complex, glenoid labrum, and the suction effect of negative intra-articular pressure.[7,8]

The pathology of anterior instability can vary based on a variety of factors. Anteroinferior labral tears (66%) and Hill-Sachs lesions (41%) represented the most common pathology seen on preoperative magnetic resonance images (MRIs) in patients who ultimately underwent surgery in the MOON (The Multicenter Orthopaedic Outcomes Network) cohort of 863 patients,[2] though arthroscopic evaluation in a separate study found 97% of first-time dislocators

suffered an anteroinferior labral tear.[9] The typical Bankart lesion involves avulsion of the anteroinferior glenohumeral ligament-labral complex with or without bony avulsion.

The anteroinferior glenohumeral ligament represents the primary restraint to anterior translation of the humerus with the arm abducted and externally rotated, the common "apprehension" position (Fig. 19.1). Humeral avulsion of the glenohumeral ligament (HAGL) is found in 9% of shoulders that require surgery for instability and can be found in the absence of other glenolabral pathology.[10] Additionally, glenoid avulsion of the glenohumeral ligament (GAGL), where the ligament is disrupted from the glenoid separate from injury to the labrum, has also been reported as a cause of recurrent instability.[11]

Bony pathology has a significant impact on the success of treatment for instability. As with Hill-Sachs lesions, glenoid bone loss affects about 40% of first-time dislocators.[6] Recurrent dislocators are twice as likely to have glenoid bone loss and the number of dislocations had a moderate correlation ($r = .56$) with the severity of glenoid bone loss in one computed tomography (CT) study of 218 patients.[6]

Patient Evaluation

Careful evaluation of the patient should begin with a detailed history and should focus on causes of instability and risk factors for recurrence. The mechanism of dislocation and the amount of trauma required are important clues to differentiate volitional dislocators and patients with hyperlaxity/multidirectional instability—two typically nonoperative pathologies that are very distinct from traumatic glenohumeral dislocation. Additionally, previous treatment should be discussed and notes (and images, if available) should be obtained from any previous surgical procedures, if applicable. Ultimately, a clear understanding of the patient's overall functional goals and other applicable details must be discussed to allow shared decision-making with regard to treatment. Of particular importance are details regarding sports participation including timing within season, position of play, and future plans for sports participation.

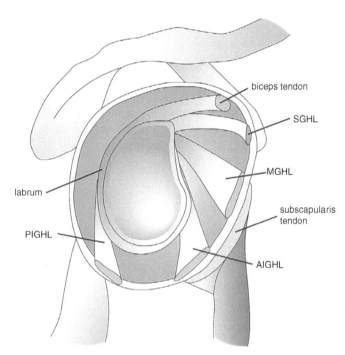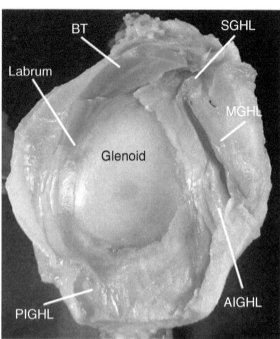

• **Fig. 19.1** Anatomy of the capsulolabral complex. Though the anteroinferior glenohumeral ligament *(AIGHL)* is the primary static restraint with the arm in a position of abduction and external rotation, the superior glenohumeral ligament *(SGHL)* plays a primary role along with the coracohumeral ligament (not pictured) with the arm at the side. The middle glenohumeral ligament *(MGHL)* plays a primary role with the arm in 45 degrees of abduction. *BT,* Biceps tendon; *PIGHL,* posteroinferior glenohumeral ligament. (Reprinted from Itoigawa Y, Itoi E. Anatomy of the capsulolabral complex and rotator interval related to glenohumeral instability. *Knee Surg Sports Traumatol Arthrosc.* 2015;24:343-349; and Krych AJ, Shindle MK, Baran S, Warren RF. Isolated arthroscopic rotator interval closure for shoulder instability. *Arthrosc Tech.* 2014;3:e35-e38.)

TABLE 19.1 Beighton Score

Joint Evaluation	Unilateral	Bilateral
At least 10 degrees of elbow hyperextension	1	2
Ability to oppose the thumb and forearm	1	2
At least 90 degrees of little finger hyperextension	1	2
At least 10 degrees of knee hyperextension	1	2
Ability to place palms flat on the floor with knees extended	1	

Points are given for unilateral or bilateral findings and the composite score calculated.

Scores >4 are considered positive for generalized joint laxity.

Adapted from Whitehead NA, Mohammed KD, Fulcher ML. Does the Beighton score correlate with specific measures of shoulder joint laxity? *Orthop J Sports Med.* 2018;6:232596711877063.

Physical Examination

A standard shoulder examination should be performed, evaluating overall range of motion and strength in addition to a neurovascular examination with a focus on the axillary nerve. Laxity should be evaluated via shoulder-specific tests such as the sulcus sign and Gagey hyperabduction sign while the Beighton Score can be used to document generalized joint laxity (Table 19.1).[12,13] Persistent pain or weakness after an instability event should prompt careful evaluation for rotator cuff injury as well, a more common finding in contact athletes and patients over 40.[14]

Several tests have been described to specifically evaluate for anterior instability. Apprehension and relocation have specificity of 96% and 92% when apprehension (not pain) and relief were used as criteria for a positive test (Fig. 19.2).[15] A positive apprehension test has also been shown to identify patients at a higher risk of recurrence after an initial instability event.[16] The test should be performed at varying levels of abduction as apprehension at lower levels of abduction may indicate higher degrees of bone loss.

Imaging

Initial X-rays can provide basic information regarding the position of the humeral head on the glenoid fractures, as well as obvious bone loss utilizing views such as the Bernageau view (for glenoid bone loss) and Stryker notch view (Hill-Sachs lesion). For treatment decisions, however, advanced imaging is highly recommended. An MRI, with arthrogram in the subacute or chronic setting, is ideal for evaluating the extent of injury to the capsuloligamentous complex, cartilage, and especially relevant for middle age and older patients—concomitant rotator cuff tears.

Quantifying glenoid bone loss or any glenoid fracture is a crucial component of informed decision-making and, though it may be noted on X-ray or MRI, it is best quantified using CT with three-dimensional

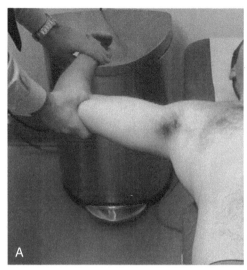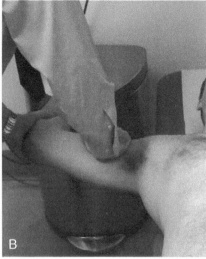

• **Fig. 19.2** The shoulder apprehension and relocation tests. (A) Apprehension test: the patient is placed supine and the arm positioned in 90 degrees of abduction and 90 degrees of external rotation. A positive test would be indicated by the patient becoming apprehensive regarding a feeling of instability. (B) Relocation test: pressure is placed on the anterior arm which should result in relief by the patient, indicating a positive test. (Reprinted from Fabricant PD, Taylor SA, McCarthy MM, et al. Open and arthroscopic anterior shoulder stabilization. *JBJS Rev.* 2015;3:e4.)

volume rendering reconstruction.[17] The most reliable measurement of glenoid bone loss is done by comparing the width of the injured glenoid with the width of the uninjured, contralateral glenoid if imaging is available.[18] More commonly, the best-fit-circle method is utilized to evaluate the extent of glenoid bone loss (Fig. 19.3).[19]

For the humeral head, the position of the bone loss and its ability to engage the glenoid are factors affecting recurrence. Intraoperative evaluation of humeral head lesions has shown that those that engage the glenoid in abduction and external rotation result in worse outcomes after arthroscopic Bankart repair.[20] As discussed below, three-dimensional volume rendering of the humerus can also be helpful to fully define the extent of the Hill-Sachs lesion and calculate the glenoid track to guide treatment (Fig. 19.4).

Natural History and Nonoperative Management

The natural history of anterior shoulder instability has been well studied and provides important information for treatment decisions. Less than 10% of adolescent patients sustaining a primary dislocation and undergoing conservative management will have a stable shoulder at 10-year follow-up.[21] Almost 50% of patients under 25 will ultimately have stabilization surgery, though this number may be even higher now given further evidence to support surgery in this younger population.[22] Though patients under 25 have the highest risk of recurrence, the risk drops by at least half after age 30.[22–24] Male sex and hyperlaxity are also known risk factors for failure of conservative treatment.[25]

While a young patient may experience disabling recurrent instability in the short term, a form of glenohumeral osteoarthritis—dislocation arthropathy—is a significant risk in the longer term. Hovelius showed that the risk of arthropathy after only one dislocation is 18%—significantly increased over the baseline rate of glenohumeral osteoarthritis.[5] Furthermore, the risk of arthropathy increases further with an increasing number of dislocations and/or increased time between the instability and surgical stabilization.[26]

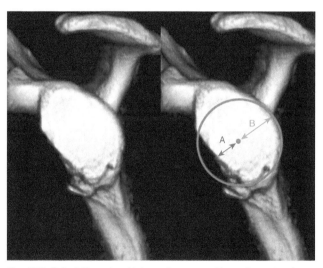

• **Fig. 19.3** Calculating glenoid bone loss on a three-dimensional computed tomography scan. A best-fit circle is created in the bottom of the glenoid. *A* = the radius from the center of the circle to the anterior edge of the glenoid. *B* = the radius from the center of the circle to the posterior edge of the glenoid. Percentage bone loss = $(B – A)/2 \times B \times 100\%$.

Functionally, patients who perform activities at or above chest level as an occupation and patients in contact or collision sports are also at higher risk of recurrence.[24] High-level contact athletes represent a unique population as nonoperative management may be pursued in-season despite a known high recurrence rate.[27] Though an athlete may be able to return to play in-season, surgery in the off-season improves the rate of return to play the next season compared to nonoperative management, independent of the number of previous instability events.[28]

In patients over 30, preadolescents, and those without high-risk functional demands, nonoperative management remains a viable option. Optimal nonoperative management for instability lacks consensus but typically involves initial immobilization after reduction. Despite numerous studies, no method,

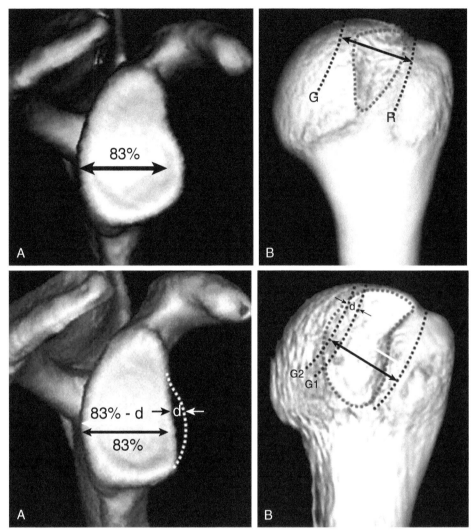

• **Fig. 19.4** Calculating the glenoid track on three-dimensional computed tomography scan. The diameter of the glenoid *(D)* is measured and multiplied by 0.83 to determine the width of the glenoid track *(top)*. If bone loss is present *(bottom)*, a measurement of the contralateral glenoid is used and multiplied by 0.83. The width of the bone loss *(d)* is then subtracted from the native estimate to give the glenoid track. The width of the glenoid track can then be superimposed on the humeral head, beginning laterally at the medial edge of the rotator cuff insertion and extending medially. A lesion contained within the glenoid track *(top)* is considered "on-track" and will not engage the glenoid. A lesion that extends beyond the glenoid track *(bottom)* is considered "off-track" and can engage the anterior edge of the glenoid. (Reprinted from Di Giacomo G, Itoi E, Burkhart SS. Evolving concept of bipolar bone loss and the Hill-Sachs lesion: from "engaging/non-engaging" lesion to "on-track/off-track" lesion. *Arthroscopy.* 2014;30:90-98.)

position, or length of immobilization has shown consistently superior outcomes.[29–32]. In our practice, we typically use a simple sling for comfort only, with the goal of ceasing immobilization as quickly as possible. Personalized physical therapy is initiated with 3–5 days of the dislocation, and a progression through passive motion, active motion, and careful strengthening is progressed as fast as the patient can tolerate without pain or apprehension. Sports-specific training is initiated once the patient has full active range of motion and restoration of normal protective strength. Individualized criterion-based progression is favored over prescribed timelines for return to activities and/or sport. An emphasis is placed on periscapular and rotator cuff strengthening to aid dynamic stabilization. Activity modification may be necessary based on specific clinical situations, but the goal is always to return the patient to their previous level of function.

In middle-aged and older patients, the evaluation and treatment may vary significantly. In patients over age 40, the risk of concomitant rotator cuff tear is reported between 28% and 38%, and thus careful physical examination of the rotator cuff and a low threshold for MRI imaging is warranted in this population.[33–35] Furthermore, these patients tend to struggle more with stiffness rather than recurrent instability. Thus first-time dislocators in this population are frequently treated nonoperatively (assuming no full-thickness rotator cuff tear) and operative stabilization is entertained if there is significant glenoid bone loss or there is a second instability event.

Just as frank dislocation is only one presentation of shoulder instability, failure of nonoperative management may not always present as a recurrent dislocation. Careful attention must be paid to subluxation, pain, and functional limitations following primary instability that may also represent failure to the patient and demonstrate a need for surgery.

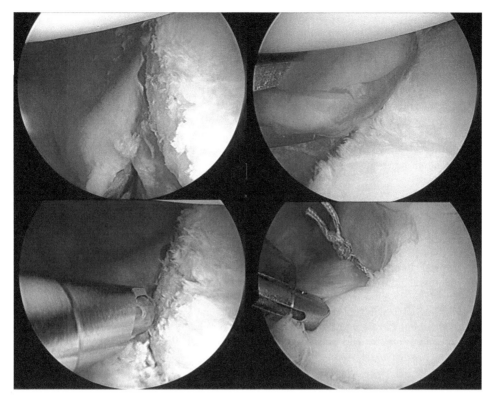

• **Fig. 19.5** Arthroscopic Bankart repair of a right shoulder with the patient in a lateral decubitus position *(top left)*. Disruption of the capsulolabral complex from the anteroinferior glenoid *(top right)*. The injured tissue is checked for quality via palpation as well as reducibility to ensure repair is possible *(bottom left)*. The anteroinferior glenoid is prepared with a bur to provide an adequate surface for healing *(bottom right)*. The drill guide is placed just on the anterior glenoid face to allow adequate reduction of the tissue. A variety of implants and techniques can be utilized for this purpose. In this case, a single limb of suture was passed under the capsulolabral tissue and knots were tied to secure the tissue back to the glenoid.

Operative Management

In patients who have failed nonoperative management or present initially with a high risk of recurrence, increasing evidence has shown the ability of surgery to improve short- and long-term outcomes. While open stabilization remains a useful option for particular patients and particular pathology, arthroscopic surgery has largely supplanted open surgery particularly in primary instability though even revision procedures, including bone augmentation procedures, are being done increasingly with arthroscopic techniques. Regardless of technique, successful operative outcomes largely depend on choosing the right procedure for the patient's pathology.

Timing of Stabilization

Recurrence after a first-time dislocation carries a variety of consequences discussed already and includes effects on the type and outcomes of surgical intervention. Recurrent instability is more likely to result in a Hill-Sachs lesion and/or Bankart lesion, has been correlated with an increased amount of glenoid bone loss specifically, and has also been found in one study to have increased biceps pathology requiring intervention.[4,6,36,37] A recent study of young athletes (mean age 19.4 years) found that the average amount of glenoid bone loss went from 6.8% in first-time dislocators to 21.8% in recurrent dislocators.[37] As a result, recurrent dislocators are less likely to undergo arthroscopic stabilization and more likely to need bone augmentation at the time of surgery.[36] Therefore in

patients at high risk of recurrence, we recommend early surgical intervention to limit recurrent instability and the associated effect on intra-articular pathology.[38,39]

Arthroscopic and Open Soft Tissue Stabilization

The vast majority of procedures performed for shoulder instability in the United States are arthroscopic soft tissue stabilizations, owing to the prevalence of this pathology within the instability population.[40,41] Excellent outcomes have been demonstrated primarily in patients with minimal bone loss and maintained quality capsular and labral tissue. However, many of the risk factors for recurrent instability overall also increase the risk for recurrent instability after arthroscopic soft tissue stabilization. These risks include patient factors such as male sex, young age, and hyperlaxity on examination as well as time from the first dislocation until surgery.[42–44] Even with a thorough preoperative evaluation, the quality of tissue and even the extent of bone loss may be more evident intraoperatively with the addition of direct visualization and tactile evaluation (Fig. 19.5). Thus plans for an isolated arthroscopic soft tissue stabilization in the setting of any bone loss or particularly recurrent dislocators, where the quality of the soft tissue is likely more compromised, should include alternative strategies for unexpected findings.

Open soft tissue stabilization, currently less commonly employed, is an important tool for any surgeon treating instability. Open stabilization through a subscapularis split allows minimal morbidity and allows direct visualization of a capsular shift done typically through a "T" capsulotomy with pants-over-vest reapproximation.[45] Though studies looking at modern arthroscopic techniques have found no difference between the outcomes of open and arthroscopic soft tissue stabilization, some prefer open techniques in certain high-risk populations.[46,47] For example, as participation in contact or overhead sports or any competitive-level sports increases the risk of failure after arthroscopic stabilization, some surgeons prefer open stabilization as a primary procedure in this population.[42] Additionally, surgeons may consider open stabilization for unique pathology such as an HAGL, poor capsulolabral tissue, or significant bone loss requiring bone grafting.

Bone Loss

Numerous studies have defined the role of glenoid bone loss in instability and the importance of addressing bone loss in preventing recurrent instability. "Critical" bone loss, which requires bone augmentation to restore stability at the time of surgery, was traditionally thought to be closer to 20%. However, that amount in recent studies has been as low as 13.5% and may be even lower in bipolar lesions.[48–50] As glenoid bone loss is a known risk factor for failure of arthroscopic stabilization, patients with any bone loss may be better candidates for open stabilization even if bone augmentation is not performed.[42]

It is important to note that, in some cases, the Bankart fragment is not "lost," but it is simply no longer attached to the anteroinferior glenoid. This situation is frequently, albeit confusingly, referred to as "bone loss" in the published literature. However, over time, the bony Bankart can resorb leading to a true bone loss situation. Whether the fractured piece of bone is present or not has implications for treatment, with at least one study showing improved outcomes in patients with glenoid rim fractures treated arthroscopically when the bony Bankart piece remained versus when it was resorbed.[51]

For patients with glenoid bone loss requiring augmentation, numerous techniques have been described and continue to be developed. Isolated bone augmentation has been performed with both open and arthroscopic means utilizing a variety of options including autograft from the distal clavicle, auto- and allograft from the iliac crest, allograft glenoid, and allograft distal tibia.[52–54] The Bristow procedure, or coracoid tip transfer, and Latarjet procedure, or whole coracoid transfer, were originally described in the 1950s and have the added benefit of dynamic soft tissue constraint from the conjoint tendon.[55] The conjoint tendon sling, static capsular reconstruction using the coracoacromial ligament, and bony augmentation of the glenoid are known as the "triple blocking effect" of the Latarjet and have resulted in low recurrence (<6%) even in long-term follow-up studies (Fig. 19.6).[56] Arthroscopic and open techniques for these procedures have shown similar clinical outcomes.[57–59]

Complications for any bone-block procedure include graft lysis, nonunion, failure of or painful fixation hardware, and neurological injury (axillary and musculocutaneous nerves) as well as long-term osteoarthritis. One study with a 20-year follow-up after Latarjet found that approximately 20% of patients develop new onset osteoarthritis while about 50% of patients with preoperative arthritis will have progression.[56] Given that patients with instability can develop the type of osteoarthritis known as glenohumeral dislocation arthropathy, and that Latarjet is often used to treat the worst instability patients, it is not clear if this represents a complication of the procedure of a progression of the natural history. In general, surgical stabilization has been found to reduce arthropathy rates overall in the long term; however, malposition of the bone graft too laterally is one modifiable risk factor for arthritic change post bone augmentation.[5]

Humeral Bone Loss

Remplissage ("to fill in" in French) describes a tenodesis of the posterior capsule and infraspinatus tendon into the humeral head defect and can be used in conjunction with Bankart repair in the setting of "off-track" Hill-Sachs lesions. Addition of remplissage to a soft tissue anterior stabilization has been shown to have a lower recurrence rate than Bankart repair alone.[60–62] Remplissage is best indicated in patients with an "off-track" lesion of the humeral head but subcritical glenoid bone loss.[63] Remplissage should be used with caution in certain populations. A majority of throwing athletes report decreased range of motion after remplissage and the Latarjet may be more effective in high-risk patients with this pathology such as collision or contact athletes, patients undergoing revision, and patients with >10% glenoid bone loss.[63,64] In humeral head defects with over 40% involvement of the articular surface, alternatives must be considered including osteochondral allograft typically in the young patient with minimal degenerative change. Metallic implants and hemiarthroplasty are often considered in older patients or patients with osteoarthritic change preoperatively.

Revision Operative Management

Many of the principles of primary instability surgery can be applied to evaluation and treatment of the patient needing revision instability surgery. Unique considerations include a critical evaluation of previous surgery, including a review of preoperative imaging and operative notes and images, to assess the adequacy of the prior procedure to address the patient's pathology. Inadequate surgery can be due to a poor procedural choice (i.e., arthroscopic Bankart repair in a patient with significant glenoid bone loss) or poor execution of the appropriate procedure (i.e., minimal fixation points below the glenoid equator in a Bankart repair). Not uncommonly, a patient may have the appropriate procedure and have it done well, but a recurrent instability event can fracture through the Bankart anchor holes leading to a glenoid rim fracture and recurrent instability.

An arthroscopic soft tissue procedure may be appropriate in a revision setting in a patient with no bone loss, preserved capsulolabral tissue quality, and inadequate fixation in the primary surgery.[65] However, given the high failure rate of arthroscopic procedures in the presence of bone loss, we believe that an open Bankart with a capsular shift is often indicated in the patient with recurrent instability and subcritical bone loss without an "off-track" Hill-Sachs lesion. In the patient with critical glenoid bone loss or bipolar lesions, a Latarjet or other bone augmentation procedure is preferred.

Summary and Clinical Decision-Making

While there is a large body of literature pertaining to anterior shoulder instability, definitive treatment protocols and recommendations remain elusive. As a result, there is wide variability in approaches to nonoperative, intraoperative, and postoperative care. The state of the art in 2020 involves a combination of patient-centered decision-making tools,[66,67] careful consideration

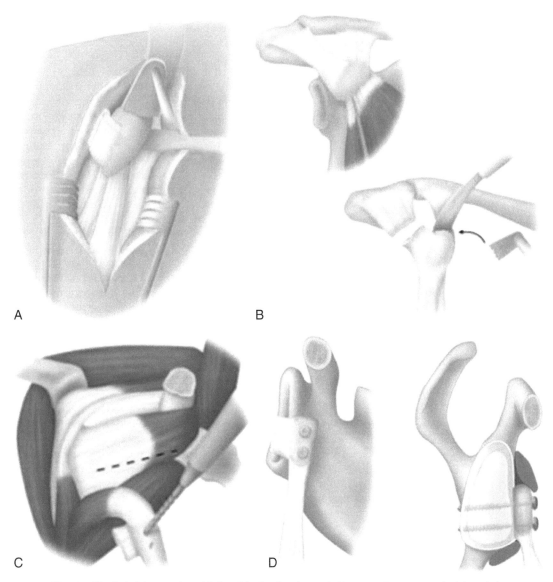

A

B

C

D

• **Fig. 19.6** The Latarjet procedure. (A) Careful retraction is needed to prevent neurovascular injury during the approach. (B) The coracoid is taken at the coracoid base (as opposed to the tip as in the Bristow procedure), preserving the conjoint tendon and a remnant of the coracoacromial ligament. (C) A subscapularis split is used and the capsule incised to expose the anterior glenoid. (D) The anterior glenoid is prepared and then the coracoid is fixed to the anterior glenoid. The coracoacromial ligament can be repaired to the capsule to constitute the third component of the "triple blocking effect." (Adapted from Bhatia S, Frank RM, Ghodadra NS, et al. The outcomes and surgical techniques of the Latarjet procedure. *Arthroscopy*. 2014;30:227-235.)

of patients' occupational and/or sports requirements and goals,[68] a careful understanding of the influence of glenoid bone loss, humeral bone loss and soft tissue quality on the outcomes of treatment,[69] and finally an honest assessment of the surgeon's position in the learning curve for some of the complex procedures required in the management of shoulder instability.[70]

Within this context, the clinician is faced with four major decisions in the management of a patient with anterior shoulder instability:

1. Does this patient need surgery?
2. If yes, then which surgery should I recommend?
3. How will I rehabilitate this patient? and finally
4. When is it safe for my patient to return to full activities/sports?

When making a decision about surgery, patients fall into three categories: those who definitely need an operation, those who definitely do not need an operation, and those who fall in the "gray zone" of decision-making. An example of a patient who definitely needs surgery would be a 17-year-old male varsity football player who has had 20 prior dislocations, is having dislocations with trivial activities such as rolling over in bed or brushing their hair, and is severely disabled by this condition. In contrast, a hypothetical 45-year-old sedentary female who sustained a first-time shoulder dislocation from a trip and fall, with fully restored motion, no apprehension, and no upper extremity athletic goals clearly does not need an operation.

Unfortunately, the majority of patients in our experience fall into the "gray zone," and a shared and informed decision about surgery needs to be discussed with the patient. We are guided in these situations by the following principles. First, we weigh athletic and occupational needs heavily in decision-making. A manual laborer who works overhead the majority of the time has much greater need for shoulder stability than a desk-based worker. Similarly, a football player has different requirements than a tennis player. Even within a single sport, position can play a large factor: for example, a wide receiver is much more likely to put their shoulder in an at-risk position than a lineman, and surgical decision-making may differ between them. Second, we heavily favor surgical intervention as quickly as possible or convenient based on data showing significantly higher failure rates of soft tissue stabilization procedures after repeated dislocations.[71] For the in-season athlete, we typically allow return to play as tolerated, with the goal of performing shoulder stabilization at the conclusion of the season, without which recurrence of instability and time lost from sport are highly likely.[28] If shoulder instability becomes a recurrent issue during the same season, we strongly encourage the athlete to consider immediate surgical stabilization. Finally, we are cautious about indicating shoulder stabilization procedures in the dominant arm of throwing athletes, and concerns about restriction of movement need to be balanced with the severity of the instability symptoms. When at all possible, addressing other factors contributing to the disabled throwing shoulder (core weakness, scapular dyskinesis, posterior capsular contracture, etc.) is preferred over surgical intervention.[72] If surgical intervention is indicated in the throwing athlete, it is critical to directly repair the labral while avoiding capsular shift or closure of the rotator interval.[72]

Once a decision has been made to proceed with surgery, evidence-based principles should be used to guide the choice of a specific operation. Beyond just synthesizing the evidence in the literature, the surgeon must also account for their own training, their own expertise, and the financial burden of the various treatment options.[73] Generally speaking, it is our preference to perform an arthroscopic anterior stabilization in the absence of contraindications. However, poorly indicated arthroscopic stabilizations clearly have inferior results.[50] As a result, our mentality when approaching the patient with anterior instability is to be aggressively looking for reasons *not* to perform an isolated arthroscopic stabilization. The clinician should have a very low threshold for gathering all diagnostic information that would help identify these contraindications, whether it is additional radiographic views, a CT scan with 3D reconstructions if there is any concern for bone loss, or simply obtaining a more thorough history and understanding of a patient's activity goals and requirements.

When performing an arthroscopic stabilization, we believe in the importance of addressing not just the anterior component but the inferior component of instability, and begin all anterior stabilizations with anchor placement in the posteroinferior quadrant to retension the PIGHL even if the tear does not extend here,[74] proceeding anteriorly from there. We believe that performing stabilization procedures in the lateral decubitus position improves access to the inferior glenoid and allows for the placement of four to five anchors between the 3:00 and 7:00 positions, thereby minimizing the risk of recurrence.[75] Additionally, we have a low

threshold for considering the addition of an arthroscopic remplissage using a knotless double-pulley technique[76] when performing an arthroscopic stabilization and encountering a Hill-Sachs lesion. In the absence of critical bone loss, this has been shown to significantly decrease recurrence rates with a minimal complication profile (though caution is advised in the dominant arm of a throwing athlete).[77] In our practice, any Hill-Sachs lesion that is easily visible while viewing from an anterolateral portal and shows any possibility of engagement on dynamic arthroscopic examination is considered for remplissage. Finally, in the setting of critical attritional glenoid bone loss (>20%), our preferred operation remains the open Latarjet coracoid transfer. While there are exciting results being published for alternative free bone-block techniques,[78–80] there are currently more data on the long-term safety and outcomes of the open Latarjet.

When it comes to rehabilitation and return to sport strategies, the clarity of the literature is poor. There is great variability in proposed rehabilitation protocols,[81] and time is the only criterion used for return to play in >75% of available studies, typically using 6 months as a safe cutoff for return to sport after surgical stabilization.[82] There is a dire need for research on scientifically and clinically valid return to play criteria after surgery for shoulder instability.[83] In the absence of reliable guidance in the literature, we have adapted to favoring an accelerated rehabilitation program. There is basic science data suggesting that labral healing should be complete within 2–3 months of surgery,[84] as well as clinical evidence of successful return to professional athletics a mean of 3 months after surgery with acceptably low redislocation rates.[85] In conjunction with our division I athletic trainers and physical therapists we have developed a criterion-based progression that mirrors evidence-based protocols on a slightly accelerated timeline (Table 19.2).[86] This has allowed us to return the majority of athletes, including collision athletes (football, lacrosse, etc.) back to full sporting activities between 4 and 5 months in the majority of cases. Future research priorities in the field include assessment of the duration of postoperative immobilization, assessment of accelerated timelines for return to strengthening and loading protocols, and prospective evaluation of the safety of accelerated return to sport programs.

Conclusion

Anterior shoulder instability represents the vast majority of shoulder instability and increasing evidence demonstrates the need for surgical intervention except in older, less active populations. Decision-making requires a careful patient evaluation including an understanding of the patient's functional activities and goals coupled with a thorough grasp of the pathology. Continued development of surgical techniques has shown the ability to prevent short- and long-term consequences through appropriate treatment of soft tissue injury with the addition of bony augmentation in populations with bone loss or in high-risk populations despite subcritical bone loss. Revision surgery requires a critical review of prior treatment and often involves escalation to an open or bone augmentation procedure.

TABLE 19.2   Criterion-Based Progression Timeline

	Range of Motion	Sling	Therapeutic Exercises
0–7 days	No shoulder motion AAROM elbow and wrist	Worn at all times	AAROM at the elbow and wrist Scapular clocks Supported pendulums
Phase 1 1–4 weeks	Motion restrictions: Forward flexion (FF): 90 degrees ER at side: 20 degrees IR: hand to stomach ABD: 45 degrees PROM → AAROM → AROM as tolerated	Begin weaning at 3 weeks if tolerated.	Cane ROM exercise: PROM → AAROM Progressive band resistance isometrics in sling until initiation of weaning. Increased resistance as tolerated, emphasis on scapular mechanics. May initiate gentle proprioceptive exercises (manual rhythmic stabilization) in neutral position as tolerated. Initiate strength and conditioning program for lower body, non-surgical UE, and core to include stationary biking. No exercise should put force through the upper trap, shoulder, elbow, or hand on the surgical side. Program to be completed in the sling.
Phase 2 4–8 weeks	Motion restrictions: FF: 160 degrees ER at side: 45 degrees ABD: 160 degrees IR: behind back to waist Week 6: Cross-body ADD ER at 90 degrees abduction: 45 degrees PROM → AAROM → AROM as tolerated	D/C at 4 weeks	Weeks 4–8: • Progressive resistance strengthening for cuff muscles and scapular stabilizers performed within AROM limitations. Guideline for progression: • Band or free weights • Start with 1–2 lbs of resistance • Increase no >1lb/level of resistance every other session as tolerated • 8–12 reps/2–3 set/3 days per week (one day of rest between sessions) • Goal: 7/10 fatigue in targeted muscles with minimal to no shoulder pain Week 6: • Start elliptical with hands stationary Week 7: • Progress proprioceptive exercises (e.g., body blade) • Initiate gentle UE closed chain weight-bearing (e.g., wall plus pushes)
Phase 3 8–12 weeks	If ROM lacking, increase to full with gentle passive stretching at end ranges.	None	Progress resistance strengthening for cuff muscles and scapular stabilizers as tolerated building on guidelines from phase 2. Incorporate eccentric movements. Week 8: • Initiate return to running program • Initiate cable presses, no shoulder extension past neutral (light to start) Week 10: • Progress UE closed chain weight-bearing progression (e.g., incline push-up/push-up plus progression). Restricted to half normal push-up depth.
Phase 4 Months 3–12	Should have full ROM, if still lacking continue with gentle passive stretching at end ranges	None	Progress UE closed chain weight-bearing progression • E.g., Horizontal push-up • E.g., Plank shoulder taps Initiate plyometric program progression as tolerated • E.g., Weighted ball toss • E.g., Plyo push-ups Begin higher effort UE ergometer Progress speed and agility drills as tolerated Begin sport-specific drills at 3 months Return to throwing at 4.5 months Throw from pitcher's mound at 6 months Return to contact sports at 4–6 months per surgeon recommendation

AAROM, Active assistive range of motion; *ABD,* abduction; *AAROM,* active range of motion; *D/C,* discontinue; *ER,* external rotation; *IR,* internal rotation; *PROM,* passive range of motion; *ROM,* range of motion; *UE,* upper extremity.

References

1. Owens BD, et al. The incidence and characteristics of shoulder instability at the United States Military Academy. *Am J Sports Med.* 2007;35:1168–1173.

2. Kraeutler MJ, et al. Descriptive epidemiology of the MOON shoulder instability cohort. *Am J Sports Med.* 2018;46:1064–1069.

3. Zacchilli MA, Owens BD. Epidemiology of shoulder dislocations presenting to emergency departments in the United States. *J Bone Joint Surg-Am.* 2010;92:542–549.

4. Yiannakopoulos CK, Mataragas E, Antonogiannakis E. A Comparison of the spectrum of intra-articular lesions in acute and chronic anterior shoulder instability. *Arthroscopy: J Arthroscop Related Surg.* 2007;23:985–990.

5. Hovelius L, Saeboe M. Neer Award 2008: arthropathy after primary anterior shoulder dislocation–223 shoulders prospectively followed up for twenty-five years. *J Shoulder Elbow Surg.* 2009;18:339–347.

6. Griffith JF, et al. Prevalence, pattern, and spectrum of glenoid bone loss in anterior shoulder dislocation: CT analysis of 218 patients. *Am J Roentgenol.* 2008;190:1247–1254.

7. Lippitt SB, et al. Glenohumeral stability from concavity-compression: a quantitative analysis. *J Shoulder Elbow Surg.* 1993;2:27–35.

8. Lee S-B, Kim K-J, O'Driscoll SW, Morrey BF, An K-N. Dynamic glenohumeral stability provided by the rotator cuff muscles in the mid-range and end-range of motion. *J Bone Joint Surg-Am.* 2000;82:849–857.

9. Taylor DC, Arciero RA. Pathologic changes associated with shoulder dislocations. *Am J Sports Med.* 1997;25:306–311.

10. Wolf EM, Cheng JC, Dickson K. Humeral avulsion of glenohumeral ligaments as a cause of anterior shoulder instability. *Arthroscopy: J Arthroscop Related Surg: Official Publication of the Arthroscopy Association of North America and the International Arthroscopy Association.* 1995;11:600–607.

11. Wolf EM, Siparsky PN. Glenoid avulsion of the glenohumeral ligaments as a cause of recurrent anterior shoulder instability. *Arthroscopy: J Arthroscop Related Surg.* 2010;26:1263–1267.

12. Whitehead NA, Mohammed KD, Fulcher ML. Does the Beighton score correlate with specific measures of shoulder joint laxity? *Orthopaedic J Sports Med.* 2018;6. 232596711877063.

13. Gagey OJ, Gagey N. The hyperabduction test. *J Bone Joint Surg. Br.* 2001;83. B:69–74.

14. Gomberawalla MM, Sekiya JK. Rotator cuff tear and glenohumeral instability. *Clin Orthopaedics Related Res.* 2013;472:2448–2456.

15. Farber AJ, Castillo R, Clough M, Bahk M, McFarland EG. Clinical assessment of three common tests for traumatic anterior shoulder instability. *J Bone Joint Surg.* 2006;88:1467–1474.

16. Safran O, Milgrom C, Radeva-Petrova DR, Jaber S, Finestone A. Accuracy of the anterior apprehension test as a predictor of risk for redislocation after a first traumatic shoulder dislocation. *Am J Sports Med.* 2010;38:972–975.

17. Bois AJ, Fening SD, Polster J, Jones MH, Miniaci A. Quantifying glenoid bone loss in anterior shoulder instability. *Am J Sports Med.* 2012;40:2569–2577.

18. Kuberakani K, et al. Comparison of best-fit circle versus contralateral comparison methods to quantify glenoid bone defect. *J Shoulder Elbow Surg.* 2020;29:502–507.

19. Walter WR, Samim M, LaPolla FWZ, Gyftopoulos S. Imaging quantification of glenoid bone loss in patients with glenohumeral instability: a systematic review. *Am J Roentgenol.* 2019;212:1096–1105.

20. Burkhart SS, De Beer JF. Traumatic glenohumeral bone defects and their relationship to failure of arthroscopic Bankart repairs. *Arthroscopy: J Arthroscop Related Surg.* 2000;16:677–694.

21. Roberts SB, Beattie N, McNiven ND, Robinson CM. The natural history of primary anterior dislocation of the glenohumeral joint in adolescence. *Bone Joint Lett J.* 2015;97-B:520–526.

22. Hovelius L, Rahme H. Primary anterior dislocation of the shoulder: long-term prognosis at the age of 40 years or younger. *Knee Surg Sports Traumatol Arthroscopy.* 2016;24:330–342.

23. Robinson CM, Howes J, Murdoch H, Will E, Graham C. Functional outcome and risk of recurrent instability after primary traumatic anterior shoulder dislocation in young patients. *J Bone Joint Surg.* 2006;88:2326–2336.

24. Sachs RA, Stone ML, Paxton E, Kuney M, Lin D. Can the need for future surgery for acute traumatic anterior shoulder dislocation be predicted? *J Bone Joint Surg.* 2007;89:1665–1674.

25. Galvin JW, Ernat JJ, Waterman BR, Stadecker MJ, Parada SA. The epidemiology and natural history of anterior shoulder instability. *Curr Rev Musculoskeletal Med.* 2017;10:411–424.

26. Buscayret F, et al. Glenohumeral arthrosis in anterior instability before and after surgical treatment. *Am J Sports Med.* 2004;32:1165–1172.

27. Dickens JF, et al. Return to play and recurrent instability after in-season anterior shoulder instability. *Am J Sports Med.* 2014;42:2842–2850.

28. Dickens JF, et al. Successful return to sport after arthroscopic shoulder stabilization versus nonoperative management in contact athletes with anterior shoulder instability: a prospective multicenter study. *Am J Sports Med.* 2017;45:2540–2546.

29. Hovelius L, et al. Primary anterior dislocation of the shoulder in young patients. A ten-year prospective study. *J Bone Joint Surg.* 1996;78:1677–1684.

30. Whelan DB, Kletke SN, Schemitsch G, Chahal J. Immobilization in external rotation versus internal rotation after primary anterior shoulder dislocation. *Am J Sports Med.* 2015;44:521–532.

31. Kuhn JE. Treating the initial anterior shoulder dislocation—an evidence-based medicine approach. *Sports Med Arthrosc Rev.* 2006;14:192–198.

32. Braun C, McRobert CJ. Conservative management following closed reduction of traumatic anterior dislocation of the shoulder. *Cochrane Database Systc Rev.* 2019. https://doi.org/10.1002/14651858.cd004962.pub4.

33. Pevney T, Hunter RE, Freeman JR. Primary traumatic anterior shoulder dislocation in patients 40 years of age and older. *Arthroscopy: J Arthroscop Related Surg.* 1997;13:379.

34. Sonnabend DH. Treatment of primary anterior shoulder dislocation in patients older than 40 years of age. Conservative versus operative. *Clin Orthop Relat Res.* 1994;304:74–77.

35. Toolanen G, Hildingsson C, Hedlund T, Knibestöl M, Öberg L. Early complications after anterior dislocation of the shoulder in patients over 40 years: an ultrasonographic and electromyographic study. *Acta Orthop Scand.* 1993;64:549–552.

36. Rugg CM, et al. Surgical stabilization for first-time shoulder dislocators: a multicenter analysis. *J Shoulder Elbow Surg.* 2018;27:674–685.

37. Dickens JF, et al. Prospective evaluation of glenoid bone loss after first-time and recurrent anterior glenohumeral instability events. *Am J Sports Med.* 2019;47:1082–1089.

38. Kirkley A, Griffin S, Richards C, Miniaci A, Mohtadi N. Prospective randomized clinical trial comparing the effectiveness of immediate arthroscopic stabilization versus immobilization and rehabilitation in first traumatic anterior dislocations of the shoulder. *Arthroscopy: J Arthroscop Related Surg.* 1999;15:507–514.

39. Bottoni CR, et al. A prospective, randomized evaluation of arthroscopic stabilization versus nonoperative treatment in patients with acute, traumatic, first-time shoulder dislocations. *Am J Sports Med.* 2002;30:576–580.

40. Bonazza NA, Liu G, Leslie DL, Dhawan A. Trends in surgical management of shoulder instability. *Orthopaedic J Sports Med.* 2017;5. 232596711771247.

41. Owens BD, Harrast JJ, Hurwitz SR, Thompson TL, Wolf JM. Surgical trends in Bankart repair. *Am J Sports Med.* 2011;39:1865–1869.

42. Phadnis J, Arnold C, Elmorsy A, Flannery M. Utility of the instability severity index score in predicting failure after arthroscopic anterior stabilization of the shoulder. *Am J Sports Med.* 2015;43:1983–1988.

43. Boileau P, et al. Risk factors for recurrence of shoulder instability after arthroscopic Bankart repair. *J Bone Joint Surg.* 2006;88:1755–1763.

44. Porcellini G, Campi F, Pegreffi F, Castagna A, Paladini P. Predisposing factors for recurrent shoulder dislocation after arthroscopic treatment. *J Bone Joint Surg.* 2009;91:2537–2542.

45. Neer 2nd CS, Foster CR. Inferior capsular shift for involuntary inferior and multidirectional instability of the shoulder. A preliminary report. *J Bone Joint Surg. Am.* 1980;62:897–908.

46. Hohmann E, Tetsworth K, Glatt V. Open versus arthroscopic surgical treatment for anterior shoulder dislocation: a comparative systematic review and meta-analysis over the past 20 years. *J Shoulder Elbow Surg.* 2017;26:1873–1880.

47. Miura K, et al. Can arthroscopic Bankart repairs using suture anchors restore equivalent stability to open repairs in the management of traumatic anterior shoulder dislocation? A meta-analysis. *J Orthop Sci.* 2018;23:935–941.

48. Shin S-J, Kim RG, Jeon YS, Kwon TH. Critical value of anterior glenoid bone loss that leads to recurrent glenohumeral instability after arthroscopic Bankart repair. *Am J Sports Med.* 2017;45:1975–1981.

49. Arciero RA, et al. The effect of a combined glenoid and Hill-Sachs defect on glenohumeral stability. *Am J Sports Med.* 2015;43:1422–1429.

50. Shaha JS, et al. Redefining 'critical' bone loss in shoulder instability. *Am J Sports Med.* 2015;43:1719–1725.

51. Mologne TS, Provencher MT, Menzel KA, Vachon TA, Dewing CB. Arthroscopic stabilization in patients with an inverted pear glenoid: results in patients with bone loss of the anterior glenoid. *Am J Sports Med.* 2007;35:1276–1283.

52. Moroder P, et al. Neer Award 2019: Latarjet procedure vs. iliac crest bone graft transfer for treatment of anterior shoulder instability with glenoid bone loss: a prospective randomized trial. *J Shoulder Elbow Surg.* 2019;28:1298–1307.

53. John R, Wong IH. Arthroscopic treatment for shoulder instability with glenoid bone loss using distal tibia allograft augmentation: two-year outcomes. *Arthroscopy: J Arthroscop Related Surg.* 2019;35:e14.

54. Kwapisz A, Fitzpatrick K, Cook J, Tokish J. Distal clavicular osteochondral autograft augmentation for glenoid bone loss: a comparison of radius of restoration versus Latarjet graft. *Arthroscopy: J Arthroscop Related Surg.* 2017;33:e2.

55. Longo UG, et al. Latarjet, Bristow, and Eden-Hybinette procedures for anterior shoulder dislocation: systematic review and quantitative synthesis of the literature. *Arthroscopy: J Arthroscop Related Surg.* 2014;30:1184–1211.

56. Mizuno N, Walch G. Long-term results of Latarjet procedure for the treatment of anterior glenohumeral instability: a 20-year follow-up study. *J Shoulder Elbow Surg.* 2012;21:e27–e28.

57. Ali J, et al. Open versus arthroscopic Latarjet procedure for the treatment of chronic anterior glenohumeral instability with glenoid bone loss. *Arthroscopy: J Arthroscop Related Surg.* 2019. https://doi.org/10.1016/j.arthro.2019.09.042.

58. Marion B, et al. A prospective comparative study of arthroscopic versus mini-open Latarjet procedure with a minimum 2-year follow-up. *Arthroscopy: J Arthroscop Related Surg.* 2017;33:269–277.

59. Horner NS, et al. Open versus arthroscopic Latarjet procedures for the treatment of shoulder instability: a systematic review of comparative studies. *BMC Muscoskel Disord.* 2018;19.

60. Longo UG, et al. Remplissage, humeral osteochondral grafts, Weber osteotomy, and shoulder arthroplasty for the management of humeral bone defects in shoulder instability: systematic review and quantitative synthesis of the literature. *Arthroscopy: J Arthroscop Related Surg.* 2014;30:1650–1666.

61. Hughes JL, Bastrom T, Pennock AT, Edmonds EW. Arthroscopic Bankart repairs with and without remplissage in recurrent adolescent anterior shoulder instability with Hill-Sachs deformity. *Orthopaedic J Sports Med.* 2018;6. 2325967118813981.

62. Camus D, et al. Isolated arthroscopic Bankart repair vs. Bankart repair with 'remplissage' for anterior shoulder instability with engaging Hill-Sachs lesion: a meta-analysis. *Orthopaedics & Traumatology, Surgery & Research: OTSR.* 2018;104:803–809.

63. Yang JS, et al. Remplissage versus modified Latarjet for off-track Hill-Sachs lesions with subcritical glenoid bone loss. *Am J Sports Med.* 2018;46:1885–1891.

64. Garcia GH, Wu H-H, Liu JN, Huffman GR, Kelly JD. IV. Outcomes of the remplissage procedure and its effects on return to sports. *Am J Sports Med.* 2016;44:1124–1130.

65. Kim S-H, Ha K-I, Kim Y-M. Arthroscopic revision Bankart repair. *Arthroscopy: J Arthroscop Related Surg.* 2002;18:469–482.

66. Streufert BD, et al. Patient preferences for treatment of a first time anterior shoulder dislocation. *J Shoulder Elbow Surg.* 2015;24:e123–e124.

67. Hutyra CA, Smiley S, Taylor DC, Orlando LA, Mather III RC. Efficacy of a preference-based decision tool on treatment decisions for a first-time anterior shoulder dislocation: a randomized controlled trial of at-risk patients. *Med Decision Making.* 2019;39:253–263.

68. Abdul-Rassoul H, Galvin JW, Curry EJ, Simon J, Li X. Return to sport after surgical treatment for anterior shoulder instability: a systematic review. *Am J Sports Med.* 2018;47:1507–1515.

69. Friedman LGM, Lafosse L, Garrigues GE. Global perspectives on management of shoulder instability. *Orthopedic Clin North Am.* 2020;51:241–258.

70. Ekhtiari S, Horner NS, Bedi A, Ayeni OR, Khan M. The learning curve for the Latarjet procedure: a systematic review. *Orthopaedic J Sports Med.* 2018;6. 232596711878693.

71. Marshall T, et al. Outcomes after arthroscopic Bankart repair: patients with first-time versus recurrent dislocations. *Am J Sports Med.* 2017;45:1776–1782.

72. Savoie III FH, O'Brien MJ. Anterior instability in the throwing shoulder. *Sports Med Arthroscopy Rev.* 2014;22:117–119.

73. Bøe B, Provencher MT, Moatshe BG. Editorial commentary: can orthopaedic surgeons agree on choice of procedure for anterior shoulder instability based on risk factors? personal and training biases confound our surgical decision making. *Arthroscopy: J Arthroscop Related Surg.* 2019;35:2026–2028.

74. Seroyer ST, Nho SJ, Provencher MT, Romeo AA. Four-quadrant approach to capsulolabral repair: an arthroscopic road map to the glenoid. *Arthroscopy: J Arthroscop Related Surg.* 2010;26:555–562.

75. Frank RM, et al. Outcomes of arthroscopic anterior shoulder instability in the beach chair vs. the lateral decubitus position: a systematic review and meta-regression analysis. *J Shoulder Elbow Surg.* 2015;24:e242.

76. Ratner DA, Rogers JP, Tokish JM. Use of a knotless suture anchor to perform double-pulley capsulotenodesis of infraspinatus. *Arthroscopy Techniques.* 2018;7:e485–e490.

77. Lazarides AL, Duchman KR, Ledbetter L, Riboh JC, Garrigues GE. Arthroscopic remplissage for anterior shoulder instability: a systematic review of clinical and biomechanical studies. *Arthroscopy: J Arthroscop Related Surg.* 2019;35:617–628.

78. Frank RM, et al. Outcomes of Latarjet versus distal tibial allograft for anterior shoulder instability repair: a prospective matched cohort analysis. *Orthopaedic J Sports Med.* 2017;5. 2325967117S0027.

79. Taverna E, Golanò P, Pascale V, Battistella F. An arthroscopic bone graft procedure for treating anterior–inferior glenohumeral instability. *Knee Surg Sports Traumatol Arthrosc.* 2008;16:872–875.

80. Amar E, Konstantinidis G, Coady C, Wong IH. Arthroscopic treatment of shoulder instability with glenoid bone loss using distal tibial allograft augmentation: safety profile and short-term radiological outcomes. *Orthopaedic J Sports Med.* 2018;6. 232596711877450.

81. DeFroda SF, Mehta N, Owens BD. Physical therapy protocols for arthroscopic Bankart repair. *Sports Health: A Multidisciplinary Approach.* 2018;10:250–258.

82. Ciccotti MC, et al. Return to play criteria following surgical stabilization for traumatic anterior shoulder instability: a systematic review. *Arthroscopy: J Arthroscop Related Surg.* 2018;34:903–913.

83. Williams III RJ. Editorial commentary: reviewing the science of our unscientific criteria for return to sports after shoulder stabilization. *Arthroscopy: J Arthroscop Related Surg.* 2018;34:914–916.

84. Abe H, et al. Healing processes of the glenoid labral lesion in a rabbit model of shoulder dislocation. *Tohoku J Exp Med.* 2012;228:103–108.

85. Gibson J, Kerss J, Morgan C, Brownson P. Accelerated rehabilitation after arthroscopic Bankart repair in professional footballers. *Shoulder Elbow.* 2016;8:279–286.

86. Ma R, Brimmo OA, Li X, Colbert L. Current concepts in rehabilitation for traumatic anterior shoulder instability. *Curr Rev Musculoskeletal Med.* 2017;10:499–506.

20

Technique Spotlight: Arthroscopic Labral Repair: Anterior and Posterior

RON GILAT, ERIC D. HAUNSCHILD, TRACY TAURO,
MICHAEL C. FU, THEODORE S. WOLFSON, AND BRIAN J. COLE

Introduction

Owing to the unique anatomy and range-of-motion (ROM) demands of the shoulder, coordination of several static and dynamic stabilizers is necessary to maintain shoulder stability. This coordination can be disrupted, most commonly secondary to acute traumatic dislocation or atraumatic laxity of the shoulder. As a result, glenohumeral instability of the shoulder is a commonly treated condition in orthopedic clinics, with reported incidence rates in the general public of 0.08 per 1000 person-years and much higher rates in military and contact athlete populations.[1] Single or recurrent dislocation events often result in tears of the capsulolabral soft tissue stabilizers around the glenoid, which, depending on location and severity, can result in posterior, multidirectional, and most commonly, anterior instability of the shoulder.

In patients with recurrent instability or, increasingly, first-time dislocators at high risk of redislocation, surgical stabilization is often indicated to minimize pain, improve shoulder function, and prevent subsequent dislocation events. Depending on the location and extent of the anterior or posterior capsulolabral tear (commonly referred to as Bankart or Kim lesions, respectively) as well as the presence of concomitant pathology, including glenohumeral bony defects, a number of different surgical approaches have been described to restore stability.

Labral tears have traditionally been repaired to the glenoid rim using open techniques, but in recent decades the use of arthroscopic repair techniques has increased significantly.[2] With the improvement in arthroscopic instrumentation, anchors, and techniques, outcomes of arthroscopic stabilization are comparable to those of open stabilization.[3–5] The purpose of this manuscript is to describe in detail a surgical technique for arthroscopic anterior and posterior labral repair using modern knotless implants. Surgical indications, preoperative planning, operative details, technical considerations, and high-yield pearls and pitfalls are highlighted to provide a practical guide to modern arthroscopic labral repair.

Preoperative Planning and Indications for Operative Managements

A thorough history and physical examination must precede and guide the treatment plan. History should be focused on the mechanism of injury, direction of instability, chronicity, degree of instability (subluxation vs. dislocation), number and frequency of instability events, risk factors for recurrence (e.g., age), presence of hyperlaxity,

and athletic participation. A thorough standard physical examination should follow, with inspection, palpation, ROM, strength, provocative tests for instability, and a peripheral neurovascular exam.[6]

Routine radiographs include the true anteroposterior, scapular, and axillary lateral view. Stryker-notch and West Point views are recommended for the evaluation of Hill-Sachs lesions and glenoid bone loss, respectively, and should be considered for screening. Magnetic resonance imaging (MRI) is critical for surgical planning to assess for the location and extent of labral pathology and rule out concomitant lesions, including humeral avulsion of the glenohumeral ligament (HAGL), anterior labral periosteal sleeve avulsion (ALPSA), and rotator cuff lesions. Computed tomography (CT) is not used routinely but should be considered if bone loss is suspected. Three-dimensional (3D) volume-rendering reconstructions with humeral subtraction are particularly valuable to quantify the glenoid bone loss.[7,8]

Indications for isolated arthroscopic labral repair is a subject of controversy (see Chapter 19). However, in our hands, we consider arthroscopic labral repair in young active patients with recurrent instability, a confirmed labral tear on MRI, and symptomatic glenohumeral instability in the absence of critical glenoid bone loss (<15%–25%). Relative contraindications to isolated arthroscopic labral repair include patients with instability that is more appropriately treated with a different operation: critical glenoid bone loss (>15%–25%), concomitant pathology including a large engaging Hill-Sachs, or the presence of a HAGL. Another, even more common relative contraindication is a labral tear in the setting of degenerative shoulder: early glenohumeral osteoarthritis without instability. These tears commonly comprise poor quality tissue, torn in an atypical and intrasubstance pattern, and are made worse with repair as this procedure can hasten the progression of stiffness and arthritis associated with their degenerative changes.

Preoperative Setup, Positioning, and Examination Under Anesthesia

We advise eligible patients to undergo interscalene block in the preoperative holding area, followed by endotracheal intubation or a laryngeal mask (LMA) in the operating room. In a patient with a suspected tear of the anterior, posterior, and/or inferior labrum, we prefer the lateral decubitus position with balanced traction. This is especially true when the pathology is suspected to be located at the more inferior section of the labrum.[9] However, this procedure can also be performed in the beach chair position, depending on the surgeon's preference and experience.

Once the patient is anesthetized, an examination under anesthesia (EUA) should be performed to assess for ROM and stability. EUA should be performed prior to positioning in the lateral decubitus position to allow comparison to the contralateral side and then repeated in the lateral decubitus position to gauge the amount of stabilization required. The load and shift maneuver can be used to assess anterior and posterior translations. While performing the load and shift maneuver in a patient with a labral tear, an audible click may be heard, particularly in cases of posterior instability with labral tear. The Sulcus sign is less appreciated in the lateral position but may be accentuated in patients with multidirectional instability (MDI).[10] The EUA is critical to quantifying the true magnitude of instability and is used to gauge the degree of stabilization to be performed.

When positioning in the lateral decubitus position, all bony prominences should be padded, an axillary roll should be placed, and a bean-bag positioning device is typically used. Once the patient is secured in the lateral decubitus position, the shoulder is then prepped and draped in a standard sterile fashion and positioned in the lateral distraction device (Lateral Decubitus Shoulder Traction Tower; Arthrex, Naples, FL). The arm is secured in the distraction device at 50 degrees shoulder abduction and 15 degrees forward flexion with 10–12 lb of in-line traction and a similar weight for lateral distraction. Balanced traction provides symmetric distraction to optimize visualization of the entire glenohumeral articulation, including the inferior aspect. Once the positioning is complete, standard landmarks are identified. A spinal needle is used to insufflate the glenohumeral joint with saline (Fig. 20.1A–B).

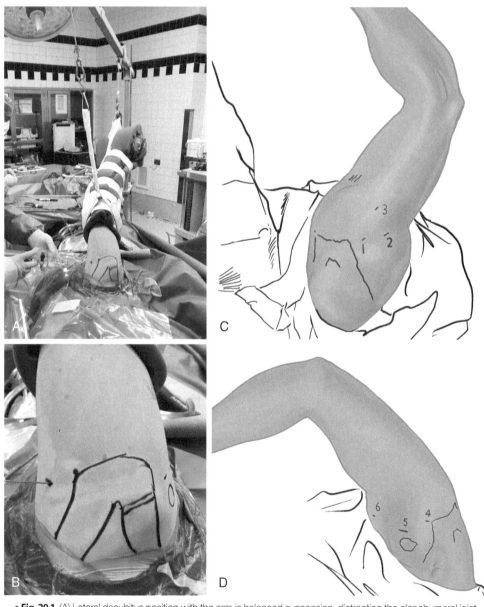

• **Fig. 20.1** (A) Lateral decubitus position with the arm in balanced suspension, distracting the glenohumeral joint. (B) The clavicle, acromion, acromioclavicular joint, and coracoid process are outlined with a marking pen. The location of the posterior portal and the estimated location of the anterior portal are also marked. A spinal needle is used to insufflate the glenohumeral joint with 60 mL of saline. We prefer not to mark the locations of other portals as their location varies and is typically identified using a spinal needle. (C) An illustration of estimated locations of the posterior viewing portal (1), posterior working portal (2), and the 7-o'clock portal (3). (D) An illustration of estimated locations of the anterosuperior viewing portal (4), anterior working portal (5), and the 5-o'clock portal (6).

Initial Portal Placement and Diagnostic Survey

Posterior portals include the standard posterior viewing portal, posterior working portal, and the 7-o'clock portal. Anterior portals include the anterosuperior viewing portal, anterior working portal, and the 5-o'clock portal (Fig. 20.1C–D). The location of the labral tear and the surgeon's preference will dictate which portals will allow the optimal view and access for repair.

Arthroscopy of the glenohumeral joint is typically initiated using a posterior viewing portal, which is made nearly in-line with the lateral edge of the acromion, and 1 cm inferior to the acromion (slightly lateral and superior to the standard posterior portal in beach chair position). This allows for the posterior portal to be angled slightly inferiorly (~15 to 20 degrees) relative to the glenoid rim, which is particularly helpful when a posterior stabilization is required, allowing improved view of the glenoid surface, avoiding portal crowding with accessory posterior portals, and can be used for posterior anchor placement. The anterosuperior viewing portal is made under direct visualization in the superior aspect of the rotator interval with the guidance of a spinal needle. A clear 5-mm cannula is inserted into the anterosuperior portal followed by a probe. In cases where the anterosuperior portal is not needed, an anterior working portal can be established instead. Once posterior and anterior portals are established, a systematic diagnostic survey of the glenohumeral joint is performed using the Southern California Orthopedic Institute (SCOI) 15-point evaluation system.[11,12] Encountered pathologies of the labrum, glenoid, humeral head, biceps tendon, and rotator cuff are comprehensively evaluated. Labral tears are typically easily detected, but some fissures (Kim lesions) resulting from repetitive microtrauma may be more subtle. Once diagnosed, the labral tear should be probed to evaluate the depth of the tear and to interrogate the chondrolabral junction. The location and extent of the tear should be documented, and a repair plan verbalized to the operating team.

An anterior (mid-glenoid) working portal is made low in the rotator cuff interval, just superior to the subscapularis tendon and lateral to the tip of the coracoid process. An 8.25-mm cannula is secured to ensure the posterior labrum can be accessed. The anterior portal will be used for anterior anchor placement, suture passage, and preparation of the posterior glenoid labrum as needed. The arthroscope is left in the posterior viewing portal for the preparation of the anterior glenoid and can then be switched to the anterosuperior portal for the preparation of the posterior glenoid as needed (Fig. 20.2A–F).

Preparation of the Glenoid Labrum

The anterior, inferior, and posterior labrum is prepared alternating viewing and working between the anterior and posterior portals

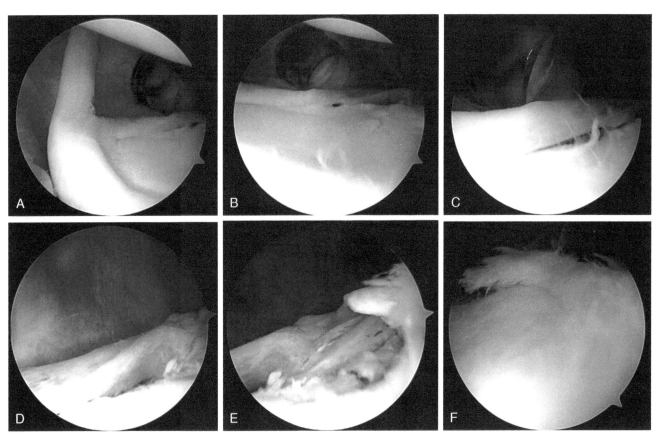

• **Fig. 20.2** Arthroscopic viewing from the posterior viewing portal of the right shoulder of a 16.5-year-old patient with recurrent instability. (A) The superior labrum and long head of biceps tendon are seen, along with a cord-like middle glenohumeral ligament. (A–C) A cannula is seen in the anterior working portal, low in the rotator cuff interval. (D–F) The labral tear is easily identified, beginning in the 3-o'clock position and continuing inferiorly and posteriorly to the 6-o'clock position. (F) Fraying of the labrum is also viewed, particularly in the inferior aspect of glenoid.

to facilitate visualization and instrument trajectory. Throughout the preparation of the glenoid, the surgeon must minimize the possibility of inadvertent iatrogenic trauma to the glenoid and humeral head cartilaginous surfaces. In our experience, this can be performed safely, utilizing the following technique.

We typically begin by debriding frayed labrum and flaps using an arthroscopic shaver. The labrum is then peeled-off and elevated from the chondrolabral junction as a sleeve of soft tissue using a Bankart elevator. Inability to achieve a sufficient mobilization and release of the medially scarred labral tear will make it impossible to achieve an anatomic labral reduction/retensioning of the glenohumeral ligaments and capsule. The glenoid rim is then decorticated using a curved and hooded bone-cutting shaver to create a bleeding bed for labral healing. A curved rasp may also be used to abrade and roughen the capsulolabral tissue and glenoid bony rim to facilitate adhesion. These steps are usually initiated in the most superior aspect of the anterior labral tear and progress inferiorly, and then posteriorly as necessary. If difficulties are encountered in preparation of the anteroinferior aspect of the labrum or a very anteroinferior anchor is contemplated, a 5-o'clock trans-scapularis portal can be established to further assist. The 5-o'clock trans-scapularis portal is established using a spinal needle, outside-in localization, approximately 2 cm inferior and slightly lateral to the anterior working portal. The portal should pass between the middle and distal thirds of the subscapularis tendon. We recommend not to insert a cannula through this portal to avoid excessive disruption of the subscapularis.[10]

If an isolated posterior labral tear is identified or if there is a posterior extension of an anterior labral tear, an additional posterior working portal is usually indicated. The optimal location for the posterior working portal location is typically identified using a spinal needle and is about 3 cm inferior to the posterolateral corner of the acromion in line with its lateral border. It is typically 2–3 cm below the posterior visualization portal. An 8.25-mm cannula is then secured to allow suture passage and anchor placement as necessary. Then, an accessory 7-o'clock portal is established using a spinal needle for localization. This portal is typically located lateral and a bit inferiorly to the posterior working portal and should pass through the teres minor muscle. In relation to the posterolateral corner of the acromion, the distance is typically 3 cm inferior and 1–2 cm lateral to the border of the posterolateral acromion. The 7-o'clock portal is relatively safe as it is a mean 39 mm superior to the axillary nerve and allows direct working access to the posteroinferior glenoid and inferior capsular recess.[13]

Posterior labral preparation may be difficult with the trajectories of the posterior portals, and while maybe counterintuitive, the anterior working portal is usually the best option. Via the anterior portal, the posterior chondrolabral junction is identified, and the labrum is peeled off and elevated using a labral elevator. The labral elevator can then be manipulated in a superior to inferior direction to complete the elevation of the labrum. Then a bone-cutting shaver can be used from the posterior or 7-o'clock portal to create the bleeding bed of the posterior glenoid. At this point, if necessary, the posterior labral preparation can be finessed using the posterior portals. Care should be taken to address incomplete tears and "marginal cracks" as these might be easily missed[14] (Fig. 20.3A–E).

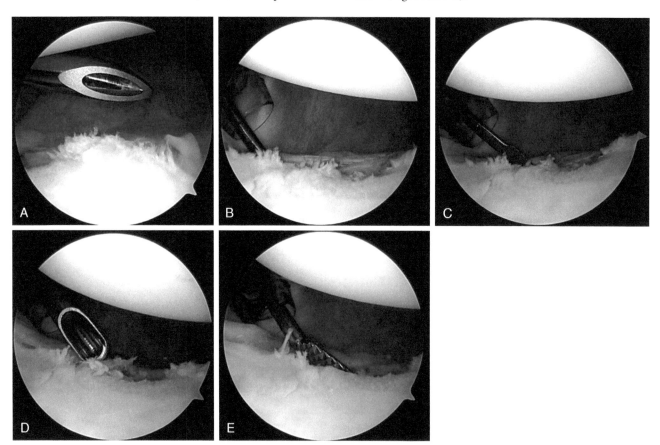

• **Fig. 20.3** Viewing from the posterior portal. (A) Preparation of the inferior labrum beginning with debridement of labral fraying using a Torpedo shaver (Arthrex, Naples, FL). (B) Elevation of the anterior capsulolabral complex using a labral elevator from the anterior working portal. (C) Use of the 7-o'clock portal to complete elevation of the inferior and posterior aspect of the capsulolabral tissue. (D) Creating the "bleeding bed" on the edge of the glenoid using a 5.0 bone cutter. (E) Final preparation using a back-curved labral rasp.

Labral Repair

Anteroinferior Labral Repair

The repair is typically performed while viewing from the posterior viewing portal and working from the anterior working (mid-glenoid) portal and the 7-o'clock portal. A curved spectrum suture passer (ConMed Linvatec, Largo, FL) loaded with a No. 1 polydioxanone (PDS) suture (Ethicon, Somerville, NJ) is inserted to the anterior working portal and the PDS suture is passed through the capsule-labral tissues.[15] The PDS suture limb that went through the tissue is then retrieved from the 7-o'clock portal and it is loaded with an ultra-high-molecular-weight polyethylene (UHMWPE) suture tape (SutureTape; Arthrex) and "shuttle-relayed" through the tissue. The PDS is then removed and the remaining limb of the SutureTape is retrieved using a loop or tape retriever via the anterior working portal. A knotless suture anchor (short, 2.9-mm PushLock; Arthrex) is then loaded with the SutureTape. A drill guide is inserted through the anterior working portal and is seated firmly on the edge of the glenoid in the corresponding location. The drill is inserted through the guide and drilling should be running all the way in and out of the guide, to avoid dislodging the guide from its position once the drill encounters the glenoid. The anchor is inserted through

the guide and secured to the glenoid after tensioning the suture limbs. The sutures are then cut with an arthroscopic suture cutter. The procedure is repeated moving from posteroinferior to anterosuperior. In many cases, the inferior aspect of the glenoid can be accessed more easily using the 5- or 7-o'clock portals.

Posterior Labral Repair

If not made beforehand, a posterior working portal and/or a 7-o'clock portal should be established. The anterosuperior portal is used for viewing. The repair is performed in a similar method to the one described for anteroinferior labral repair. The repair should start inferiorly and proceed in a posterior direction. The 7-o'clock portal can be used as the working portal for the more inferior aspects of the glenoid, and the posterior working portal for the more posterior aspects. A spectrum suture passer is used to pass a PDS suture through the capsule-labral tissue and is later retrieved from the anterior working portal. A SutureTape is shuttle-relayed using the PDS and then retrieved through the posterior working portal. A PushLock anchor is loaded with the SutureTape and screwed to the glenoid at the appropriate position. Care must be taken at all times to avoid iatrogenic cartilage damage and "collision" between adjacent anchors (Fig. 20.4A–D).

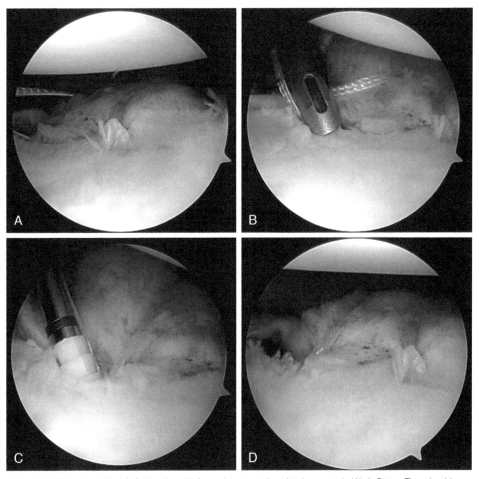

• **Fig. 20.4** Viewing of the inferior glenoid from the posterior viewing portal. (A) A SutureTape had been passed through the capsulolabral tissue. (B) A drill guide is placed on the edge of the glenoid to facilitate drilling through the 7-o'clock portal. (C) A 3.5-mm PushLock anchor is inserted and the sutures are tightened. (D) The inferior capsulolabral tissue following complete repair.

Bony Bankart Repair

Repair of a bony Bankart or management of glenoid bone loss is beyond the scope of this chapter. However, typically if a bony Bankart lesion is encountered it is generally repaired in a similar fashion, unless the bony fragment is large enough to accommodate screw fixation. Alternative techniques have also been described with double-row fixation.[16] Reduction and internal fixation of a large bony Bankart fragment can be performed arthroscopically or via an open approach as indicated and according to the surgeon's preference.

Postoperative Protocol

Anterior Stabilization

The shoulder is immobilized in a shoulder abduction sling day and night for 2 weeks, then only during daytime from 2 to 6 weeks. Passive ROM is initiated at 3 weeks postoperatively, allowing up to 90 degrees flexion, 45 degrees abduction, and 20 degrees extension. Active and active-assisted ROM is initiated at 6 weeks, with full active ROM expected by 12–16 weeks postoperatively. Return to full activity is based on the individual situation but is expected at 5–7 months postoperatively.[17]

Posterior Stabilization

The shoulder is immobilized in a shoulder abduction sling day and night for 2 weeks, then only at daytime from 2 to 6 weeks. Passive ROM is initiated at 3 weeks postoperatively, allowing up to 90 degrees flexion, 90 degrees abduction, and 45 degrees internal brace. Active and active-assisted ROM is initiated at 6 weeks, with full active ROM expected by 12–16 weeks postoperatively. Return to full activity is individual but expected at 5–7 months postoperatively.[18]

PEARLS AND PITFALLS

Pearls

The lateral decubitus position allows better distraction of the glenohumeral joint and optimizes visualization and access to the inferior glenoid. Make sure the patient is fastened securely to the table.

The assistant should be instructed to maintain the cannula in its position when instrumentation is utilized within the cannula to avoid cannula pullout.

The accessory 5- and 7-o'clock portals enable direct access to the anteroinferior and posteroinferior glenoid, respectively, and can facilitate an easier repair.

The drill should be running all the way up and down the drill guide to avoid dislodging the drill guide.

Pitfalls

When performing a concomitant open procedure or if a transition to an open procedure is required, the patient needs to be repositioned in a beach chair position.

Cannula pullout can result in disorientation, time lost, and extravasation of arthroscopic fluid into soft tissue.

Use of accessory portals should be performed with care to avoid injury to neurovascular structures, particularly the axillary nerve, which is at risk when manipulations are performed around the 6-o'clock position.

Inadequate visualization or access during labral preparation with a labral elevator or a bone-cutter can result in iatrogenic cartilage injury.

PEARLS AND PITFALLS

Pearls

In order to avoid cartilage injury when drilling, the surgeon should look for the appearance of bone marrow bubbles, movement of the glenoid cartilage, or movement of an adjacent anchor. Drilling should be stopped immediately if any of these are encountered.

Pitfalls

Iatrogenic cartilage injury is common and should be avoided at all times. Risk is high during labral preparation and drilling for anchor placement.

Summary

This technique is a reliable, safe, and efficient arthroscopic labral repair technique for shoulder instability. The use of accessory portals and following the pearls and pitfalls presented herein may aid in achieving excellent results in technically challenging cases. Although this is our preferred approach, many other reliable techniques are available and should be utilized based on the surgeon's preference and experience.

References

1. Galvin JW, Ernat JJ, Waterman BR, Stadecker MJ, Parada SA. The epidemiology and natural history of anterior shoulder instability. *Curr Rev Musculoskel Med.* 2017;10:411–424.
2. Owens BD, Harrast JJ, Hurwitz SR, Thompson TL, Wolf JM. Surgical trends in Bankart repair: an analysis of data from the American Board of Orthopaedic Surgery certification examination. *Am J Sports Med.* 2011;39:1865–1869.
3. Bottoni CR, Smith EL, Berkowitz MJ, Towle RB, Moore JH. Arthroscopic versus open shoulder stabilization for recurrent anterior instability: a prospective randomized clinical trial. *Am J Sports Med.* 2006;34:1730–1737.
4. Hohmann E, Tetsworth K, Glatt V. Open versus arthroscopic surgical treatment for anterior shoulder dislocation: a comparative systematic review and meta-analysis over the past 20 years. *J Shoulder Elbow Surg.* 2017;26:1873–1880.
5. Chalmers PN, Mascarenhas R, Leroux T, et al. Do arthroscopic and open stabilization techniques restore equivalent stability to the shoulder in the setting of anterior glenohumeral instability? A systematic review of overlapping meta-analyses. *Arthrosc J Arthrosc Relat Surg.* 2015;31:355–363.
6. Hendawi T, Milchteim C, Ostrander R. Bankart repair using modern arthroscopic technique. *Arthroscopy Tech.* 2017;6:e863–e870.
7. Rerko MA, Pan X, Donaldson C, Jones GL, Bishop JY. Comparison of various imaging techniques to quantify glenoid bone loss in shoulder instability. *J Shoulder Elbow Surg.* 2013;22:528–534.
8. Bishop JY, Jones GL, Rerko MA, Donaldson C, Group MS. 3-D CT is the most reliable imaging modality when quantifying glenoid bone loss. *Clini Orthopaed Related Res.* 2013;471:1251–1256.
9. Provencher MT, Romeo AA, Solomon DJ, Bach Jr BR, Cole BJ. Arthroscopic preparation of the posterior and posteroinferior glenoid labrum. *Orthopedics.* 2007;30:904–905.
10. Cvetanovich GL, Hamamoto JT, Campbell KJ, McCarthy M, Higgins JD, Verma NN. The use of accessory portals in Bankart repair with posterior extension in the lateral decubitus position. *Arthroscopy Techniques.* 2016;5:e1121–e1128.
11. Snyder S. A complete system for arthroscopy and bursoscopy of the shoulder. *Surg Rounds Orthop.* 1989;3:57–65.
12. Snyder SJ, Wuh HC. Arthroscopic evaluation and treatment of the rotator cuff and superior labrum anterior posterior lesion. *Operative Tech Orthopaed.* 1991;1:207–220.

13. Davidson PA, Rivenburgh DW. The 7-o'clock posteroinferior portal for shoulder arthroscopy. *Am J Sports Med.* 2002;30:693–696.
14. Kim S-H, Ha K-I, Yoo J-C, Noh K-C. Kim's lesion: an incomplete and concealed avulsion of the posteroinferior labrum in posterior or multidirectional posteroinferior instability of the shoulder. *Arthrosc J Arthrosc Relat Surg.* 2004;20:712–720.
15. Driscoll MD, Burns JP, Snyder SJ. Arthroscopic transosseous bony Bankart repair. *Arthroscopy Techniques.* 2015;4:e47–e50.
16. Millett PJ, Braun S. The "bony Bankart bridge" procedure: a new arthroscopic technique for reduction and internal fixation of a bony Bankart lesion. *Arthroscopy.* 2009;25:102–105.
17. Cole BJ. *Arthroscopic Anterior Stabilization Rehabilitation Protocol*; 2020. https://www.briancolemd.com/wp-content/themes/ypo-theme/pdf/arthroscopic-anterior-stabilization.pdf
18. Cole BJ. *Posterior Stabilization Rehabilitation Protocol*; 2020. https://www.briancolemd.com/wp-content/themes/ypo-theme/pdf/posterior-stabilization.pdf

21

Technique Spotlight: Technical Aspects of the Arthroscopic Remplissage

JOHN M. TOKISH

Introduction

The treatment of the significant Hill-Sachs lesion (HSL) continues to evolve. One option that has gained popularity is a transfer of the infraspinatus/posterior capsule directly into the Hill-Sachs defect. Originally described by Connolly in 1972[1] as an open procedure, the transferred infraspinatus and capsule may exclude the defect from the intra-articular aspect of the joint and effectively prevent engagement of the HSL with the glenoid. This technique may also act as a check-rein, limiting the head from translating anteriorly during abduction/external rotation, further limiting the potential for engagement. Purchase et al.[2] described the arthroscopic version and coined the term "remplissage" from the French "to fill in." The arthroscopic remplissage has gained popularity as an adjunct to arthroscopic Bankart repair.

Indications

Systematic reviews have reported overall recurrence rates of 5.4% to 5.8%.[3,4] Some reviews have noted that Rowe scores have improved from an average of 36 to 88 points, without significant loss of motion.[3,4] Others have reported small losses of motion of questionable clinical significance—up to 14 degrees of external rotation with the arm at the side.[4–6] The ideal remplissage indication is in the setting of a large HSL with minimal to no glenoid bone loss (Fig. 21.1). It remains a source of active debate regarding when, on the small end, the Hill-Sachs can be ignored and the anteroinferior labral injury addressed with a Bankart repair or a Latarjet/bony procedure to lengthen the arc length. On the larger end, it is likewise unclear when the Hill-Sachs is too large for the remplissage to be effective and when the humeral head articular defect is best addressed with a humeral or talar osteochondral allograft versus a hemiarthroplasty. I have become more aggressive with this technique, now employing it in most cases of significant HSLs, except those in a thrower, or overhead athlete.

Technical Keys

The arthroscopic remplissage is a relatively simple procedure that can be performed with minimal adjustments to standard arthroscopic techniques. I prefer to perform this procedure with a knotless, passless double-pulley technique which we described

previously.[7] This technique allows the entire procedure to be performed with the camera intra-articular and requires neither suture passage, nor knot tying. The technique uses two suture anchors placed at the anterior and posterior edges of the HSL. The key to the procedure is to make a single skin incision and portal, which can be used to direct two separate passes through the cuff to reach both the anterior and posterior limits of the HSL. The passage of the anchor through the cuff is the tissue grab, and I pass the suture from each anchor through the anchor of the other, giving a double mattress, double-pulley technique that is reproducible, simple, and effective. There are, however, several keys to making this procedure smooth and efficient that will be discussed below.

Positioning

While the remplissage can be performed in either the beach chair or lateral decubitus position, the latter provides significant advantages for visualization. The lateral traction afforded can

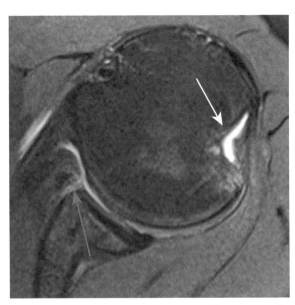

• **Fig. 21.1** Axial magnetic resonance imaging Hill-Sachs lesion. The *red arrow* points to the Bankart lesion; the *yellow arrow* points to the Hill-Sachs lesion.

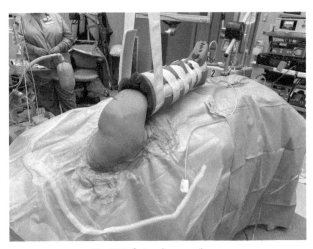

• **Fig. 21.2** Setup for remplissage.

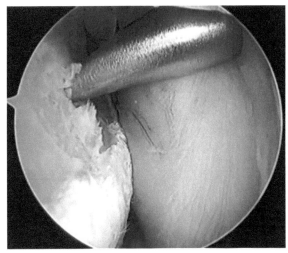

• **Fig. 21.3** Switching stick to anterior Hill-Sachs lesion.

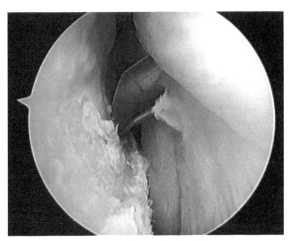

• **Fig. 21.4** Sled guide for drill.

significantly aid in the concomitant Bankart repair, and abduction of the arm, which is far easier to maintain in the lateral position, is a critical step in visualization and performance of the procedure. In our hands, the arm is placed in 20 to 30 degrees of abduction for the standard Bankart procedure, and the remplissage is performed with the arm around 60 degrees of abduction without lateral traction (Fig. 21.2). This position allows complete visualization of the rotator cuff insertion and HSL, as well as approximating the proper portion of the infraspinatus footprint to the defect itself.

Portal Position

Standard posterior, anterosuperior, and mid-glenoid portals are used to perform the Bankart operation. I prefer to perform the Bankart operation first, and then move to the remplissage. I have not found any incidence of this increasing the technical difficulty of the case, nor have I found any instance of Bankart repair compromise by this approach. The arm is then placed into abduction, and the lateral traction strap is removed. I have found that the optimal viewing portal is variable, with the anterosuperior portal and posterior portal often being correct depending on the size and location of the lesion. The HSL is identified and biologically prepared with the use of a rasp or shaver or burr until punctate bleeding bone is encountered. The remplissage is performed with one additional portal. In this technique, the camera remains intra-articular throughout the entire procedure. A spinal needle is used to penetrate the skin and enter the joint near the midpoint of the lateral acromial border, approximately 1 to 2 cm lateral to the acromion. Care is taken to ensure that the spinal needle can easily reach the anterior and posterior limits of the Hill-Sachs defect, and that the angle taken by the spinal needle gives a relatively perpendicular approach to the humeral head such that the anchor will not penetrate the articular surface. I prefer to place the anchors toward the articular surface so as to "exclude" the defect when possible. This may or may not be critical, however, as I believe the primary effect of the remplissage procedure is to translate the head posteriorly, rather than to "exclude" the HSL. Once the correct position and trajectory of the spinal needle are determined, a skin incision is placed around the spinal needle and it is replaced with a narrow switching stick and proper angle of approach is confirmed. An 8-mm arthroscopic cannula is established through the skin and deltoid down to, but not through, the infraspinatus.

The position of the lateral portal is critical. It must be near the midpoint of the remplissage lesion, so that the anchors can be directed to both the posterior and anterior aspects of the HSL, and with sufficient separation between cuff passes to allow adequate tissue spanning of the defect. Its depth is also critical, as it must be into the subacromial space, just adjacent to the bursal surface of the rotator cuff. This ensures that the construct will not tether the deltoid fascia and ensures that appropriate spanning distance between anchors exists to span, but not overconstrain the remplissage. Lastly, the lateral approach ensures that the anchors pass through the tendinous portion of the rotator cuff to avoid the error of passing through the medial, muscular portion of the rotator cuff, which can lead to rotator cuff tear and an overaggressive capsulodesis.

Anchor Placement

Once the anterior switching stick is placed to ensure it can reach the anterior aspect of the lesion (Fig. 21.3), a drill guide is placed over it and positioned at the anterior aspect of the HSL (Fig. 21.4). While this is held in place, a drill is advanced (Fig. 21.5) and followed by a suture anchor (Fig. 21.6). The trajectory of the switching stick is critical. Where it passes through the cuff will determine the point of fixation between the cuff and HSL. If this pierce point is too medial, it can result in an overaggressive shift and may limit motion. The ideal point of penetration is adjacent to the medial edge of the HSL, through the tendinous portion

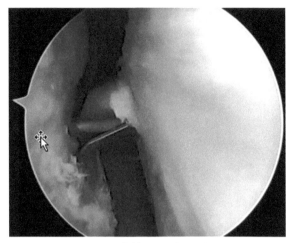

• **Fig. 21.5** Drilling anterior anchor.

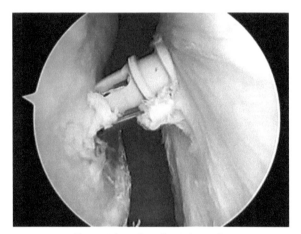

• **Fig. 21.6** Insertion of anterior anchor.

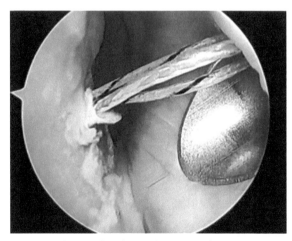

• **Fig. 21.7** Anterior knotless anchor inserted.

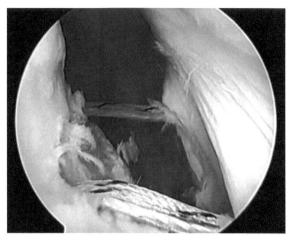

• **Fig. 21.8** After posterior anchor placed.

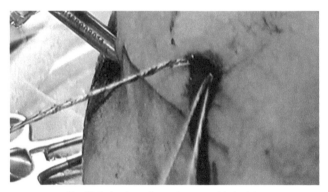

• **Fig. 21.9** Anchors through same skin incision.

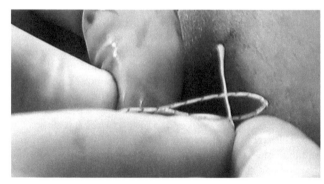

• **Fig. 21.10** Placing one anchor through a loop of the other.

it can reach the posterior edge of the HSL. The steps of anchor drilling are repeated, and the guide is again removed, leaving one anchor at each of the anterior and posterior borders of the HSL, with the sutures exiting with similar spacing through the capsule and tendon (Fig. 21.8).

Reduction and Securing of the Remplissage Into the Defect

The sutures are kept separate, although they emerge from the same lateral portal (Fig. 21.9). Using a 3.9-mm knotless corkscrew suture anchor (Arthrex, Naples, FL), the suture from the posterior anchor is passed through the reduction loop of the anterior anchor (Fig. 21.10). The reduction suture (nonlooped) side of the

of the infraspinatus (Fig. 21.7). The guide is then removed from the cannula, leaving this posterior anchor with sutures exiting through the posterior capsule and infraspinatus. The same narrow switching stick is reintroduced through the cannula, but it is redirected posteriorly and the tissue of the infraspinatus and capsule is indented bluntly until it is at the most posterior aspect of the Hill-Sachs defect. At this position, the switching stick is advanced through the tendon and capsule, and care is taken to ensure that anterior anchor reduction suture is then pulled, until the posterior anchor is passed through the anterior anchor and retrieved (Fig. 21.11). This process is repeated, such that the anterior anchor's suture is passed through the posterior reduction suture loop, and it is, in turn, passed through the posterior anchor and retrieved. Both sutures are tensioned, and the capsule and tendon are pulled down such that the lesion is completely excluded (Fig. 21.12A–B). A knot pusher can be used to reduce the cuff down to the HSL, excess suture length is trimmed, and the remplissage is examined through a gentle range of motion to ensure that it remains reduced. The final construct completely excludes the HSL from the joint

Alternative methods of performing the remplissage are possible. Instead of one portal being used, the anchors can be placed through separate percutaneous insertions. This may have the advantage of allowing better spacing through the posterior capsule and tendon between the anchors, and a broader area of tendon and capsule incorporated into the repair. If this technique is done, however, the subacromial space must be entered and the sutures retrieved into a single cannula for tying to avoid a tissue bridge. This requires some additional subacromial bursal clearance and suture retrieval—extra steps that inhibit operative efficiency.

PEARLS AND PITFALLS

While the arthroscopic remplissage can be a useful and efficient technique in the surgeon's approach to instability, there are several technical pitfalls that must be avoided to ensure its success.

- The first is visualization. Prior to beginning the procedure, care should be taken to ensure that the entire HSL can be visualized with working space between the lesion and the edge of the rotator cuff. This is optimized by removal of any lateral traction used to perform the Bankart repair, and the placement of the arm into abduction. Rotation can aid in visualization, but I recommend that the entirety of the lesion be visualized without requiring movement of the arm during this portion of the procedure. This allows for a consistent position of piercing the capsule and infraspinatus tendon. Normally the entire procedure can be accomplished by viewing from the posterior portal with a 30-degree arthroscope, and using the anterior portal and lateral subacromial portals as the working portals, but I do not hesitate to change to view from the posterior portal or to employ a 70-degree arthroscope, if it affords better visualization of the anterior edge of the HSL.

- Order of the operation can also be a critical step in ensuring a smooth procedure. Repair of the Bankart can diminish the space to view the HSL, and vice versa. Thus many recommend that one begin the operation by placing the Bankart anchors and sutures, but to leave them untied and parked through the mid-glenoid portal. The remplissage is then performed as described, and once complete, the Bankart is revisited, and its sutures are securely tied. I have found this unnecessary in most cases and generally proceed with the Bankart repair with the arm in lateral traction and relative adduction first, and once complete, I remove the lateral traction, place the arm into abduction, and proceed with the remplissage as described.

- Anchor placement can be challenging to visualize, and the choice of anchor and method of insertion can help to avoid pitfalls. Choosing an anchor that can be inserted through a drill guide allows the surgeon to accomplish this step with one pass. Once the switching stick is through the correct insertion point in the capsule and tendon, the case can proceed all the way to anchor placement without reinserting or adjusting the anchor position. Minimizing the number of steps, particularly when they involve passing instruments through the capsule and cuff, is more efficient and protects the repair tissue from additional insertional trauma.

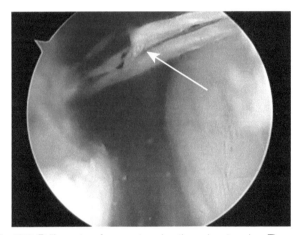

• **Fig. 21.11** Pulling suture from post anchor through ant anchor. The *yellow arrow* shows the passed stitch looped through the passing suture of the anchor. As the passing suture is pulled, the stitch goes through the anchor mechanism, creating a one-way self-locking construct, which enables knotless fixation.

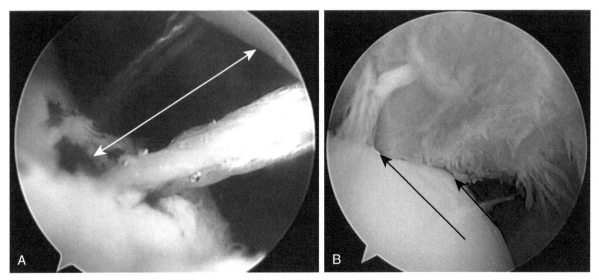

• **Fig. 21.12** Hill-Sachs lesion prior to reduction. (A) This demonstrates the Hill-Sachs lesion with anchors placed in the defect before reduction of the posterior capsule to the defect. The *yellow arrow* represents the space between the defect and the capsule. (B) The same shoulder after the remplissage has been completed. The *black arrows* point to the intimate contact between the posterior capsule and the humeral head.

- Location of penetration of the capsule and infraspinatus is the critical step for this remplissage technique. The sutures should be introduced through the tendon, and not the muscle, to avoid over-tensioning the capsule. Over-tensioning can also be a risk with very large HSLs, if attempts are made to bring the capsule and tendon to the medial edge of the defect. In these cases, consider placing the suture anchor off the medial edge and into the defect. Elkinson et al.[8] demonstrated that anchor placement in the valley of the defect was no different than sutures on the edge, but that more medialized sutures resulted in increased range of motion restrictions.

Conclusion

The addition of the remplissage has proven to be a valuable adjunct in anterior shoulder instability in the setting of a large HSL. This procedure can be reproducibly performed with improved results in patients with this condition. Meticulous attention to detail can make this technique efficient and simple to perform.

References

1. Connolly JF. Humeral head defects associated with shoulder dislocation—their diagnostic and surgical significance. *Instr Course Lect.* 1972;21:42–54.
2. Purchase RJ, Wolf EM, Hobgood ER, Pollock ME, Smalley CC. Hill-Sachs "remplissage": an arthroscopic solution for the engaging Hill-Sachs lesion. *Arthroscopy.* 2008;24(6):723–726.
3. Buza 3rd JA, Iyengar JJ, Anakwenze OA, Ahmad CS, Levine WN. Arthroscopic Hill-Sachs remplissage: a systematic review. *J Bone Joint Surg Am.* 2014;96(7):549–555.
4. Lazarides AL, Duchman KR, Ledbetter L, Riboh JC, Garrigues GE. Arthroscopic remplissage for anterior shoulder instability: a systematic review of clinical and biomechanical studies. *Arthroscopy.* 2019;35(2):617–628.
5. Boileau P, O'Shea K, Vargas P, et al. Anatomical and functional results after arthroscopic Hill-Sachs remplissage. *J Bone Joint Surg Am.* 2012;94(7):618–626.
6. Merolla G, Paladini P, Di Napoli G, Campi F, Porcellini G. Outcomes of arthroscopic Hill-Sachs remplissage and anterior Bankart repair: a retrospective controlled study including ultrasound evaluation of posterior capsulotenodesis and infraspinatus strength assessment. *Am J Sports Med.* 2015;43(2):407–414.
7. Ratner DA, Rogers JP, Tokish JM. Use of a knotless suture anchor to perform double-pulley capsulotenodesis of infraspinatus. *Arthrosc Tec.* 2018;7(5):E485–E490.
8. Elkinson I, Giles JW, Boons HW, et al. The shoulder remplissage procedure for Hill-Sachs defects: does technique matter? *J Shoulder Elbow Surg.* 2013;22(6):835–841.

22

Technique Spotlight: Arthroscopic Latarjet

M. CHRISTIAN MOODY, LEONARD ACHENBACH, THIBAULT LAFOSSE, AND LAURENT LAFOSSE

Indications for Arthroscopic Latarjet

Contraindications to arthroscopic Latarjet include presence of breast implants (due to the position and trajectory of the M portal) and prior coracoid harvest. The procedure is more challenging after prior open shoulder surgery due to the scar tissue but, with experience, can be performed safely in such a setting as well.

Once a detailed history, clinical examination, and radiological investigations are performed, an intraoperative assessment of the ligamentous stability can determine the appropriate operation. The following scenarios will provide examples of different surgical indications.

Glenoid Bone Loss

Many authors have reported failure of soft tissue repairs in the setting of glenoid bone loss.[1,2] The mechanical consequences of anteroinferior glenoid erosion are significant, and even a relatively small amount of bone loss can significantly affect the recurrence rate after arthroscopic or open soft tissue (Bankart) repair. A detailed discussion of the different options for assessment of the glenoid and humeral lesions is found in Chapter 19. In summary, assessment of the degree of bone loss can be made through a variety of methods including plain radiographs, specific magnetic resonance imaging (MRI) sequences, computed tomography (CT) scan with 3D volume rendering, arthroscopic assessment and measurement.[3,4] CT reconstructions provide a robust static measurement of bone loss. Arthroscopically, the distance from the glenoid rim as measured from the bare spot can assist the surgeon in identifying an inverted pear glenoid confirming substantial bone loss and the likely failure of an isolated soft tissue repair.

In some cases, the bony fragment can be replaced and arthroscopically repaired by anchors and sutures. However, this fragment is often comminuted, partially or completely resorbed over time, and may have poor healing potential. Furthermore, suture fixation is not as rigid as two screws with solid, cortical fixation. In these cases, a bone reconstruction as performed by the Latarjet procedure should be considered.

Humeral Bone Loss

The location and the depth of the Hill-Sachs lesion is variable with each case: sometimes small and superficial, sometimes large and/or deep, and rarely double. Its location and depth is responsible for persistent instability, even in cases of a well done Bankart repair.[5,6] Its precise assessment is difficult but can be approached by simple X-ray in internal rotation and 2D or 3D CT scan. The "remplissage" of the infraspinatus tendon has been described with satisfactory results but external rotation may be limited and long-term results have not been reported.[7]

The location and size of the Hill-Sachs lesion determines whether the articular arc is reduced and whether this will engage on the glenoid.[8] A dynamic arthroscopy with the shoulder in abduction and external rotation will demonstrate whether the lesion is engaging even within an athletic overhead range of movement. A bone block procedure here will increase the arc of the anterior glenoid thereby increasing the degree of external rotation that can be achieved before the Hill-Sachs lesion approaches the glenoid rim. We believe that by enlarging the glenoid articular arc with a bone graft, stability can be achieved without addressing the Hill-Sachs lesion directly.[9]

Bipolar Bone Loss

The "bipolar lesion" is responsible for many cases of recurrent instability.[8] This combination of two lesions usually occurs with varying degrees of severity for each individual lesion. These can be assessed before the procedure by examination, plain radiographs, and CT scan. It is critical to look for both lesions during the diagnostic portion of the arthroscopy under dynamic visualization.

Poor Capsular Tissue

A humeral avulsion of the glenohumeral ligaments (HAGL) lesion is sometimes possible to diagnose by an MRI or CT arthrography, but in most cases is discovered during the diagnostic arthroscopy. Different techniques of humeral reattachment by suture and anchor are possible depending on the location of the detachment, but our results with this technique have been disappointing due to the stiffness after repair.

Furthermore, in patients with multiple dislocations, collagen hyperlaxity syndromes (e.g., Ehlers-Danlos syndrome, Marfan's syndrome), or capsular damage secondary to attempted thermal capsulorrhaphy, the intrinsic structure of the glenohumeral ligaments is deranged although this may not be evident

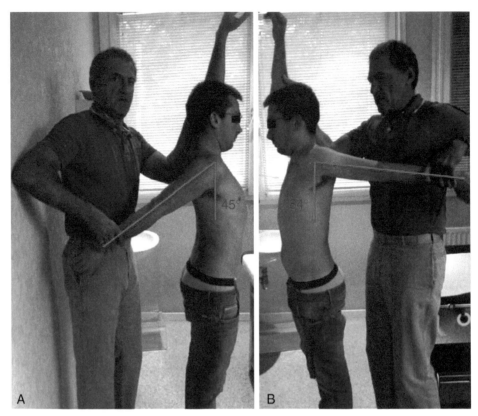

• **Fig. 22.1** Hyper extension-internal rotation (HERI) test examination.

macroscopically. Simply repairing this damaged tissue to the glenoid does not restore stability to the shoulder. This has been likened to rehanging a baggy or incompetent hammock. In these situations, we believe that relying on a soft tissue repair of this incompetent capsule is not as reliable as Latarjet bone block.

Revision of Bankart Repair

After an open or arthroscopic Bankart repair, success is often measured by the absence of recurrent dislocations. In some cases, the joint is incompletely stabilized but may allow function for a more sedentary lifestyle without overt symptoms of instability. This can, in part, explain the excellent results seen in series with a short follow-up. After 5 to 7 years we find this particular group of patients can go on to develop instability and/or arthritis. In these cases, the initial operation was considered successful although the pathological lesion was never truly corrected and the glenoid subsequently becomes increasingly eroded. Again, these patients can be successfully managed with a Latarjet procedure.

Preoperative Evaluation

There is no substitute for a complete history and physical examination when making surgical decisions for patients with anterior shoulder instability. Important details that are obtained in each patient who presents with instability include age, number of dislocations, direction of dislocation, previous procedures or treatments, level of sport participation, and level of risk of sport/work for redislocation.

Physical examination should include inspection for atrophy, deformity, and any prior surgical scars, assessment of active and passive range of motion, neurovascular evaluation including strength and sensation, apprehension examination, and finally the hyper extension-internal rotation (HERI) examination (Fig. 22.1). The HERI test assesses the integrity of the inferior glenohumeral ligament (IGHL) and inferior capsule complex without causing apprehension for patients (Fig. 22.2).[10]

For preoperative imaging, we obtain plain radiographs with Grashey anteroposterior (AP), internal and external rotation, and axillary views. Standard AP X-rays may show a fracture or a more subtle loss of contour of the anteroinferior glenoid rim. A decrease in the apparent density of the inferior glenoid subchondral line often signifies an erosion of the glenoid rim between 3 and 6 o'clock. An axillary view or better, a Bernageau view, may show flattening of this area of the glenoid when bone loss has occurred.[11] Computed tomographic arthrogram (CTA) provides a more detailed imaging modality that is essential to quantify the bone loss preoperatively.

Positioning and Equipment

The patient should be intubated with a general endotracheal anesthesia as we find muscle paralysis critical to avoid "jumping," especially during the muscular split with electrocautery.

We use the beach chair position with the use of an arm holder/positioner. To facilitate relaxation of the anterior deltoid and the conjoint tendon, the position of the arm can be changed depending on the steps of the procedure in order to increase the workspace in the shoulder. The arm can thus be held with an articulating arm holder or by an assistant.

Our preferred equipment and instrumentation is included in the DePuy Latarjet Experience tray (DePuy, Warsaw, IN), which includes all items described in the following technique text.

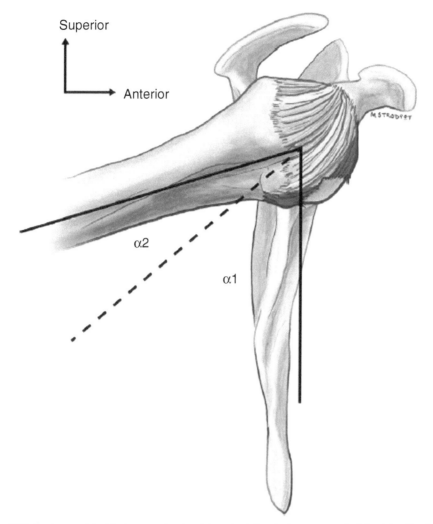

Superior

Anterior

α2

α1

• **Fig. 22.2** Anatomy related to hyper extension-internal rotation test assessment of the integrity of the inferior glenohumeral ligament and inferior capsule complex.

Technique for the Arthroscopic Latarjet

The arthroscopic Latarjet technique can be divided into five steps.[12] These include joint evaluation and exposure, harvesting of the coracoid process, subscapularis split, coracoid transfer, and fixation of the coracoid process.

The following seven portals are used in our practice (Fig. 22.3):

- Portal A: Standard posterior
- Portal E: Standard anterior to access the rotator interval (RI)
- Portal D: Anterolateral at the level of the anterolateral corner of the acromion
- Portal I: Aligned with the coracoid process, just above the axillary fold
- Portal J: Between I and D portal, parallel to the subscapularis fibers
- Portal M: The most medial and anterior portal through the pectoralis major, aligned with the glenoid face
- Portal H: Anterosuperior portal just above and slightly medial to the coracoid

Step 1: Joint Evaluation and Exposure

The arthroscopy commences by establishing and viewing through the standard A posterior portal. The anterior E portal is established using an outside-in technique and a probe is introduced through the RI. With the probe, a diagnostic arthroscopic examination including a dynamic stability assessment is performed, specifically looking for bony glenoid lesions, humeral defects (Fig. 22.4A), and soft tissue lesions, such as an HAGL.

Opening of the RI, Exposure of Both Sides of Subscapularis, and Preparation of the Glenoid Neck

The glenohumeral joint is opened by removing the capsule of the RI at the upper border of subscapularis. At this step, the coracoacromial (CA) ligament can be detached from the coracoid if it helps to expose the workspace. However, it can also be performed later during the procedure. Next, we work posterior to the subscapularis to detach the anteroinferior labrum and medial glenohumeral ligament (MGHL) between 2 and 5 o'clock to expose the glenoid neck. The intended graft site is exposed and the capsule between glenoid neck and subscapularis is resected. We detach the pathological anterior capsule and remove any medially healed bony Bankart fragments. A pituitary rongeur is helpful to remove the soft-encountered suture material from prior failed soft tissue repairs.

A spinal needle is inserted parallel to the upper border of the subscapularis tendon to ensure the best positioning of the D portal that will allow a trajectory to reach anterior and posterior to the subscapularis. The arthroscope is placed in the D portal and instruments are then used in the E portal. To provide a healthy base for graft healing, the glenoid neck is abraded with the burr. Both sides of the subscapularis tendon are then exposed, with particular attention to the articular side of subscapularis. These releases are necessary to facilitate the transfer of the coracoid graft. In case of any further intra-articular pathology, it should be addressed at this stage, for example, a posterior labral repair. The intra-articular preparation is now completed.

Coracoid Soft Tissue Preparation

While viewing through the D portal and working through the E portal, complete the skeletonization of the inferior and lateral portions of the coracoid by removing any remaining bursa and fatty tissue under the coracoid and any remnants of the CA ligament (Fig. 22.4B). The anterior surface of the conjoint tendon is exposed. Next, the clavipectoral fascia is released on the lateral side of the conjoint tendon/short head of biceps all the way down to the level where it is crossed by the pectoralis major.

Posterior to the conjoint tendon and anterior to the subscapularis is a medial tissue barrier that separates the brachial plexus

from the subcoracoid bursa. This is gently divided to reveal the axillary nerve. If not readily apparent, the anterior humeral circumflex artery and its venae comitantes ("the three sisters") can be followed medially and the axillary nerve can be found where it dives between the inferior edge of the subscapularis and the three sisters. It is important to visualize this nerve and appreciate its location when it comes to splitting the subscapularis muscle and placing the graft. Any further soft tissue attachments to the coracoid in the bursa are released to free the coracoid for its later transfer.

If not performed earlier during the procedure, the CA ligament should be located at its coracoid insertion site and subsequently detached. Attention must be paid to coagulate the terminal branch of the acromiothoracic artery. The anterior aspect of the conjoint tendon is liberated from the deltoid fascia, if this release was not performed sufficiently priorly. The inferior limit of this release should be the pectoralis major tendon. Splitting the deltoid fascia anterior of the coracoid process facilitates visualization.

Split the adhesions between the pectoralis minor (PM) and pectoralis major. The upper border of PM tendon on the medial border of the coracoid is now released taking care to keep the

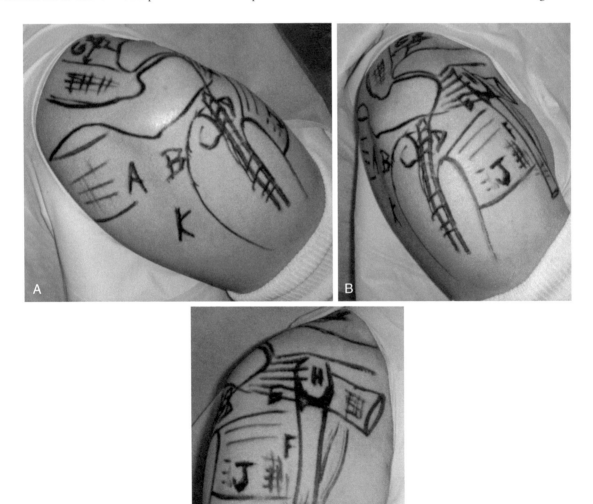

• **Fig. 22.3** Arthroscopic portals used for the arthroscopic Latarjet. See text for portal descriptions.

electrocautery on bone during this step. Finalize the preparation of the coracoid process by completely debriding its superior part from any soft tissue back to the anterior edge of the coracoclavicular (CC) ligaments. With the dissection of the coracoid and the conjoint tendon completed, and having an awareness of the position of the nerves, we can proceed with the knowledge that everything lateral to the conjoint tendon is safe.

Step 2: Harvesting the Coracoid

Preparation of the anterior portals. Establish the I, J, and M portals.

Using an outside-in technique, the I portal is placed above the axillary fold, aligned with the axis of the coracoid process. Manipulation of the needle used to localize this portal should anticipate visualizing the four sides of the coracoid when the arthroscope is introduced through this I portal. The J portal is placed midway on an arc between the I and the D portals. The J portal gives a more "head-on" view of the coracoid whereas the D portal gives a better lateral view. Two perpendicular views are necessary to ensure optimum coracoid preparation. The I portal facing the coracoid directly is used for the coracoid preparation and to work on the split of the subscapularis. The J portal allows a complementary visualization of the coracoid, particularly during the bony preparation of the coracoid, once harvested, before its transfer through the subscapularis.

The M portal is the most medial. It should be aligned with the glenoid surface and should provide for management of the coracoid fixation parallel to the glenoid. Despite its very medial location, this portal is not dangerous as long as the PM is not penetrated. Once this muscle is detached, the plexus is in line with the M portal, and close attention should be emphasized with the use of this portal.

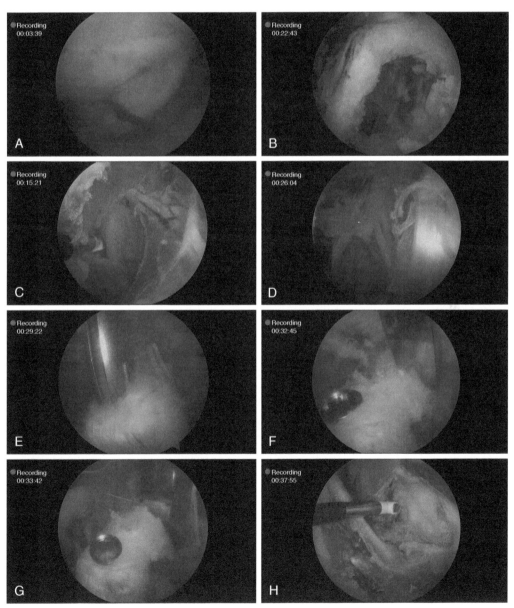

• **Fig. 22.4** (A) Large engaging Hill-Sachs lesion, (B) clearance around coracoid, (C) locating the axillary nerve, (D) locating the musculocutaneous nerve, (E) guide for drilling coracoid, (F) osteotomy starting with medial and lateral one-third cortex cuts with lateral osteotomy shown here, (G) middle one-third cut shown here, (H) subscapularis split between inferior one-third and upper two-thirds of tendon,

Continued

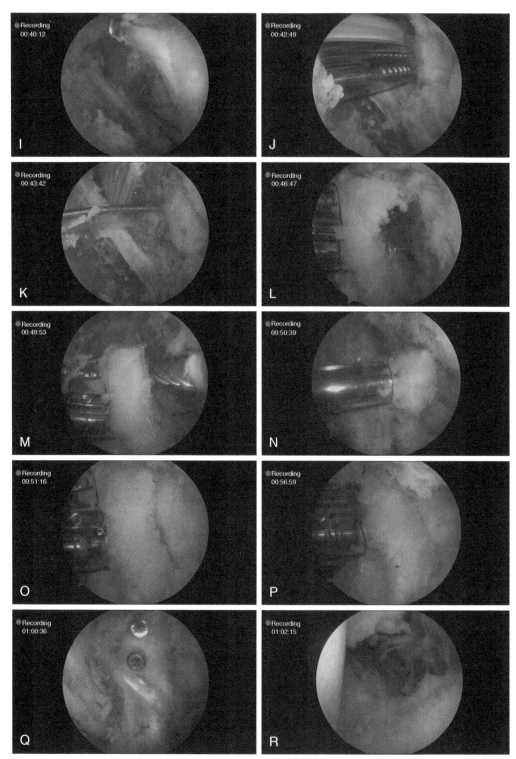

• **Fig. 22.4, cont'd** (I) retraction of the subscapularis split, (J) guidewire placement, (K) guidewire placement part 2, (L) lining up graft with handle over guidewire, (M) sculpting graft, (N) turn graft to guide through subscapularis split, (O) lining up graft against anterior glenoid, (P) screw placement, (Q) final graft placement from the anterior view, and (R) final graft placement from the posterior view.

PM detachment. Once the arthroscope is introduced in the I portal, the electrocautery is introduced into the M portal and the upper and lower parts of PM are located. It is difficult but crucial to separate PM from the conjoint tendon. The electrocautery should remain superficial and the split should proceed very cautiously until the musculocutaneous nerve is located (Fig. 22.4D).

PM is then totally detached from the coracoid process. Failure to complete this release can lead to bleeding during the coracoid transfer due to the richly vascularized tissue in this location or, postoperatively, a form of iatrogenic PM syndrome with compression on the neurovascular structures if the PM remains intact and then is "tightened" by the coracoid transfer. The brachial plexus can be visualized at this stage, but it is not necessary or advisable to dissect the plexus for this procedure.

Define the H portal. At this point the arthroscope is in the J portal and the electrocautery in the I portal. An arthroscopic switching stick is used through the D portal as a retractor to elevate the deltoid away from the coracoid. I like to place the other end through the plastic fluid collection bag on the drapes to keep this "retractor" in the same position as long as I need it there. Locate the coracoid's midpoint again with a long spine needle perpendicular to the axis. This will serve to guide the position of the coracoid drill guide. The typical error is to be too lateral or too anterior with the portal given the way the coracoid twists laterally and hooks inferiorly. Once satisfied, make a superior incision for the H portal.

Drilling the coracoid and inserting the anterior top hat. Place the 15 degrees coracoid drill guide flush on top of the coracoid. It is important to regularly change the viewing angle of the scope by rotation to ensure mediolateral alignment of the now inserted coracoid drill guide. Place the guide over the junction of lateral two-thirds and medial one-third of the coracoid. Use the 7-mm distance device—included in the new drill guides (DePuy-Synthes)—to ensure proper alignment to the lateral aspect of the coracoid process (Fig. 22.4E).

Drill the Alpha-hole (inferior and distal) with a K-wire. It is important while doing this to visualize inferior to the coracoid to verify that the direction of the K-wires is perpendicular to the superior surface of the coracoid and to avoid penetrating too deep into the brachial plexus. Locate the final position of the Beta-hole relative to the axis. Rotationally align the coracoid drill guide and then drill the Beta (proximal) K-wire.

Remove the drill guide, leave the K-wires and check the wire positions from all vantage points. Overdrill both holes with the coracoid step drill. To ensure drilling is bicortical, place a clamp at the end of the K-wire while drilling. When the clamp (and thus the wire) begin rotating, the second cortex has been passed. Remove the clamp and the drill but keep the K-wires.

The drill holes are now tapped to prepare for the top hat and glenoid screws. The posterior Beta K-wire is removed. The anterior top hat is now inserted in the anterior Alpha drill hole and the K-wire is removed.

Coracoid osteotomy. Once the coracoid is prepared, we are now ready to make the osteotomy through the H portal. First, the osteotome is placed on the medial most proximal aspect just anterior to the CC ligaments. Here, osteotomy of the medial quarter of the coracoid is performed. The same is done on the lateral aspect (Fig. 22.4F). Then, in a third step, a controlled complete osteotomy is performed by placing the osteotome in the line connecting the two previous osteotomies (Fig. 22.4G).

At this stage, the retro-coracoid fascia is usually still attached to the coracoid, between the coracoid and the upper border and anterior aspect of the subscapularis, preventing any coracoid mobilization. It is necessary to release this fascia paying attention to locate, visualize, and preserve the axillary nerve just behind.

Step 3: Subscapularis Split

Determine the level of the subscapularis split. Viewing through the I portal, remove any remaining bursa on the anterior aspect of the subscapularis by introducing the shaver in the J portal. Hemostasis by the electrocautery introduced in the M portal is managed at the same time. Locate the three sisters (one artery and two veins) and the axillary nerve (Fig. 22.4C) running along the muscle to avoid neurovascular injury. Determine the upper two-thirds and lower one-third of the subscapularis muscle-tendon unit (Fig. 22.4H). Care is taken in our practice to always respect the position of the split in the subscapularis.

Subscapularis split. The arm is placed in a little external rotation without causing anterior translation of the humeral head and 30 degrees forward flexion. Create the split by using electrocautery. The split is completed down to the glenoid neck in the line of fibers of subscapularis, extending from the lateral insertion of subscapularis on the lesser tuberosity, passing medially close to the axillary nerve. Expert Tip: *Start medial by the axillary nerve and moving lateral in line with the fibers of the muscle, use a switching stick through the E or J portal to elevate the upper edge of the split muscle to provide counter tension while moving to the deeper layers of muscle. A probe is introduced through the A portal and can be used to depress the inferior edge of the split to keep the subscapularis window open (Fig. 22.4I).*

Step 4: Preparation of Glenoid Bed and Graft Trimming

The shoulder is manipulated with the arm holder in slight internal rotation with scapula retropulsion in order to decrease the subscapularis tension and to facilitate the screw orientation. The scapula retropulsion is facilitated by a slight change of position of the patient. The table is changed from a beach chair to a supine position. Use this chance to view the anterior glenoid neck and assure that the surface is flat and ready to accept the coracoid process (CP) graft. Additional bony abrasion with a burr can be performed by introducing the burr in the M portal for this task.

Graft trimming. Move the scope to the J portal. Insert the 15 degrees Coracoid Process Guide (CPG) through the M portal and thread the now-freed coracoid onto the CPG. Secure it to the CPG by manually screwing the coracoid positioning cannula into the top hat. The freshly harvested graft is mobilized and all remaining adhesions of the PM and the medial fascia are removed. Particular attention must be paid to avoid the musculocutaneous nerve while this is done. The mobile coracoid usually has a medial spike arising from its base that must be trimmed to permit good bony contact with the glenoid.

In order to stabilize the coracoid while the burr is introduced through the D portal, a K-wire is introduced into the Alpha coracoid screw hole, through the subscapularis split and then drilled unicortically into the glenoid bone approximately at the definitive location. This K-wire will ensure that the coracoid does not move during its preparation and protect the plexus which is in close proximity. The guide should be placed at 5 o'clock and approximately 7 mm medial to the glenoid articular surface. A 5-mm probe can assist with this placement. The probe is introduced through the A portal and positioned with the tip against the anterior inferior surface of the glenoid. The 5 mm plus the 2 mm between the edge of the guide and the K-wire tip within the guide will allow precise placement (Fig. 22.4J–K). Note that this position can always be adjusted at a later step if the graft is either too lateral or medial. To facilitate trimming, the arthroscope is held by an assistant, and—using a two-handed technique—the graft can be controlled on the cannula with one hand and trimmed with the burr (D portal) with the other hand (Fig. 22.4M). The graft should be flat to the glenoid and its upper part should be smaller than the lower part in order to anticipate and limit the upper resorption. The graft is now ready for transfer and fixation to the glenoid.

Step 5: Coracoid Transfer and Coracoid Fixation

Manipulate the coracoid on the coracoid positioning cannula to the glenoid neck along the K-wire (Fig. 22.4L). This is made easier by elevating the subscapularis split with the switching stick. Pass the graft horizontally through the subscapularis, then turn 90 degrees around the K-wire for its desired position on the glenoid (Fig. 22.4N). The graft itself can be used to depress the inferior leaflet of the subscapularis split. The coracoid graft is positioned low on the glenoid, with the inferior portion of the graft in line with the inferior glenoid (Fig. 22.4O) and should not be prominent compared to the glenoid surface but flush with the subchondral bone.

To achieve the best position of the graft, we recommend a two-step approach. First, the upper part of the graft is positioned flush at the optimal and desired position. Then a K-wire is passed through the Beta-hole and drilled bicortically to fix this position. The wire will emerge through the skin of the posterior shoulder, at which stage, a clamp is placed on it. A minimal angulation between the K-wires and the glenoid surface is optimal to engage the longest screw in the best bone and avoid a more medial trajectory which can leave prominent screw heads anteriorly and potentially injure the suprascapular nerve in the spinoglenoid notch posteriorly. Expert Tip: *Proper orientation of the K-wires will typically exit the skin approximately 2–3 cm medial to the A portal.*

In the second step, if the position of the coracoid graft and the first K-wire are desirable with regard to the graft placement, then a second K-wire in the Alpha-hole is then inserted unicortically. If the graft position is medial or lateral, the K-wire in the Alpha-hole is repositioned prior to bicortical drilling. With the inferior K-wire removed, the graft can be manipulated and rotated around the upper Beta-hole K-wire into the desired position. The K-wire in the Alpha-hole is then also drilled bicortically and through the posterior skin. The second K-wire should emerge at close proximity to the first K-wire. This wire will also be clamped. The Alpha wire should emerge inferior to the Beta wire and the wires should be relatively parallel. If they are not parallel, then the eventual screw trajectory will be off and there may be inferior fixation strength. If wires are not oriented correctly or not parallel, simply remove the Alpha wire and replace it with a different trajectory to correct the issue. That can be difficult as there is typically extensive swelling at this point in the case, yet perfect relaxation of the patient and perfect visualization are needed. It is important to place the K-wires in the perfect position before moving to the next step.

Overdrill the glenoid Beta K-wire with the cannulated glenoid 3.2 drill bicortically from anterior. Remove the drill. The K-wires will stay in place as held by the posterior clamps. If needed, insert the cannulated measurement device from posterior until resistance of the cortex is felt to determine screw lengths. Then remove the cannulated measurement device. Place the Beta screw (Fig. 22.4P) without fully tightening and then overdrill the Alpha K-wire. The screws are inserted and alternately tightened to reduce the graft using compression onto the glenoid neck. The K-wires can then be removed posteriorly.

Final checks. The graft and screw position are visually inspected through the D (Fig. 22.4Q), and J and A (Fig. 22.4R) portals and any final trimming can be done at this stage with the burr. Any prominence of the graft thereafter can be burred flush to the glenoid. Ensure that no soft tissue is entrapped under the graft that would impede motion or bone to bone healing. We also ensure that we can get full external rotation and that the graft is

not tethering the subscapularis. Lastly, we examine the conjoint tendon and ensure that there are no medial fascial bands that could compress neurovascular structures.

After portal closure, the patient is placed in a slight resting abduction pillow.

Postoperative X-rays should demonstrate that the graft is properly fixed. Only 3D CT can assess the graft positioning accurately, which we order at 3 months in routine postoperative courses. We order plain films for patients at 6 weeks and 3 months postoperatively (Fig. 22.4).

PEARLS AND PITFALLS

Visualization is the theme for this pearl section. Excellent visualization will lead to success with every step of the procedure.

- The key to visualization starts with anesthesia. Optimal control of bleeding through pressure control along with precise arthroscopic cauterization will allow for optimal visualization.
- Taking time to free up adhesions and connective tissue will allow you to work in a cathedral size space in the anterior compartment of the shoulder rather than a closet. These areas include the space along the anterior aspect of the conjoint tendon, the interval between pectoralis major and minor, the subcoracoid space anterior to the subscapularis muscle, and the interval between the subscapularis muscle and the anterior glenoid.
- As with any procedure that involves neurovascular exposure, know where the nerves at all times are and recheck at each step.

Complications and Management

Perioperative complications are essentially coracoid breakage and neurovascular injury.[13,14] When encountering excessive arthroscopic difficulties (uncontrolled bleeding, excessive swelling, difficulties for screw positioning), these conditions should lead to an open conversion at any stage.

Early postoperative complications are extremely rare, but it is important to control and monitor swelling. Hematomas, though rare, need to be closely watched to detect any sign of possible vascular injury.

Graft nonunion occurs rarely and this complication has decreased with the use of the top hat washer. The top hat allows greater compression to be applied to the graft.

When compression is accomplished, successful union usually occurs within 6 weeks. Long-term graft resorption, however, has been a more common problem, leading to uncovering of the screw heads anteriorly. This has resulted in pain and tendon impingement in some patients that later resolved with arthroscopic removal of the screws.

Recurrent instability is uncommon[14] but is a difficult problem to manage; however, arthroscopic revision bone grafting with an iliac crest graft (Eden-Hybinette) has resulted in good outcomes with restored stability.[15]

Expert Advice

The arthroscopic Latarjet technique is our preferred treatment option, especially for lesions with significant bone loss and for athletes involved in contact sports or throwing. It is important to note that this procedure should be reserved for surgeons with extensive arthroscopy expertise. We recommend becoming familiar with the anterior shoulder compartment, including the subcoracoid space when possible during routine arthroscopic procedures. Then, in a laboratory setting use a cadaver to perform the full procedure for the first time. Finally, asking a local mentor to assist in the live setting can provide tips and troubleshooting assistance that is second to none. We also strongly recommend to start with open Latarjet and once that becomes reliable, to proceed arthroscopically and convert to the open technique if necessary. This allows safe and stepwise progression through the skills of arthroscopic steps and a constant exit strategy.

References

1. Boileau P, Villalba M, Héry J-Y, et al. Risk factors for recurrence of shoulder instability after arthroscopic Bankart repair. *JBJS*. 2006;88-A(8):1755–1763.
2. Walch G, Boileau P, Levigne C, et al. Arthroscopic stabilization for recurrent anterior shoulder dislocation: results of 59 cases. *Arthroscopy*. 1995;11:173–179.
3. Burkhart S, De Beer J. Traumatic glenohumeral bone defects and their relationship to failure of arthroscopic Bankart repairs: significance of the inverted-pear glenoid and the humeral engaging Hill-Sachs lesion. *Arthroscopy*. 2000;88(8):677–694.
4. Wellmann M, Petersen W, Zantop T, et al. Open shoulder repair of osseous glenoid defects: biomechanical effectiveness of the Latarjet procedure versus a contoured structural bone graft. *Am J Sports Med*. 2009;37(1).
5. Gill T, Micheli L, Gebhard F, et al. Bankart repair for anterior instability of the shoulder. Long-term outcome. *J Bone Joint Surg Am*. 1997;79(6):850–857.
6. Latarjet M. Treatment of recurrent dislocation of the shoulder. *Lyon Chir*. 1954;49:994–997.
7. Expert Shoulder Panel. *French Arthroscopic Society Meeting*; 2015. December. Grenoble, Rhone-Alpes
8. Itoi E. 'On-track' and 'off track' shoulder lesions. *EFORT Open Reviews*. 2017;2:343–351.
9. Itoi E, Yamamoto N, Muraki T, et al. Stabilizing mechanism in bone grafting of a large glenoid defect. *J Bone Joint Surg*. 2010;92(1):2059–2066.
10. Lafosse T, Fogerty S, Idoine J, Gobezie R, Lafosse L. 2016 Hyper extension-internal rotation (HERI): a new test for anterior gleno-humeral instability. *J Orthop Traumatol: Surgery and Research*. 2016;102:3–12.
11. Bernageau J, Patte D, Debeyre J, et al. Value of the glenoid profile in recurrent luxations of the shoulder. *Rev Chir Orthop Reparatrice Appar. Mot.* 1976;62:142–147.
12. Lafosse L,LE. The arthroscopic Latarjet procedure for the treatment of anterior shoulder instability. *Arthrosc J Arthrosc Relat Surg*. 2007;23:1242.e1–1242.e5.
13. Gartsman G, Edwards B, Elkousy H, et al. Immediate and early complications of the open Latarjet procedure: a retrospective review of a large consecutive case series. *J. Shoulder Elbow Surgery*. 2017;26:68–72.
14. Walch G, Leuzinger J, Nourissat G, et al. Complications of arthroscopic Latarjet: a multicenter study of 1555 cases. *J Shoulder Elbow Surg*. 2017; 26(5):e148.
15. Lafosse L, Giannakos A, Schwartz D, et al. All-Arthroscopic revision Eden-Hybinette procedure for failed instability surgery: technique and preliminary results. *Arthroscopy*. 2017;33:39–48.

23

Posterior Shoulder Instability

ELOY TABEAYO AND ANSHU SINGH

Introduction

Posterior shoulder dislocations are uncommon and potentially challenging traumatic injuries. Their incidence is around 1.1 per 100,000 population per year, which accounts for about 2% to 5% of all shoulder dislocations.[1–3] Traumatic injuries such as falls, motor vehicle accidents, or sports injuries, followed by seizures, are the most common causes of posterior shoulder dislocation, and, more rarely, electrocution can be also implicated.[2,3]

Some historical series report a missed or delayed diagnosis in 75% of cases,[2] although a recent systematic review reported a lower, but still deeply concerning, 51% incidence of misdiagnosis.[4] When orthogonal anteroposterior (AP) and Velpeau (or axillary) views are used, the rate of accurate diagnosis in the emergency room rises to 90%.[3] Most of the misdiagnosed cases happen due to lack of experience of the clinician, poor radiographic imaging, or concomitant injuries confounding the presentation. However, a high index of suspicion, an adequate physical examination, and, most importantly, the appropriate radiographic evaluation with orthogonal views to include an axillary or Velpeau view are adequate to detect most acute injuries. This is particularly important in a setting of seizures, due to altered consciousness and limited nociceptive stimuli response in the postictal state.[5]

Posterior glenohumeral instability—both dislocations and subluxations—can be seen both in an acute scenario and with recurrent instability. Careful evaluation of the posterior structures including the capsulolabral complex and the bony anatomy will be key to adequately diagnose and treat these patients.

Pathoanatomy

The primary static stabilizer against posterior translation of the humeral head is the inferior glenohumeral ligament complex. It is comprised of three structures: anterior band, axillary pouch, and posterior band (Fig. 23.1). It becomes taut in internal rotation, limiting posterior translation, but it also provides stability to inferior translation in abduction and to anterior translation in external rotation.[6] In addition, the structures of the rotator interval have been proven to be a significant static restraint of posterior and inferior translation of the humeral head. In a cadaveric study, increased posterior translation was demonstrated upon transection of the coracohumeral ligament and joint capsule at the level of the rotator interval, while anterior translation remained stable.[7] The joint capsule is also a restraint to translation. It is thinnest on the posterior aspect, superior to the posterior band of the inferior glenohumeral ligament (PIGHL). This portion of the capsule does not have ligamentous reinforcements. Damage to both the anterior and posterior capsules is necessary to allow posterior dislocation.[8] Other major static posterior stabilizers of the glenohumeral joint are the asymmetric cartilage layer, which is thickest around the periphery of the joint, increasing the concavity of the glenoid, as well as the posterior labrum.

Traumatic acute posterior labral injuries can be seen after an acute dislocation. These can be detachments of the labrum similar to those seen after an anterior shoulder dislocation (reverse Bankart lesions). However, frequently, a concealed tear, known as the Kim lesion, can be identified as a superficial crack between the articular cartilage and the posteroinferior labrum. When probed, the deep portion of the posteroinferior quadrant of the labrum is found to be detached off the surface of the medial glenoid.[9] Posterior labrum injuries are also common in overhead athletes with repetitive subluxation events. This is often related to a contracture in the posterior capsule and PIGHL, which can be seen in those throwers with glenohumeral internal rotation deficit (GIRD). In this scenario, when the arm is abducted and externally rotated, the tight PIGHL causes superior translation of the humeral head, allowing increased external rotation. This abnormal position alters the vector of the long head of the biceps tendon into a more posterior and vertical angle, with resulting torsional forces that are transmitted to the labrum, which ultimately cause a "peel-back" mechanism of the posterior and superior labrum.[10]

Beyond the static effect of the soft-tissue stabilizers, an individual's particular bony anatomy may affect glenohumeral stability. Specifically, excessive glenoid retroversion may play a role in posterior shoulder instability. Eichinger et al. tested the effect of glenoid version in a cadaveric model of shoulder instability and found that over one half of the shoulders with a retroversion of 15 degrees auto-dislocated posteriorly, compared with those models between 10 degrees of anteversion and 10 degrees of retroversion.[11] This finding had already been suggested in multiple studies with atraumatic posterior shoulder instability patients.[12–15] Despite these associations, the role of glenoid version in acute *traumatic* posterior shoulder dislocation or subluxation remains more controversial in the literature.

Muscles that produce concavity compression forces across the glenohumeral joint are considered dynamic stabilizers. Specifically, the infraspinatus, supraspinatus, teres minor, coracobrachialis, and anterior deltoid contribute to posterior glenohumeral

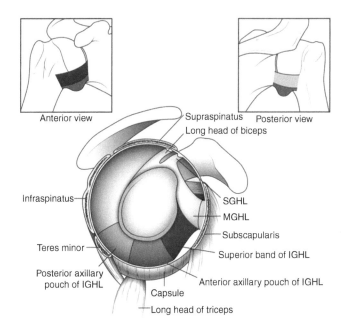

• **Fig. 23.1** Illustration of the dynamic and static stabilizers of the shoulder. *IGHL,* Inferior glenohumeral ligament; *MGHL,* middle glenohumeral ligament; *SGHL,* superior glenohumeral ligament. (From Rouleau DM, Hebert-Davies J, Robinson CM. Acute traumatic posterior shoulder dislocation. *J Am Acad Orthop Surg.* 2014;22(3):145-152.)

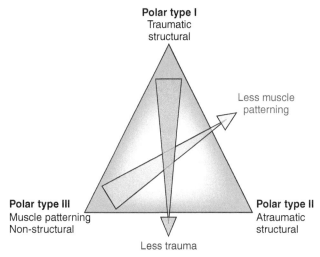

• **Fig. 23.2** Stanmore's triangle for shoulder instability is a graphic representation of the interplay between traumatic, ligamentous, and muscle firing aspects of shoulder instability. Individuals may fall mostly on one point (e.g., forceful traumatic mechanism) or be a blend of several factors, each of which bears consideration. (From Lewis A, Kitamura T, Bayley JIL. (ii) The classification of shoulder instability: new light through old windows! *Curr Orthop.* 2004;18(2):97-108.)

stability.[16] The stabilizing effect of the rotator cuff, in particular, is the most important stabilizer of the glenohumeral joint. The strength and accurate neuromuscular control this requires is the impetus behind physical therapy programs that work to improve these factors as a mechanism of improving posterior instability.

It should be noted that patients with hyperlaxity syndromes (Ehlers-Danlos syndrome, multidirectional instability, etc.) can have posterior shoulder dislocation or subluxation without discreet trauma. The patulous posterior capsule in these patients does not sufficiently restrain posterior translation and, if the delicate neuromuscular control of the rotator cuff is lost, these patients will suffer recurrent instability events with little or no trauma.

There are several possible mechanisms that can lead to a posterior shoulder instability event—either subluxation or dislocation. The most frequent scenario is a posteriorly directed, high-energy force with the shoulder adducted, flexed, and internally rotated.[2] Examples of this mechanism are a driver in an auto accident with hands on the steering wheel, awkwardly bench pressing a heavyweight, a football lineman sustaining a blocking injury, or a boxer at the moment of impact while punching.[2] Forceful, imbalanced, and unopposed contraction of the shoulder muscles can also cause a posterior dislocation. This can happen during seizures or electrocution, where the strong internal rotators (pectoralis major, latissimus dorsi, and teres major) overpower the relatively weak external rotators (infraspinatus and teres minor), causing superior migration, posterior displacement, and internal rotation of the humeral head.[5] Bilateral shoulder dislocation is also not uncommon, and almost universally caused by seizures.[17] Furthermore, recurrent posterior dislocation is common in this patient population, due to attritional bone loss, more severe impaction defects caused by increased muscle tone during seizures, and metabolic bone disorders, such as altered vitamin D metabolism caused by antiepileptic drugs.[5,18,19] In the setting of seizure-induced instability, involvement of a neurologist is important to avoid recurrent seizures. In cases of chronic reconstruction after posterior instability, surgery should be delayed until the neurologist and the surgeon are satisfied that the seizures are controlled.[20,21]

Alcoholism can pose a risk factor for posterior shoulder dislocation, either in the setting of acute intoxication[22] or due to seizures in a withdrawal scenario.[23] It can be difficult to obtain a reliable history in this patient population, and therefore careful attention must be paid to imaging findings to determine the chronicity of the injury, as neglected posterior dislocations are, unfortunately, not as rare as one would wish. Although there are no studies showing outcomes of posterior dislocation in patients with alcoholism, some studies raise concerns of poorer prognosis with respect to dislocation arthropathy after an anterior shoulder dislocation event in this population.[24] In the experience of the authors, compliance with postoperative restrictions and rehabilitation are often challenging, compromising the outcomes. Therefore it is our standard practice to manage alcoholism prior to any complex reconstructive procedure for chronic dislocations. In addition, when cirrhosis is present, attention must be paid to correct possible coagulopathies[25] and minimize the risk of anesthetic complications.[26]

Classification

There is a lack of a definitive, uniform classification system for posterior shoulder instability, although several authors have proposed systems. The Stanmore Classification applies to anterior and posterior instability and considers structural and muscle patterning that contributes to instability in a fluid manner (Fig. 23.2).[27] May created a simple classification that included categories of habitual, traumatic, and obstetric posterior shoulder dislocation or subluxation.[28] Detenbeck classified dislocations based on timing: acute, chronic (>3 weeks), and recurrent (traumatic and atraumatic).[29] Hawkins and Bell added the presence of an anterior defect lesion (reverse Hill-Sachs); voluntary versus habitual (deliberate) versus involuntary dislocations; and recurrent versus locked, missed, chronic dislocations.[30] More recently, Heller

TABLE 23.1	Stability Tests					
Test	Sensitivity (%)	Specificity (%)	PPV	NPV		
Kim test	80	94	0.73	0.96		Patient is in a sitting position, 90 degrees of abduction, axial loading, and 45-degree diagonal elevation applied to the distal arm, with inferior and posterior force applied to the proximal arm. Test is positive if patient reports pain.
Jerk test	73	98	0.88	0.95		Patient is in a sitting position, the examiner stabilizes the scapular spine and the clavicle with one hand and holds the elbow with the other hand. Then the patient's arm is abducted to 90 degrees, internally rotated to 90 degrees, an axial force and horizontal adduction is applied. Test is positive if patient reports pain or if a clunk or click is felt.
Posterior stress test	–	–	–	–		Patient is in a sitting position. The examiner stabilizes the posterior border of the scapula and with his other hand applies a posterior force to the arm while in 90 degrees of forward flexion, adduction, and internal rotation. The test is positive if it elicits pain or apprehension.
Load and shift test	37.5	89.2	0.25	0.94		The patient is supine. The arm is placed in abduction and 20 degrees of forward flexion. Then the humeral head is loaded and a posterior directed force is applied. The amount of translation is then graded.

NPV, Negative predictive value; *PPV*, positive predictive value.

proposed a classification based on different parameters: traumatic, atraumatic, acute, persistent, recurrent, and voluntary, based on an extensive review of 300 publications.[31]

Several authors put the threshold between acute and chronic (also known as neglected or locked) dislocations at 6 weeks. This number is arbitrary, but clearly with diagnostic or treatment delay, the shoulder becomes more difficult to relocate and reduction is more challenging to maintain. The posteriorly dislocated, internally rotated position leads to a complete lack of balance of the soft tissue envelope with contracture of the anterior capsule and patulous posterior capsule with a posterior capsulolabral disruption. In addition, with a neglected dislocation, the humeral head defect becomes progressively larger. Defects of <40% of the articular surface may have a more favorable prognosis compared with larger lesions.[32]

Finally, posterior shoulder dislocations can also be classified according to the location of the humeral head, as the humerus may dislocate in a subacromial (posterior to the glenoid and inferior to the acromion), subglenoid (posterior and inferior to the glenoid), or subspinous (beneath the spine of the scapula) position. Subacromial dislocations are the most common.[33]

Physical Examination

The physical examination of posterior shoulder dislocation differs significantly from the more typical anterior dislocation and therefore may be missed in an acute setting if the provider does not consider the diagnosis. These patients may not be able to provide a thorough history if inebriated, postictal, or post electrocution. Thus it is paramount to have a high index of suspicion, and to know the most common findings on physical examination, as these are constant and unequivocal.[2]

On visual inspection, the arm is usually held in internal rotation. This is best seen with the elbow flexed at 90 degrees.[34] A prominent coracoid, fullness of the posterior shoulder, and squaring of the anterior and lateral acromion are common visual

findings, although displacement of the humeral head or alteration of the axis of the humerus can be subtle and sometimes missed.[2,22,34] Limited forward elevation and supination can also be present in these cases, with a constant and very characteristic fixed internal rotation deformity, and a lack of external rotation. This should not be confused with adhesive capsulitis in an acute setting.[22]

In the evaluation of recurrent posterior dislocation, the provider may perform specific instability tests. These include the jerk test,[35] the Kim test,[36] the posterior stress test,[37] and the load and shift test (Table 23.1; Fig. 23.3).[38,39] In addition, the Beighton score should be considered as a validated and reproducible means of evaluating hyperlaxity that may be a primary or secondary driver of recurrent posterior instability (Fig. 23.4).[40]

Imaging

Several findings have been described on AP radiographs of the glenohumeral joint in a posterior dislocation setting. These include the "light bulb sign," a circular appearance of the humeral head caused by the internal rotation of the proximal humerus that alters the view of the tuberosities; "the trough sign," a line within the humeral head representing an impaction fracture or reverse Hill-Sachs lesion; and "the rim sign," a widened articular distance of over 7 mm from the medial humeral head to the anterior glenoid rim (Fig. 23.5).[41,42]

The most reliable confirmatory radiographic study is the axillary view. Standard axial views may be difficult to perform in the setting of acute posterior shoulder instability due to the patient's inability to abduct the shoulder and/or pain. Modifications of the technique allow a reliable radiographic examination while the patient remains comfortably in a sling. Several techniques have been described: the Velpeau axillary view, angle-up view,[43] apical-oblique projection,[44] or modified axial radiograph.[45]

For patients for whom an adequate radiograph cannot be obtained and for aid in the surgical planning and defining

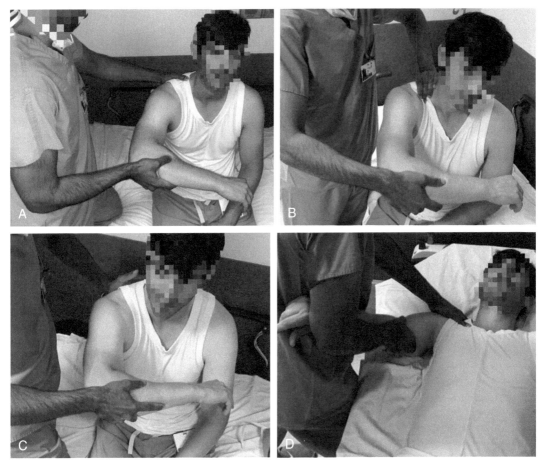

• **Fig. 23.3** These images demonstrate (A) the jerk test, (B) the Kim test, (C) the posterior stress test, and (D) the load and shift test.

Specific joint laxity	YES		NO
1. Passive apposition of thumb of forearm	☐ Left	☐ Right	☐
2. Passive hyperextension of V-MCP>90°	☐ Left	☐ Right	☐
3. Active hyperextension of elbow>10°	☐ Left	☐ Right	☐
4. Active hyperextension of knee>10°	☐ Left	☐ Right	☐
5. Ability to flex spine placing palms to floor without bending knees	☐		☐

'Each "YES" is 1 point A score ≥ 4 out 9 is generally considered an indication of JH, (MCP; metacarpophalangeal),

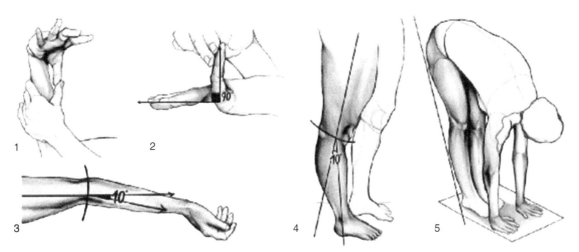

• **Fig. 23.4** Beighton's score for joint hyperlaxity (JH). (From Folci M, Capsoni F. Arthralgias, fatigue, paresthesias and visceral pain: can joint hypermobility solve the puzzle? A case report. *BMC Musculoskelet Disord*. 2016;17(1):58.)

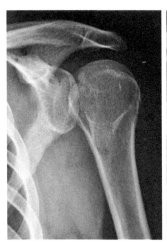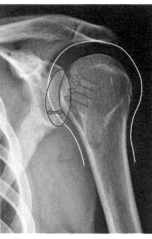

• **Fig. 23.5** In these images we can appreciate the light bulb sign, with the humeral head contour resembling that of a light bulb due to the internal rotation of the humerus, that hides the greater tuberosity *(yellow line)*; the rim sign, as a widened space >7 mm between the anterior rim of the glenoid and the humeral head surface *(blue arrow)*; and the trough sign, a compression fracture of the humeral head, or Hill-Sachs lesion *(red arrows)*.

associated fracture planes, computed tomography (CT) is very helpful. This imaging modality offers an accurate delineation of the bony anatomy, including characterization of reverse Hill-Sachs lesions, fractures, bony fragments, or glenoid morphologic parameters such as retroversion and bone loss. In addition, a CT scan can provide hints as to the chronicity of the injury with the presence of sclerosis, callus, or remodeling indicating a chronic picture. Separate 3D CT volume renderings of the humerus and glenoid can also provide the clinician with a better understanding of the clinical scenario.[1,32,46,47] In a systematic review, Rouleau reported that 65% of posterior glenohumeral dislocations had associated injuries, the most common being a reverse Hill-Sachs lesion (29% of the cases), followed by humeral neck fractures (18.5%), and lesser tuberosity fractures (14.3%). They recommended a CT scan prior to performing reduction maneuvers.[48]

Magnetic resonance imaging (MRI) is useful to evaluate the extent of soft tissue injuries. The most common are posterior labrum tears (reverse Bankart lesions), posterosuperior tears, and posterior labrocapsular periosteal sleeve avulsions (POLPSA), which are found in 52% of the cases.[49] Rotator cuff tears have five times higher risk in the absence of a Hill-Sachs lesion, with a reported incidence of 13%.[48] Other associated injuries include labrum tears and biceps tendon pathology. Although typically more useful in a chronic or recurrent setting, MRI can be useful in certain scenarios, such as in an irreducible dislocation with an incarcerated long head of the biceps tendon.[50,51] A recent meta-analysis showed that 3-tesla magnetic resonance arthrogram (MRA) had greater sensitivity (0.90 vs. 0.83) but similar specificity (1.00 vs. 1.00) for posterior labral tears, when compared with MRI.[52]

Treatment Options and Approaches

Chronic posterior shoulder dislocation can be surprisingly well tolerated in elderly, low-demand patients, or those with an unacceptably high surgical risk. In this patient population, "supervised neglect" is an option, provided individuals are willing to accept significantly decreased range of motion. Often these patients

regain enough functional forward flexion to be able to perform many activities of daily living.[47,53,54] Hawkins reported an average of 105 degrees of forward flexion, 40 degrees of internal rotation deformity, and internal rotation to the 12th thoracic vertebra in a series of 41 locked posterior shoulder dislocations.[22]

In 12 shoulders that had been dislocated for fewer than 6 weeks, in the previously mentioned series, Hawkins reported a successful closed reduction as a definitive treatment in only 3 of them, all of which had been dislocated for <4 weeks, and whose bone defect involved <20% of the articular surface of the humeral head. Larger defects resulted in recurrent glenohumeral dislocation in internal rotation.[22]

A spontaneous or self-reduction of a chronic dislocation is possible, but less likely than in an acute shoulder dislocation. More often, manipulation is needed, and general anesthesia is usually required to achieve the necessary level of muscle relaxation.[32]

Prior to any forceful maneuver, associated fractures must be ruled out, and therefore a CT scan is recommended.[48] Reduction of a dislocation with an occult anatomic neck fracture can lead to further displacement of the fragments, increasing the likelihood of an adverse event, such as osteonecrosis of the humeral head. In addition, a CT scan will allow for better evaluation of the bone defect, which ultimately dictates treatment options.

Once fractures have been ruled out and the bone defect has been deemed smaller than 40% to 50% of the articular surface of the humeral head,[32] a trial of closed reduction can be performed. Gentle traction alone was successful in 33% of the 112 patients in a series published by Robinson.[3] If this maneuver fails, adding forward flexion and adduction can be tried and is often enough to achieve reduction of the glenohumeral joint. The addition of an anterior force at the posterior humeral head can facilitate the maneuver.[55,56] Occasionally, when the glenoid rim is impacted into the reverse Hill-Sachs, gentle internal rotation and lateral traction may disimpact the humeral head. Once the defect has been disengaged, external rotation will relocate the joint, but care must be taken to prevent forceful external rotation before clearing the glenoid rim, as this can cause a fracture of the humerus.[3,32,54] The Stimson technique can also be tried when no associated fractures or significantly engaged Hill-Sachs lesions are found. The patient is positioned prone on the table with the affected arm hanging outside of the table and 5 to 10 pounds of longitudinal traction are applied to the hand. As the patient relaxes, the muscle spasm is overcome with the weight and the shoulder self-reduces.[57,58]

Indications for surgery include a displaced lesser tuberosity fracture, a significant posterior glenoid fracture, an irreducible dislocation with closed manipulation, an open dislocation, or an unstable reduction.[33] Open reduction is indicated if closed reduction fails to relocate the glenohumeral joint. This happens more often with larger bone defects or in dislocations that have been neglected for longer than 6 weeks.[22,32,53] In this situation, different approaches are available. A standard deltopectoral approach is the most common,[2,22] but it provides limited access to the posterior structures. With the head lying deeper than usual, the rotator interval can be opened to allow the introduction of a finger or instrument which will manually help reduce the joint. Working through the rotator interval is typically successful, but if further exposure is still required, the alternatives are a subscapularis peel, a subscapularis tenotomy, a lesser tuberosity osteotomy, or even working through the fracture plane of preexisting lesser tuberosity fracture. In a posterior shoulder dislocation scenario, identifying the subscapularis tendon may be challenging, as the humeral head will be deep and in internal rotation, and a tight conjoint tendon can make structures difficult to visualize. A useful anatomic landmark is the long head of the biceps tendon, as it will be located just lateral to the insertion of the subscapularis tendon. We routinely perform a biceps tenodesis as this allows us to identify the bicipital groove and open the rotator interval completely without concern for postoperative iatrogenic biceps instability issues. Care must be taken not to injure the anterior circumflex vessels, as this may cause disruption of the vascular supply to the humeral head, leading to osteonecrosis.[57] Furthermore, the posterior dislocation tensions the axillary nerve, causing it to be tightly opposed to the subscapularis and requiring extra care during the approach.

Occasionally, a second posterior approach may be necessary if reduction cannot be achieved. This can be done by splitting the deltoid fibers at the raphe between the posterior and the middle head, from the posterolateral corner of the acromion, and dividing the infraspinatus and posterior capsule about 1 cm from its lateral insertions as described by Cheng et al.[59]

For the deep portion of the exposure, Shaffer described an open infraspinatus splitting approach that allows good exposure of the posterior capsule, labrum, and glenoid without compromising neurovascular structures or tendon integrity, with improved visualization of the glenoid. To achieve this, the split of the infraspinatus tendon has to be performed at the raphe level and should not be carried medially more than 15 mm to avoid iatrogenic injury to any interval-crossing branches of the suprascapular nerve.[60] Alternatively, we have had good success splitting the interval between the infraspinatus and the teres minor, with the advantage that this interval can be carried medially if the posterior glenoid needs to be addressed.

The deltoid-splitting superior subacromial approach is another option that is essentially a variation of an open approach used to expose the rotator cuff. The supraspinatus tendon is split 5 mm behind the rotator cuff interval, offering exposure to the proximal humerus and the glenoid from above. During this approach, if the deltoid split is carried distally, the axillary nerve is at risk. Therefore exposure of the proximal humeral shaft is limited with this technique.[61]

With closed or open reduction, stability should be dynamically assessed to evaluate how much internal rotation is safe before the anterior humeral defect engages the posterior glenoid rim. If the reduction is maintained throughout a functional rotation, then the shoulder should be immobilized in a neutral abduction wedge pillow and sling. Patients are typically cautioned not to reach across the midline and certainly not to reach behind the back as internal rotation is the position of instability for this injury. If further external rotation is needed for stability, the shoulder can be immobilized in a shoulder spica or a brace that will allow more rigid external rotation such as a gunslinger. This position will be maintained for 4 to 6 weeks to allow for healing of the posterior capsulolabral complex, which is invariably disrupted in these patients.[3,53,62] Scougall demonstrated that these structures reliably healed without repair in a monkey model of surgically detached posterior capsule and labrum.[63]

If the shoulder is deemed unstable despite immobilization in external rotation, an adjunctive stabilization procedure will be necessary.

The McLaughlin procedure was described in 1952 to fill in smaller reverse Hill-Sachs lesions, generally <20% of the articular surface. The shoulder is approached through a deltopectoral interval, and an arthrotomy is performed by peeling off the subscapularis tendon from its attachment to the lesser tuberosity. Then the glenohumeral joint is reduced, and a bleeding bone bed

is prepared by debriding the defect. Afterwards, the subscapularis tendon is repaired to a more medial position, directly into the bone defect, with transosseous sutures. The circumflex vessels need to be preserved by leaving a small sleeve of the tendon attached to the humeral insertion.[2] An alternative to this technique was described by Spencer. In their modification, the arthrotomy is performed through a longitudinal split of the subscapularis. They use that window to assess and reduce the joint, clean it from debris, and prepare the bony surface of the impaction fracture. Then they use three suture anchors to tenodese the subscapularis tendon over the bone defect, without violating its original insertion.[64] Recently, arthroscopic techniques have been described to perform this modification.[65–67]

The modified McLaughlin technique was described by Neer for patients with an impression defect involving 20% to 45% of the humeral head (Fig. 23.6). A lesser tuberosity osteotomy is elevated just medial to the biceps tendon, taking care to preserve the insertion of the subscapularis and capsule to expose the glenoid fossa. The impaction fracture is debrided, and the osteotomy is medialized and secured into the defect with one or two malleolar screws.[22]

Disimpaction and elevation of the depressed cartilage and subchondral bone grafting has been proposed as a joint-preserving treatment for residual instability in acute dislocations with bone defects >20% (see Chapter 24).[68–70] Osteochondral bone grafting has also been described as an alternative in larger bone defects or more chronic defects where disimpaction is not feasible, but case series and reports are scarce in the literature. Physiologically younger patients with good healing potential may benefit from this technique. However, older individuals with osteoarthritic changes or osteoporosis may have an unacceptable risk of adjacent bone collapse and graft prominence.[71] Gerber reported a series of four cases with humeral defects between 40% and 55% treated with femoral head allograft (three frozen, one fresh), shaped to the defect, and secured with countersunk screws. Three out of four patients had a satisfactory outcome, although one progressed to osteoarthritis with poor functional results. Similarly, in the largest series to date, Diklic reported no pain or restrictions in 9 out of 13 patients treated with a fresh-frozen femoral head allograft for locked, chronic posterior shoulder dislocations.[72] Other alternatives, such as fresh or fresh-frozen size-matched humeral head allografts, have also been explored with good results.[73,74] Fresh allograft has the advantage of having living cartilage, with a theoretically decreased risk of arthritic changes. A meta-analysis by Saltzman et al. of the relatively sparse osteochondral allograft literature reported a substantial complication rate of 30% and a resorption of the graft in 36% of the cases. In addition, when compared with fresh-frozen allografts, fresh humeral head grafts might have an inferior resorption rate, although this needs further research.[73] Due to difficulties in procuring proximal humeral allografts, some authors have explored the use of fresh talar dome allograft for Hill-Sachs defects, as it can offer excellent surface congruency with the humeral head,[75] but there are very few studies reporting patient outcomes using this graft in reverse Hill-Sachs lesions.[76,77]

Defects larger than 40% to 50% are usually found in older patients with osteoporosis or in missed or delayed diagnosis. In a chronic dislocation with a high degree of bone loss, in patients mid-50s and older, or in poor candidates for graft incorporation, shoulder arthroplasty is an option to lengthen the arc of the humeral head to avoid any defect engagement over the posterior rim of the glenoid.[32,33,57] Hemiarthroplasty is typically used if there are minimal to no arthritic changes on the glenoid and

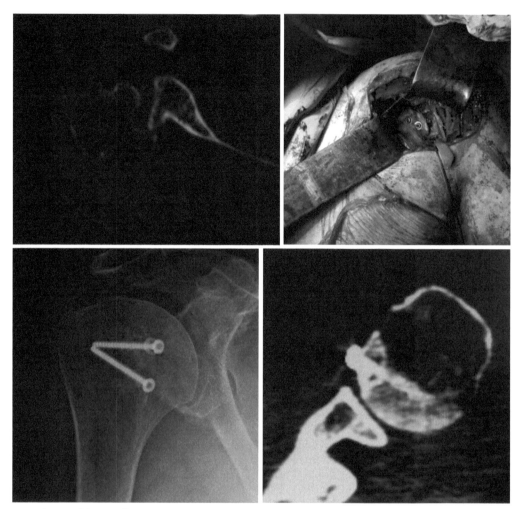

• **Fig. 23.6** The modified McLaughlin procedure is indicated in cases with a humeral head defect of 20%–40%. Through a deltopectoral incision, an osteotomy of the lesser tuberosity is performed and the bone block is transferred into the humeral head defect. (From Demirel M, Erşen A, Karademir G, Atalar AC, Demirhan M. Transfer of the lesser tuberosity for reverse Hill-Sachs lesions after neglected posterior dislocations of the shoulder: a retrospective clinical study of 13 cases. *Acta Orthop Traumatol Turc*. 2017;51(5):362-366. doi.org/10.1016/j.aott.2017.07.004.)

because there is concern that the frequently visualized residual posterior-inferior subluxation may lead to early glenoid loosening (Fig. 23.7).[22,32,78,79] It has been suggested that the version of the humeral component is a key factor in the success of this procedure, as standard retroversion of 20 degrees may be excessive in some chronic patients, and the treating surgeon should consider partial anterior correction of this parameter. According to Hawkins, the longer the dislocation has been present, the less retroversion should be used to reduce the risk of posterior subluxation or dislocation.[22] However, anterior capsular release together with standard retroversion has been favored by other authors.[32,54,80]

More recently, reverse total shoulder arthroplasty has emerged as an option as the semiconstrained design provides a stabilizing force in patients with chronic dislocations. Furthermore, especially with a lateralized glenosphere center of rotation design, stability may be afforded by the reverse architecture even when the chronically retracted anterior capsule/subscapularis cannot be fully released to the point where it is repairable. In older patients, patients with concomitant arthritis, or those with a concomitant rotator cuff tear, reverse total shoulder replacement can be considered (Fig. 23.8).[33]

In cases of acute posterior shoulder dislocation, while repair of posterior capsulolabral structures has been described,[81] it is thought that many heal without intervention.[1] However, in the cases who do experience recurrent posterior instability and/or pain after dislocation, or in the vastly more common scenario of patients with a more subtle subluxation injury mechanism (very often in throwing athletes, weightlifters, or football linemen), posterior capsulolabral procedures may be necessary. These techniques are especially helpful when there is little to no humeral head bone loss. For these cases, we prefer an arthroscopic repair of the posterior labrum with suture anchors (Fig. 23.9). Open techniques of capsular shift, repair, and augmentation can be performed through a posterior approach and an infraspinatus split. A recent meta-analysis of 53 studies collected 815 cases of arthroscopic and 314 cases of open management of posterior glenohumeral instability. They reported superior outcomes with arthroscopic procedures compared with open techniques in terms of recurrent instability (8% vs. 19%), subjective stability (91% vs. 80%), patient satisfaction (94% vs. 86%), return to sports at any level (92% vs. 66%), and return to the previous level of play (67% vs. 37%).[82] Therefore we advocate for an arthroscopic repair

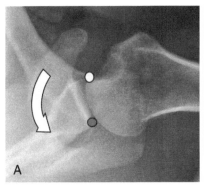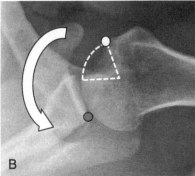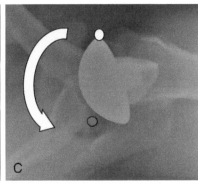

• **Fig. 23.7** (A) Large reverse Hill-Sachs defect and small posterior bony Bankart after posterior instability event. During internal rotation *(yellow arrow)* when the edge of the defect *(yellow dot)* meets the edge of the glenoid *(red dot)*, a recurrent dislocation will occur. Treatment options include (B) osteochondral allograft *(dotted wedge)* to increase the arc length of the humeral head and thus the range before dislocation or (C) humeral head hemiarthroplasty which works in the same way. (Images courtesy Grant E. Garrigues, MD.)

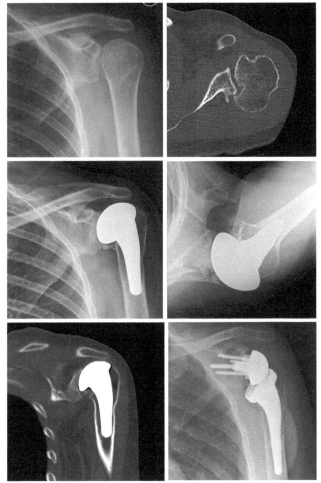

• **Fig. 23.8** A 48-year-old female with a chief complaint of pain and stiffness 4 months after falling off a bicycle. Initially diagnosed with a contusion. When presenting to us, she had an active elevation of 0 degrees, with a 10-degree internal rotation deformity, and 30% humeral head bone loss and a 20% of posterior glenoid bone loss. Although matched humeral head allograft was available, when debriding the lesion, more than half of the subchondral bone in the humeral head was impacted, necessitating hemiarthroplasty. Posterior subluxation is noted on postoperative radiographs. She developed progressive posterior glenoid erosion and superior rotator cuff tear. Nine years after her index procedure, she was converted to a reverse shoulder arthroplasty.

of the posterior capsulolabral complex to restore the stability of the glenohumeral joint in patients with recurrent instability or subluxation events and <20% of humeral bone defect.

Other treatment options that have been described in a setting of chronic, recurrent posterior instability are posterior bone block augmentation of the glenoid[83], glenoid osteotomies,[33] and rotational osteotomies of the humerus.[84]

Regardless of the treatment, the shoulder is immobilized in slight abduction and external rotation for 4 to 6 weeks, with immediate pendulum exercises encouraged. Motion behind the back and across the midline is discouraged for the first 6 weeks. Progression to unlimited range of motion and isometric posterior rotator cuff strengthening are started upon discontinuation of the immobilization. Patients can resume noncontact sports at 3 months and contact activities between 4 and 6 months.[57]

Relevant Complications

Complications are not uncommon, but prevalence is difficult to quantify due to the rarity of this condition, the wide range of treatment options, and the variety of reporting instruments used between series.

Redislocation may occur after closed reduction or a stabilization procedure. McLaughlin reported no recurrent dislocations after closed reduction in four out of five patients without bone loss. The fifth patient had persistent episodes of locking for 3 years after the index injury, which eventually ceased without further treatment.[2] Detenbeck treated 10 acute dislocations with closed reduction with no recurrence of dislocation.[29] However, Wilson,[55] Dimon,[85] and Roberts[86] reported recurrent events in 36%, 33%, and 37% of their cases, in small case series. In a more recent study including 120 posterior dislocations, Robinson reported a 19% recurrence of either dislocation or subluxation, with over 90% of the recurring events happening <1 year after the index injury. Of the 23 recurrent dislocations, 16 had a seizure as the cause of the initial event.[3] These data indicate that if treated acutely, traumatic posterior shoulder dislocations do not typically recur other than select cases with a very powerful mechanism.

Avascular necrosis (AVN) of the humeral head is a rare complication, and often iatrogenic. Robinson reported no cases of AVN in their series of 120 patients with acute posterior shoulder

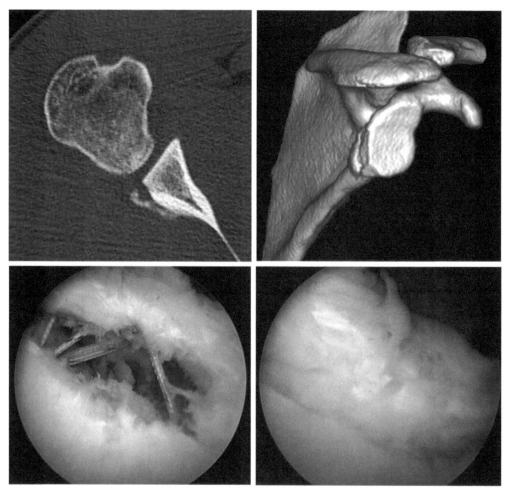

• **Fig. 23.9** A 17-year-old male who complained of recurrent posterior shoulder pain and clunking after a trauma during football practice 1 year ago. The computed tomography scan demonstrates a reverse bony Bankart and reverse Hill-Sachs lesion. The intraoperative pictures of arthroscopic repair of the posterior glenoid lesion with anchors and horizontal mattress sutures.

dislocations.[3] A recent systematic review reported a 5% and 2% rate of AVN in 124 cases of acute and 104 cases of chronic locked posterior dislocations.[4] However, in this study they also included posterior fracture-dislocations, which are known risk factors for osteonecrosis.[33] They reported that all the cases that sustained AVN underwent an open surgical procedure.

Posttraumatic osteoarthrosis is an uncommon finding after posterior shoulder dislocation, but it has been reported that when it occurs, it has a tendency to be more severe than after anterior shoulder dislocation. Total shoulder replacement can be performed if the severity of pain and stiffness warrants intervention.[87]

As discussed above, anatomic shoulder arthroplasty with a nonaugmented glenoid for posterior shoulder dislocation has a high incidence of complications and poorer outcomes when compared with the same procedure for other diagnoses. Wooten,[79] Cheng,[59] and Sperling[78] reported recurrent instability after an arthroplasty for locked posterior dislocation in 3 of 32 patients, 2 of 12 patients, and 1 of 7 patients, respectively. Furthermore, Wooten reported a reoperation rate of 31% for various reasons, including infection, glenoid wear, component loosening, or recurrent dislocation.[79] Augmented anatomic glenoids that allow posterior defects to be corrected (Fig. 23.10) and reverse total shoulder arthroplasty are expected to give superior results but data are lacking.

Review of Treatment Outcomes

Generally worse outcomes are expected with a delayed diagnosis, larger bone defects, associated fractures, presence of arthritic changes, if open reduction is necessary, or if an arthroplasty is required. In cases with a trivial bone defect with acute, stable closed reduction, subsequent stability of the glenohumeral joint can be expected in 63% to 100% of the cases.[3,29,55,85,86] The functional outcome in these patients is very good, with the largest series reporting a deficit in Disability of the Arm, Shoulder and Hand (DASH) score and Western Ontario Shoulder Instability Index (WOSI) of 18% and 5% decrease versus a perfect score, respectively, and a deficit of range of motion compared with the contralateral shoulder of <5% of abduction, flexion and external rotation in abduction, 8.5% of external rotation in adduction, and 11.7% of internal rotation in abduction. In this series, the group of patients that developed instability had similar outcomes in terms of range of motion and WOSI and DASH scores.[3]

The modified McLaughlin technique is a good option when dealing with a bone defect of <50% of the humeral head. Khira reported good outcomes for this procedure, with UCLA scores averaging 30 points, and average forward flexion, internal rotation, external rotation, and abduction of 165, 75, 50, and 150 degrees in a series of 12 cases of locked posterior dislocations with

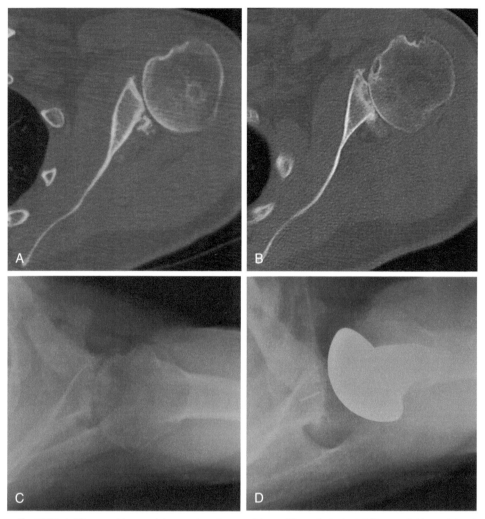

• **Fig. 23.10** A 48-year-old man status post motocross injury with posterior instability event. He sustained (A) posterior glenoid fracture with humeral head subluxation into the defect that (B) went on to rapid osteoarthritis after it was neglected for 4 months. He underwent anatomic total shoulder arthroplasty with a posterior augmented glenoid component (Perform+, Wright/Tornier) which corrected his (C) preoperative posterior subluxation visible on the axillary lateral and (D) the correction remained durable at 5-year follow-up. (Image courtesy Grant E. Garrigues, MD.)

a bone defect between 20% and 45%. In their technique, they supplemented their lesser tuberosity transfer with added iliac crest bone graft.[88] Shams reported nine good and excellent results in 11 patients who underwent a lesser tuberosity transfer to treat a defect of 25% to 50% of the humeral head.[89] In their series of seven patients, Banerjee obtained an excellent result in six cases and a good result in one, with a mean Constant score of 92, forward flexion of 175 degrees, and external rotation to 54 degrees, although internal rotation was restricted between the waist and the thoracic vertebra in all of their patients.[90] Kokkalis had good outcomes in five patients treated with morselized femoral head bone allograft and lesser tuberosity transfer, with a mean Constant score of 84% and 100% of patient satisfaction.[91]

Patients undergoing anatomic arthroplasty for larger defects have mixed outcomes in the literature. In his series of 32 patients undergoing shoulder arthroplasty for locked posterior dislocation, Wooten reported 12 excellent or satisfactory results in 18 patients undergoing a hemiarthroplasty, and only 7 satisfactory results in 14 cases of anatomic total shoulder arthroplasty. They concluded that arthroplasty in this setting can lead to decreased pain, but it is associated with a significant rate of complications.[79] Cheng reported improved function, American Shoulder and Elbow Surgeons (ASES) score, and pain levels, with continued decreased strength in a series of five patients with locked posterior fracture-dislocations treated with an anatomic total shoulder arthroplasty. He concludes that this procedure provides good pain relief, but overhead activities and heavy lifting remain challenging after surgery.[59] Sperling had four satisfactory results and two unsatisfactory results with hemiarthroplasty for locked posterior dislocation, and three excellent or satisfactory results versus three unsatisfactory results with anatomic total shoulder arthroplasty. Checchia found worse outcomes in his series of five cases treated with a hemiarthroplasty after an acute posterior fracture-dislocation (two good results, three unsatisfactory results), compared with the group of eight shoulders that received the same treatment in a chronic scenario (five good or excellent results, three unsatisfactory results). Out of five shoulders treated with an anatomic total shoulder replacement, only one was classified as good.[80] Overall, all the authors conclude that anatomic total shoulder arthroplasty with a nonaugmented glenoid in this setting can be technically challenging, has higher reoperation rates, and the outcomes are worse than the same treatment for other indications. Although it can reliably reduce shoulder pain, range of motion and strength are usually limited compared with the contralateral, normal shoulder.

There are scattered case reports of reverse total shoulder arthroplasty for posterior shoulder dislocation[92] or posterior fracture-dislocation[93] in the literature, showing promising short-term outcomes regarding joint stability and scores. To our knowledge, there are no reports of anatomic total shoulder arthroplasty with a posterior glenoid bone block augmentation.

Conclusion

Posterior shoulder instability has a spectrum of presentation and treatment options that must be tailored to the individual pathology and demands. The most critical aspect to avoid a poor outcome is to make an early, accurate diagnosis based on the presenting history, physical, and imaging.

References

1. Kowalsky MS, Levine WN. Traumatic posterior glenohumeral dislocation: classification, pathoanatomy, diagnosis, and treatment. *Orthop Clin North Am.* 2008;39(4):519–533.
2. McLaughlin HL. Posterior dislocation of the shoulder. *J Bone Jt Surg.* 1952;34-A(3):584–590.
3. Robinson CM, Seah M, Akhtar MA. The epidemiology, risk of recurrence, and functional outcome after an acute traumatic posterior dislocation of the shoulder. *J Bone Jt Surg - Ser A.* 2011;93-A(17):1605–1613.
4. Basal O, Dincer R, Turk B. Locked posterior dislocation of the shoulder: a systematic review. *EFORT Open Rev.* 2017;3(1):15–23.
5. Goudie EB, Murray IR, Robinson CM. Instability of the shoulder following seizures. *J Bone Jt Surg - Ser B.* 2012;94 B(6):721–728.
6. Levine WN, Flatow EL. The pathophysiology of shoulder instability. *Am J Sports Med.* 2000;28(6):910–917.
7. Harryman DT, Sidles JA, Harris SL, Matsen FA. The role of the rotator interval capsule in passive motion and stability of the shoulder. *J Bone Jt Surg.* 1992;74-A(1):53–66.
8. Pagnani MJ, Warren RF. Stabilizers of the glenohumeral joint. *J Shoulder Elb Surg.* 1994;3(3):173–190.
9. Kim S-H, Ha K-I, Yoo J-C, Noh K-C. Kim's lesion: an incomplete and concealed avulsion of the posteroinferior labrum in posterior or multidirectional posteroinferior instability of the shoulder. *Arthrosc J Arthrosc Relat Surg.* 2004;20(7):712–720.
10. Imhoff AB, Savoie III FH, eds. *Shoulder Instability across the Life Span.* Springer-Verlag: Berlin; 2017.
11. Eichinger JK, Massimini DF, Kim J, Higgins LD. Biomechanical evaluation of glenoid version and dislocation direction on the influence of anterior shoulder instability and development of Hill-Sachs lesions. *Am J Sports Med.* 2016;44(11):2792–2799.
12. Wirth MA, Seltzer DG, Rockwood CA. Recurrent posterior glenohumeral dislocation associated with increased retroversion of the glenoid. *Clin Orthop Relat Res.* 1994;308:98–101.
13. Brewer BJ, Wubben RC, Carrera GF. Excessive retroversion of the glenoid cavity. A cause of non-traumatic posterior instability of the shoulder. *J Bone Jt Surg - Ser A.* 1986;68-A(5):724–731.
14. Di Giacomo G, Piscitelli L, Pugliese M. The role of bone in glenohumeral stability. *EFORT Open Rev.* 2018;3(12):632–640.
15. Weishaupt D, Zanetti M, Nyffeler RW, Gerber C, Hodler J. Posterior glenoid rim deficiency in recurrent (atraumatic) posterior shoulder instability. *Skeletal Radiol.* 2000;29:204–210.
16. Mulla DM, Hodder JN, Maly MR, Lyons JL, Keir PJ. Glenohumeral stabilizing roles of the scapulohumeral muscles: implications of muscle geometry. *J Biomech.* 2020;100:1–8.
17. Shaw JL. Bilateral posterior fracture-dislocation of the shoulder and other trauma caused by convulsive seizures. *J Bone Joint Surg Am.* 1971;53(7):1437–1440.
18. Beerhorst K, Schouwenaars FM, Tan IY, Aldenkamp AP. Epilepsy: fractures and the role of cumulative antiepileptic drug load. *Acta Neurol Scand.* 2012;125(1):54–59.
19. Pack AM, Olarte LS, Morrell MJ, Flaster E, Resor SR, Shane E. Bone mineral density in an outpatient population receiving enzyme-inducing antiepileptic drugs. *Epilepsy Behav.* 2003;4(2):169–174.
20. Bühler M, Gerber C. Shoulder instability related to epileptic seizures. *J Shoulder Elb Surg.* 2002;11(4):339–344.
21. Raiss P, Lin A, Mizuno N, Melis B, Walch G. Results of the Latarjet procedure for recurrent anterior dislocation of the shoulder in patients with epilepsy. *J Bone Jt Surg - Ser B.* 2012;94 B(9):1260–1264.
22. Hawkins RJ, Neer II CS, Pianta RM, Mendoza FX. Locked posterior dislocation of the shoulder. *J Bone Jt Surg.* 1987;69-A(1):9–18.
23. Sunku N, Kalaiah K, Marulasidappa G, Gopinath P. Bilateral anterior fracture-dislocation of shoulder joint-a rare case with delayed presentation. *J Orthop Case Reports.* 2012;2(4):7–9.
24. Hovelius L, Saeboe M. Neer Award 2008: arthropathy after primary anterior shoulder dislocation-223 shoulders prospectively followed up for twenty-five years. *J Shoulder Elb Surg.* 2009;18(3):339–347.
25. O'Leary JG, Greenberg CS, Patton HM, Caldwell SH. AGA clinical practice Update: coagulation in cirrhosis. *Gastroenterology.* 2019;157(1):34–43.e1.
26. Rahimzadeh P, Safari S, Reza Faiz SH, Alavian SM. Anesthesia for patients with liver disease. *Hepat Mon.* 2014;14(7).
27. Lewis A, Kitamura T, Bayley JIL. (ii) the classification of shoulder instability: new light through old windows! *Curr Orthop.* 2004;18(2):97–108.
28. May VR. Posterior dislocation of the shoulder: habitual, traumatic and obstetrical. *Orthop Clin North Am.* 1980;11(2):271–285.
29. Detenbeck LC. Posterior dislocations of the shoulder. *J Trauma.* 1972;12(3):183–192.
30. Hawkins RJ, Belle R. Posterior instability of the shoulder. *Instr Course Lect.* 1989;38(211):215.
31. Heller K, Forst J, Forst R, Cohen B. Posterior dislocation of the shoulder: recommendations for a classification. *Arch Orthop Trauma Surg.* 1994;113:228–231.
32. Robinson CM, Aderinto J. Posterior shoulder dislocations and fracture-dislocations. *J Bone Jt Surg.* 2005;87-A(3):639–650.
33. Rockwood CA, Matsen III FA, Wirth MA, Lippitt SB, Fehringer E V., Sperling JW, eds. *Rockwood and Matsen's the Shoulder.* 5th ed. Philadelphia, PA: Elsevier; 2017.
34. Rowe CR, Zarins B. Chronic unreduced dislocations of the shoulder. *J Bone Jt Surg.* 1982;64-A(4):494–505.
35. Blasier RB, Soslowsky LJ, Malicky DM, Palmer ML. Posterior glenohumeral subluxation: active and passive stabilization in a biomechanical model. *J Bone Jt Surg.* 1997;79-A(3):433–440.
36. Kim SH, Park JS, Jeong WK, Shin SK. The Kim test: a novel test for posteroinferior labral lesion of the shoulder - a comparison to the Jerk test. *Am J Sports Med.* 2005;33(8):1188–1192.
37. Pollock RG, Bigliani LU. Recurrent posterior shoulder instability. *Clin Orthop Relat Res.* 1993;291:85–96.
38. Gerber C, Ganz R. Clinical assessment of instability of the shoulder. With special reference to anterior and posterior drawer tests. *J Bone Joint Surg Br.* 1984;66(4):551–556.
39. Morey VM, Singh H, Paladini P, Merolla G, Phadke V, Porcellini G. The Porcellini test: a novel test for accurate diagnosis of posterior labral tears of the shoulder: comparative analysis with the established tests. *Musculoskelet Surg.* 2016;100(3):199–205.
40. Smits-Engelsman B, Klerks M, Kirby A. Beighton score: a valid measure for generalized hypermobility in children. *J Pediatr.* 2011;158(1):119–123. e4.
41. Cisternino SJ, Rogers LF, Stufflebam BC, Kruglik GD. The trough line: a radiographic sign of posterior shoulder dislocation. *AJR Am J Roentgenol.* 1978;130(5):951–954.

42. Arndt JH, Sears AD. Posterior dislocation of the shoulder. *Am J Roentgenol Radium Ther Nucl Med.* 1965;94:639–645.

43. Bloom MH, Obata WG. Diagnosis of posterior dislocation of the shoulder with use of Velpeau axillary and angle-up roentgenographic views. *J Bone Joint Surg Am.* 1967;49-A(5):943–949.

44. Garth WP, Slappey CE, Ochs CW. Roentgenographic demonstration of instability of the shoulder: the apical oblique projection. *J Bone Jt Surg - Ser A.* 1984;66(9):1450–1453.

45. Wallace WA, Hellier M. Improving radiographs of the injured shoulder. *Radiography.* 1983;49(586):229–233.

46. Frank RM, Romeo AA, Provencher MT. Posterior glenohumeral instability: evidence-based treatment. *J Am Acad Orthop Surg.* 2017;25(9):610–623.

47. Kirtland S, Resnick D, Sartoris DJ, Patel D, Greenway G. Chronic unreduced dislocations of the glenohumeral joint: imaging strategy and pathologic correlation. *J Trauma.* 1988;28(12):1622–1631.

48. Rouleau DM, Hebert-Davies J. Incidence of associated injury in posterior shoulder dislocation. *J Orthop Trauma.* 2012;26(4):246–251.

49. Saupe N, White LM, Bleakney R, et al. Acute traumatic posterior shoulder dislocation: MR findings. *Radiology.* 2008;248(1):185–193.

50. Hottya GA, Tirman PFJ, Bost FW, Montgomery WH, Wolf EM, Genant HK. Tear of the posterior shoulder stabilizers after posterior dislocation: MR imaging and MR arthrographic findings with arthroscopic correlation. *Am J Roentgenol.* 1998;171(3):763–768.

51. Allard JC, Bancroft J. Irreducible posterior dislocation of the shoulder: MR and CT findings. *J Comput Assist Tomogr.* 1991;15(4):694–696.

52. Ajuied A, McGarvey CP, Harb Z, Smith CC, Houghton RP, Corbett SA. Diagnosis of glenoid labral tears using 3-tesla MRI vs. 3-tesla MRA: a systematic review and meta-analysis. *Arch Orthop Trauma Surg.* 2018;138(5):699–709.

53. Loebenberg MI, Cuomo F. The treatment of chronic anterior and posterior dislocations of the glenohumeral joint and associated articular surface defects. *Orthop Clin North Am.* 2000;31(1):23–34.

54. Cicak N. Posterior dislocation of the shoulder. *J Bone Jt Surg - Ser B.* 2004;86(3):324–332.

55. Wilson JC, McKeever FM. Traumatic posterior (retroglenoid) dislocation of the humerus. *J Bone Jt Surg.* 1949;31-A(1):160–180.

56. Duralde XA, Fogle EF. The success of closed reduction in acute locked posterior fracture-dislocations of the shoulder. *J Shoulder Elb Surg.* 2006;15(6):701–706.

57. Rouleau DM, Hebert-Davies J, Robinson CM. Acute traumatic posterior shoulder dislocation. *J Am Acad Orthop Surg.* 2014;22(3):145–152.

58. Court-Brown CM, McQueen MM, Tornetta P. *Orthopaedic Surgery Essentials: Trauma.* Philadelphia: Lippincott Williams & Wilkins; 2006:68–88.

59. Cheng SL, Mackay MB, Richards RR. Treatment of locked posterior fracture-dislocations of the shoulder by total shoulder arthroplasty. *J Shoulder Elb Surg.* 1997;6(1):11–17.

60. Shaffer BS, Conway J, Jobe FW, Kvitne RS, Tibone JE. Infraspinatus muscle-splitting incision in posterior shoulder surgery. An anatomic and electromyographic study. *Am J Sports Med.* 1994;22(1):113–120.

61. Stableforth PG, Sarangi PP. Posterior fracture-dislocation of the shoulder. A superior subacromial approach for open reduction. *J Bone Joint Surg Br.* 1992;74(4):579–584.

62. Cautilli RA, Joyce MF, Mackell JV. Posterior dislocations of the shoulder: a method of postreduction management. *Am J Sports Med.* 1978;6(6):397–399.

63. Scougall S. Posterior dislocation of the shoulder. *J Bone Jt Surg.* 1957;39B(4):726–732.

64. Spencer EE, Brems JJ. A simple technique for management of locked posterior shoulder dislocations: report of two cases. *J Shoulder Elb Surg.* 2005;14(6):650–652.

65. Martetschlager F, Padalecki JR, Millett PJ. Modified arthroscopic McLaughlin procedure for treatment of posterior instability of the shoulder with an associated reverse Hill-Sachs lesion. *Knee Surg Sports Traumatol Arthrosc.* 2013;21(7):1642–1646.

66. Bernholt DL, Lacheta L, Goldenberg BT, Millett PJ. Arthroscopic knotless modified McLaughlin procedure for reverse Hill–Sachs lesions. *Arthrosc Tech.* 2020;9(1):e65–e70.

67. Matthewson G, Wong IH. Posterior glenohumeral capsular reconstruction with modified McLaughlin for chronic locked posterior dislocation. *Arthrosc Tech.* 2019;8(12):e1543–e1550.

68. Gerber C. L'instabilite posterieure de l'epaule. *Cah d'enseignement la SOFCOT - Paris,* Expans Sci Fr. 40:223-245.

69. Gerber C. Chronic, locked anterior and posterior dislocations. In: Warner JJP, Ianotti J, Gerber C, eds. *Complex and Revision Problems in Shoulder Surgery.* Philadelphia: Lippincott-Raven; 1997:99–116.

70. Griggs S, Holloway B, Williams G, Iannotti J. Treatment of locked anterior and posterior dislocations of the shoulder. In: Iannotti J, Williams G, eds. *Disorders of the Shoulder: Diagnosis and Management.* Philadelphia: Lippincott Williams & Wilkins; 1999:335–359.

71. Gerber C, Lambert SM. Allograft reconstruction of segmental defects of the humeral head for the treatment of chronic locked posterior dislocation of the shoulder. *J Bone Jt Surg - Ser A.* 1996;78(3):376–382.

72. Diklic ID, Ganic ZD, Blagojevic ZD, Nho SJ, Romeo AA. Treatment of locked chronic posterior dislocation of the shoulder by reconstruction of the defect in the humeral head with an allograft. *J Bone Jt Surg - Ser B.* 2010;92(1):71–76.

73. Saltzman BM, Riboh JC, Cole BJ, Yanke AB. Humeral head reconstruction with osteochondral allograft transplantation. *Arthrosc J Arthrosc Relat Surg.* 2015;31(9):1827–1834.

74. Black LO, Ko JWK, Quilici SM, Crawford DC. Fresh osteochondral allograft to the humeral head for treatment of an engaging reverse Hill-Sachs lesion: technical case report and literature review. *Orthop J Sport Med.* 2016;4(11):1–5.

75. Chan CM, LeVasseur MR, Lerner AL, Maloney MD, Voloshin I. Computer modeling analysis of the talar dome as a graft for the humeral head. *Arthrosc J Arthrosc Relat Surg.* 2016;32(8):1671–1675.

76. Mitchell JJ, Vap AR, Sanchez G, et al. Concomitant reverse Hill-Sachs lesion and posterior humeral avulsion of the glenohumeral ligament: treatment with fresh talus osteochondral allograft and arthroscopic posterior humeral avulsion of the glenohumeral ligament and labrum repair. *Arthrosc Tech.* 2017;6(4):e987–e995.

77. Provencher MT, Sanchez G, Schantz K, et al. Anatomic humeral head reconstruction with fresh osteochondral talus allograft for recurrent glenohumeral instability with reverse Hill-Sachs lesion. *Arthrosc Tech.* 2017;6(1):e255–e261.

78. Sperling JW, Pring M, Antuna SA, Cofield RH. Shoulder arthroplasty for locked posterior dislocation of the shoulder. *J Shoulder Elb Surg.* 2004;13(5):522–527.

79. Wooten C, Klika B, Schleck CD, Harmsen WS, Sperling JW, Cofield RH. Anatomic shoulder arthroplasty as treatment for locked posterior dislocation of the shoulder. *J Bone Jt Surg.* 2014;e19:1–6.

80. Checchia SL, Santos PD, Miyazaki AN. Surgical treatment fracture-dislocation of acute and chronic of the shoulder. *J Shoulder Elb Surg.* 1998;7(1):53–65.

81. Karachalios T, Bargiotas K, Papachristos A, Malizos KN. Reconstruction of a neglected posterior dislocation of the shoulder through a limited posterior deltoid-splitting approach. A case report. *J Bone Joint Surg Am.* 2005;87(3):630–634.

82. Delong JM, Jiang K, Bradley JP. Posterior instability of the shoulder: a systematic review and meta-analysis of clinical outcomes. *Am J Sports Med.* 2015;43(7):1805–1817.

83. Servien E, Walch G, Cortes ZE, Edwards TB, O'Connor DP. Posterior bone block procedure for posterior shoulder instability. *Knee Surg Sports Traumatol Arthrosc.* 2007;15(9):1130–1136.

84. Surin V, Blader S, Markhede G, Sundholm K. Rotational osteotomy of the humerus for posterior instability of the shoulder. *J Bone Jt Surg.* 1990;72A(2):181–186.

85. Dimon 3rd JH. Posterior dislocation and posterior fracture dislocation of the shoulder: a report of 25 cases. *South Med J.* 1967;60(6):661–666.

86. Roberts A, Wickstrom J. Prognosis of posterior dislocation of the shoulder. *Acta Orthop Scand.* 1971;42(4):328–337.

87. Samilson RL, Prieto V. Dislocation arthropathy of the shoulder. *J Bone Jt Surg - Ser A.* 1983;65(4):456–460.

88. Khira YM, Salama AM. Treatment of locked posterior shoulder dislocation with bone defect. *Orthopedics.* 2017;40(3):e501–e505.

89. Shams A, Osama ME, Mohamed G, et al. Modified technique for reconstructing reverse Hill-Sachs lesion in locked chronic posterior shoulder dislocation. *Eur J Orthop Surg Traumatol.* 2016;26(8):843–849.

90. Banerjee M, Balke M, Bouillon B, et al. Excellent results of lesser tuberosity transfer in acute locked posterior shoulder dislocation. *Knee Surg Sports Traumatol Arthrosc.* 2013;21:2884–2888.

91. Kokkalis ZT, Mavrogenis AF, Ballas EG, Papanastasiou J, Papagelopoulos PJ. Modified McLaughlin technique for neglected locked posterior dislocation of the shoulder. *Orthopedics.* 2013;36(7):912–916.

92. Hasler A, Fornaciari P, Jungwirth-Weinberger A, Jentzsch T, Wieser K, Gerber C. Reverse shoulder arthroplasty in the treatment of glenohumeral instability. *J Shoulder Elb Surg.* 2019;28(8):1587–1594.

93. Wendling A, Vopat ML, Yang SY, Saunders B. Near-simultaneous bilateral reverse total shoulder arthroplasty for the treatment of bilateral fracture dislocations of the shoulder. *BMJ Case Rep.* 2019;12(10):10–13.

24

Technique Spotlight: Open Reduction and Bone Grafting of Reverse Hill-Sachs Lesions

BRYANT P. ELRICK, PHILIP C. NOLTE, AND PETER J. MILLETT

Conflicts of Interest: The position of PCN at the Steadman Philippon Research Institute is supported by Arthrex. PJM is a consultant for and receives royalties from Arthrex, Medbridge, and Springer; owns stock in VuMedi; receives support from the Steadman Philippon Research Institute and Vail Valley Medical Center; and has corporate sponsorship from the Steadman Philippon Research Institute, Smith & Nephew, Arthrex, Siemens, and Össur. BPE reports no conflicts of interest.

Indications

Surgical intervention for reverse Hill-Sachs (rHS) lesions is dependent upon the clinical significance of the lesion and symptoms of instability.[1] Considerations include size of the defect, engagement, location, orientation, extent of glenoid bone loss, bone quality, timing (acute vs. chronic), persistent instability, displaced fractures (e.g., lesser tuberosity, glenoid), and the general medical condition of the patient.[1,2] Conservative management is generally trialed and can be effective in patients with small nonengaging lesions, and older, less active patients with substantial defects affecting >40% of the humeral head usually require arthroplasty.[1] Treatment decision-making is more challenging for mid-sized defects. Although these lesions have been successfully managed with multiple treatment options including the McLaughlin procedure and associated modified techniques that tenodese the subscapularis into the defect either with[3] or without[4,5] the lesser tuberosity, bone allograft reconstruction of the humeral head[6] and rotational humeral osteotomy,[7] clear surgical and technical indications remain ill-defined in the literature.

Anatomic restoration techniques are usually reserved for acute lesions, but have been indicated for lesions presenting up to 6 months post injury.[8] Restorative techniques have been used to treat defects between 20% and 50% of the humeral head. The authors prefer using open reduction and bone disimpaction technique (Fig. 24.1) to treat young, active patients without significant glenoid bone loss who have suffered an rHS impaction fracture subsequent to an acute posterior dislocation with good bone stock, preserved articular cartilage, and humeral head defect between 20% and 40%.

Preoperative Evaluation

Posterior glenohumeral (GH) dislocation has been reportedly missed on initial evaluation in up to 60%–79% of cases[9]; therefore, a thorough history and physical examination is imperative, in combination with orthogonal radiographs to include an axillary lateral. If the humeral head remains dislocated, the injured extremity is typically held locked in internal rotation with deficits in both passive and active range of motion (ROM).[10] For cases with a history concerning posterior instability who are not currently dislocated, the posterior drawer, Kim, and Jerk tests can be used to assess posterior instability.[11] Axillary nerve injury is a well-known complication of GH dislocation, with a wide range of reported incidence (3%–40%).[12,13] Although these injuries commonly resolve without intervention, prompt identification and management of nerve injury are important to avoid potential long-term functional deficits. Posterior GH dislocation is frequently caused by first seizure and should raise suspicion for an underlying diagnosis of epilepsy[14]; therefore, history of these symptoms should be assessed and, if present, consultation of a neurologist should be sought to avoid a postoperative seizure that may compromise treatment.

A complete radiographic shoulder series should be ordered (three views: true anteroposterior [AP], axillary, and scapular Y view). Axillary radiographs are imperative to evaluate GH relationships, visualize glenoid rim and lesser tuberosity fractures, and help estimate the size of the defect[2] (Fig. 24.2A). If this is not possible due to patient discomfort, a Velpeau view can be obtained. Computed tomography (CT) imaging with or without three-dimensional reconstruction is an invaluable tool in the assessment of osseous morphology and should be obtained to assess for a concentrically reduced GH joint, evaluate posterior bone loss, identify fractures (especially nondisplaced fractures of the anatomic neck and lesser tuberosity), and quantify anterior humeral head defects,

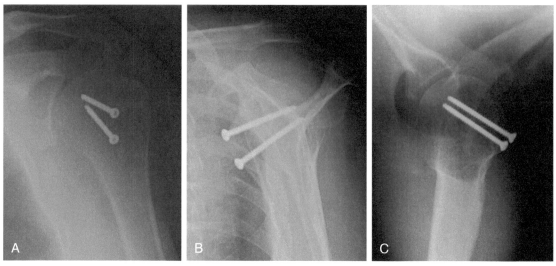

• **Fig. 24.1** Postoperative (A) anteroposterior, (B) scapular Y, and (C) axial radiographs of a left shoulder after open reduction and fracture disimpaction to treat an acute reverse Hill-Sachs defect.

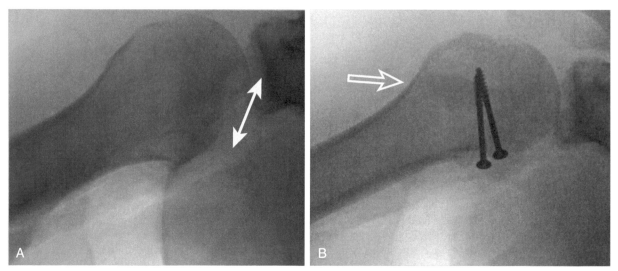

• **Fig. 24.2** Intraoperative axillary images of a (A) right shoulder immediately after open reduction showing the impacted reverse Hill-Sachs lesion *(double arrow)* and (B) after anatomic reduction of the articular surface, backfilling with bone graft along the indicated trajectory *(arrow)*, and placement of rafter screws.

including size and location (Fig. 24.3). Magnetic resonance imaging (MRI) can be a helpful adjunct to assess soft tissue pathology including labral tears and capsular injury and laxity[11] especially in chronic or recurrent cases. Practically, the authors typically order a CT scan if the GH joint remains dislocated ("locked dislocation") to assess for associated fractures that may complicate reduction and an MRI for posterior instability that has been reduced to assess for associated soft tissue injuries.

Positioning and Equipment

The procedure is typically carried out with both general endotracheal anesthesia (to allow muscle relaxation for difficult/muscular patients) as well as a regional nerve block for postoperative pain control. The patient is placed into the beach chair position and a pneumatic arm holder is used. If the patient has a locked posterior dislocation that was not previously reducible with attempts in the emergency room, the shoulder is carefully reduced under general anesthesia, facilitated by muscle relaxation or with an interscalene

block. An examination under anesthesia is performed to assess stability and engagement of the defect on the posterior glenoid rim. Examination may demonstrate high-grade posterior translation and locked-positioning if the rHS catches on the posterior glenoid. If the GH joint is not amenable to closed reduction under anesthesia, open reduction must be performed. A full list of equipment and materials used in the surgical technique is shown in Table 24.1.

Surgical Technique

Following closed reduction of the shoulder, a standard posterior viewing portal is established 2 cm medial and 2 cm inferior to the posterolateral acromion. A diagnostic arthroscopy is performed using a standard 30-degree arthroscope and the humeral cartilage, posterior glenoid, and posterior capsulolabral complex are carefully evaluated for injury. A dynamic evaluation allows for characterization of rHS lesion (e.g., size, depth, location, engagement) (Fig. 24.4). An anterosuperior working portal is established

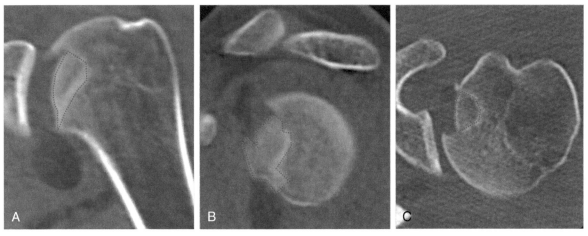

• **Fig. 24.3** Preoperative (A) coronal, (B) sagittal, and (C) transverse computed tomography of a left shoulder outlining the anterosuperior humeral impaction fracture *(red-dotted line)*. (Image courtesy Grant E. Garrigues, MD.)

TABLE 24.1	Procedural Equipment and Material
Positioning	• Pneumatic arm holder
Diagnostic arthroscopy	• Standard 30-degree arthroscope +/− arthroscopic instrumentation based on intra-articular pathology (e.g., radiofrequency cautery device, shaver)
Cortical window	• 8-mm anterior cruciate ligament reamer
Fragment reduction	• Curved bone tamp • Elevator or small osteotome
	• Two 4.0 cannulated fully threaded screws
	• Bone graft chips (autograft or allograft)
Imaging	• Fluoroscope

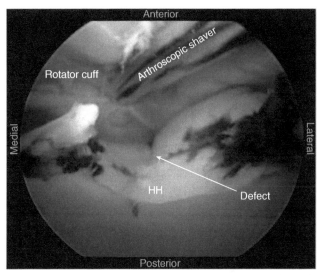

• **Fig. 24.4** Arthroscopic view of the osteochondral impression defect (reverse Hill-Sachs impaction fracture) in the humeral head *(HH)* of a right shoulder.

through the rotator interval, as well as an anteroinferior portal near the level of the coracoid, under direct visualization. Concomitant pathology should be treated arthroscopically.

Following the arthroscopic part of the surgery, or in cases that were not amenable to closed reduction, a standard deltopectoral incision is made and the deltopectoral interval is established. The conjoint tendon is identified and retracted medially. Dissection is carried out and the rotator interval is opened to visualize the rHS. Approximately 1 cm of the superior subscapularis may also be reflected inferiorly to visualize the anterior humeral surface if visualization through the rotator interval is inadequate. If the humerus remains posteriorly dislocated and locked on the glenoid rim, full takedown of the subscapularis may be necessary (either with a tenotomy or lesser tuberosity osteotomy). Open reduction can then be accomplished with adduction and internal rotation of the arm and applied lateral traction to the humeral head to disengage it from the posterior glenoid rim. The long head of the biceps tendon (LHBT) is typically tenodesed if the subscapularis is tenotomized. Takedown of the subscapularis is more commonly

needed in chronic locked dislocations, which is not the subject of this chapter.

Disimpaction of Reverse Hill-Sachs

The arm is internally rotated to allow visualization and an 8-mm cortical window is created posterolaterally in the greater tuberosity with the use of an 8-mm reamer to gain retrograde access to the defect (Fig. 24.5A). The window should be positioned to allow the appropriate trajectory for the bone tamp to access the impaction fracture. The shoulder can be articulated through external and internal rotation to aid in proper placement of the window while allowing visualization of the defect through the rotator interval.[2] Under direct visualization, a curved bone tamp is placed through the cortical window and used to disimpact the fracture (Fig. 24.5B), while reduction is simultaneously controlled with palpation through the rotator interval. In chronic cases, a small osteotome or elevator can be used to free the depressed cartilage before elevation.[15] Again, the shoulder can be rotated during disimpaction to appropriately visualize the lesion

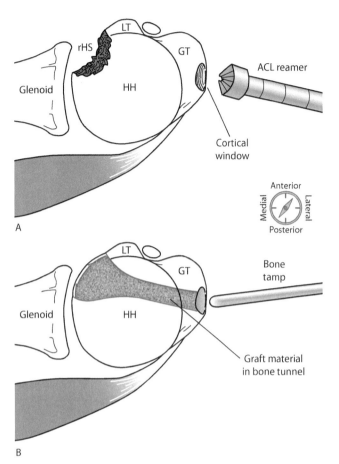

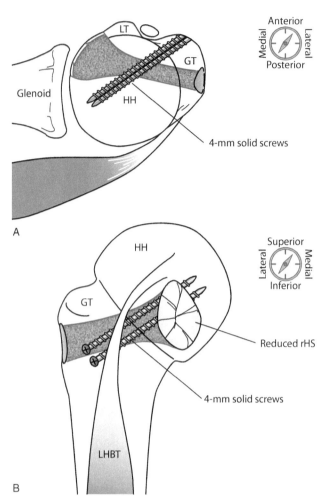

• **Fig. 24.5** Illustration of key procedural steps in a right shoulder. (A) A cortical window is established posterolaterally in the greater tuberosity (GT) and retrograde access to the reverse Hill-Sachs (rHS) lesion is obtained using an anterior cruciate ligament (ACL) reamer. (B) A bone tamp is utilized through the cortical window to disimpact the fracture and osseous chips are used to fill the defect. *HH*, Humeral head; *LT*, lesser tuberosity.

• **Fig. 24.6** Illustration of key procedural steps in a right shoulder. (A) Two 4.0-mm cannulated screws are placed beneath the reverse Hill-Sachs lesion as subchondral support. (B) Final setting with reduced fracture, osseous chip filling, and supportive screw placement. *GT*, Greater tuberosity; *HH*, humeral head; *LT*, lesser tuberosity; *LHBT*, long head of biceps tendon; *rHS*, reverse Hill-Sachs.

and aid in restoring the joint surface. Although it is important not to overaggressively tamp the bone and risk a perforation of the tamp, slight over-reduction is acceptable due to settling as the fracture heals.[2]

Bone graft is used to support the subchondral regions beneath the rHS impaction fracture (Fig. 24.5B). Either allograft[16] or autograft[15] material can be used with satisfactory results; the authors typically prefer mineralized cancellous allograft due to reduced morbidity. Approximately 15 cc of mineralized cancellous allograft bone chips are impacted underneath the defect, acting as a subchondral and subcortical buttress. Two 4.0-mm cannulated fully threaded unicortical cancellous screws are placed through the greater tuberosity, directly beneath the fracture, for additional subchondral support (Fig. 24.6). The authors of this chapter prefer extra-articular screws directed from anterolateral to posteromedial, while the editors of this book frequently use two screws placed anterior to posterior through the lesser tuberosity—either method leads to the same effect. Palpation through the rotator interval confirms that there is no intra-articular screw penetration. The cortical window is filled with bone graft and the previously made cortical window is tamped back into place. AP and axillary fluoroscopic views are obtained to confirm proper screw placement, adequate reduction, and to ensure that the normal convexity of the humeral articular surface

has been restored before wound irrigation and layered-closure (Fig. 24.2B).

Postoperative Care

Approach to postoperative rehabilitation varies and is highly based on the surgeon's preference. Typically, patients are placed in an immobilization sling or brace in neutral rotation for 3–6 weeks postsurgery.[15,17] External rotation and internal rotation should be limited to 30 degrees and to the body, respectively, in order to protect the subscapularis repair and prevent fracture reimpaction.[16] Internal rotation that would engage the reduced articular surface and cause both recurrent posterior instability and loss of articular reduction should be strictly avoided until bony healing is complete at approximately 6 weeks. More aggressive rehabilitation approaches may allow patients to begin pendulum and passive ROM exercises immediately,[16,17] while others may delay passive ROM for 2–3 weeks.[15,18] Overhead activity and posterior loading of the shoulder should be avoided for approximately 5–6 weeks.[15–18] Active-assisted and active range of motion are typically begun around 4–6 weeks[16] with a full return to activity and sport at approximately 6 months.[17]

PEARLS AND PITFALLS

Pearls

- Appropriate portal placement is key to adequately visualize the reverse Hill-Sachs defect.
- Graft material should be firmly impacted to prevent collapse of the reduced fragment.
- External and internal rotation of the operative extremity can aid in visualization and reduction of the impacted fracture.
- Mild over-reduction of the bony fragment is well tolerated due to natural settling with movement.
- Anatomic restoration of the joint surface is important to prevent onset of osteoarthritis.

Pitfalls

- Establishing the cortical window too inferior can result in iatrogenic injury to the axillary nerve.
- Overaggressive tamping can lead to substantial over-reduction of the bony fragment and subsequent osteoarthritis.
- Insufficient bone stock due to chronic dislocation or osteoporosis puts elevation and fixation of the fragment at risk for failure.

References

1. Provencher MT, Frank RM, Leclere LE, et al. The Hill-Sachs lesion: diagnosis, classification, and management. *J Am Acad Orthop Surg.* 2012;20(4):242–252.
2. Ponce BAMP, Warner JP. *Management of Posterior Glenohumeral Instability with Large Humeral Head Defects.* Philadelphia: Lippincott Williams & Wilkins; 2004.
3. Banerjee M, Balke M, Bouillon B, et al. Excellent results of lesser tuberosity transfer in acute locked posterior shoulder dislocation. *Knee Surg Sports Traumatol Arthrosc.* 2013;21(12):2884–2888.
4. Bernholt DL, Lacheta L, Goldenberg BT, Millett PJ. Arthroscopic knotless modified McLaughlin procedure for reverse Hill-Sachs lesions. *Arthroscopy Techniques.* 2019;9(1):e65–e70.
5. Martetschlager F, Padalecki JR, Millett PJ. Modified arthroscopic McLaughlin procedure for treatment of posterior instability of the shoulder with an associated reverse Hill-Sachs lesion. *Knee Surg Sports Traumatol Arthrosc.* 2013;21(7):1642–1646.
6. Black LO, Ko JK, Quilici SM, Crawford DC. Fresh osteochondral allograft to the humeral head for treatment of an engaging reverse Hill-Sachs lesion: technical case report and literature review. *Orthop J Sports Med.* 2016;4(11). 2325967116670376.
7. Weber BG, Simpson LA, Hardegger F. Rotational humeral osteotomy for recurrent anterior dislocation of the shoulder associated with a large Hill-Sachs lesion. *J Bone Joint Surg Am.* 1984;66(9):1443–1450.
8. Neer 2nd CS. Displaced proximal humeral fractures: part I. Classification and evaluation. 1970. *Clin Orthop Relat Res.* 2006;442:77–82.
9. Kokkalis ZT, Iliopoulos ID, Antoniou G, et al. Posterior shoulder fracture-dislocation: an update with treatment algorithm. *Eur J Orthop Surg Traumatol: Orthop Traumatol.* 2017;27(3):285–294.
10. Kowalsky MS, Levine WN. Traumatic posterior glenohumeral dislocation: classification, pathoanatomy, diagnosis, and treatment. *Orthop Clin N Am.* 2008;39(4):519–533 (viii).
11. Tannenbaum E, Sekiya JK. Evaluation and management of posterior shoulder instability. *Sports Health.* 2011;3(3):253–263.
12. Atef A, El-Tantawy A, Gad H, Hefeda M. Prevalence of associated injuries after anterior shoulder dislocation: a prospective study. *Int Orthop.* 2016;40(3):519–524.
13. Visser CP, Coene LN, Brand R, Tavy DL. The incidence of nerve injury in anterior dislocation of the shoulder and its influence on functional recovery. A prospective clinical and EMG study. *J Bone Joint Surg Br.* 1999;81(4):679–685.
14. Langenbruch L, Rickert C, Gosheger G, et al. Seizure-induced shoulder dislocations - case series and review of the literature. *Seizure.* 2019;70:38–42.
15. Bock P, Kluger R, Hintermann B. Anatomical reconstruction for reverse Hill-Sachs lesions after posterior locked shoulder dislocation fracture: a case series of six patients. *Arch Orthop Trauma Surg.* 2007;127(7):543–548.
16. Euler SA, Spiegl UJA, Millett PJ. Posterior shoulder instability with a reverse Hill-Sachs defect: repair with use of combined arthroscopic labral repair and fracture disimpaction: a case report. *JBJS Case Connect.* 2014;4(3):e86.
17. Khayal T, Wild M, Windolf J. Reconstruction of the articular surface of the humeral head after locked posterior shoulder dislocation: a case report. *Arch Orthop Trauma Surg.* 2009;129(4):515–519.
18. Assom M, Castoldi F, Rossi R, Blonna D, Rossi P. Humeral head impression fracture in acute posterior shoulder dislocation: new surgical technique. *Knee Surg Sports Traumatol Arthrosc: Official Journal of the ESSKA.* 2006;14(7):668–672.

25

Treatment Algorithm for Proximal Humerus Fractures

BETTINA HOCHREITER, BERNHARD JOST, AND CHRISTIAN SPROSS

Introduction

Proximal humeral fractures (PHFs) account for nearly 6% of all fractures.[1] They have an overall incidence of 40 in 100,000 patients. This number is predicted to triple by 2030 with a growing elderly population leading to an increase in age-related osteoporosis.[2–4] As such, management of these fractures will continue to pose challenges on many fronts. From fracture characterization to treatment options and personalized treatment decisions, there is limited guidance from the literature. The individuality of affected patients, fracture pattern, and vascular impairment as well as bone quality makes uniform treatment difficult. Therefore it is particularly important to develop clear evidence and treatment algorithms for the various patient subgroups.

At the beginning of the 20th century, conservative treatment was the mainstay of treatment by default as there were no viable alternatives. With the foundation of the Arbeitsgemeinschaft für Osteosynthesefragen (AO) in 1958, new treatment options with devices for open reduction internal fixation (ORIF) were developed. In 1970 Charles Neer presented his results of hemiprosthetic replacements for proximal humerus fractures.[5] Subsequently, more fractures were treated operatively and with the development of anatomically contoured, angular stable (locking) implants at the beginning of the 21st century, ORIF became the "gold standard" for the surgical treatment of PHFs. The success of these treatments, however, does not just depend on the implants themselves but also upon appropriate patient selection and surgical expertise. More recently there have been some reports of high complication and revision rates.[6–10] The PROFHER trial,[11] being the largest randomized trial to date on PHFs, has provided high-quality evidence to justify nonsurgical treatment for the majority of low-energy injuries. Understandably, this trial has divided opinion and stimulated vigorous debate. At one end of the spectrum with an undisplaced fracture in an elderly patient, few would dispute the role of conservative treatment. While at the other end with a comminuted fracture-dislocation in a young patient, there is obviously a role for operative intervention. However, a number of more or less displaced fractures in a highly variable spectrum of patients exists in between. The management of those situations currently remains controversial. In this group, the advantage of ORIF over nonsurgical treatment would be weighed against the risk of potentially significant complications.

In addition, the considerations go beyond nonsurgical versus surgical management as the latter encompasses a vast array of shifting and nuanced management options. Within ORIF there are different plate designs, intramedullary (IM) nails, augments with allograft struts and bone graft substitutes, and beyond. More recently, the reverse total shoulder arthroplasty (rTSA) has become a valuable option for treating comminuted proximal humerus fractures, particularly, in elderly patients.[12,13] While reports of improved function with low revision rates are promising, long-term follow-up studies have not yet been published. At this time, however, rTSA does appear to provide better outcomes than ORIF for elderly patients with certain displaced fractures.[14]

The aim of any fracture treatment should be to bring patients back as near as possible to their preinjury function and quality of life. Given the variety of individuals, vocations, avocations, and fracture types, there is not one solution for all patients but may be a best individualized solution for each patient. Thus the whole range of treatment options should be considered for each individual. Therefore an evidence-based treatment algorithm, including patient-specific factors like functional demands and bone quality, may be helpful to the orthopedic surgeon faced with these common treatment decisions.

This chapter contains the first clinical results of the evidence-based treatment algorithm published in the sixth edition of *Skeletal Trauma: Basic Science, Management, and Reconstruction*.[15] Based on these results, the algorithm has been updated and simplified with a new version, which will be further described in this chapter as well.[15a]

Anatomy

In this section, anatomic parameters that have important implications for imaging, repair, and reconstruction of the proximal humerus are briefly depicted.

The mean humeral head retrotorsion ranges from 18 to 30 degrees (total range is 10–55 degrees) relative to the epicondylar axis.[16,17] The average adult humeral head has a radius of curvature of 22–25 mm.[5] Humeral head inclination ranges from 132 to 141 degrees.[18] The most cephalad surface of the articular segment is on average 8 mm above the greater tuberosity, The size of the humeral head determines the lateral displacement of the greater tuberosity and the rotator cuff insertions and has an effect on the kinematics of the glenohumeral joint. Considerable variations are seen with neurovascular structures.[19] The axillary nerve crosses on average 5.4 cm in females and 6.2 cm in males from the midportion of the acromion.[20] The musculocutaneous nerve enters the coracobrachialis muscle at 5 cm from the coracoid on average. The vascular supply of the shoulder girdle is derived from the subclavian artery and the rich arborization of arteries that originate from the axillary artery (Fig. 25.1). The most important vessels for proximal humeral blood supply are the circumflex anterior and posterior humeral arteries. Even today, controversy exists regarding which of these arteries is more important for the blood supply of the humeral head. Initially, Gerber and colleagues[21] showed in a cadaver study that the humeral head was perfused by the anterolateral ascending branch of the anterior circumflex artery in all specimens. That vessel ran parallel to the lateral aspect of the tendon of the long head of the biceps and entered the humeral head where the proximal end of the intertubercular groove met the greater tuberosity. When the intraosseous (terminal) part of the anterolateral branch, the so-called arcuate artery, had

been perfused, almost the entire epiphysis was radiopaque. The posterior circumflex artery vascularized only the posterior portion of the greater tuberosity and a small posteroinferior part of the head. Anastomoses between the different arteries were abundant, but vascularization of all of the humeral head was possible only through the anterolateral branch of the anterior circumflex artery. More recently, Hettrich and colleagues[22] found that the posterior humeral circumflex artery provides 64% of the blood supply to the humeral head. This finding is a possible explanation for the relatively low rates of osteonecrosis seen in association with displaced fractures of the proximal part of the humerus where the anterior blood supply is frequently disrupted.

Tingart and colleagues[23] measured total, trabecular, and cortical volumetric bone mineral density (BMD) in the humeral head. The greater tuberosity was divided into three regions, and the lesser tuberosity and articular surface were each divided into two regions. The proximal head showed a significantly higher trabecular (+46%) and cortical BMD (+15%) than the distal one. The mean trabecular BMD of the articular surface was significantly higher (+80%), and the cortical BMD was significantly lower (−11%) than that of the tuberosities. In the proximal half of the greater tuberosity, trabecular BMD was higher in the posterior than in the middle and anterior regions. Cortical BMD was higher in the middle region than in the anterior and posterior ones. In the distal half of the greater tuberosity, trabecular BMD was significantly higher in the posterior than in the middle region, and cortical BMD was significantly higher in the anterior than in the middle region. In the proximal half of the articular surface, trabecular BMD was significantly higher in the posterior region than in the anterior one. Their results point to bone sites that may provide stronger fixation for implants and reduce the risk of implant loosening.

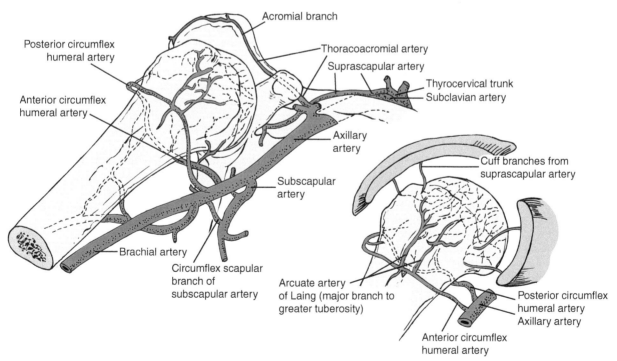

• **Fig. 25.1** Vascular supply to the shoulder region. (From Browner B, Jupiter J, Krettek C, Anderson P. *Skeletal Trauma: Basic Science, Management, and Reconstruction.* 6th ed. Philadelphia: Elsevier; 2019: Fig. 47.4.)

Classification

Since Neer's fundamental writings in 1970,[5,24] many attempts have been made to quantify or classify PHFs or fracture patterns more precisely to improve treatment and patient outcomes. Consequently, it has been difficult to compare the results of the historical with the current literature. Despite ample experience with these fractures, their treatment based on classifications remains controversial.

Early classification schemes described the anatomic location of the fracture and the mechanism of injury but did not consider the importance of fracture anatomy or displacement of the fracture. Codman[25] noted that most PHFs occur along the lines of the former physes of the proximal end of the humerus and described four possible fracture fragments: greater tuberosity, lesser tuberosity, anatomic head, and shaft. Based on this description, Neer[24] proposed the four-segment classification system, which included his clinical and operative findings.

The classification of proximal humerus fractures is commonly based on anteroposterior (AP) and lateral radiographs but can be difficult and unreliable.[26,27] Therefore if additional information is needed, we have a low threshold for a computed tomography (CT) scan with three-dimensional (3D) reconstructions in our institution which undoubtedly gives more accurate information with regard to fracture pattern and certainly allows better planning if surgery is intended.[28,29]

The Neer Classification

In his study of the classification and evaluation of proximal humerus fractures,[24] Neer originally described six groups. A segment (greater, lesser tuberosity, anatomical, surgical neck) is defined as a "part" if its displacement is >1 cm or 45 degrees.

Neer himself adapted his classification and focused on the four segments and their displacement.[30,31] The major modification was the use of a "one-part" fracture type despite the former group I. Therein all fractures with <1 cm or 45 degrees of displacement of any segment or combination of segments were included. The two- to four-part fractures were used as mentioned in his primary description (Fig. 25.2). Later, the valgus-impacted four-part fracture was also included in this revised classification system.[30] The adapted Neer classification has been used since its introduction and is still the most referenced classification for fractures of the proximal humerus.[5,32–35]

AO/ASIF Classification System

The AO/American Society for Internal Fixation (AO/ASIF) organization proposed a new classification, which was an expansion and modification of the Neer classification.[36] The main difference was that they paid special attention to the impaction or displacement of the fracture parts and described them in a more detailed way to include the important aspect of the vascular impairment. Basically, the AO/ASIF system differentiates three types of fractures (Fig. 25.3A–C): extra-articular unifocal, extra-articular bifocal, and intra-articular. Each of these groups is divided into further subgroups depending on fracture location and complexity. Since the original publication of the AO/OTA Fracture Classification in 1996, there has been a lot of progress in fracture classification. Therefore a compendium was recently published updating the prior editions.[37]

Hertel's Classification and Predictors of Humeral Head Ischemia

Hertel and colleagues[38] designed a "LEGO" classification system (Fig. 25.4) based on Codman's original drawings. In this fracture description, five fracture planes are combined, which render 12 basic fracture patterns (+2 additional head-split patterns). Fracture planes lie between the greater tuberosity and the head, the greater tuberosity and the shaft, the lesser tuberosity and the head, the lesser tuberosity and the shaft, and the lesser tuberosity and the greater tuberosity. They found that a dorsomedial metaphyseal head extension of <8 mm and >2 mm of displacement of the medial periosteal hinge in fractures with isolated articular segments were good predictors for intraoperative head ischemia. However, these findings did not correlate with postoperative avascular necrosis (AVN) in a later follow-up study.[39,40]

Role and Reliability of Classifications

The AO/ASIF system, which is more detailed and also widely accepted, has not replaced the Neer classification. The most recent edition of the AO/ASIF fracture compendium has integrated the Neer classification to facilitate the clinical comprehension (Fig. 25.3A–C).

However, the main limitation in the Neer classification is the measurement of 1 cm and 45 degrees on standard radiographs, which is fundamental for the decision whether a fractured segment becomes a "part" with subsequent surgical consequences. Therefore the reproducibility, or lack thereof, of the Neer classification has been the subject of many studies.[41–44] In most of these studies, the inter- and intrarater reliability were only moderate. The experience of the observer and also the quality of radiographs are important factors influencing the reliability. Also, the benefit of the addition of CT to plain radiography has been studied, and a slight increase in intraobserver but no change in interobserver reliability was found.[45] Comparisons of the reliability of the AO/ASIF system with the Neer classification showed advantages for the latter.[26,28,44] Brunner and colleagues could improve their inter- and intrarater reliability from moderate to good or excellent after the use of 3D volume–rendered CT scans.[28] Additional information from CT scans plays a more important role in modern fracture classification of the proximal humerus and has, therefore, been used in recent studies.[33,34] As mentioned before, the authors have a low threshold for a CT scan with 3D reconstructions to obtain information with regard to fracture pattern, segment dislocation, and treatment decision.

Authors' Preferences and Fractures With Special Interest

Multiple, recently performed prospective randomized studies on conservative versus operative fracture treatment in elderly patients with three- or four-part fractures consistently have shown no functional benefit with surgery.[33,34,46,47] Therefore it seems that in the setting of elderly or unfit patients, the discussion of fracture classification becomes secondary because the consequences for further treatment are questionable. However, in younger patients with high demand, a clear understanding of the fracture remains critical to restore full shoulder functionality.[40] Shrader showed that the understanding of complex fracture patterns rather than their classification should be focused on.[48] Therefore in the

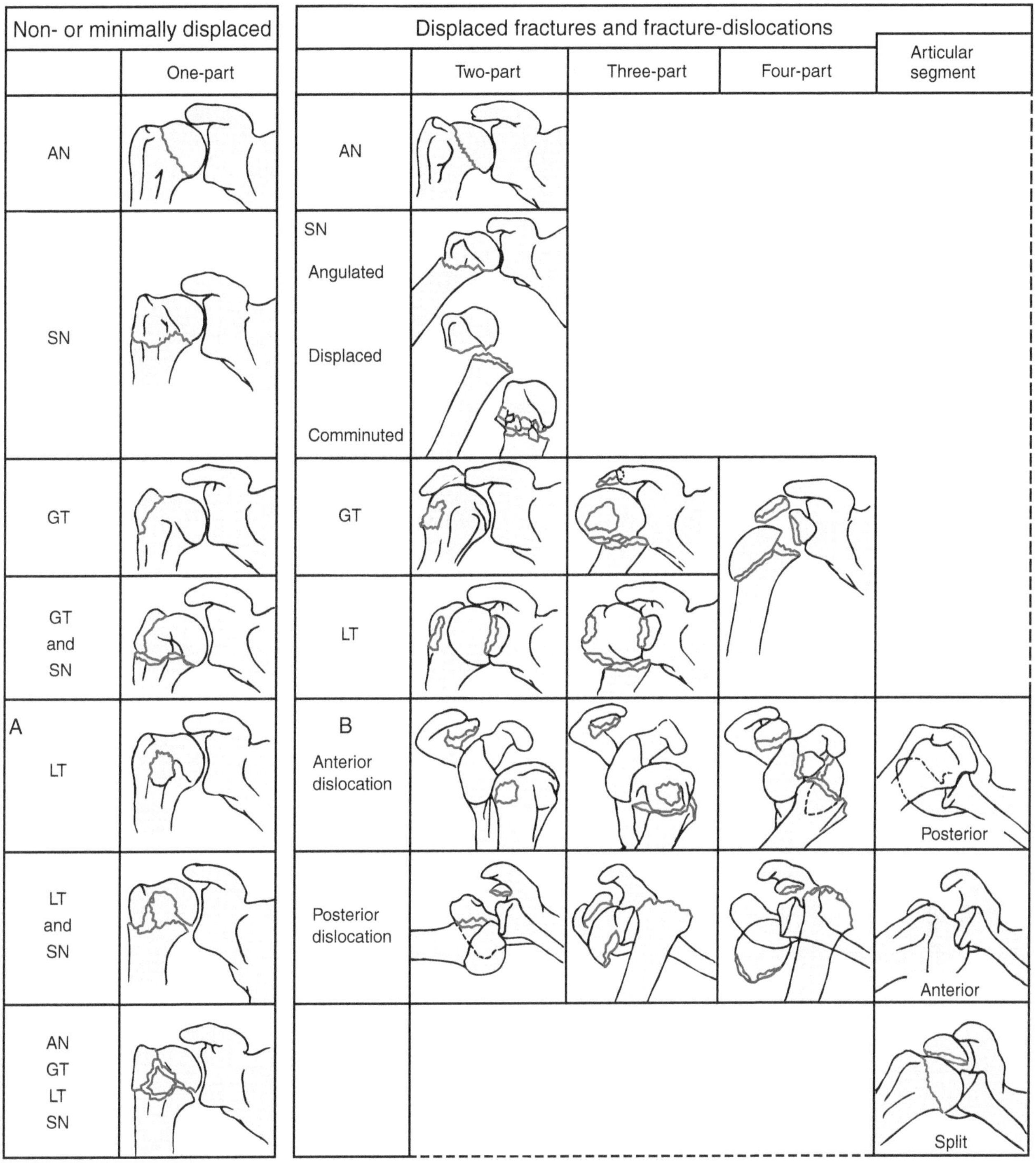

Non- or minimally displaced		Displaced fractures and fracture-dislocations				
	One-part		Two-part	Three-part	Four-part	Articular segment
AN		AN				
SN		SN Angulated Displaced Comminuted				
GT		GT				
GT and SN		LT				
A LT		B Anterior dislocation				Posterior
LT and SN		Posterior dislocation				Anterior
AN GT LT SN						Split

• **Fig. 25.2** Four-part classification for fractures and fracture-dislocations. *AN,* Anatomic neck; *GT,* greater tuberosity; *LT,* lesser tuberosity; *SN,* surgical neck. (From Browner B, Jupiter J, Krettek C, Anderson P. *Skeletal Trauma: Basic Science, Management, and Reconstruction.* 6th ed. Philadelphia: Elsevier; 2019: Figs. 47.24 and 47.25.)

authors' institution, CT scans are used for a better understanding of fractures with subtle but potentially relevant displacement and for fractures where surgical treatment is planned. Based on that, the authors use the Neer classification and pay special attention to certain fracture patterns and configurations that have been found to behave in a particular manner and are described in the following section.

Two-Part Greater Tuberosity Fracture

In an epidemiologic study on 1027 proximal humerus fractures, a 19% incidence of isolated greater tuberosity fractures was found[1] and 5% thereof were fracture-dislocations. These fractures need special mention because their classification as well as treatment remains controversial. Mutch and colleagues[49] have described a classification of greater tuberosity fractures that is based on

Extra-articular, unifocal, 2-part 11A

Subgroup 1

Greater tuberosity fracture 11A1.1

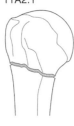

Subgroup 2

Simple fracture 11A2.1

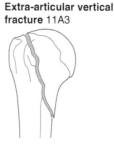

Subgroup 3

Extra-articular vertical fracture 11A3

Lesser tuberosity fracture 11A1.2

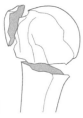

Wedge fracture 11A2.2

Mutlifragmentary fracture 11A2.3

A

Extra-articular, bifocal, 3-part, surgical neck fracture 11B

Subgroup 1

With greater tuberosity fracture 11B1.1

Subgroup 2

With lesser tuberosity fracture 11B1.2

B

Articular or 4-part fracture 11C

Subgroup 1
"anatomical neck fracture"

Valgus impacted with greater and/or lesser tuberosity fracture 11C1.1

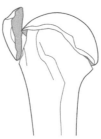

Isolated anatomical neck 11C1.3

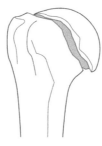

Subgroup 2
"anatomical neck and metaphyseal fracture"

Intact articular surface 11C3.1

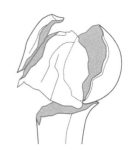

Articular surface fracture 11C3.2

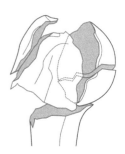

Articular surface fracture and diaphyseal extension 11C3.3

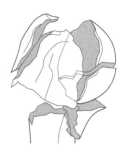

C

• **Fig. 25.3** (A–C) Description of the Arbeitsgemeinschaft für Osteosynthesefragen/American Society for Internal Fixation fracture classification of the proximal humerus. Copyright by AO Foundation, Switzerland. (Adapted from Meinberg EG, Agel J, Roberts CS, Karam MD, Kellam JF. Fracture and Dislocation Classification Compendium—2018. *J Orthop Trauma*. 2018;32(1):S1-S70.)

fracture morphology. It separates fractures into three types: avulsion, split, and depression. They found a significantly greater number of glenohumeral dislocations in the depression (46%) compared with the avulsion (21%) and split (25%) fracture types. Neer[24] suggested treating isolated greater tuberosity fractures with >1 cm of displacement operatively. Park[50] introduced a strategy depending on the patient's activity level. Given concerns for subacromial impingement–related pain and decreased function, he recommended surgical fixation in young and active patients with a displacement of >5 mm and in athletes and overhead laborers with >3 mm. This strategy has been supported by the findings of a biomechanical study performed by Bono and colleagues.[51] They found significantly increased abduction forces of the deltoid muscle with a superior displacement of the greater tuberosity of 5 mm and 1 cm. Also, other authors agreed with the surgical treatment with a displacement of >5 mm.[52,53] Recently,

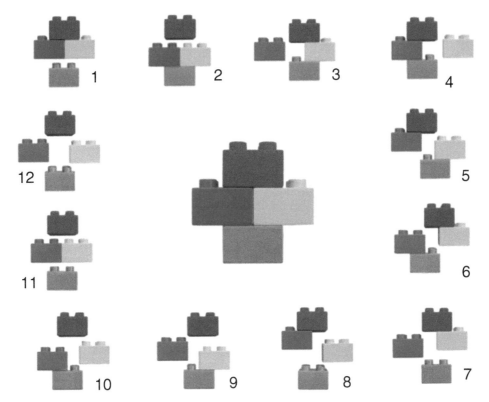

• **Fig. 25.4** (A) Binary (LEGO) description system with 12 basic fracture patterns (*red*, head; *yellow*, lesser tuberosity; *blue*, greater tuberosity; *green*, shaft). (B) Length of the medial metaphyseal head extension. The longer the extension, the more likely the head is perfused. (C) Integrity of the medial hinge. (From Hertel RW. Fractures of the proximal humerus in osteoporotic bone. *Osteoporos Int.* 2005;16(Suppl 2):S65–S72; and Browner B, Jupiter J, Krettek C, Anderson P. *Skeletal Trauma: Basic Science, Management, and Reconstruction.* 6th ed. Philadelphia: Elsevier; 2019: Fig. 47.27.)

Nyffeler et al.[54] developed a measurement method, which allows predicting a possible subacromial conflict on standard AP radiographs, considering not only the displacement of the fragment, but also the width of the subacromial space. A so-called Impingement-Index was calculated and biomechanically validated. They conclude that reduction of a displaced greater tuberosity fragment should be considered if the Impingement-Index is ≥0.7. Parsons et al.[55] found difficulties in evaluating the exact displacement of the greater tuberosity on plain radiographs and recommended the use of an AP view with the arm in 30 degrees of external rotation. Depending on the radiographic projection, about 50% of their involved experts would have recommended surgery for 5-mm displaced fractures. The evidence on this topic is not strong, and the treatment therefore mainly depends on the surgeon's preference. In active patients, the authors use CT scans to determine the exact direction and amount of displacement and consider arthroscopic or open surgical reduction in cases with >5 mm of displacement. In elderly patients with low bone quality, the threshold for conservative treatment is higher and at least up to 1 cm of displacement.

Fracture morphology significantly influences the technical aspects of surgical management. Avulsion-type fractures involve a small fragment of bone and the fracture line is horizontal. The mechanism is probably similar to rotator cuff tears with the tendon avulsing a fragment of bone rather than causing a cuff tear. These fractures usually can be treated conservatively. Should fixation be required for displaced fractures, an (arthroscopic) double-row suture or suture bridge technique can be performed.

Split-type fractures involve a large fragment with a vertical fracture line. For surgical fixation of this type of fracture, a low-profile suture plate may be used but other techniques including suture fixation, tension band, screws, and conventional plate fixation have also been described.

Depression-type fractures involve a fragment that is displaced inferiorly. This lesion is essentially a very lateral Hill-Sachs-type lesion due to impaction of the entire greater tuberosity beneath the inferior surface of the glenoid during glenohumeral dislocation. The authors usually treat these fractures conservatively. If pain or functional impairment persists, a magnetic resonance imaging (MRI) to assess the rotator cuff should be performed.

Head-Split Fractures and Fracture-Dislocations

Since Neer's[24] definition, head-split and head-impression fractures are also mentioned together with fracture-dislocations. The incidence was found to be about 6% anterior, 0.4% posterior, and 0.7% of articular surface fractures.[1] The term "head-split" is often associated with the development of AVN, even though this condition can only be considered a poor-to-moderate predictor of humeral head ischemia.[38] In general, a clear definition and classification of head-split fractures are lacking in the literature and historically have been based on plain radiographs.[38,56,57] This makes the already scarce number of outcome reports even more difficult to interpret. Peters and colleagues[58] recently proposed a classification system of four distinct head-split fracture patterns, based on the available evidence and their own clinical experience:

Type I: Head-split fracture with the fracture line within the posterior half of the humeral head with the larger head fragment located anteriorly.

Type II: Head-split fracture with the fracture line within the anterior half of the humeral head with the larger head fragment located posteriorly.

Type III: Head-split fracture with a loose or free-floating central fragment.

Type IV: Comminuted head-split fracture.

In a recently published paper by the same group, 30 patients with a head-split fracture were retrospectively evaluated, with a mean follow-up of 49 ± 18 months (range: 12–83 months). Of those 30, 24 were treated with ORIF, 4 with rTSA, and 2 with HA. The complication rate was 83% overall and 88% for primary ORIF, 75% for primary rTSA, and 50% for HA. The revision rate was 29% for ORIF (excluding the three cases of implant removal) and 0% for primary rTSA and hemiarthroplasty (HA). No factor was found to be associated with clinical failure except for a trend for worse outcomes in patients with higher BMI; the above-mentioned classification could not predict clinical outcome. However, patients who underwent revision procedures had worse clinical outcome scores overall. rTSA may be the most predictable treatment option for head-split fractures in elderly patients.

Fracture-dislocations need emergent treatment and special attention should be paid to locked anterior greater tuberosity and posterior lesser tuberosity fracture-dislocations. Hersche and Gerber[59] described a series of these fractures with additional occult anatomic or surgical neck fractures. During the reposition maneuver, the head fragment stayed in its primary locked anterior or posterior position and the occult fracture line was displaced. All of these patients developed AVN. Therefore the authors first rule out such an obscure fracture by CT scan when the radiograph is suspicious. When a neck fracture is excluded, a careful try of closed reduction under general anesthesia can be made. If a fracture of the anatomic or surgical neck is detected on the CT scan, one careful try of closed reduction under fluoroscopy can be done with standby for ORIF in the operating room. In situ ORIF before reduction may be considered if there is not much fracture displacement; otherwise, the head needs to be carefully reduced through the rotator interval (which can be extended into a subscapularis tenotomy if needed). If the fracture is not displaced, the plate can be used as reduction-aid only and be removed afterwards with "conservative" fracture treatment (Fig. 25.5).

Neer[5] proposed primary prosthetic replacement for four-part fracture-dislocations and articular fracture involvement of >50% of the humeral head. However, posterior fracture-dislocations should be mentioned separately. Despite their rarity, Robinson et al. described a series of 26 younger patients with posterior fracture-dislocations. They were treated with ORIF and had excellent functional results after 2 years.[60] Please see Technique Spotlight: Open Reduction and Bone Grafting of reverse Hill Sachs (Chapter 24) for a detailed description of one way to manage these challenging injuries in the acute setting.

Management

Despite voluminous literature on the treatment of fractures of the proximal humerus, there is still no standard of care, and a lot of controversies remain. The highly variable nature of this injury, the difficult classification of the fractures, and the high number of treatment strategies with new implants (that are promoted by manufacturers and surgeons) are possible reasons for these disagreements. Prospective randomized studies comparing different treatment options for specific fracture types are relatively rare,[61] and the management and especially the surgical technique are mainly based on the surgeon's experiences and preferences. This section gives a general view on the nonoperative and operative management of fractures of the proximal humerus based on the current literature.

Emergency Treatment

Open fractures are rare but need rapid treatment. Prophylactic antibiotics and tetanus prophylaxis (if indicated) are administered immediately in the emergency department, followed by a primary débridement and irrigation of an adequately exposed wound, and, finally, skeletal stabilization with either temporary external fixation or definitive internal fixation, if direct soft tissue closure is possible. If a vascular injury is suspected, emergency angiography and vascular repair are recommended. Depending on the fracture type, nerve involvement was found in the electromyography in up to 82%.[62] The axillary nerve was most frequently injured and therefore must be tested at the time of first treatment (check for deltoid muscle fibrillations when the patient is asked to slightly abduct the shoulder to indicate that the axillary nerve is intact). The second most often affected nerve is the suprascapular nerve. A traumatic nerve palsy in this scenario is generally not an indication for an emergent treatment because the majority of cases are due to traction injuries and resolve spontaneously. However, special care must be taken in case of high-energy trauma or worsening pain and nerve palsy. In such cases, vascular injury with subsequent damage to the brachial plexus must be ruled out by emergent angiography.

Evaluation of BMD and Its Influence on Fracture Management

The age and sex distribution and the high incidence of low-energy trauma highlight the role of osteoporosis in fractures of the proximal humerus. Low BMD has shown to be an important risk factor for fractures of the proximal humerus with significant influence on their treatment.[63–67] Regarding this association, elderly patients with fractures of the proximal humerus should undergo a fragility workup, including an assessment of previous fractures in their skeletal history.[68] Dual-energy X-ray absorptiometry (DXA) is the gold standard for assessing osteoporosis in patients. However, it is valid only for specific anatomic sites which do not include the proximal humerus. There is evidence, however, that the BMD of the upper limb (distal radius) is less than that of typically measured sites (such as the proximal femur and lumbar spine) in patients with proximal humerus fractures.[3] Nevertheless, the assessment of bone quality should be part of the decision-making process for the treatment of PHFs.

Several options may be used to quantify osteoporosis in the proximal humerus. However, one of the limiting factors until recently was the lack of validated measurement methods. Tingart et al.[69] introduced a cortical thickness measurement concept that correlated to local BMD of the (nonfractured) proximal humerus. On an AP radiograph, two levels were defined to calculate the cortical thickness. The first one is chosen at the level where the endosteal borders of the diaphyseal cortex become parallel and the second level is 2 cm distal to the first one. The combined cortical thickness is calculated as a mean of the medial and lateral cortical thickness at the two levels and adjusted for the magnification error of the radiograph. They found a combined cortical thickness of <4 mm to be a reliable and reproducible predictor for low BMD of the proximal humerus. In a later study, the combined cortical thickness showed a strong correlation to the DXA of the femur and lumbar spine. However, the threshold value of 6 mm resulted in a better sensitivity and a specificity for predicting osteoporosis.[70]

Peripheral quantitative CT (pQCT) also provides a good method to assess BMD of the proximal humerus, as shown by Krappinger et al.[29] This method can be combined with the CT scan, which is often used for definitive fracture classification and planning of surgery.[69]

In a study performed in our institution, we defined the deltoid tuberosity index (DTI), a simple one-level measurement on the AP radiograph.[71] The index is calculated just proximal to

the deltoid tuberosity, where the outer cortical border become parallel for the first time. This structure usually is well outlined on the AP fracture radiograph because of the internally rotated relieving posture of the arm. At this level, the outer cortical diameter is divided by the inner endosteal diameter resulting in a ratio, which does not need to be corrected for the magnification error (Fig. 25.6). A further upside of this measurement is that this region of the humerus is hardly involved by proximal humerus fractures, in contrast to the Tingart region. In an initial study, the correlation between the DTI and the BMD of the (nonfractured and fractured) humeral head (measured with pQCT) was strong ($r = .8$, $P < .001$).[71] Furthermore, the clinical relevance of low bone quality (DTI < 1.4) for complications after locking plate ORIF surgical treatment of proximal humerus fractures was evident. Patients younger than 65 years

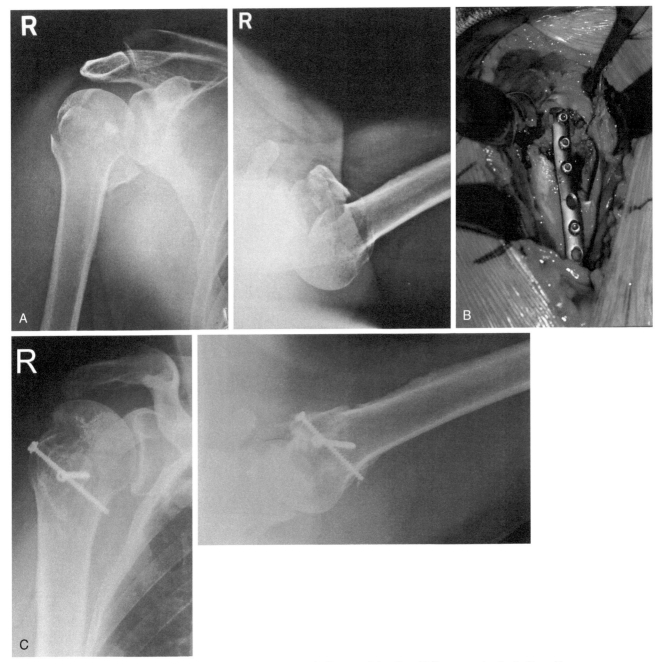

• **Fig. 25.5** (A) A 56-year-old man with a posterior fracture-dislocation. (B) Temporary in situ fixation with one-third tubular plate. (C) Definitive fixation of lesser tuberosity with screws, radiographic follow-up 4 years postoperatively. (D and E) Clinical follow-up 4 years postoperatively.

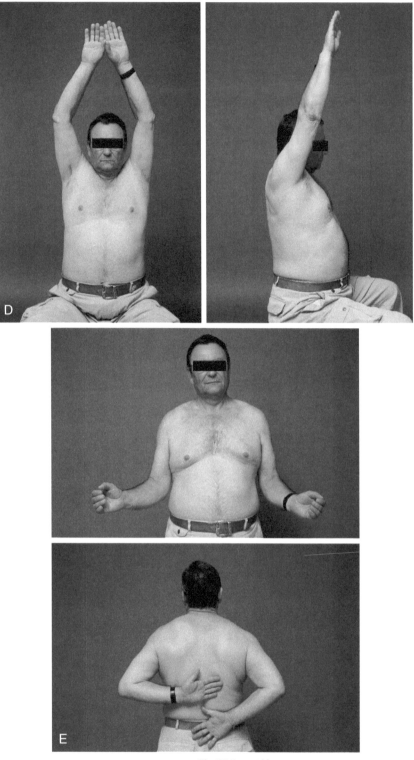

• Fig. 25.5, cont'd

with a DTI >1.4 had the best chance of avoiding head screw cut-out (94%).[67] Preoperative assessment of local BMD should be part of the treatment plan for patients with proximal humerus fractures.[72,73]

In addition to understanding the effects of osteoporosis on the proximal humerus, aiding the diagnosis and treatment of

this disease can also help prevent other fractures and the morbidity and mortality associated with them. Many risk factors for primary osteoporosis have been identified, including increased age, tobacco smoking, sedentary lifestyle, and alcoholism. Secondary osteoporosis has been linked to metabolic disorders, malabsorptive diseases, rheumatism, and hypogonadism. In

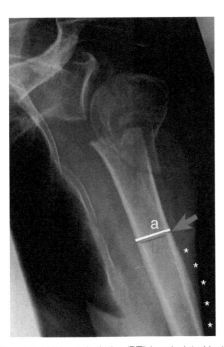

• **Fig. 25.6** The deltoid tuberosity index (DTI) is calculated just proximal to the deltoid tuberosity (*asterisks*), where the outer cortical borders become parallel for the first time. At this level, the outer cortical diameter (*a*) is divided by the inner endosteal diameter (*b*) resulting in a ratio, which does not need to be corrected for the magnification error. DTI values of <1.4 have been found to correlate very well with low bone quality of the humeral head.

general, the more risk factors that are present, the greater is the risk of fracture.[74] Decreased serum vitamin D is common, with reported rates ranging from 40% to 90% in adults, and is strongly associated with bone loss in patients with known osteoporosis. Hypovitaminosis D has been shown to strongly correlate with fracture risk.[75]

The World Health Organization (WHO) and US National Osteoporosis Foundation recommend that women aged >65 years and men aged >70 years as well as all patients >50 years based on their risk profile undergo BMD screening. According to the WHO definition, any patient who sustains a fragility fracture is assumed to have underlying osteoporosis and therefore should undergo BMD screening as well. Prevention is the most important principle in the management of osteoporosis and cannot be overemphasized.[76] The surgeon must recognize risk factors for osteoporosis that may adversely affect surgical outcomes and consider referral for preventive strategies. Adequate caloric intake, appropriate dietary calcium and vitamin D intake, and resistance exercise are methods of increasing peak bone mass.[76] Cigarette smoking should be discouraged or discontinued completely, and alcohol should be consumed only in moderation. Since the majority of osteoporosis-related fractures result from falls, it is also important to evaluate risk factors for falling. Treatment of osteoporosis should be considered for patients with low BMD (a *T*-score of −1.0 to −2.5) and either a 10-year risk of hip fracture >3%, or a 10-year risk of any osteoporotic fracture >20%.[77] The US Food and Drug Administration (FDA) recommends that postmenopausal women diagnosed with osteoporosis should receive 1500 mg of calcium and 400 IU of vitamin D daily, while the US National Osteoporosis Foundation recommends 800–1000 IU of vitamin D daily for adults older than age 50 years.[74]

Nonoperative Treatment

Indications and Outcome

Since Neer[24] suggested conservative treatment for one-part (non-displaced or minimally displaced) fractures, they have been the scope of only a few studies. However, most found good functional results in the majority of treated patients.[78–80] While displaced two-, three- and four-part fractures used to be treated operatively, they have become the scope of conservative treatment now.[11,33,34,47] This might be due to relatively high complication rates after ORIF[8,81,82] or to the consistently restricted functional results after fracture HA.[83–85]

In recent years, several prospective randomized studies looked at conservative treatment compared with surgical intervention. A recent multicenter, prospective, randomized clinical trial (the PROFHER trial) was performed in the United Kingdom.[11] The authors concluded that there is no statistically significant benefit of surgery versus conservative treatment after 2 years. This study has been heavily criticized for the selection bias in its methodology (i.e., all patients who "met clear indication for surgery" were excluded), inappropriate scoring (Oxford Shoulder Score, SF-12, EQ-5D), involvement of too many surgeons, too many surgical techniques, and no trial-related clinical assessment or radiological follow-up.[86,87] There is no doubt, however, this study was an impressive undertaking that has stimulated discussion and has paved the way for further studies on this topic.

In studies performed by Olerud et al.,[33,34] patients with valgus-impacted three- or four-part fractures were not included because they were treated conservatively anyway. However, they looked at the conservative treatment of patients over 55 years with displaced three- and four-part fractures compared with angular stable ORIF or HA. Overall, they found no significant difference in terms of function. The conservatively treated patients with three-part fractures reached a mean Constant score (CS) of 58 points compared with 61 points in the ORIF group and the conservatively treated patients with four-part fractures of 49 points compared with 48 points in patients with hemiarthroplasties. However, the quality of life (EQ-5D) was in favor of the surgical groups at the costs of a higher complication and revision rate.[33,34] The authors concluded that the tendency of better functional results or quality of life after a surgical procedure of these fractures has to be balanced against the higher risk of revision rates. They found that the overall acceptable outcome and limited need for surgical intervention might justify a conservative treatment of elderly, low-demand patients with three- or four-part fractures.

Recent prospective randomized studies also looked at conservative treatment versus rTSA in patients over 70 years. Even here the differences in outcome are subtle. One study found no significant clinical difference,[88] whereas the other one found a significantly better functional outcome after rTSA.[89] The CSs are between 50 and 60 points in both groups after 1 or 2 years with better ROM in the rTSA group. The authors conclude that rTSA should probably only be offered to elderly patients with high demands.

Given the results of all these randomized controlled trials (RCTs), it seems that the randomization of the patients only based on age and fracture type brings the results to a similar but relatively low level in both the conservative and the operative groups. If we look for examples in older reports on conservative treatment for displaced proximal humerus fractures, we can find 80% of good or excellent results for valgus and varus-impacted fractures.[90,91] Randomization leads undoubtedly to the highest level of evidence but it may not lead to the best functional outcome for the individual patient.

In our opinion, a more individual treatment concept can help to choose the right patient for the right treatment. Such an individual treatment strategy can be based on age, individual demands, and bone quality. These factors seem to be important for the functional outcome after the treatment of proximal humerus fractures and are difficult to include in RCTs as groups would become too small.

Nonoperative Treatment Protocol

Lefevre-Colau[92] showed in his prospective RCT that physiotherapy with early mobilization is safe for conservative treatment of patients with stable impacted proximal humerus fractures.

In a recently published double-blind RCT, Carbone et al.[93] showed that, in contrast to the strict "five times a week physiotherapy regimen" proposed by Lefevre-Colau, two sessions of physiotherapy a week showed comparable results.

In St. Gallen, we use the same protocol for all of our nonoperative and operatively treated proximal humerus fractures. The arm is supported in a sling for 6 weeks. No therapy for the first 2 weeks, then physiotherapy may be started with pendulum exercises for weeks 3 and 4. Finally, in the 5 and 6 postoperative weeks, the patients can begin unrestricted passive ROM.[33,34,47] At week 6, active-assisted to active ROM progression is initiated with a continued emphasis on regaining full passive ROM.

Complications After Nonoperative Treatment

For one-part fractures, the most frequent complication is limited ROM, especially internal and external rotation.[80] A markedly limited shoulder function, mainly caused by stiffness, has occurred in up to 10% of patients.[79] We find that patients who are unwilling or unable to prioritize stretching after union of the fracture due to chronic pain or other impediments are at risk of this complication. Late arthroscopic capsular release with release of subacromial adhesions is an option for patients who have recalcitrant stiffness due to capsular contracture and adhesions who fail to progress with physical therapy.[94]

In a recently published systematic review and meta-analysis on operative and nonoperative treatment of PHFs,[95] the following reinterventions for conservatively treated fractures were mentioned: arthroplasty for displacement and malunion, open reduction and internal plate fixation for displacement, and acromioplasty for impingement complaints. In the included studies, there was no significant difference in the rate of AVN between operative and nonoperative treatment of PHFs.[79,80] The rate of nonunion and AVN, however, depends on the fracture type.[90,91,96] Initial manipulations and smoking are predictors for nonunions in nonoperatively treated patients.[96]

Surgical Treatment

Despite the abundance of literature on surgical treatment of proximal humerus fractures, there is still no standard of care, and the main question of which patient and fracture are suitable for which surgical treatment remains unanswered. Surgeon's preference, patient's individuality, the high variety of fracture configurations, the difficulty in classification, and the high number of different implants are the main reasons for these disagreements. Also, prospective studies comparing different treatment options for specific fracture types are relatively rare and the management and especially the surgical technique are mainly based on the surgeon's experience and preferences. However, with the large choice of different implants, there may not be a gold standard and it may be reasonable that each surgeon chooses the implant, which works best in their hands.

After the indication for a surgical treatment is made, the preoperative planning consists of a precise understanding of the fracture pattern, preferably with the help of an additional CT scan. Furthermore, the surgeon should choose the implant with which he has the most experience. But the treating surgeon must also be experienced with variable devices because the treatment may change during surgery, for example, when internal fixation is not stable enough or the fracture cannot be reduced anatomically and primary hemi- or reverse arthroplasty is needed.

Conventional Versus Locking Plate ORIF

Despite the voluminous reports on locking plates, there are not many studies comparing their clinical outcome with conventional plate ORIF. Their biomechanical advantage has been proven in cadaver studies.[97] Handschin et al.[98] retrospectively compared the outcome of 30 patients treated with angular stable ORIF with a matched group of 60 patients who were treated with one-third tubular plates. Both groups included mainly three- and four-part fractures, and the mean age of the patients was 62 years. The mean CS of both groups was 60 points. Furthermore, they found no differences between the two groups concerning complication and revision rate, but the implant costs were significantly higher for the locking plate.

Locking Plate ORIF and Intramedullary Nailing

Despite the anatomic shape and multiple options for head screw placement of newer implants, ORIF is still demanding, and especially complex fracture types must not be underestimated.[99] It seems that along with the broad use of precontoured locking plates, their indications have been expanded to more complex fracture patterns. This might be a reason why there is an increasing number of reports about high complication rates found in the literature.[6,8–10,82] A subgroup analysis showed that displaced articular segment fractures and fracture-dislocations or head splits as well as varus displaced fractures were all prone to complications, revision surgeries, and diminished clinical outcomes.[6,7,82] Further predictors for impaired outcome were found to be low BMD (<95 mg/cm^3, or DTI < 1.4), increasing age, nonanatomic reduction of the medial hinge, and smoking.[6,64,67,100] These factors should be kept in mind when considering an angular stable ORIF (locking plate) for a proximal humerus fracture.

The complication rate after the use of angular stable implants varies between 10% and 60% with revision rates up to 50%.[6,8–10,101,102] The complications can be divided into "implant" and "nonimplant related." AVN, malreduction, primary screw cutout, and infection are the most common complications, which are unrelated to the implant. In larger series or systematic reviews, the rate of AVN is reported to be between 4% and 54%, depending on fracture types (highest for fracture-dislocations and head splits).[7,9,10,102,103] Secondary loss of reduction, secondary screw cut-out with or without destruction of the glenoid, and failure of the screws or plate are reported complications, which are classified as "implant related." The rate of secondary varus displacement is reported to be up to 25% and this is felt to be related to an impaired clinical outcome.[8,9] Secondary screw cut-out with penetration of the joint occurs because of the angular stability of the implant, which does not allow any slipback of the screws (unlike conventional screws) in case of head collapse or AVN.

The appearance of this complication is consistently reported to be between 6% and 11%.[6,9,10,101,102] It should be of special interest because the screws can severely and rapidly impair the glenoid cartilage and bone stock, which limits the options of later revision surgery.[99]

A further complication, which is primarily related to the deltoid-split approach used in the minimally invasive plate osteosynthesis (MIPO) technique, is an axillary nerve injury. It is reported to be between 0% and 4%.[101,104] In a systematic review of three RCTs and three prospective cohort studies comparing the deltoid-split with the deltopectoral approach including 426 patients, no axillary nerve injuries were reported.[105] The anterolateral deltoid-split puts the crossing, anterior motor branch of the axillary nerve at risk. The nerve can either be approached directly from superficial to deep or once the proximal split is large enough, it can be palpated on the undersurface of the deep deltoid. If a low surgical neck fracture is present, care should be taken to ensure the nerve is not entrapped at the fracture site.[106]

Locked intramedullary nailing (IMN) with or without tension band sutures, although technically demanding, has shown comparable results to locking plate ORIF.[107,108] It has potential advantages of improved medial column support and a more minimally invasive approach that leads to less disturbance of the healing biology. On the other hand, poor results have been reported with first- and second-generation nails with up to 73% rotator cuff problems[109] and high rates of nonunion.[110] Meanwhile, third-generation humeral IM nails with a small core diameter, short length, and straight design are available. These features allow and facilitate a percutaneous approach through the supraspinatus muscle fibers to avoid the tendinous insertion at the footprint (comparable to a cannula inserted during arthroscopy for rotator cuff repair). In a retrospective review[111] of 41 patients with two-part surgical neck fractures treated with IMN, all fractures went on to union and no screw migration or articular perforation was found. One patient had asymptomatic AVN and two patients underwent revision. Only in one patient the nail had to be removed due to rotator cuff irritation and shoulder pain due to a high placement of the nail. While some excellent results have been reported and the latest techniques are presented here, a systematic review suggested that the indications for nailing should be limited to two-part surgical neck and three-part fractures as the complication rate of four-part fractures was found to be up to 63%. We agree that two-part displaced surgical neck fractures are an excellent indication for an IM device.[112]

Primary HA Versus Locking Plate ORIF

HA is notorious for poor outcomes due to the high rate (~50%) of greater tuberosity nonunion or resorption, along with the further risk of tuberosity nonunion.[83,113] On the other hand, the revision rate of hemiarthroplasties for fracture is low as, even with a poor functional result, the pain is typically minimal. Therefore this approach has served as a good solution for low-demand patients with complex fracture types since the 1970s. In a study comparing HA and angular stable ORIF in elderly patients (mean age 75 years) with fracture-dislocations or head-split fractures, we found clinically better results in the ORIF group especially if they had no complication (mean 72 points in CS). However, the complication rate in the ORIF group was high with an AVN rate over 50% in these complex fractures and the revision rate was clearly in favor of the HA group (4% vs. 45%).[7] These findings are comparable to other studies[82,114] that compared HA with angular stable (locking plate) ORIF also for three- and four-part fractures.

With the rise of rTSA for successful fracture treatment in the elderly, HA has lost ground in this patient group. The big question remains how to treat younger and active patients or elderly patients with high demands if the fractures cannot be reduced in a stable manner. Should they be treated with an HA knowing the risk of secondary displacement of the greater tuberosity and an unsatisfying clinical result is 50%? Or should we implant primary rTSA in younger patients with irreducible fractures and accept the risk of later challenging revision surgeries? With our treatment algorithm (see following section), we attempt to answer these questions.

Primary Locking Plate ORIF Versus Primary rTSA

Recently, first results of the DelPhi trial,[14] a multicenter, single-blinded RCT, comparing ORIF and rTSA for treating displaced proximal humerus fractures in the elderly was published. Patients between 65 and 85 years with three- or four-part proximal humerus fractures (OTA/AO B2 and C2) were included. At 2-year follow-up, 57 patients who received rTSA and 47 patients who received ORIF were evaluated. The patients in the rTSA group scored significantly better than the ORIF group in the overall comparison of the CS. The CS was 68.0 points for the rTSA group compared with 54.6 points for the ORIF group. Furthermore, the CS stratified by age indicated that both age groups (65–74 and 75–85) profited from rTSA. The subscores of the CS showed that the benefit of rTSA was mainly due to better ROM (except for internal rotation) and strength. In the rTSA group, four patients had a secondary surgical procedure. In the ORIF group, seven patients had a secondary surgical procedure, four patients were converted to reverse TSA, and three patients had implants removed. The data suggest an advantage of rTSA over ORIF in the treatment of displaced three- and four-part PHFs in elderly patients.

Primary rTSA Versus Primary HA

With the increasing interest in primary rTSA for the treatment of proximal humerus fractures, some recent comparative reports have been published with mainly small numbers of included patients and medium-term follow-up.[115–118]

A systematic review and meta-analysis by Austin et al.[119] analyzed all RCTs and cohort studies reporting on rTSA in comparison with HA for geriatric (>65 years) proximal humerus fractures. Fifteen studies including 421 patients treated with rTSA and 492 treated with HA were included. Compared with HA, the rTSA group had significantly improved pain scores, outcome scores, and forward flexion. The HA group had a significantly increased risk of reoperation (relative risk = 2.8). Multiple studies reported on HA patients being converted to an rTSA to improve function or pain.[117,120,121] The authors conclude that there is no outcome evaluated in their study in which HA outperforms rTSA underlining an important role for rTSA as a first-line arthroplasty option for PHFs in a patient population older than 65 years.

Delayed rTSA for Failed Conservative Treatment

A recent systematic review,[122] including four comparative cohort studies[123–126] as well as 12 case series, found no differences in forward flexion, clinical outcome scores, or all-cause reoperation comparing acute versus delayed rTSA. These findings suggest that rTSA performed in a delayed fashion for the treatment of PHF sequelae does not result in relevant inferior outcomes or more complications, making initial conservative treatment, with the possibility of delayed rTSA if symptomatic sequelae develop, a reasonable treatment strategy without compromising the ultimate outcome. The similar outcomes for acute primary rTSA and delayed primary rTSA provide the surgeon flexibility with surgical timing. Some patients with PHF may have comorbidities and other injuries. A "wait-and-see" approach to elderly patients with PHF can reduce surgical intervention for those patients who do well with conservative management while providing good functional outcomes with delayed rTSA to those who remain symptomatic. Given the risks associated with surgery, this option seems to be especially important and has to be considered in geriatric patients.

This strategy is one of the mainstays of our treatment algorithm for elderly patients (see below) and the above-mentioned clinical results reflect our experience. However, one has to be aware that delayed rTSA is technically more demanding than primary rTSA. In addition, there are particular fracture patterns that may theoretically do poorly with delayed rTSA. There is no actionable data on these subgroups but in our experience, these include fracture-dislocations where the dislocated head fragment will lead to an imbalance in the soft tissue envelope that may lead to an unstable arthroplasty if performed late. In addition, fractures of the proximal humerus that also involve the humeral shaft may be more challenging late as stem placement may be more complex. Lastly, fractures where the metadiaphysis becomes incarcerated deep within the deltoid tend to get stiff and also make the late dissection challenging to avoid injury to the axillary nerve and deltoid.

rTSA for Failed Operative Treatment

Limited evidence is available for the use of rTSA for failed operative treatment of proximal humerus fractures as salvage option.[122,127,128] Nevertheless, this is an important topic as rTSA is often the only remaining option for improvement of shoulder function in these patients.

We reported on a negatively selected series of 121 patients with complications after ORIF with locking plates.[99] Complications resulted in secondary arthroplasties in over 50% of the patients. rTSA improved the mean CS from 25 to 48 points. Nevertheless, these outcome scores are worse than the results after primary rTSA for fracture or delayed rTSA for fracture sequelae after nonoperative treatment.

Ernstbrunner et al.[127] evaluated a cohort of 30 patients with a mean age of 52 years (30–59 years) who received rTSA after failed ORIF (23%) or conversion from failed HA to rTSA (77%). The main reason for salvage rTSA was painful shoulder dysfunction, which was mainly associated with screw cut-out and humeral head collapse in ORIF patients and with glenoid erosion in or rotator cuff dysfunction in HA patients. In 63% of the patients, >1 previous shoulder operation other than rTSA had been performed. With the available data, the number of previous surgical procedures, infection prior to salvage rTSA, and failed HA were significantly associated with postoperative complications. At a minimum of 8-year follow-up, the shoulder function significantly improved compared to preoperatively. The authors conclude that salvage rTSA for failed operative treatment of PHFs in patients younger than 60 years is associated with a high complication rate of approximately one-third. Revision of hemiarthroplasties is associated with inferior overhead function compared with revision of failed ORIF, and an inability to anatomically reinsert the greater tuberosity is associated with inferior overall shoulder function. Nonetheless, salvage rTSA ultimately leads to reliable and durable improvement in function and pain in these painful and severely disabled shoulders for which no other treatment method has proved to be comparably successful.

Holschen et al.[128] reported on 28 patients, in whom an HA, as a treatment for a PHF, had failed and underwent conversion into an rTSA. Final follow-up was at a mean of 61 months postoperatively. Mean ASES (American Shoulder and Elbow Surgeons) and adjusted CSs improved significantly to 59 points and 63%, respectively. The visual analogue scale (VAS) pain score decreased significantly. The mean forward flexion and abduction were 104 and 98 degrees, respectively. Nine patients (32%) had a complication. In conclusion, conversion to rTSA leads to a significant reduction in pain as well as a considerable improvement in shoulder function. However, the complication rate of one-third is relatively high and needs to be considered.

Postoperative Rehabilitation Protocol

Independent from the surgical procedure, the postoperative treatment mainly depends on the degree of stability achieved. Stable reductions and fixations may be passively mobilized immediately after surgery, and a sling can be used for 4–6 weeks. Active ROM exercises are usually started after 6–8 weeks and strengthening after 3 months. However, the above-mentioned relatively high rate of reduction failures, even with the use of rigid, angular stable, locking implants, has questioned early mobilization after this procedure.[129]

In cases with an unstable medial hinge after any type of fixation, where the humeral head blood supply is most tenuous, passive mobilization should be delayed for at least 2–4 weeks because this has shown to be successful in terms of motion at final follow-up as well as risk reduction of loss of fixation and collapse.[129] It may take 9–12 months to regain maximal range of shoulder motion, strength, and endurance.[130]

A neutral or external rotation brace should be used for 6 weeks after ORIF of a posterior fracture-dislocation and internal rotation should be avoided during rehabilitation because internal rotation prior to posterior soft tissue healing is a position of instability.

The aftercare of primary HA or rTSA is limited by the healing of the tuberosities to the stem and to each other. In general, we believe a stiff shoulder is more easily treated and tolerated than a shoulder with displaced tuberosities; thus we use a conservative mobilization algorithm for all patients with proximal humerus fractures (including the entire range from nonoperative treatment to ORIF to HA to rTSA).[33] Patients wear a sling for 6 weeks with strict rest for 2 weeks (only passive ROM for elbow and hand). Pendulum exercises are started from week 3 and free passive mobilization from week 5 after surgery. After the first clinical and radiographic assessment at 6 weeks, free active and passive ROM is allowed. Strengthening is usually started after 3 months, when the tuberosities have healed and a reasonable ROM has been achieved.

The Development of the Treatment Algorithm

The consideration of the aforementioned controversies on the different treatment strategies for fractures of the proximal humerus led us to develop an evidence-based patient-adapted treatment algorithm for proximal humerus fractures. Our goals were (1) to find the best possible evidence for the treatment of each patient and fracture group and (2) to restore patients back to their quality of life before the trauma. Therefore we separate young and healthy patients <65 years (usually working age), who need maximal shoulder functionality to return to work as soon as possible from elderly, retired patients ≥65 years. In the latter group, there is a huge range in demands and in state of health. Thus we separate here patients who live in nursing homes or need help for their daily living from independent elderly patients with high demands. As the latter group of independent, active elderly may have the same demands as the young patients, they need a maximum shoulder function as well. However, as it is difficult to draw a clear line at a certain age, we assess the local bone quality to estimate the biological age of these patients. Finally, we adapt the treatment to the fracture types in all these groups of patients. Since 2014 we have used this algorithm in our clinic and have followed up all patients with isolated proximal humerus fractures in a prospective analysis. The development of the first version of the algorithm was published in the fifth and sixth editions of *Skeletal Trauma*.[15,131] We also published the clinical 1-year results of the first 192 patients and found mainly good clinical results with the same quality of life (EQ-5D) before and 1 year after the injury.[132] As a direct consequence of our experience using Version 1.0 of this algorithm, we modified the algorithm to simplify and improve it (Version 2.0) (Figs. 25.7 and 25.8).

Young and Active Patients <65 Years

This group of patients contains mainly younger men because they have their peak incidence for PHFs between the ages of 30 and 60 years. These patients usually have good bone quality and need to return to work as soon as possible. The authors' treatment pathways to regain maximal shoulder function is depicted in the algorithm (Fig. 25.7).

As mentioned previously, the literature is scarce on conservative treatment for proximal humerus fractures in young patients. Therefore the range of nonoperative treatment in these patients is limited to one-part fractures with the exception of isolated fractures of the tuberosities. The authors use CT scans to assess the exact amount of displacement and prefer operative treatment in case of more than 5 mm of superior and/or posterior displacement of the greater or more than 5 mm of medial displacement of the lesser tuberosity (see the "Authors' Preferences and Fractures With Special Interest" section). Small avulsions are usually treated arthroscopically with a double-row or a suture bridge technique. For large fractures of the greater tuberosity, the authors use a lateral one-third tubular buttress plate with tension band sutures of the cuff to the plate. Two-, three-, or four-part fractures as well as fracture-dislocations and head-split fractures are usually treated with ORIF in young patients. Here we used to separate valgus-impacted fractures as they are known to have a better prognosis than varus fracture patterns after ORIF.[73,133] For these fractures we used a simple one-third tubular plate for buttress with tension band sutures of the tuberosities in Version 1.0. For all other displaced fractures, we used an angular stable implant (NCB; Zimmer, Warsaw, IN, USA) for ORIF. If a stable reduction was not possible or the head showed no intraoperative borehole bleeding, we converted intraoperatively to HA (Zimmer; Anatomical Shoulder Fracture System) in these young patients. The advantage of this implant is the modularity, which allows a later conversion to an rTSA without the need for stem removal. All open surgeries are performed via a deltopectoral approach in our institution, except displaced greater tuberosity fractures which are fixed through a limited anterolateral deltoid-split approach.

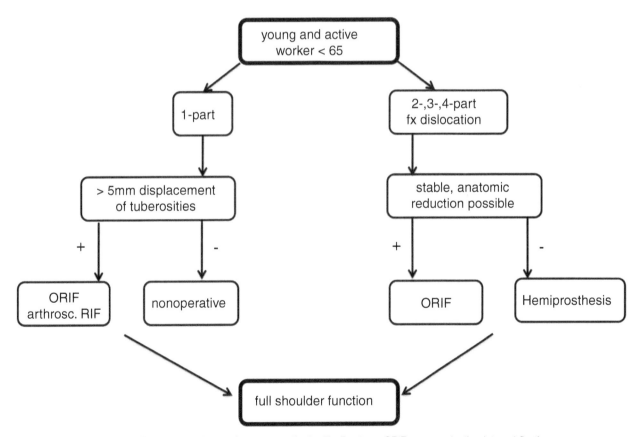

• **Fig. 25.7** Treatment pathways for young patients. *Fx*, Fracture; *ORIF*, open reduction internal fixation. (From Spross C, Farei JM, Manser M, Jacxsens M, Zdravkovic V, Jost B. Outcome of management of proximal humerus fractures using a patient-specific, evidence-based treatment algorithm. Accepted March 2021. *J Bone J Surg*.)

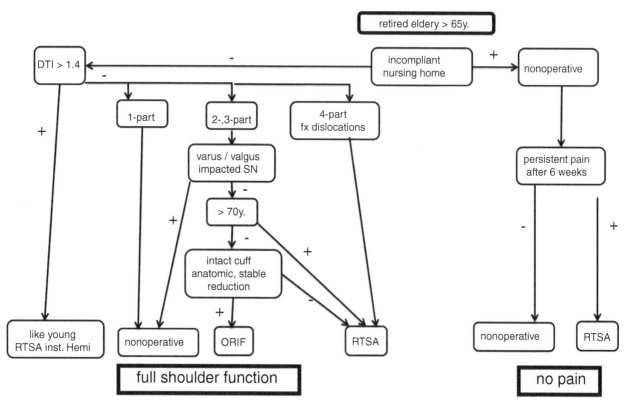

• **Fig. 25.8** Treatment pathways for elderly patients. *DTI,* Deltoid tuberosity index; *Fx,* fracture; *Hemi,* hemiarthroplasty; *ORIF,* open reduction internal fixation; *rTSA,* reverse total shoulder arthroplasty; *SN,* surgical neck. (From Spross C, Farei JM, Manser M, Jacxsens M, Zdravkovic V, Jost B. Outcome of management of proximal humerus fractures using a patient-specific, evidence-based treatment algorithm. Accepted March 2021. *J Bone J Surg.*)

Elderly Patients ≥65 Years

After the age of 50 years, the incidence of PHFs rises with a 4:1 female-to-male ratio. Osteoporosis is an important factor that influences the incidence and the outcome of these fractures in elderly patients (see the "Evaluation of BMD and Its Influence on Fracture Management" section). Furthermore, the demands and the daily activities of these patients are very individual, and therefore the treatment strategy cannot be reduced to a cutoff at a certain age. The literature shows that elderly patients do not need full shoulder function for a good quality of life, and nearly all fracture types can be treated nonoperatively with acceptable function and patient satisfaction (see the "Nonoperative Treatment: Indications and Outcome" section). However, the treatment of older patients with osteoporotic bone and high demands on shoulder function present a challenging clinical scenario to the surgeon treating PHFs. Angular stable ORIF with a locking plate does not completely solve the problem of construct stability in osteoporotic bone and leads to new complications including head screw cutout with possible damage to the glenoid. In addition, the limited shoulder function and the problems with the greater tuberosity after primary HA remain unsolved, especially for patients with osteoporotic bone. Therefore primary rTSA has gained interest in this group of patients, but there is still a lack of long-term follow-up (which might not be as important in the elderly where the prosthesis usually survives the patient). However, as mentioned, conservative treatment can yield satisfying results also in certain displaced fractures in the right patients. If conservative treatment fails, there is still secondary rTSA with promising results in the quiver of the

treating surgeon. Thus the threshold for conservative treatment in more complex fractures can be lower for elderly patients.

In the algorithm, we generally differentiate between elderly patients with high and low demands (Fig. 25.8). Patients who do regular exercises (e.g., walking, swimming, skiing, golf, tennis) and live independently without any help are classified as high demand with the need for maximal shoulder function (Fig. 25.8, left side). On the other hand, patients who need regular help for activities of daily living are classified as low demand without mandatory need for full shoulder function. We treat these patients conservatively whenever possible. Usually, pain can be controlled quickly with the use of a simple sling. The only indications of surgery in these patients would be fracture-dislocation, neurovascular injury, or persistent pain during the follow-up. If surgery is performed, we usually use an rTSA for pain relief (Fig. 25.8, right side).

Elderly patients with high demands are further assessed for osteoporosis using the DTI (Fig. 25.6). If there is good bone quality (DTI > 1.4), they are treated in the same manner as young patients with the exception of primary rTSA instead of HA in patients older than 70 years. For active patients with osteoporosis, the indication for nonoperative treatment is broader and includes all one-part fractures, up to 1-cm displacement of the tuberosities. Also, varus- or valgus-impacted two-part and three-part surgical neck fractures are treated conservatively. These fractures have been the scope of specific studies on conservative treatment with generally good functional results (see the "Nonoperative Treatment: Indications and Outcome" section). For active patients with osteoporosis, we used ORIF only in the specific circumstance of severely displaced (<50% of head/shaft contact) surgical neck fractures, <70 years of age, when the anatomical reduction was possible. However, we use primary rTSA if a stable ORIF is not possible or in four-part fractures, fracture-dislocations, and head-split fractures.

Results of Version 1.0

Starting in January 2014, all patients who suffered isolated proximal humerus fractures and were treated in our institution were eligible for the prospective enrollment in the study. Exclusion criteria were age <18 years, inability (even with support) to fill out the EQ-5D questionnaire, patients refusing to take part in the study, fracture >14 days old, initial treatment elsewhere, pathologic fractures, and concomitant fractures or injuries. In the emergency department, we assessed the demands and quality of life before the trauma (EQ-5D) and the level of independence was estimated. Local bone quality (DTI; Fig. 25.6) and the Neer fracture type were assessed on AP and lateral radiographs. A CT scan was performed if the fracture pattern was unclear or any surgical treatment was planned. The consultant orthopedic surgeon in charge defined the treatment strategy according to the algorithm. However, the algorithm was meant to guide the treatment decision and was not compulsory. Thus the assigned and effectively chosen pathways were not always the same; both were noted for further analysis. Follow-up appointments were scheduled after 3 and 12 months. A specifically trained physiotherapist examined all patients clinically including EQ-5D, CS, and Subjective Shoulder Value (SSV). Radiographic examination included AP views in internal and neutral rotation as well as axial and lateral views. Any complications or unplanned surgery were noted in the protocol. Patients unable to attend the 12-month follow-up were interviewed by phone to assess EQ-5D and SSV.

Adherence to Algorithm

A total of 192 consecutive patients with a complete 1-year follow-up were included for our first analysis.[132] Overall, the adherence to the algorithm was high and 83% of the patients were treated according to the algorithm. The main reasons for deviation from it were preferred conservative treatment in elderly patients, preferred rTSA rather than HA in patients between >65 and <70 years of age, and preferred angular stable ORIF instead of one-third tubular ORIF. In nearly one-third of the patients who were not treated according to the algorithm, the reason for deviation was patient related (e.g., patient's wish). Especially in the conservative group, patients treated according to the algorithm achieved significantly better results compared with patients who were not treated according to the algorithm.

Outcome of Treatment Groups

Totally 132 (69%) patients have been treated conservatively, 36 (19%) with ORIF, 20 (10%) with rTSA, and 4 (2%) with HA. The conservative treatment of one-part fractures worked very well for young and elderly patients (Table 25.1). Clinical results were excellent after 1 year, and unplanned surgery due to secondary displacement was rarely needed (Fig. 25.9A–B). Also, conservative treatment of varus- or valgus-impacted two- or three-part fractures in elderly patients with low bone quality was successful (Figs. 25.10A–B and 25.11A–C). We chose conservative treatment, regardless of the fracture type (apart from fracture-dislocations), for dependent low-demand patients who live in nursing homes (Fig. 25.12A–C). None of these patients needed late surgery.

ORIF achieved very satisfying clinical results after 1 year (Table 25.1), especially if the treatment was according to the algorithm. Compared with other studies, we had fewer severe complications like AVN or head screw cut-outs[6,9] which may be the result of our very specific patient selection. However, we had a higher total rate

TABLE 25.1 Outcome of Patients Treated According to the Algorithm

Treatment Group (n)	Conservative	ORIF	HA	rTSA
Mean EQ-5D preop (points)	0.9	0.9	0.89	0.8
Mean EQ-5D 1 year (points)	0.91	0.86	0.79	0.87
Mean absolute CS 1 year (points)	78.2	68.2	44	65.6
Pain	14	13	14.6	13.9
Flexion (degrees)	147.2	128	70	120.5
Mean relative CS 1 year (%)	101.4	90.2	49.8	93.3
Mean SSV 1 year (%)	82.9	77.9	45	78.3
Unplanned surgery	0	11	2	0

CS, Constant score; HA, hemiarthroplasty; ORIF, open reduction internal fixation; rTSA, reverse total shoulder arthroplasty; SSV, Subjective Shoulder Value.

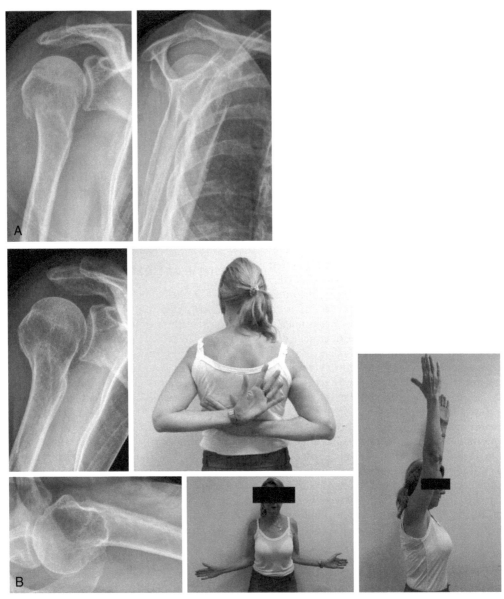

• **Fig. 25.9** (A) A 59-year-old woman with a one-part fracture. Initial radiographs, anteroposterior, and lateral views. (B) Radiographic and clinical follow-up after 6 months with anatomic healing of the fracture and good functional result (absolute Constant score: 80 points; SSV 71%; EQ-5D pretrauma: 0.89 after 6 months: 0.79).

of unplanned surgeries with a particularly high rate of implant removal in our cohort (31%). This may partially be explained by the more prominent implant we used in the beginning compared with most other studies[6,10] but also by the exclusive selection of high-demand patients for this surgical procedure.

HA was considered for patients <70 years where the fracture could not be reduced in a stable manner. It was used only in four cases; they resulted in limited function and a 50% revision rate (Table 25.1), which is unsatisfying and more or less reflects the findings of a recent study with the same implant.[134]

rTSA showed very satisfying functional outcomes after 1 year without requiring revision surgery (Table 25.1). Although the age limit was set at 70 years, we found that most of the patients between 65 and 70 years, previously considered for HA, were

treated with rTSA. Apparently, these patients were very active and the surgeons wanted to offer them the best possible solution, which they felt was rTSA rather than HA. The age cutoff for rTSA is still under debate with the increasing tendency to lower it as long-term rTSA data (not for fracture treatment) are promising[135] and the results after HA consistently unpredictable.[134]

Consequences and Conclusions

Looking at the low revision rate after conservative treatment, this selection of treatment seems to work well with a high patient satisfaction and restoration of the same quality of life after 1 year. Especially for conservative treatment, it seems important to choose the right patient with the right fracture to achieve such

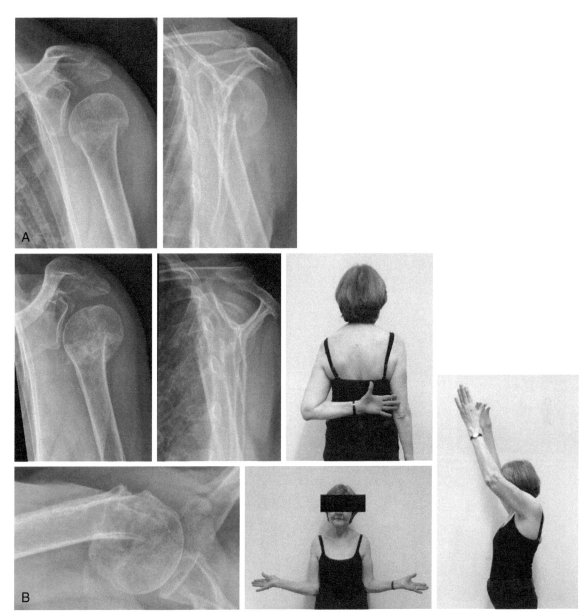

• **Fig. 25.10** (A) A 72-year-old active woman with poor bone quality and a dorsally tilted two-part fracture. Initial radiographs, anteroposterior, and lateral views. (B) Radiographic and clinical follow-up 6 months after conservative treatment showing malunion of the head fragment but a good functional result and satisfied patient (absolute Constant score: 68 points; SSV 80%; EQ-5D pretrauma: 1 after 6 months: 0.85).

good results. This becomes clear if we compare our clinical outcome of conservatively treated patients to the clinical outcome of randomized trials.[11,33,34] Results of humerus fractures treated conservatively according to our algorithm are better with regard to function as well as patient satisfaction. On the other hand, it is possible that even a broader spectrum of patients could be treated successfully with conservative treatment. Thus we expanded the indications for conservative treatment in Version 2.0 (Fig. 25.8).

Even though the overall outcome of patients treated with angular stable ORIF was successful, the high rate of unplanned surgeries, especially implant removal, was still unsatisfying. Thus we changed to a lower profile implant (PHILOS; DePuy Synthes, West Chester, PA, USA) and became even more specific with indications for ORIF in elderly patients with low bone quality (Fig. 25.8). The one-third tubular plate pathway for valgus-impacted fractures in Version 1.0 of the algorithm[132] has been omitted as, while this technique was once a mainstay, more surgeons feel comfortable with the technique for locking plate ORIF (Fig. 25.7).

The age threshold for primary rTSA is still under debate but we now lowered it from 70 years old in Version 1.0 to 65 years in Version 2.0 as the results are clearly favorable compared to ORIF or HA and long-term rTSA data for other indications are promising.[134,135]

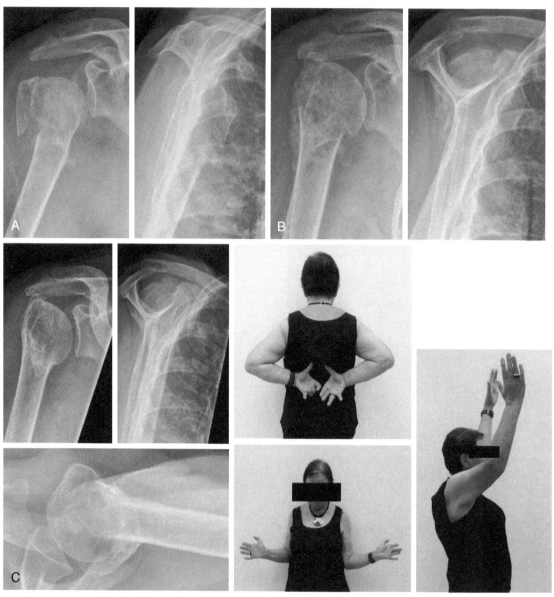

• **Fig. 25.11** (A) A 72-year-old active woman with poor bone quality and a three-part fracture. Initial radiographs, anteroposterior, and lateral views. (B) Radiographs 6 weeks posttrauma show varus impaction and callus formation. (C) Radiographic and clinical follow-up after 1 year with malunion of the head fragments but unimpaired shoulder function (absolute Constant score: 68 points, SSV 100%; EQ-5D pretrauma: 1 after 1 year: 1).

Conclusion

Despite the relatively high incidence of fractures of the proximal humerus, there is still not enough evidence to give definitive recommendations for treatment. Some quality evidence exists for the conservative treatment of one-part fractures with early mobilization. However, the acceptable displacement of the tuberosities, especially in active patients, is still unclear in this group of fractures. The newer and broadly used angular stable implants did not solve the long-standing problems of insult to the humeral head vascular supply and construct stability in osteoporotic bone for displaced three- and four-part fractures. Therefore

these fracture types were moved toward nonoperative treatment and prosthetic replacement again, especially in elderly patients. Primary HA has proven to result in good pain relief with a 50:50 chance of tuberosity healing and subsequently satisfying clinical result. Therefore rTSA has been considered for the treatment of elderly patients with high demands. These implants tend to have a better functional outcome and similar revision rates compared with HA. However, there is not enough long-term experience of their use for fracture treatment to answer all relevant questions regarding longevity and the ideal patients for these implants. Thus we believe rTSA should still be restricted to patients older than 65 years of age. In conclusion, the individuality of the patients

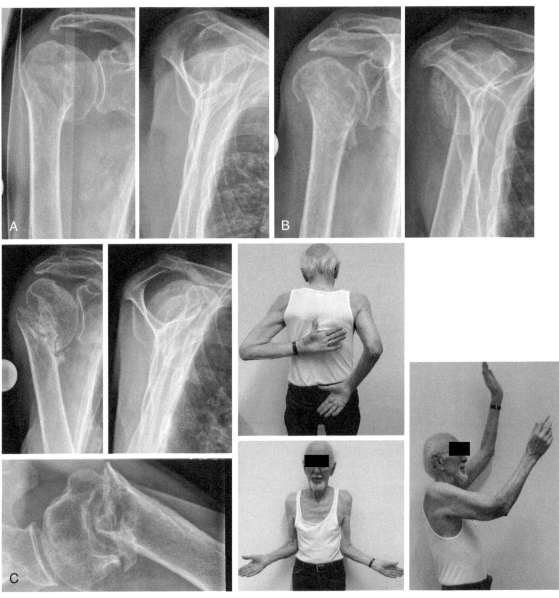

• **Fig. 25.12** (A) A 90-year-old, dependent, low-demand patient who lives in a nursing home. Initial radiographs, anteroposterior, and lateral views show a varus displaced two-part fracture. (B) Radiographs 6 weeks posttrauma show dorsally tilted secondary displacement of the head fragment. (C) Radiographic and clinical follow-up after 1 year showing a happy patient satisfied with the function of his shoulder despite fracture malunion (absolute Constant score: 37 points; SSV 70%; EQ-5D pretrauma: 0.59 after 1 year: 0.58).

with fractures of the proximal humerus and the variety of different fracture types demand a guide for versatile treatments ranging from nonoperative to rTSA. Our published algorithm has resulted in satisfying clinical results and a relatively low revision rate and we continue to strive for refinements with our ongoing evaluation of the next iteration of our algorithm.

References

1. Court-Brown CM, Caesar B. Epidemiology of adult fractures: a review. *Inj.* 2006;37(8):691–697. https://doi.org/10.1016/j.injury.2006.04.130.
2. Rose SH, Melton LJ, Morrey BF, Ilstrup DM, Riggs BL. Epidemiologic features of humeral fractures. *Clin Orthop Relat R.* 1982 Aug; (168):24-30. https://doi.org/10.1097/00003086-198208000-00003.
3. Wilson J, Bonner TJ, Head M, Fordham J, Brealey S, Rangan A. Variation in bone mineral density by anatomical site in patients with proximal humeral fractures. *Bone Joint Lett J.* 2009;91-B(6):772–775. https://doi.org/10.1302/0301-620x.91b6.22346.
4. Palvanen M, Kannus P, Niemi S, Parkkari J. Update in the epidemiology of proximal humeral fractures. *Clin Orthop Relat R.* 2006;442:87–92. https://doi.org/10.1097/01.blo.0000194672.79634.78.
5. Neer CS. Displaced proximal humeral fractures. II. Treatment of three-part and four-part displacement. *J Bone Jt Surg Am Volume.* 1970;52(6):1090–1103. https://doi.org/10.2106/00004623-197052060-00002.
6. Spross C, Platz A, Rufibach K, Lattmann T, Forberger J, Dietrich M. The PHILOS plate for proximal humeral fractures—risk factors for complications at one year. *J Trauma Acute Care Surg.* 2012;72(3):783–792. https://doi.org/10.1097/ta.0b013e31822c1b5b.

7. Spross C, Platz A, Erschbamer M, Lattmann T, Dietrich M. Surgical treatment of Neer Group VI proximal humeral fractures: retrospective comparison of PHILOS® and hemiarthroplasty. *Clin Orthop Relat R.* 2011;470(7):2035–2042. https://doi.org/10.1007/s11999-011-2207-1.

8. Owsley KC, Gorczyca JT. Fracture displacement and screw cutout after open reduction and locked plate fixation of proximal humeral fractures [corrected]. *J Bone Jt Surg Am Volume.* 2008;90(2):233–240. https://doi.org/10.2106/jbjs.f.01351.

9. Sproul RC, Iyengar JJ, Devcic Z, Feeley BT. A systematic review of locking plate fixation of proximal humerus fractures. *Inj.* 2011;42(4):408–413. https://doi.org/10.1016/j.injury.2010.11.058.

10. Südkamp N, Bayer J, Hepp P, et al. Open reduction and internal fixation of proximal humeral fractures with use of the locking proximal humerus plate. *J Bone Jt Surg.* 2009;91(6):1320–1328. https://doi.org/10.2106/jbjs.h.00006.

11. Handoll HH, Keding A, Corbacho B, Brealey SD, Hewitt C, Rangan A. Five-year follow-up results of the PROFHER trial comparing operative and non-operative treatment of adults with a displaced fracture of the proximal humerus. *Bone Jt J.* 2017;99-B(3):383–392.https://doi.org/10.1302/0301-620x.99b3.bjj-2016-1028.

12. Chun Y-M, Kim D-S, Lee D-H, Shin S-J. Reverse shoulder arthroplasty for four-part proximal humerus fracture in elderly patients: can a healed tuberosity improve the functional outcomes? *J Shoulder Elb Surg.* 2017;26(7):1216–1221. https://doi.org/10.1016/j.jse.2016.11.034.

13. Grubhofer F, Wieser K, Meyer DC, et al. Reverse total shoulder arthroplasty for acute head-splitting, 3- and 4-part fractures of the proximal humerus in the elderly. *J Shoulder Elb Surg.* 2016;25(10):1690–1698. https://doi.org/10.1016/j.jse.2016.02.024.

14. Fraser AN, Bjørdal J, Wagle TM, et al. Reverse shoulder arthroplasty is superior to plate fixation at 2 years for displaced proximal humeral fractures in the elderly: a multicenter randomized controlled trial. *J Bone Jt Surg Am.* 2020;102(6):477–485. https://doi.org/10.2106/jbjs.19.01071.

15. Browner B, Jupiter J, Krettek C, Anderson P. In: *Skeletal Trauma: Basic Science, Management, and Reconstruction.* 6th ed. Philadelphia: Elsevier; 2019.

15a. Spross C, Farei JM, Manser M, Jacxsens M, Zdravkovic V, Jost B. Outcome of management of proximal humerus fractures using a patient-specific, evidence-based treatment algorithm. *J Bone J Surg.* Accepted March 2021.

16. Boileau P, Walch G. The three-dimensional geometry of the proximal humerus: implications for surgical technique and prosthetic design. *J Bone Jt Surg.* 1997;79(5):857–865. https://doi.org/10.1302/0301-620x.79b5.7579.

17. Pearl ML, Volk AG. Retroversion of the proximal humerus in relationship to prosthetic replacement arthroplasty. *J Shoulder Elb Surg.* 1996;5(2):S89. https://doi.org/10.1016/s1058-2746(96)80397-1.

18. Sintini I, Burton WS, Sade P, Chavarria JM, Laz PJ. Investigating gender and ethnicity differences in proximal humeral morphology using a statistical shape model. *J Orthop Res Official Publ Orthop Res Soc.* 2018;36(11):3043–3052. https://doi.org/10.1002/jor.24070.

19. Eglseder WA, Goldman M. Anatomic variations of the musculocutaneous nerve in the arm. *Am J Orthop Belle Mead N J.* 1997;26(11):777–780.

20. Burkhead WZ, Scheinberg RR, Box G. Surgical anatomy of the axillary nerve. *J Shoulder Elb Surg Am Shoulder Elb Surg Et Al.* 1992;1(1):31–36. https://doi.org/10.1016/s1058-2746(09)80014-1.

21. Gerber C, Schneeberger AG, Vinh TS. The arterial vascularization of the humeral head. An anatomical study. *J Bone Jt Surg.*1990;72(10):1486–1494.https://doi.org/10.2106/00004623-199072100-00009.

22. Hettrich CM, Boraiah S, Dyke JP, Neviaser A, Helfet DL, Lorich DG. Quantitative assessment of the vascularity of the proximal part of the humerus. *J Bone Jt Surgery-American.* 2010;92(4):943–948. https://doi.org/10.2106/jbjs.h.01144.

23. Tingart MJ, Bouxsein ML, Zurakowski D, Warner JP, Apreleva M. Three-dimensional distribution of bone density in the proximal humerus. *Calcified Tissue Int.* 2003;73(6):531–536. https://doi.org/10.1007/s00223-002-0013-9.

24. Neer CS. The Classic: displaced proximal humeral fractures: part I. Classification and evaluation. *Clin Orthop Relat R.* 2006;442:77–82. https://doi.org/10.1097/01.blo.0000198718.91223.ca.

25. Codman E. *The Shoulder.* Boston: Company KP; 1934.

26. Siebenrock KA, Gerber C. The reproducibility of classification of fractures of the proximal end of the humerus. *J Bone Jt Surg.* 1993;75(12):1751–1755. https://doi.org/10.2106/00004623-199312000-00003.

27. Gracitelli MEC, Dotta TAG, Assunção JH, et al. Intraobserver and interobserver agreement in the classification and treatment of proximal humeral fractures. *J Shoulder Elb Surg.* 2017;26(6):1097–1102. https://doi.org/10.1016/j.jse.2016.11.047.

28. Brunner A, Honigmann P, Treumann T, Babst R. The impact of stereo-visualisation of three-dimensional CT datasets on the inter- and intraobserver reliability of the AO/OTA and Neer classifications in the assessment of fractures of the proximal humerus. *J Bone Jt Surg Br Volume.* 2009;91-B(6):766–771. https://doi.org/10.1302/0301-620x.91b6.22109.

29. Krappinger D, Roth T, Gschwentner M, et al. Preoperative assessment of the cancellous bone mineral density of the proximal humerus using CT data. *Skeletal Radiol.* 2012;41(3):299–304. https://doi.org/10.1007/s00256-011-1174-7.

30. Neer CS. Four-segment classification of proximal humeral fractures: purpose and reliable use. *J Shoulder Elb Surg.* 2002;11(4):389–400. https://doi.org/10.1067/mse.2002.124346.

31. Neer CS. Four-segment classification of displaced proximal humeral fractures. In: *Chapter 9, Instructional Course Lectures of the American Academy of Orthopaedic Surgeons.* St. Louis: Mosby; 1975:160–168.

32. Mills HJ, Horne G. Fractures of the proximal humerus in adults. *J Trauma Inj Infect Critical Care.* 1985;25(8):801–805. https://doi.org/10.1097/00005373-198508000-00013.

33. Olerud P, Ahrengart L, Ponzer S, Saving J, Tidermark J. Internal fixation versus nonoperative treatment of displaced 3-part proximal humeral fractures in elderly patients: a randomized controlled trial. *J Shoulder Elb Surg.* 2011;20(5):747–755. https://doi.org/10.1016/j.jse.2010.12.018.

34. Olerud P, Ahrengart L, Ponzer S, Saving J, Tidermark J. Hemiarthroplasty versus nonoperative treatment of displaced 4-part proximal humeral fractures in elderly patients: a randomized controlled trial. *J Shoulder Elb Surg.* 2011;20(7):1025–1033. https://doi.org/10.1016/j.jse.2011.04.016.

35. Olerud P, Ahrengart L, Söderqvist A, Saving J, Tidermark J. Quality of life and functional outcome after a 2-part proximal humeral fracture: a prospective cohort study on 50 patients treated with a locking plate. *J Shoulder Elb Surg Am Shoulder Elb Surg Et Al.* 2010;19(6):814–822. https://doi.org/10.1016/j.jse.2009.11.046.

36. Müller ME, Koch P, Nazarian S, Schatzker J. *The Comprehensive Classification of Fractures of Long Bones (Published Online)* Berlin, Heidelberg: Springer; 1990. ISBN: 978-3-642-61261-9.

37. Meinberg EG, Agel J, Roberts CS, Karam MD, Kellam JF. Introduction: fracture and dislocation classification compendium-2018: International comprehensive classification of fractures and dislocations Committee. *J Orthop Trauma.* 2018;32(suppl 1):S1–S10. https://doi.org/10.1097/bot.0000000000001063.

38. Hertel R, Hempfing A, Stiehler M, Leunig M. Predictors of humeral head ischemia after intracapsular fracture of the proximal humerus. *J Shoulder Elb Surg.* 2004;13(4):427–433. https://doi.org/10.1016/j.jse.2004.01.034.

39. Bastian JD, Hertel R. Initial post-fracture humeral head ischemia does not predict development of necrosis. *J Shoulder Elb Surg Am*

Shoulder Elb Surg Et Al. 2008;17(1):2–8. https://doi.org/10.1016/j.jse.2007.03.026.

40. Bastian JD, Hertel R. Osteosynthesis and hemiarthroplasty of fractures of the proximal humerus: outcomes in a consecutive case series. *J Shoulder Elb Surg.* 2009;18(2):216–219. https://doi.org/10.1016/j.jse.2008.09.015.

41. Brien H, Noftall F, MacMaster S, Cummings T, Landells C, Rockwood P. Neer's classification system. *J Trauma Inj Infect Critical Care.* 1995;38(2):257–260. https://doi.org/10.1097/00005373-199502000-00022.

42. Kristiansen B, Andersen ULS, Olsen CA, Varmarken J-E. The Neer classification of fractures of the proximal humerus. *Skeletal Radiol.* 1988;17(6):420–422. https://doi.org/10.1007/bf00361661.

43. Sidor ML, Zuckerman JD, Lyon T, Koval K, Cuomo F, Schoenberg N. The Neer classification system for proximal humeral fractures. An assessment of interobserver reliability and intraobserver reproducibility. *J Bone Jt Surg.* 1993;75(12):1745–1750. https://doi.org/10.2106/00004623-199312000-00002.

44. Sjödén GOJ, Movin T, Güntner P, et al. Poor reproducibility of classification of proximal humeral fractures: additional CT of minor value. *Acta Orthop Scand.* 1997;68(3):239–242. https://doi.org/10.3109/17453679708996692.

45. Bernstein J, Adler LM, Blank JE, Dalsey RM, Williams GR, Iannotti JP. Evaluation of the Neer system of classification of proximal humeral fractures with computerized tomographic scans and plain radiographs. *J Bone Jt Surg.* 1996;78(9):1371–1375. https://doi.org/10.2106/00004623-199609000-00012.

46. Boons HW, Goosen JH, van Grinsven S, van Susante JL, van Loon CJ. Hemiarthroplasty for humeral four-part fractures for patients 65 years and older: a randomized controlled trial. *Clin Orthop Relat R.* 2012;470(12):3483–3491. https://doi.org/10.1007/s11999-012-2531-0.

47. Fjalestad T, Hole MØ, Hovden IAH, Blücher J, Strømsøe K. Surgical treatment with an angular stable plate for complex displaced proximal humeral fractures in elderly patients: a randomized controlled trial. *J Orthop Trauma.* 2012;26(2):98–106. https://doi.org/10.1097/bot.0b013e31821c2e15.

48. Shrader MW, Sanchez-Sotelo J, Sperling JW, Rowland CM, Cofield RH. Understanding proximal humerus fractures: image analysis, classification, and treatment. *J Shoulder Elb Surg.* 2005;14(5):497–505. https://doi.org/10.1016/j.jse.2005.02.014.

49. Mutch J, Laflamme GY, Hagemeister N, Cikes A, Rouleau DM. A new morphological classification for greater tuberosity fractures of the proximal humerus: validation and clinical implications. *Bone Joint J.* 2014;96-B(5):646–651.

50. Park TS, Choi IY, Kim YH, Park MR, Shon JH, Kim SI. A new suggestion for the treatment of minimally displaced fractures of the greater tuberosity of the proximal humerus. *Bulletin Hosp Jt Dis New York N Y.* 1997;56(3):171–176.

51. Bono CM, Renard R, Levine RG, Levy AS. Effect of displacement of fractures of the greater tuberosity on the mechanics of the shoulder. *Bone Joint Lett J.* 2001;83-B(7):1056–1062. https://doi.org/10.1302/0301-620x.83b7.10516.

52. Platzer P, Thalhammer G, Oberleitner G, et al. Displaced fractures of the greater tuberosity: a comparison of operative and nonoperative treatment. *J Trauma Inj Infect Critical Care.* 2008;65(4):843–848. https://doi.org/10.1097/01.ta.0000233710.42698.3f.

53. Gruson KI, Ruchelsman DE, Tejwani NC. Isolated tuberosity fractures of the proximal humerus: current concepts. *Inj.* 2008;39(3):284–298. https://doi.org/10.1016/j.injury.2007.09.022.

54. Nyffeler RW, Seidel A, Werlen S, Bergmann M. Radiological and biomechanical assessment of displaced greater tuberosity fractures. *Int Orthop.* 2018;43(6):1479–1486. https://doi.org/10.1007/s00264-018-4170-x.

55. Parsons BO, Klepps SJ, Miller S, Bird J, Gladstone J, Flatow E. Reliability and reproducibility of radiographs of greater tuberosity displacement. *J Bone Jt Surg.* 2005;87(1):58–65. https://doi.org/10.2106/jbjs.c.01576.

56. Guix JMM, Gonzalez AS, Brugalla JV, Carril EC, Baños FG. Proposed protocol for reading images of humeral head fractures. *Clin Orthop Relat R.* 2006;448:225–233. https://doi.org/10.1097/01.blo.0000205899.28856.98.

57. Audigé L, Bhandari M, Kellam J. How reliable are reliability studies of fracture classifications? A systematic review of their methodologies. *Acta Orthop Scand.* 2004;75(2):184–194. https://doi.org/10.1080/00016470412331294445.

58. Peters P-M, Plachel F, Danzinger V, et al. Clinical and radiographic outcomes after surgical treatment of proximal humeral fractures with head-split component. *J Bone Jt Surg.* 2020;102(1):68–75. https://doi.org/10.2106/jbjs.19.00320.

59. Hersche O, Gerber C. Iatrogenic displacement of fracture-dislocations of the shoulder. A report of seven cases. *J Bone Jt Surg Br Volume.* 1994;76-B(1):30–33. https://doi.org/10.1302/0301-620x.76b1.8300677.

60. Robinson CM, Akhtar A, Mitchell M, Beavis C. Complex posterior fracture-dislocation of the shoulder. *J Bone Jt Surg.* 2007;89(7):1454–1466. https://doi.org/10.2106/jbjs.f.01214.

61. Handoll HH, Brorson S. Interventions for treating proximal humeral fractures in adults. *Cochrane Db Syst Rev.* 2015;11(11):CD000434. https://doi.org/10.1002/14651858.cd000434.pub4.

62. Visser CPJ, Coene LNJEM, Brand R, Tavy DLJ. Nerve lesions in proximal humeral fractures. *J Shoulder Elb Surg.* 2001;10(5):421–427. https://doi.org/10.1067/mse.2001.118002.

63. Fankhauser F, Schippinger G, Weber K, et al. Cadaveric-biomechanical evaluation of bone-implant construct of proximal humerus fractures (Neer type 3). *J Trauma Inj Infect Critical Care.* 2003;55(2):345–349. https://doi.org/10.1097/01.ta.0000033139.61038.ef.

64. Krappinger D, Bizzotto N, Riedmann S, Kammerlander C, Hengg C, Kralinger FS. Predicting failure after surgical fixation of proximal humerus fractures. *Inj.* 2011;42(11):1283–1288. https://doi.org/10.1016/j.injury.2011.01.017.

65. Lee SH, Dargent-Molina P, Bréart G, EGE de l'Osteoporose S. Risk factors for fractures of the proximal humerus: results from the EPIDOS prospective study. *J Bone Mineral Res Official J Am Soc Bone Mineral Res.* 2002;17(5):817–825. https://doi.org/10.1359/jbmr.2002.17.5.817.

66. Seebeck J, Goldhahn J, Städele H, Messmer P, Morlock MM, Schneider E. Effect of cortical thickness and cancellous bone density on the holding strength of internal fixator screws. *J Orthopaed Res.* 2004;22(6):1237–1242. https://doi.org/10.1016/j.orthres.2004.04.001.

67. Spross C, Zeledon R, Zdravkovic V, Jost B. How bone quality may influence intraoperative and early postoperative problems after angular stable open reduction–internal fixation of proximal humeral fractures. *J Shoulder Elb Surg.* 2017;26(9):1566–1572. https://doi.org/10.1016/j.jse.2017.02.026.

68. Namdari S, Voleti PB, Mehta S. Evaluation of the osteoporotic proximal humeral fracture and strategies for structural augmentation during surgical treatment. *J Shoulder Elb Surg.* 2012;21(12):1787–1795. https://doi.org/10.1016/j.jse.2012.04.003.

69. Tingart MJ, Apreleva M, Stechow D von, Zurakowski D, Warner JJP. The cortical thickness of the proximal humeral diaphysis predicts bone mineral density of the proximal humerus. *Bone Joint Lett J.* 2003;85-B(4):611–617. https://doi.org/10.1302/0301-620x.85b4.12843.

70. Mather J, MacDermid JC, Faber KJ, Athwal GS. Proximal humerus cortical bone thickness correlates with bone mineral density and can clinically rule out osteoporosis. *J Shoulder Elb Surg.* 2013;22(6):732–738. https://doi.org/10.1016/j.jse.2012.08.018.

71. Spross C, Kaestle N, Benninger E, et al. Deltoid tuberosity index: a simple radiographic tool to assess local bone quality in proximal humerus fractures. *Clin Orthop Relat R.* 2015;473(9):3038–3045. https://doi.org/10.1007/s11999-015-4322-x.

72. Nho SJ, Brophy RH, Barker JU, Cornell CN, MacGillivray JD. Management of proximal humeral fractures based on current

literature. *J Bone Jt Surg.* 2007;89(suppl 1):44–58. https://doi.org/10.2106/jbjs.g.00648.

73. Hertel R. Fractures of the proximal humerus in osteoporotic bone. *Osteoporosis Int.* 2005;16(suppl 2):S65–S72. https://doi.org/10.1007/s00198-004-1714-2.

74. Forstein DA, Bernardini C, Cole RE, Harris ST, Singer A. Before the breaking point: reducing the risk of osteoporotic fracture. *J Am Osteopath Assoc.* 2013;113(2 suppl 1):S5–S24. quiz S25.

75. Cherniack EP, Levis S, Troen BR. Hypovitaminosis D: a widespread epidemic. *Geriatrics.* 2008;63(4):24–30.

76. Lane JM, Nydick M. Osteoporosis: current modes of prevention and treatment. *J Am Acad Orthop Sur.* 1999;7(1):19–31. https://doi.org/10.5435/00124635-199901000-00003.

77. Unnanuntana A, Gladnick BP, Donnelly E, Lane JM. The assessment of fracture risk. *J Bone Jt Surg Am Volume.* 2010;92(3):743–753. https://doi.org/10.2106/jbjs.i.00919.

78. Clifford PC. Fractures of the neck of the humerus: a review of the late results. *Inj.* 1980;12(2):91–95. https://doi.org/10.1016/0020-1383(80)90129-1.

79. Kovalk KJ, Gallagher MA, Marsicano JG, Cuomo F, Mcshinawy A, Zuckerman JD. Functional outcome after minimally displaced fractures of the proximal part of the humerus. *J Bone Jt Surg.* 1997;79(2):203–207. https://doi.org/10.2106/00004623-199702000-00006.

80. Tejwani NC, Liporace F, Walsh M, France MA, Zuckerman JD, Egol KA. Functional outcome following one-part proximal humeral fractures: a prospective study. *J Shoulder Elb Surg.* 2008;17(2):216–219. https://doi.org/10.1016/j.jse.2007.07.016.

81. Agudelo J, Schürmann M, Stahel P, et al. Analysis of efficacy and failure in proximal humerus fractures treated with locking plates. *J Orthop Trauma.* 2007;21(10):676–681. https://doi.org/10.1097/bot.0b013e31815bb09d.

82. Solberg BD, Moon CN, Franco DP, Paiement GD. Locked plating of 3- and 4-part proximal humerus fractures in older patients: the effect of initial fracture pattern on outcome. *J Orthop Trauma.* 2009;23(2):113–119. https://doi.org/10.1097/bot.0b013e31819344bf.

83. Boileau P, Krishnan SG, Tinsi L, Walch G, Coste JS, Molé D. Tuberosity malposition and migration: reasons for poor outcomes after hemiarthroplasty for displaced fractures of the proximal humerus. *J Shoulder Elb Surg.* 2002;11(5):401–412. https://doi.org/10.1067/mse.2002.124527.

84. Kralinger F, Schwaiger R, Wambacher M, et al. Outcome after primary hemiarthroplasty for fracture of the head of the humerus. *Bone Joint Lett J.* 2004;86-B(2):217–219. https://doi.org/10.1302/0301-620x.86b2.14553.

85. Mighell MA, Kolm GP, Collinge CA, Frankle MA. Outcomes of hemiarthroplasty for fractures of the proximal humerus. *J Shoulder Elb Surg.* 2003;12(6):569–577. https://doi.org/10.1016/s1058-2746(03)00213-1.

86. Krieg JC. Surgical and nonsurgical treatment produced similar outcomes for proximal humeral fractures. *J Bone Jt Surg.* 2015;97(22):1890. https://doi.org/10.2106/jbjs.9722.ebo102.

87. Steinhaus ME, Dare DM, Gulotta LV. Displaced proximal humerus fractures: is a sling as good as a plate? *HSS J.* 2016;12(3):287–290. https://doi.org/10.1007/s11420-015-9479-z.

88. Lopiz Y, Alcobía-Díaz B, Galán-Olleros M, García-Fernández C, Picado AL, Marco F. Reverse shoulder arthroplasty versus nonoperative treatment for 3- or 4-part proximal humeral fractures in elderly patients: a prospective randomized controlled trial. *J Shoulder Elb Surg.* 2019:Dec;28(12):2259–2271. https://doi.org/10.1016/j.jse.2019.06.024.

89. Chivot M, Lami D, Bizzozero P, Galland A, Argenson J-N. Three- and four-part displaced proximal humeral fractures in patients older than 70 years: reverse shoulder arthroplasty or nonsurgical treatment? *J Shoulder Elb Surg.* 2019;28(2):252–259. https://doi.org/10.1016/j.jse.2018.07.019.

90. Court-Brown CM, Cattermole H, McQueen MM. Impacted valgus fractures (B1.1) of the proximal humerus: the results of non-operative treatment. *J Bone Jt Surg.* 2002;84(4):504–508. https://doi.org/10.1302/0301-620x.84b4.12488.

91. Court-Brown C, McQueen M. The impacted varus (A2.2) proximal humeral fracture prediction of outcome and results of nonoperative treatment in 99 patients. *Acta Orthop Scand.* 2004;75(6):736–740. https://doi.org/10.1080/00016470410004111.

92. Lefevre-Colau M, Babinet A, Fayad F, et al. Immediate mobilization compared with conventional immobilization for the impacted nonoperatively treated proximal humeral fracture. *J Bone Jt Surgery-American Volume.* 2007;89(12):2582–2590. https://doi.org/10.2106/jbjs.f.01419.

93. Carbone S, Razzano C, Albino P, Mezzoprete R. Immediate intensive mobilization compared with immediate conventional mobilization for the impacted osteoporotic conservatively treated proximal humeral fracture: a randomized controlled trial. *Musculoskelet Surg.* 2017;101(suppl 2):137–143. https://doi.org/10.1007/s12306-017-0483-y.

94. Karas V, Riboh JC, Garrigues GE. Arthroscopic management of the stiff shoulder. *JBJS Rev.* 2016;4(4):1. https://doi.org/10.2106/jbjs.rvw.o.00047.

95. Beks RB, Ochen Y, Frima H, et al. Operative versus nonoperative treatment of proximal humeral fractures: a systematic review, meta-analysis, and comparison of observational studies and randomized controlled trials. *J Shoulder Elb Surg.* 2018;27(8):1526–1534. https://doi.org/10.1016/j.jse.2018.03.009.

96. Hanson B, Neidenbach P, de Boer P, Stengel D. Functional outcomes after nonoperative management of fractures of the proximal humerus. *J Shoulder Elb Surg.* 2009;18(4):612–621. https://doi.org/10.1016/j.jse.2009.03.024.

97. Hessmann MH, Sternstein W, Hansen M, Krummenauer F, Pol TF, Rommens M. Locked plate fixation and intramedullary nailing for proximal humerus fractures: a biomechanical evaluation. *J Trauma Inj Infect Critical Care.* 2005;58(6):1194–1201. https://doi.org/10.1097/01.ta.0000170400.68994.ab.

98. Handschin AE, Cardell M, Contaldo C, Trentz O, Wanner GA. Functional results of angular-stable plate fixation in displaced proximal humeral fractures. *Inj.* 2008;39(3):306–313. https://doi.org/10.1016/j.injury.2007.10.011.

99. Jost B, Spross C, Grehn H, Gerber C. Locking plate fixation of fractures of the proximal humerus: analysis of complications, revision strategies and outcome. *J Shoulder Elb Surg.* 2013;22(4):542–549. https://doi.org/10.1016/j.jse.2012.06.008.

100. Osterhoff G, Hoch A, Wanner GA, Simmen H-P, Werner CML. Calcar comminution as prognostic factor of clinical outcome after locking plate fixation of proximal humeral fractures. *Inj.* 2012;43(10):1651–1656. https://doi.org/10.1016/j.injury.2012.04.015.

101. Acklin YP, Stoffel K, Sommer C. A prospective analysis of the functional and radiological outcomes of minimally invasive plating in proximal humerus fractures. *Inj.* 2013;44(4):456–460. https://doi.org/10.1016/j.injury.2012.09.010.

102. Brunner F, Sommer C, Bahrs C, et al. Open reduction and internal fixation of proximal humerus fractures using a proximal humeral locked plate: a prospective multicenter analysis. *J Orthop Trauma.* 2009;23(3):163–172. https://doi.org/10.1097/bot.0b013e3181920e5b.

103. Thanasas C, Kontakis G, Angoules A, Limb D, Giannoudis P. Treatment of proximal humerus fractures with locking plates: a systematic review. *J Shoulder Elb Surg.* 2009;18(6):837–844. https://doi.org/10.1016/j.jse.2009.06.004.

104. Röderer G, Erhardt J, Graf M, Kinzl L, Gebhard F. Clinical results for minimally invasive locked plating of proximal humerus fractures. *J Orthop Trauma.* 2010;24(7):400–406. https://doi.org/10.1097/bot.0b013e3181ccafb3.

105. Xie L, Zhang Y, Chen C, Zheng W, Chen H, Cai L. Deltoid-split approach versus deltopectoral approach for proximal humerus fractures: a systematic review and meta-analysis. *Orthop Traumatology Surg Res.* 2019;105(2):307–316. https://doi.org/10.1016/j.otsr.2018.12.004.

106. Gardner MJ. Proximal humerus fracture plating through the extended anterolateral approach. *J Orthop Trauma.* 2016;30:S11–S12. https://doi.org/10.1097/bot.0000000000000586.

107. Wheeler DL, Colville MR. Biomechanical comparison of intramedullary and percutaneous pin fixation for proximal humeral fracture fixation. *J Orthop Trauma.* 1997;11(5):363–367. https://doi.org/10.1097/00005131-199707000-00012.

108. Williams GR, Copley LA, Iannotti JP, Lisser SP. The influence of intramedullary fixation on figure-of-eight wiring for surgical neck fractures of the proximal humerus: a biomechanical comparison. *J Shoulder Elb Surg.* 1997;6(5):423–428. https://doi.org/10.1016/s1058-2746(97)70048-x.

109. Lopiz Y, Garcia-Coiradas J, Garcia-Fernandez C, Marco F. Proximal humerus nailing: a randomized clinical trial between curvilinear and straight nails. *J Shoulder Elb Surg.* 2014;23(3):369–376. https://doi.org/10.1016/j.jse.2013.08.023.

110. Boileau P, d'Ollonne T, Hatzidakis AM, Morrey ME. Intramedullary locking nail fixation of proximal humerus fractures: rationale and technique. In: *Proximal Humerus Fractures (Published Online).* Springer International Publishing; 2014:73–98. https://doi.org/10.1007/978-3-319-08951-5_5.

111. Boileau P, d'Ollonne T, Bessière C, et al. Displaced humeral surgical neck fractures: classification and results of third-generation percutaneous intramedullary nailing. *J Shoulder Elb Surg.* 2018;28(2):276–287. https://doi.org/10.1016/j.jse.2018.07.010.

112. Wong J, Newman JM, Gruson KI. Outcomes of intramedullary nailing for acute proximal humerus fractures: a systematic review. *J Orthop Traumatology Official J Italian Soc Orthop Traumatology.* 2015;17(2):113–122. https://doi.org/10.1007/s10195-015-0384-5.

113. Boileau P, Winter M, Cikes A, et al. Can surgeons predict what makes a good hemiarthroplasty for fracture? *J Shoulder Elb Surg.* 2013;22(11):1495–1506. https://doi.org/10.1016/j.jse.2013.04.018.

114. Cai M, Tao K, Yang C, Li S. Internal fixation versus shoulder hemiarthroplasty for displaced 4-part proximal humeral fractures in elderly patients. *Orthopedics.* 2012;35(9):e1340–1346. https://doi.org/10.3928/01477447-20120822-19.

115. Boyle MJ, Youn S-M, Frampton CMA, Ball CM. Functional outcomes of reverse shoulder arthroplasty compared with hemiarthroplasty for acute proximal humeral fractures. *J Shoulder Elb Surg.* 2013;22(1):32–37. https://doi.org/10.1016/j.jse.2012.03.006.

116. Gallinet D, Clappaz P, Garbuio P, Tropet Y, Obert L. Three or four parts complex proximal humerus fractures: hemiarthroplasty versus reverse prosthesis: a comparative study of 40 cases. *Orthop Traumatology Surg Res Otsr.* 2009;95(1):48–55. https://doi.org/10.1016/j.otsr.2008.09.002.

117. Garrigues GE, Johnston PS, Pepe MD, Tucker BS, Ramsey ML, Austin LS. Hemiarthroplasty versus reverse total shoulder arthroplasty for acute proximal humerus fractures in elderly patients. *Orthopedics.* 2012;35(5):e703–708. https://doi.org/10.3928/01477447-20120426-25.

118. Young SW, Segal BS, Turner PC, Poon PC. Comparison of functional outcomes of reverse shoulder arthroplasty versus hemiarthroplasty in the primary treatment of acute proximal humerus fracture. *ANZ J Surg.* 2010;80(11):789–793. https://doi.org/10.1111/j.1445-2197.2010.05342.x.

119. Austin DC, Torchia MT, Cozzolino NH, Jacobowitz LE, Bell J-E. Decreased reoperations and improved outcomes with reverse total shoulder arthroplasty in comparison to hemiarthroplasty for geriatric proximal humerus fractures. *J Orthop Trauma.* 2019;33(1):49–57. https://doi.org/10.1097/bot.0000000000001321.

120. Sebastia-Forcada E, Lizaur-Utrilla A, Cebrian-Gomez R, Miralles-Muñoz FA, Lopez-Prats FA. Outcomes of reverse total shoulder arthroplasty for proximal humeral fractures. *J Orthop Trauma.* 2017;31(8):e236–e240. https://doi.org/10.1097/bot.0000000000000858.

121. Repetto I, Alessio-Mazzola M, Cerruti P, Sanguineti F, Formica M, Felli L. Surgical management of complex proximal humeral fractures: pinning, locked plate and arthroplasty: clinical results and functional outcome on retrospective series of patients. *Musculoskelet Surg.* 2017;101(2):153–158. https://doi.org/10.1007/s12306-017-0451-6.

122. Torchia MT, Austin DC, Cozzolino N, Jacobowitz L, Bell J-E. Acute versus delayed reverse total shoulder arthroplasty for the treatment of proximal humeral fractures in the elderly population: a systematic review and meta-analysis. *J Shoulder Elb Surg.* 2019;28(4):765–773. https://doi.org/10.1016/j.jse.2018.10.004.

123. Nikola M, Hrvoje K, Nenad M. Reverse shoulder arthroplasty in acute fractures provides better results than in revision procedures for fracture sequelae. *Int Orthop.* 2015;39(2):343–348. https://doi.org/10.1007/s00264-014-2649-7.

124. Roberson TA, Granade CM, Hunt Q, et al. Nonoperative management versus reverse shoulder arthroplasty for treatment of 3- and 4-part proximal humeral fractures in older adults. *J Shoulder Elbow Surg.* 2017;26(6):1017–1022.

125. Seidl A, Sholder D, Warrender W, et al. Early versus late reverse shoulder arthroplasty for proximal humerus fractures: does it matter? *Archives Bone Jt Surg.* 2017;5(4):213–220. https://doi.org/10.22038/abjs.2017.20040.1522.

126. Dezfuli B, King JJ, Farmer KW, Struk AM, Wright TW. Outcomes of reverse total shoulder arthroplasty as primary versus revision procedure for proximal humerus fractures. *J Shoulder Elb Surg.* 2016;25(7):1133–1137. https://doi.org/10.1016/j.jse.2015.12.002.

127. Ernstbrunner L, Rahm S, Suter A, et al. Salvage reverse total shoulder arthroplasty for failed operative treatment of proximal humeral fractures in patients younger than 60 years: long-term results. *J Shoulder Elb Surg.* 2020 Mar;29(3):561–570. https://doi.org/10.1016/j.jse.2019.07.040.

128. Holschen M, Siemes M-K, Witt K-A, Steinbeck J. Five-year outcome after conversion of a hemiarthroplasty when used for the treatment of a proximal humeral fracture to a reverse total shoulder arthroplasty. *Bone Jt J.* 2018;100-B(6):761–766. https://doi.org/10.1302/0301-620x.100b6.bjj-2017-1280.r1.

129. Schulte LM, Matteini LE, Neviaser RJ. Proximal periarticular locking plates in proximal humeral fractures: functional outcomes. *J Shoulder Elb Surg.* 2011;20(8):1234–1240. https://doi.org/10.1016/j.jse.2010.12.015.

130. Inauen C, Platz A, Meier C, et al. Quality of life after osteosynthesis of fractures of the proximal humerus. *J Orthop Trauma.* 2013;27(4):e74–e80. https://doi.org/10.1097/bot.0b013e3182693cac.

131. Browner B, Jupiter J, Krettek C, Anderson P. *Skeletal Trauma: Basic Science, Management, and Reconstruction.* 5th ed. Philadelphia: Elsevier; 2014.

132. Spross C, Meester J, Mazzucchelli RA, Puskás GJ, Zdravkovic V, Jost B. Evidence-based algorithm to treat patients with proximal humerus fractures—a prospective study with early clinical and overall performance results. *J Shoulder Elb Surg.* 2019;28(6):1022–1032. https://doi.org/10.1016/j.jse.2019.02.015.

133. Jakob R, Miniaci A, Anson P, Jaberg H, Osterwalder A, Ganz R. Four-part valgus impacted fractures of the proximal humerus. *J Bone Jt Surg Br Volume.* 1991;73-B(2):295–298. https://doi.org/10.1302/0301-620x.73b2.2005159.

134. White JJE, Soothill JR, Morgan M, Clark DI, Espag MP, Tambe AA. Outcomes for a large metaphyseal volume hemiarthroplasty in complex fractures of the proximal humerus. *J Shoulder Elb Surg.* 2017;26(3):478–483. https://doi.org/10.1016/j.jse.2016.08.004.

135. Bacle G, Nové-Josserand L, Garaud P, Walch G. Long-term outcomes of reverse shoulder arthroplasty: a follow-up of a previous study. *JBJS.* 2017;99(6):454–461.

26

Technique Spotlight: Nonoperative Rehabilitation for Proximal Humeral Fractures

JUNE KENNEDY

Proximal humeral fractures (PHFs) represent ~5% of all fractures and are the second most common fracture in adults over 65 years of age.[1] For communication, we frequently use the Neer classification system given its common use and ability to guide surgical versus nonsurgical treatment.[2] The majority of PHF in the >65-year-old population are minimally displaced and stable (44%) or two-part surgical neck fractures (39%).[3] Nonoperative management is recommended for fractures that are nondisplaced or minimally displaced with two or three fragments in any age group; two-, three-, or four-part nondisplaced fractures in older patients; and displaced fractures in patients who are poor surgical candidates due to comorbidities.[4] Approximately 75% to 78% of all PHFs are managed nonoperatively with sling immobilization and physical therapy.[1,5]

Clinical decision-making throughout rehabilitation for PHF is guided by the need to maintain stability of the fracture segments. Patient-specific factors such as age, dependence on assistive device for safe mobility, comorbidities, and ability to comply with rehabilitation precautions should be considered. An important component of the patient assessment should include balance since the majority of PHFs occur secondary to a fall in the elderly.

A scoping review of the literature regarding rehabilitation following PHF revealed heterogeneity of low-quality studies, therefore concluding that there is insufficient evidence to inform practice regarding different PHF interventions.[6] One particular fracture pattern where there are supportive data and consensus is the impacted two-part PHF. Two prospective trials of early versus 3-week delayed mobilization for patients with impacted two-part PHF found that patients immobilized longer had more pain and a slower recovery at 3 to 4 months compared with those with early motion.[7,8] Proposed rehabilitation guidelines in Table 26.1 are based on expert opinion, the timing of bone healing, and the results of two surveys on practice patterns in Canada and the UK.[1,9] A slower rehabilitation approach is suggested for complex fractures compared with stable, nondisplaced, or minimally displaced fractures. However, once osseous union is achieved (typically around 6 weeks), no matter the fracture pattern, frequent stretching in all planes without limitations should begin in an attempt to regain passive range of motion. It is of paramount importance that full range of motion is achieved before the scar tissue becomes recalcitrant to stretching. Strengthening can proceed in due time as there is no outer limit on when this phase must be completed.

Common exercises prescribed for rehabilitation after PHF are shown in Figs. 26.1–26.3 and may be most comfortable in a seated position early in rehabilitation. Elevation and external rotation performed in a seated position with the arm supported as demonstrated in Figs. 26.1 and 26.2 offer patients a convenient method of integrating range of motion throughout the day which may enhance compliance. The active stage of recovery of elevation can be progressed from supine, to inclined, to upright position as shown in Fig. 26.3, and load can be increased by initially having a bent then straight elbow. This active elevation progression has been shown to gradually advance electromyographic activity in upper extremity muscles.[10]

PEARLS AND PITFALLS

- A pitfall in therapy for patients with PHF is the initiation of strength challenges prior to optimizing glenohumeral range of motion. Passive range of motion must be optimized prior to beginning active motion, and active range of motion with good mechanics should be attained prior to the initiation of resistive training to prevent poor mechanics with exercises.[11]
- Motion recovery should be pain-free in any shoulder rehabilitation process.[11] Aggressive physical therapy results in increased muscle guarding which ultimately decreases range of motion, erodes patient trust and satisfaction, and discourages compliance.
- Recalcitrant stiffness can be managed with low-load long-duration stretching and should be communicated to providers if unresponsive to interventions. When it comes to stretching, frequency is even more important than intensity.

TABLE 26.1	Rehabilitation Guidelines Following Proximal Humeral Fractures Managed Nonoperatively for Stable and Complex Patterns		
	Stable	Complex	Suggested Exercises
Sling	3 weeks	6 weeks	
Pendulum, distal circulation, and posture	1 week	2 weeks	• Pendulum • Elbow, wrist, and hand AROM • Seated active scapular retraction
Elevation			
PROM	Begin at 2 weeks to 90 degrees After 4 weeks as tolerated	Begin at 4 weeks to 90 degrees After 6 weeks as tolerated	• Table slide or step back (Fig. 26.1) • Supine partner or well-arm assisted
AAROM	4–6 weeks as tolerated	6 weeks as tolerated	• Rope and pulley • Supine dowel assisted
AROM	6 weeks when P/AAROM restored	8 weeks when P/AAROM restored	• Reverse pendulum in supine • Supine to reclined to upright AROM (Fig. 26.3)
Resisted	8–12 weeks when AROM normalized with good biomechanics	12 weeks when AROM is normalized with good mechanics	1–3-pound dumbbell or band resistance in reclined or upright position
External Rotation—Arm at Side			
PROM	Begin at 3 weeks to 30 degrees After 6 weeks progress as tolerated	Begin at 6 weeks slow progression as tolerated	• Seated well-arm assisted—keeping arm supported and back against chair (Fig. 26.2) • Partner assisted in supine-scapular plane • Doorframe
AAROM	6 weeks as tolerated	8 weeks as tolerated	Supine dowel assisted—scapular plane
AROM	8 weeks or when P/AAROM restored	10 weeks or when P/AAROM restored	• Seated unassisted ER (gravity eliminated; Fig. 26.2) • Side-lying ER (against gravity)
Resisted	10 weeks when AROM = PROM	12 weeks when AROM = PROM	• 1–3-pound dumbbell in side-lying • Band resistance
External rotation—90 degrees abduction	After 6 weeks	After 8 weeks	• Supine dowel assisted—scapular plane • Doorframe
Internal Rotation			
AROM	After 6 weeks	After 6 weeks	Hand slide up back gently
Resisted	10 weeks	12 weeks	Band resistance
Scapula	4–6 weeks—prone unweighted Add resistance 8 weeks	6–8 weeks prone unweighted Add resistance 10–12 weeks	• Prone unweighted: extension to hip + scapular depression retraction • Prone horizontal abduction • Add light dumbbell to above • Band resistance: low row with elbows straight and bent

Recommendations are intended to serve as a guideline and should be tailored to specific patients with close communication with the provider regarding progression based on radiographic evidence of healing. Movement as tolerated means that the patient pain level is <3/10.

AROM, active range of motion; *AAROM,* active-assisted range of motion; *ER,* external rotation; *PROM,* passive range of motion.

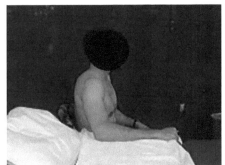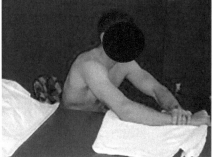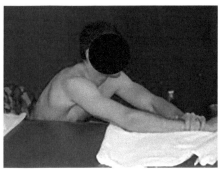

• **Fig. 26.1** Table slide exercise for supported shoulder flexion/elevation.

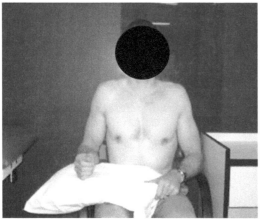
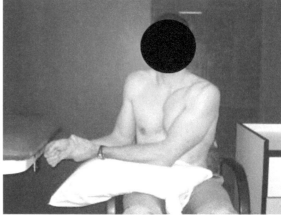

• **Fig. 26.2** Well-arm-assisted external rotation in seated position.

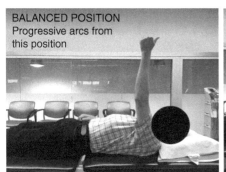

BALANCED POSITION
Progressive arcs from
this position

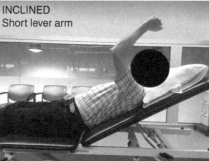

INCLINED
Short lever arm

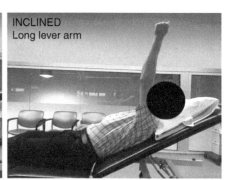

INCLINED
Long lever arm

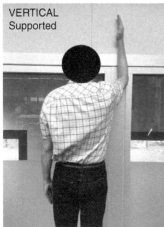

VERTICAL
Supported

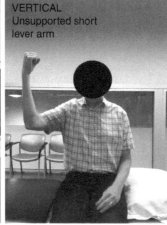

VERTICAL
Unsupported short
lever arm

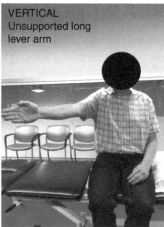

VERTICAL
Unsupported long
lever arm

• **Fig. 26.3** The active range-of-motion progression from supine, to reclined, to upright with short (bent elbow), and then long (straight elbow) lever arm to graduate load.

References

1. Kwan LL, MacIntyre NJ. Rehabilitation of Proximal Humerus Fractures: An Environmental Scan of Canadian Physiotherapy Practice Patterns. *J Nov Physiother Rehabil.* 2017;1:104–119.
2. Kancherla VK, Singh A, Anakwenze OA. Management of acute proximal humeral fractures. *J Am Acad Orthop Surg.* 2017;25(1): 42–52.
3. Clement ND, Duckworth AD, McQueen MM, Court-Brown CM. The outcome of proximal humeral fractures in the elderly: predictors of mortality and function. *Bone Joint Lett J.* 2014;96-B(7):970–977.
4. Misra S, Vaishya R, Trikha V, Maheshwari J. Practice guidelines for proximal humeral fractures. *J Clin Orthop Trauma.* 2019;10(3):631–633.
5. Beks RB, Ochen Y, Frima H, et al. Operative versus nonoperative treatment of proximal humeral fractures: a systematic review, meta-analysis, and comparison of observational studies and randomized controlled trials. *J Shoulder Elbow Surg.* 2018;27(8):1526–1534.
6. Slobogean GP, Johal H, Lefaivre KA, et al. A scoping review of the proximal humerus fracture literature. *BMC Musculoskelet Disord.* 2015;16:112.
7. Hodgson SA, Mawson SJ, Stanley D. Rehabilitation after two-part fractures of the neck of the humerus. *J Bone Joint Surg Br.* 2003;85(3):419–422.

8. Lefevre-Colau MM, Babinet A, Fayad F, et al. Immediate mobilization compared with conventional immobilization for the impacted nonoperatively treated proximal humeral fracture. A randomized controlled trial. *J Bone Joint Surg Am.* 2007;89(12): 2582–2590.

9. Hodgson S. Proximal humerus fracture rehabilitation. *Clin Orthop Relat Res.* 2006;442:131–138.

10. Wise MB, Uhl TL, Mattacola CG, Nitz AJ, Kibler WB. The effect of limb support on muscle activation during shoulder exercises. *J Shoulder Elbow Surg.* 2004;13(6):614–620.

11. Gaunt B. Core principles of the systematic approach to shoulder rehabilitation. In: Gaunt BW, McCluskey GM, eds. *A Systematic Approach to Shoulder Rehabilitation.* Columbus, GA: HPRC. 2012:156–168.

27

Technique Spotlight: ORIF Proximal Humerus Fracture with Deltopectoral Approach

MATTHEW R. COHN, WILLIAM M. CREGAR, JOSEPH B. COHEN, AND JOEL C. WILLIAMS

Indications

Several options exist for the management of proximal humerus fractures including nonoperative care, closed reduction and percutaneous pinning, open reduction and internal fixation (ORIF) with a plate and screw construct, intramedullary nailing, and arthroplasty. The majority of these injuries are nondisplaced or minimally displaced and may be managed nonoperatively with positive functional outcomes.[1,2] However, a subset of patients presenting with displaced proximal humerus fractures are deemed surgical candidates based on a myriad of considerations including both fracture characteristics and patient-related factors (see Chapter 25: Treatment Algorithm for Proximal Humerus Fractures). Fracture characteristics that should be taken into consideration include the degree of displacement, fracture complexity, bone quality, size of the humeral head fragment, history of rotator cuff deficiency or rotator cuff arthropathy, presence of fracture-dislocations, chondral damage/head-split, and risk for future avascular necrosis.

The Neer classification is the most widely used classification system for proximal humerus fractures.[1] Fractures are described based on the number of displaced fragments (one-, two-, three-, or four-part), which include the humeral shaft, greater tuberosity, lesser tuberosity, and articular segment. Fragments displaced >1 cm or angulated >45 degrees are considered truly "displaced" segments based on the classification scheme.[1] Despite the fairly low intraobserver reliability and reproducibility, we find it a helpful tool to communicate a general idea of fracture morphology.[3,4]

Patient characteristics such as physiologic age, past medical history, preinjury level of activity, functional demands, occupation, handedness, home living condition and support system, and ability to participate in and comply with a structured physical therapy program should all be considered in deciding management.

Appropriate patient selection criteria for surgical management have been a topic of much debate, and a consensus on optimal management remains poorly defined. Results from the Proximal Fracture of the Humerus Evaluation by Randomization (PROF-HER) trial, which suggested that operative intervention provides no benefit over nonoperative treatment, further clouds decisional management of these injuries.[5] The validity of this study's results has been questioned due to a number of methodologic limitations and poorly defined surgical indications.

Generally, we prefer management with ORIF for substantially displaced proximal humerus fractures in active, healthy, physiologically "young" patients, with adequate bone stock and no contraindications to surgery. This includes significantly displaced two-part tuberosity and surgical neck fractures as well as most three-part fractures, four-part fractures, and fracture-dislocations, where adequate reduction and stability can be achieved and healing potential remains adequate. Patients presenting with unreconstructable humeral heads, unacceptably high risk of osteonecrosis (i.e., delayed presentation of head-split or fracture-dislocations), rotator cuff deficiency, or significant glenoid arthrosis may be better suited with primary arthroplasty.

On the other side of the spectrum, patients may be better suited for nonoperative management or primary versus delayed arthroplasty if they are physiologically "elderly," low-demand, have low potential to heal tuberosity fragments, have poor bone quality, or suffer from comorbidities such as diabetes, vascular disease, metabolic disorders, or poor nutritional status[6] that risk bone failure around the fixation construct and screw cutout. Recent literature suggests inferior outcomes in elderly patients who undergo revision arthroplasty following failed ORIF attempts when compared with delayed arthroplasty following failed nonoperative attempts.[3] This highlights the concept that ORIF should be performed in a select patient population on an individualized basis where a multitude of factors are taken into consideration and a patient-involved decision is reached.

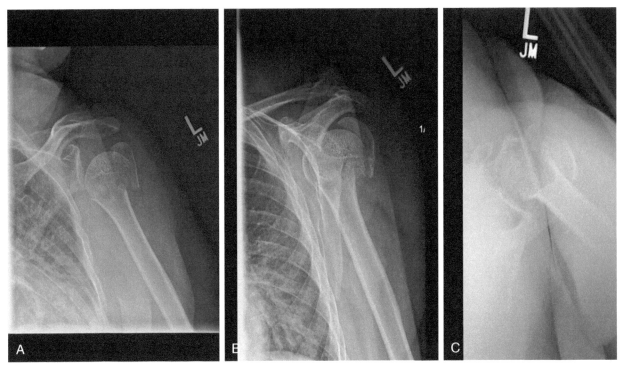

• **Fig. 27.1** Shoulder trauma series including **(A)** Grashey, **(B)** scapula Y, and **(C)** axillary views demonstrating a three-part proximal humerus fracture.

Preoperative Evaluation

Pertinent information to be obtained from a patient's history include the mechanism of injury, antecedent pain, history of malignancy, and history of previous injuries and/or surgeries to the operative extremity. A low-energy mechanism such as a ground-level fall or history of other fragility fractures should clue the clinician into the patient's overall poor bone quality. This can present as an opportunity for the orthopedic surgeon to diagnose and guide treatment for low bone density disorders in order to prevent future fragility fractures.[7,8]

In the setting of high-energy injuries, physical examination should begin with the advanced trauma life support protocol. All other extremities should be evaluated, including the spine and chest wall, with a combination of palpation and range of motion to screen for concomitant injuries prior to performing a focused examination of the suspected injured extremity. Focused physical examination begins with evaluation of the soft tissues and skin surrounding the shoulder and axilla to rule out the presence of an open fracture. A careful neurovascular examination should be performed with particular attention to the motor and sensory function of the axillary nerve. Evaluation of the axillary nerve is performed by assessing independent muscle contraction of the posterior, lateral, and anterior divisions of the deltoid muscle and proximal lateral arm sensation.

A complete radiographic shoulder series should be obtained, including a true glenoid anteroposterior (AP) or *Grashey* view, axillary lateral view, and scapula Y lateral view (Fig. 27.1A–C). The axillary lateral view defines the humeral head-glenoid relationship and is imperative in evaluating for glenohumeral dislocation or glenoid articular surface involvement.[9] Lesser tuberosity displacement can also be further evaluated with this view. Alternatively, if the patient is unable to

tolerate positioning for an axillary lateral, a Velpeau view can be obtained.[10] The scapula Y view provides information on the head-shaft angulation and displacement in the sagittal plane, whereas the Grashey AP view provides information on coronal (varus/valgus) fracture alignment and tuberosity displacement. Computed tomography (CT) imaging with or without three-dimensional (3D) reconstructions is not always indicated for proximal humerus fractures; however, it can provide more detailed information regarding tuberosity displacement, nondisplaced fracture lines, degree of comminution, articular surface involvement, and definitive glenohumeral relationship especially when an axillary lateral radiograph is of poor quality or unable to be obtained.[9] Generally, the authors obtain a CT scan in settings where the degree of tuberosity displacement is not well visualized on standard radiographs, axillary lateral views cannot be obtained to evaluate for fracture-dislocations, and if the fracture pattern is poorly visualized on radiographs in operative fractures for the purpose of surgical planning.

Position and Equipment

The procedure is typically performed under general endotracheal anesthesia to allow for adequate muscle relaxation to aid in reduction. Regional anesthesia such as an interscalene block may be performed for postoperative pain control. The patient is positioned supine with his or her head on the cantilever end of a radiolucent table. Following intubation, the table is rotated 90 degrees with the operative shoulder facing the center of the operating room. A plexiglass, radiolucent board is placed under the pad of the table such that an approximately one-foot by one-foot area beyond the edge of the table can support the patient's upper arm. The patient's torso is positioned so the operative shoulder is over the lateral edge of the bed to maximize access to the proximal

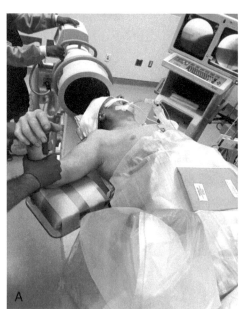
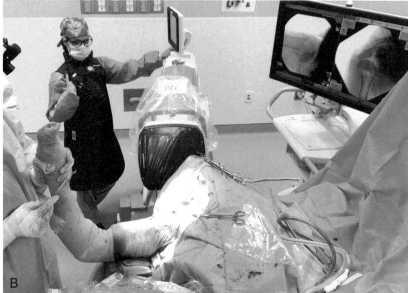

• **Fig. 27.2** Positioning of the C-arm for axillary fluoroscopy view while (**A**) positioning and (**B**) intraoperatively.

humerus and to allow for an adequate axillary fluoroscopic view. At this point, AP and axillary fluoroscopic views with the C-arm positioned at the head of the OR table may be obtained to ensure that adequate orthogonal fluoroscopic images are accessible. An AP view of the humerus will be used to determine coronal plane alignment, cranial-caudal plate position, and screw lengths. The arm should be externally rotated 20 to 30 degrees to view the humeral head and neck in profile while accounting for native retroversion. An axillary view is performed with the beam parallel to the floor and the patient with the arm in 30 to 90 degrees of abduction (Fig. 27.2A–B). This view will be used to assess sagittal plane deformity, version, reduction of the glenohumeral joint and tuberosities, anterior-posterior placement of the plate, and screw lengths and trajectories.

Foam pads or towels are placed on the arm board to match the height of the table's padding (Fig. 27.2A). Foam padding is placed under the heels and blankets are placed under the patient's knees to provide hip and knee flexion (Fig. 27.3). All other bony prominences are well padded. The patient's head may be secured with tape and a towel placed over the forehead or a foam head holder. A U-shaped drape is placed within the axilla from the scapula posteriorly ending just above the nipple line medially. A straight drape is placed along the neck and mid-clavicular line.

The prep and drape is finalized with sterile towels and two U-shaped drapes with the aperture secured with strips of Ioban (3M; Saint Paul, MN, USA). A stockinette and Coban (3M) are placed over the ipsilateral upper extremity ending just distal to the supracondylar region of the humerus. A sterile drape to allow passage of the C-arm is placed distal to the operative extremity. The Mayo stand and back table are located lateral to the operative extremity (Fig. 27.4A–B). A summary of procedural equipment is presented in Table 27.1.

Exposure

The coracoid process is marked and the incision is marked from 1 cm lateral to the coracoid toward the midline of the arm, oriented

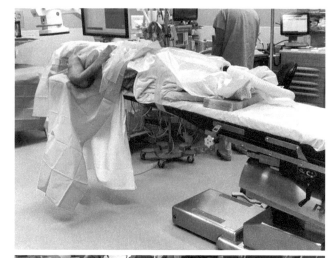
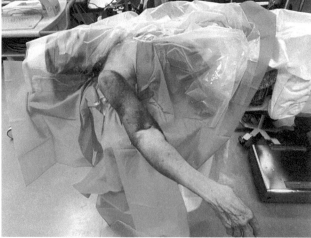

• **Fig. 27.3** Supine position on a cantilever table with the arm resting on a short radiolucent plexiglass arm board.

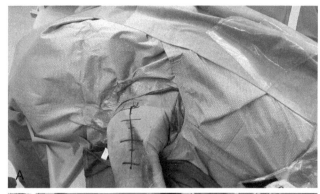

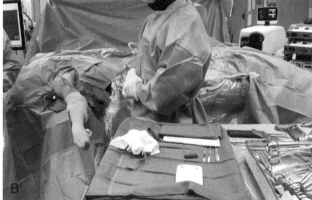

• **Fig. 27.4** (**A**) Coracoid process and incision for deltopectoral exposure marked. (**B**) Positioning of the Mayo stand and back table in relation to the primary surgeon.

TABLE 27.1	Procedural Equipment and Material
Positioning	• Cantilever radiolucent table, plexiglass radiolucent arm board • Impervious stockinette, 4-inch elastic self-adherent wrap • Foam padding under heels • Pillow under knees • Bilateral calf SCDs
Exposure Biceps tenodesis	• Gelpi, Langenbeck, Army-Navy, Chandler, Hohmann retractors • Heavy nonabsorbable suture
Reduction	• Cobb elevator, narrow AO elevator, Hohmann retractor, large and small pointed reduction clamps, 1.6 and 2.0-mm K-wires, 2.5 and 4.0-mm terminally threaded Schanz pins • Wire driver/drill
Fixation	• Anatomically contoured 3.5 mm proximal humerus locking compression plate • Minifragmentary plates and screws • Fibular strut allograft, calcium phosphate cement, cancellous allograft as needed
Imaging	• Fluoroscope

AO, Arbeitsgemeinschaft für Osteosynthesefragen; *SCDs,* sequential compression devices.

laterally toward the deltoid tuberosity. The incision is more laterally based compared to a traditional deltopectoral exposure to allow easier access to the lateral aspect of the proximal humerus for plate and screw placement (Fig. 27.4A). The distal extent of the incision is dictated by fracture extension down the humeral shaft and planned plate length.

Skin and subcutaneous tissues are incised sharply while being careful not to injure the cephalic vein. Gelpi retractors are placed to help with maintaining exposure. The cephalic vein marks the deltopectoral interval and is mobilized with forceps and Metzenbaum scissors medially or laterally, depending on the surgeon's preference. We generally mobilize the vein laterally to maintain the tributaries from the deltoid. Others prefer mobilizing the vein medially, as the majority of the reduction and fixation will occur on the lateral aspect of the operative field.

The cephalic vein is usually marked by a "fat-stripe." If there is difficulty locating the cephalic vein, it is often more easily identified proximally toward Mohrenheim's fossa, which is an inverted triangle formed by borders of the clavicle, deltoid, and the clavicular head of the pectoralis major. After the deltopectoral interval is defined, the deltoid muscle is retracted laterally and the pectoralis major medially with Langenbeck or self-retaining retractors. The proximal aspect of the incision is retracted with a Richardson retractor or a Hohmann retractor placed under the coracoacromial ligament in the subacromial space (Fig. 27.5A–B).

A Hohmann retractor is placed underneath the deltoid over the lateral humerus to retract the deltoid laterally, and the subdeltoid bursa is bluntly released. Additionally, the anterolateral portion of the deltoid insertion is released to mobilize the deltoid and to create space for the plate. The deltoid insertion has been reported to

be approximately 7 cm in length and 2 cm in width at the proximal border.[11] We typically release 1–2 cm of the deltoid insertion with a shield-tipped elevator to allow the distal aspect of the plate to sit on the lateral humerus. The clavipectoral fascia is incised lateral to the conjoint tendon and muscle fibers of the short head of the biceps.

We prefer to perform a soft tissue tenodesis of the long head of the biceps tendon (LHBT) at this point. The LHBT is dissected from its groove by pulling tension with forceps and freeing it from its sheath with Metzenbaum scissors. The LHBT is followed into the rotator interval and transected as it approaches its intra-articular glenoid origin. A soft tissue tenodesis to the upper portion of the pectoralis major tendon is performed using nonabsorbable heavy suture in a figure-of-eight fashion (Fig. 27.6).

Reduction

The proximal humerus has several deforming forces that must be considered when performing reduction. The humeral shaft is often translated anteromedially by the pull of the pectoralis major, while the supraspinatus, infraspinatus, and teres minor provide moments that lead to external rotation, posteromedial displacement, and varus positioning of the greater tuberosity and any attached articular segment. The subscapularis provides an internal rotation force that rotates the entire articular segment if unopposed—for example, in the case of a three-part fracture where the lesser tuberosity is intact to the articular segment. Metaphyseal impaction resulting in valgus alignment is common. Varus patterns may be observed, often with the humeral shaft telescoped into the articular segment.

Obtaining a high-quality reduction is associated with lower complication rates and improved patient-reported outcomes.[12–14] Primary goals of the reduction include anatomic alignment of the

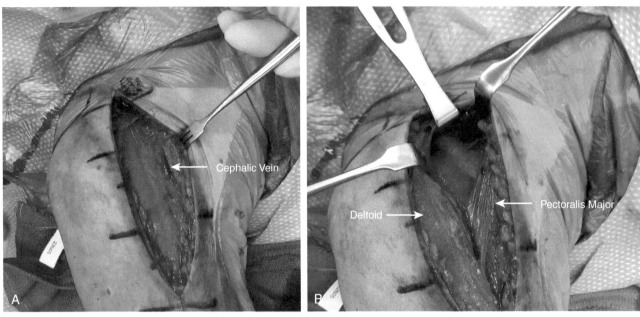

• **Fig. 27.5** (**A**) Identification of the cephalic vein at the deltopectoral interval. (**B**) Retraction of the deltoid laterally and pectoralis major medially, revealing the clavipectoral fascia.

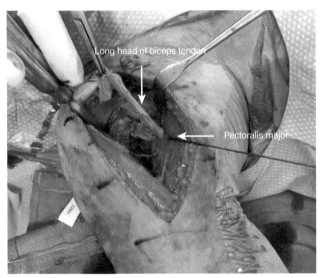

• **Fig. 27.6** Soft tissue tenodesis of the long head of the biceps tendon to the upper border of the pectoralis major.

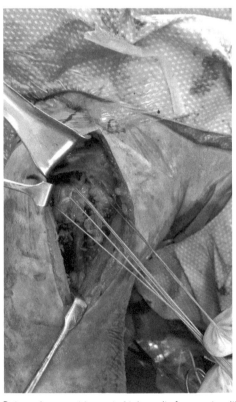

• **Fig. 27.7** Suture placement to control tuberosity fragments with #5 Fiberwire (Arthrex, Naples, FL, USA) or #5 Ethibond (Johnson & Johnson, New Brunswick, NJ, USA).

calcar and avoidance of varus malalignment. Failure to achieve these goals may result in varus collapse and articular screw penetration.[15,16] The ideal head-shaft angle has been reported to be between 120 and 150 degrees in the coronal plane and <25 degrees in the sagittal plane.[13,14]

A number of reduction maneuvers may be used depending on the fracture pattern. In patients with a fracture-dislocation, some have advocated in situ fixation prior to reduction to avoid endangering the tenuous blood supply.[17] However, we prefer careful reduction of the glenohumeral joint first. The humeral head may be reduced simply with manual manipulation and a Cobb elevator. A 2.0-mm K-wire or 2.5-mm terminally threaded Schanz pin placed within the humeral head may be used as joysticks for more direct control.

To control the tuberosity fragments, heavy nonabsorbable traction sutures are placed through the rotator cuff tendons in a figure-of-eight fashion (Fig. 27.7). These are secured to the drapes with a clamp until needed for reduction of the tuberosities.

Next, reduction of the humeral head is performed with a focus on restoring humeral inclination, offset, version, and the medial calcar. If valgus impaction is present, a narrow elevator or K-wire

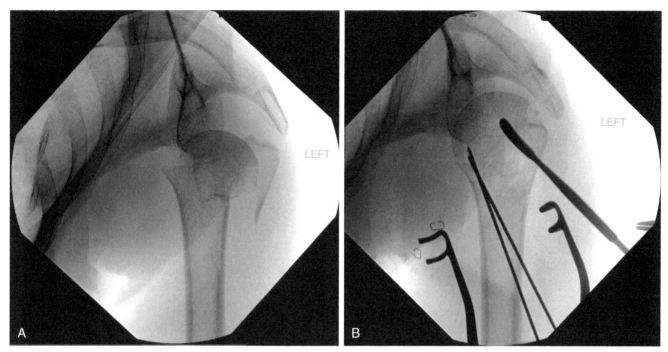

• **Fig. 27.8** (**A**) and (**B**) Elevation of the humeral head from a valgus position using an elevator.

is placed through the lateral aspect of the fracture directed at the apex of the articular segment and elevated to lever the head out of valgus (Fig. 27.8A–B).

The plate may also be used as a reduction tool. This is done by placing the plate in the proper position on the proximal segment and securing the proximal segment with locking screws. The plate and proximal segment are then anatomically aligned on the lateral fluoroscopic image. A gap is intentionally left between the plate and the proximal shaft adjacent to the fracture on the AP fluoroscopic image. The most distal hole in the plate is then secured with a nonlocking screw. A second nonlocking screw is then placed adjacent to the fracture to pull the shaft laterally, thereby creating mismatch compression. Additional fixation may be added as needed (Fig. 27.9A–D).

Contouring of the plate may be necessary to avoid malreduction. The reduction of the calcar may be assessed by looking for continuity of Shenton's line of the shoulder. If varus deformity is present, a narrow Hohmann retractor is placed into the fracture toward the medial side to shoehorn the head segment into a more valgus position. Provisional fixation is held using multiple 2.0-mm K-wires driven across the fracture site. Of note, these should be placed strategically to avoid blocking appropriate lateral placement of the plate. They may be directed from distal to proximal from the anterior shaft to the posterior humeral head. Alternatively, they can be placed from proximal to distal from the rotator interval and lesser tuberosity into the posterior humeral shaft (Fig. 27.10A–C).

After the humeral head is adequately reduced and provisionally fixed, the tuberosity fragments are reduced with the traction sutures, pointed reduction clamps, and/or K-wires. Reduction of the tuberosities can help maintain an elevated position of the reduced humeral head in valgus-impacted fractures.

Fixation

Locking plates are most commonly used for fixation. We prefer using an anatomically contoured 3.5-mm locking compression plate. If there is calcar comminution with lack of medial support or volumetric metaphyseal defects, we will also consider using an intramedullary fibular allograft to augment our fixation (Fig. 27.11A–D). Cement augmentation may be used for large metaphyseal defects. We prefer to use calcium phosphate cement, which can be drilled and improves humeral head locking screw purchase.

The rotator cuff sutures are passed through the plate prior to positioning it on the humerus. On the AP fluoroscopic view, the plate is positioned so the most inferior humeral head screw abuts the medial calcar. This screw acts as a buttress to resist varus collapse (Fig. 27.11D). It is important to avoid placing the plate too proximally because the calcar screw will become less effective and risks impingement of the proximal plate against the acromion with abduction. On the axillary view, the plate should be placed in the midline of the humerus (Fig. 27.12). We typically place a minimum of two nonlocking screws distally, which brings the plate flush with the shaft followed by placement of proximal locking screws. When placing the locking screws in the humeral head, we prefer to drill in a unicortical fashion to only open the lateral cortex. We then place the depth gauge through the locking guide in the same trajectory and gently push to subchondral bone to create a path for the screw while removing minimal bone and reducing the chance for articular surface penetration. We typically insert a screw 2 to 4 mm less than the depth gauge reads at the subchondral bone. After humeral head locking screws are placed, AP and axillary views are scrutinized to ensure no screws enter the glenohumeral joint. Because the humeral head is a convex surface, any fluoroscopic view with a protruding screw indicates articular penetration and should be revised to a shorter screw.

After plate placement, the tuberosity sutures are tied down to the plate. If a lesser tuberosity fracture is present, minifragment screws can be placed independently or through a one-quarter tubular plate for additional fixation (Fig. 27.12). Similar constructs may be used for fixation of a large greater tuberosity fragment.

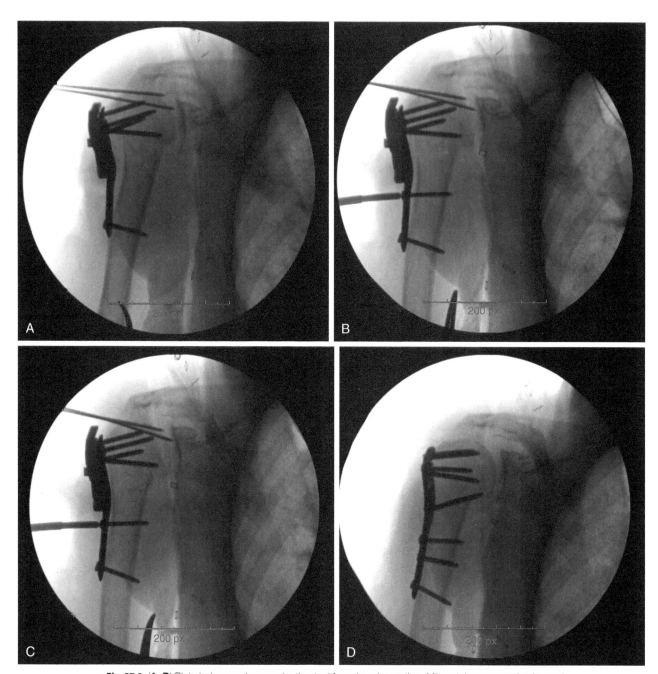

• **Fig. 27.9** (**A–D**) Plate being used as a reduction tool for valgus impaction. Mismatch compression is used to compress the shaft into the proximal segment. Note how the plate is "off bone" of the humeral shaft in the upper left figure and the head translated laterally. As the plate is compressed to bone, the fracture alignment improves.

Closure

A drain is used sparingly when there was difficulty with hemostasis during the case. The deltopectoral fascia is closed with 0 braided absorbable sutures followed by closure of subcutaneous tissue with 2-0 braided absorbable sutures and skin with 3-0 nylon sutures in tensionless vertical mattress fashion.

Postoperative Care

We generally prefer aspirin 81 mg daily for deep vein thrombosis prophylaxis for 3 weeks unless another anticoagulant is indicated for medical purposes. The patient is usually made non—weight-bearing with their operative arm in a sling for comfort. Crutch mobilization is sometimes permitted in the polytraumatized patient with excellent fixation. The progression of activity and physical therapy is dependent on fracture pattern, stability following fixation, bone quality, and physiologic age of the patient. If stable fixation is achieved, pendulum exercises and passive range of motion are often permitted starting postoperative day 1. By 2 weeks postoperatively, patients may be progressed to lift up to the weight of a coffee-cup. At 6 weeks postoperatively, patients are typically permitted to begin active range-of-motion exercises. Strengthening exercises begin at 12 weeks postoperatively.

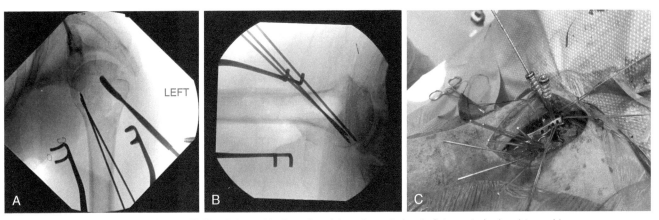

• **Fig. 27.10** (**A**) and (**B**) The 2.0-mm K-wires placed from the anterior shaft to posterior head to avoid impeding lateral plate placement. (**C**) Plate placed lateral to K-wires.

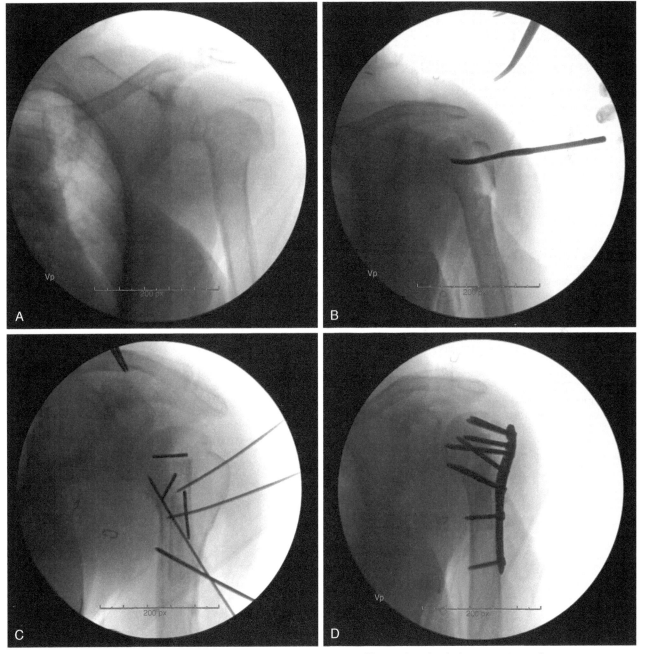

• **Fig. 27.11** (**A**) Valgus-impacted proximal humerus fracture, (**B**) elevation of articular segment revealing volumetric metaphyseal bone loss, (**C**) intramedullary fibular allograft and fracture provisionally fixed with 2.0-mm K-wires, and (**D**) final fixation construct.

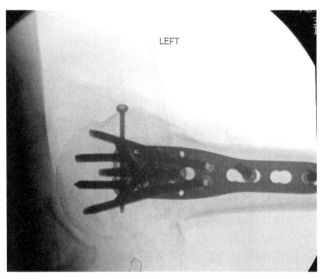

• **Fig. 27.12** Lesser tuberosity fixation using a 2.7-mm cortical screw.

PEARLS AND PITFALLS

Pearls

- Open reduction internal fixation (ORIF) utilized for patients with moderate to high functional demands with (1) degree of displacement that will limit function if treated nonoperatively, (2) bone quality that will allow stable fixation, (3) pattern that appears amenable to healing without high risk of avascular necrosis (AVN), (4) younger age and/or functional demands render arthroplasty undesirable
- Ensure satisfactory Anteroposterior (AP) and axillary fluoroscopic views are able to be obtained prior to prepping and draping
- Supine position with plexiglass arm board allows a high degree of freedom to manipulate arm during reduction
- Release of proximal deltoid insertion allows proper plate placement
- Major goals of reduction are to restore head-shaft angle (120–150 degrees in the coronal plane and <25 degrees in the sagittal plane) and alignment of the calcar
- K-wires should be placed from anterior shaft to posterior head to allow proper plate placement
- Augmentation with fibular strut allograft, calcium phosphate cement, or cancellous allograft may be necessary in cases of severe metaphyseal impaction

Pitfalls

- Inadequate fluoroscopic imaging may risk detection of screw penetration into the glenohumeral joint
- Avoid placing the plate too proximal, as this may result in impingement or an ineffective calcar screw
- Ensure sutures placed in rotator cuff are tied through holes in plate

References

1. Neer 2nd CS. Displaced proximal humeral fractures. I. Classification and evaluation. *J Bone Joint Surg Am*. 1970;52:1077–1089.
2. Hasty EK, Jernigan 3rd EW, Soo A, Varkey DT, Kamath GV. Trends in surgical management and costs for operative treatment of proximal humerus fractures in the elderly. *Orthopedics*. 2017;40:e641–e647.
3. Brien H, Noftall F, MacMaster S, Cummings T, Landells C, Rockwood P. Neer's classification system: a critical appraisal. *J Trauma*. 1995;38:257–260.
4. Siebenrock KA, Gerber C. The reproducibility of classification of fractures of the proximal end of the humerus. *J Bone Joint Surg Am*. 1993;75:1751–1755.
5. Rangan A, Handoll H, Brealey S, et al. Surgical vs nonsurgical treatment of adults with displaced fractures of the proximal humerus: the PROFHER randomized clinical trial. *J Am Med Assoc*. 2015;313:1037–1047.
6. Bishop JA, Palanca AA, Bellino MJ, Lowenberg DW. Assessment of compromised fracture healing. *J Am Acad Orthop Surg*. 2012;20:273–282.
7. Dang DY, Zetumer S, Zhang AL. Recurrent fragility fractures: a cross-sectional analysis. *J Am Acad Orthop Surg*. 2019;27:e85–e91.
8. Cohn MR, Gianakos AL, Grueter K, Rosen N, Cong G-T, Lane JM. Update on the comprehensive approach to fragility fractures. *J Orthop Trauma*. 2018;32:480–490.
9. Rothberg D, Higgins T. Fractures of the proximal humerus. *Orthop Clin North Am*. 2013;44:9–19.
10. Khoriati AA, Antonios T, Bakti N, Mohanlal P, Singh B. Outcomes following non operative management for proximal humerus fractures. *J Clin Orthop Trauma*. 2019;10:462–467.
11. Rispoli DM, Athwal GS, Sperling JW, Cofield RH. The anatomy of the deltoid insertion. *J Shoulder Elbow Surg*. 2009;18:386–390.
12. Schnetzke M, Bockmeyer J, Porschke F, Studier-Fischer S, Grützner PA, Guehring T. Quality of reduction influences outcome after locked-plate fixation of proximal humeral type-C fractures. *J Bone Joint Surg Am*. 2016;98:1777–1785.
13. Liskutin T, Harkin E, Summers H, Cohen J, Bernstein M, Lack W. The influence of biplanar reduction and surgeon experience on proximal humerus fractures treated with ORIF. *Injury*. 2020;51:322–328.
14. Schnetzke M, Bockmeyer J, Porschke F, Studier-Fischer S, Grützner PA, Guehring T. Quality of reduction influences outcome after locked-plate fixation of proximal humeral type-C fractures. *J Bone Joint Surg Am*. 2016;98:1777–1785.
15. Gardner MJ, Weil Y, Barker JU, Kelly BT, Helfet DL, Lorich DG. The importance of medial support in locked plating of proximal humerus fractures. *J Orthop Trauma*. 2007;21:185–191.
16. Lee CW, Shin SJ. Prognostic factors for unstable proximal humeral fractures treated with locking-plate fixation. *J Shoulder Elbow Surg*. 2009;18:83–88.
17. Hersche O, Gerber C. Iatrogenic displacement of fracture-dislocations of the shoulder. A report of seven cases. *J Bone Joint Surg Br*. 1994;76:30–33.

28

Technique Spotlight: ORIF Proximal Humerus Fracture with IMN

BENJAMIN W. SEARS AND ARMODIOS M. HATZIDAKIS

Intramedullary Fixation for Proximal Humerus Fractures

Indications

Proximal humeral fractures continue to increase in frequency with projected rates of emergency visits in the United States alone annually to exceed 275,000 by 2030 and well over a million visits worldwide.[1] Although many fractures can be treated nonoperatively, significantly displaced or angulated fractures in certain patients may benefit from surgical intervention. Intramedullary nail fixation has gained interest in conjunction *with* evolution of implant design. This surgical technique with modern devices allows for the predictable healing of two-part surgical neck fractures,[2] capture of tuberosity fracture fragments, the option for percutaneous device placement, and protection of vascularity to the fracture and head segment as a result of minimally invasive exposure and insertion.[3] As a result, almost all two-part fractures and an increasing number of three- and four-part fractures can predictably be managed with intramedullary fixation.[4,5]

Preoperative Evaluation (Examination and Imaging)

Preoperative evaluation mandates close neurovascular examination as some patients can present with an associated axillary nerve or brachial plexus neuropraxic injury.[6] Serious vascular complications have been reported with even minimally displaced fractures.[7] Routine images include Grashey, Scapular-Lateral, and axillary views of the injured shoulder to evaluate fracture pattern and displacement, and confirm humeral head location. Computed tomography (CT) imaging including 2D and 3D reconstructions can be valuable for preoperative planning as it may allow improved appreciation of calcar comminution, three- and four-part tuberosity fracture segment displacement, and nondisplaced fracture planes. If patients report preinjury shoulder pain or weakness, preoperative magnetic resonance imaging (MRI) is indicated to evaluate for preexisting rotator cuff pathology that may shift treatment options toward arthroplasty.

Positioning and Equipment

Intramedullary nailing of two-part surgical neck fractures may be accomplished in either a "lazy lateral" position on a bean

bag with a radiolucent trauma table (Fig. 28.1) or in the beach chair position. In the beach chair position, the head of the bed is raised approximately 35–45 degrees allowing access for imaging, unobstructed implant insertion, and improved ease of conversion to arthroplasty in multipart fractures (Fig. 28.2). Fluoroscopy is positioned on the contralateral side and preoperative radiographs are confirmed prior to draping. Reproducible imaging is critical for achieving anatomic fracture reduction and appropriate nail position, particularly with the percutaneous technique. A Grashey view is taken with the C-arm tilted horizontally to match the semirecumbent orientation of the patient and orbiting the machine 30–45 degrees to obtain a parallel view of the glenoid face (Fig. 28.3). With the arm in neutral rotation, this image will reproduce a view of the proximal humerus that profiles the lateral greater tuberosity and humeral head, guiding

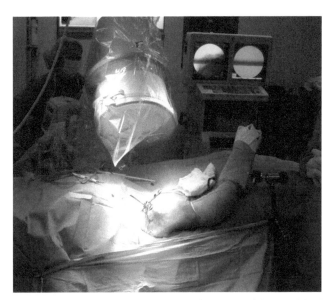

• **Fig. 28.1** "Lazy lateral" position. With the patient on a radiolucent table, the fracture side is rotated up 30 degrees and a bean bag is placed under the fracture. The fluoroscope is brought in from the opposite side and the monitor typically positioned at the foot of the bed. An arm holder is attached to the bed distally to keep the arm in a position of neutral rotation and light traction.

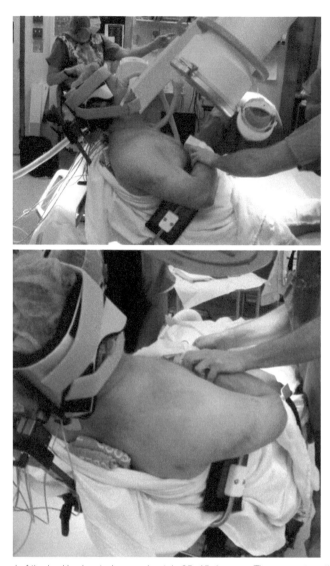

• **Fig. 28.2** Beach chair position. The head of the bed is elevated approximately 35–45 degrees. The support on the side of the fracture is dropped out to allow radiolucency for Grashey and scapular Y-lateral radiographs.

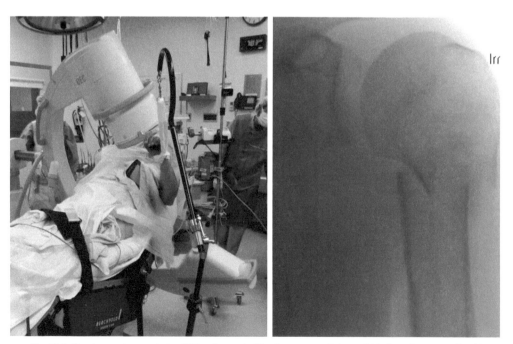

• **Fig. 28.3** Grashey anteroposterior (AP) radiograph. The fluoroscope is brought in from the opposite side of the fracture and rotated back 30–50 degrees to obtain a Grashey (true AP) view of the shoulder. The glenoid and greater tuberosity are brought into profile in the coronal plane.

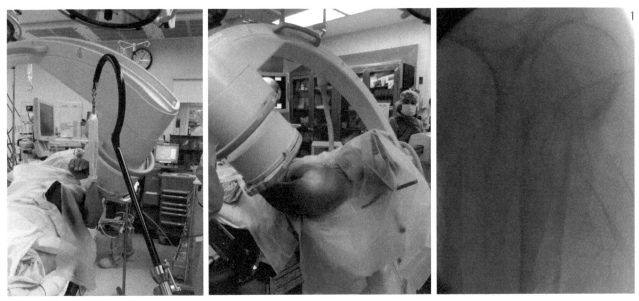

• **Fig. 28.4** Scapular Y-lateral view. The fluoroscope is brought in from the opposite side of the fracture and rotated forward 30–40 degrees to obtain a scapular Y-lateral view of the shoulder.

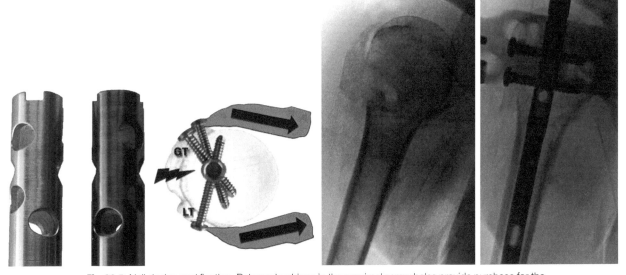

• **Fig. 28.5** Nail design and fixation. Polymer bushings in the proximal screw holes provide purchase for the proximal screws, allowing compression and buttressing of the tuberosities and humeral head. Wide screw spread enhances tuberosity fixation and compression of the tuberosities in the sagittal plane as seen on the scapular lateral view.

entry of the nail in the coronal plane. The complimentary radiograph to the Grashey view is the scapular Y-lateral in which the C-arm is orbited over the patient to approximately 30–45 degrees (Fig. 28.4). This view allows for interpretation of the position of the lesser tuberosity and infraspinatus/teres minor tubercles of the greater tuberosity. From this view, the correct position of the guide pin in the anterior to posterior direction is determined as well as optimal tuberosity screw position. The patient's arm should be secured in neutral rotation (gunslinger position) throughout the procedure to ensure consistency of intraoperative radiographic evaluation and to prevent malreduction and/or loss of fixation.

Our current approach is to utilize a straight implant delivered into the proximal humerus via an antegrade approach through a small reamed opening in the most superior portion of the humeral head. This removes a small amount of superior humeral head articular cartilage in a non–weight-bearing area of the humeral head located medial to the rotator cuff tendon and footprint. The device allows for tuberosity screws to be placed through an extramedullary guide into the implant where fixation is achieved via intraimplant polyethylene bushings thereby reducing reliance on bone quality for tuberosity screw fixation (Figs. 28.5 and 28.6). Distally, antirotation screws can be placed in a dynamic or static fashion after achieving compression at the fracture site.

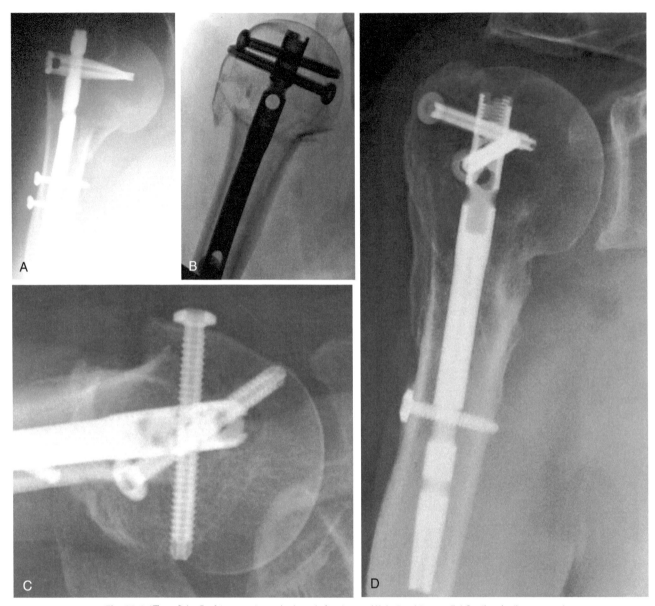

• **Fig. 28.6** "Transfixion" of two-part surgical neck fractures. (A) Lateral to medial fixation in the coronal plane can lead to loss of fixation and recurrent varus angulation. (B–D) Widely angulated screws transfix the proximal segment in the sagittal plane, preventing varus displacement and resulting in predictable healing in anatomic alignment.

Detailed Technique Description

Open Technique

As opposed to plate fixation which requires implant position along the lateral proximal humerus, intramedullary implants are delivered from a superior approach. As a result, an open delto-pectoral or extended lateral approach to the fracture site is not required for intramedullary fracture management. In our experience, either a percutaneous, limited anterolateral, or an extended anterior deltoid sleeve with lateral deltoid split approach is sufficient for reduction and fixation of most proximal fractures using an intramedullary nail. These approaches limit exposure and potential disruption of the vascular supply to the fracture site. In addition, the vascular anastomosis between the deltoid branch of the thoracoacromial artery and anterolateral anterior circumflex artery inserting into the anterolateral proximal humerus is preserved, potentially leading to improved healing after this approach (Fig. 28.7).[8]

Most fractures can be managed via an anterolateral acromial approach which utilizes an incision following Langer's lines along the lateral acromion. A split is made in the raphe between the anterior and middle heads of the deltoid. Care is taken not to continue the split beyond 4-5 cm distal to the anterolateral acromion to protect the axillary nerve. A stay suture can be placed in the deltoid fascia at this location if there is concern that the split may propagate. For more complex fractures, the deltoid and coracoacromial ligament can be completely released off of the acromion and acromioclavicular joint, creating an anterior "sleeve" of deltoid that can be easily repaired to the acromion (Fig. 28.8). A rongeur

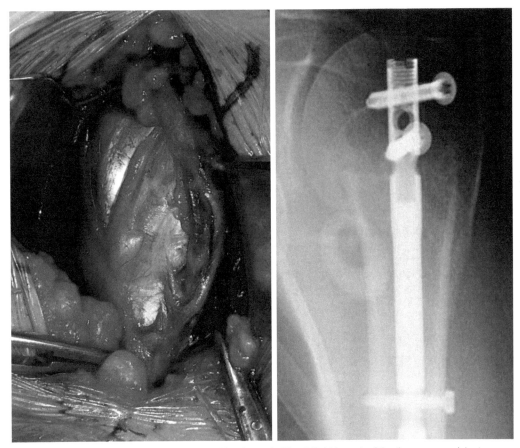

• **Fig. 28.7** Anterolateral proximal humerus blood supply. The deltoid branch of the thoracoacromial artery, as described by Gerber et al., usually provides a large anastomosis to the anterior circumflex artery and humeral neck. A superior approach leaves this collateral circulation unviolated, resulting in rapid callus formation and robust healing after intramedullary nailing of proximal humerus fractures.

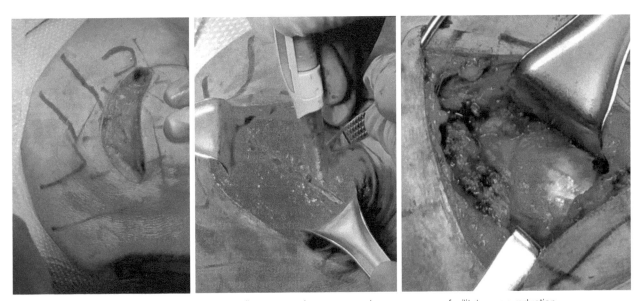

• **Fig. 28.8** Anterior deltoid "sleeve" exposure. An open superior exposure can facilitate open reduction of complex fractures without disrupting the anterolateral blood supply to the humeral head and fracture fragments. A vertical incision along Langer's lines followed by a horizontal incision of the deltotrapezial aponeurosis allows for excellent visualization and manipulation of the rotator cuff and fracture fragments. A "sleeve" of anterior deltoid is elevated off of the tenterior clavicle and acromion and deltoid split no more than 4-5 cm distal to the lateral acromion. This sleeve is easily repaired to the acromion and aponeurosis at the end of the procedure and heals predictably.

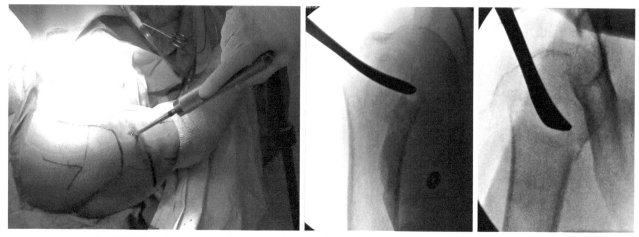

• **Fig. 28.9** Percutaneous reduction of a surgical neck fracture. A small incision is made slightly proximal to the fracture site to provide optimal leverage for reduction of the proximal segment. The skin and deeper tissues are spread and a round-tipped instrument, such as a small Cobb elevator is inserted into the fracture site. Position of the elevator is confirmed on the anteroposterior (AP) and lateral views prior to attempted manipulation of the proximal segment.

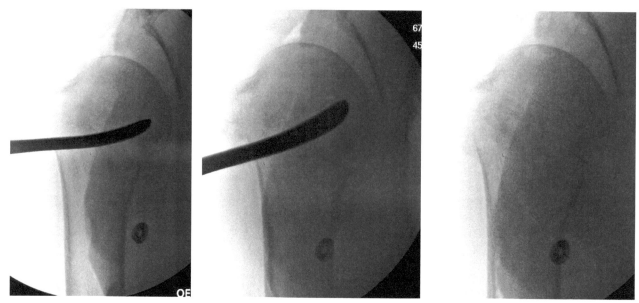

• **Fig. 28.10** Percutaneous "head lift." Once the Cobb elevator is in the appropriate position, the humeral head is brought out of varus and slightly overreduced in valgus. The Cobb is removed, resulting in anatomic angulation of the humeral neck. The humeral shaft is manually manipulated to optimize the reduction.

can be used to remove a small amount of anterior acromion to complete an acromioplasty which can facilitate access to the superior aspect of the humerus and decorticate the anterior-inferior acromion to facilitate later suture passage during the deltoid repair.

Percutaneous Technique

Percutaneous nail insertion is most commonly used for displaced two-part fractures that involve the surgical neck, but can be utilized for some three- and four-part fracture patterns. This technique is dependent on reliable and reproducible intraoperative imaging. Evaluation of fracture reduction and identification of

the nail starting point is most consistently achieved using the two intraoperative radiographs described above, including a Grashey view and a scapular Y-lateral view. Reduction of the fracture is obtained prior to implant placement by placing a blunt-tipped instrument (Cobb or Joker) through a percutaneous stab incision along the anterolateral proximal humerus just distal to the fracture (Fig. 28.9). Soft tissues are carefully spread using a Kelly clamp or hemostat prior to placement of the instrument. The instrument is advanced into the fracture site and is used to manipulate the head segment into an anatomic neck-shaft angle and version with confirmation of reduction on Grashey and lateral imaging (Fig. 28.10). If there is a tuberosity fracture component requiring

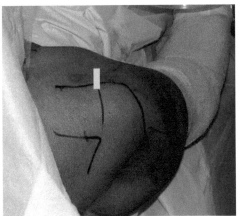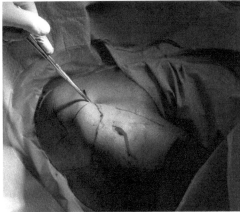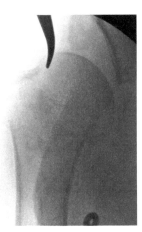

• **Fig. 28.11** Location of entry portal (percutaneous). Ideal trajectory of the guide pin into the proximal humerus usually starts immediately anterior to the acromioclavicular joint. The humerus is held in slight extension to optimize the guide path of the nail. A tonsil clamp is utilized to locate the superior articular surface and lightly spread the muscular fibers of the supraspinatus or rotator interval.

reduction, a K-wire or ball spike pusher can be positioned on the infraspinatus tubercle to guide the fracture piece anteriorly under the humeral head. Once an anatomic reduction of the fracture is obtained, the guide pin starting position is confirmed with intraoperative imaging and the nail and locking screws implanted via small percutaneous incisions.

A starting point for guidewire placement is localized just anterior to the acromioclavicular joint and medial to the coracoacromial ligament (Fig. 28.11). A straight antegrade nail is utilized with the desired entry point at the zenith of the humeral head on the Grashey view and centered in the anteroposterior (AP) direction on the Y-lateral view ensuring preservation of the rotator cuff tendon and footprint. After a 9-mm starting cortical hole is reamed, the nail is then advanced over the guidewire (Fig. 28.12). Proximal locking fixation is dependent on the degree of tuberosity comminution and the complexity of the fracture pattern. If possible, greater tuberosity screw fixation is directed at the infraspinatus and teres minor tubercles optimizing screw fixation where there is increased bone density. This is most reliably seen on the Y-lateral view as is lesser tuberosity screw fixation which is directed at the lesser tuberosity prominence. Identifying accurate nail depth should be verified on both AP and lateral imaging. The starting reaming device and implant can be placed percutaneously without direct visualization of the rotator cuff or articular surface as the device should be placed medial to the footprint through rotator cuff muscle and not tendon. If utilizing an open approach, the reaming device and implant can also be placed directly through the rotator cuff muscle or the tendon and muscle can be split longitudinally along its fibers in order to visualize the humeral head for articular surface fracture reduction or for direct visualizing of the starting point. In these cases, violation of the cuff insertion on the greater tuberosity footprint should be avoided and the cuff can be repaired with side-to-side suture using #2 nonabsorbable suture.

Fracture-Specific Technique

Two-Part

Reduction is commonly obtained via distal arm traction with an arm holder and gentle manipulation of the humeral diaphysis.

Maintaining the arm in modest extension will also help facilitate nail placement immediately anterior to the acromion. Standard reduction includes gentle arm traction with lifting of the humeral head utilizing a Cobb or Joker through a lateral stab incision to correct valgus or varus angulation and rotational malalignment.

Following nail insertion, compression at the fracture site is most commonly accomplished via hand-applied pressure at the elbow to compress the fracture site prior to distal screw fixation. Another option, requiring accurate nail depth, is by obtaining initial fixation in the distal fracture segment and gentle retrograde impaction via the jig. Most nailing systems also have dynamic screw options allowing for compression with axial load postoperatively.

Three- and Four-Part

With the evolution of nail design, an increasing number of three- and four-part fractures can be managed with intramedullary fixation. After reducing the humeral head, greater tuberosity reduction can be facilitated with either a K-wire insertion into the fracture fragment and utilized as a joystick, or use of a ball spike pusher placed on the teres tubercle in order to push the tuberosity anteriorly and under the head segment (Fig. 28.13). The head is lifted up and then allowed to "rest" on the reduced tuberosity fracture segment, maintaining the reduction. Commonly, one or multiple K-wires are utilized to hold reduction during nail placement. An open approach can facilitate reduction of tuberosities with sutures.

Postoperative Rehabilitation

Postoperative rehabilitation is dependent on the fracture type and fixation stability but typically includes sling protection with early rehabilitation including passive forward elevation to 90 degrees and external rotation to 30 degrees. Sling immobilization is discontinued at 4–6 weeks postoperatively and active motion is initiated upon visualization of tuberosity and surgical neck callus. Once healing is confirmed, usually at 2–3 months postoperatively, more aggressive stretching and light strengthening are permitted.

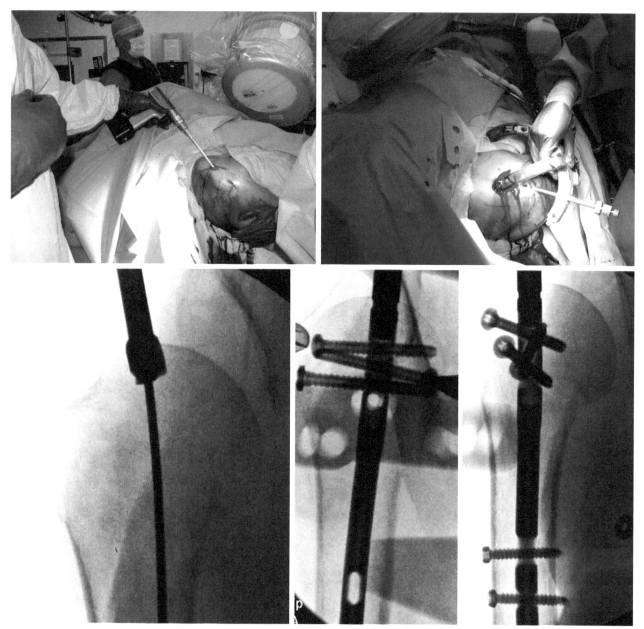

• **Fig. 28.12** Nail and screw placement. The guidewire is advanced from the superior humeral head into the proximal humeral shaft with proper position confirmed in the coronal and sagittal planes. After reaming, the nail is placed over the guidewire, buried below the articular surface followed by placement of greater and lesser tuberosity screws. An inferior humeral head support screw can be helpful to support the humeral head in multifragment fractures but is usually not necessary for surgical neck fractures.

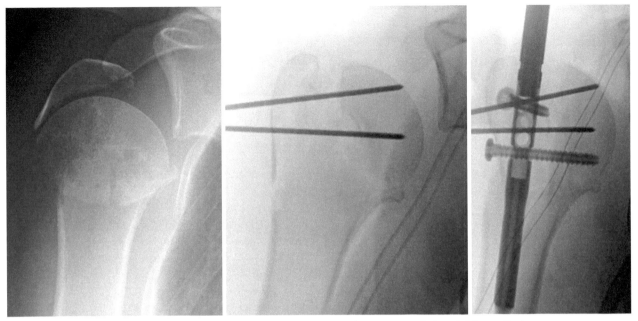

• **Fig. 28.13** Reduction and fixation of multipart fractures. One or two well-placed 4.5-mm K-wires are usually sufficient, even in this four-part fracture, to maintain the reduction during nail and screw placement.

PEARLS AND PITFALLS

- The choice to proceed with intramedullary fixation requires a detailed preoperative understanding of the fracture pattern so that the surgeon can choose the best strategy for approach, reduction maneuvers, and fixation.

- Intraoperatively, the setup of the procedure is as important as the procedure itself. Patient positioning and image intensification alignment require stringent attention to detail and communication with the radiology technician has to be optimal to ensure that radiographs that could be obtained before the procedure can be reproduced during the procedure accurately.

- Open and percutaneous reduction maneuvers require understanding and finesse during the procedure, as the fracture fragments are often delicate and can be prone to fragmentation. Utilization of the intact rotator cuff for ligamentotaxis during reduction can maintain reduction with little and sometimes no provisional fixation. A well-placed K-wire is often all that is needed to maintain reduction of the humeral head and greater tuberosity during placement of the nail.

- The nail should be of straight design and needs to be inserted medially in the apex of the humeral head to optimize nail fixation of the head fragment as well as to maximize screw spread in the proximal segment and tuberosities. Lateral insertion of the nail should be avoided as this technique will damage the supraspinatus insertion and compromise overall fixation. Widely directed screw spread in the proximal segment is desirable to fix the tuberosities with maximal stability while resisting the deforming forces of the rotator cuff.

- Care should be taken to ensure proper depth of the nail to prevent rotator cuff damage and subacromial impingement. Conversely, burying the nail too deeply in the proximal humerus can compromise fixation of the proximal segment and lead to nonunion.

- The judicious use of injectable bone graft substitutes can augment fixation, particularly in valgus impaction fracture patterns where there is compaction of proximal humerus metaphyseal bone.

References

1. Kim SH, Szabo RM, Marder RA. Epidemiology of humerus fractures in the United States: nationwide emergency department sample, 2008. *Arthritis Care Res.* 2012;64(3):407–414. https://doi.org/10.1002/acr.21563.

2. Hatzidakis AM, Shevlin MJ, Fenton DL, Curran-Everett D, Nowinski RJ, Fehringer EV. Angular-stable locked intramedullary nailing of two-part surgical neck fractures of the proximal part of the humerus. A multicenter retrospective observational study. *J Bone Joint Surg Am.* 2011;93(23):2172–2179. https://doi.org/10.2106/JBJS.J.00754.

3. Wong J, Newman JM, Gruson KI. Outcomes of intramedullary nailing for acute proximal humerus fractures: a systematic review. *J Orthop Traumatol.* 2016;17(2):113122. https://doi.org/10.1007/s10195-015-0384-5.

4. Lin J. Effectiveness of locked nailing for displaced three-part proximal humeral fractures. *J Trauma.* 2006;61(2):363–374.

5. Kloub M, Holub K, Polakova S. Nailing of three- and four-part fractures of the humeral head — long-term results. *Injury.* 2014;45(suppl 1):S29–S37. https://doi.org/10.1016/j.injury.2013.10.038.

6. Visser CP, Tavy DL, Coene LN, Brand R. Electromyographic findings in shoulder dislocations and fractures of the proximal humerus: comparison with clinical neurological examination. *Clin Neurol Neurosurg.* 1999;101:86–91.

7. Sungalo MA, Sears BW. Delayed radial nerve injury from a brachial artery pseudoaneurysm following a four-part proximal humerus fracture. *JBJS Case Conn.* 2019;9(3). e0165.

8. Gerber C, Schneeberger AG, Vinh TS. The arterial vascularization of the humeral head. An anatomical study. *J Bone Joint Surg Am.* 1990;72:1486–1494.

29

Technique Spotlight: RSA for Fracture

ROBERT J. GILLESPIE AND SUNITA MENGERS

For a patient sustaining a proximal humerus fracture, the goal of treatment is to maximize functional outcome and patient satisfaction. While no clear consensus exists as to the optimal management of these injuries, and the results of closed treatment are frequently adequate in this patient population, certain fracture patterns and patient characteristics may help direct surgeons in selecting an appropriate plan of care.[1,2]

Current practice suggests reverse total shoulder arthroplasty (rTSA) is best suited in the treatment of elderly patients sustaining proximal humerus fractures with complex fracture patterns who desire the maximum achievable functional result. Specifically, patients suffering from severely displaced three- or four-part fractures or fracture-dislocations, those presenting in a delayed fashion, or individuals found to have poor bone quality are considered optimal candidates for treatment with rTSA. While nonoperative treatment is frequently an option, these fracture patterns are subject to a number of potential complications with nonoperative treatment including malunion, nonunion, and avascular necrosis.[2,3] Additionally, individuals found to have poor bone quality, including those with osteoporosis, are at increased risk of failure and hardware loosening with open reduction and fixation and should therefore be identified as candidates for rTSA.[1,4,5] While hemiarthroplasty may be considered for the rare, unreconstructable younger patients with proximal humerus fracture or patients where a glenoid fracture makes secure baseplate fixation unattainable, rTSA is generally preferred in patients aged 65 and older due to improved postrehabilitation results of forward elevation and functional outcomes.[2,6–8] Finally, rTSA is indicated for complex proximal humerus fractures with concomitant irreparable rotator cuff pathology, as the use of the reverse prosthesis alters the center of rotation at the joint such that the arm is reliant on the function of the deltoid muscle rather than a deficient rotator cuff for range of motion.[1,9]

For patients where the medical comorbidities are severe and the potential benefit of an rTSA over closed treatment only comes with unacceptable anesthetic and surgical risks, closed treatment is preferred. Furthermore, patients must be willing and able to undergo a rehabilitation program postoperatively, have no active infection, have a functioning deltoid/axillary nerve, and a glenoid sufficient for stable glenoid component fixation. Lastly, patients who use the arm as a weight-bearing shoulder, for example, using a walker to assist with ambulation, are relatively contraindicated.

Preoperative Examination

A thorough preoperative history and examination is critical to identify optimal candidates for rTSA following proximal humerus fracture. Elderly female patients are most at risk of proximal humerus fracture. Therefore younger patients presenting with fractures secondary to low-impact trauma necessitate further workup to rule out pathologic causes of injury.[10] Preinjury functional status and hand dominance are also crucial to establishing appropriate expectations of postoperative recovery. Patient medical history including a diagnosis of osteoporosis, anticoagulation use, or other comorbidities will provide insight into infection risk and fitness for surgery. A detailed description of mechanism of injury will offer clues into need for additional workup to identify concurrent trauma to head, neck, shoulder girdle, forearm, or hand.[10]

As with any traumatic injury, physical examination should entail close examination of the affected area and surrounding structures. With a suspected proximal humerus fracture, evaluation of the wrist, forearm, elbow, and shoulder girdle is warranted.[1] Skin examination includes investigation for previous surgical scars, areas of skin tenting, distribution of ecchymosis, and open wounds. Gross deformity may

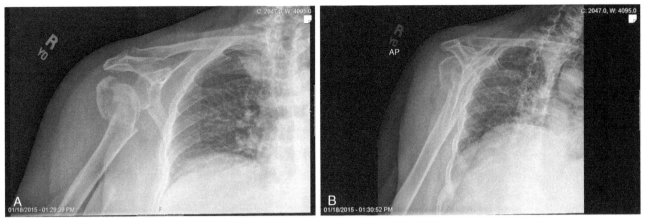

• **Fig. 29.1** (A) Anteroposterior and (B) scapula Y views of proximal humerus fracture.

indicate concurrent dislocation of the humeral head.[1,10] A detailed neurologic examination is crucial, with particular attention focused on the integrity of axillary nerve, as this is the most frequently injured nerve during proximal humerus fracture.[1,10] For patient comfort, we recommend testing the posterior head of the deltoid by having the patient, with their arm hanging at the side, push the elbow posteriorly against the examiner's one hand while the examiner's other hand palpates for firing of the muscle. While motor assessment may be limited by patient intolerance secondary to pain. However, sensory function can be evaluated through light touch. Finally, adequate perfusion should be assessed, and signs of vascular compromise including weak distal pulses, slow capillary refill, and hypoesthesia require immediate attention.[10]

Typical radiographic imaging includes a complete trauma series consisting of true anteroposterior, scapular-Y, and axillary views (Fig. 29.1).[1–3,10] Whenever possible, plain radiographic images should be obtained with the patient in the upright position to appreciate the effect of gravity upon the fracture alignment.[1] Computed tomography may be necessary to better evaluate complex fracture patterns and assess the integrity of the rotator cuff musculature.[2,3] Magnetic resonance imaging (MRI) is rarely indicated.[1] Imaging should be evaluation for alignment, fragmentation of the humeral head or tuberosities, and bone quality as osteoporotic bone is at greater risk of ultimate failure with attempts at reduction with internal fixation.[1,4,5] The humerus is the second most common site for long bone metastases, with 8%–10% of lytic lesions progressing to impending or established fracture.[11] Therefore great care must be taken to avoid missing a pathologic fracture secondary to a neoplasm. Furthermore, the presence of an associated glenoid fracture, though rarely described in the literature in limited case reports,[12] may compromise the integrity of reverse baseplate fixation, and thus the glenoid should be carefully scrutinized.

Positioning and Equipment

Appropriate positioning and equipment are of utmost importance to ensure visualization of the surgical site during

the procedure. A 60-degree seated "beach chair" position is ideal to allow manipulation of the shoulder through a full range of motion as necessary and to achieve adequate exposure throughout the operation. Particularly, the posterior aspect of the shoulder must remain unencumbered to allow full extension and adduction for access to the humeral canal. All bony prominences should be padded to protect the patient from injury during the surgery. The authors typically use an arm holder, though a padded Mayo stand can also be used to support the limb during the case.

Detailed Technique Description

A standard deltopectoral incision is made extending from the coracoid to the tip of the deltoid insertion to gain adequate exposure to the fracture site along with the greater and lesser tuberosities.[9] The cephalic vein is identified and retracted laterally along with the deltoid muscle, where the vessel is protected throughout the operation (Fig. 29.2A). The clavipectoral fascia is excised along the lateral border of the conjoint tendon to gain exposure to the fracture site (Fig. 29.2B). Typically, there is hematoma and soft callus filling the area of the subacromial and subdeltoid bursa that must be removed to expose the fracture fragments and the rotator cuff. The axillary nerve is identified with palpation using the tug test at the posterior aspect of the quadrilateral space and the inferior border of the subscapularis. At this point, tenotomy or tenodesis of the biceps tendon is frequently performed.[9] We prefer a soft tissue tenodesis to the upper border of the pectoralis major.

The greater and lesser tuberosities are exposed and separated at the fracture site. The fracture plane for the greater tuberosity is typically 5–7 mm posterior to the bicipital groove and thus approximately 5–7 mm of supraspinatus may traverse the fracture and attach to the fragment with the lesser tuberosity, bicipital groove, and a small portion of the greater tuberosity. This tissue must be released to allow separation and control of the tuberosities. Heavy nonabsorbable sutures are placed through each tuberosity at the bone-tendon interface to be utilized for the later repair. Three sutures should be placed around the greater tuberosity and two around the lesser tuberosity. Suture management is absolutely critical.

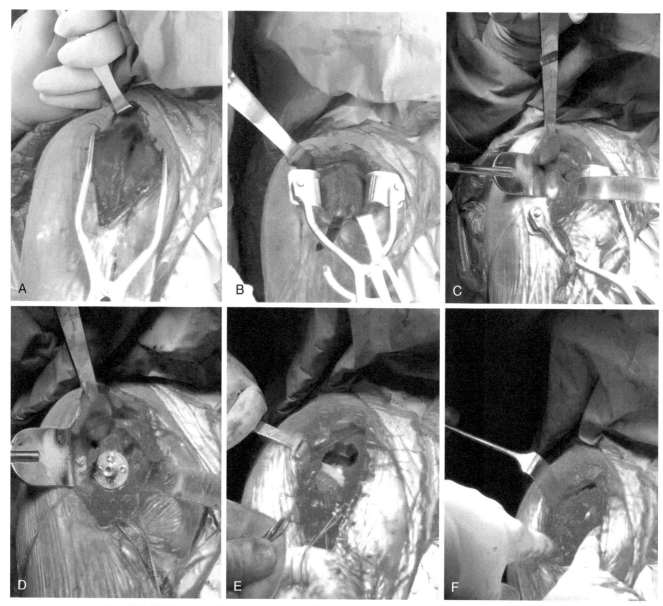

• **Fig. 29.2** (A) Standard deltopectoral incision, (B) exposure of the fracture site, (C) glenoid exposure and tagging of tuberosities, (D) insertion of the glenoid baseplate with inferior tilt, (E) reduction of tuberosities, and (F) anchoring of vertical and horizontal sutures.

We recommend using different colors of high tensile suture, using different types of snaps (Kelly, Tonsil, straight snap, mosquito, etc.), and marking every other suture with a sterile marking pen to aid in suture management. The humeral head and any comminuted fragments of the humeral head are carefully removed and saved as a potential graft source during the reconstruction. Copious irrigation is used to clean the wound and decrease the incidence of heterotopic ossification.

Next, attention is turned to the glenoid. A full release of the rotator interval is performed, and the labrum is released circumferentially to allow visualization of the true edges of the glenoid (Fig. 29.2C). Particular focus is placed on exposure to the inferior aspect of the glenoid to ensure the implant lays flush during insertion. The glenoid is prepared with reaming, and a baseplate is inserted and secured according to the technique recommended by the manufacturer (Fig. 29.2D).

A glenosphere is then selected and inserted with careful consideration to achieve appropriate fit. To reduce complications such as dislocation, use of a larger glenosphere should be considered. In the shoulder system used by the authors, this usually means a 36-mm glenosphere (vs. 32 mm used in other diagnoses such as cuff tear arthropathy) with 6 mm of lateralization. The final glenosphere is impacted into place. Alternatively, a trial glenosphere can be utilized to ensure proper soft tissue tensioning, but this is not our standard practice.

Following this, the humerus is similarly prepared using reamers and broaches. A humeral stem is selected, taking into account any retroversion necessary to obtain correct fit. With fractures extending into the metaphysis or diaphysis, a longer humeral stem is preferred.[9] For severe comminution, imaging of the contralateral humerus can be useful to be sure correct height is used for the implant. In patients with an intact calcar, appropriate height can be obtained with this valuable anatomic landmark. Appropriate selection of implants is confirmed using a trial reduction and moving the arm through a full range of motion to ensure stability and proper deltoid tension. Alternatively, the editor recommends reducing the trial stem/liner to the glenosphere, holding the stem/liner coated to the glenosphere, and then pulling down on the arm to "telescope" the humerus out along the stem. The proper height of the stem can then be marked on the trial. Once final components have been determined, the shoulder is re-dislocated, trial implants are removed, and two drill holes are made for vertical sutures for the later tuberosity and rotator cuff repair. If a trial glenosphere has been used, the definitive implant can now be impacted into place.

The humeral component is prepared via a black and tan method which uses a bone graft buffer between cement to protect the proximal humerus bone from thermal necrosis and improve healing.[13,14] In this technique, cement is injected into the distal humeral canal, and the proximal 2 cm are subsequently removed. A cancellous bone graft is placed in the void, and the humeral stem is inserted, resulting in a "black and tan" appearance (Fig. 29.3). Nonabsorbable suture should then be placed through appropriate suture holes on the implant for later tuberosity repair. The final humeral polyethylene insert is impacted into place, and shoulder is reduced.

Attention is then turned toward repair of the greater and lesser tuberosities as previously described (Fig. 29.4).[15]

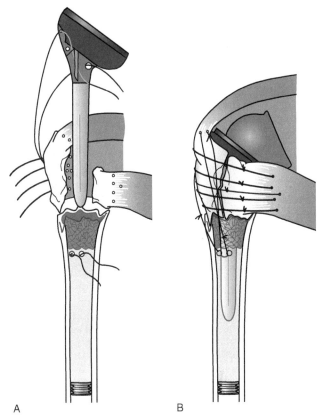

A   B

• **Fig. 29.3** Black and tan technique. (From Formaini NT, Everding NG, Levy JC, Rosas S. Tuberosity healing after reverse shoulder arthroplasty for acute proximal humerus fractures: the "black and tan" technique. *J Shoulder Elbow Surg.* 2015;24(11):e299–306.)

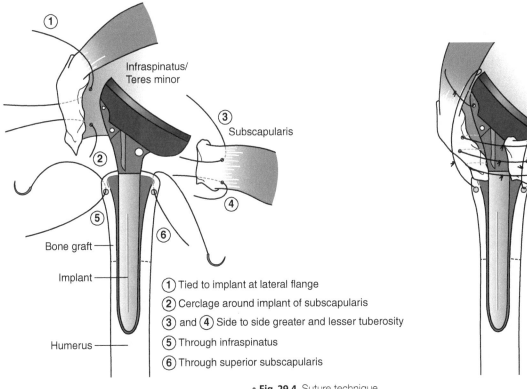

Infraspinatus/
Teres minor

③ Subscapularis

②

Bone graft

Implant

⑤

⑥

Humerus

① Tied to implant at lateral flange
② Cerclage around implant of subscapularis
③ and ④ Side to side greater and lesser tuberosity
⑤ Through infraspinatus
⑥ Through superior subscapularis

• **Fig. 29.4** Suture technique.

One of the original greater tuberosity sutures is brought around the implant and through the subscapularis to function as a cerclage and another will be positioned directly to the lateral portion of the implant, reducing the greater tuberosity to the lateral aspect of the implant (Fig. 29.2E). The two sutures initially placed around the lesser tuberosity and the final from the greater tuberosity are then used for side-to-side sutures between tuberosity, achieving a reduction of the tuberosities to each other. Next, the vertical sutures previously placed in the humerus are subsequently passed through the subscapularis and infraspinatus musculature, ensuring the sutures remain flush with the greater and lesser tuberosity, and the sutures are tied down (Fig. 29.2F). The arm is brought through a full range of motion to evaluate the shoulder for stability and any signs of impingement. The wound is copiously irrigated, and a drain is placed in the subdeltoid space when necessary. The deltopectoral interval is closed followed by superficial layers, and the patient is placed in a sling.

Postoperative rehabilitation involves immobilization in a sling with an abduction pillow for at least 4–6 weeks to allow adequate tuberosity healing. Patients are advised to begin pendulum exercises with the first few days postoperatively. Gentle active assisted and passive range of motion in the scapular plane can be initiated with advancement of therapy once radiographic evidence of healing is obtained. Typically, rehabilitation is completed at 5 months with the full recovery and optimal outcomes seen 1 year after injury.[16]

PEARLS AND PITFALLS

Pearls

- Glenoid preparation: it all starts with a solid foundation.
  - Maintain neutral or inferior tilt: superior tilt associated with component notching and implant loosening.[9,17,18]
  - The convex shape of the glenoid, inferior positioning of the baseplate, and reaming frequently lead to a "subchondral smile" of reaming just beyond the cancellous layer at the inferior aspect of the glenoid. However, the majority of the subchondral bone should be preserved as it leads to more secure glenoid implant fixation.[9]
  - Limit retroversion to <10 degrees: reduces risk of humeral component impingement on the acromion/spine.[9]
- Tuberosity healing: critical for restoring range of motion, particularly external rotation, and for avoiding prosthetic instability.[19]
  - Black and tan technique: protects tuberosities from thermal necrosis via a layer of bone graft.[13,14]

Pitfalls

- Beware of associated glenoid fractures or pathologic fractures secondary to neoplasm—these will dramatically change your management and can be subtle. They are uncommon, but given the large number of proximal humerus fractures, there is a good chance these situations will arise in your practice.
- Dislocation: avoid the leading cause of repeat intervention.[20]
  - Incidence: 4.7% of all rTSAs; 38% of repeat interventions after rTSA.
  - Risk factors: inadequate tissue tension, failed soft tissue repair, tuberosity malunion, implant malpositioning, improper glenosphere selection.

- Consider larger glenosphere for potential increase in stability.
  - Early (<3 months): closed reduction, immobilization.
  - Late (>3 months): surgical intervention to correct tissue tension and component selection.[20,21]
- Beware of pressfit humeral stems for this indication.
  - Sometimes the humerus can be press fit and the prosthesis has stable fixation in the bone at exactly the right height. However, this is uncommon. Typically, the loss of proximal humeral bone leads to a lack of bony support, especially in rotation and especially in this population of elderly patients with poor bone quality. The error is to implant the stem too deep in a foolhardy attempt to obtain adequate press fit. Unfortunately, this shortens the deltoid and leads to an unstable prosthesis. Cement allows the surgeon to cement at the appropriate height for deltoid tension and tuberosity reconstruction.
- Infection: may require antibiotics, open lavage, or removal of hardware.
- Scapular notching: due to particulate polyethylene debris.
  - Risk factors: use of traditional "Grammont-style" implants with 155-degree humerosocket inclination and placement of glenosphere with superior tilt.[17,18,21]
  - Evaluate for impingement prior to final component placement.

Despite known pitfalls, management of complex proximal humerus fracture with rTSA offers improved functional outcomes in elderly patients when compared with alternative surgical interventions. With tuberosity healing and appropriate implant selection, satisfactory patient results can be seen predictably.

References

1. Jo MJ, Gardner MJ. Proximal humerus fractures. *Curr Rev Musculoskelet Med.* 2012;5(3):192–198.
2. Jones KJ, Dines DM, Gulotta L, Dines JS. Management of proximal humerus fractures utilizing reverse total shoulder arthroplasty. *Curr Rev Musculoskelet Med.* 2013;6(1):63–70.
3. Schumaier A, Grawe B. Proximal humerus fractures: evaluation and management in the elderly patient. *Geriatr Orthop Surg Rehabil.* 2018;9. https://doi.org/10.1177/2151458517750516.
4. Jung SW, Shim SB, Kim HM, Lee JH, Lim HS. Factors that influence reduction loss in proximal humerus fracture surgery. *J Orthop Trauma.* 2015;29(6):276–282.

5. Spross C, Zeledon R, Zdravkovic V, Jost B. How bone quality may influence intraoperative and early postoperative problems after angular stable open reduction-internal fixation of proximal humeral fractures. *J Shoulder Elbow Surg.* 2017;26(9):1566–1572.

6. Mata-Fink A, Meinke M, Jones C, Kim B, Bell JE. Reverse shoulder arthroplasty for treatment of proximal humeral fractures in older adults: a systematic review. *J Shoulder Elbow Surg.* 2013;22(12):1737–1748.

7. Ferrel JR, Trinh TQ, Fischer RA. Reverse total shoulder arthroplasty versus hemiarthroplasty for proximal humeral fractures: a systematic review. *J Orthop Trauma.* 2015;29(1):60–68.

8. Schairer WW, Nwachukwu BU, Lyman S, Craig EV, Gulotta LV. Reverse shoulder arthroplasty versus hemiarthroplasty for treatment of proximal humerus fractures. *J Shoulder Elbow Surg.* 2015;24(10):1560–1566.

9. Werthel JD, Sirveaux F, Block D. Reverse shoulder arthroplasty in recent proximal humerus fractures. *Orthop Traumatol Surg Res.* 2018;104(6):779–785.

10. Khmelnitskaya E, Lamont LE, Taylor SA, Lorich DG, Dines DM, Dines JS. Evaluation and management of proximal humerus fractures. *Adv Orthop.* 2012;2012:861598.

11. Moura DL, Alves F, Fonseca R, Freitas J, Casanova J. Treatment of pathological humerus-shaft tumoral fractures with rigid static interlocking intramedullary nail-22 years of experience. *Rev Bras Ortop (Sao Paulo).* 2019;54(2):149–155.

12. Königshausen M, Mempel E, Rausch V, Gessmann J, Schildhauer TA, Seybold D. Combined fractures of the humeral head and the glenoid. *Obere Extremität.* 2019;14(2):118–126.

13. Levy JC. Avoiding cement bone necrosis effect on tuberosity healing. *Tech Shoulder Elbow Surg.* 2013;14(3):81–84.

14. Formaini NT, Everding NG, Levy JC, Rosas S. Tuberosity healing after reverse shoulder arthroplasty for acute proximal humerus fractures: the "black and tan" technique. *J Shoulder Elbow Surg.* 2015;24(11):e299–306.

15. Boileau P, Walch G, Krishnan SG. Tuberosity osteosynthesis and hemiarthroplasty for four-part fractures of the proximal humerus. *Tech Shoulder Elbow Surg.* 2000;1(2):96–109.

16. Cabarcas BC, Gowd AK, Liu JN, et al. Establishing maximum medical improvement following reverse total shoulder arthroplasty for rotator cuff deficiency. *J Shoulder Elbow Surg.* 2018;27(9):1721–1731.

17. Laver L, Garrigues GE. Avoiding superior tilt in reverse shoulder arthroplasty: a review of the literature and technical recommendations. *J Shoulder Elbow Surg.* 2014;23(10):1582–1590.

18. Gutierrez S, Walker M, Willis M, Pupello DR, Frankle MA. Effects of tilt and glenosphere eccentricity on baseplate/bone interface forces in a computational model, validated by a mechanical model, of reverse shoulder arthroplasty. *J Shoulder Elbow Surg.* 2011;20(5):732–739.

19. Gallinet D, Adam A, Gasse N, Rochet S, Obert L. Improvement in shoulder rotation in complex shoulder fractures treated by reverse shoulder arthroplasty. *J Shoulder Elbow Surg.* 2013;22(1):38–44.

20. Boileau P. Complications and revision of reverse total shoulder arthroplasty. *Orthop Traumatol Surg Res.* 2016;102(1 Suppl):S33–S43.

21. Cheung E, Willis M, Walker M, Clark R, Frankle MA. Complications in reverse total shoulder arthroplasty. *J Am Acad Orthop Surg.* 2011;19(7):439–449.

30

Technique Spotlight: Endosteal Allograft for Complex Proximal Humeus Fracture Reconstruction

L. HENRY GOODNOUGH, MALCOLM R. DEBAUN, AND MICHAEL J. GARDNER

Indications

Proximal humerus fractures are common injuries, and in certain patients, surgical fixation can restore anatomy, provide stability, improve pain, and restore function.[1] Mitigating the risk of postoperative complications is critical for optimizing patient outcomes,[2] and multiple studies have demonstrated reoperation rates of 14%–24%,[2-5] with preoperative varus deformity in particular having high rates of postoperative failure. Reduction and support of the medial calcar improve maintenance of reduction postoperatively.[6,7] Restoration of the inferomedial calcar with a customized fibular allograft as an adjunct to a laterally based locking plate (Fig. 30.1A–C) is a modern technique which has yielded promising results with reoperation rates as low as 4.4%.[8-14, 21-25] The senior author's relative indications include displaced three- and four-part fractures, osteoporotic bone, varus deformity, or calcar comminution.

Preoperative Evaluation

Evaluation of the patient includes identifying the patient's age, dominant arm, functional status, occupation, as well as comorbidities and involves a comprehensive neurovascular evaluation of the injured extremity. Imaging of the injured extremity begins with a full radiographic shoulder series to identify displacement, coronal plane deformity, and presence of tuberosity involvement (Fig. 30.1D–E). An axillary or Velpeau view is mandatory to demonstrate a concentrically reduced glenohumeral joint. Computed tomography with three-dimensional reconstruction is recommended for complex patterns to guide preoperative planning and to delineate intra-articular fracture lines ("head-split" component).

Positioning and Equipment

Preoperatively, requested equipment includes pointed reduction clamps, threaded and nonthreaded K-wires (2.0–3.2 mm) and Schanz pins for manipulative reduction. Implants include precontoured lateral locking plates for proximal humerus fixation, heavy suture for tuberosity reduction and fixation, as well as a freeze-dried fibular allograft (~5 cm in length). A power saw and a high-speed burr are available to prepare the graft, and a bone tamp and mallet should be available for graft insertion.

The patient is positioned supine on a reverse cantilevered table with a padded radiolucent plexiglass under the injured shoulder (Fig. 30.1F). The torso is translated laterally to facilitate intraoperative fluoroscopy. The endotracheal tube with its holder (Christmas tree) should face away from the operative shoulder. An arthroscopic arm holder positions the injured extremity in space and allows controlled manipulation of the arm (Fig. 30.1G). The table is turned 90 degrees, and the C-arm is brought in from the head of the patient to allow for anteroposterior (AP) and axillary views (Fig. 30.1H–J) to judge reduction quality and implant placement.

Detailed Technique Description

The authors prefer an anterolateral acromial approach.[15,16] After sterile preparation of the skin and draping, the location of the axillary nerve distally is estimated by drawing a transverse line 65 mm distal to a point just posterior to the palpable anterolateral border of the acromion[15,16] (Fig. 30.1K). Subsequently, an incision is made from the anterolateral border of acromion, longitudinally, down the lateral border of the arm. The raphe between anterior and lateral heads of deltoid is identified and split (Fig. 30.1L–M). The dissection is carried down to the acromion proximally. The location of the axillary nerve is again estimated 65 mm directly from the exposed acromion (Fig. 30.2). Proximally, the subdeltoid bursa is incised, which typically reveals the intertuberosity fracture line. Blunt dissection proximal and distal identifies the soft tissue sling containing the axillary nerve, which is protected with a vessel loop (Fig. 30.1N). The fracture is identified and cleaned. Tuberosity fragments, if identified, are tagged and controlled with heavy suture.

The cryopreserved fibular allograft is thawed in warm saline. Appropriate size can be initially estimated with fluoroscopy: The graft should be small enough for intraosseous positioning by allowing

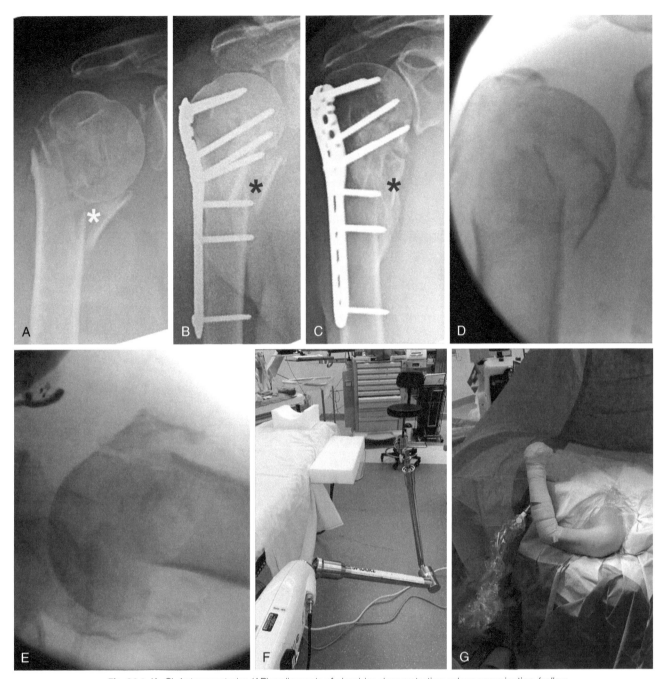

• **Fig. 30.1** (A–C) Anteroposterior (AP) radiograph of shoulder demonstrating calcar comminution *(yellow asterisk)*, (B) postoperative film with calcar restoration with fibular allograft *(blue asterisk)*, and (C) healed fracture *(blue asterisk)*. (D) and (E) Preoperative AP and axillary X-ray. (F–H) OR setup. (I) and (J) C-arm setup. (K–N) Anterolateral approach to acromion.

it to "tilt" medially into the inferior humeral head, yet an insufficiently sized graft will not effectively couple the surgical neck to the intact metaphysis.[14] After templating, a power saw can be used on the back table to cut the graft to size; distally, the graft can be beveled laterally, and the edges smoothened with a high-speed burr (Fig. 30.3A), for ease of positioning within the metaphysis. A K-wire is inserted in the proximal portion of allograft as a manipulative aid. The graft is inserted antegrade through the fracture line. Reduction aids are utilized to realign the humeral head fragment to the intact metaphysis (Fig. 30.3D). A bone tamp and mallet is typically used to impact the fibula into the inferomedial humeral head and potentially improve the calcar reduction (Fig. 30.3E). Care must be taken to ensure that the fibula does not fall too far into the intramedullary

space. A K-wire in the graft can be helpful in this regard as a joystick, and a second K-wire can be placed through the humeral metaphysis and into the graft to affix it in place. Lastly, the graft should be placed medially in a position to provide calcar substitution, and into the medial subchondral bone of humeral head, but not too distally down the canal where it may complicate future arthroplasty procedures.

The fracture is reduced and provisionally stabilized with K-wires proximal to the eventual plate position (Fig. 30.3F). A proximal humerus locking plate is inserted antegrade, deep to the sling of soft tissue containing axillary nerve. Plate positioning is confirmed on orthogonal views and provisionally stabilized with K-wires or fixed with screws proximally. The plate should be positioned to accommodate an oblique screw abutting the calcar and not impinge the

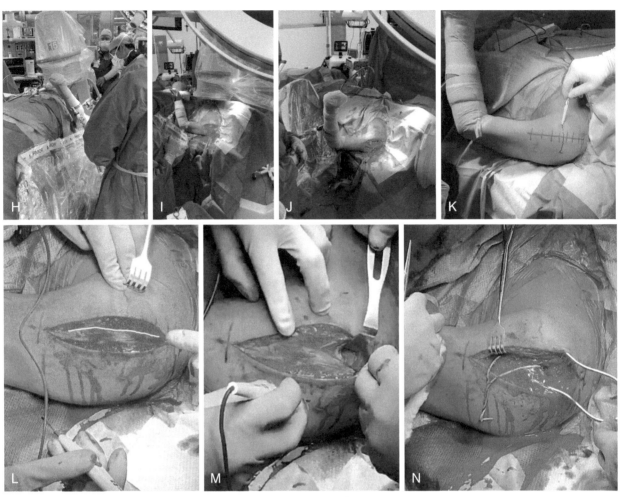

• **Fig. 30.1, cont'd**

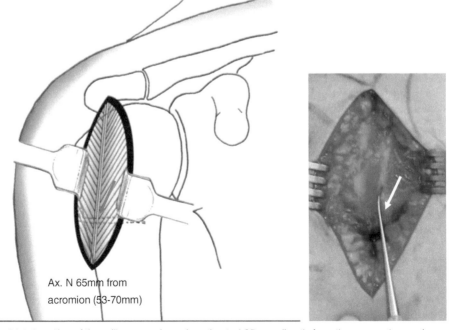

Ax. N 65mm from
acromion (53-70mm)

• **Fig. 30.2** Location of the axillary nerve is again estimated 65 mm directly from the exposed acromion.

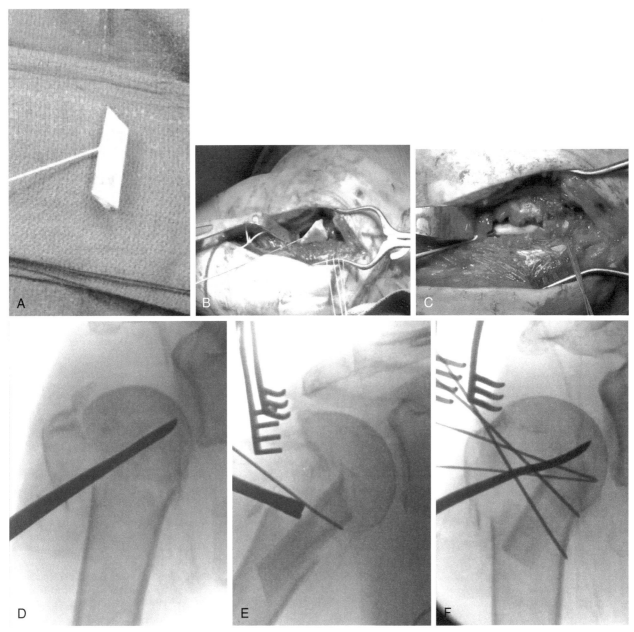

• **Fig. 30.3** Endosteal fibula allograft preparation/insertion. (A) Graft is prepared and beveled on back table. (B) and (C) Graft insertion. (D) and (E) Provisional reductions aids for manipulation of fracture and insertion of graft. (F–H) Graft insertion. (I) and (J) Plate and allograft can be used to fine tune reduction. (K) and (L) Final anteroposterior and axillary radiographs with endosteal allograft and lateral locking plate.

subacromial space (Fig. 30.3G–H). Distally, a nonlocking screw is placed to oppose the plate to the bone. Residual varus-valgus deformity can be corrected via the plate and allograft (Fig. 30.3I–J). Valgus deformity can be corrected with a bicortical screw, distally pulling the metaphysis to the plate. Slight residual varus deformity can be corrected with a cortical screw drilled through the lateral cortex which, upon insertion, pushes the allograft against the medial calcar and provides a valgus force. Fixation is completed

with a bicortical screw distally through the allograft, and multiple locking screws proximally, including a calcar locking screw (Fig. 30.3K–L). Screw lengths are checked with either live fluoroscopy or advance-withdrawal techniques in the convex humeral head. Suture fixation of the tuberosities is tensioned and tied through the plate. The wound is irrigated, local antibiotics may be administered, the axillary nerve is again examined, and the wound, including the deltoid fascia, is closed in layers.

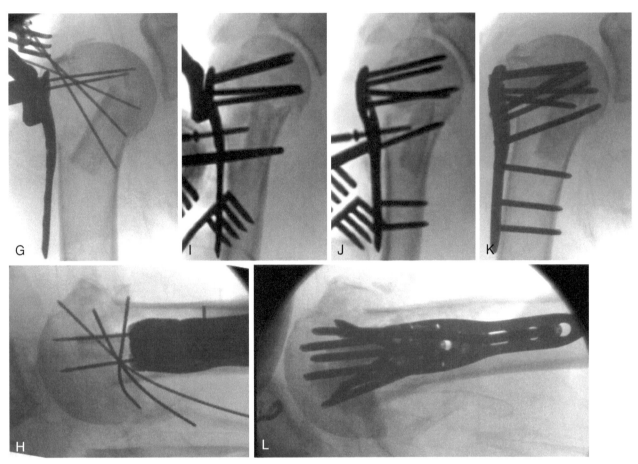

• **Fig. 30.3, cont'd**

PEARLS AND PITFALLS

- Inherent pitfalls include limited supply of allografts, a learning curve associated with shaping and customizing each allograft, difficulties removing the graft when ingrown.
- There are pitfalls associated with graft sizing. In particular, if the graft is too big, it can become incarcerated in the diaphysis, making it difficult to maneuver.[8]
- Avoid an excessively long extension of graft down the humeral canal as this will complicate later arthroplasty options, should this become necessary.
- While the technique described here is frequently used to provide medial column support to resist varus displacement with the graft placed medially along the calcar, for a valgus displaced pattern the graft should be placed in a vertical orientation to strut the lateral column and prevent redisplacement.

References

1. Hessmann MH, Hansen WSM, Krummenauer F, et al. Locked plate fixation and intramedullary nailing for proximal humerus fractures: a biomechanical evaluation. *J Trauma*. 2005;58(6):1194–1201.
2. Spross C, Platz A, Rufibach K, et al. The PHILOS plate for proximal humeral fractures—risk factors for complications at one year. *J Trauma Acute Care Surg*. 2012;72(3):783–792.
3. Gardner MJ, Weil Y, Barker JU, et al. The importance of medial support in locked plating of proximal humerus fractures. *J Orthop Trauma*. 2007;21(3):185–191.
4. Erhardt JB, Stoffel K, Kampshoff J, et al. The position and number of screws influence screw perforation of the humeral head in modern locking plates: a cadaver study. *J Orthop Trauma*. 2012;26(10):e188–192.
5. Sproul RC, Iyengar JJ, Devcic Z, et al. A systematic review of locking plate fixation of proximal humerus fractures. *Injury*. 2011;42(4):408–413.
6. Südkamp N, Bayer J, Hepp P, et al. Open reduction and internal fixation of proximal humeral fractures with use of the locking proximal humerus plate. Results of a prospective, multicenter, observational study. *J Bone Joint Surg Am*. 2009;91(6):1320–1328.
7. Brunner F, Sommer C, Bahrs C, et al. Open reduction and internal fixation of proximal humerus fractures using a proximal humeral locked plate: a prospective multicenter analysis. *J Orthop Trauma*. 2009;23(3):163–172.
8. Hirschmann MT, Quarz V, Audigé L, et al. Internal fixation of unstable proximal humerus fractures with an anatomically pre-shaped interlocking plate: a clinical and radiologic evaluation. *J Trauma*. 2007;63(6):1314–1323.
9. Gardner MJ, Lorich DG, Werner CML, et al. Second-generation concepts for locked plating of proximal humerus fractures. *Am J. Orthop*. 2007;36(9):460–465.
10. Gardner MJ, Boraiah S, Helfet DL, et al. Indirect medial reduction and strut support of proximal humerus fractures using an endosteal implant. *J Orthop Trauma*. 2008;22(3):195.

11. Gardner MJ, Boraiah S, Helfet DL, et al. The anterolateral acromial approach for fractures of the proximal humerus. *J Orthop Trauma.* 2008;22(2):132–137.

12. Palmer A K. Techniques for using a novel intramedullary cage technology for fixation of proximal humeral fractures. *Journal of Exercise, Sports & Orthopedics.* 2016;3(2):1–6.

13. Meinberg EG, Agel J, Roberts CS, et al. Fracture and dislocation classification compendium-2018. *J Orthop Trauma.* 2018;32(suppl 1):S1–S170.

14. Moonot P, Ashwood N, Hamlet M. Early results for treatment of three- and four-part fractures of the proximal humerus using the PHILOS plate system. *J Bone Joint Surg Br.* 2007;89(9):1206–1209.

15. Agudelo J, Schürmann M, Stahel P, et al. Analysis of efficacy and failure in proximal humerus fractures treated with locking plates. *J Orthop Trauma.* 2007;21(10):676–681.

16. Koukakis A, Apostolou CD, Taneja T, et al. Fixation of proximal humerus fractures using the PHILOS plate: early experience. *Clin Orthop Relat Res.* 2006;442:115–120.

17. Jost B, Spross C, Grehn H, et al. Locking plate fixation of fractures of the proximal humerus: analysis of complications, revision strategies and outcome. *J Shoulder Elbow Surg.* 2013;22(4):542–549.

18. Owsley KC, Gorczyca JT. Fracture displacement and screw cutout after open reduction and locked plate fixation of proximal humeral fractures [corrected]. *J Bone Joint Surg Am.* 2008;90(2):233–240.

19. Solberg BD, Moon CN, Franco DP, et al. Locked plating of 3- and 4-part proximal humerus fractures in older patients: the effect of initial fracture pattern on outcome. *J Orthop Trauma.* 2009;23(2):113–119.

20. Gerber C, Werner CML, Vienne P. Internal fixation of complex fractures of the proximal humerus. *J Bone Joint Surg Br.* 2004;86(6):848–855.

21. Saltzman BM, Erickson BJ, Harris JD, et al. Fibular strut graft augmentation for open reduction and internal fixation of proximal humerus fractures. *Orthop J Sports Med [Internet].* 2016. [cited 2019 Jul 9];4(7). Available from: https://www.ncbi.nlm.nih.gov/pmc/articles/PMC4962341/.

22. Little MTM, Berkes MB, Schottel PC, et al. The impact of preoperative coronal plane deformity on proximal humerus fixation with endosteal augmentation. *J Orthop Trauma.* 2014;28(6):338–347.

23. Tan E, Lie D, Wong MK. Early outcomes of proximal humerus fracture fixation with locking plate and intramedullary fibular strut graft. *Orthopedics.* 2014;37(9):e822–827.

24. Matassi F, Angeloni R, Carulli C, et al. Locking plate and fibular allograft augmentation in unstable fractures of proximal humerus. *Injury.* 2012;43(11):1939–1942.

25. Neviaser AS, Hettrich CM, Beamer BS, et al. Endosteal strut augment reduces complications associated with proximal humeral locking plates. *Clin Orthop Relat Res.* 2011;469(12):3300–3306.

31

Humeral Shaft Fractures

REZA OMID AND LUKE T. NICHOLSON

Introduction

Fractures of the humeral shaft represent 1% to 3% of all fractures and have an annual incidence of 4.5 per 100,000 patients.[1] The distribution of fractures follows a bimodal distribution with peaks occurring in the seventh and third decades of life commonly due to ground-level falls in elderly females and high-energy trauma in young males, respectively.[2] The nonoperative management of humeral shaft fractures has historically resulted in very high union rates and a high degree of patient satisfaction, with deformity of the humerus well accommodated by the large arc of motion at the shoulder and elbow. Wider indications for fixation and lower union rates with nonoperative management described in recent literature have expanded the role of operative management for humeral shaft fractures in recent years.[3] Operative techniques include open reduction and plate fixation, minimally invasive plate osteosynthesis (MIPO), intramedullary nailing, and external fixation.

Relevant Anatomy

The management of humeral shaft fractures requires an in-depth understanding of humerus anatomy, the surrounding neurovascular structures, and, in particular, the relationship of the radial nerve to the humerus. The humeral shaft is defined as the region distal to the surgical neck and proximal to the medial and lateral epicondyles of the humerus. Proximally, the humerus is cylindrical; distally, it becomes triangular with posterior, anterolateral, and anteromedial surfaces.[4] The humerus is supplied by a nutrient vessel located about the medial aspect of the distal aspect of the middle third of the humeral shaft (Fig. 31.1).[5] The deltoid tuberosity is an osseous elevation on the humerus that serves as the insertion for the three heads of the deltoid muscle[6]; it is a deforming force for humeral shaft fractures and serves as an important anatomic landmark for the radial nerve, which passes the posterior midline of the humerus within 0.1 cm of the distal-most aspect of the tuberosity (Fig. 31.2).[7] The spiral groove is a feature that separates the origins of the medial and lateral heads of the triceps, between which the radial nerve passes as it descends from proximal to distal through the posterior arm.[7]

The radial nerve is of particular importance when managing humeral shaft fractures because it lies in direct contact with the posterior humerus from 17.1 to 10.9 cm proximal to the lateral epicondyle.[7] The nerve enters the brachium anterior to the subscapularis and latissimus dorsi and descends with the profunda brachii artery through the triangular interval, defined as the anatomic space between the long head of the triceps and the humerus below the teres major. The nerve is maintained between the medial and lateral heads of the triceps as it courses adjacent to, but not within, the spiral groove of the humerus. Importantly, at this level, the nerve trifurcates into its main trunk, a branch to the medial head of the triceps, and the posterior antebrachial cutaneous nerve.[7] All three branches travel together along the posterior humerus; if a single branch is mistaken to be "the radial nerve" in this region, injury may occur as other branches are not properly identified and protected (Fig. 31.3). Distally, the nerve passes through the lateral intermuscular septum 10.2 cm proximal to the lateral epicondyle. As it passes across the lateral intermuscular septum, the nerve is focally tethered. This tether point is thought to be responsible for

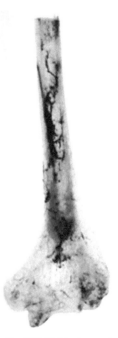

• **Fig. 31.1** Nutrient vessel.

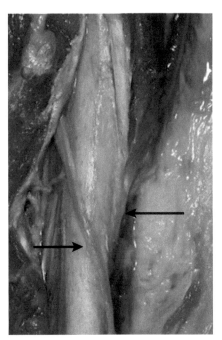

• **Fig. 31.2** Spiral groove deltoid relationship. *Left arrow:* radial nerve within spiral groove; *right arrow:* deltoid insertion.

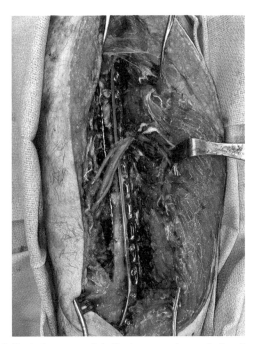

• **Fig. 31.3** Posterior approach to the humerus demonstrating the relationship of the radial nerve which contacts the humerus 10-17 cm proximal to the lateral epicondyle.

the high incidence of radial nerve palsy with mid to distal humeral shaft fractures; the eponymous Holstein-Lewis fracture is a distal third spiral fracture that was historically thought to put the radial nerve at particularly high risk for injury, although more recent literature has downplayed this association.[8] In the anterior compartment, the nerve courses between the brachialis muscle, to which it provides partial innervation, and the brachioradialis muscle, before passing anterior to the lateral epicondyle into the forearm.

The ulnar nerve passes posterior to the pectoralis major and descends medial to the axillary artery in the anterior compartment of the brachium. It becomes of particular interest during the exposure of

the distal humerus as it pierces the medial intermuscular septum 8 cm proximal to the medial epicondyle. In the posterior compartment, it descends anterior and medial to the medial head of the triceps until it passes posterior to the medial epicondyle to enter the cubital tunnel.

The median nerve and brachial artery are located anteromedial to the humerus throughout the brachium and travel in close proximity to one another. The median nerve travels lateral to the brachial artery in the interval between the brachialis and biceps until the level of the coracobrachialis insertion, when the nerve crosses anterior to the brachial artery and subsequently descends medial to the artery in the distal brachium and antecubital fossa.

The musculocutaneous nerve pierces the coracobrachialis muscle and then descends the length of the brachium in the interval between the biceps and brachialis, where it provides innervation to each muscle. It continues distally as the lateral antebrachial cutaneous nerve, which pierces the deep fascia lateral to the biceps tendon at the intercondylar line. The nerve is at risk of injury during a brachialis splitting anterior approach to the humerus if not properly identified and protected.

The axillary nerve passes in close proximity to the inferior glenoid before passing with the posterior humeral circumflex vessels through the quadrilateral space, defined by the long head of the triceps and the humerus medially and laterally, respectively, and the teres minor and teres major superiorly and inferiorly, respectively. The axillary nerve splits into anterior and posterior branches at the 6 o'clock position on the glenoid; the anterior branch courses laterally around the surgical neck of the humerus 4–6 cm distal to the acromion[9] to provide innervation to the anterior and middle heads of the deltoid, while the posterior branch continues posteriorly to provide innervation to the posterior head of the deltoid and teres minor muscle. The posterior branch additionally gives off the superior lateral brachial cutaneous nerve.[10] The axillary nerve serves as the proximal extent of the exposure of the humerus through a posterior approach.

Classification

The most widely used classification system for humeral shaft fractures is the AO/OTA (AO Foundation/Orthopaedic Trauma Association) classification. The humeral shaft is identified as bone number 1, fracture location 2, or AO/OTA 12 (Fig. 31.4). As with other diaphyseal fractures, the AO/OTA system subdivides humeral shaft fractures into subtypes A for simple fractures, B for wedge fractures, and C for complex fractures. Subtype A fractures are further divided into spiral, oblique, and transverse patterns. Subtype B fractures are further divided into spiral wedge, bending wedge, and fragmented wedge patterns. Subtype C fractures are further divided into spiral, segmental, and irregular patterns.

Treatment Options

Treatment options for humeral shaft fractures vary broadly; choice in the management of select humeral shaft fractures must be carefully guided by patient factors, associated injuries, fracture characteristics, and patient preferences. Indications for nonoperative versus operative management of select humeral shaft fractures are discussed in detail in the following section. Techniques for surgical management include open reduction and internal fixation, MIPO, and intramedullary nailing.

Nonoperative Treatment With Fracture Brace

Nonoperative treatment is appropriate for many patients presenting with isolated spiral or oblique humeral shaft fracture. Patients

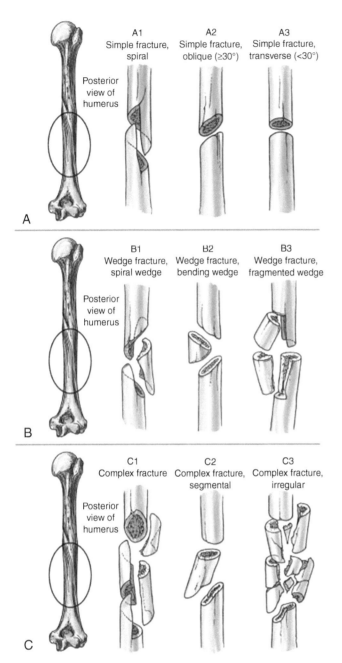

A1 Simple fracture, spiral
A2 Simple fracture, oblique (≥30°)
A3 Simple fracture, transverse (<30°)

Posterior view of humerus

A

B1 Wedge fracture, spiral wedge
B2 Wedge fracture, bending wedge
B3 Wedge fracture, fragmented wedge

Posterior view of humerus

B

C1 Complex fracture
C2 Complex fracture, segmental
C3 Complex fracture, irregular

Posterior view of humerus

C

• **Fig. 31.4** AO/OTA classification of humeral shaft fractures.

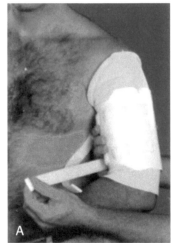
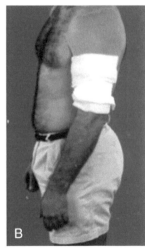

A   B

• **Fig. 31.5** Fracture brace.

are initially placed in a coaptation splint or hanging arm cast for 1 to 2 weeks after injury. A custom fracture brace is fabricated using two plastic sleeves encircled with two adjustable Velcro straps (Fig. 31.5). For fractures of the proximal diaphysis, an over-the-shoulder addition is applied to the brace. Patients are instructed to maintain the brace at all times except for bathing and must tighten the straps several times daily to allow for swelling subsidence and muscle atrophy. Gravity-assisted pendulum exercises and elbow range of motion are encouraged. Radiographs are obtained at the time of brace application, at 6 weeks post injury, and every 6 weeks thereafter to assess for union.[11] Patients are examined clinically at 6 weeks; gross fracture site mobility at 6 weeks is an independent predictor of nonunion formation and should be discussed with the patient as a possible indication for transition to surgical care.[12]

Open Reduction and Plate Osteosynthesis

Open reduction and plate osteosynthesis is considered to be the most practical means of surgical treatment for most humeral shaft fractures. Because of the high rotational forces through the humerus and propensity for nonunion, strict adherence to sound orthopedic principles is especially important in the management of humeral shaft fractures. In particular, careful soft tissue handling and avoidance of periosteal stripping are critical to successful outcome. The ultimate goal is to obtain an anatomic reduction with absolute stability for most simple fracture patterns. Oblique and spiral fractures are ideally managed with single or multiple lag screw fixation and neutralization plating. Transverse fractures are optimally suited for compression plating with a carefully under-contoured plate (Fig. 31.6). Comminuted fractures not amenable to anatomic reduction are best treated with relative stability via bridging plate constructs with long working lengths or intramedullary nailing (Fig. 31.7). Large fragment 4.5-mm broad plates are often preferred due to their biomechanical superiority over 4.5-mm narrow plates and small fragment 3.5-mm plates[13] and are optimal for supporting early weight-bearing or crutch use.[14] Broad plates of 4.5 mm also typically have staggered holes which may decrease the risk of a linear stress riser. In certain cases, the narrow 4.5-mm plate may be optimal to allow for plate contouring in more complex anatomical areas such as the distal aspect of the humerus. Eight cortices of screw purchase are desired on either side of the fracture whenever possible. Locking screw fixation has not been shown to be biomechanically superior to nonlocking screw fixation for diaphyseal humerus fractures,[15] although it is recommended to use locking screws in the setting of pathologic fracture, osteoporotic bone, or humerus nonunion. When desired, dual plating has been advocated by some authors to increase construct stiffness, and orthogonal plating has been shown to be superior to side-by-side plating (Fig. 31.8). For fractures of the proximal humeral diaphysis, 3.5-mm anatomic proximal humerus plates are ideally suited to obtaining purchase in the humeral head but may require elevation of a portion of the anterior deltoid insertion. For fractures of the distal humeral diaphysis, a stout 3.5-mm posterolateral extra-articular distal humerus plate is commonly used but is frequently prominent on the posterior aspect of the lateral column of the elbow resulting in symptomatic hardware. If the patient desires a late hardware removal, the radial nerve must be elevated to remove the plate safely which can result in a radial nerve palsy.

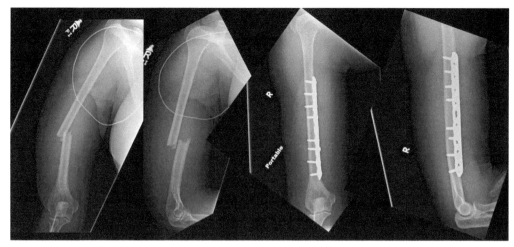

• **Fig. 31.6** Transverse fractures are typically treated with compression plating.

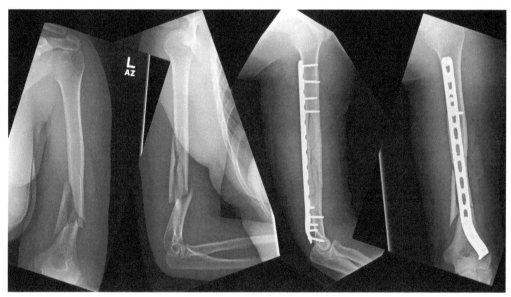

• **Fig. 31.7** Highly comminuted fractures are best treated with relative stability via bridging plate constructs with long working lengths.

For this reason, our preferred technique for most supracondylar distal humerus fractures that have at least 3 to 4 cm of bone proximal to the olecranon fossa is to use a long proximal humerus flipped upside down along the anterior humerus (Fig. 31.9).[16]

Minimally Invasive Plate Osteosynthesis

MIPO is an alternative to open reduction internal fixation for certain fracture patterns and can be performed from an anterior or posterior approach. The anterior technique utilizes two 4 to 5 cm incisions, one just proximal to the elbow flexion crease and lateral to the biceps muscle, and one at the distal extent of the deltopectoral interval (Fig. 31.10). The posterior approach utilizes one 4 to 5 cm incision lateral to the olecranon fossa and one larger proximal incision to allow adequate visualization and protection of the radial nerve (Fig. 31.10). Most authors recommend the use of a contoured large fragment 4.5-mm narrow plate passed submuscularly with great care to pass the plate deep to the radial nerve. The primary benefit of the MIPO technique is minimization of soft tissue disruption at the fracture site by passing the plate through

two incisions following an indirect reduction. The main limitation of the technique is the inability to obtain absolute stability for simple fracture patterns (Fig. 31.11).

Antegrade Intramedullary Nailing

Intramedullary nailing of humeral shaft fractures is a minimally invasive option typically utilized for comminuted or pathologic fractures of the humerus. It should also be considered in the setting of a highly traumatized soft tissue envelope where an open plating approach may carry increased risk of wound complications. Complex fracture patterns including those with extensive comminution and segmental patterns are most appropriate for this fixation strategy. Although retrograde nailing options are available, this strategy is limited to middle third or proximal fractures and is relatively contraindicated in patients with narrow intramedullary canals. As a result, an antegrade approach is typically performed. Injury to the rotator cuff and risk of shoulder dysfunction are the primary concern in antegrade nailing; however, with proper technique, this potential risk can be minimized. Further details on this technique can be found in Chapter 32.

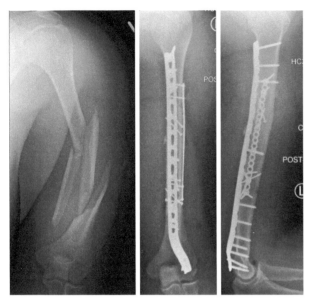

• **Fig. 31.8** Dual plating with mini-fragment hardware can allow for fragment-specific reconstruction while minimizing soft tissue disruption.

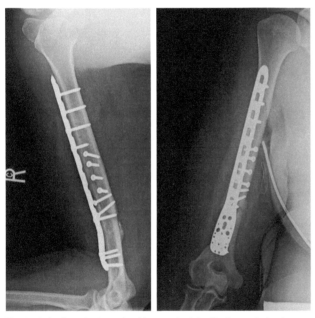

• **Fig. 31.9** An inverted proximal humeral plate fits the anterior humerus and is well-suited for plating a distal third shaft fracture.

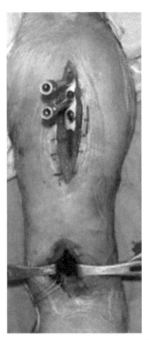

• **Fig. 31.10** Minimally invasive plate osteosynthesis from an anterior approach.

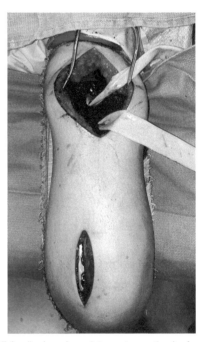

• **Fig. 31.11** Minimally invasive plate osteosynthesis from a posterior approach.

Indications for Surgical Treatment

Indications for surgical intervention include both strong and relative indications. Strong indications include open fracture, compartment syndrome, vascular injury requiring repair, complete radial nerve palsy after closed fracture manipulation, and ipsilateral both bone forearm fracture causing a "floating elbow." Brachial plexus injury may be considered a strong indication because of a high rate of nonunion with fracture brace application to a flaccid arm; however, the extent of the brachial plexus injury should be considered in following this guideline. Relative indications for surgical stabilization include multiple extremity injury, pathologic fracture, obesity, pendulous breasts in a female patient, soft tissue injury precluding use of a fracture brace, and certain fracture characteristics that increase the risk of a nonunion, such as a displaced proximal diaphyseal fracture, transverse fracture, and a fracture that is mobile at 6 weeks.[12] It should be noted that degree of angulation or deformity is not a reliable indication for surgical management because neither has been shown to correlate with functional outcome.[17]

Surgical Approaches

The vast majority of humeral shaft fractures can be managed through the anterolateral or posterior approaches. Additional surgical approaches include the minimally invasive anterior approach, the minimally invasive posterior approach, the direct medial approach, and the direct lateral approach.

Anterolateral Approach

The anterolateral approach is ideal for access to proximal and mid-shaft humeral fractures but can be used for distal humerus fractures as well. Advantages of the anterolateral approach include proximal extension through the deltopectoral interval, supine patient positioning, and avoidance of the radial nerve for proximal shaft fractures. The patient is positioned supine with a radiolucent arm board. The surgeon should confirm adequate fluoroscopic visualization of the proximal humerus prior to draping the patient, particularly if planning to place screws into the humeral head.

The internervous interval lies between the pectoral nerves and axillary nerve proximally, and musculocutaneous and radial nerves distally. The incision is centered at the level of the fracture and extended proximally toward the coracoid process and distally toward the lateral ridge of the distal humerus. The subcutaneous tissues are divided in line with the incision until the deep fascia of the arm is encountered and incised along the lateral border of the biceps muscle. The cephalic vein is identified and protected between the deltoid and pectoralis major muscles. For all but the most proximal of fractures, the radial nerve should be identified and protected in the distal incision. It is most easily found between the brachialis and brachioradialis muscle bellies in the distal arm and traced proximally to its passage across the lateral intermuscular septum. Care should be taken to ensure all branches of the nerve are protected. If necessary for proximal exposure, the deltopectoral interval is utilized. If a standard proximal humerus plate is selected for fracture management, the anterior border of the deltoid insertion on the deltoid tuberosity may be elevated; this is accommodated by the broad insertion of the deltoid.[6] Similarly, if proximal exposure of the humerus is necessary, release of the pectoralis major tendon may be necessary but it should be repaired. Distally, the musculocutaneous nerve can be identified as it passes between the biceps and brachialis muscle bellies; its continuation as the lateral antebrachial cutaneous nerve should be protected. Attention should be paid to the anatomy of the brachialis muscle, which has a large superficial head originating proximolaterally and a smaller deep head originating along the anterior humeral metaphysis. The deep head is safely split in its midline of the humerus given its dual innervation by the musculocutaneous and radial nerves (Fig. 31.12).

Posterior Approach

The posterior approach is ideal for access to distal humeral shaft fractures. Advantages of the posterior approach include visualization of the posterior distal humerus and exposure of the radial nerve when indicated for nerve exploration. The posterior approach requires that the plate be placed directly deep to the nerve; while this is technically straightforward during primary fixation, it puts the nerve at risk of injury during secondary procedures, such as hardware removal. For this reason, one should consider an anterior approach for supracondylar distal humerus fractures.

For the posterior approach, the patient is positioned prone or lateral with the arm draped over a post or bolster. A sterile tourniquet may be used for dissection of the radial nerve. The incision is centered over the fracture site and extended distally toward the tip of the olecranon and proximally toward the posterolateral corner of the acromion. The subcutaneous tissues are divided in line with the incision until fascia is encountered and incised longitudinally. Identification of the radial nerve can either be done proximally in the midline by developing the interval between the long and lateral heads of the triceps, or distally by retracting the lateral head

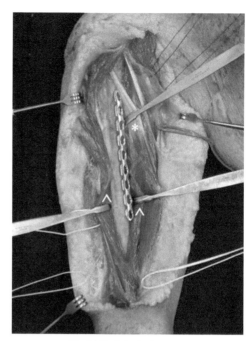

• **Fig. 31.12** Anterior humerus.

of the triceps medially and identifying the radial nerve as it pierces the lateral intermuscular septum. Care should be taken to ensure all branches of the nerve are protected. Exposure of the fracture site can either be done through a trans-tricipital or paratricipital approach as described by Gerwin.[18] The trans-tricipital approach utilizes a triceps split to expose both the radial nerve and fracture site and allows visualization of approximately 15 cm of humerus. The paratricipital approach involves retracting the triceps medially and opening the lateral intermuscular septum to mobilize the radial nerve. The medial and lateral heads of the triceps can then be elevated to allow more proximal exposure (Fig. 31.13).[18]

Relevant Complications

The most relevant complications associated with the management of humeral shaft fractures are nonunion, radial nerve palsy, infection, and shoulder site morbidity specific to antegrade intramedullary nailing. Union rates and radial nerve palsy management for nonoperatively treated fractures are discussed in detail in the following section. Nonunion rates in operatively managed fractures range from 4% to 17.5%, with few large series providing high-level data on union rate following internal fixation.[3,19] Radial nerve palsy following operative management of humeral shaft fractures is of particular relevance during the posterior approach to the humerus and during revision surgery, when the nerve is commonly encased in scar tissue overlying the posterior plate.

Review of Treatment Outcomes

Large, historical series have demonstrated exceptional results with nonoperative management of humeral shaft fractures. Most notable is Sarmiento's work reporting 97.5% union of all humeral shaft fractures and 98% union of closed humeral shaft fractures managed with a fracture brace.[20] By modern standards, these series are impressive not just for their high rates of union but also for the treatment of all fractures, including open fractures, with functional bracing. Modern treatment of humeral shaft fractures incorporates the knowledge gained by these early studies with contemporary

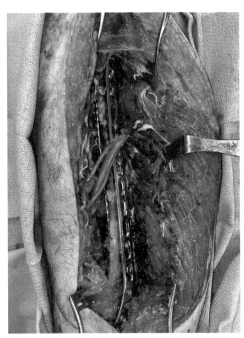

• **Fig. 31.13** The medial and lateral heads of the triceps can then be elevated from the posterior humerus to allow for more proximal humeral exposure.

surgical indications and treatment goals, including early return to functional activity. Few high-quality studies guide the decision between nonoperative and operative management, with a 2012 Cochrane review determining that there is no evidence available from randomized controlled trials to ascertain whether surgical or nonoperative management results in a superior outcome.[21]

Union Rate With Nonoperative Management

High union rates have been reported with nonoperative management of humeral shaft fractures in retrospective historical case series. In Sarmiento's original 1977 series of 51 fractures, 50 (98%) healed successfully and one, a pathologic fracture, went on to nonunion. In a follow-up study in 2000, Sarmiento later reported on 620 patients in whom 97.5% of all fractures went on to successful union, including 98% of closed fractures. Zagorski and Ostermann each separately reported a union rate of 98% in separate series of 170 and 191 fractures in 1988 and 1993, respectively. These studies have since been criticized for their high loss to follow-up, including a 33% loss to follow-up in Sarmiento's 2000 series, and the imprecise description of follow-up in patients who were followed up to complete union. In a 2010 review of 18 clinical studies that included historical case series, Papasoulis reported a union rate of 94.5% with functional brace treatment.[22] In more recent literature, Ali et al. reported a union rate of 83% in 138 fractures treated with functional bracing in 2015.[23] Similarly, Harkin reported a 33% nonunion rate at 6 months in 2017.[19] In the largest multicenter series to date on the nonoperative management of humeral shaft fractures, Serrano et al. most recently reported a 29% conversion to surgical intervention in 1182 patients, 60% of whom were converted due to persistent nonunion (overall 17.5% nonunion rate at 6 months).[3]

Fracture Location and Morphology

Fracture morphology and location play a prominent role in determining likelihood of union with nonoperative management.

Fractures of the proximal third of the humerus, in particular, have a predilection to nonunion. Rutgers and Ring reported a 29% nonunion rate in proximal third fractures versus 4% and 0% nonunion rates in middle and distal third fractures, respectively.[24] In the series by Ali et al., the nonunion rate for proximal third fractures was 24% compared with 12% and 15% for middle and distal third fractures, respectively.[23] In their series on 1182 patients, Serrano et al. reported a statistically significant association between proximal shaft fracture and nonunion on univariate analysis.[3] Castella reported specifically on a nonunion pattern in nine patients that occurred at the junction of the middle and proximal third of the humerus with a long lateral butterfly fragment attached to the deltoid, which is thought to predispose fractures in this region to nonunion.[25] For fractures of the distal third of the humerus, nonoperative management results in very high rates of union with an increased risk of varus malunion of minimal functional significance.[26] Operative treatment has been found to improve alignment and allow for a quicker return to function with an increased risk of iatrogenic radial nerve injury and need for reoperation (Jawa).[26]

In comparing fracture morphology, the majority of series have identified simple fracture patterns, particularly transverse patterns, as at risk of nonunion, due to the decreased surface area available for callus generation.[27,28] Ring et al. did identify a decreased union rate in spiral fractures; however, the small sample size in this series is a limitation that should be assessed in light of numerous other publications supporting the opposite finding.[29]

Radial Nerve Palsy

Radial nerve palsy can be separated into primary or secondary nerve palsy, occurring either at the time of injury or during the surgical management of humeral shaft fracture, respectively. Observation is generally recommended for primary radial nerve palsy that accompanies low-energy humeral shaft fractures being managed nonoperatively given a high rate of spontaneous radial nerve recovery. The literature does, however, support early intervention in specific scenarios, including open injury, high-energy trauma, and in settings where patients have a strong preference for early intervention. In a meta-analysis on the management of radial nerve palsy associated with humeral shaft fracture, Shao et al. found an overall incidence of 11.8% in 4517 fractures. The overall rate of recovery was 88.1%, while spontaneous recovery was 70.7% in patients managed without exploration. Because it is not possible to know how many patients who were explored would have recovered without an operation, the true incidence of recovery without intervention is unknown but presumed to be somewhere between 70% and 88%. Compared with patients explored late (>3 months after injury), those explored early (within 3 weeks of injury) did not show a greater chance for recovery, and the authors, therefore advocate for expectant management of primary radial nerve palsy.[30] Similarly, in a decision analysis model, Bishop and Ring came to the conclusion that initial observation is the preferred strategy for closed radial nerve palsies associated with humeral shaft fractures, with exceptions in the settings of low likelihood of recovery and high patient desire for early intervention.[31] In an evaluation of injury mechanism in 18 patients, Venouziou et al. identified an association between severe nerve injury and high-energy trauma and concluded that high-energy injury patterns may warrant exploration while low-energy patterns have a high likelihood of recovery without exploration.[32] Advocates for early exploration cite the ease of dissection and the ability to identify nerve incarceration or laceration at the time of exploration in favoring early exploration.[33]

Operative Outcomes

Few high-level studies compare outcomes of operatively treated and nonoperatively treated humeral shaft fractures. The only completed randomized controlled trial to date compares MIPO with fracture bracing and demonstrates decreased nonunion rate in patients managed surgically (0% vs. 15%), and improved alignment in patients managed surgically.[34] When comparing functional bracing with open reduction internal fixation for extra-articular distal third diaphyseal humeral shaft fractures, surgery has been shown to achieve more predicable alignment and quicker return of function at the expense of increased risk of infection and radial nerve palsy.[26] With respect to union rates, several retrospective cohort studies have found decreased delayed union and nonunion in humeral shaft fractures treated surgical versus closed management.[19,35]

In comparing MIPO and ORIF (open reduction internal fixation), a prospective randomized trial of 67 fractures found similar union rates and excellent functional outcomes in each group.[36] A subsequent meta-analysis of two randomized trials and three nonrandomized trials found no difference in union rate, delayed union, malunion, infection, operative time, or clinical outcome measures between the two techniques, but did identify an increased risk of radial nerve palsy in the ORIF group compared with the MIPO group.[37]

Intramedullary nailing has been shown in multiple systematic reviews and meta-analyses to result in similar outcomes to open reduction and plate fixation, including similar rates of union, infection, and radial nerve palsy but with a higher incidence of shoulder complications and reoperation.[38,39] Shoulder complications have been shown to include decreased range of motion, impingement, and persistent pain. Furthermore, reoperation rate has been shown to be higher with intramedullary nails, with one study reporting that one reoperation could be prevented for every 10 patients treated with plates.[40] The incidence of intramedullary nailing for humeral shaft fractures has subsequently decreased, with ABOS Part II Boards Candidates reporting a decrease from 42.9% in 2004 to 21.2% in 2013.[41] In a systematic review comparing conventional plating with MIPO and intramedullary nailing, Tetsworth et al. concluded that MIPO results in better clinical outcomes with a lower rate of nonunion compared with standard plating and intramedullary nailing, although there was noted heterogeneity among studies analyzed limiting these conclusions.[42]

References

1. Ekholm R, Adami J, Tidermark J, Hansson K, Törnkvist H, Ponzer S. Fractures of the shaft of the humerus. An epidemiological study of 401 fractures. *J Bone Joint Surg*. 2006;88(11):1469–1473.
2. Tytherleigh-Strong G, Walls N, McQueen MM. The epidemiology of humeral shaft fractures. *J Bone Joint Surg*. 1998;80(2):249–253.
3. Serrano R, Mir HR, Sagi HC, et al. Modern results of functional bracing of humeral shaft fractures: a multicenter retrospective analysis. *J Orthopaed Trauma*. 2020;34(4):206–209.
4. Goldberg SH, Omid R, Nassr AN, Beck R, Cohen MS. Osseous anatomy of the distal humerus and proximal ulna: implications for total elbow arthroplasty. *J Shoulder Elbow Surg/Am Shoulder Elbow Surg*. 2007;16(3 Suppl):S39–S46.
5. Carroll SE. A study of the nutrient foramina of the humeral diaphysis. *J Bone Joint S*. 1963;45-B:176–181.
6. Rispoli DM, Athwal GS, Sperling JW, Cofield RH. The anatomy of the deltoid insertion. *J Shoulder Elbow Surg/Am Shoulder Elbow Surg*. 2009;18(3):386–390.
7. Carlan D, Jeffrey P, Megan MPJ, Weiland AJ, Boyer MI, Gelberman RH. The radial nerve in the brachium: an anatomic study in human cadavers. *J Hand Surg*. 2007;32(8):1177–1182.
8. Shao YC, Grotz MRW, Limb D, Giannoudis P. Radial nerve palsy associated with fractures of the shaft of the humerus: a systematic review. *Bone Joint Lett J*. 2005;87(12):1647–1652. https://doi.org/10.1302/0301-620X.87B12.
9. Cetik O, Uslu M, Acar HI, Comert A, Tekdemir I, Cift H. Is there a safe area for the axillary nerve in the deltoid muscle? A cadaveric study. *J Bone Joint Surg*. 2006;88(11):2395–2399.
10. Leechavengvongs S, Teerawutthichaikit T, Witoonchart K, et al. Surgical anatomy of the axillary nerve branches to the deltoid muscle. *Clin Anat*. 2015;28(1):118–122.
11. Crespo AM, Konda SR, Egol KA. Set it and forget it: diaphyseal fractures of the humerus undergo minimal change in angulation after functional brace application. *Iowa Orthopaed J*. 2018;38:73–77.
12. Driesman AS, Fisher N, Raj K, Sanjit K, Egol KA. Fracture site mobility at 6 weeks after humeral shaft fracture predicts nonunion without surgery. *J Orthopaed Trauma*. 2017;31(12):657–662.
13. Patel R, Neu CP, Curtiss S, Fyhrie DP, Yoo B. Crutch weightbearing on comminuted humeral shaft fractures: a biomechanical comparison of large versus small fragment fixation for humeral shaft fractures. *J Orthopaed Trauma*. 2011;25(5):300–305.
14. Tingstad EM, Wolinsky PR, Shyr Y, Johnson KD. Effect of immediate weightbearing on plated fractures of the humeral shaft. *J Trauma*. 2000;49(2):278–280.
15. O'Toole RV, Andersen RC, Vesnovsky O, et al. Are locking screws advantageous with plate fixation of humeral shaft fractures? A biomechanical analysis of synthetic and cadaveric bone. *J Orthopaed Trauma*. 2008;22(10):709–715.
16. Sohn HS, Shin SJ. Modified use of a proximal humeral internal locking system (PHILOS) plate in extra-articular distal-third diaphyseal humeral fractures. *Injury*. 2019;50(7):1300–1305.
17. Shields E, Sundem L, Childs S, et al. The impact of residual angulation on patient reported functional outcome scores after non-operative treatment for humeral shaft fractures. *Injury*. 2016;47(4):914–918.
18. Gerwin M, Hotchkiss RN, Weiland AJ. Alternative operative exposures of the posterior aspect of the humeral diaphysis with reference to the radial nerve. *J Bone Joint Surg*. 1996;78(11):1690–1695.
19. Harkin FE, Large RJ. Humeral shaft fractures: union outcomes in a large cohort. *J Shoulder Elbow Surg/Am Shoulder Elbow Surg*. 2017;26(11):1881–1888.
20. Sarmiento A, Zagorski JB, Zych GA, Latta LL, Capps CA. Functional bracing for the treatment of fractures of the humeral diaphysis. *J Bone Joint Surg Am*. 2000;82(4):478–486.
21. Gosler MW, Testroote M, Morrenhof JW, Janzing HMJ. Surgical versus non-surgical interventions for treating humeral shaft fractures in adults. *Cochrane Database Sys Rev*. 2012;1:CD008832.
22. Papasoulis E, Drosos GI, Ververidis AN, Verettas DA. Functional bracing of humeral shaft fractures. A review of clinical studies. *Injury*. 2010;41(7):e21–27.
23. Ali E, Griffiths D, Obi N, Tytherleigh-Strong G, Van Rensburg L. Nonoperative treatment of humeral shaft fractures revisited. *J Shoulder Elbow Surg/Am Shoulder Elbow Surg*. 2015;24(2):210–214.
24. Rutgers M, Ring D. Treatment of diaphyseal fractures of the humerus using a functional brace. *J Orthopaed Trauma*. 2006;20(9):597–601.
25. Castellá FB, Garcia FB, Berry EM, Perelló EB, Sánchez-Alepuz E, Gabarda R. Nonunion of the humeral shaft: long lateral butterfly fracture—a nonunion predictive pattern? *Clin Orthopaed Related Res*. 2004;424:227–230.
26. Jawa A, McCarty P, Doornberg J, Harris M, Ring D. Extra-articular distal-third diaphyseal fractures of the humerus. A comparison of functional bracing and plate fixation. *J Bone Joint Surg*. 2006;88(11):2343–2347.
27. Koch PP, Gross DFL, Gerber C. The results of functional (Sarmiento) bracing of humeral shaft fractures. *J Shoulder Elbow Surg/Am Shoulder Elbow Surg*. 2002;11(2):143–150.

28. Ekholm R, Tidermark J, Törnkvist H, Adami J, Ponzer S. Outcome after closed functional treatment of humeral shaft fractures. *J Orthopaed Trauma*. 2006;20(9):591–596.

29. Ring D, Chin K, Taghinia AH, Jupiter JB. Nonunion after functional brace treatment of diaphyseal humerus fractures. *J Trauma*. 2007;62(5):1157–1158.

30. Shao YC, Harwood P, Grotz MRW, Limb D, Giannoudis PV. Radial nerve palsy associated with fractures of the shaft of the humerus: a systematic review. *J Bone Joint Surg*. 2005;87(12):1647–1652.

31. Bishop J, Ring D. Management of radial nerve palsy associated with humeral shaft fracture: a decision analysis model. *J Hand Surg*. 2009;34(6):991–996.e1.

32. Venouziou AI, Dailiana ZH, Varitimidis SE, et al. Radial nerve palsy associated with humeral shaft fracture. Is the energy of trauma a prognostic factor? *Injury*. 2011;42(11):1289–1293.

33. Chang G, Ilyas AM. Radial nerve palsy after humeral shaft fractures: the case for early exploration and a new classification to guide treatment and prognosis. *Hand Clin*. 2018;34(1):105–112.

34. Matsunaga FT, Marcel JST, Marcelo HM, Nicola AN, Flavio F, Joao CB. Minimally invasive osteosynthesis with a bridge plate versus a functional brace for humeral shaft fractures: a randomized controlled trial. *J Bone Joint Surg*. 2017;99(7):583–592.

35. Westrick E, Hamilton B, Toogood P, Henley B, Firoozabadi R. Humeral shaft fractures: results of operative and non-operative treatment. *Int Orthopaed*. 2017;41(2):385–395.

36. Kim JW, Chang-Wug O, Young-Soo B, Jung JK, Chul Park K. A prospective randomized study of operative treatment for noncomminuted humeral shaft fractures: conventional open plating versus minimal invasive plate osteosynthesis. *J Orthopaed Trauma*. 2015;29(4):189–194.

37. Yu BF, Liu LL, Yang GJ, Zhang L, Lin XP. Comparison of minimally invasive plate osteosynthesis and conventional plate osteosynthesis for humeral shaft fracture: a meta-analysis. *Medicine*. 2016;95(39). e4955.

38. Kurup H, Munier H, Andrew JG. Dynamic compression plating versus locked intramedullary nailing for humeral shaft fractures in adults. *Cochrane Database Sys Rev*. 2011;6:CD005959.

39. Ouyang H, Xiong J, Xiang P, Cui Z, Chen L, Yu B. Plate versus intramedullary nail fixation in the treatment of humeral shaft fractures: an updated meta-analysis. *J Shoulder Elbow Surg/Am Shoulder Elbow Surg*. 2013;22(3):387–395.

40. Bhandari M, Devereaux PJ, McKee MD, Schemitsch EH. Compression plating versus intramedullary nailing of humeral shaft fractures—a meta-analysis. *Acta Orthop*. 2006;77(2):279–284.

41. Gottschalk MB, Carpenter W, Hiza E, Reisman W, Roberson J. Humeral shaft fracture fixation: incidence rates and complications as reported by American Board of Orthopaedic Surgery Part II Candidates. *JBJS*. 2016;98(17):e71.

42. Tetsworth K, Erik H, Glatt V. Minimally invasive plate osteosynthesis of humeral shaft fractures: current state of the art. *J Am Acad Orthopaed Surg*. 2018;26(18):652–661.

32

Technique Spotlight: Radial Nerve Identification in the Upper Extremity

REZA OMID AND LUKE T. NICHOLSON

The radial nerve is of particular interest in the management of upper extremity orthopedic trauma due to its circuitous course, close proximity to bone, and sensitivity to injury. Proximal to the brachium, it may be identified through a deltopectoral approach by releasing the pectoralis minor from its insertion on the coracoid process to expose the infraclavicular brachial plexus. In the brachium, the nerve wraps circumferentially around the humerus in a predictable manner and can be identified posteriorly in the midline of the humerus at the level of the distal deltoid tuberosity[1] between the long and lateral heads of the triceps (Fig. 32.1). Exposure in the brachium is accomplished with a standard longitudinal posterior midline incision centered between the long and lateral heads of the triceps. The deep investing fascia of the triceps is opened longitudinally and the raphe between the medial and lateral heads is identified. In thin patients, the radial nerve can be palpated deep to the raphe as it courses obliquely through the posterior compartment. The long and lateral heads of the triceps are bluntly separated until the radial nerve and profunda brachii artery are encountered (Fig. 32.2). An alternative to identifying the radial nerve between the heads of the triceps is to identify it lateral to the triceps in the distal posterior brachium as described by Gerwin et al.[2] The incision is extended from the proximal midline of the brachium towards the lateral epicondyle. Distally, the triceps muscle is bluntly retracted off of the lateral intermuscular septum. The radial nerve can be identified proximal to its passage through the intermuscular septum an average of 10.2 cm proximal to the lateral epicondyle. The posterior antebrachial cutaneous nerve is typically encountered first when dissecting from distal to proximal (Fig. 32.3) and can be traced back to the radial nerve proper which lies medial and anterior to it (Fig. 32.4). Because the nerve is tethered at the lateral intermuscular septum, it is recommended that the septum be released for several centimeters distal to the nerve. The nerve can then be traced proximally and the triceps reflected medially to allow visualization of approximately 26 cm of humeral diaphysis.[2]

After passing through the lateral intermuscular septum, the nerve enters the anterior compartment of the arm and passes between the origins of the superficial and deep heads of the brachialis muscle. The superficial head originates off of the anterolateral aspect of the mid-humerus and lateral intermuscular septum. The smaller deep head originates off of the distal third of the anterior aspect of the humerus.[3] Using a standard anterolateral approach centered on the lateral aspect of the biceps muscle, the radial nerve is identified distally in the interval between the brachialis and brachioradialis muscles (Fig. 32.5). Identification of the nerve in this interval is frequently challenging, particularly in patients with muscular arms as the interval between these muscles is not always readily identifiable. The authors recommend a slow and careful blunt dissection with a focus on looking deep and medial to the brachioradialis muscle belly. Spreading in line with the anticipated course of the nerve is paramount to avoiding inadvertent injury. Distally, the nerve courses directly anteriorly and medially to the capitellum at the level of the ulnohumeral joint while staying anterior to the fibers of the brachialis, with which it is intimately associated.[4]

The radial nerve divides into the posterior interosseous nerve (PIN) and superficial radial sensory nerve (SRN) approximately 8 cm distal to the lateral intermuscular septum and 3.6 cm proximal to the leading edge of the supinator muscle (Fig. 32.6).[5] The SRN travels along the undersurface of the brachioradialis as it descends into the forearm before emerging between the brachioradialis and first extensor compartment 9 cm proximal to the radial styloid.[6] The PIN crosses the radial shaft 33 mm (in supination) to 52 mm (in pronation) distal to the capitellum.[7] It may be accessed in the proximal forearm most easily between the brachioradialis and extensor carpi radialis longus (ECRL) proximal to the supinator. The "L" in longus can help the surgeon remember that the fascia overlying the ECRL is lighter than the brachioradialis fascia in identifying this interval. Blunt dissection in this plane will reveal recurrent vessels from the radial artery that need to be ligated to access the underlying PIN. If the nerve is to be identified within or distal to the supinator as is commonly required during exposure of a proximal radius fracture, the Thompson approach between the extensor carpi radialis brevis (ECRB) and extensor digitorum communis (EDC) is utilized. After bluntly developing the interval between these two, the supinator fascia is encountered and split. The PIN travels perpendicular to the fibers of the supinator muscle between its superficial and deep heads directly towards the ulnar styloid. Once identified, the PIN can be protected while the supinator muscle is elevated from the proximal radius to allow for fracture fixation.

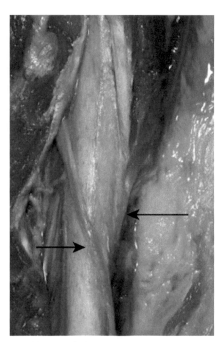

• **Fig. 32.1** The radial nerve (*left arrow*) passes the posterior midline of the humerus within 0.1 cm of the distal aspect of the deltoid tuberosity (*right arrow*).

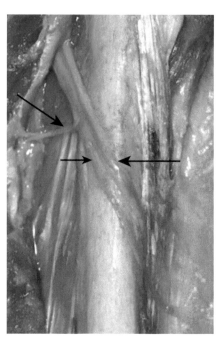

• **Fig. 32.2** Posterior approach to the humerus demonstrating the relationship of the radial nerve which contacts the humerus 10-17 cm proximal to the lateral epicondyle.

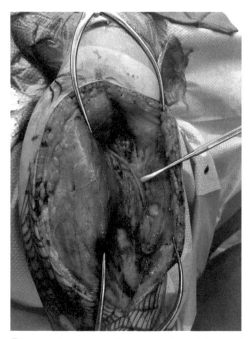

• **Fig. 32.3** The posterior antebrachial cutaneous nerve is typically encountered first when dissecting from distal to proximal and can be traced back to the radial nerve.

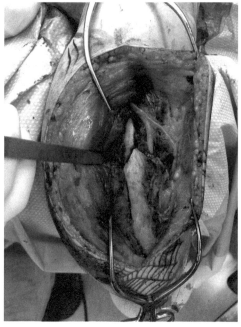

• **Fig. 32.4** The posterior antebrachial cutaneous nerve and its relationship to the radial nerve.

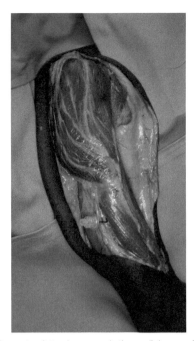

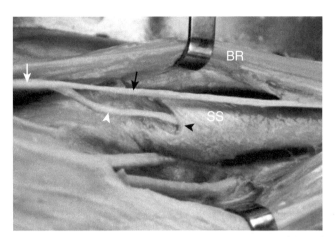

• **Fig. 32.6** The radial nerve (*large white arrow*) divides into superficial radial nerve (*large black arrow*) and the posterior interosseous nerve (PIN). The superficial radial nerve travels along the undersurface of the brachioradialis *(BR)* as it descends into the forearm before emerging between the BR and first extensor compartment 9 cm proximal to the radial styloid.[6] The PIN (*small white arrow*) crosses the radial shaft distal to the capitellum and travels through the superficial head of the supinator muscle (*SS; short black arrow*).

• **Fig. 32.5** In the anterolateral approach the radial nerve is identified distally in the interval between the brachialis and brachioradialis muscles. This clinical image demonstrates the radial nerve (pinned) deep to the superficial head of the brachialis.

References

1. Carlan D, Pratt J, Patterson JMM, Weiland AJ, Boyer MI, Gelberman RH. The radial nerve in the brachium: an anatomic study in human cadavers. *J Hand Surg Am.* 2007;32(8):1177–1182.
2. Gerwin M, Hotchkiss RN, Weiland AJ. Alternative operative exposures of the posterior aspect of the humeral diaphysis with reference to the radial nerve. *J Bone Joint Surg Am.* 1996;78(11):1690–1695.
3. Leonello DT, Galley IJ, Bain GI, Carter CD. Brachialis muscle anatomy. A study in cadavers. *J Bone Joint Surg Am.* 2007;89(6):1293–1297.
4. Omid R, Hamid N, Keener JD, Galatz LM, Yamaguchi K. Relation of the radial nerve to the anterior capsule of the elbow: anatomy with correlation to arthroscopy. *Arthroscopy.* 2012;28(12):1800–1804.
5. Thomas SJ, Yakin DE, Parry BR, Lubahn JD. The anatomical relationship between the posterior interosseous nerve and the supinator muscle. *J Hand Surg Am.* 2000;25(5):936–941.
6. Abrams RA, Brown RA, Botte MJ. The superficial branch of the radial nerve: an anatomic study with surgical implications. *J Hand Surg Am.* 1992;17(6):1037–1041.
7. Diliberti T, Botte MJ, Abrams RA. Anatomical considerations regarding the posterior interosseous nerve during posterolateral approaches to the proximal part of the radius. *J Bone Joint Surg Am.* 2000;82(6):809–813.

33

Technique Spotlight: Nonoperative Management of Humeral Shaft Fractures

KYLE M. ALTMAN, GREGORY K. FAUCHER, AND
M. CHRISTIAN MOODY

Indications

The majority of isolated humeral shaft fractures can be managed nonoperatively. It is widely accepted that acute, closed, isolated fractures in a cooperative, ambulatory patient will achieve union with nonoperative management without a significant angular deformity or any functional limitations. However, while indications for nonoperative management of humeral shaft fractures are a continual debate, it is widely accepted that the humerus can tolerate 15–20 degrees of angular deformity, 30 degrees of rotational malalignment, and 2–3 cm of shortening without compromising function.

Sarmiento et al. published the most notable study supporting nonoperative management of humeral shaft fractures in 2000. Humeral shaft fractures in 620 patients were treated nonoperatively with functional bracing including those with open fractures, segmental fractures, ipsilateral shoulder dislocation, and radial nerve palsies. They reported a union rate of 98% for closed fractures and 94% for open fractures. Eighty-seven percent healed in <16 degrees of varus angulation, and 98% of patients had a shoulder range-of-motion deficit of <25 degrees.[1]

Toivanen et al. reviewed 93 consecutive patients with closed, humeral shaft fractures managed nonoperatively with functional bracing and reported nonunion rates based on fracture location and AO (Arbeitsgemeinschaft für Osteosynthesefragen) classification. They noted a higher rate of nonunion in fractures of the proximal one-third (54%) and AO type A fractures (23%).[2]

More recently, Papasoulis et al. reviewed 18 case series and reported nonunion rates based on location, AO type, and fracture configuration. They also observed higher nonunion rates in fractures of the proximal one-third (8.2%), AO type A fractures (15.4%), and long, oblique fractures (17.5%) (Fig. 33.1), although these findings were not statistically significant. They also reported an overall union rate of 95% with an average time to union of 10–11 weeks. Varus malunion was the most common complication; however, the residual deformity was usually <20 degrees and did not affect cosmetic or functional outcome. They observed deficits in range of motion, most notably shoulder abduction, external rotation, and elbow extension; however, this rarely exceeded 10 degrees.[3] Similar findings have been demonstrated in several other studies.[4–6]

Despite historically high union rates and satisfactory functional outcomes reported with nonoperative treatment of humeral shaft fractures, more recent literature may contradict this paradigm. Serrano et al. recently published a multicenter retrospective review of 1182 patients initially treated with functional bracing for humeral shaft fractures and noted a 29% failure rate requiring surgical intervention.[7] They showed that females and alcoholics were more likely to be converted to surgery. Proximal shaft, comminuted, segmental, and butterfly fractures were also linked with higher rate of conversion.[7]

Likewise, two recently published prospective, randomized trials suggest higher union rates and better functional outcomes with surgical fixation compared with functional bracing. Khameneh et al. compared ORIF (open reduction internal fixation) with functional bracing and found a significantly faster time to union with operative treatment compared with functional bracing (13.9 vs. 18.7 weeks).[8] Similarly, Matsunaga recently published results of minimally invasive osteosynthesis with bridge plating compared with functional bracing and reported lower nonunion rates (0% vs. 15%) and less coronal plane angulation (2 vs. 10.5 degrees) (Table 33.1).[9]

Techniques

Coaptation/U-Slab Splinting

Coaptation splinting is widely used for immediate immobilization in the acute setting, oftentimes in the emergency room. This technique involves passing plaster from the medial side of the arm in the axilla distally around the elbow, ascending up the lateral side over the acromion with the elbow at 90 degrees of flexion. Plaster is then secured to the arm with an ace wrap and allowed to harden.

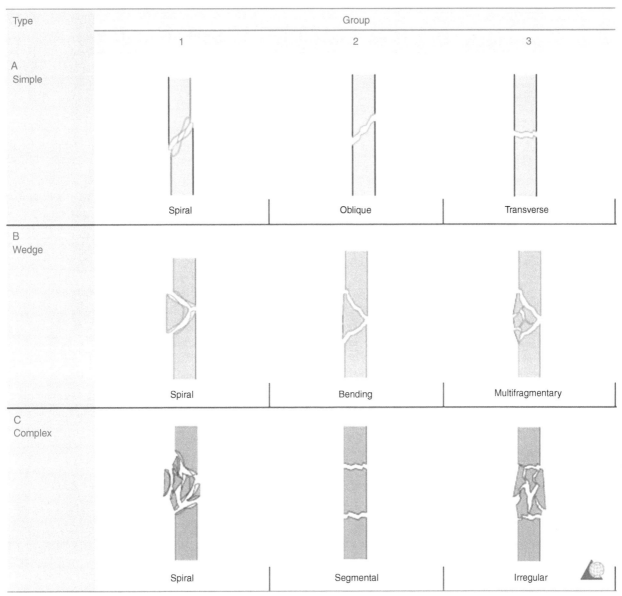

Type	Group		
	1	2	3
A Simple	Spiral	Oblique	Transverse
B Wedge	Spiral	Bending	Multifragmentary
C Complex	Spiral	Segmental	Irregular

• **Fig. 33.1** Humeral shaft fractures. [A, From Updegrove GF, Mourad W, Abboud JA. Humeral shaft fractures. *J Shoulder Elbow Surg.* 2018; 27(4):e87-e97. © 2017. B, Reproduced with permission from AO Surgery Reference, www.aosurgery.org. Copyright by AO Foundation, Switzerland. Arbeitsgemeinschaft für Osteosynthesefragen (AO)/Orthopaedic Trauma Association (OTA) classification of diaphyseal fractures.]

TABLE 33.1   Indications for Nonoperative Management of Humeral Shaft Fractures

Strong indications	Closed, isolated fracture in a compliant, ambulatory patient
Relative indications	AO/OTA type A fracture Proximal one-third or long oblique patterns Segmental fracture Open fracture without neurovascular injury
Relative contraindications	Patient with polytrauma Additional injuries to ipsilateral arm Persisting or increasing nerve dysfunction Periprosthetic fracture
Strong contraindications	Vascular injury Nonunion Pathologic fracture

AO, Arbeitsgemeinschaft für Osteosynthesefragen; *OTA*, Orthopaedic Trauma Association.

A cuff-and-collar is then placed around the wrist to support the weight of the injured extremity (Fig. 33.2).

POSITIONING AND EQUIPMENT

- The patient should be upright with their body towards the edge of the bed so that the injured extremity can be easily accessed
- 10–12 sheets of 4-inch plaster or 4-inch fiberglass
- 6-inch stockinette
- 4-inch ACE wrap × 3
- Cuff-and-collar

PEARLS AND PITFALLS

- Pad the injured extremity with at least two layers of splint padding with extra layers over boney prominences. The medial and lateral epicondyles and olecranon are particular areas that require supplemental padding.

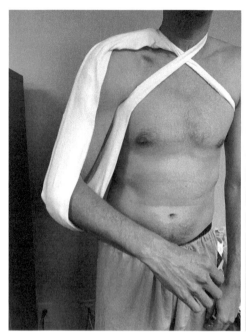
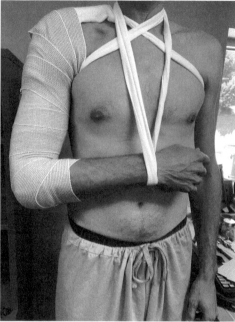

• **Fig. 33.2** Methods of nonoperative immobilization: coaptation splint.

- Pass 8–10 sheets of wet, 4-inch plaster or fiberglass inside a 6-inch stockinette leaving approximately 2 ft of free stockinette on either side of the plaster. Split the stockinette longitudinally from either end to the level of the plaster leaving two limbs on either side that can be tied around the body. After placing your splint, tie the axillary end over the contralateral shoulder and the lateral limb under the contralateral axilla to mitigate the risk of the splint propagating distally.
- Wrap the splint snugly with multiple 4-inch elastic bandages and conform the splint to the arm. This can be loosened to the patient's comfort after the splint has solidified.
- If not secured and contoured properly, the splint can migrate distally resulting in functional instability, especially with more proximal fractures.
- Insufficient padding in the axilla can cause irritation and pressure sores.
- If the lateral limb of splint does not extend proximally enough to immobilize the shoulder, the fracture may remain unstable.
- Patients with larger body habitus are at risk of varus angulation. To counteract this, a valgus mold to the coaptation splint may be necessary.

Hanging Arm Cast

The hanging arm cast was introduced by Caldwell in 1933 and was the standard of care for nonoperative management of humeral shaft fractures until Sarmiento introduced functional bracing in 1977. The technique involves stabilizing the fracture by wrapping the extremity in plaster from above the fracture site to the wrist with the elbow maintained at 90 degrees of flexion (Fig. 33.3). This technique is particularly successful in treating oblique, spiral, and shortened fractures; however, it does require more routine surveillance to monitor for fracture distraction.[10]

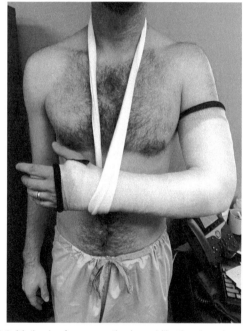

• **Fig. 33.3** Methods of nonoperative immobilization: hanging arm cast.

POSITIONING AND EQUIPMENT

- Sit the patient upright at the edge of the bed to allow for unimpeded access to the injured extremity
- 4-inch stockinette
- 4-inch cast padding
- 4-inch plaster
- Cuff-and-collar

PEARLS AND PITFALLS

- A lightweight cast should be used whenever possible.
- The cast should extend from 2 cm proximal to the fracture to the wrist with the elbow in 90 degrees of flexion and neutral rotation.
- The cast must be suspended by a strap that hangs around the patient's neck and holds the fracture in the appropriate alignment.
- The arm must be held in a dependent position at all times, including sleep.
- Over distraction at the fracture site can lead to nonunion.
- Prolonged immobilization of the elbow can lead to stiffness.

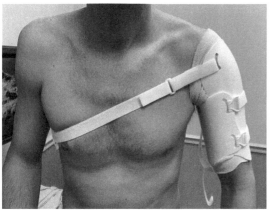 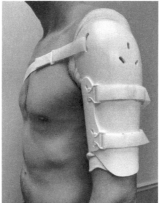 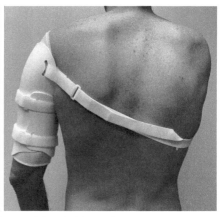

• **Fig. 33.4** Methods of nonoperative immobilization: functional Sarmiento brace pictured with proximal extension.

Functional Bracing

Initially described by Sarmiento in 1977, functional bracing has become the standard of care for definitive nonoperative management of humeral shaft fractures. Provisional immobilization is initially achieved with one of the above techniques until acute swelling has resolved, typically 10–14 days. At that time, a prefabricated polyethylene brace consisting of two sleeves is placed over the fractured humerus and secured with two Velcro straps. A cuff-and-collar is then placed with the elbow at 90 degrees of flexion to support the injured extremity (Fig. 33.4). Soft tissue compression and muscle contraction provide rotation and angular control through the "hydraulic effect," and gravity keeps the distal fragment out to length. Patients are instructed to remove the cuff-and-collar and initiate pendulum exercise with the elbow in full extension to prevent stiffness of the elbow and shoulder joints. They are also instructed to limit active abduction or flexion of the shoulder and avoid resting the elbow on a chair, table, or their lap to mitigate the risk of varus angulation during the initial healing phase. Radiographs are obtained at 1-week intervals in the brace initially for 3 weeks to ensure acceptable alignment of the fracture[11] (Fig. 33.5).

- Positioning and Equipment
  - Sarmiento brace with Velcro straps
  - 4-inch stockinette
  - Cuff-and-collar

PEARLS AND PITFALLS

- Tighten the Velcro straps daily as swelling subsides to achieve maximum control of the fracture.
- The patient should be instructed to perform daily pendulum and elbow range-of-motion exercises to prevent shoulder and elbow stiffness.
- Active elbow motion should be encouraged to exert dynamic pressure at the fracture site to maintain reduction and assist with stabilization.
- Do not use sling to support the weight of the extremity because this will prevent gravity from providing longitudinal traction of the fracture.
- Difficult to treat short and obese patients using this technique particularly with fractures that involve the proximal third of the humerus.
- At approximately 8 weeks, the patient can wean from the brace as comfort allows for household activities excluding overhead activities. At 12 weeks, the patient can completely discontinue the brace if doing well clinically and there is no gross motion at the fracture site. At this point, the patient may begin strength training and increasing activity level.

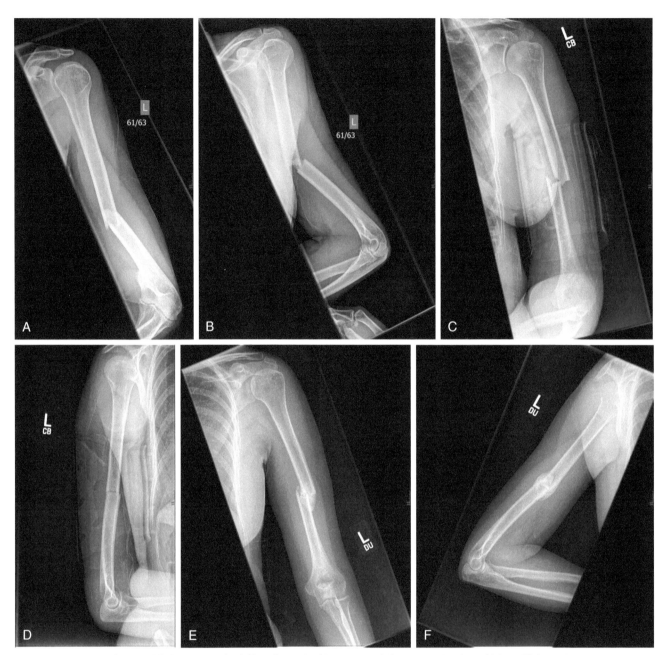

• **Fig. 33.5** (A) Anteroposterior (AP) radiograph of humeral shaft fracture at the time of injury. (B) Lateral radiograph of humeral shaft fracture at the time of injury. (C) AP radiograph of humeral shaft fracture 2 weeks after transition to functional brace. (D) Lateral radiograph of humeral shaft fracture 2 weeks after transition to functional brace. (E) AP radiograph of healed humeral shaft fracture after 4 months of treatment with functional brace demonstrating robust bridging callus indicating radiographic union. (F) Lateral radiograph of healed humeral shaft fracture after 4 months of treatment with functional brace demonstrating robust bridging callus indicating radiographic union. (Updegrove, GF, Mourad, W. Humeral shaft fractures. *Shoulder Elbow Surg.* 2018; 27(4):e87-e97.)

References

1. Sarmiento A, Zagorski JB, Zych GA, Latta LL, Capps CA. Functional bracing for the treatment of fractures of the humeral diaphysis. *JBJS*. 2000;82(4):478.

2. Toivanen JAK, Nieminen J, Laine HJ, Honkonen SE, Järvinen MJ. Functional treatment of closed humeral shaft fractures. *Intl Orthop*. 2005;29(1):10–13.

3. Papasoulis E, Drosos GI, Ververidis AN, Verettas DA. Functional bracing of humeral shaft fractures. A review of clinical studies. *Injury*. 2010;41(7):e21–e27.

4. Ekholm R, Tidermark J, Törnkvist H, Adami J, Ponzer S. Outcome after closed functional treatment of humeral shaft fractures. *J Orthop Trauma*. 2006;20(9):591–596.

5. Ali E, Griffiths D, Obi N, Tytherleigh-Strong G, Van Rensburg L. Nonoperative treatment of humeral shaft fractures revisited. *J Shoulder Elbow Surg*. 2015;24(2):210–214.

6. Decomas A, Kaye J. Risk factors associated with failure of treatment of humeral diaphyseal fractures after functional bracing. *J La State Med Soc: Official Organ of the Louisiana State Medical Society*. 2010;62(1):33–35.

7. Serrano R, Mir HR, Sagi HC, et al. Modern results of functional bracing of humeral shaft fractures: a multicenter retrospective analysis. *J Orthop Trauma*. 2020;34(4):206–209.

8. Khameneh SMH, Abbasian M, Abrishamkarzadeh H, et al. Humeral shaft fracture: a randomized controlled trial of nonoperative versus operative management (plate fixation). *Orthop Res Rev*. 2019;11:141.

9. Matsunaga FT, Tamaoki MJS, Matsumoto MH, Netto NA, Faloppa F, Belloti JC. Minimally invasive osteosynthesis with a bridge plate versus a functional brace for humeral shaft fractures: a randomized controlled trial. *JBJS*. 2017;99(7):583–592.

10. Caldwell JA. Treatment of fractures in the Cincinnati General Hospital. *Ann Surg*. 1933;97(2):161.

11. Sarmiento A, Kinman PB, Galvin EG, Schmitt RH, Phillips JG. Functional bracing of fractures of the shaft of the humerus. *J Bone Joint Surg Am*. 1977;59:596–601.

34

Technique Spotlight: Minimally Invasive Plate Osteosynthesis in Humeral Shaft Fractures

DANIEL E. HESS AND JULIAN McCLEES ALDRIDGE III

Indications

Surgical treatment of humeral shaft fractures is indicated after inadequate closed reduction, polytrauma, open fractures, bilateral injuries, and ipsilateral forearm fractures requiring surgical intervention.[1] Excessive body mass index (BMI) or habitus forces the humerus into an unacceptable varus posture in a patient who otherwise would be best treated initially in a functional brace (i.e., smoker, diabetes).

It should be noted that the majority of humeral shaft fractures will meet criteria for nonoperative, conservative management. These fractures tolerate a great deal of deformity and malunion before becoming functionally limiting. This includes ≤20 degrees of anterior angulation, ≤30 degrees of varus/valgus coronal alignment, and ≤3 cm of shortening.[2] Because the humerus possesses such anatomic forgiveness, establishing rigid stability with absolute anatomic reduction of the fracture site is not critical. Furthermore, an overly aggressive soft tissue dissection in an effort to perfectly align the fracture may be detrimental to the healing of the fracture.

When surgical intervention is indicated, traditional open reduction with internal fixation through an extensile approach has been the gold standard. However, this surgical approach is also associated with increased operative time, risk of triceps denervation, as well as increased risk of iatrogenic radial nerve injury. Minimally invasive plate osteosynthesis (MIPO) is a technique where plate fixation is achieved through minimized incisions, submuscular placement, and avoidance of fracture site exposure. This is an attractive option that minimizes soft tissue disruption while preserving humeral shaft union rates. Historically, intramedullary nailing (IMN) has been an attractive option due to its ease of application through a minimally invasive technique; however, the attendant rotator cuff morbidity and increased risk of neurovascular injury with distal interlocking screw placement have led to a decline in its use.

There have been numerous studies that have compared the various surgical fixation techniques for humeral shaft fractures. In direct comparison studies, MIPO compares favorably with ORIF (open reduction internal fixation) and IMN.[3–5] MIPO also carries a high union rate with decreased risk of iatrogenic radial nerve injury[5–7] compared with ORIF and IMN. MIPO plating, with less triceps dissection and soft tissue disruption, can allow for early elbow motion and weight-bearing which is especially beneficial in the polytrauma scenario. This technique has also been shown to decrease operative time and blood loss when compared with ORIF.[3,8–10] While ORIF aims for rigid fixation and primary bone healing, the goal of MIPO fixation is relative stability and secondary bone healing with a long plate "working length." It utilizes intact soft-tissue envelopes and indirect reduction techniques to achieve acceptable alignment, minimizing disruption of developing callus and periosteal vascularization. This technique is similar to the goals of an IMN technique but avoids the shoulder complications (rotator cuff injury, shoulder pain, etc.) seen in humeral nailing.[7]

There are specific indications and contraindications for MIPO. It is indicated for diaphyseal humeral shaft fractures (Fig. 34.1A–B) from the surgical neck of the humerus to 10–12 cm proximal to the distal articular surface.[11] There is no role for MIPO plating with intra-articular fractures where an anatomic reduction is necessary. Contraindications include pathologic fractures, active infection, soft-tissue injuries that preclude appropriate incisions, vascular injury requiring exploration and repair, and radial nerve dysfunction. The latter two conditions require extensive exposure, thereby limiting the benefits of the minimally invasive technique. Radial nerve palsy in a blunt, closed, or gunshot wound injury does not absolutely preclude the MIPO technique, although once the decision has been made to operate, most upper extremity surgeons favor identifying and establishing the degree of nerve injury to predict and guide postoperative expectations and management.

A relative contraindication remains surgeon comfort and level of experience with this technique.

Preoperative Evaluation

Mechanism of injury (blunt, sharp, penetrating trauma), concomitant injuries, status of the soft tissues, and a thorough

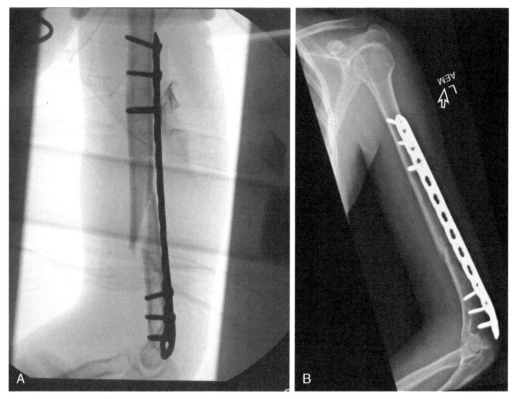

• **Fig. 34.1** (A) and (B) Anteroposterior and lateral radiographs of a patient who successfully underwent humeral plating using minimally invasive plate osteosynthesis technique for a distal one-third humeral shaft fracture.

neurovascular examination are of paramount importance in the initial survey. Often the degree of energy in an injury can predict the amount of periosteal disruption as well as distinguishing the degree of radial nerve injury (neurapraxia vs. neurontomesis).

One should obtain a thorough medical history including previous injuries to ipsilateral shoulder and/or elbow that may limit the range of motion after fixation. Previous injuries to neurovascular structures may influence the preoperative examination and should be noted. It is also important to determine the patient's ability to rehabilitate and readiness for surgical intervention.

The physical examination of this patient should include a detailed neurovascular examination, paying close attention to radial nerve function (motor and sensory). Assessing contralateral external rotation and internal rotation arcs of the shoulder is also imperative and will aid in your intraoperative decision-making.

Radiographic anteroposterior (AP) and lateral views of the humerus are obtained to include the shoulder and elbow joint. A particular fracture pattern to be aware of is the eponymic Holstein-Lewis fracture, which is a distal one-third spiral diaphyseal fracture. Distal and middle-third humeral shaft fractures have the highest rate of radial nerve palsy at 23.2% and 15.2%, respectively.[12,13] Transverse and spiral fractures have been found to have significantly higher rates of radial nerve palsy compared with oblique or comminuted fractures.[13] A transthoracic lateral can be helpful to characterize the sagittal deformity while limiting rotation through the fracture site. Traction views, while not routinely obtained, can be beneficial if there is significant comminution or shortening but we do not routinely obtain these views. Shortening at the fracture site and varus coronal alignment, especially in obese patients, are the most common deformities seen on radiographs.

Radiographic AP and lateral views of the contralateral uninjured humerus can provide a wealth of information relevant to the reconstruction, including the patient's preinjury length and rotation. Computed tomography (CT) and magnetic resonance imaging (MRI) are not typically utilized for an initial injury, but advanced imaging (CT) can be helpful in cases of rotational malunion or evaluation of delayed/nonunions. We do not routinely obtain contralateral imaging to gauge rotation and length, as this is best measured intraoperatively with anatomic landmarks and rotation of the proximal segment. Achieving the exact length in these cases is not typically necessary as the humerus can tolerate up to 2 cm of shortening without functional impact and some degree of shortening may actually encourage osteosynthesis.[14]

Positioning and Equipment

The authors recommend utilization of a plate with locking capabilities as described by Jiang et al.[15] For midshaft fractures, this is typically a straight 3.5-mm or narrow 4.5-mm locking compression plate (LCP). For more distal one-third or proximal one-third fractures, precontoured plates are available from several implant companies (Fig. 34.2).

We prefer lateral positioning and a posterior approach for midshaft to distal one-third diaphyseal fractures (Fig. 34.3). This allows for the easiest posterior exposure, identification, exploration, and protection of the radial nerve. The patient should be placed in the lateral decubitus position with the operative arm closest to the ceiling and all bony prominences well-padded. A beanbag-positioning device or hip positioners can be used to maintain the patient's lateral position. The operative arm is then draped over an L-shaped arm positioner. It should be noted that if the arm holder is placed at or proximal to the level of the fracture, a flexion deformity will be introduced and will need to be accounted for during the reduction. If the arm holder is distal to

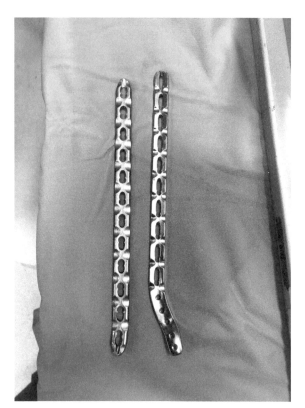

• **Fig. 34.2** Clinical photograph of the precontoured plates used for a case utilizing minimally invasive plate osteosynthesis technique for a distal one-third humeral shaft fracture.

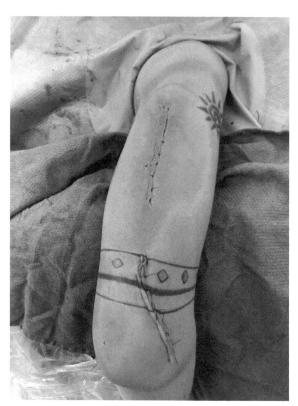

• **Fig. 34.3** Clinical photograph of the incision locations for a right distal one-third humeral shaft fracture. Note the patient is in lateral decubitus positioning with an arm holder beneath the upper arm. Proximal is to the top of the picture and distal is to the bottom.

the fracture, an extension deformity will result and will need to be corrected. Alternatively, the arm could be placed onto a sterile padded Mayo stand with a towel bump placed at the apex of the fracture. This places the elbow in extension, relaxes the triceps, and can improve a paratricipital exposure.

If the fracture location allows for it, we prefer to use a sterile tourniquet or a HemoClear tourniquet to limit draping out our exposure site. If the fracture is too proximal to provide sufficient exposure with a tourniquet, none is used. In these cases, where medically allowable, we inject 1% lidocaine with epinephrine in the anticipated surgical incision sites.

For proximal or midshaft fractures or in a patient with cervical spine injuries, where an anterior approach is planned, we prefer the beach chair position, with the head of the bed raised approximately 30 degrees from the horizontal and the operative arm resting on a sterile, padded Mayo stand. Supine positioning with the arm extended onto a radiolucent table with the elbow in mild flexion to relax the biceps has also been well described.

Technique[11,16]

It is important to remember that the goal of MIPO technique is for relative stability and secondary bone healing. In that sense, the LCP is being used as an "internal external-fixator," providing enough stability to encourage callus formation. The plate can be placed either anteriorly or posteriorly, depending on the location of the fracture in the diaphysis and/or soft tissue issues. Distal one-third fractures are typically approached posteriorly, while proximal one-third fractures are typically approached anteriorly.

For an anterior approach, two incisions are planned, each approximately 3–5 cm in length. The proximal incision is the distal extent of the deltoid-pectoral intermuscular plane. The goal in the proximal

incision is to expose the humeral diaphysis lateral to the long head of the biceps tendon. Distally, an incision is made lateral to the biceps muscle belly, ending approximately 1–2 cm from the antecubital crease. The biceps is retracted medially, and the underlying brachialis is split longitudinally in its midline, taking advantage of the dual innervation of this muscle (lateral-radial; medial-musculocutaneous), to expose the distal humeral diaphysis. The fracture is reduced provisionally through closed and indirect means. Elevators (Cobb are preferable due to their rounded nature) are used to tunnel from the proximal incision distally and from the distal incision proximally, maintaining contact with bone the entire way, creating a potential space for the plate to pass. This pathway is submuscular, but ideally extraperiosteal, to avoid damage to the blood supply. A trick to maintain this submuscular and extraperiosteal plane is to pass the Cobb elevator inverted with the rounded edge against the periosteum. As it is typically easier to control the shorter end of the fracture segment, we recommend initial fixation into the distal fragment for distal fractures and proximal fragment for more proximal fractures. For midshaft fractures, either direction of fixation will suffice. If we have a contour match between the plate and the bone surface, we will start by placing a single nonlocking bicortical screw to pull the plate down to the bone, followed by two to three locking bicortical screws in the same fragment. The plate is then used as a reduction tool as the opposite fragment is reduced to the plate with axial traction and appropriate rotation. The fragment is held in place with a large reduction clamp and fixed in a similar technique as described above. Ideally, at least six cortices both proximally and distally will be achieved.

For distal one-third fractures and some midshaft fractures, we prefer a posterior approach. We recommend making two incisions to facilitate plate placement and fixation (Fig. 34.4). However, we recommend increasing the size of the proximal incision to

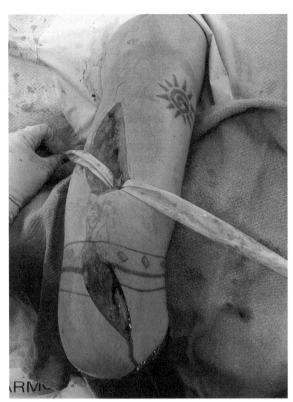

• **Fig. 34.4** Intraoperative photograph with the two incisions made for a right distal one-third humeral shaft fracture with the patient in lateral decubitus positioning. The 1-inch Penrose drain is around the radial nerve in the proximal incision.

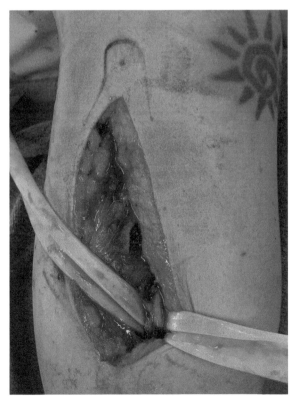

• **Fig. 34.5** Intraoperative photograph with a close-up of the proximal incision over the midshaft of the right humerus showing a 1-inch Penrose drain around the radial nerve in the spiral groove of the humerus.

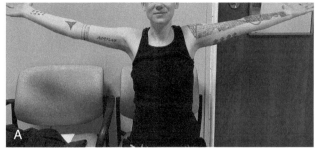

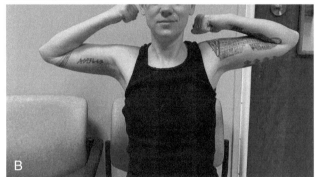

• **Fig. 34.6** (A) and (B) 6-month postoperative clinical photograph of a patient demonstrating elbow motion comparable to her contralateral extremity.

approximately 8–12 cm to identify the radial nerve in the spiral groove in addition to exposure for plate fixation in the proximal safe zone. The proximal incision is made over the posterior surface of the humerus. The triceps fascia is sharply incised, then the interval between the long and lateral heads of the triceps is bluntly dissected to expose the radial nerve in the spiral groove (Fig. 34.5). We prefer a Penrose drain around the nerve to better spread out the tension on the nerve and do not affix any clamp to the Penrose drain in order to prevent any unintended stretch. Distal exposure is made just proximal to the olecranon fossa in midshaft fractures or along the posterior-lateral column in more distal one-third fractures. If there is a concern for a radial nerve entrapment or a Holstein-Lewis type fracture pattern, this distal incision can also be utilized to visualize the radial nerve deep to the brachialis at this level.[17] Once a submuscular pathway has been created with elevators connecting the two incisions, the plate is passed in a distal to proximal direction. There is direct visualization of the plate passing deep to the radial nerve. Direct visualization of the nerve in the spiral groove is maintained throughout the remainder of the case. We typically recommend distal fixation first and then using the plate as a reduction tool proximally as described in the anterior approach technique.

Postoperatively, we provide the patient with a sling for comfort but encourage immediate passive and active-assisted range-of-motion exercises of the shoulder and elbow. The sling is discontinued after 2 weeks. Ideally, we limit weight-bearing to two pounds until bridging callus is seen radiographically. If the patient needs the arm to help with activities of daily living and balance assistance, we will allow weight-bearing with a platform walker as long as there is some cortical contact at the fracture site and locking screws both proximal and distal. Platform weight-bearing can encourage healing by loading directly axially without significant rotational or torsional stresses. Once bridging bone is seen on radiographs, activities can advance as tolerated, aiming for a full activity return by 3–6 months, depending on demand. Fig. 34.6 demonstrates a patient with near full elbow flexion and extension 6 months postoperatively

PEARLS AND PITFALLS

- Lay the plate over the skin to plan your incisions and to choose proper plate length (Fig. 34.7).

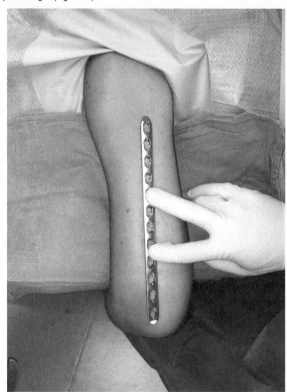

• **Fig. 34.7** Intraoperative photograph with our planned plate overlying the patient's left upper arm to best plan out our incision locations.

- Draw out cutaneous landmarks, including medial and lateral epicondyles, olecranon tip, and the expected course of the radial nerve as it decussates across the humerus through the spiral groove, entering and exiting at approximately 18 and 12 cm from the medial joint line, respectively, for posterior approaches[18] (Fig. 34.8).

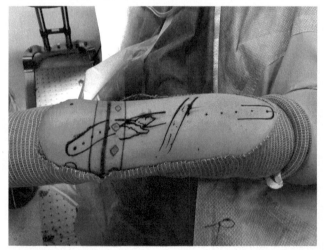

• **Fig. 34.8** Intraoperative photograph after our plate was traced out with surgical marker on the skin as well as important landmarks such as the radial nerve in the spiral groove, the medial and lateral humeral epicondyles, and the fracture location.

- Carefully avoid injury to the lateral antebrachial cutaneous nerve, which often appears in the distal incision for an anterior plating. It is easily located running lateral to the biceps between the biceps tendon and the brachialis, and often runs in parallel with the cephalic vein.
- Limit lateral retraction of the brachialis in the distal anterior approach to avoid neurapraxia to the radial nerve as it passes into the anterior compartment between the brachialis and brachioradialis.
- A locking guide engaged within the plate's screw hole(s) serves as a helpful handle for insertion and two locking guides provide better rotational control when directing the plate.
- Try to avoid passing the plate subperiosteally as this will disrupt blood supply and any initial callus formation.
- If the straight plate to bone-surface interface does not adequately match up, use a table-top plate bender to adjust the contour appropriately (Fig. 34.9).

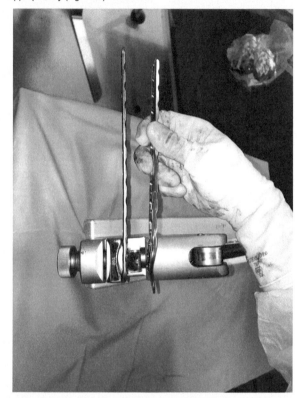

• **Fig. 34.9** Table-top plate benders are occasionally used intraoperatively to better match the patient's humeral anatomy.

- If there is concern about the bone quality or the plate malreducing the fracture, an all-locking screw construct is helpful and reasonable, as long as the working length (i.e., screw spread from fracture) is sufficient to allow for enough micromotion at the fracture site to encourage secondary bone healing.
- Maintain the forearm in supination to protect the radial nerve from the distal end of the anterior plate.[16]
- Avoid restriction in elbow flexion by making sure the distal end of the plate is superior to the coronoid fossa if the plate is placed anteriorly.[19]
- Aim for a long "working length" and avoid putting screws near the fracture site to encourage secondary bone healing (Fig. 34.10A–C). Typically, the fracture site is not directly visualized with this technique.

Continued

PEARLS AND PITFALLS—CONT'D

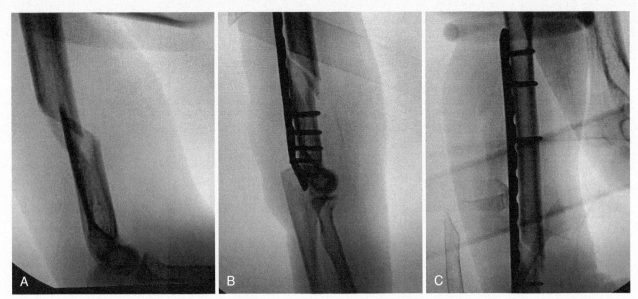

• **Fig. 34.10** (A)–(C) Fluoroscopic images of lateral view of a right distal one-third humeral shaft fracture. The long "working length" is highlighted with the final views.

- When bridging across comminution, it is not necessary to obtain the exact preinjury length of the humerus as up to 2 cm of shortening is well tolerated without functional impact.[14] Pull gentle axial traction to encourage ligamentotaxis and observe the tension on the soft tissues, especially the triceps and biceps. Provisionally fix with serrated reduction clamps over the plate on both the proximal and distal fragments and check fluoroscopy and clinical appearance before "buying" your length with screws.

- After provisional plate fixation, gently range the arm through an external and internal rotation arc to confirm the fracture is not rotationally misaligned and is comparable to the contralateral side. If the contralateral humerus is atraumatic, then comparative radiographs can give an estimate of proper length. However it is important to remember that cortical contact is more important than restoring exact length.

References

1. Carroll EA, Schweppe M, Langfitt M, Miller AN, Halvorson JJ. Management of humeral shaft fractures. *J Am Acad Orthop Surg.* 2012;20(7):423–433. https://doi.org/10.5435/JAAOS-20-07-423.

2. Sarmiento A, Zagorski JB, Zych GA, Latta LL, Capps CA. Functional bracing for the treatment of fractures of the humeral diaphysis. *J Bone Jt Surg - Ser A.* 2000;82(4):478–486. https://doi.org/10.2106/00004623-200004000-00003.

3. Oh C-W, Byun Y-S, Oh J-K, et al. Plating of humeral shaft fractures: comparison of standard conventional plating versus minimally invasive plating. *Orthop Traumatol Surg Res.* 2012;98(1):54–60. https://doi.org/10.1016/j.otsr.2011.09.016.

4. Davies G, Yeo G, Meta M, Miller D, Hohmann E, Tetsworth K. Case-match controlled comparison of minimally invasive plate osteosynthesis and intramedullary nailing for the stabilization of humeral shaft fractures. *J Orthop Trauma.* 2016;30(11):612–617. https://doi.org/10.1097/BOT.0000000000000643.

5. An Z, Zeng B, He X, Chen Q, Hu S. Plating osteosynthesis of mid-distal humeral shaft fractures: minimally invasive versus conventional open reduction technique. *Int Orthop.* 2010;34(1):131–135. https://doi.org/10.1007/s00264-009-0753-x.

6. Qiu H, Wei Z, Liu Y, et al. A Bayesian network meta-analysis of three different surgical procedures for the treatment of humeral shaft fractures. *Medicine (Baltim).* 2016;95(51). e5464. https://doi.org/10.1097/MD.0000000000005464.

7. An Z, He X, Jiang C, Zhang C. Treatment of middle third humeral shaft fractures: minimal invasive plate osteosynthesis versus expandable nailing. *Eur J Orthop Surg Traumatol.* 2012;22(3):193–199. https://doi.org/10.1007/s00590-011-0827-5.

8. Lin T, Xiao B, Ma X, Fu D, Yang S. Minimally invasive plate osteosynthesis with a locking compression plate is superior to open reduction and internal fixation in the management of the proximal humerus fractures. *BMC Musculoskelet Disord.* 2014;15:206. https://doi.org/10.1186/1471-2474-15-206.

9. Kim JW, Oh CW, Byun YS, Kim JJ, Park KC. A prospective randomized study of operative treatment for noncomminuted humeral shaft fractures: conventional open plating versus minimal invasive plate osteosynthesis. *J Orthop Trauma.* 2015;29(4):189–194. https://doi.org/10.1097/BOT.0000000000000232.

10. Hadhoud M, Darwish A, Mesriga MK. Minimally invasive plate osteosynthesis versus open reduction and plate fixation of humeral shaft fractures. *Menoufia Med J.* 2015;28(1):154. https://doi.org/10.4103/1110-2098.155974.

11. Tetsworth K, Hohmann E, Glatt V. Minimally invasive plate osteosynthesis of humeral shaft fractures: current state of the art. *J Am Acad Orthop Surg.* 2018;26(18):652–661. https://doi.org/10.5435/JAAOS-D-17-00238.

12. Holstein A, Lewis GM. Fractures of the humerus with radial-nerve paralysis. *J Bone Joint Surg Am.* 1963;45:1382–1388. https://doi.org/10.2106/00004623-196345070-00004.

13. Shao YC, Harwood P, Grotz MRW, Limb D, Giannoudis PV. Radial nerve palsy associated with fractures of the shaft of the humerus. A

systematic review. *J Bone Jt Surg - Ser B.* 2005;87(12):1647–1652. https://doi.org/10.1302/0301-620X.87B12.16132.

14. Hughes RE, Schneeberger AG, An KN, Morrey BF, O'Driscoll SW. Reduction of triceps muscle force after shortening of the distal humerus: a computational model. *J Shoulder Elbow Surg.* 1997;6(5):444–448. https://doi.org/10.1016/S1058-2746(97)70051-X.

15. Jiang R, Luo CF, Zeng BF, Mei GH. Minimally invasive plating for complex humeral shaft fractures. *Arch Orthop Trauma Surg.* 2007;127(7):531–535. https://doi.org/10.1007/s00402-007-0313-z.

16. Apivatthakakul T, Phornphutkul C, Laohapoonrungsee A, Sirirungruangsarn Y. Less invasive plate osteosynthesis in humeral shaft fractures. *Oper Orthop Traumatol.* 2009;21(6):602–613. https://doi.org/10.1007/s00064-009-2008-9.

17. Zogbi DR, Terrivel AM, Mouraria GG, Mongon MLD, Kikuta FK, Zoppi Filho A. Fracture of distal humerus: MIPO technique with visualization of the radial nerve. *Acta Ortop Bras.* 2014;22(6):300–303. https://doi.org/10.1590/1413-78522014220601003.

18. Zlotolow DA, Catalano LW, Barron OA, Glickel SZ. Surgical exposures of the humerus. *J Am Acad Orthop Surg.* 2006; 14(13):754–765. https://doi.org/10.5435/00124635-200612000-00007.

19. Kobayashi M, Watanabe Y, Matsushita T. Early full range of shoulder and elbow motion is possible after minimally invasive plate osteosynthesis for humeral shaft fractures. *J Orthop Trauma.* 2010;24(4):212–216. https://doi.org/10.1097/BOT.0b013e3181c2fe49.

35

Technique Spotlight: Intramedullary Fixation for Midshaft Humerus Fractures

BENJAMIN W. SEARS AND ARMODIOS M. HATZIDAKIS

Indications

Most humeral shaft fractures can be effectively managed without surgery utilizing functional bracing. However, displaced or comminuted humeral shaft fractures, fractures with extension into the proximal humerus, and patients following polytrauma with multiple extremity fractures may benefit from surgical fixation. Intramedullary fixation for midshaft humerus fractures can be a valuable option for the management of complex, comminuted, and segmental fractures. This method of fixation should also be considered in a compromised soft tissue envelope where large surgical exposure should be avoided (Fig. 35.1). These implants are typically placed antegrade by insertion through a small hole in the humeral head articular cartilage into the intramedullary canal and thereby can provide stabilization to most of the humeral shaft. Fractures that extend into the distal humeral metaphysis or articular surface are typically not amenable to intramedullary fixation as the intramedullary canal terminates 2–3 cm proximal to the olecranon fossa. Retrograde nailing can also be utilized to avoid iatrogenic injury to the humeral head articular surface but is typically limited to middle-third diaphyseal fractures and is relatively contraindicated in patients with small intramedullary canals or who are younger in age.[1] Additionally, primary fixation with plating remains the recommended treatment choice for simple transverse or short oblique humeral shaft fractures as the nonunion rate has been shown to be significantly higher in these fracture types treated with antegrade nailing compared with plate osteosynthesis.[2]

Preoperative Evaluation (Imaging, Examination, etc.)

Preoperative evaluation mandates a close neurovascular examination as the incidence of radial nerve neuropraxia following humeral shaft fracture has been reported at 11.8%[3] and up to 22% in patients with distal-third diaphysis spiral fractures.[4] Routine images should include anteroposterior (AP) and transthoracic lateral imaging of the humeral shaft with inclusion of the elbow articulation. Additionally, Grashey, Y-lateral, and axillary views of the shoulder can be helpful to evaluate for proximal fracture extension as well as for congruency of the glenohumeral articulation. Dedicated elbow radiographs are utilized for distal-third fractures to further characterize fracture extension and to ensure intramedullary nailing would provide sufficient fixation. Humeral rotation should also be assessed preoperatively. This can be achieved through an internal and external shoulder rotation examination of the noninjured side. Additionally, radiographic assessment can be performed comparing the contralateral bicipital groove contour at various degrees of humeral rotation.

Positioning and Equipment

A beach chair positioner is utilized with the head of bed raised 30–40 degrees allowing for improved imaging access and easier implant insertion. We prefer to secure the operative limb in an arm positioner held in neutral rotation with slight shoulder extension, which helps to limit variability while interpreting intraoperative fluoroscopic images. Alternatively, the patient can be positioned supine with a radiolucent arm board. Fluoroscopy is positioned on the contralateral side and preoperative radiographs are confirmed prior to draping. Reproducible imaging is critical for achieving anatomic fracture reduction as well as appropriate nail placement. Our preference is to use two specific intraoperative radiographs allowing for reproducible and readily interpretable images (Fig. 35.2). The first radiograph is a Grashey view taken with the C-arm tilted horizontally to match the semirecumbent orientation of the patient and orbiting the machine 30–45 degrees to obtain an exact perpendicular view of the glenoid face. With the arm in neutral rotation, this image will reproduce the standard AP view of the humeral head. The second radiograph is the Y-lateral view in which the C-arm is orbited the other way over the patient to approximately 30–45 degrees. This view allows for interpretation of the position of the tuberosities as the profile of the lesser tuberosity and the infraspinatus and teres minor tubercles of the greater tuberosity should be identifiable if reduced anatomically. From this view, correct position of the guide pin in the anterior to posterior direction is determined as well as optimal tuberosity screw position. All intraoperative images are obtained via rotation of the C-arm with the patient's arm secured in neutral

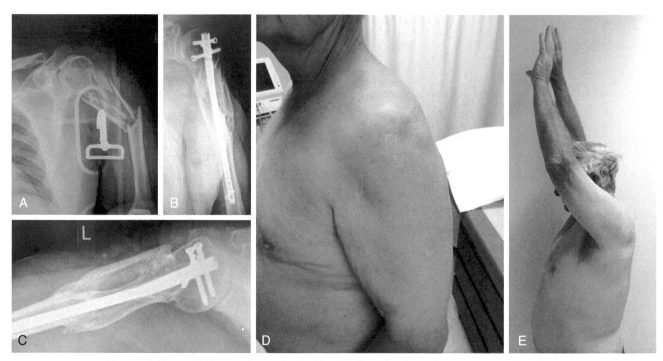

• **Fig. 35.1** A 62-year-old farmer who was involved in a significant farming accident presented with a Gustilo III open degloving injury and fracture to his humeral shaft. He was treated with urgent open irrigation and debridement and (A) intramedullary fixation and primary soft tissue repair. An intramedullary implant was utilized to bridge the highly comminuted fracture and to avoid placement of hardware into the zone of open injury. (B) and (C) Final anteroposterior and axillary radiographs taken at 3 years from injury demonstrate complete union with a (D and E) well-healed soft tissue envelope and excellent clinical function.

rotation (gunslinger position) during the entirety of the procedure, limiting positional intraoperative variables.

The most commonly used current generation intramedullary fixation options are straight implants delivered into the proximal humerus via an antegrade approach through a small reamed opening in the most superior portion of the humeral head. Although this violates the articular cartilage, it positions the entry point medial to the rotator cuff tendon attachment allowing for implant insertion through rotator cuff muscle rather than the cuff tendon or footprint. Older implants designed with a proximal bend to avoid the articular cartilage were found to have unacceptable rates of cuff pathology and postoperative shoulder pain.[5,6]

Alternatively, retrograde implants may be considered for middle-third and some proximal third diaphyseal fractures which avoid iatrogenic injury to the rotator cuff or humeral articular cartilage. The patient is positioned in the prone or lateral position and the implants are inserted through a supracondylar entry portal in the posterior distal humerus via a split through the triceps muscle. Insertion of the implant in a retrograde fashion has been associated with fracture at the insertion site and increased risk for fracture in patients with small intramedullary canals.[7]

Technique

For humeral shaft fractures that do not involve the proximal humerus, our preference is to begin with appropriate placement of the guide pin for the planned intramedullary implant prior to fracture reduction (Fig. 35.2). Often, the implant can be placed predictably via a percutaneous technique in which the starting position is identified utilizing fluoroscopic imaging and typically

correlates with just anterior to the acromion at the level of the acromioclavicular joint. Long intramedullary implants are designed as straight nails delivered in antegrade fashion with the desired entry point at the zenith of the humeral head on the Grashey view and centered in the AP direction on the Y-lateral view. The guide pin is delivered to the distal portion of the proximal fracture segment stopping just proximal to the fracture site. If necessary, the starting point can also be identified with an open approach utilizing an incision along the lateral acromion in the same fashion as the incision used for an open rotator cuff repair. A deltoid split is made in the raphe between the anterior and middle heads of the deltoid and the rotator cuff is opened medial to its insertion in line with muscle fibers at the level of the insertion point.

If the guide pin can traverse the fracture segments without the assistance of an open approach, it should be delivered to the distal end of the intramedullary canal and confirmed that it remained in the intramedullary canal with perpendicular fluoroscopic views. This can be facilitated with placement of traction on the limb, held with the arm positioner, along with associated percutaneous manipulation of the fracture segments with a towel wrap, mallet, or K-wire joystick. In our experience, most fractures require a small incision to reduce the fracture and maneuver the guide pin into the distal fracture segment. The appropriate level of the incision is confirmed via initial fluoroscopy, and a small to moderate incision is utilized to avoid extensive soft tissue and disruption of fracture biology. Fracture reduction is then performed utilizing joystick maneuvers, pointed reduction clamps, or cerclage sutures or wire. If placing cerclage hardware at the level of the middle or distal third humerus, great care should be employed in order to protect the radial nerve (Fig. 35.3). Under direct visualization, the guide pin is placed past the fracture site into the distal intramedullary canal. After adequate position of the guide pin is confirmed, a starting cortical hole is reamed at the starting point and appropriate nail length is confirmed. The intramedullary canal is then reamed with handheld flexible reamers to a size 0.5–1.0 mm greater than the planned nail diameter and the final implant is then advanced over the guidewire. Distally, the nail should extend past the fracture by a minimum of two cortical widths. Proximally, the nail should be countersunk to just under the humeral cortex, which typically correlates with the proximal interlocking screws directed at the teres minor and infraspinatus tubercles of the greater tuberosity.

If the fracture does not extend into the proximal humerus, typically two unicortical locking screws are utilized to secure the proximal segment. If there is fracture extension into the calcar region or the tuberosities, appropriate screws are used to reduce and secure the head segment and tuberosity fractures (Fig. 35.4). Distally, two bicortical screws are typically utilized as torque on the distal segment is higher with arm motion than seen in the proximal segment. This can be performed either via perfect circle technique or with an extramedullary guide that is available with some implant designs. Either way, care should be taken to protect the radial nerve and median nerve during placement of the distal screws. If using a perfect circle technique, a larger more formal incision is recommended to directly visualize the humeral cortex and protect the surrounding soft tissues. If an extramedullary guide is available, a soft tissue protector can be placed through the guide to protect the surrounding structures. Adjacent fixation including lag screws or cerclage fixation can be utilized to secure and compress the fracture; however, primary fixation is often not achievable and therefore placement of allograft into the fracture zone can be helpful to stimulate healing following surgery. Assessing rotation can be challenging in highly comminuted or displaced fractures. For these cases, our preference is to maintain

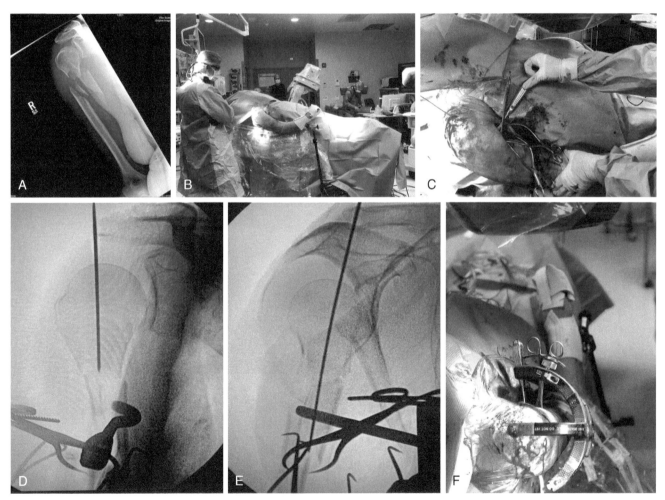

• **Fig. 35.2** A 78-year-old male with a history of diabetes and chronic obstructive pulmonary disease following a fall from standing with a displaced segmental humeral shaft fracture. He was treated with an intramedullary nail in order to limit requirement for open surgical dissection. The segmental fracture piece was reduced and secured with cerclage sutures. Allograft was placed at the fracture through the incision after nail placement. (A) Segmental humeral shaft fracture. (B) Patient positioning in beach chair position. (C) Reduction of fracture through a small incision after appropriate position of guide pin in proximal fracture segment. (D) Anteroposterior (AP) fluoro image of guide pin placed down to the level of fracture. (E) The fracture has been reduced through an open incision. (F) Lateral fluoro image of pin placement through reduced fracture position of jig and reduction clamps. At 6 months postoperatively, this patient demonstrates robust callus formation, (G) postoperative AP, (H) postoperative lateral image, (I) and (J) as well as excellent clinical function.

Continued

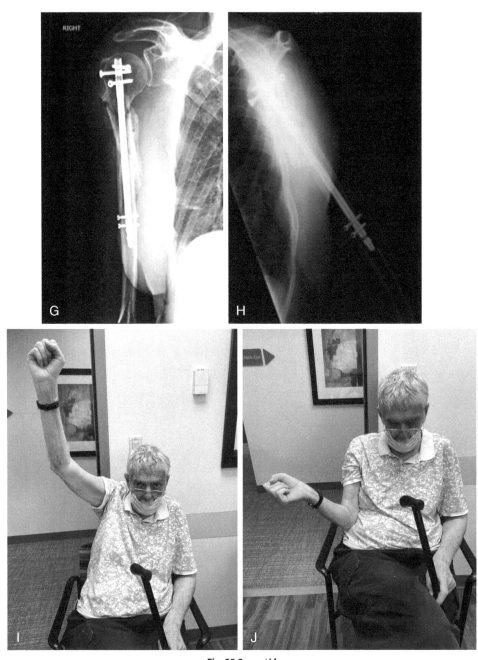

• Fig. 35.2, cont'd

the arm in an arm positioner in the gunslinger position which maintains the distal fracture segment in a neutral rotation. Proper rotation of the proximal segment is assessed via intraoperative Grashey fluoroscopic images in which the profile of the proximal humerus should be seen correlating to an appropriate retroversion of the humeral head in relationship to the glenoid (typically 30 degrees retroversion) with the distal humerus in neutral rotation.

Postoperative rehabilitation is dependent on the fracture type and fixation stability but typically includes sling protection with immediate passive forward elevation and external rotation. Sling immobilization is discontinued at 4–6 weeks postoperatively and active motion is initiated upon visualization of callus. Once healing is confirmed, usually at 3–4 months postoperatively, more aggressive stretching and strengthening are initiated.

PEARLS AND PITFALLS

- Careful preoperative neurovascular examination is key as concomitant radial nerve injury is common.
- Small open approach at the nail start point can be performed to mobilize and protect rotator cuff during nail placement. Alternatively, the nail can be placed via a percutaneous approach proximally.
- If open reduction is needed, soft tissue dissection should be minimized to preserve fracture blood supply.
- Shanz pins and K-wires may be placed percutaneously for fracture manipulation and reduction.
- If using a perfect circle technique for placement of distal interlock screws, an open incision should be utilized to find and protect crossing neurovascular structures.

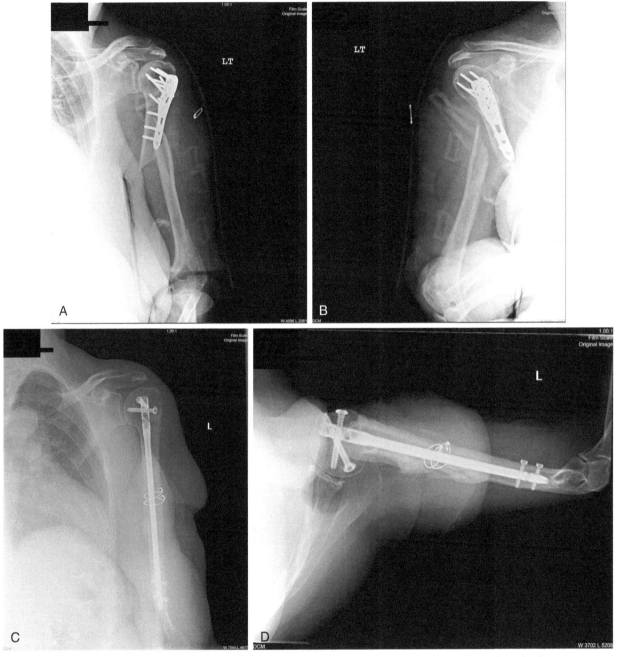

• **Fig. 35.3** A 67-year-old female with a midshaft humerus fracture below a previously placed proximal humeral locking plate. She was treated with removal of the plate, placement of a long intramedullary nailing, and a cerclage wire at the level of the fracture. (A) Anteroposterior (AP) humerus with shaft fracture below a previously placed locking plate. (B) Lateral view. (C) 7-month postoperative AP view, cerclage wire visible at the level of fracture. (D) 7-month postoperative axillary view.

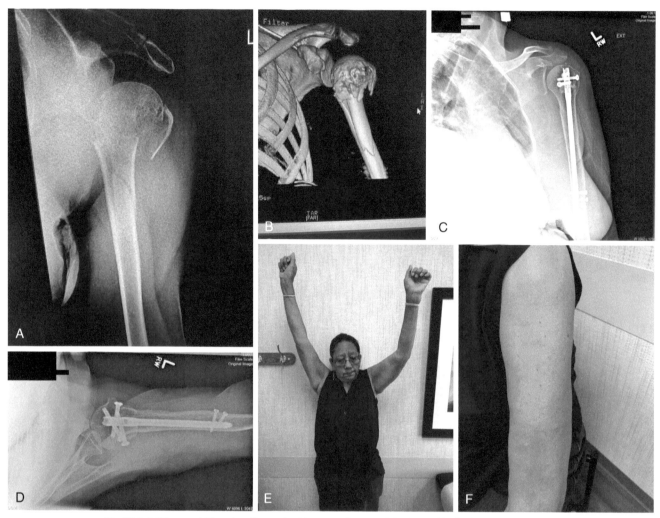

• **Fig. 35.4** A 68-year-old female with proximal humerus three-part fracture with diaphyseal extension into the humeral shaft. She was treated with a long intramedullary nail and greater tuberosity reduction and fixation utilizing a completely percutaneous technique. (A) Anteroposterior (AP) radiograph demonstrating a displaced three-part proximal humerus fracture with diaphyseal extension. (B) Computed tomography scan demonstrating diaphyseal extension. (C) 4-year postoperative AP. (D) 4-year postoperative axillary view. (E) Postoperative elevation. (F) Postoperative evaluation of the arm demonstrating limited surgical incisions.

References

1. Cheng HR, Lin J. Prospective randomized comparative study of antegrade and retrograde locked nailing for middle humeral shaft fracture. *J Trauma*. 2008;65:94–102.
2. Wen H, Zhu S, Li C, Chen Z, Yang H, Xu Y. Antegrade intramedullary nail versus plate fixation in the treatment of humeral shaft fractures: an update meta-analysis. *Medicine (Baltim)*. 2019;98(46). https://doi.org/10.1097/MD.0000000000017952. e17952.
3. Shao YC, Harwood P, Grotz MR, Limb D, Giannoudis PV. Radial nerve palsy associated with fractures of the shaft of the humerus: a systematic review. *J Bone Jt Surg Br*. 2005;87(12):1647–1652.
4. Schwab TR, Stillhard PF, Schibli S, Furrer M, Sommer C. Radial nerve palsy in humeral shaft fractures with internal fixation: analysis of management and outcome. *Eur J Trauma Emerg Surg*. 2018;44(2):235–243.
5. Lopiz Y, Garcia-Coiradas J, Garcia-Fernandez C, Marco F. Proximal humerus nailing: a randomized clinical trial between curvilinear and straight nails. *J Shoulder Elbow Surg*. 2014 Mar;23(3):369–376. https://doi.org/10.1016/j.jse.2013.08.023.
6. Nolan BM, Kippe MA, Wiater JM, Nowinski GP. Surgical treatment of displaced proximal humerus fractures with a short intramedullary nail. *J Shoulder Elbow Surg*. 2011;20(8):1241–1247. https://doi.org/10.1016/j.jse.2010.12.010.
7. Garnavos C. Diaphyseal humeral fractures and intramedullary nailing: can we improve outcomes? *Indian J Orthop*. 2011;45(3):208–215.

36

Adult Distal Humerus Fractures

RACHEL HONIG, JOAQUIN SANCHEZ-SOTELO, AND
JONATHAN BARLOW

Introduction

While rare, fractures of the distal humerus are complex and have always created unique challenges for orthopedic surgeons. Until the second half of the 20th century, most of these fractures could not be reliably fixed and therefore were treated nonoperatively. Complications including nonunion, malunion, neurovascular injury, and joint stiffness were common. Subsequently with nonoperative management, patients often could not return to employment and the psychosocial effects were substantial. With the development of principle-based internal fixation of distal humerus fractures and the advancements of total elbow arthroplasty (TEA) over the past several decades, there has been substantial improvement in the prognosis after injury. While these fractures remain a challenge for modern-day surgeons, most patients can now expect a functional elbow at the conclusion of treatment, allowing improved quality of life and contribution to society.

Relevant Anatomy

The elbow joint functions as a constrained hinge. The distal humerus consists of a widened portion of the metaphysis forming the medial and lateral supracondylar ridges and the corresponding articular surfaces of the humerus. Conceptually, the articular surface of the distal humerus can be divided into two separate components: ulnohumeral and radiocapitellar. The ulnohumeral joint is responsible for flexion and extension. The radiocapitellar joint supports the radius during forearm axial rotation. These joints are anatomically part of the same synovial complex, but may be viewed as functionally independent.

The ulnohumeral hinge joint can also be referred to as the ulnotrochlear joint. The trochlea forms the center of the hinge and it is supported by the medial and lateral columns. The word *trochlea* is Latin for pulley and the trochlea is truly shaped like a pulley. It has a 300-degree arc of thick cartilage that articulates with the semilunar notch of the ulna. This articulation is what provides the highly constrained relationship between humerus and olecranon, with substantial contributions to the bony stability of the elbow. Because of this, the integrity of the trochlea is an important part of the classification system discussed later in the chapter.

The radiocapitellar joint is the articulation between radial head and the capitellum, on the anterior aspect of the lateral column

of the humerus. This is a far less constrained joint, allows for axial rotation, and accommodates flexion and extension. The capitellum is covered with thick hyaline cartilage and is spheroidal in shape. There is a groove that separates the capitellum from the trochlea. This is where the radial head articulates with the humerus throughout pronation, supination, and flexion.[1,2]

Biomechanically, in the coronal plane, the trochlea and the medial and lateral columns represent a mechanical triangle.[3] The columns are triangular in cross section and the apices of the triangles point toward the central fossa. Because these columns support the articular surface, it is critical to restore both the medial and lateral columns when performing fracture fixation. While the medial column is entirely extra-articular, the capitellum forms part of the lateral column. The medial column ends as the medial epicondyle (Fig. 36.1A–B).

The ulnohumeral joint is also constrained by ligamentous supports. Medially, the medial ulnar collateral ligament (mUCL or MCL) originates on the distal aspect of the medial epicondyle and attaches to the ulna at the sublime tubercle (Fig. 36.2).[4] The medial epicondyle also functions as the origin of the flexor/pronator mass. The MCL is a major contributor to valgus and posteromedial rotary restraint. Thus, due to the ligamentous contribution of the MCL to elbow stability, anatomic reduction of the bone origin of this structure is important. The lateral column terminates as the lateral supracondylar ridge and epicondyle, which provide origins for the lateral collateral ligament and extensor mass (Fig. 36.3). These soft tissue structures also contribute to elbow stability.

The olecranon and coronoid fossa are located proximal to the trochlea between the medial and lateral columns. These fossae accommodate the proximal ulna during extension and flexion (Fig. 36.4). Impingement of the proximal ulna into these fossae, which can occur with inadequate fracture reduction, supracondylar shortening, or inadvertent insertion of screws through these fossae, will impede elbow range of motion (ROM) postoperatively.[3–6]

To safely manage distal humerus fractures, understanding the anatomy of the neurovascular structures in the elbow region and their precise locations is required. The radial nerve enters the spiral groove of the humerus 20 cm proximal to the medial condyle and then circles around the posterior humeral shaft. It exits the spiral groove approximately 10–15 cm proximal to the lateral epicondyle. The lateral antebrachial cutaneous nerve and the motor branches to the triceps and anconeus branch were off at

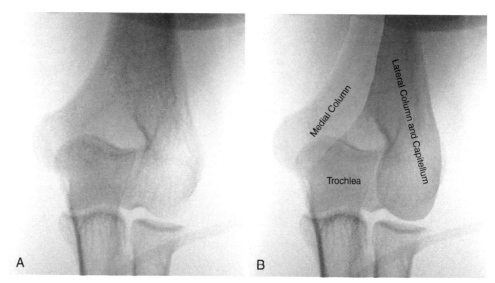

• **Fig. 36.1** (A) and (B) Normal anteroposterior radiographs of a left elbow. The lateral column extends distally and includes the capitellum. The medial column extends to the medial epicondyle and is connected to the trochlea by a thin corridor of bone.

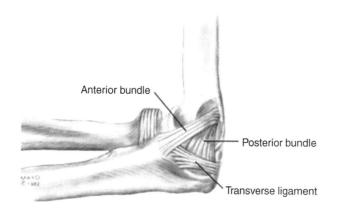
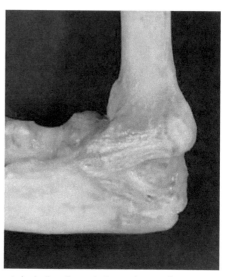

• **Fig. 36.2** The classic orientation of the medial collateral ligament, including the anterior and posterior bundles, and the transverse ligament. This last structure contributes relatively little to elbow stability. (Copyright © 2018 Mayo Foundation for Medical Education and Research, Published by Elsevier Inc., All rights reserved. Morrey BF, Sanchez-Sotelo J, Morrey ME. *Morrey's The Elbow and Its Disorders*. Philadelphia: Elsevier; 2018; Fig. 2.21.)

this location. The radial nerve then courses anteriorly through the lateral intramuscular septum. While the nerve courses between the brachialis and the brachioradialis, it bifurcates into the posterior interosseous nerve (PIN) and the radial sensory nerve. The radial nerve is at risk when there is proximal extension of fractures into the spiral groove, with excessive traction, and when using longer lateral plates during fixation (Fig. 36.5).

In the anteromedial aspect of the arm, the median nerve and brachial artery travel together between the biceps and brachialis muscles, with the median nerve lying medial (Fig. 36.6). They both course anterior to the medial intermuscular septum and then under the bicipital aponeurosis into the medial antecubital fossa. They then course between the heads of pronator teres and distally under flexor digitorum superficialis. Injury to these structures has been reported infrequently, likely due to the protection provided by the brachialis muscle.

The ulnar nerve travels anterior to the medial intermuscular septum in the upper arm until reaching the arcade of Struthers. It then pierces the intermuscular septum and enters the posterior compartment, where it travels with the medial head of the triceps. The ulnar nerve then courses behind the medial epicondyle and into the cubital tunnel, where it rests on the MCL. The ulnar nerve enters the anterior forearm between the two heads of flexor carpi ulnaris (Fig. 36.7). Injury to the ulnar nerve can occur either as a consequence of the injury or secondary to nerve manipulation at the time of surgery during initial injury or iatrogenically during open reduction internal fixation (ORIF) and occurs in 20% of patients postoperatively.[6]

Management of the ulnar nerve during distal humerus fixation remains a controversial topic. While identification and protection of the nerve are required for safe surgical management,

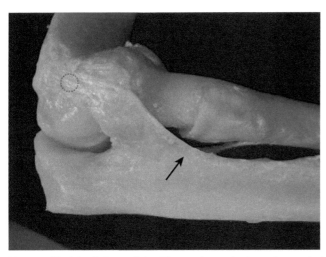

• **Fig. 36.3** The lateral ulnar collateral ligament complex has a humeral origin at the axis of rotation and inserts into the tubercle of the supinator crest *(arrow)*. Due to its site of origin on the flexion axis *(circle)*, it is taut both in extension and in flexion. (Copyright © 2018 Mayo Foundation for Medical Education and Research, Published by Elsevier Inc., All rights reserved. Morrey BF, Sanchez-Sotelo J, Morrey ME. *Morrey's The Elbow and Its Disorders*. Philadelphia: Elsevier; 2018; Fig. 2.25.)

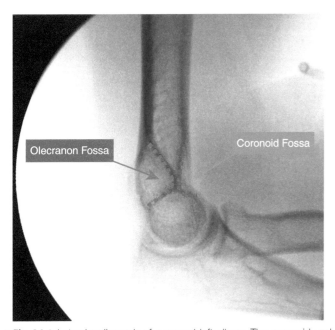

Olecranon Fossa

Coronoid Fossa

• **Fig. 36.4** Lateral radiograph of a normal left elbow. The coronoid and olecranon fossa are shown. These can be challenging to see after the placement of distal humerus hardware. Careful avoidance of hardware or bony fragments in these fossae is critical.

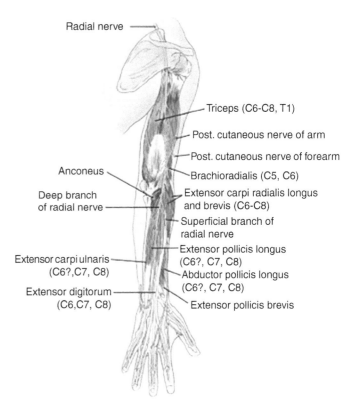

Radial nerve

Triceps (C6-C8, T1)

Post. cutaneous nerve of arm

Post. cutaneous nerve of forearm

Brachioradialis (C5, C6)

Anconeus

Deep branch of radial nerve

Extensor carpi radialis longus and brevis (C6-C8)

Superficial branch of radial nerve

Extensor pollicis longus (C6?, C7, C8)

Extensor carpi ulnaris (C6?,C7, C8)

Abductor pollicis longus (C6?, C7, C8)

Extensor digitorum (C6,C7, C8)

Extensor pollicis brevis

• **Fig. 36.5** The muscles innervated by the right radial nerve. *Post.*, Posterior. (Redrawn from Langman J, Woerdeman MW. *Atlas of Medical Anatomy*. Philadelphia: WB Saunders; 1976. Copyright © 2018 Mayo Foundation for Medical Education and Research, Published by Elsevier Inc., All rights reserved. Morrey BF, Sanchez-Sotelo J, Morrey ME. *Morrey's The Elbow and Its Disorders*. Philadelphia: Elsevier; 2018; Fig. 2.34.)

medial, lateral, and posterior arcades. These arcades receive blood supply from a variety of arteries around the elbow. Perforating vessels from these three arcades contribute to the interosseous blood supply. The rich local blood supply facilitates revascularization of large fracture fragments, and with the exception of capitellar shear fractures, osteonecrosis is relatively rare after internal fixation of distal humerus fractures.[2]

Pathoanatomy

The age distribution of distal humerus fractures follows a trimodal pattern. The age of the patient and the nature of the injury affect fracture patterns, comminution, and bone loss. Pediatric supracondylar fractures, which are very common, exceed the scope of this chapter. In the young/middle-age adult population, high-energy distal humerus fractures are most commonly the consequence of motor vehicle accidents or other high-energy trauma. The most common type of adult distal humerus fracture, however, occurs in elderly patients with underlying osteopenia or osteoporosis after a mechanical fall from standing. The increasing independence and longevity afforded by modern lifestyles and health care have increased the frequency of these fractures in the elbow surgeon's practice.

A careful assessment of the pathoanatomy of distal humerus fractures by the treating surgeon is critical. Anteroposterior (AP) and lateral X-ray of distal humerus fractures are routinely obtained as a basic imaging modality (Figs. 36.8 and 36.9).

there is controversy about the value of transposition. Transposition decompresses the nerve and allows it to run a new course safely away from internal fixation devices and fracture fragments. However, the extent of dissection necessary to transpose the ulnar nerve can devascularize the nerve and contribute to unintended iatrogenic injury. The data do not clearly support transposition or in situ nerve placement and thus remain based on the surgeon's preference.[7]

The blood supply of the distal humerus is another factor to consider. The distal humerus has an extensive anastomotic blood supply. The extraosseous blood supply can be categorized into

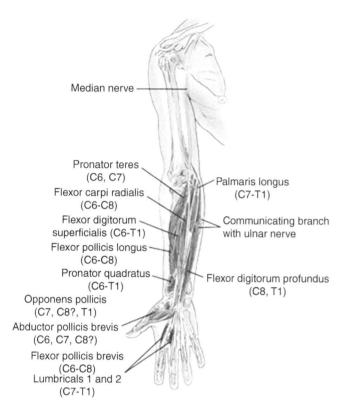

• **Fig. 36.6** The median nerve innervates the flexor pronator group of muscles about the elbow, but there are no branches above the joint. (Redrawn from Langman J, Woerdeman MW. *Atlas of Medical Anatomy*. Philadelphia: WB Saunders; 1976. Copyright © 2018 Mayo Foundation for Medical Education and Research, Published by Elsevier Inc., All rights reserved. Morrey BF, Sanchez-Sotelo J, Morrey ME. *Morrey's The Elbow and Its Disorders*. Philadelphia: Elsevier; 2018; Fig. 2.33.)

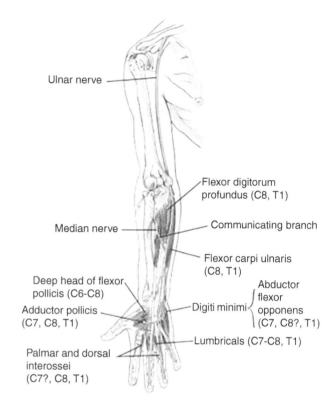

• **Fig. 36.7** Muscles innervated by the right ulnar nerve. There are no muscular branches of this nerve above the elbow joint. (Redrawn from Langman J, Woerdeman MW. *Atlas of Medical Anatomy*. Philadelphia: WB Saunders; 1976. Copyright © 2018 Mayo Foundation for Medical Education and Research, Published by Elsevier Inc., All rights reserved. Morrey BF, Sanchez-Sotelo J, Morrey ME. *Morrey's The Elbow and Its Disorders*. Philadelphia: Elsevier; 2018; Fig. 2.35.)

When patient features and fracture complexity suggest the use of elbow arthroplasty, plain radiographs may be sufficient. On the contrary, in the majority of fractures considered for internal fixation, plain radiographs are inadequate to assess the complex geometry of the distal humerus and its fractures. Furthermore, in our practice, we prefer three-dimensional computed tomography (3D CT) to traction views based on the ability to accurately interpret fracture fragments. For this reason, we almost always obtain a CT scan after application of a temporary splint. Obtaining the CT scan with the patient's arm over their head allows substantially improved visualization of fracture fragments and bony detail, especially in larger patients. This can typically be done without substantial increase in patient discomfort. 3D rendering can contribute greatly to the surgeon's understanding of the fracture pattern and is requested in essentially all of these injuries. Using the 3D CT scan, a more complete understanding of the extent and severity of the injury can be obtained (Figs. 36.10 and 36.11).[8]

A careful physical examination can help determine whether neurovascular structures are injured. The skin should be assessed for possible open fractures; abrasions should be cleaned and investigated to avoid missing an open fracture (Fig. 36.12). The radial pulse should be palpated and compared to the contralateral limb. A wrist and hand examination should be completed to assess for wrist pain and distal radioulnar joint (DRUJ) instability and pain. This is especially advisable in the setting of associated proximal

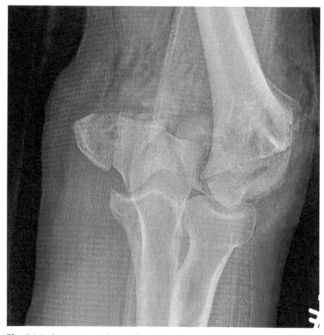

• **Fig. 36.8** Anteroposterior radiograph of a comminuted left intercondylar humerus fracture. Detailed assessment of fracture fragments is limited on radiographs.

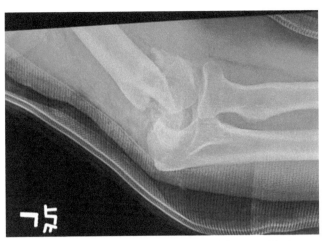

• **Fig. 36.9** Lateral radiograph of a comminuted left intercondylar humerus fracture. Detailed assessment of fracture fragments is limited on radiographs.

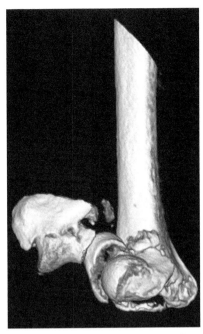

• **Fig. 36.10** Three-dimensional computed tomography reconstructions allow image manipulation to better understand the fracture fragments. View of the case from Figs. 36.3 and 36.4 shown. Lateral comminution and a fracture between the medial epicondyle and trochlea are apparent.

ulna and/or radius fractures. In the setting of high-energy distal humerus fractures, a thorough secondary and tertiary survey should be completed to assess for associated injuries.

Several main pathoanatomical factors differentiate the severity of the injury and can help guide decision-making and treatment. First, intra-articular involvement (and the degree of intra-articular involvement) is critical. Extra-articular fractures requiring surgery can typically be repaired through a "triceps-on" approach. These fractures seem to be associated with a lower rate of posttraumatic contracture and typically have a more predictable postoperative outcome. Intra-articular fractures, particularly those with intra-articular comminution and segmental intra-articular involvement, typically necessitate additional distal exposure, through some variation of a triceps-reflecting approach (most commonly olecranon osteotomy). It is our opinion that intra-articular fractures with a fracture line separating the medial epicondyle from the medial trochlea are especially challenging (Figs. 36.13 and 36.14).

A second critical factor is whether the fracture is open or closed. In most cases of open distal humerus fracture, the distal humerus is driven through the triceps posteriorly and out through the skin. This typically leaves a substantial defect in the triceps tendon and, in some cases, can be associated with bone loss (Fig. 36.15). In these cases, early parenteral antibiotics, aggressive debridement of the open fracture, and sometimes staged management are indicated. Antibiotic-eluting cement beads may be inserted at the fracture site, which may be temporarily stabilized with a splint or external fixator.

One additional factor that should be scrutinized in preoperative imaging is the degree of supracondylar comminution. In young patients, with good bone quality and minimal comminution, a direct extra-articular reduction can often facilitate anatomic reduction of the intra-articular portion of the fracture. However, in older patients, or in patients with profound supracondylar comminution, the narrow column structure of the distal humerus can preclude an accurate extra-articular read. In cases of substantial supracondylar comminution, a nonanatomic reduction is accepted, utilizing supracondylar shortening, in order to get bony apposition and compression.

Finally, although rare, some patients can have associated fractures to the proximal radius and ulna. These fractures will necessitate additional treatment plans to address them. In some cases,

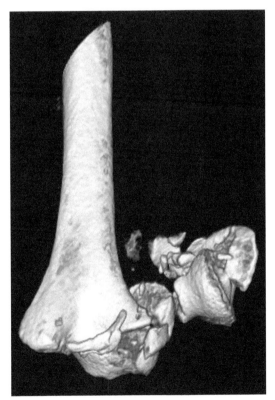

• **Fig. 36.11** Second three-dimensional computed tomography view of the case from Figs. 36.3 and 36.4.

an olecranon fracture can be utilized as the olecranon osteotomy. In other cases, radial head pathology or ligament injuries need to be addressed in addition to the distal humerus. All these structures should be carefully scrutinized on preoperative imaging.

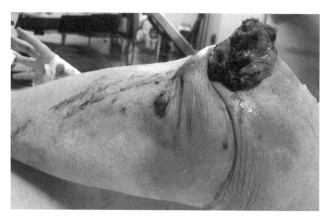

• **Fig. 36.12** Clinical image of the patient from Figs. 36.3 and 36.4 demonstrates a segmental open injury, with two open wounds. There is bone loss associated with this open fracture. This fracture was treated with initial debridement followed by staged repair. The incision incorporated these open wounds to avoid skin bridges and additional tissue trauma.

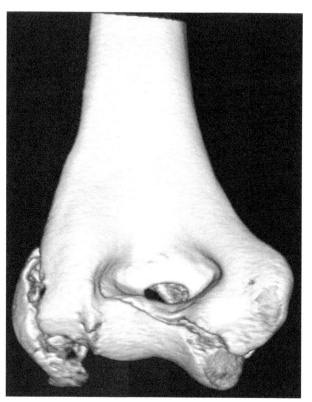

• **Fig. 36.14** Three-dimensional computed tomography reconstruction of a complex intercondylar distal humerus fracture, posterior view, demonstrating an impacted fracture between the medial epicondyle and trochlea.

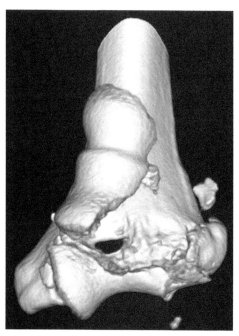

• **Fig. 36.13** Three-dimensional computed tomography reconstruction of a complex intercondylar distal humerus fracture. There is an articular fracture of the capitellum and lateral trochlea, as well as the lateral epicondyle.

Classification

Due to increasing acceptance of operative treatment, multiple classification systems have been created. A useful classification system should reliably describe the pattern of the injury, guide treatment, predict prognosis, and facilitate research. As is true for many other anatomic areas, a comprehensive and effective classification system remains elusive for distal humerus fractures. No classification scheme has had high rates of inter- and intraobserver agreement.

The AO/OTA (AO Foundation/Orthopaedic Trauma Association) classification system provides an effective framework for discussing and treating distal humerus fractures (Fig. 36.16). Similar to classification systems for other periarticular fractures, these fractures are first classified as extra-articular (Fig. 36.16A),

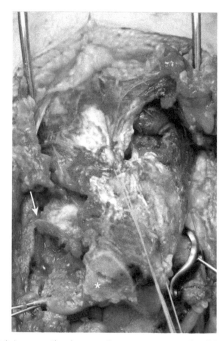

• **Fig. 36.15** Intraoperative image of a severe, open distal humerus fracture. The *star* marks the olecranon osteotomy. The lateral aspect of the distal humerus is marked with an *arrow*. There is profound bone loss. In addition, the triceps has been nearly transected by the bone, from the trauma. The tendon is marked with sutures and is being pulled distally. These tendon injuries are repaired in addition to the repairing the olecranon osteotomy.

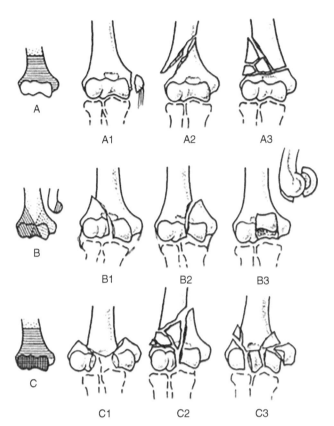

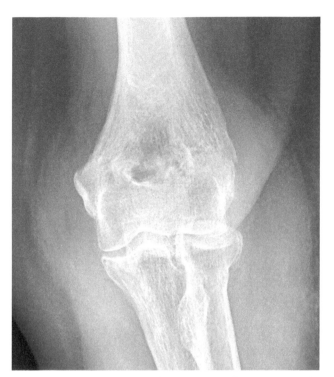

• **Fig. 36.17** Anteroposterior X-ray of a transcondylar fracture without distal extension.

• **Fig. 36.16** The AO/OTA (AO Foundation/Orthopaedic Trauma Association) classification system provides an effective framework for discussing and treating distal humerus fractures. (Wong A, Baratz M. Elbow Fractures. Distal Humerus. *J Hand Surg.* 2009;34(1):176–190.)

partial intra-articular-single column (Fig. 36.16B), or complex intra-articular-both columns (Fig. 36.16C). The increasing complexity and location of comminution are further used to subdivide each category of fracture. These subdivisions become increasingly complex and unwieldy. However, understanding the patterns and concepts outlined by the AO/OTA classification system can assist surgical decision-making and communication.[9]

Other commonly used classification schemes are the Milch and the Jupiter classification schemes. At our institution, we typically divide fractures as described in the most recent edition of *Morrey's The Elbow and Its Disorders.*[10] First, fractures are divided into extra-articular fractures and intra-articular fractures. Extra-articular fractures include (1) transcondylar fractures (transverse fractures through the condyles at or below the top of the olecranon fossa) (Figs. 36.17 and 36.18), (2) supracondylar fractures (Figs. 36.19 and 36.20), and (3) epicondyle fractures (avulsions of the lateral or medial epicondyle). Intra-articular fractures are divided into either (1) intercondylar fractures (fractures of the columns with intra-articular involvement) (Figs. 36.21–36.23) or (2) purely articular fractures, which are typically isolated articular shear fracture of the capitellum. Further fracture classification is provided descriptively.

Treatment Options

Broadly, treatment can be divided into three categories: nonoperative management, ORIF, and TEA. Nonoperative management is considered for nondisplaced fractures and, particularly, in the elderly and infirm population. In select patients, conservative

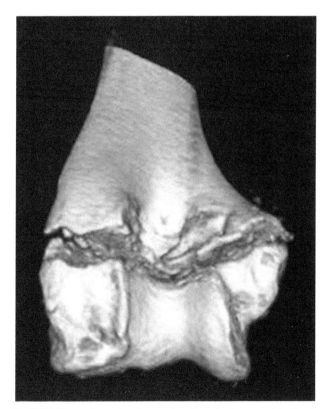

• **Fig. 36.18** Three-dimensional reconstruction of a transcondylar fracture without distal extension.

treatment may lead to an acceptable outcome, even in the absence of bony union.[11] ORIF is the treatment of choice for the vast majority of distal humerus fractures, particularly in the young and healthy. Modern fixation methods have made this

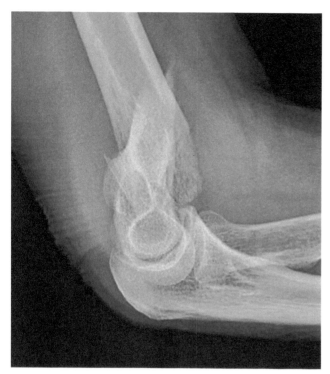

• **Fig. 36.19** Lateral X-ray of a supracondylar humerus fracture. The lateral fracture exits just proximally to the lateral epicondyle. The fracture does not extend into the joint. This fracture is amenable to a "triceps-on" approach, working on both sides of the triceps.

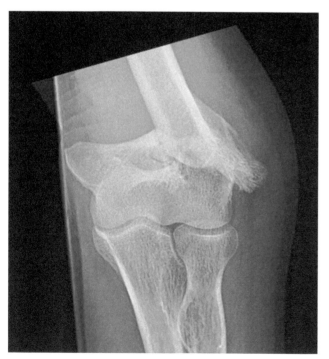

• **Fig. 36.20** Anteroposterior X-ray of supracondylar humerus fracture from Fig. 36.19.

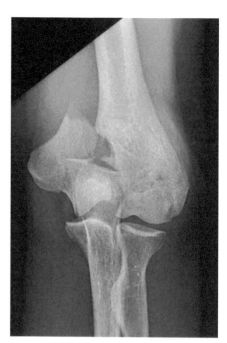

• **Fig. 36.21** Anteroposterior X-ray, of a comminuted, intercondylar humerus fracture.

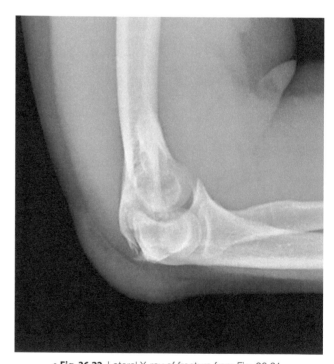

• **Fig. 36.22** Lateral X-ray of fracture from Fig. 36.21.

treatment regimen more reliable and have decreased the risk of catastrophic failure. In elderly patients presenting with a complex fracture pattern, elbow arthroplasty is a reasonable option for the primary treatment of comminuted intercondylar distal humerus fractures.

Indications for Surgical Treatment

Surgical management should be considered for the vast majority of distal humerus fractures. Exceptions include truly nondisplaced fractures, as well as fractures in the elderly and infirm. Truly nondisplaced fractures can be treated with a short period of casting (1–3 weeks) followed by early, protected ROM. Follow-up radiographs and early physical examination should be carefully scrutinized, to assess for motion at the fracture

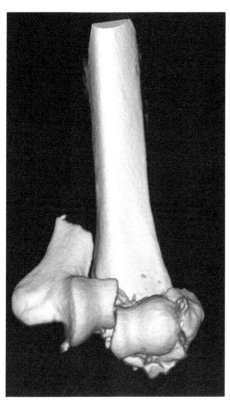

• **Fig. 36.23** Three-dimensional (3D) reconstruction image of fracture from Figs. 36.21–36.22, showing comminution of the lateral column.

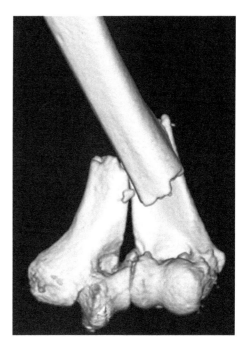

• **Fig. 36.24** Three-dimensional reconstruction of a displaced distal humerus fracture in an 89-year old patient. In addition to the supracondylar fracture and intercondylar split, there is a fracture line between the epicondyles and the trochlea with impaction.

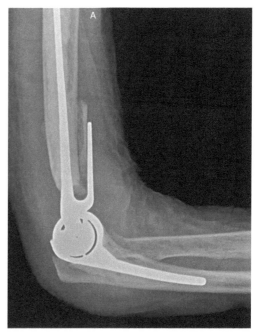

• **Fig. 36.25** Lateral radiograph of cemented total elbow arthroplasty in the patient from Fig. 36.18. A longer stem is used given the loss of the condyles distally.

site. This can be a harbinger of an impending nonunion. However, in certain low-demand patients, nonunions may be well tolerated.

ORIF is the treatment of choice for most displaced distal humerus fractures. Exceptions to this rule would be patients in whom TEA may be advantageous. A well-done randomized controlled trial demonstrated improved outcomes with TEA compared with ORIF in elderly patients.[6] These results were durable at long-term follow-up (average 12.5 years).[12] In our practice, we prefer TEA for closed, intercondylar fractures in high-functioning elderly patients (Figs. 36.24–36.26). We still consider ORIF for open fractures, and for obese elderly patients, particularly those who use their arms extensively for mobilization. Recent data seem to indicate that patients who had a previous ORIF do not have a substantial increase in complication rates when converted to TEA.[13] For this reason, when we have concerns about the durability of TEA, we favor ORIF.

Surgical Approaches

Distal humerus fracture fixation approaches need to vary based on the pathoanatomy of the fracture. Epicondyle fractures in isolation can be exposed through a direct medial or lateral approach. Purely articular fractures, particularly articular shear fractures of the capitellum, are typically addressed through a lateral approach, or increasingly with arthroscopic approaches. Intercondylar, transcondylar, and supracondylar fractures are most commonly exposed using a number of posterior approaches that are tailored to maximize access to the fractures, while minimizing complications.

The two main families of posterior approaches are the so-called "triceps-on" approaches and "triceps-off" approaches. Both approaches are performed through a posterior skin incision. The

ulnar nerve is identified and protected. For a "triceps-on" exposure, the triceps is elevated off the posterior humerus and access to the medial and lateral columns can be obtained. Distal visualization of the articular fragments is impeded by the intact triceps tendon and olecranon tip. For this reason, we typically use a "triceps-on" approach for supracondylar fractures without intercondylar involvement, and in certain transcondylar fractures in which distal fixation can be obtained without the need for triceps reflection.

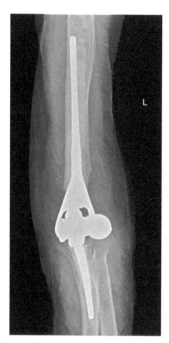

• **Fig. 36.26** Anteroposterior radiograph of cemented total elbow arthroplasty in the patient from Fig. 36.18.

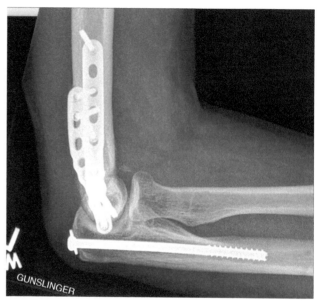

• **Fig. 36.27** A 6.5 mm cannulated screw with a washer provides strong, low-profile fixation, with a lower rate of hardware removal than pins and wires. This osteotomy has united in a good position.

The biggest advantage of this approach is that the extensor mechanism is left undisturbed and the risk of complications related to olecranon osteotomy nonunion, the need for hardware removal from the olecranon, and triceps weakness are reduced.

"Triceps-off" approaches can be completed by detaching the triceps from the olecranon, or through an olecranon osteotomy. The Bryan-Morrey triceps–reflecting approach involves reflecting the triceps subperiosteally off the olecranon and the anconeus off of the ulna. The tip of the olecranon can be partially removed to allow better access to the distal humeral articular surface and decrease extension deficits. However, only the posterior aspect of the distal humerus can be well visualized. Alternatively, a V-shaped triceps tenotomy may be used, which allows tendon-to-tendon repair of the triceps at the completion of the procedure. These two approaches have the advantage of avoiding olecranon hardware and avoiding violation of the ulnar canal, which may be advantageous in older patients at risk of needing elbow arthroplasty. However, the amount of joint visualized is less than with an olecranon osteotomy. We typically utilize this approach for low transcondylar (with or without simple intercondylar involvement) fractures in older patients, particularly those with preexisting arthritis.

The olecranon osteotomy exposure is the most popular exposure and is widely used for intercondylar distal humerus fractures. It allows extensive access to the distal humerus articular exposure to the joint surface. Details of the surgical technique are outlined in the accompanying technique article to this chapter. This approach is utilized in intercondylar fractures, particularly those with articular comminution. Various techniques have been described for fixation of the olecranon osteotomy. We have found fixation with a 6.5-mm cannulated screw and washer to be quick, safe, and have a low risk of complications (Fig. 36.27). Nonunion and subsequent failure of fixation of the osteotomy may occur, although it is rare. Overall, a posterior approach with an olecranon osteotomy remains the workhouse of distal humerus fracture internal fixation surgery.

Complications

Hardware Failure

As techniques for "principle-based" fixation of distal humerus fractures have evolved, and plate technology has improved, the rate of hardware failure has decreased substantially. Some early studies documented up to 25% failure rate of ORIF in the elderly.[14] A series of 34 patients, however, using a "principle-based" technique had no hardware failures and had more predictable outcomes than nonoperative management. This may be related to changes in plate technology, in addition to an evolution in principles of fracture reduction and plate application in this patient population.[15,16] Furthermore, there has been a linear correlation shown between bone mineral density and the holding power of screws. Thus hardware failure is more common in older osteoporotic women. Locking compression plates create a fixed-angle construct, which may be advantageous for these osteoporotic fractures.

Infection/Wound Complications

Wound complications and infection continue to occur after both ORIF and TEA for distal humerus fractures. This may be related to the trauma to the skin over the posterior aspect of the elbow and the need to raise subcutaneous flaps in order to obtain adequate exposure. One study from Mayo Clinic using modern internal fixation techniques reported a 16% rate of major wound healing complications. Almost half of these (7%) required plastic surgery assistance for closure. Other studies have documented similar rates of superficial and deep wound infections.[17] In our practice, we immobilize the elbow in extension for 1–2 weeks postoperatively to reduce the risk of postoperative wound healing issues. We also have a low threshold to apply negative pressure wound therapy applied to the surgical incision.

Neurovascular Injury

The ulnar nerve is the most commonly affected nerve in the surgical treatment of distal humerus fractures. Ulnar nerve dysfunction may be traumatic or iatrogenic. Symptoms can range from paresthesia to complete ulnar nerve palsy. Postoperative ulnar

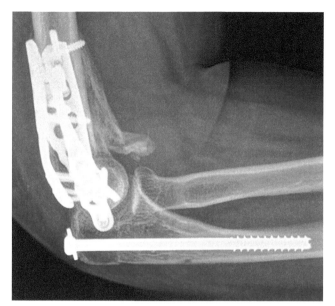

• **Fig. 36.28** Lateral radiographs of a 26-year-old woman with a distal humerus who underwent open reduction internal fixation (ORIF), with subsequent motion limiting heterotopic ossification. She had a closed head injury and delay to diagnosis, undergoing ORIF at 18 days post injury.

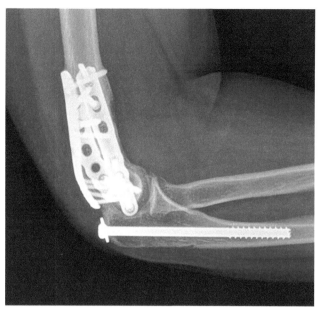

• **Fig. 36.29** Lateral radiographs 6 months after injury, heterotopic bone has been removed (patient in Fig. 36.22). Motion was restored to normal at the time of release and has improved postoperatively.

neuropathy has been reported in roughly 20% of patients, even with adequate release and transposition. Fortunately, the same series reported a very low incidence of permanent nerve dysfunction.[18] The need for multiple revision internal fixation surgeries is correlated with a higher level of permanent ulnar nerve dysfunction, another reason to emphasize meticulous surgical technique at the time of primary fixation.[19]

Heterotopic Ossification

The incidence of heterotopic ossification (HO) after ORIF for distal humerus fractures is around 40%. Delayed surgery, the use of bone graft, extended immobilization, and concomitant central nervous system injury are all factors that reportedly increase the risk of HO.[20] Both nonsteroidal anti-inflammatory drugs (NSAIDs) and radiation therapy have been used for HO prophylaxis. Radiation therapy was associated with an increased risk of olecranon osteotomy nonunion and is therefore no longer advocated by our group.[21] There is an ongoing debate about the use of NSAIDs as prophylaxis for the development of HO, but at this time the literature is equivocal. In our practice, we use 14 days of indomethacin for patients at increased risk of HO (delay to surgery, head injury, bone graft, and other risk factors). Depending on the location of HO formation, there can be variable functional consequences. Therefore the indication for surgical resection of ectopic bone needs to be considered on a case-by-case basis (Figs. 36.28 and 36.29).[2,22,23]

Posttraumatic Arthritis

Posttraumatic arthritis has been infrequently reported following distal humerus ORIF. In a series of 47 patients treated with ORIF for distal humerus by Flinkkilä et al., no patients went on to develop symptomatic arthritis and need elbow arthroplasty.[24] In a series of 32 patients at our institution, only two patients (6%) had substantial posttraumatic arthritis, and neither underwent further surgery by the time of publication.[15] While unclear from the literature, it may be that the low rates of delayed surgery for arthritis

are related to the unforgiving nature of the surgery (malreductions and malunions lead to early failure), and acceptance of functional limitations by patients after elbow trauma.

Prominent Hardware

While prominence of hardware applied to the distal humerus is relatively rare, issues with olecranon osteotomy hardware are common. A recent review of screw and washer fixation in comparison with plate and screw fixation or traditional "tension band" constructs (typically K-wires with a tension band wire) demonstrated that the screw and washer construct had lower hardware removal rates (15% with screw alone) than tension band wiring (40%) or plate fixation (30%).[25] While the risk of hardware prominence should be discussed with patients preoperatively, it is fairly uncommon that patients require an additional surgery to remove the hardware.[22] However, proceeding with hardware removal after union has occurred is a reasonable option for patients with symptomatic hardware.

Review of Treatment Outcomes

Outcomes of distal humerus fracture ORIF are dependent on the fracture type and the surgery performed. For extra-articular fractures, union and restoration of elbow motion are reliable. Nonoperative management has been shown to provide adequate outcomes for frail, elderly patients when operative management is not a viable option.[11] However, ORIF and TEA are usually indicated for these fractures and provide overall better outcomes. With more distal, transcondylar variants, the complication rate does increase, as does the difficulty in fixation. Sanchez-Sotelo et al. reported a series of transcondylar fractures, with reasonable outcomes (95-degree arc of motion) and relatively low complication rate (29% reoperation rate).[26]

Regarding intra-articular fractures, both ORIF and TEA have the potential to provide good results. A recent systematic review compared almost 300 elderly patients treated with ORIF or TEA for distal humerus fracture. Functional outcomes were similar for both groups (flexion: 100 degrees ORIF, 101 degrees TEA; extension: 20 degrees ORIF, 25 degrees TEA; Mayo Elbow Performance Score [MEPS]: 87.5 ORIF, 90 TEA). The complication rate was 38% for TEA (11% major complications) and 34% for ORIF (14% major complications). These differences were not statistically significant.[27] This may reflect selection bias, as randomized controlled trials have shown improved outcomes with TEA for more severe fractures.[6]

Whether selecting nonoperative management, ORIF, or TEA for comminuted distal humerus fractures, current outcomes are acceptable with a relatively low risk of complications and reoperations. Careful preoperative examination and imaging are critical to surgical planning and indications. Meticulous surgical technique, with special attention being paid to a "principle-based" approach to fixation, and avoidance of complications, is critical to optimize outcomes.

References

1. Tornetta P. *Rockwood and Green's Fractures in Adults*, 9th ed. Philaelphia: Lippincott Williams & Wilkins; 2020: Chapter 38.
2. Galano GJ, Ahmad CS, Levine WN. Current treatment strategies for bicolumnar distal humerus fractures. *Am Acad Orthopaedic Surgeon*. 2010;18(1):20–30.
3. Youssef B, Youssef S, Ansara S, et al. Fractures of the distal humerus. *Trauma*. 2008;10(2):125–132.
4. Labott JR, Aibinder WR, Dines JS, Camp CL. Understanding the medial ulnar collateral ligament of the elbow: review of native ligament anatomy and function. *World J Orthopedics*. 2018;9(6):78–84.
5. O'Driscoll SW. Current concepts in fractures of the distal humerus. In: Morrey BF, Sanchez-Sotelo J, eds. *The Elbow and its Disorders*. Philadelphia: Saunders Elsevier; 2009:337–348.
6. McKee MD, Veillette CJH, Hall JA, et al. A multicenter, prospective, randomized, controlled trial of open reduction—internal fixation versus total elbow arthroplasty for displaced intra-articular distal humeral fractures in elderly patients. *J Shoulder Elbow Surg*. 2009;18(1):3–12.
7. Shearin JW, Chapman TR, Miller A, et al. Ulnar nerve management with distal humerus fracture fixation. *Hand Clin*. 2018;34(1):97–103.
8. Doornberg J, Lindenhovius A, Kloen P, et al. Two and three-dimensional computed tomography for the classification and management of distal humeral fractures. *J Bone Joint Surg-Am*. 2006;88(8):1795–1801.
9. Hazra R-OD, Helmut L, Gunnar J, et al. Fracture-pattern-related therapy concepts in distal humeral fractures. *Obere Extremität*. 2018;13(1):23–32.
10. Morrey BF, Sanchez-Sotelo J, Morrey ME. *Morrey's the Elbow and its Disorders*. Philadelphia: Elsevier; 2018.
11. Batten TJ, Sin-Hidge C, Brinsden MD, Guyver PM. Non-operative management of distal humerus fractures in the elderly: a review of functional outcomes. *Euro J Orthopaedic Surg Traumatol*. 2017;28(1):23–27.
12. Dehghan N, Furey M, Schemitsch L, et al. Long-term outcomes of total elbow arthroplasty for distal humeral fracture: results from a prior randomized clinical trial. *J Shoulder Elbow Surg*. 2019;28(11):2198–2204.
13. Logli AL, Shannon SF, Boe CC, Morrey ME, O'Driscoll SW, Sanchez-Sotelo J. Total elbow arthroplasty for distal humerus fractures provided similar outcomes when performed as a primary procedure or after failed internal fixation. *J Orthopaedic Trauma*. 2020;34(2):95–101.
14. Frankle MA, Herscovici D, Dipasquale TG, Vasey MB, Sanders RW. A comparison of open reduction and internal fixation and primary total elbow arthroplasty in the treatment of intraarticular distal humerus fractures in women older than age 65. *J Orthopaedic Trauma*. 2003;17(7):473–480.
15. Sanchez-Sotelo J, Torchia M, O'Driscoll SW. Principle-based internal fixation of distal humerus fractures. *Tech Hand Upper Extremity Surg*. 2001;5(4):179–187.
16. Jupiter JB, Neff U, Holzach P, et al. Intercondylar fractures of the humerus. An operative approach. *J Bone Joint Surg*. 1985;67(2):226–239.
17. Sharma S, John R, Dhillon MS, Kishore K. Surgical approaches for open reduction and internal fixation of intra-articular distal humerus fractures in adults: a systematic review and meta-analysis. *Injury*. 2018;49(8):1381–1391.
18. Shin SJ, Sohn HS, Do NH. A clinical comparison of two different double plating methods for intraarticular distal humerus fractures. *J Shoulder Elbow Surg*. 2010;19:2–9.
19. Svernlov B, Nestorson J, Adolfsson L. Subjective ulnar nerve dysfunction commonly following open reduction, internal fixation (ORIF) of distal humeral fractures and in situ decompression of the ulnar nerve. *Strategies Trauma Limb Reconstr*. 2017;12:19–25.
20. Foruria AM, Lawrence TM, Augustin S, Morrey BF, Sanchez-Sotelo J. Heterotopic ossification after surgery for distal humeral fractures. *Bone Joint Lett J*. 2014;96-B(12):1681–1687.
21. Hamid N, Ashraf N, Bosse MJ, et al. Radiation therapy for heterotopic ossification prophylaxis acutely after elbow trauma. *J Bone Joint Surg-Am*. 2010;92(11):2032–2038.
22. Gofton WT, Macdermid JC, Gofton WT, et al. Functional outcome of AO type C distal humeral fractures, *J Hand Surg*. 2003;28(2):294–308.
23. Savvidou O, Zampeil F, Koutsouradis P, et al. Complications of open reduction and internal fixation of distal humerus fractures. *EFORT Open Rev*. 2018;3(10):558–567.
24. Flinkkilä T, Toimela J, Sirniö K, Leppilahti J. Results of parallel plate fixation of comminuted intra-articular distal humeral fractures. *J Shoulder Elbow Surg*. 2014;23(5):701–707.
25. Woods BI, Rosario BL, Siska PA, Gruen GS, Tarkin IS, Evans AR. Determining the efficacy of screw and washer fixation as a method for securing olecranon osteotomies used in the surgical management of intraarticular distal humerus fractures. *J Orthopaedic Trauma*. 2015;29(1):44–49.
26. Simone JP, Streubel PN, Sanchez-Sotelo J, Morrey BF. Low transcondylar fractures of the distal humerus: results of open reduction and internal fixation. *J Shoulder Elbow Surg*. 2014;23(4):573–578.
27. Chen H, Li D, Zhang J, Xiong X. Comparison of treatments in patients with distal humerus intercondylar fracture: a systematic review and meta-analysis. *Ann Med*. 2017;49(7):613–625.

37

Technique Spotlight: Principle-Based Internal Fixation of Distal Humerus Fractures

JONATHAN BARLOW, RACHEL HONIG, AND JOAQUIN SANCHEZ-SOTELO

Indications

Open reduction and internal fixation (ORIF) is recommended for the majority of medically stable patients with displaced distal humerus fractures. In selected cases, nonsurgical management or total elbow arthroplasty (TEA) may be preferred.

Preoperative Evaluation

Initial presentation of a distal humerus fracture typically includes pain, swelling, and deformity. These fractures can be the result of a low-energy injury in osteoporotic patients or a high-energy injury in younger patients. A comprehensive neurovascular examination should be completed. When these fractures are open, traumatic wounds tend to open posteriorly and can commonly partially rupture the triceps tendon in the process. In these cases, the location of the soft-tissue wound can affect the positioning of the skin incision. Anteroposterior (AP) and lateral radiographs should be obtained (Figs. 37.1 and 37.2). In addition, computed tomography (CT) scans are extremely useful for preoperative planning. Three-dimensional reconstructions allow for subtraction of the radius and ulna, which can further demonstrate the location and degree of comminution, articular involvement, and column involvement (Fig. 37.3). Preoperatively, patients must be counseled about the risks of nonunion/malunion, wound issues, nerve injury, hardware prominence, stiffness, and posttraumatic arthritis, as well as the potential for multiple surgeries if complications do occur.

Positioning and Equipment

The patient may be positioned supine, lateral, or prone. Author preferences are for the supine position or the lateral decubitus position with the arm at 90 degrees in a radiolucent padded armrest. Supine positioning is easier for the operating room (OR) staff and allows easy conversion to TEA if necessary. The

lateral positioning is more cumbersome and could be difficult in a trauma patient with spine precautions. However, the imaging is straightforward and the padded armrest allows a more stable base for the proximal humerus to rest. A trial of fluoroscopic imaging prior to prepping and draping can ensure appropriate positioning and accurate imaging. Vessel loops or Penrose drain should be available for gentle manipulation and protection of the ulnar nerve after mobilization. There are a number of commercially available plates specifically designed for distal humerus fracture fixation. Our preference is to use precontoured

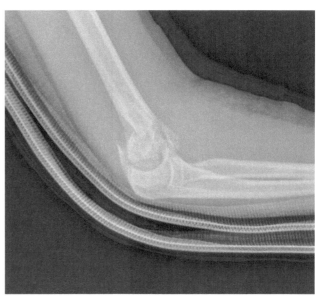

• **Fig. 37.1** Lateral radiograph of a displaced intercondylar distal humerus fracture. While helpful in the initial evaluation of a distal humerus fracture, radiographs do not allow detailed understanding of intra-articular fracture lines.

distal humerus locking plates with an option for medial extension onto the trochlea. If an olecranon osteotomy is performed, utilization of a 6.5-mm cannulated screw with washer provides a low-profile yet strong repair (Table 37.1).

Technique Description

Begin with a single midline posterior approach to expose both columns of the distal humerus. When treating an open fracture, the incision is commonly modified to incorporate the traumatic

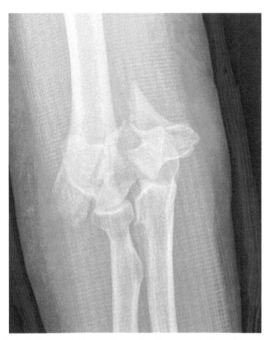

• **Fig. 37.2** Anteroposterior radiograph of same displaced intercondylar distal humerus fracture in Fig.37.1.

wound. Then, carry dissection down to the triceps tendon. Visualize the ulnar nerve and dissect proximally and distally. A subcutaneous flap superficial to the flexor-pronator mass can be developed to transpose the ulnar nerve to allow safe surgical access to the entire distal humerus. Using the floor of the ulnar nerve as a landmark, identify the posterior aspect of the distal humerus. Slide a Cobb or Young elevator across the posterior aspect of the humerus to identify where to split along the lateral aspect of the triceps. Dissect down to the "bare area" between the olecranon articular facet and the coronoid articular facet for the olecranon osteotomy. This should be visualized from both the medial and lateral sides to ensure appropriate placement. Place a guidewire for a 6.5-mm cannulated screw through the tip of the olecranon (Figs. 37.4 and 37.5). After tapping, place the final screw until it is nearly down. This will confirm appropriate fit and length. If unable to achieve appropriate screw purchase, one can consider increasing size of screw and trial with a corresponding larger tap. Then, using an oscillating saw, make a chevron osteotomy exiting into the bare area and complete the cut with an osteotome. We make the chevron nearly "flat" to avoid having the cut exit into the coronoid. The olecranon fragment can then be reflected to provide excellent visualization.

Internal fixation of distal humerus fractures should follow five basic steps (Table 37.2). The process typically proceeds in a distal to proximal direction. Attention should first be directed to the intra-articular fragments. Save small unsalvageable fragments for bone grafting. Fix the articular fragments together with small K-wires until a complete articular fracture can be converted to a partial articular fracture by reduction to a column. If some of these wires will be used for definitive fixation of small fragment, they should be threaded. As a rule, all of these wires should be placed close to the subchondral bone (distal) so that they will not interfere with later screw placement in the main articular fragments. If possible, reconstruct the articular surface so that a portion of the joint surface is reapproximated to its associated column. It is best

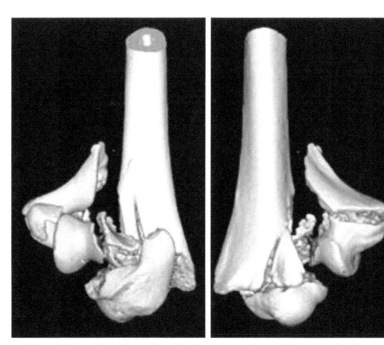

• **Fig. 37.3** Selected images from three-dimensional reconstructions of the same distal humerus fracture. Through image manipulation, one can gain a better understanding of the fracture lines and mechanisms for reduction and fixation.

TABLE 37.1	Five Steps of Internal Fixation of Distal Humerus Fractures

1. Articular reduction
2. Provisional fixation and plate application
3. Distal fixation
4. Supracondylar compression
5. Final fixation

TABLE 37.2	O'Driscoll's Technical Objective Checklist for Principle-Based Fixation of Distal Humerus Fractures

- Every screw in the distal segment to pass through plate.

- Engage a fragment on the opposite side that is also fixed to a plate.

- As many screws as possible should be placed in the distal fragments.

- Each screw should be as long as possible.

- Each screw should engage as many articular fragments as possible.

- To link the columns together, screws in the distal fragments should be locked together by interdigitation to create a fixed-angle construct.

- Plates should be applied such that compression is achieved at the supracondylar level for both columns.

- Plates must be strong and stiff enough to resist breaking or bending before union occurs at the supracondylar level.

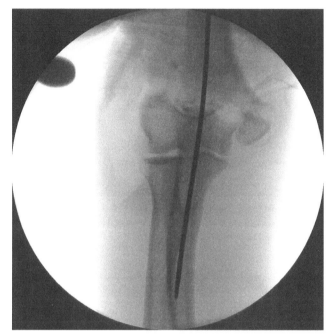

• **Fig. 37.4** Prior to creating the olecranon osteotomy, a guide pin for a 6.5-mm cannulated screw can be placed. Given the shape and curve of the proximal ulna, the pin will engage first on the anteroposterior view. In this view, we can see the tip of the pin just engaging the far cortex of the ulna. This would be a good length to ensure stable fixation of the screw.

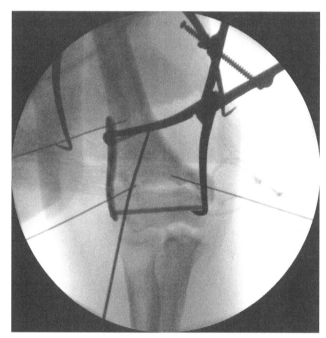

• **Fig. 37.6** The intra-articular fracture and lateral column have been reduced and fixed with a plate, based on cortical reads. This allows an anatomic reduction of the distal humerus. Now, compression is being applied across the medial column, in anticipation of plate application.

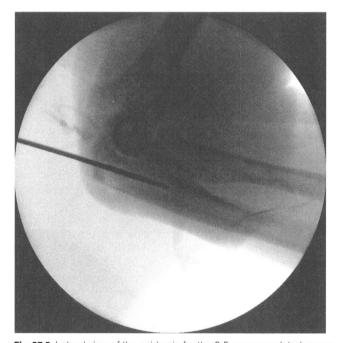

• **Fig. 37.5** Lateral view of the guide pin for the 6.5-mm cannulated screw. The pin should aim down the medullary canal. If the starting point is too ventral, the fragment will tend to translate dorsally with final seating.

to begin with the column that is easiest to get an anatomic reduction (Fig. 37.6). After one column is reduced, the remaining portion of the articular surface can be reconstructed to the repaired segment (Figs. 37.7 and 37.8). Occasionally, minifragment screws are also used to support the reduction. With multiple intra-articular pieces, they can even be placed intraosseously. It is important to maintain bone corridors for screws through plates, as these are the more powerful/important screws. In the setting of profound comminution in the supracondylar region, the articular reduction can be obtained, followed by supracondylar shortening to create bony contact and direct compression in the supracondylar region.

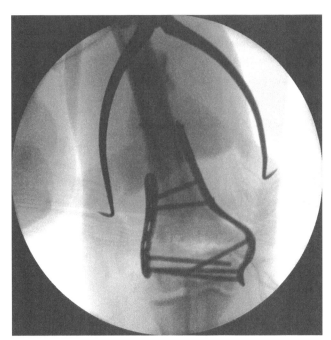

• **Fig. 37.7** Final fluoroscopic view of the fracture from Fig. 37.6. Supracondylar compression has been created with pointed reduction clamps and using the glide holes of the plate. Distal hardware interdigitates in the articular segment, creating a strong construct.

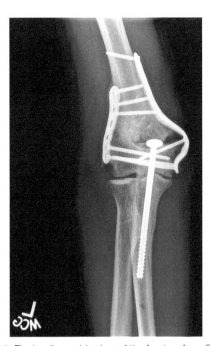

• **Fig. 37.8** Final radiographic view of the fracture from Fig. 37.6.

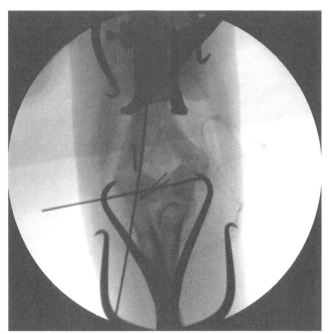

• **Fig. 37.9** The articular segment has been reduced. A large pointed reduction clamp can add additional compression to the articular fractures. Plates can be applied, and distal locking screws can be placed through the compressed articular segment. Clinical photos demonstrate the excellent visualization afforded by an olecranon osteotomy. Soft tissue attachments are preserved distally where possible to aid in fracture healing and as the attachments of the ligaments.

As provisional fixation, pin the medial and lateral columns to the humeral shaft and shift focus to plate application.

Dual plating is the gold standard for fixation, but there are no consensuses about whether parallel or orthogonal positioning is the optimal configuration. Recent meta-analyses indicated better biomechanical parameters with parallel plating and similar clinical outcomes with faster union time with parallel plating. Parallel plating does seem to be superior for the more complex fractures (extensive supracondylar comminution, poor bone

quality).[1,2] Regardless of the plate configuration selected, the goal is to achieve stable fixation of both columns and obtain maximal supracondylar compression. In some cases, parallel plating with a third posterior lateral plate is also advantageous. Specifically, low capitellar fractures can be minimally captured with a lateral plate. Fixation from the medial plate is the main fixation into the fragment, but an additional posterolateral plate can be advantageous for increased fixation along the distal lateral column.

When reconstructing the articular surface to the proximal metaphysis, first begin using the distal screws in the plate and fix the distal articular surface. Compression of the articular surface can be completed with clamps or with nonlocking screws applied through the plates in compression mode. We typically prefer clamp application, followed by locking screw fixation if the compression has been maximized with the clamp or nonlocking screw fixation in an eccentric position through a plate hole if further compression is desired (Fig. 37.9). Then, place clamps or screws in the compression side of the plate to add additional supracondylar compression. It may be necessary to work from one side to the other to obtain adequate bilateral compression. When both columns are compressed and stabilized, additional screws should be added to complete the construct with consideration of the technical objective checklist (Figs. 37.10–37.13) (Table 37.3). For cases of extensive metaphyseal comminution, an accessory minifragment plate can be helpful to hold the reduction. These are typically placed orthogonally to the planned precontoured plate position and are particularly helpful when carefully spanning multiple length unstable fragments. These plates have a small footprint that minimizes periosteal compromise and potential fracture healing impairment (Figs. 37.14–37.16).

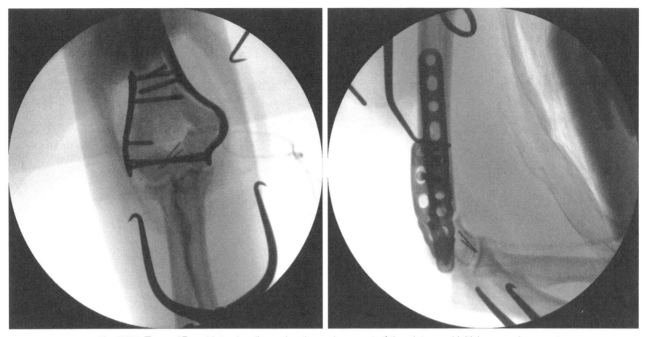

• **Fig. 37.10** These AP and lateral radiographs show placement of the plates and initial screw placement once the articular segment was reduced.

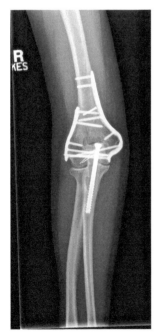

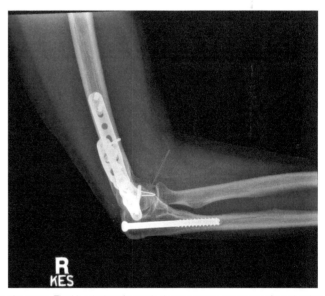

• **Fig. 37.12** Final healed radiograph demonstrates an anatomic reduction. Small threaded K-wires *(arrow)* captured an osteochondral fragment too small to capture with the plate and screw construct.

• **Fig 37.11** Final healed anteroposterior radiograph shows excellent distal fixation obtained into the articular segment with parallel fixation.

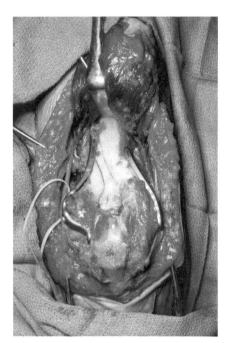

• **Fig. 37.13** Clinical photograph after hardware placement using parallel plating technique.

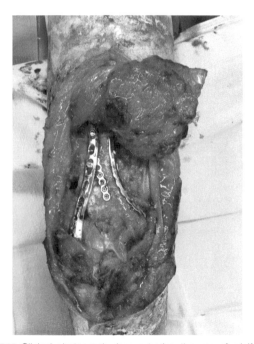

• **Fig. 37.14** Clinical photograph demonstrating the use of minifragment fixation to span metaphyseal comminution. Typically, these plates are best placed orthogonal to the corresponding precontoured column plates.

TABLE 37.3	Procedural Equipment Checklist
Positioning	• Surgeon preference
	• Can be supine, lateral, or prone
	• Sterile tourniquet with arm surgically prepared up to the shoulder
Imaging	• Fluoroscopy
Approach/ulnar nerve transposition	• Cobb or Young elevator
	• Vessel loops or Penrose drain
Olecranon osteotomy	• Oscillating saw
	• Osteotome
	• 6.5-mm cannulated screw with washer and appropriate guidewire and tap
Fracture reduction	• Drill
	• 0.62- and 0.45-mm K-wires (both threaded and unthreaded)
	• Pointed reduction clamps
Final fixation	• Precontoured distal humerus locking plates with both locking and nonlocking screws
Closure	• High-tensile nonabsorbable suture for repair of triceps tenotomy
	• 0-PDS for reinforcement and for triceps fascia
	• 2-0 and 3-0 monocryl for final skin closure

PDS, polydioxanone.

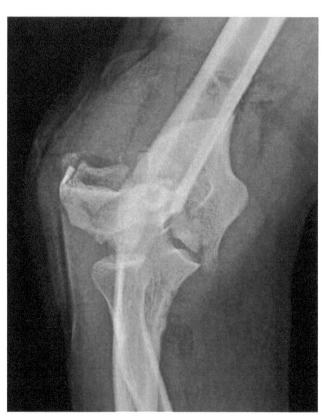

• **Fig. 37.15** Lateral radiograph of fracture.

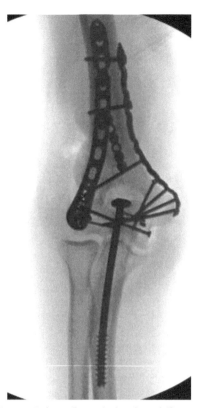

• **Fig. 37.16** Anteroposterior radiograph showing minifragment fixation and precontoured column plates.

PEARLS AND PITFALLS

- Careful patient positioning will facilitate stable access to the fracture fragments and adequate intraoperative imaging.
- Have a low threshold for olecranon osteotomy to enable direct reduction, compression, and anatomic fixation of intra-articular fractures. A 6.5-mm cannulated screw along the ulnar intramedullary canal can allow simple, strong, low-profile fixation of olecranon osteotomy fragments (Fig. 37.4).
- Direct articular reduction is usually the first step, followed by supracondylar compression. Both plates should contribute to fixation of the articular fragments and supracondylar compression.
- Once the construct is complete, range the elbow through its full range of motion to assess for stability and hardware impingement before closure.

References

1. Shih C-A, Su W-R, Lin W-C, Tai T-W. Parallel versus orthogonal plate osteosynthesis of adult distal humerus fractures: a meta-analysis of biomechanical studies. *Int Orthop*. 2018;43(2):449–460. https://doi.org/10.1007/s00264-018-3937-4.
2. Yu X, Xie L, Wang J, Chen C, Zhang C, Zheng W. Orthogonal plating method versus parallel plating method in the treatment of distal humerus fracture: a systematic review and meta-analysis. *Int J Surg*. 2019;69:49–60. https://doi.org/10.1016/j.ijsu.2019.07.028.

38

Technique Spotlight: Total Elbow Arthroplasty for Distal Humerus Fracture

MARK E. MORREY

Introduction

Articular fractures of the distal humerus are treated most successfully with operative intervention in order to restore function. Despite advances in plating constructs, these fractures can be difficult to fix and failures can result in a high reoperation rate. Therefore in unreconstructable distal humerus fractures, total elbow arthroplasty (TEA) has arisen as a viable treatment option.

Indications

Unreconstructable distal humeral fractures—those fractures in which open reduction internal fixation (ORIF) is not possible due to the size of the fragments, severe comminution, and/or poor bone quality where screw purchase is not possible (Fig. 38.1A–D).

Relative Indications

- Osteoporotic bone stock in an elderly patient
- Low-demand patient
- Distal humeral articular fracture in rheumatoid or preexisting arthrosis

Contraindications

- Infection
- Neurologic compromise affecting hand function
- Noncompliant patient

Relative Contraindications

- Open fracture
- Need for weight-bearing through the upper extremity

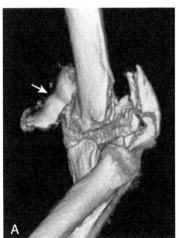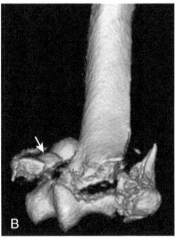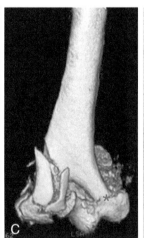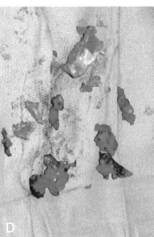

• **Fig. 38.1** (A) Lateral oblique, (B) anteroposterior, and (C) posterior views of a three-dimensional computed tomography reconstruction shows an unreconstructable distal humerus fractures with multiple comminuted fragments, a complete articular shear *(arrow)* fracture with little subchondral bone, and supracondylar comminution of both the medial and lateral columns *(asterisk)*. (D) The intraoperative picture of the multiple comminuted fracture fragments unable to reliably receive fixation.

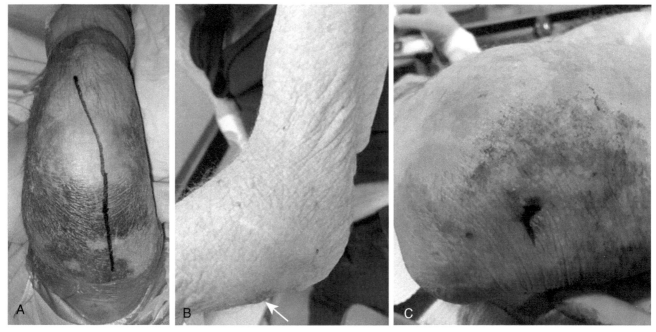

• **Fig. 38.2** Skin examination after distal humerus fracture shows (A) marked ecchymosis, (B) swelling and subtle abrasions *(arrow)*, or (C) puncture wounds and open fractures. The skin should also be examined for prior incisions which may alter the surgical approach.

Preoperative Evaluation

With a history of trauma to the upper extremity, attention should be paid to whether a low- or high-energy injury occurred as this can serve as a surrogate for bone quality. The patient should be questioned for the presence of antecedent joint pain prior to injury (as in the case of inflammatory arthropathy) and their activity level and demands. A very careful neurovascular examination should be conducted to ensure a functional hand and no prior injury to the neurovascular structures. The skin should always be examined for ecchymosis, swelling, fracture blisters, tenuous skin, prior surgery, or open fracture (Fig. 38.2A–C).

Imaging studies include the use of standard radiographs and a computed tomography (CT) scan which can be particularly helpful in fractures with comminution. Two-dimensional (2D) and three-dimensional (3D) CT reconstructions are very beneficial for planning and decision-making for either ORIF or arthroplasty when contemplating the two surgical options (Fig. 38.3A–I). If prior radiographs are available, this may also help guide treatment if joint pathology existed a priori, as in the case of rheumatoid arthritis, and TEA would provide a more favorable outcome. Coupled with the history, the physical examination, imaging studies, and intraoperative findings, the decision to perform a TEA for fracture can be individualized to wisely provide the best patient outcome.

Setup and Positioning

We prefer to place the patient in the supine position over an arm bolster which can afford the surgeon the possibility of performing ORIF or TEA (Fig. 38.4). The patient should be moved to the edge of the bed to allow for fluoroscopic examination if needed during instrumentation. The bed is tilted 10 degrees to the contralateral side of the injury to allow for an assistant to help manage the upper extremity during the surgery (Fig. 38.4). Instruments, trials, and imaging studies are set up accordingly at the periphery

and are readily available (Fig. 38.4), and the use of a magnetic pad helps increase safety and efficiency with frequent instrument changes (Fig. 38.4). For fracture setting , a tourniquet is frequently not necessary; however, a sterile tourniquet may be employed during cementation or if bleeding is encountered.

Technique

For TEA in the acute fracture setting, we prefer a posterior incision with careful consideration for any skin defects which would signify an open fracture (Fig. 38.5A–C). Typical landmarks are identified including the location of the ulnar nerve and the tip of the olecranon and subcutaneous border of the ulna (Fig. 38.5B). Depending on the location of skin defects they may be incorporated into the incision (Fig. 38.5C) and carried laterally or medially to the tip of the olecranon as necessary. The typical length of the incision is 5–8 cm distal and 10–12 cm proximal to the tip of the olecranon depending on the size of the patient and level of the fracture fragments. Dissection is then carried down to the investing fascia of the triceps without violating the triceps tendon proper (Fig. 38.6A–C). In open fractures, the triceps will oftentimes have been violated by the sharp proximal humerus and punctured (Fig. 38.7A). If this is the case, exposure through this interval can be completed after triceps mobilization and elevation from the posterior aspect of the humerus (Fig. 38.7B) and the ends of the humerus inspected for gross contamination, debridement, and fixation or TEA (Fig. 38.7C–D).

Approach

If the triceps mechanism has not been violated, dissection is carried around the investing fascia of the medial triceps to the intermuscular septum to identify the ulnar nerve (Fig. 38.8A–C). This is facilitated with the use of a self-retaining retractor on the medial tendon of the triceps lateral and the investing fascia medial to the

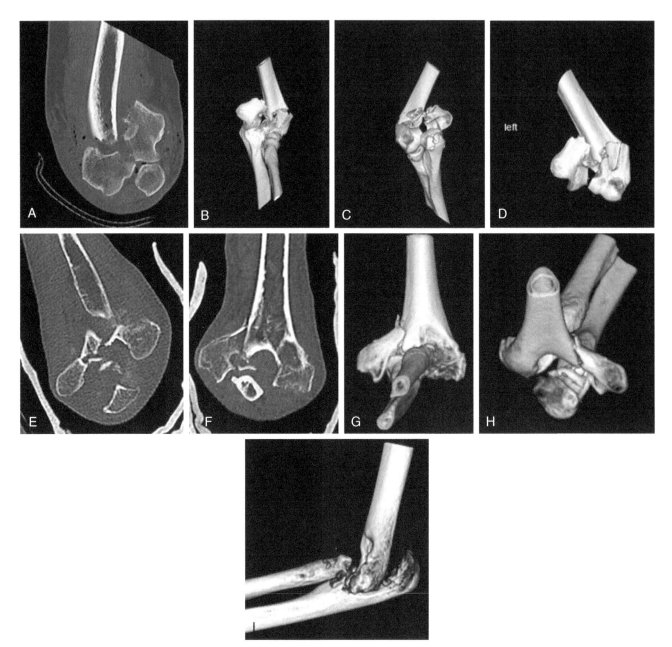

• **Fig. 38.3** *The top panel* shows the (A) two-dimensional (2D) and (B-C) three-dimensional (3D) reconstruction in the anterior (B), posterior (C) and with subtraction view of the forearm (D) of a T-type distal humerus fracture involving both columns but with excellent bone quality and the large fragments amenable to fixation. The *bottom panel* (E–I) shows a different patient with a bicolumnar distal humerus fracture with intra-articular comminution of the articular elements with poor bone quality, cystic change, and an antecedent rheumatoid change with expanded sigmoid fossa and loss of articular congruity. The patient was treated successfully with total elbow arthroplasty.

nerve (Fig. 38.8B–C). The nerve is then unroofed and dissected free with a vessel loop which is placed around the nerve and knotted to facilitate gentle retraction without traction injury which could be caused by the weight of a clamp (Fig. 38.8D). The nerve is gently mobilized medially and laterally to release the adventitial tissue or adhesions which often surround it after trauma (Fig. 38.8C–D). The articular branches are sacrificed with bipolar cautery as they are pain generators and the nerve dissected to the first motor branch, which is also sacrificed if it cannot be mobilized effectively. The intermuscular septum is released to allow for ulnar nerve transposition at the end of the case. The triceps can

be mobilized with a periosteal elevator to the medial or lateral direction with removal of the fat pad and release of the posterior capsule and well-placed retractors or a 1-inch Penrose drain with a paratricipital approach. This approach maintains the entire triceps attachment to the olecranon and anconeus to the ulna and can provide access for ORIF or TEA. A lateral skin flap is elevated to Kocher's interval between the anconeus and extensor carpi ulnaris distally and the lateral margin of the triceps proximally.

After debridement, the fracture fragments are assessed beginning with the articulation. It is at this time that we determine whether or not ORIF is a viable option or TEA needs to be performed. In most

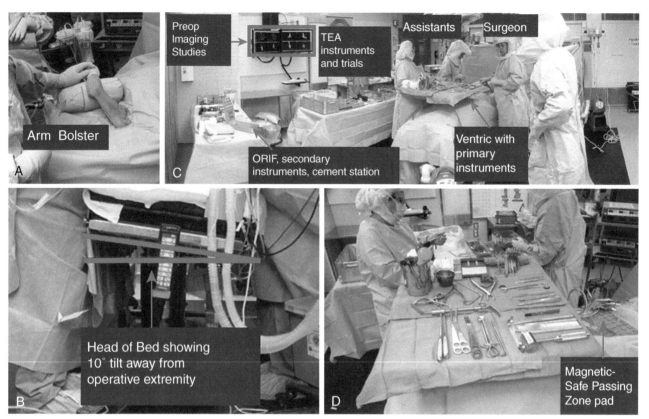

• **Fig. 38.4** Photographs showing the operating room setup for surgical efficiency. An arm bolster (A) is used to allow the assistant to easily control the upper extremity. The head of the bed is tilted 10° away from the operative extremity (B) which allows gravity to help with arm positioning. The imaging studies and instruments are readily available and assistance positioned and to help with retraction (C). A magnetic pad is used for a safe passing zone to avoid injury to the operative team (D). *ORIF*, Open reduction and internal fixation; *TEA*, total elbow arthroplasty.

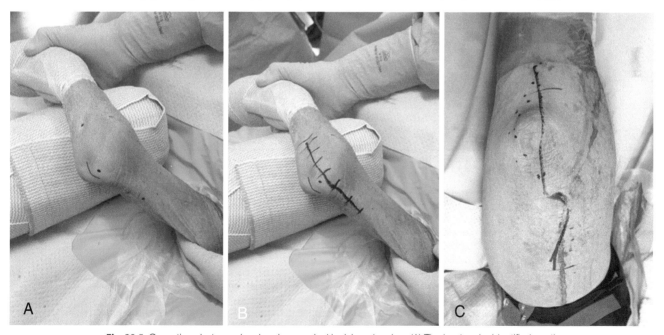

• **Fig. 38.5** Operative photographs showing surgical incision planning. (A) The landmarks identified are the tip of the olecranon, subcutaneous border of the ulna, and mid triceps. Incisions in both cases are to the lateral side of the olecranon and straight in (B) and curved to incorporate the skin puncture defect of the open fracture in (C). A sterile tourniquet can be placed in the event of blood loss and during cementation but, in general, is not used for most parts of the procedure.

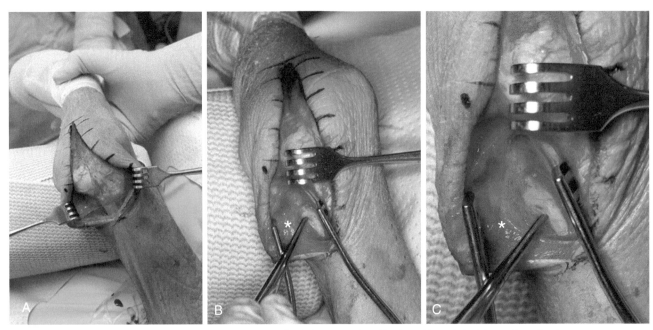

• **Fig. 38.6** Intraoperative photographs (A–C) of ulnar nerve identification. After skin incisions, dissection is carried to the investing fascia of the triceps (A), which is incised and traced medially to the ulnar nerve in the wide-angle photograph (B) and closeup (C) photographs of the location of the ulnar nerve. By utilizing the investing fascia *(asterisk)* of the triceps, dissection of the nerve (identified by the pick-up) is facilitated by placing a self-retaining retractor on the triceps tendon laterally and the investing fascia medially, which brings the nerve into view for release.

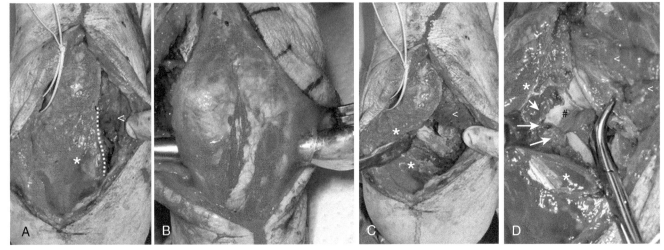

• **Fig. 38.7** (A) After the ulnar nerve is protected *(blue vessiloop)*, the fracture can be assessed by mobilizing the triceps from the posterior aspect of the humerus and can utilize the defect in the triceps created by the fracture *(dashed line)*. (B) A periosteal elevator is introduced below the triceps from medial to lateral to elevate and protect the triceps. (C) In this case, a lateral para-olecranon approach is created by the fracture and exploited taking the anconeus *(arrowhead)* laterally and triceps *(asterisk)* medial to the arthrotomy. (D) After excision of the fat pad and posterior capsule *(arrows)*, the joint surface *(hatch)* can be evaluated by mobilizing the triceps to the medial (as in this case) or lateral side to determine whether open reduction and internal fixation or total elbow arthroplasty (TEA) is needed if the decision is still in question. The flexor pronator mass and anterior band of the medial collateral ligament on the medial side and lateral collateral ligament and extensors from the epicondyle remain intact until the decision for TEA is made definitively.

B2 and some type C fractures, the triceps can be mobilized enough to allow for visual inspection of the posterior joint and an adequate articular read. This reduces the need for hardware and subsequent complications due to olecranon osteotomy and fixation after TEA. If it is determined that reconstruction is impossible after olecranon osteotomy, it is still possible to perform TEA and subsequent

olecranon fixation with a tension band construct; however, we prefer to make this decision prior to osteotomy (Fig. 38.9A–D).

Next, the fascia of the ulnar attachment of the flexor carpi ulnaris is identified on the ulna and incised to elevate the flexor carpi ulnaris from the medial aspect of the ulna, relax the nerve, and allow for exposure into the joint. We then tag the medial collateral ligament

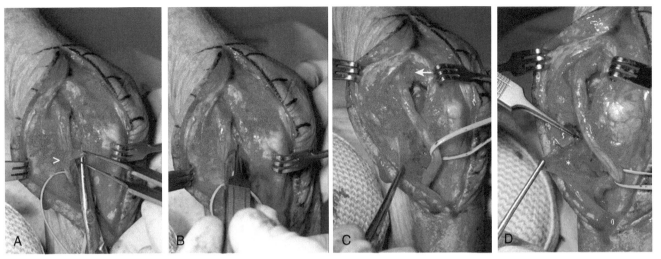

• **Fig. 38.8** After the nerve is unroofed all the way between the two head of the flexor carpi ulnaris, a vessiloop is placed on the nerve and tied instead of clamped to avoid a traction injury from a heavier hemostat. The nerve is gently mobilized by working on the (B) medial and (C) lateral sides of the nerve to release adhesions to the intramuscular septum *(asterisk)*. The articular branches *(arrowhead* in A) are isolated and cauterized (B) and the nerve is dissected fully to the first motor branch *(arrow)* in (C) and intermuscular septum *(asterisk)* removed (D).

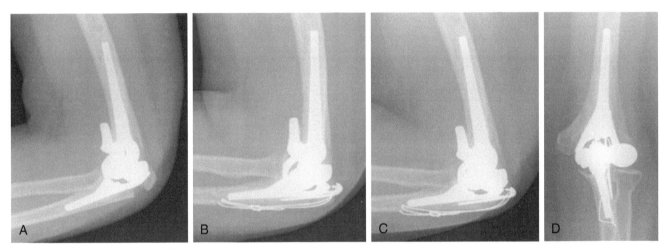

• **Fig. 38.9** (A) Radiograph of an olecranon osteotomy after total elbow arthroplasty has been performed. (B) The osteotomy can be fixed with K-wires driven into the ulna posterior to the implant with the addition of a tension band construct distal to the implant. (C) Lateral and (D) anteroposterior radiographs 14 months after surgery showing a healed olecranon osteotomy.

with a suture and elevate the medial collateral ligament along with the overlying flexor group and soft tissue from the fracture fragments and remove them (Fig. 38.10A–C). Typically, at this point, the elbow can be subluxated to the medial side and remaining muscle, tendon, and remaining capsular attachments released from the bone (Fig. 38.11A–C). The entire lateral soft tissue envelope is raised laterally off of the distal humerus after tagging sutures are placed, which both provide a ripstop and identification of the extensor wad and lateral ulnar collateral ligament at the completion of the case for closure to the lateral soft tissue structures. The elbow can then be completely dislocated in the anterior humerus prepared to later accept the bone graft which will be placed behind the total elbow humeral flange.

Humeral Preparation

Next, the humerus is prepared to accept the cutting jigs for the placement of the humeral implant. We begin this preparation by

"unroofing" the olecranon fossa with a rongeur in soft bone and a bur if the bone is of better quality. The canal of the humerus is opened with a bur. It is important to keep in mind that the bone of the olecranon fossa is in line with the humeral canal and, therefore, enough posterior bone must be removed in order to enter the humeral canal with a straight shot. We typically will not remove a large portion of cancellous bone by reaming but prefer to keep the cancellous bone intact and expand it for cement interdigitation with broaches. The starting broach is placed after reaming and the cutting jig is supplied to complete the cuts of the distal humerus (Fig. 38.12A). Oftentimes there is missing bone and not all the cuts are typically made if there is significant bone loss from the fracture (Fig. 38.12B–C). To the extent possible, the medial or lateral epicondyle should be retained for later soft tissue healing. A bur is utilized to ease the edges and cut marks left by the micro sagittal saw to avoid a stress riser and propagation of a columnar fracture (Fig. 38.13A). The broaches are then

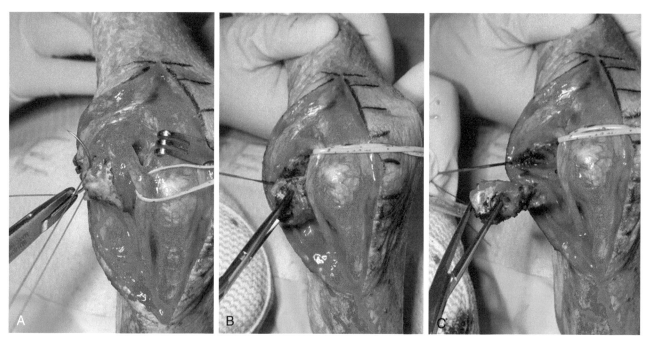

• **Fig. 38.10** (A) A tagging suture is placed in the medial collateral ligament and medial flexors for later repair. (B) The soft tissues are then released from the medial fracture fragment and (C) a window into the joint is created to remove the large fracture fragment.

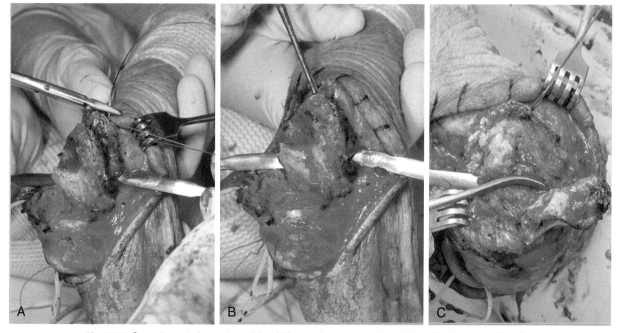

• **Fig. 38.11** Once the anterior and medial soft tissues have been released from the humerus, the elbow can be dislocated laterally and the lateral ulnar collateral ligament and lateral extensor musculature tagged for later repair in (A). The entire distal humerus is then exposed in (B), and retractors placed around the medial and lateral columns and the anterior aspect of the humerus is prepared with a periosteal elevator or osteotome (C) to later accept the bone graft which is placed behind the flange of the implant.

introduced into the canal (Fig. 38.13B) in the proper rotation (Fig. 38.13C–D) using the anterior cortex as a guide when large amounts of posterior bone are missing. It is important to place the implant in the proper rotation to avoid an off-axis line of pull of the triceps or biceps which would lead to undue stresses across the implant and potential early loosening. We have found the anterior humeral apex to be a reliable landmark for rotational alignment.

Once the humerus has been prepared, the shortest trial component is inserted into the humeral canal (Fig. 38.14A) and elbow provisionally reduced without preparation of the ulnar component in order to have a quick check of whether or not the depth of insertion is appropriate (Fig. 38.14B–C). If the implant is placed distally, the elbow will not fully extend and additional preparation and depth of insertion is necessary to gain extension (Fig. 38.14B). Additionally,

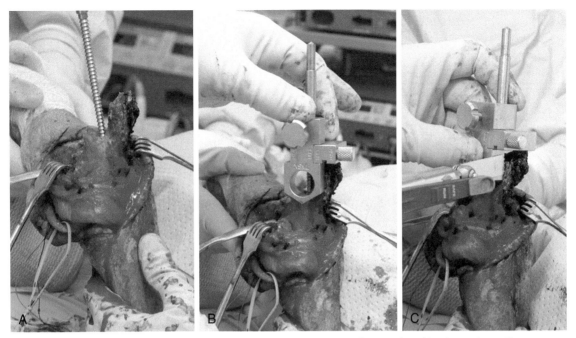

• **Fig. 38.12** A starting broach (A) is placed into the humeral canal after opening with a bur and a cutting jig (B) applied and a microsagittal saw is used to complete the remaining distal humeral cuts (C) for the implant. It is not uncommon to have areas of significant missing bone in the fracture setting.

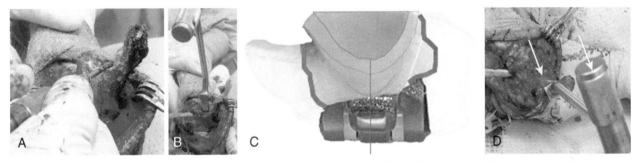

• **Fig. 38.13** After the initial cuts are made with a microsagittal saw, (A) a bur is used to round the cuts made from the saw to avoid any stress risers and potential propagation of additional fracture. (B) The broaches are then introduced sequentially in the proper rotation as illustrated in the intraoperative picture (C) and illustration (D) where the anterior humeral apex is used to align the broach and subsequent placement of the implant.

impinging bone can be easily assessed anteriorly and removed later in the procedure during the ulnar preparation (Fig. 38.14C).

A bur is utilized to allow the humeral component to be placed more proximally if necessary to gain extension (Fig. 38.15A–D). The operating surgeon must take great care to avoid thinning the columnar bone too much which may cause an iatrogenic or intraoperative fracture with excessive proximal placement of the implant. The elbow can then be reduced again for a trial range of motion and assessment of impingement (Fig. 38.16A–B). At this point if the radial head impinges or abuts the humeral yoke, the radial head can be resected; however, we prefer to leave it intact if there is no impingement as it can be used for bone graft in a revision setting if necessary in the future.

Ulnar Preparation

Next, with the forearm dislocated to the medial aspect of the humerus, retractors are placed to rotate and "present" the ulna to allow for preparation for the ulnar component (Fig. 38.17A). As

with the humerus, proper entry trajectory into the ulna is critical for proper ulnar component positioning. The base of the coronoid is located and the ulna is squeezed between the operating surgeon's fingers to localize the trajectory for entry of the bur (Fig. 38.17B). The hard cortical bone of the ulna at the entry point is widened with the bur in order to avoid off-axis injury and perforation of the ulna (Fig. 38.17C).

Once the entry point has been determined, a guide rod can be inserted into the ulna to confirm the intramedullary position. If the guide pin has undue flexion, the tip of the olecranon is removed and a trough can be created to take the implant out of flexion and avoid violating the posterior cortex with reaming or subsequent preparation. The canal can be reamed at this point. In very small canals, however, we prefer to utilize the broach to allow for as much cement interdigitation into the cancellous bone as possible. It is important to ensure the proper rotation and depth of insertion of the broach and sequentially broach until the appropriate size of the implant has been reached. Again, we prefer not to remove bone and attempt to get a very tight fit of the ulnar

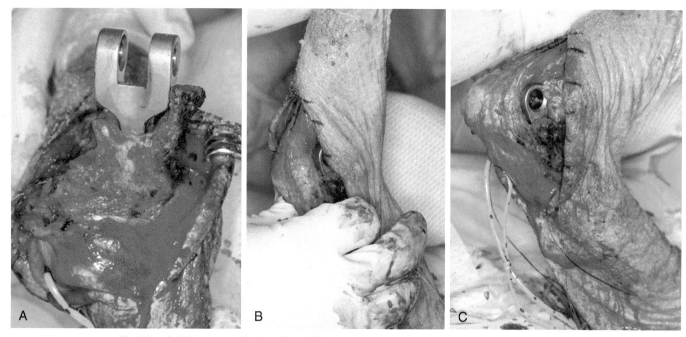

• **Fig. 38.14** A trial component is then placed in the distal humerus (A) and the elbow is relocated momentarily for a quick assessment of the range of motion in extension (B) and flexion (C) which will help to determine whether or not additional depth of insertion for extension or removal of impinging bone in flexion is needed to achieve full range of motion.

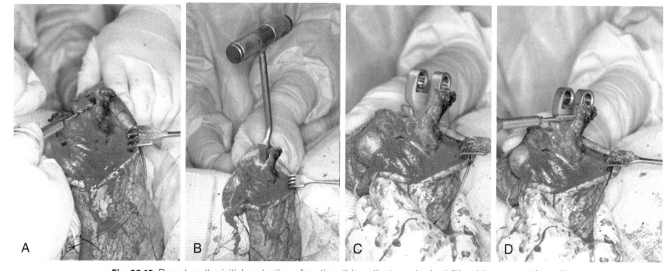

• **Fig. 38.15** Based on the initial evaluation of motion, this patient required additional bone resection with the bur (A) in order to seat the implant further to gain full extension. The broach is then reintroduced (B) and the trial implant (C) is placed and additional bone removed (D) in order to allow the implant to be seated fully. As the implant is "sunk" more fully into the humerus, the remaining columns can become thinned and great care is required to avoid fracture.

component. The posterior aspect of the ulna is a useful landmark to determine rotation, and if the radial head is intact the axis of rotation should fall through the center of the radial head and at the center of the greater sigmoid notch.

The trial ulna can then be used to determine the proper depth of insertion and rotation (Fig. 38.18A). The proximal-most aspect of the implant should not protrude beyond the olecranon tip to avoid over-stressing the triceps tendon and as with the broaches should be centered within the greater sigmoid notch. If greater depth is needed in extremely tight canals in which a perforation is

likely to happen, the implant can be modified by cutting the tip. If this is done, we prefer to roughen the distal portion to allow for better cement bonding and then its use as a subsequent trial without cement as well (Fig. 38.18B–C).

After the implant has been trialed, the humerus can again be inserted for range-of-motion check, and if acceptable cementation of the components can then commence. We typically prefer to cement the ulna first and start by placing a cement restrictor within the ulna. This can be a commercial restrictor if the canal size will allow or in cases of an extremely small canal, small pieces

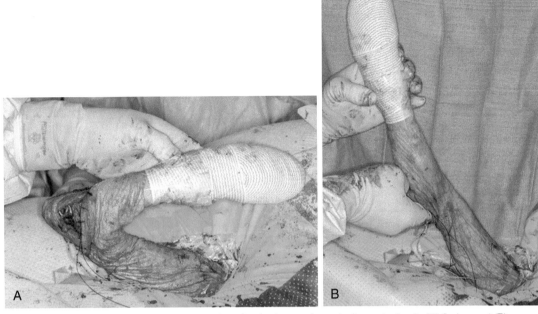

• **Fig. 38.16** A subsequent trial range of motion is then performed after reduction in (A) flexion and (B) extension, confirming the depth of insertion is appropriate.

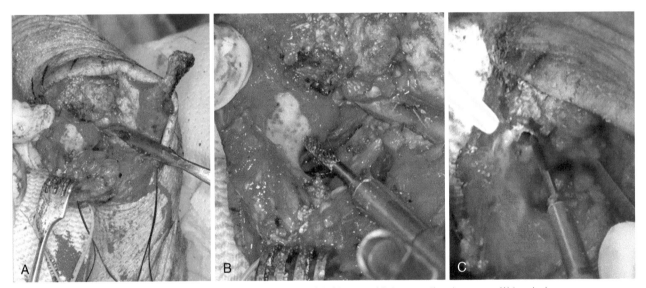

• **Fig. 38.17** The ulna is then dislocated to the medial side to avoid stress on the ulnar nerve (A) by placing a retractor on the coronoid and retracting the humerus anteriorly and the ulna posteriorly to expose the greater sigmoid fossa to allow the entry and preparation of the ulna through the base of the coronoid with a bur (B) which is expanded at the cortical bone entrance (C) into the canal to avoid malpositioning of the ulnar component. The dorsal cortex of the ulna is pinched between the thumb and forefinger to ensure proper trajectory into the ulnar canal.

of cancellous bone could be inserted and impacted with the trial or a tamp to provide a cement restrictor which will allow for thumb pressurization. We attempt to have very little cement beyond the tip of the implant if revision is needed later. A cement restrictor is also placed within the humerus and the canals thoroughly irrigated with a pulse lavage and dried with an opened sponge.

After thoroughly drying the canals, the tip of the cement gun is cut to the approximate length of the humeral component, the ulna is cemented first utilizing thumb pressurization, and the ulnar component impacted into place slowly in the correct rotation

(Fig. 38.19A). We prefer to use 1.5 batches of cement with a gram of vancomycin in the cement and always utilize a gun and vacuum preparation. Because of the normal distal bend of the ulna, the ulnar component does have a tendency to rotate upon insertion and this can be mitigated with the use of a tamp inserted through the implant to control rotation as it is seated (Fig. 38.19B–C).

The humerus is then prepared in a similar fashion with slow introduction of the cement (Fig. 38.20A) followed by thumb pressurization (Fig. 38.20B–C) and slow impaction of the humeral component in the proper rotation using the anterior cortex as a

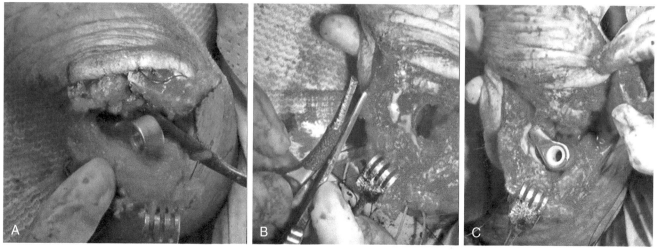

• **Fig. 38.18** After broaching, the trial is inserted into the ulna and is too proud in (A) requiring additional preparation and modification of the implant by cutting the tip in (B) to avoid fracture. Malrotation must be avoided by aligning the axis parallel to the flat of the ulna (C). If the radial head is intact, the axis of rotation should fall through the center of the radial head.

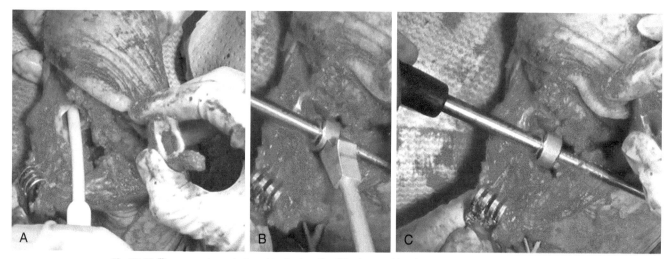

• **Fig. 38.19** The cement nozzle is cut to the length of the humeral implant and then placed into the ulnar canal and cement deployed (A) and finger pressurized and the ulna impacted into place in the correct rotation (B). (C) A tamp can be used to ensure the rotation is held as the bow of the ulna can cause rotation of the implant upon its insertion.

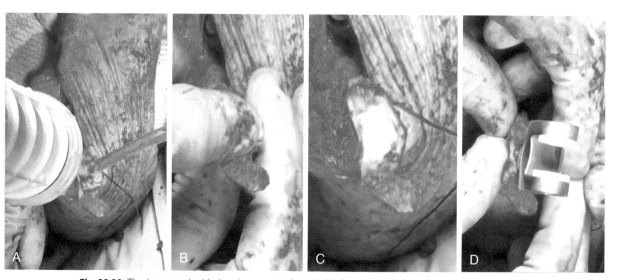

• **Fig. 38.20** The humerus is dried and cemented in a similar fashion again filling the canal (A) followed by finger pressurizing (B) to fill the canal (C), and the implant placed with the bone graft just posterior to the flange (D) and impacted in place.

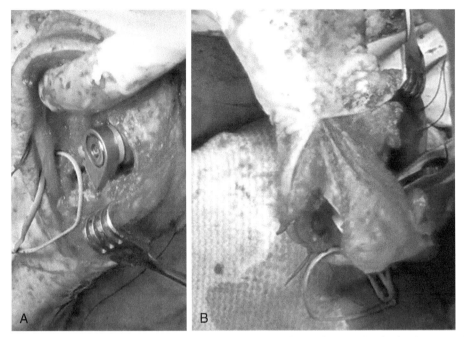

• **Fig. 38.21** A final check for impinging bone is made after coupling the implants by viewing from the (A) medial and (B) lateral sides and removed if necessary with a rongeur or osteotome. The ulnar nerve is transposed anteriorly at the end of the case bringing the medial and lateral soft tissues back to the medial and lateral margins of the triceps to cover the implant.

guide for rotation and placement of the bone graft as previously prepared (Fig. 38.20D). The bone graft is placed behind the flange prior to full seating of the humeral component and will wedge behind the flange as the humerus is impacted into place.

After the cement is cured, the elbow is reduced and the bushing pins are inserted opposite one another and coupled. With the Coonrad-Morrey prosthesis, the bushing pin tines at the end of the prosthesis should be expanded to ensure that it is fully seated.

At this point, a final check for impinging bone can be carried out and removed if necessary (Fig. 38.21A–B) and the ulnar nerve formally transposed into a subcutaneous pocket anteriorly. The soft tissues are then brought up to the margin of the triceps in order to close around the implant and the wounds closed in layers with monofilament sutures.

Postoperative Care

An anterior slab splint is applied with the arm in approximately 60 degrees of flexion to allow the soft tissues to heal for 1–2 weeks with an incisional wound VAC (vacuum-assisted closure) after closure. Postoperative X-rays are reviewed to provide a baseline within the splint. After 1 week the splint is removed, and if the incision is well-healed the patient may begin motion immediately. Because the triceps is not formally released, active extension can begin immediately. We recommend that patients do not stress the implant by lifting heavy loads (>10 lb at any one time) or performing activities with repetitive motion under a load (>2 lb). We follow-up patients routinely for the life of the implant and have routine postoperative visits at 3-month, 1-year, 3-year, and 5-year intervals for surveillance (Fig. 38.22A–B).

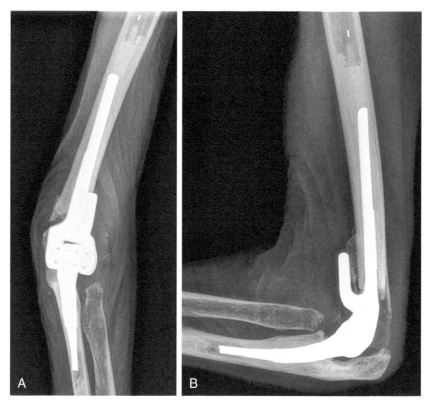

• **Fig. 38.22** (A) Anteroposterior and (B) lateral postoperative X-rays at 1 year showing incorporation of the bone graft behind the anterior flange and well-fixed components.

39

Traumatic Elbow Ligamentous Injury

ADAM C. WATTS

Introduction

The elbow is the second most commonly dislocated joint in the human body after the shoulder joint. This is likely to be due to the relatively small surface area of the joint, the short working length of stabilizing structures, and the large moment arms on either side of the articulation that magnify the forces applied to the limb. Stability of the elbow comes from the interplay between static stabilizers (the bones and ligaments) and dynamic neuromuscular stabilizers. While dislocation may be the result of violent trauma, there is a spectrum of injury that may occur to the elbow depending on the energy applied, the direction of forces, and possibly individual factors such as collagen properties, bone density, and reaction times. Isolated ligament injuries can be difficult to diagnose without a high index of suspicion, and if missed may result in chronic instability issues, elbow stiffness, or rapid chondral damage and arthritis. This chapter will review the anatomy, useful imaging, diagnosis, and management of traumatic ligament injuries around the elbow.

Anatomy

The elbow is a complex asymmetrical articulation between the humerus, ulna, and radius. The radius and ulna are related throughout their length within the forearm joint and neither the elbow nor the forearm can be considered in isolation. Neuromuscular structures crossing the joint act to pull the forearm onto the end of the humerus and to generate angular displacement (joint movement). This action brings the coronoid process of the ulna and radial head into apposition with the trochlea and capitellum, anteriorly when the elbow is flexed and distally when the elbow is extended. The coronoid process is fundamental to stability of the ulnohumeral joint and consists of the anteromedial facet, the anterolateral facet, and a medial projection, the sublime tubercle, into which the anterior band of the medial collateral inserts (Fig. 39.1). The fulcrum for varus and valgus moments across the elbow lies between the two facets. The surface area of the anteromedial facet is much greater than that of the anterolateral facet and is almost equal to that of the radial head.[1] When the forearm goes into valgus, a greater load is shared by the anterolateral facet and the radial head. Conversely, a varus load is transmitted to the

anteromedial coronoid facet. The olecranon process, which meets the coronoid process at the bare area of the articulation to form the greater sigmoid notch, contributes to elbow stability in extension when it will engage with the olecranon fossa of the humerus and resist varus and valgus moment. On the medial side of the elbow, the greater sigmoid notch covers the medial trochlea through an arc of 170 degrees, whereas the radial head only covers a 90-degree arc of the capitellum so the relative contribution of the osseous elements is unbalanced. On the lateral side of the elbow, the ligaments and neuromuscular elements must compensate to provide adequate stability.[2]

The lateral ligament complex is a broad interwoven thickening of the lateral capsule that is considered as four separate elements. The annular ligament (AL) arises from the anterior lip of the lesser sigmoid notch, wraps around the radial head, and inserts into the supinator crest. The radial collateral ligament (RCL) arises from the anterior part of a small elevation on the lateral condyle, the lateral epicondyle, and passes distally to blend with the AL. The lateral ulna collateral ligament (LUCL) arises from the anteroinferior portion of the lateral epicondyle to pass dorsally and distally to the supinator crest and blends with the AL, and the accessory LUCL made up of superficial fibers passing from the LUCL to the AL and supinator crest distally. The relative importance of each of these elements is debated in the literature, but in truth they are all interdependent, with disruption of one element affecting the function of another.[3] Recent studies have indicated an additional posterolateral ligament (Osborn-Cotterill ligament) arising from the inferior part of the lateral epicondyle that passes dorsally to attach to the rim of the greater sigmoid notch and produces a sling dorsal to the radial head.[4] This ligament appears to provide stability to the radial head in posterior drawer, performed by applying a posterior force to the radial head that is gripped between the examiner's finger and thumb with the elbow relaxed in a posture between 30 and 90 degrees of elbow flexion (Fig. 39.2). In a positive test, the radial head can be felt to subluxate dorsally. Comparison can be made to the uninjured elbow.

On the medial side, the medial ligament has three elements. The anterior bundle of the medial collateral ligament (aMCL) arises from the anteroinferior part of the medial epicondyle (ME), a much larger osseous protuberance that arises from the medial condyle. The origin of the ligament is roughly midway between the base on the trochlea and the tip of the ME. The aMCL passes distally to insert into the sublime tubercle of the coronoid process of the ulna. The posterior band of the medial collateral ligament (pMCL) arises from the inferior border of the ME and fans out to insert into the rim of the greater sigmoid notch of the ulna. The transverse or oblique medial ligament passes from the medial side of the olecranon to the ulna just dorsal to the sublime tubercle and does not appear to contribute to elbow stability. The anterior band of the ligament is tighter in extension and the posterior band in flexion.

The origin of both medial and lateral ligament complexes is often thought to lie in the center of the distal humeral spool.

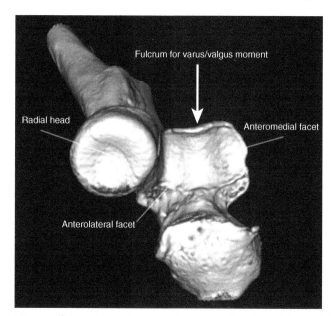

• **Fig. 39.1** Osseous stability comes from the articulation of the distal humerus articular surface with the radial head and coronoid. The antero-medial facet is an important varus stabilizer with a surface area almost equivalent to that of the radial head. (Copyright A. Watts.)

Anatomical footprint studies appear to indicate that on both the medial and the lateral sides of the humerus the center of the ligament footprint on the humerus lies 2 mm posterior to the center of the spool. The reason for this is not clear. It may be to give a cam effect such that the ligaments tighten in flexion increasing stability when carrying objects in this position, but it is important when considering repair or reconstruction of the medial ligaments (Fig. 39.3). Although the ligaments act as static restraints, they also contain the important sensory organs for proprioception of the elbow.[5] The anterior and posterior capsules are relatively deficient in these receptors, which means injury to the ligaments can have a detrimental effect on joint movement.

The third layer of stability comes from the neuromuscular elements around the elbow. Anteriorly and posteriorly there are three principle flexors and extensor elements. Anteriorly, the brachialis is muscular almost to its insertion and has a short moment arm lying close to the joint line, and the short and long head of biceps have a long tendinous insertion to the bicipital tuberosity on the radius with a longer moment arm for elbow flexion forces. Posteriorly, the triceps has three heads, the medial head lies close to the joint line, has a short moment arm, and is muscular almost to its insertion. Additionally, the long and lateral heads have a lengthy tendon and insert further from the joint line to the olecranon process. It is the tendinous insertions that are most prone to rupture. Medially, the pronator teres, flexor carpi radialis, flexor digitorum superficialis, palmaris longus, and flexor carpi ulnaris contribute to valgus stability, particularly in the absence of a functional MCL. Laterally, the brachioradialis, extensor carpi radialis longus and brevis, extensor digitorum communis, and extensor carpi ulnaris all contribute to varus stability, particularly in the absence of a functional lateral ligament complex. Anconeus is thought to be a dynamic stabilizer on the lateral side of the joint although the contribution is debated.[6,7] The resultant moment from all these elements acts to pull the forearm bones proximally and dorsally onto the end of the humerus. Loss of the medial or lateral secondary stabilizers in the presence of ligament injuries can result in significant instability of the elbow.

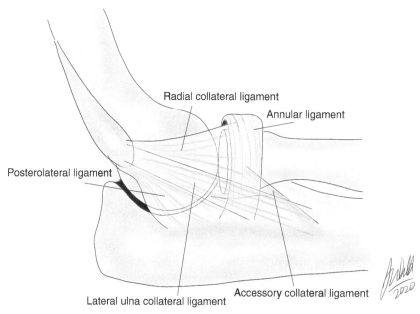

• **Fig. 39.2** Ligamentous anatomy of the lateral elbow. (Copyright A. Watts.)

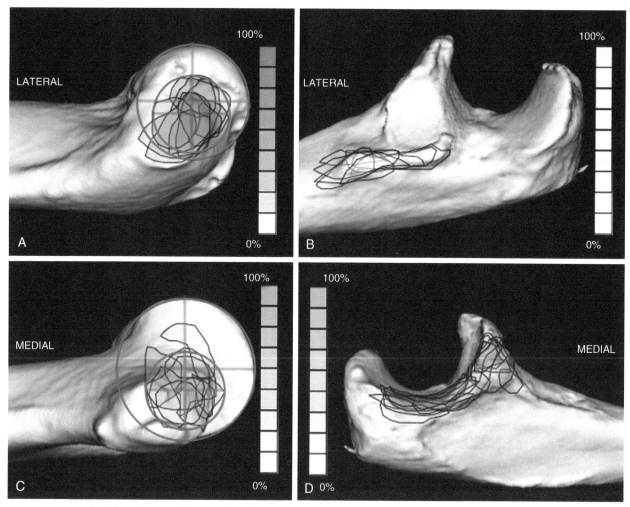

• **Fig. 39.3** Ligament footprints. (A) Lateral humerus, (B) lateral ulna (posterolateral ligament not shown), (C) medial humerus, (D) medial ulna. Note the center of the footprint lies dorsal to the center of the articular spool. (Copyright A. Watts.)

Diagnosis and Imaging

The diagnosis of acute ligament injury requires an index of suspicion based on the history of the injury and reported symptoms. In complete elbow dislocation, the diagnosis is rarely challenging with obvious deformity following a fall or high-energy injury. Usually the skin is intact but evidence of an open injury typically necessitates urgent surgical management. It is important to examine for neurological and vascular compromise and document the presence of any deficit. Prompt reduction is essential to relieve pain, limit the extent of cartilage compromise, and reduce the risk of neurovascular or cutaneous damage. Ideally, at the time of elbow reduction an assessment would be made of elbow stability looking at joint gapping with a fluoroscope on varus and valgus stress of the joint and assessing congruency of the elbow in full extension.[8] Widening of the usually parallel joint line of >10 degrees has been associated with a five-fold increase in the risk of recurrent instability.[9] The standard teaching of stability at 30 or 60 degrees of flexion determining the need for surgical intervention carries no scientific basis or obvious logic. The elbow should be stable through a full arc to confidently allow active mobilization.

In most cases, the patient will have had the elbow reduced in the emergency department and present to the specialist with a congruent elbow. The extent of the soft tissue injury is difficult to determine on clinical grounds. A history of a high-energy injury,

extensive soft tissue injury, neurological compromise, or significant displacement on plain radiographs may all suggest more significant injury but do not precisely identify which of the stabilizers are damaged. The elbow will be swollen and painful and assessment of stability is unlikely to yield additional useful information. The clinician can, therefore, take a view that the overall likelihood of recurrent instability is low and treat accordingly or may choose to try to stratify the injury using radiographic imaging.[10,11]

Plain X-rays will confirm that the elbow remains satisfactorily reduced and that there is no bony injury. Flakes of bone from the lateral or ME may indicate a ligamentous avulsion. A "drop sign," with gapping between the ulna and the distal humerus, may be visible in the early stages after injury but does not in itself mandate surgical intervention.[12] Possible causes for this appearance include hemarthrosis, temporary muscle inhibition, or ligament injury. An isolated coronoid fracture, with radial head intact, indicates a posteromedial rotatory instability (PMRI) fracture-dislocation and needs further investigation. This is not a minor avulsion injury but suggests an impaction or punch injury of the trochlea through the coronoid process.

Computed tomography (CT) is not usually indicated in simple dislocation as by definition the skeleton should be intact. It can be helpful, however, if there is any doubt about the diagnosis and is often used in cases of PMRI to assess the amount of bone lost from the coronoid and the presence of ulnohumeral joint subluxation.[13]

TABLE 39.1   Grading System for Soft Tissue Injury in Posterolateral Elbow Dislocation

Grade of Injury	SOFT TISSUE INJURY			
	Medial Ligament	Lateral Ligament Complex	Common Flexor Origin	Common Extensor Origin
1	Avulsed	Functional	Functional	Functional
2	Avulsed	Avulsed	Functional	Functional
3	Avulsed	Avulsed	Avulsed	Functional
4	Avulsed	Avulsed	Avulsed	Avulsed

Copyright A Watts.

Magnetic resonance imaging (MRI) is a useful investigation in the dislocated elbow as it can be used to identify torn structures and stratify the injury.[11] Simple elbow dislocation is graded from 1 to 4 based on the presence of avulsion of the medial ligament, lateral ligament, common flexor origin, and common extensor origin according to the scheme in Table 39.1. Those patients with grade 4 injuries where all the soft tissues have been avulsed from the epicondyles are thought to be at greatest risk of recurrent instability.[14] MRI can also be used to identify the presence of ligament injury with a PMRI with particular attention paid to the lateral ligament complex, common extensor origin, and pMCL.

Isolated ligament avulsion injuries can be diagnosed using MRI where there is an index of suspicion. Hyperextension injuries of the elbow can result in a spectrum of injury similar to a simple dislocation and at the lower end of the scale isolated injuries to the anterior band of the MCL are seen.[15] Bruising over the ME, with tenderness over the anterior band and pain from the medial ligament on valgus stress testing or modified milking maneuver will indicate a need for further investigation.[16] The moving valgus stress test is usually reserved for chronic injuries.[17]

Isolated lateral ligament injuries or injuries to the posterolateral ligament are more challenging to diagnose and many go unnoticed leading to chronic posterolateral rotatory instability (PLRI). Lateral ligament injury should be considered in any patient presenting with lateral elbow pain and a history of trauma. Some patients will report a clunk or click on the lateral side of the joint on mobilization and very occasionally the patient will be aware of frank instability of the radial head on the capitellum. Persistent stiffness after elbow trauma, particularly segmental radial head fractures with no or minimal displacement that fail to recover normal function in the usual time period, should raise a suspicion of ligamentous injury, as elbow instability is one of the hidden causes of posttraumatic stiffness. The presence of bruising over the lateral side of the elbow may indicate a high-grade injury, as it suggests that the tough lateral fascia has been torn, allowing hematoma to escape to the subdermal layers. The pivot shift test is difficult to perform in the acutely injured elbow but as the swelling settles a posterior drawer test may indicate posterolateral instability.[2,18]

Particular attention should be paid to the patient falling backwards on to the hand, sometimes ending up with their arm stuck underneath them, who reports that they can straighten their elbow but cannot flex beyond 90 degrees. This is highly suggestive of a PMRI fracture-dislocation pattern. They may have a visible cubitus varus on elbow extension.[19]

MRI is a useful tool to investigate a suspected ligament injury. Arthrography is not usually required in the acute setting because of hemarthrosis but injectable contrast or saline injection can be

TABLE 39.2   Grading System for Medial Ligament Injury

ULNA COLLATERAL LIGAMENT INJURY CLASSIFICATION ON MAGNETIC RESONANCE IMAGING	
Classification	Description
Type I	Edema in UCL only, low-grade partial tear
Type II	Partial tear of UCL, no extravasation of fluid on arthrogram, high-grade partial tear
Type III	Complete full-thickness tear of the UCL with extravasation of fluid on arthrogram
Type IV	Tear/pathology in >1 location on UCL (i.e., ulna and humerus)
Subset	H (humerus), U (ulna), M (midsubstance)

UCL, Ulnar collateral ligament.

From Joyner PW, Bruce J, Hess R, Mates A, Mills FB, Andrews JR. Magnetic resonance imaging–based classification for ulnar collateral ligament injuries of the elbow. *J Shoulder Elbow Surg.* 2016;25(10):1710-1716.

used to enhance the imaging if necessary.[20] On the medial side the anterior band is most easily visualized on coronal T1 and T2 slices passing from the ME to the sublime tubercle. Fluid between the ligament and tubercle, the "T" sign, is suggestive of a medial ligament injury but can be a normal appearance in some. As a result, clinical correlation and the presence of edema are required to confirm diagnosis.[21] The ligament may tear from the tubercle, the humerus, or there may be a "Z"-shaped tear starting anteriorly from the sublime tubercle, passing up the ligament and then posteriorly off the humerus (Table 39.2).[22] This may give the impression of a midsubstance tear. Posterior ligament injuries can be visualized on the axial slices and will normally be avulsed from the humerus. MRI will identify fracture or contusion to the coronoid process and radial head. The sagittal images should be inspected for joint subluxation with incongruence of the trochlea in the greater sigmoid notch. On the lateral side, the ligament is usually avulsed from the humeral origin. The tear may extend into the common extensor origin which makes persistent instability more likely. This is best seen on coronal slices. Avulsion of the posterolateral ligament, with or without a bony ossicle, from the posterior capitellum can be identified on sagittal slices and can occur as an isolated injury or as part of a lateral ligamentous complex tear. Ultrasound can be used to perform a dynamic assessment of acute ligament injury. It is, however, limited by the comfort of the patient and the availability of skilled practitioners in the acute setting. Joint gapping medially on valgus stress may indicate a torn MCL. Assessment of lateral instability is more challenging because of the variability of the position of the radial head on the capitellum in the normal population. Soft tissue avulsion injury can be demonstrated in skilled hands.

Pathlogy

Simple Elbow Dislocation

Simple elbow dislocation by definition is a dislocation of the elbow without bony injury. The etiology, pathoanatomy, and management are the subject of debate in the literature but it is certain that there is a spectrum of injury to the soft tissue stabilizers. Some patients are at greater risk of recurrent instability than others.[23] The title "simple" might lead to the conclusion that this is a benign injury; however, between 5% and 10% of patients will experience recurrent elbow instability symptoms and 40% will have elbow stiffness.[10,24] The cause of this may be related to the care received and in particular the period of immobilization, but persistent instability of the elbow may also be a causal factor. Simple elbow dislocation can be classified according to the direction of dislocation; posterolateral is most common (80%), followed by posteromedial (5%), posterior, or most uncommonly, anterior, or divergent.

There are two models of injury described in the literature. The first is a valgus compression supination mechanism on a flexed elbow. In this scenario, the soft tissue stabilizers are torn sequentially from lateral to medial with a principle focus on the involvement of capsuloligamentous structures. In this model, the injury starts with an avulsion of the lateral ligamentous complex, extends through the anterior and posterior capsule, and ultimately results in avulsion of the medial ligament, the so-called Horii circle.[25] This model fits with the PLRI pattern of injury. Importantly, it has been shown that the elbow can dislocate with the medial ligament intact.

The alternative mechanism is a valgus hyperextension injury model in which the elbow opens on the medial side first, tearing the medial ligament, (Fig. 39.4) and then the lateral ligament fails.[26] In this model, as the forearm continues to displace from the distal humerus, the musculotendinous origins are also avulsed first on the medial side and then on the lateral side.[23,27,28]

MRI assessment of a consecutive series of simple dislocations has shown that a full spectrum of injury is seen in simple dislocations.[11] The most common posterolateral dislocations appear to follow the valgus hyperextension model with a higher frequency, and higher grade, of medial structure injury than lateral. Although the numbers are small, the same study indicates that posteromedial dislocation may follow the valgus compression supination model with more significant soft tissue disruption seen laterally than medially in this group. Importantly, the extent of the soft tissue disruption is variable in simple elbow dislocation, some with isolated ligament tears through to complete soft tissue stripping of the distal humerus, and therefore it can be expected that the prognosis is quite heterogeneous.

It seems reasonable to consider that those with most soft tissue damage might be at the greatest risk of ongoing instability, and further that, because of the importance of the lateral soft tissue stabilizers on the osseously unstable lateral side of the joint,

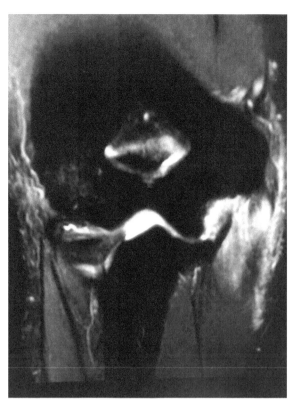

• **Fig. 39.4** Coronal magnetic resonance imaging of elbow hyperextension injury showing avulsion of the anterior band of the medial ligament from the humerus. The lateral ligament structure was intact. (Copyright A. Watts.)

high-grade lateral-sided injury is a particular risk factor. If the models suggested are correct, then ongoing instability is only likely to be a problem in a small proportion of posterolateral dislocations in whom the injury is of such a high grade that the lateral ligament and common extensor tendon have been avulsed; conversely patients with posteromedial dislocation are likely to be at greater risk of instability because the primary pathology is to the lateral soft tissues.

This hypothesis is supported by the observations of Josefsson et al. who showed that stability of the joint after simple dislocation is dependent not on the ligament injury but the injury to the musculotendinous units, and second by Adolfsson et al. showing the majority of recurrent dislocations will result from a previous posteromedial dislocation, and when it does follow a posterolateral dislocation the patient typically has torn the ligaments and tendons on the medial and lateral sides of the elbow in the initial injury.[14,27] Recurrent dislocation is the most overt sign of persistent instability but there are a number of patients for whom the elbow fails to recover satisfactory function with ongoing pain and stiffness, and in these patients too an assessment of the soft tissue stabilizers can be informative.

Management of Simple Elbow Dislocation

The acutely dislocated elbow needs prompt reduction with appropriate analgesia and sedation by a suitably trained practitioner. Ideally, assessment of stability will be undertaken at the time of reduction with fluoroscopic measurement of varus and valgus joint gapping on an anteroposterior view with the elbow in extension, and joint congruency on the lateral projection with the elbow in full extension. Once reduced the elbow can be supported in a sling or collar and cuff. The use of a splint or cast has been shown to be unnecessary and may have a negative impact on the outcome. If the elbow has been shown to be stable with fluoroscopy after reduction, immediate active mobilization should be encouraged. This is best performed with the patient lying supine, shoulder flexed to 90 degrees, and forearm in neutral.[29] This position not only places less strain on the ligaments, it also reduces biceps activity, allowing better elbow extension.[30,31]

In cases where elbow stability has not been assessed at the time of reduction, or there is uncertainty, a decision needs to be made with the patient about continuing with nonoperative treatment and accepting low risk of persistent instability and greater risk of stiffness, or to assess the elbow further with an MRI scan, to stratify the injury and decide on the need for surgical intervention if a high-grade soft tissue injury is identified.

In cases with instability identified on examination with fluoroscopy, defined as joint gapping of >10 degrees, at the time of reduction or grade 4 lesions on MRI (complete stripping of soft tissues from distal humerus), acute surgical stabilization should be discussed.[8,9] There is an argument to consider surgery in all cases of posteromedial dislocation.

Acute surgical stabilization can be performed arthroscopically or more usually as an open procedure. Open stabilization is performed through separate medial and lateral approaches with the patient in a lateral position with the elbow over a support. Anchors can be used to re-attach the ligaments and tendon origins. It is the author's usual practice to stabilize the lateral side first, to downgrade the injury, then reassess and stabilize the medial side if the elbow remains unstable.[32] Arthroscopic lateral ligament repair is an advanced skill. A number of techniques have been described either using two lateral portals or an anteromedial and accessory lateral portal.[33,34] These techniques use anchors placed under arthroscopic vision sometimes with fluoroscopic confirmation. Arthroscopic suture passers are helpful to grasp the lateral ligament. While arthroscopic medial ligament repair has been described, it is a procedure that carries significant risk due to the proximity of the ulnar nerve to the ligament. Postoperative rehabilitation is the same as for the acutely injured "stable" dislocation.

Outcome of Simple Elbow Dislocation

Simple dislocation will result in a satisfactory outcome for the majority of patients. A randomized controlled trial has not shown a difference in the outcome between nonoperative and early operative treatment in an unstratified series of patients.[35] No study has examined the benefits of early surgery in those with high-grade lesions only. Early mobilization has been shown to lead to a superior outcome in those with "stable" elbow after simple dislocation.[9]

Acute Medial Collateral Ligament Tear

MCL problems are often related to specific sporting activities and as a result there are significant variations in the prevalence between countries and cultures. Many injuries are chronic or acute on chronic failure which will not be addressed in this chapter. Acute injuries to the MCL typically involve the anterior bundle as a result of hyperextension of the elbow.[15] Activities such as judo, rugby, wrestling, gymnastics, and goalkeeping in soccer in which sudden hyperextension loads are applied through the ligament can lead to avulsion injuries either from the humeral origin or from the ulna insertion. In other activities more commonly associated with chronic injury such as pitching, javelin throwing, and bowling, acute injuries can be seen with sudden loads. True valgus

injuries can occur rarely and may be associated with triceps avulsion and radial head fracture.[36]

As with simple elbow dislocation, a spectrum of medial ligament injury can be seen from strains, through partial tears to complete ligament disruption. The presence of a common flexor tendon injury is an indicator of the energy of the injury and greater likelihood of instability symptoms.[22]

The treatment depends on the nature of the injury. Strain and minimal partial tear of the ligament is usually treated nonoperatively with good recovery. Instability symptoms would not be expected until 100% of the ligament is torn.[31] Pain, however, can be a debilitating issue. Activity modification, pain relief, and physiotherapy are recommended. In those patients with persistent symptoms, injection around the ligament may be of benefit. Recovery of symptoms has been observed after platelet-rich plasma injection; however, without a control arm it is not possible to confirm effectiveness.[37,38]

If pain remains or the patient has a complete tear with instability symptoms, ligament repair is indicated. Instability may cause a "popping sensation" on the medial side of the elbow with pain and increased laxity on valgus stress testing and often, in the acute injury, fibrillation of the flexor-pronator muscles. Bruising will often be found on the medial side of the elbow. The milking maneuver and the moving valgus stress test will usually produce pain. MRI scan will identify the pattern of any tear and will aid preoperative planning. Arthrography would not normally be needed.

Open repair is the usual treatment in an athlete that requires integrity of the aMCL.[39] This can be performed through a medial approach to the elbow with the patient supine on the operating table with the arm on an arm board. The approach can be made through a straight incision extending distally from the ME or through a curvilinear incision posterior to the ME and extending distally across the forearm. The deep approach is either through the bed of the ulnar nerve, which gives direct access to the sublime tubercle but with a risk of neural adhesion, or in the internerve interval between flexor carpi ulnaris and palmaris longus.[40] This latter approach can be done as a muscle split but can be extended proximally if necessary and has the advantage of preserving the bed of the ulnar nerve. An in situ decompression of the nerve can be performed to ensure it is protected through the case. When undertaking a repair, it is important to understand the anatomy of the tear. Many aMCL avulsions will be from the sublime tubercle and a whip stitch can be placed in the ligament and secured to the bone through drill holes or an anchor. Care must be taken with anchors placed into the ME that they do not perforate dorsally into the bed of the ulnar nerve, where they can cause irritation. Midsubstance failure is rare, and in most cases actually indicates a "Z"-shaped tear. This is characterized as an avulsion of the anterior part of the anterior band from the sublime tubercle, extension proximally up the ligament, and then posteriorly from the humerus into the pMCL (Fig. 39.5). These require fixation at both ends. Some surgeons choose to protect their repair with a synthetic augment with bone anchorage on either side of the joint. Posterior MCL injury, as seen in a posteromedial fracture dislocation, is usually an avulsion from the humeral origin.

The outcome of surgery is usually good with recovery of around 8–12 weeks. The patient should be warned of the risks of infection, nerve injury, heterotopic ossification, repair failure, and ongoing instability. Rehabilitation progresses through immediate active range-of-movement exercises with the patient lying supine, shoulder flexed to 90 degrees, and forearm in neutral, to

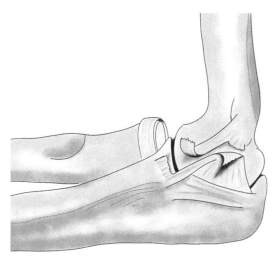

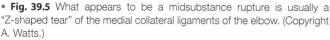

• **Fig. 39.5** What appears to be a midsubstance rupture is usually a "Z-shaped tear" of the medial collateral ligaments of the elbow. (Copyright A. Watts.)

active open and closed chain movement exercises, to inline loading, varus/valgus loading, plyometric exercises, and a return to sports–specific program. A sling can be used between exercises to protect the repair in the first 6 weeks. A hinged brace has not been shown to be of benefit and has been shown to put abnormal forces across the joint.[41]

Acute Posterolateral Ligament Tear

The capsule attaching to the posterior capitellum has been shown to play an important role in stability of the radial head in mid-flexion.[4] This posterolateral ligament can be torn in isolation, as part of a lateral ligament complex injury, or as part of an osseoligamentous injury to the elbow, from minor radial head rim fractures to elbow fracture dislocations. Frequently the ligamentous avulsion is associated with a bone fragment avulsion from the posterior capitellum. This fragment can be a minor flake avulsion or a large bone defect that has been either avulsed or sheared off by the subluxating radial head. This lesion, first described by Osborne and Cotterill and commonly bearing their names, is not well recognized (Fig. 39.6).[42,43] The incidence is unknown and relevance to management currently uncertain. Over-investigation is likely to lead to overtreatment and a pragmatic approach is recommended. There are currently two scenarios in which acute or subacute posterolateral ligament repair is indicated. The first are patients with fracture-dislocation in whom radial head instability is still present on posterior drawer after satisfactory lateral ligament repair. The other scenario is the patient with an otherwise innocuous injury who fails to recover as expected. An example of this is a patient with a Mason 1 radial head fracture still complaining of significant lateral elbow pain and elbow stiffness at 6 weeks with no evidence of nonunion of the fracture. Assessment of posterior drawer may reveal increased laxity compared to the contralateral side and an MR arthrogram can demonstrate avulsion of the posterolateral ligament (Fig. 39.7).

Acute symptomatic posterolateral ligament avulsions can be managed with arthroscopic or open repair using proximal and direct lateral portals or an arthrotomy posterior to the capitellum. Bare bone between the articular cartilage and posterolateral joint capsule is pathological indicating soft tissue stripping and this can be repaired with sutures and a bone anchor. Arthroscopic signs of

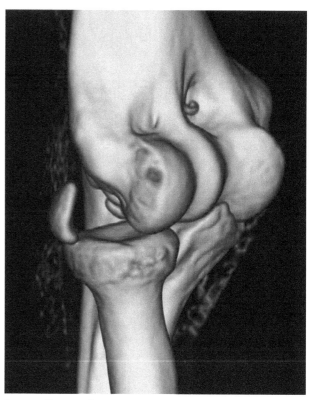

• **Fig. 39.6** Osborne-Cotterill lesion with avulsion of bone fragment from the posterior capitellum in association with elbow luxation. The size of the fragment is variable and in some cases the posterolateral ligament will be avulsed without a bone fragment. (Copyright A. Watts.)

lateral instability include lateral joint line gapping between the olecranon and trochlea when viewed from the posterior compartment as the forearm is supinated, and uncovering of the radial head when viewed from the proximal lateral portal in forearm supination and elbow extension such that the anterior edge of the radial head becomes visible. The drive-through sign, in which the arthroscope can readily pass between the ulna and the humerus in the greater sigmoid notch, may not be positive, as it would be if the lateral ligament complex is torn.

In delayed cases, posterolateral capsular reefing is an alternative to repair or reconstruction. This is performed as an arthroscopic procedure with absorbable heavy polydioxanone (PDS) sutures passed through the capsule from the origin of the ligament on the humerus to the distal insertion near the supinator crest, and then subcutaneously around anconeus to be tied to themselves. This procedure described by Van Riet appears to improve instability symptoms either through tightening the lateral structures or through improving proprioception.[44]

Acute Lateral Ligament Tear

Lateral ligament avulsion injuries can occur in isolation as part of a valgus compression supination injury, or as part of a more extensive injury. Valgus compression supination injury can extend to include the common extensor origin, radial head fracture, and anterolateral facet coronoid fracture. Lateral ligament avulsion is seen in posteromedial simple elbow dislocation and higher grade posterolateral dislocations. Posteromedial elbow fracture dislocation is associated with lateral ligament avulsion, anteromedial facet fracture with or without involvement of the sublime tubercle, and avulsion of the

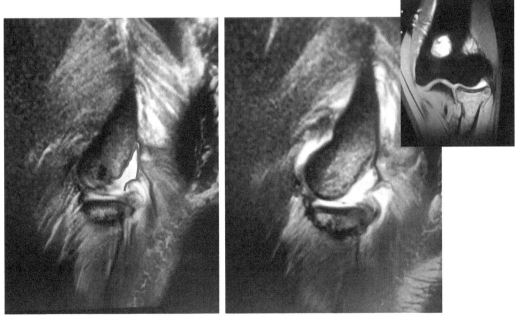

• **Fig. 39.7** Posterolateral ligament avulsion without bony injury seen on magnetic resonance imaging scan in a patient with positive posterior draw but negative pivot shift. Note the intact lateral ligament complex. (Copyright A. Watts.)

pMCL. In all of these situations, the lateral ligamentous complex and common extensor origin are an important contributor to the instability that is observed because of the primary importance of the soft tissues to stability on the lateral side of the joint.

Not all isolated lateral ligament avulsions will be symptomatic and many go unrecognized. If the patient has low or routine daily functional demands, is comfortable, and is moving the elbow well without mechanical symptoms, then a trial of nonoperative treatment is reasonable. In those patients with lateral elbow pain, bruising, locking, or elbow stiffness unimproved with therapy, further investigation with MRI or MR arthrography is helpful in making the diagnosis. In cases of PMRI, an MRI scan may be more useful than a CT as the extent of soft tissue disruption is more easily determined. Both MRI and CT will identify the extent of the fracture and the congruency of the ulnohumeral joint.

Posterolateral Rotatory Instability

PLRI is a valgus compression external rotation (supination) instability of the elbow as a result of insufficiency of the lateral soft tissue stabilizers of the elbow, which allow the radial head to subluxate dorsally and laterally on the capitellum.[18] It is the most common chronic instability seen in the elbow. It is typically caused by trauma such as a fall onto an outstretched hand, but other causes include chronic cubitus varus and iatrogenic causes, including steroid injections or surgery such as tennis elbow release or distal humerus osteosynthesis.[45] The patient will typically present with complaints of lateral elbow pain and clicking or locking of the elbow. The posterior drawer test is typically painful and shows an increase in posterior displacement of the radial head on the capitellum.[46,47] The tabletop test and push-up test are positive in which the patient has more pain in forearm supination than pronation when pushing up from a table or chair, respectively.[48] The tabletop relocation test is performed by asking the patient to repeat the tabletop bench press in pronation with the examiner's thumb supporting the posterior radial head, thus should prevent

subluxation and relieve pain.[49] In the acute setting, only the posterior draw is likely to be tolerated and even here the instability may be masked by swelling and guarding.

MRI is the most reliable tool to assess the injury in the acute setting and in most cases will show peel back of the lateral ligament complex from the distal humerus, sometimes extending into the common extensor origin (Fig. 39.8). In 5%–10% of cases, the ligament complex will be avulsed from the supinator crest, often with a sliver of bone that may be identified on CT scan.[50]

When recognized in the acute setting, repair can be performed as an open or arthroscopic procedure. The open repair can be done with the patient supine with the arm on an arm table, or in a lateral decubitus position with the elbow over a bolster. A straight incision is made over the lateral epicondyle. There will frequently be a rent in the tough lateral fascia. If not present, a straight incision through this layer will reveal the tendon and ligament avulsion that can be easily repaired back to the lateral epicondyle with sutures and a bone anchor or bone tunnels. The forearm should be held in pronation at around 45 degrees of flexion without any varus force as the repair is undertaken in order to ensure that the radial head subluxation is reduced. Recheck the posterior drawer to ensure that the stability is restored. If it is not, it may be necessary to examine the posterior capitellum for a posterolateral ligament avulsion and repair this where necessary. Any additional bony injury should be addressed as necessary.

Arthroscopic repair can be performed using a proximal lateral and direct lateral portal or with a 70-degree arthroscope viewing from the anteromedial portal and instrumenting through an accessory lateral portal placed just posterior to the capitellum. Sutures can be passed through the avulsed ligament with the aid of a suture passer and loaded onto an anchor that is placed in the center of the lateral condyle. Positioning of this anchor is challenging and can be aided by the use of fluoroscopy. Radial head fractures and coronoid fractures can be managed arthroscopically in experienced hands. Fractures of the anterolateral coronoid facet, associated with a radial head fracture, that do not extend to involve the

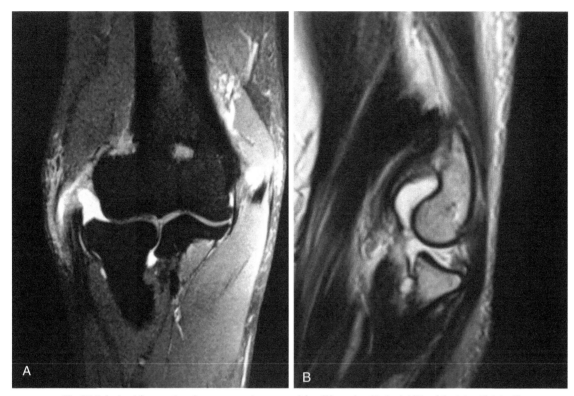

• **Fig. 39.8** Lateral ligament and common extensor avulsion (A) can lead to instability of the lateral joint with dorsal subluxation of the radial head (B). (Copyright A. Watts.)

anteromedial coronoid facet do not need to be addressed as long as radial head and lateral ligament complex function are restored.[51] Complications of surgery include persistent instability, elbow stiffness, heterotopic ossification, and nerve injury.

Chronic injuries, those presenting >6 weeks after the trauma, can be addressed with direct repair if, with careful dissection, the lateral ligament can be mobilized back to the lateral epicondyle. However, more frequently the insufficiency of the lateral soft tissues requires reconstruction with a graft.[52] The choice of graft and technique for reconstruction is open to the surgeon as there is no evidence of superiority of one over the other. The options are to use autograft, allograft, synthetic graft, or composites. Fixation can be through bone tunnels, with anchors, buttons, or interference screws. This procedure is performed through a lateral anconeus interval approach. Rehabilitation is as for a direct repair with immediate active mobilization with the patient lying supine, shoulder flexed to 90 degrees, and forearm in neutral. The arm can be rested in a sling after surgery for up to 6 weeks. There is no proven benefit from the use of splints or braces. The recovery period to return to competitive sport is between 4 and 6 months.

Recurrent instability occurs in 0%–15% of cases.[53,54] In these cases, consider the possible causes including primary surgical technique, the choice of graft, loss of graft fixation, associated bone loss to radial head and coronoid, associated posterolateral ligament avulsion with or without posterior capitellum bone defect (Osborne-Cotterill lesion), and reinjury. A large Osborne-Cotterill lesion can be addressed with remplissage using an anchor to secure the posterolateral capsule into the floor of the bone defect.

Posteromedial Rotatory Instability

PMRI, better termed posteromedial elbow fracture dislocation, is an osseoligamentous injury with a fracture of the anteromedial

facet of the coronoid process with or without extension into the sublime tubercle, lateral ligament complex sleeve avulsion, and possible posterior band of the medial ligament avulsion injury.[46] This is a Type A injury in the Wrightington classification of elbow fracture dislocation (Fig. 39.9).[55] As with all fracture-dislocations, there is variability in the extent of the involvement of the coronoid and the soft tissue stabilizers depending on the injury mechanism and energy applied to the elbow. The injury is sustained as a result of a fall backwards onto a pronated hand such that the forearm subluxates into varus and internal rotation on the humerus driving the medial trochlea ridge through the anteromedial facet of the coronoid process. The patient will often report that they landed on top of their arm which was stuck behind their back. The unstable PMRI will present with an ability to extend the elbow but an inability to flex beyond 90 degrees. With the shoulder held in abduction at 90 degrees, active elbow flexion and extension is frequently associated with a palpable crepitus.[56,57] In extension, the elbow may have a varus carrying angle. Plain lateral elbow radiographs will demonstrate a coronoid fracture with intact radial head. Careful interpretation of the anteroposterior elbow radiograph will often reveal a "delta sign" with narrowing of the joint space between the coronoid and medial trochlea condyle due to joint subluxation (Fig. 39.10). In some instances, the elbow joint may be dislocated but with a telltale coronoid fragment sitting anterior to the trochlea. These are often reported as "a simple dislocation with a flake avulsion of the coronoid" but this is a misinterpretation and these elbows are at risk of severe persistent instability that can result in rapid cartilage damage and arthrosis.[58]

There is little consensus on the management, not all will require surgical stabilization, but identification of those that do is problematic. Clearly, a joint that is subluxated or dislocated after closed reduction will require surgical stabilization. Foruria et al. report assessing the stability based on the congruity of the

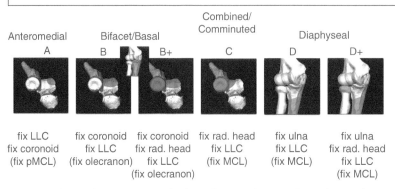

| Wrightington Classification Elbow Fracture Dislocation |

| Anteromedial | Bifacet/Basal | | Combined/
Comminuted | Diaphyseal | |
| A | B | B+ | C | D | D+ |

fix LLC
fix coronoid
(fix pMCL)

fix coronoid
fix LLC
(fix olecranon)

fix coronoid
fix rad. head
fix LLC
(fix olecranon)

fix rad. head
fix LLC
(fix MCL)

fix ulna
fix LLC
(fix MCL)

fix ulna
fix rad. head
fix LLC
(fix MCL)

• **Fig. 39.9** The Wrightington classification of elbow fracture-dislocation. *LLC*, lateral ligament complex; *MCL*, medial collateral ligament; *pMCL*, posterior band of the medial collateral ligament. (Copyright A. Watts.)

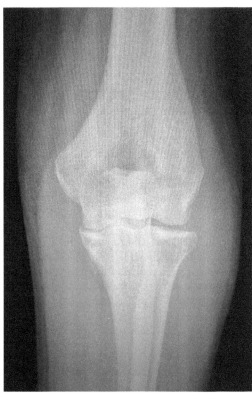

• **Fig. 39.10** Typical X-ray appearance of a posteromedial rotatory instability pattern injury (Wrightington A) with anteromedial facet fracture and intact radial head. Note the apparent widening of the joint from medial to lateral (delta sign) caused by subluxation of the joint into varus. (Copyright A. Watts.)

ulnohumeral joint on CT scan.[13] If the joint is not subluxated, then they advocate nonoperative treatment and report satisfactory outcomes in the majority of these patients. The CT, however, is a snapshot static image of a dynamic instability and it is not clear how reliable this approach is. An alternative is to perform MRI examination to assess the degree of soft tissue disruption, the size of the coronoid defect, and the joint incongruity. If the scan indicates disruption of the soft tissue stabilizers, particularly the lateral ligamentous complex, and the coronoid anteromedial facet, then surgical stabilization would be indicated to avoid persistent instability leading to rapid arthrosis for which there is no simple

solution. In cases where the ligaments are intact and the joint is congruent, these patients can be managed nonoperatively with a concomitant coronoid fracture.

Stabilization can be performed as an open or arthroscopic procedure in a stepwise fashion from the lateral ligament to the anteromedial coronoid process and lastly the posterior band of the medial ligament, until stability is restored. In some cases. with small bone fragments, repair of the lateral ligament alone will suffice.[29,34] With the patient supine on the operating table and arm on an arm table, open repair of the lateral ligament complex can be performed through a straight lateral incision over the lateral epicondyle as described previously. A separate medial incision is made to approach the coronoid using a Hotchkiss approach or an approach through the bed of the ulnar nerve. The latter approach is directed towards the sublime tubercle but can make access to the anteromedial facet more challenging and carries a risk of adhesion of the ulnar nerve that can result in neuropathy or neurogenic joint stiffness. The "over-the-top" Hotchkiss approach between flexor carpi ulnaris and palmaris longus exploits an internervous plane but does not have a clean plane of dissection, instead the muscle fibers have to be split and elevated from the medial ligament and joint capsule (Fig. 39.11). The interval for dissection is indicated by a fascial condensation, and a perforation vessel can often be found piercing the fascia at this interval. The dissection is limited distally by the recurrent ulnar artery but proximally the dissection can be continued through the common flexor origin proximally up the humeral shaft, if required, to give good exposure of the coronoid. Fixation with a buttress plate or screws can be performed. If the coronoid is multifragmentary, it is preferable to perform an extracapsular dissection and to use a buttress plate over the top of the fragments and capsule to maintain stability and vitality of the bone fragments. In rare cases, the coronoid may not be amenable to osteosynthesis in which case reconstruction can be performed with allograft or autograft harvested from the olecranon process, iliac crest, or rib costochondral junction.[59–61]

Smaller anteromedial coronoid fragments can be fixed arthroscopically using threaded K-wires, cannulated screws, or headless compression screws passed over a guidewire from the dorsal ulna cortex aimed proximally and ventrally towards the fracture fragment (Fig. 39.12).[62,63] The fragment is held reduced using a probe as the wire is advanced. The lateral ligament complex can be repaired arthroscopically using the techniques previously described in this chapter.[34]

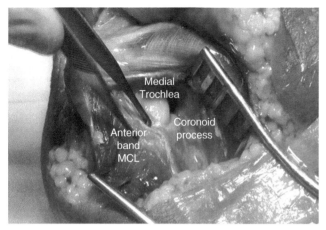

• **Fig. 39.11** The "over-the-top" Hotchkiss approach to the coronoid through a muscle split between flexor carpi ulnaris and palmaris longus. The forceps are holding the anterior band of the medial collateral ligament (MCL) that is usually intact in a posteromedial rotatory instability pattern of elbow fracture-dislocation. (Copyright A. Watts.)

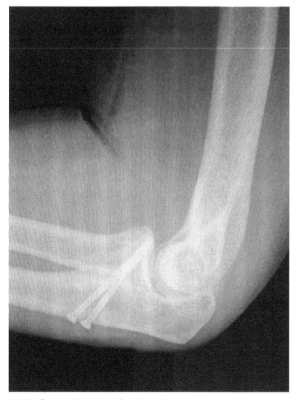

• **Fig. 39.12** Coronoid fracture fixation with two cannulated screws passed from the dorsal cortex ventrally and proximally for maximum purchase and biomechanical advantage. (Copyright A. Watts.)

References

1. Shin S-H, Jeon I-H, Kim H-J, et al. Articular surface area of the coronoid process and radial head in elbow extension: surface ratio in cadavers and a computed tomography study in vivo. *J Hand Surg.* 2010;35(7):1120–1125.
2. O'Driscoll SW, Jupiter JB, King GJW, Hotchkiss RN, Morrey BF. The unstable elbow. *J Bone Jt Surg.* 2000;82(5):724.
3. Dunning CE, Zarzour ZDS, Patterson SD, Johnson JA, King GJW. Ligamentous stabilizers against posterolateral rotatory instability of the elbow. *J Bone Jt Surg-Am.* 2001;83(12):1823–1828.
4. Edwards DS, Arshad MS, Luokkala T, Kedgley AE, Watts AC. The contribution of the posterolateral capsule to elbow joint stability: a cadaveric biomechanical investigation. *J Shoulder Elbow Surg.* 2018;27(7):1178–1184.
5. Petrie S, Collins JG, Solomonow M, Wink C, Chuinard R, D'Ambrosia R. Mechanoreceptors in the human elbow ligaments. *J Hand Surg.* 1998;23(3):512–518.
6. Basmajian JV, Griffin WR. Function of anconeus muscle. An electromyographic study. *J Bone Joint Surg Am.* 1972;54(8):1712–1714.
7. Miguel-Andres I, Alonso-Rasgado T, Walmsley A, Watts AC. Effect of anconeus muscle blocking on elbow kinematics: electromyographic, inertial sensors and finite element study. *Ann Biomed Eng.* 2017;45(3):775–788.
8. Schnetzke M, Aytac S, Studier-Fischer S, Grützner P-A, Guehring T. Initial joint stability affects the outcome after conservative treatment of simple elbow dislocations: a retrospective study. *J Orthop Surg [Internet].* 2015;10(1):128. http://josr-online.biomedcentral.com/articles/10.1186/s13018-015-0273-x.
9. Schnetzke M, Aytac S, Keil H, et al. Unstable simple elbow dislocations: medium-term results after non-surgical and surgical treatment. *Knee Surg Sports Traumatol Arthrosc.* 2017;25(7):2271–2279.
10. Anakwe RE, Middleton SD, Jenkins PJ, McQueen MM, Court-Brown CM. Patient-reported outcomes after simple dislocation of the elbow. *J Bone Jt Surg-Am.* 2011;93(13):1220–1226.
11. Luokkala T, Temperley D, Basu S, Karjalainen TV, Watts AC. Analysis of magnetic resonance imaging–confirmed soft tissue injury pattern in simple elbow dislocations. *J Shoulder Elbow Surg.* 2019;28(2):341–348.
12. Coonrad RW, Roush TF, Major NM, Basamania CJ. The drop sign, a radiographic warning sign of elbow instability. *J Shoulder Elbow Surg.* 2005;14(3):312–317.
13. Foruria AM, Gutiérrez B, Cobos J, Haeni DL, Valencia M, Calvo E. Most coronoid fractures and fracture-dislocations with no radial head involvement can be treated nonsurgically with elbow immobilization. *J Shoulder Elbow Surg.* 2019;28(7):1395–1405.
14. Adolfsson LE, Nestorson JO, Scheer JH. Extensive soft tissue lesions in redislocated after simple elbow dislocations. *J Shoulder Elbow Surg.* 2017;26(7):1294–1297.
15. Tyrdal S, Olsen BS. Hyperextension of the elbow joint: patho-anatomy and kinematics of ligament injuries. *J Shoulder Elbow Surg.* 1998;7(3):272–283.
16. Hariri S, Safran MR. Ulnar collateral ligament injury in the overhead athlete. *Clin Sports Med.* 2010;29(4):619–644.
17. O'Driscoll SWM, Lawton RL, Smith AM. The "moving valgus stress test" for medial collateral ligament tears of the elbow. *Am J Sports Med.* 2005;33(2):231–239.
18. O'Driscoll SW, Bell DF, Morrey BF. Posterolateral rotatory instability of the elbow. *J Bone Joint Surg Am.* 1991;73(3):440–446.
19. O'Driscoll SW, Jupiter JB, Cohen MS, Ring D, McKee MD. Difficult elbow fractures: pearls and pitfalls. *Instr Course Lect.* 2003;52:113–134.
20. Schwartz ML, al-Zahrani S, Morwessel RM, Andrews JR. Ulnar collateral ligament injury in the throwing athlete: evaluation with saline-enhanced MR arthrography. *Radiology.* 1995;197(1):297–299.
21. Timmerman LA, Andrews JR. Undersurface tear of the ulnar collateral ligament in baseball players: a newly recognized lesion. *Am J Sports Med.* 1994;22(1):33–36.
22. Joyner PW, Bruce J, Hess R, Mates A, Mills FB, Andrews JR. Magnetic resonance imaging–based classification for ulnar collateral ligament injuries of the elbow. *J Shoulder Elbow Surg.* 2016;25(10):1710–1716.
23. Robinson PM, Griffiths E, Watts AC. Simple elbow dislocation. *Shoulder Elb.* 2017;9(3):195–204.
24. Eygendaal D, Verdegaal SH, Obermann WR, van Vugt AB, Pöll RG, Rozing PM. Posterolateral dislocation of the elbow joint. Relationship to medial instability. *J Bone Joint Surg Am.* 2000;82(4):555–560.

25. O'Driscoll SW, Morrey BF, Korinek S, An KN. Elbow subluxation and dislocation. A spectrum of instability. *Clin Orthop.* 1992;280:186–197.

26. Rhyou IH, Kim YS. New mechanism of the posterior elbow dislocation. *Knee Surg Sports Traumatol Arthrosc.* 2012;20(12):2535–2541.

27. Josefsson PO, Johnell O, Wendeberg B. Ligamentous injuries in dislocations of the elbow joint. *Clin Orthop.* 1987;(221):221–225.

28. Schreiber JJ, Potter HG, Warren RF, Hotchkiss RN, Daluiski A. Magnetic resonance imaging findings in acute elbow dislocation: insight into mechanism. *J Hand Surg.* 2014;39(2):199–205.

29. Schreiber JJ, Paul S, Hotchkiss RN, Daluiski A. Conservative management of elbow dislocations with an overhead motion protocol. *J Hand Surg.* 2015;40(3):515–519.

30. Lee AT, Schrumpf MA, Choi D, et al. The influence of gravity on the unstable elbow. *J Shoulder Elbow Surg.* 2013;22(1):81–87.

31. Ferreira LM, King GJW, Johnson JA. In-vitro quantification of medial collateral ligament tension in the elbow. *J Appl Biomech.* 2017;33(4):277–281.

32. Watts AC. Primary ligament repair for acute elbow dislocation. *JBJS Essent Surg Tech.* 2019;9(1):e8.

33. Savoie III FH, O'Brien MJ, Field LD, Gurley DJ. Arthroscopic and open radial ulnohumeral ligament reconstruction for posterolateral rotatory instability of the elbow. *Clin Sports Med.* 2010;29(4):611–618.

34. Rashid A, Copas D, Granville-Chapman J, Watts A. Arthroscopically-assisted fixation of anteromedial coronoid facet fracture and lateral ulnar collateral ligament repair for acute posteromedial rotatory fracture dislocation of the elbow. *Shoulder Elb.* 2017;11(5):378–383. https://doi.org/10.1177/1758573217738138.

35. Josefsson PO, Gentz CF, Johnell O, Wendeberg B. Surgical versus non-surgical treatment of ligamentous injuries following dislocation of the elbow joint. A prospective randomized study. *J Bone Joint Surg Am.* 1987;69(4):605–608.

36. Yoon MY, Koris MJ, Ortiz JA, Papandrea RF. Triceps avulsion, radial head fracture, and medial collateral ligament rupture about the elbow: a report of 4 cases. *J Shoulder Elbow Surg.* 2012;21(2):e12–e17.

37. Podesta L, Crow SA, Volkmer D, Bert T, Yocum LA. Treatment of partial ulnar collateral ligament tears in the elbow with platelet-rich plasma. *Am J Sports Med.* 2013;41(7):1689–1694.

38. Dines JS, Williams PN, ElAttrache N, et al. Platelet-rich plasma can be used to successfully treat elbow ulnar collateral ligament insufficiency in high-level throwers. *Am J Orthop Belle Mead NJ.* 2016;45(5):296–300.

39. Norwood LA, Shook JA, Andrews JR. Acute medial elbow ruptures. *Am J Sports Med.* 1981;9(1):16–19.

40. Hotchkiss RN, Kasparyan GN. The medial "over the top" approach to the elbow. *Tech Orthop.* 2000;15(2):105–112.

41. Manocha RH, King GJW, Johnson JA. In vitro kinematic assessment of a hinged elbow orthosis following lateral collateral ligament injury. *J Hand Surg.* 2018;43(2):123–132.

42. Osborne G, Cotterill P. Recurrent dislocation of the elbow. *J Bone Joint Surg Br.* 1966;48(2):340–346.

43. Jeon I-H, Micic ID, Yamamoto N, Morrey BF. Osborne-Cotterill lesion: an osseous defect of the capitellum associated with instability of the elbow. *Am J Roentgenol.* 2008;191(3):727–729.

44. van Riet RP. Arthroscopic lateral collateral ligament imbrication. In: Bain G, Eygendaal D, van Riet RP, eds. *Surgical Techniques for Trauma and Sports Related Injuries of the Elbow [Internet].* Berlin, Heidelberg: Springer; 2020:263–267. http://link.springer.com/10.1007/978-3-662-58931-1_35.

45. O'Driscoll SW, Spinner RJ, McKee MD, et al. Tardy posterolateral rotatory instability of the elbow due to cubitus varus. *J Bone Jt Surg-Am.* 2001;83(9):1358–1369.

46. O'Driscoll SW, Jupiter JB, King GJ, Hotchkiss RN, Morrey BF. The unstable elbow. *Instr Course Lect.* 2001;50:89–102.

47. Anakwenze OA, Kancherla VK, Iyengar J, Ahmad CS, Levine WN. Posterolateral rotatory instability of the elbow. *Am J Sports Med.* 2014;42(2):485–491.

48. Regan W, Lapner PC. Prospective evaluation of two diagnostic apprehension signs for posterolateral instability of the elbow. *J Shoulder Elbow Surg.* 2006;15(3):344–346.

49. Arvind CHV, Hargreaves DG. Table top relocation test—new clinical test for posterolateral rotatory instability of the elbow. *J Shoulder Elbow Surg.* 2006;15(4):500–501.

50. Schmidt-Horlohé K, Wilde P, Kim Y-J, Bonk A, Hoffmann R. Avulsion fracture of the supinator crest of the proximal ulna in the context of elbow joint injuries. *Int Orthop.* 2013;37(10):1957–1963.

51. Papatheodorou LK, Rubright JH, Heim KA, Weiser RW, Sotereanos DG. Terrible triad injuries of the elbow: does the coronoid always need to be fixed? *Clin Orthop Relat Res.* 2014;472(7):2084–2091.

52. Daluiski A, Schrumpf MA, Schreiber JJ, Nguyen JT, Hotchkiss RN. Direct repair for managing acute and chronic lateral ulnar collateral ligament disruptions. *J Hand Surg.* 2014;39(6):1125–1129.

53. Kim BS, Park KH, Song HS, Park S-Y. Ligamentous repair of acute lateral collateral ligament rupture of the elbow. *J Shoulder Elbow Surg.* 2013;22(11):1469–1473.

54. Sanchez-Sotelo J, Morrey BF, O'Driscoll SW. Ligamentous repair and reconstruction for posterolateral rotatory instability of the elbow. *J Bone Joint Surg Br.* 2005;87(1):54–61.

55. Watts AC, Singh J, Elvey M, Hamoodi Z. Current concepts in elbow fracture dislocation. *Shoulder Elb.* 2019;13. 175857321988401.

56. Ramirez MA, Stein JA, Murthi AM. Varus posteromedial instability. *Hand Clin.* 2015;31(4):557–563.

57. Pollock JW, Brownhill J, Ferreira L, McDonald CP, Johnson J, King G. The effect of anteromedial facet fractures of the coronoid and lateral collateral ligament injury on elbow stability and kinematics. *J Bone Jt Surg-Am.* 2009;91(6):1448–1458.

58. Bellato E, Fitzsimmons JS, Kim Y, et al. Articular contact area and pressure in posteromedial rotatory instability of the elbow. *J Bone Jt Surg.* 2018;100(6):e34.

59. Papandrea RF, Morrey BF, O'Driscoll SW. Reconstruction for persistent instability of the elbow after coronoid fracture-dislocation. *J Shoulder Elbow Surg.* 2007;16(1):68–77.

60. Alolabi B, Gray A, Ferreira LM, Johnson JA, Athwal GS, King GJ. Reconstruction of the coronoid process using the tip of the ipsilateral olecranon. *J Bone Jt Surg-Am.* 2014;96(7):590–596.

61. Bain G, Doornberg JN. Coronoid process reconstruction. In: Bain G, Eygendaal D, van Riet RP, eds. *Surgical Techniques for Trauma and Sports Related Injuries of the Elbow [Internet].* Berlin, Heidelberg: Springer; 2020:313–320. http://link.springer.com/10.1007/978-3-662-58931-1_41.

62. Adams JE, Merten SM, Steinmann SP. Arthroscopic-assisted treatment of coronoid fractures. *Arthrosc J Arthrosc Relat Surg.* 2007;23(10):1060–1065.

63. Hausman MR, Klug RA, Qureshi S, Goldstein R, Parsons BO. Arthroscopically assisted coronoid fracture fixation: a preliminary report. *Clin Orthop.* 2008;466(12):3147–3152.

40

Technique Spotlight: Lateral Ulnar Collateral Ligament Repair

ZACHARY J. FINLEY, MICHAEL J. O'BRIEN, AND FELIX H. SAVOIE

Introduction

Injuries to the lateral ulnar collateral ligament (LUCL) of the elbow can be caused by simple elbow dislocations as well as complex trauma, or unfortunately, from iatrogenic injury. Simple elbow dislocations can often be treated successfully with bracing and rehabilitation.[1] However, failure of the LUCL to heal can lead to varus and posterolateral rotatory instability (PLRI) of the elbow. Simple activities of daily living, such as pushing up from a chair or lifting objects with the elbow extended, become painful and difficult, not to mention the more demanding forces exerted across the elbow in sports such as wrestling, gymnastics, and football.[1,2]

Indications

Indications for surgical treatment of an LUCL injury include pain and functional impairment despite appropriate nonoperative management.[3,4] In cases where initial radiographs reveal a bony avulsion of the LCL complex proximally off of the posterior lateral epicondyle of the humerus, acute surgical treatment may be indicated. Acute repair may also be indicated in high-level athletes who cannot afford to miss large portions of the athletic season. In the chronic setting, the LUCL is unlikely to heal in its native origin making bracing a less effective treatment option. As a result, surgical repair is typically indicated. This can be performed either open or arthroscopically. While arthroscopic repair can be technically challenging, it can provide excellent visualization of the LCL complex and articular surfaces as repair is performed.

Arthroscopic Repair

In the elbow with an acute PLRI, repair of the avulsed LUCL complex can be efficacious in restoring stability. This repair can be performed arthroscopically, our preferred method, or open. Arthroscopy of the acutely injured elbow demands efficiency and precision, as tearing of the capsule will allow fluid extravasation and swelling. A concrete preoperative plan must be formulated and followed with adjustments made for arthroscopic findings. We perform this procedure in the prone position with a nonsterile tourniquet on the upper arm. The operative extremity is positioned with the elbow flexed over an arm board attached to the side of the bed, with the upper arm resting on a bump of rolled sheets (Fig. 40.1). A list of equipment used can be found in Table 40.1. The procedure begins with the establishment of a proximal anterior medial portal and a diagnostic arthroscopy of the anterior compartment. Fractures of the radial head or coronoid can be identified. In the acute setting, abundant hematoma will be encountered in the joint and tearing of

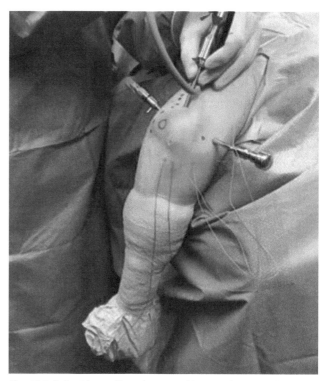

• **Fig. 40.1** Patient is positioned prone with operative extremity over an arm board. The arthroscope is positioned in a posterior transtendinous portal, with water inflow in an anteromedial portal and a cannula in a lateral soft-spot portal.

TABLE 40.1	Equipment for Arthroscopic Treatment
• Sterile tourniquet	
• 18-gauge spinal needle	
• Motorized shaver	
• Rasp	
• Hewson suture passer	
• No. 2 braided, nonabsorbable suture	
• Double- or triple-loaded suture anchors	
• 4-mm 30-degree arthroscope	
• Interchangeable arthroscopic cannulas	
• Retrograde suture retriever	
• Suture grasper	
• Arthroscopic knot pusher	
• Suture for skin closure (surgeon's preference)	
• Dressing and splint material	

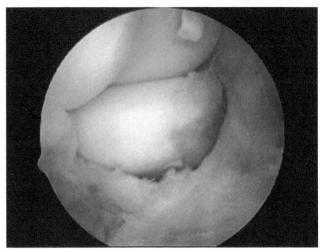

• **Fig. 40.3** View of the radiocapitellar joint in the anterior compartment from a proximal anteromedial viewing portal, demonstrating laxity of the annular ligament. The annular ligament droops down to the radial neck with gapping between the ligament and radial head, signifying incompetence of the lateral ulnar collateral ligament complex. This finding is present in every case of posterolateral rotatory instability. Tightening of the annular ligament following repair is one sign of an adequate repair.

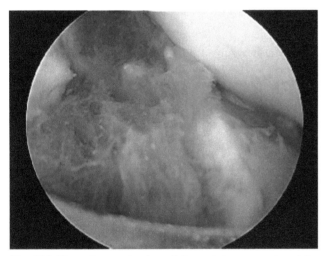

• **Fig. 40.2** The arthroscopic view of the anterior compartment from the proximal anteromedial portal demonstrating the tip of the coronoid and subluxated ulnohumeral articulation, with torn anterior capsule and exposed brachialis muscle as often noted in acute dislocations.

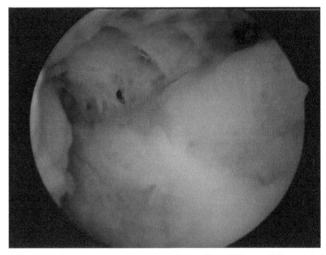

• **Fig. 40.4** After an elbow dislocation, the tearing of the medial capsule is evidence of acute instability. The view is of the posteromedial gutter from a posterior viewing portal.

the anterior capsule is readily apparent. One can often see the damage to the brachialis muscle through the torn capsule (Fig. 40.2). A proximal anterior lateral portal can be positioned to clean out the associated hematoma.

On the lateral side, laxity of the annular ligament and LCL complex will be evident in every case (Fig. 40.3). Occasionally, the LCL complex will be flipped into the radiocapitellar joint. It is important to view the annular ligament for damage and place a suture in it if necessary. Valgus load and forearm supination demonstrates PLRI with the radial head subluxating off the capitellum, indicative of injury to the LUCL. On the medial side, an arthroscopic valgus stress test can be performed to evaluate the incompetence of the medial ulnar collateral ligament. During evacuation of the hematoma, great care is taken not to resect or damage the LCL complex.

The arthroscope is then placed into the posterior central portal, and the hematoma in the posterior compartment of the elbow is evacuated via a proximal posterior lateral portal. Both of these portals need to be relatively proximal to allow for the later repair of the ligament, usually at least 3 cm above the olecranon tip. A view of the medial gutter will show hemorrhage and occasional tearing of the capsule near the posterior aspect of the medial epicondyle (Fig. 40.4).

One common finding is the ability to move an arthroscope placed down the posterolateral gutter from the posterior central portal straight across the ulnohumeral articulation into the medial gutter. This maneuver is not possible in a stable elbow and is termed the "drive-through sign of the elbow" (Fig. 40.5). It is somewhat analogous to the "drive-through sign" in shoulder instability. The elimination of the laxity that allows this maneuver is one of the key aspects of confirming an adequate arthroscopic repair in patients with PLRI.

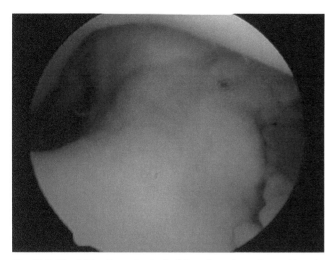

• **Fig. 40.5** The "drive-through sign" of the elbow is performed by placing the arthroscope into the posterolateral gutter and moving it straight across the ulnohumeral articulation into the medial gutter. In this view, the arthroscope is in the ulnohumeral articulation from a posterior transtendon portal, with the distal humerus at the top of the image, and the articular cartilage of the olecranon at the bottom of the image.

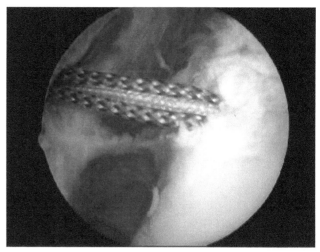

• **Fig. 40.7** A suture anchor is placed percutaneously at the avulsion site of the lateral ulnar collateral ligament (LUCL) on the posterior aspect of the lateral epicondyle of the humerus. The humeral origin of the LUCL is just lateral and distal to the olecranon fossa of the humerus. The arthroscope is in a posterior transtendon viewing portal.

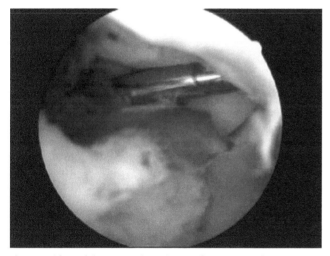

• **Fig. 40.6** View of the posterolateral gutter from a posterior transtendon portal, demonstrating the lateral ulnar collateral ligament (LUCL) avulsed from the lateral epicondyle of the humerus and sitting posterior to the radiocapitellar joint. The shaver is coming in through a soft-spot portal. Great care must be taken when using the shaver so as not to damage or resect the LUCL.

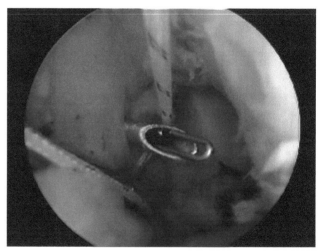

• **Fig. 40.8** This image demonstrates passing sutures through the healthy portion of the lateral ulnar collateral ligament during arthroscopic repair. The view is of the posterolateral gutter from a posterior transtendon viewing portal, with a suture passer entering through the soft-spot portal and piercing the healthy portion of the ligament.

The lateral gutter and capsule are evaluated next. The arthroscope is easily advanced down the lateral gutter, owing to incompetence of the LCL complex. It is very important to stay close to the ulna as the lateral gutter is evaluated and the hematoma debrided, as the avulsed ligament and bone fragments are displaced distally and may inadvertently be removed by the shaver. The origin of the LCL complex on the posterior aspect of the lateral epicondyle can be visualized as a bare area where the ligament has avulsed off of the humerus. It is usually directly lateral and slightly inferior to the center of the olecranon fossa. This area on the posterior humerus should be lightly debrided with a motorized shaver (Fig. 40.6).

Once the area of damage has been defined, an arthroscopic anchor may be placed into the humerus at the site of origin of the LUCL (Fig. 40.7). We do not use fluoroscopy for anchor placement in this setting as the arthroscope allows direct visualization of the LUCL origin. A percutaneous suture passer is placed through a "soft-spot" portal to retrieve the sutures. The limbs of the suture are retrieved to place two horizontal mattress sutures through the noninjured part of the ligament (Fig. 40.8). In the case of a bony avulsion, place one set of sutures around the bone fragment and the other distal to the fragment. The sutures are tensioned while viewing with the arthroscope down the lateral gutter, which should have the effect of pushing the arthroscope out of the lateral gutter as tension is restored to the LCL complex. The elbow is extended to approximately 30 degrees and the sutures are tied beneath the anconeus muscle, tightening the ligament. Motion and stability are evaluated with the arthroscope back in the anterior compartment, confirming that tension has been restored to the annular ligament (Fig. 40.9).

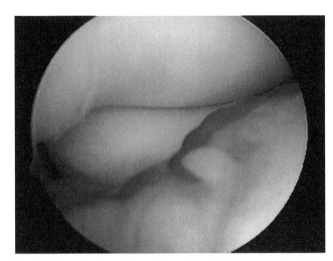

• **Fig. 40.9** Anterior view of the radiocapitellar joint from a proximal antero-medial viewing portal following lateral ulnar collateral ligament repair, demonstrating the tension has been restored to the annular ligament. The arthroscope should routinely be placed back in the anterior compartment following repair to confirm adequate tension to the annular ligament.

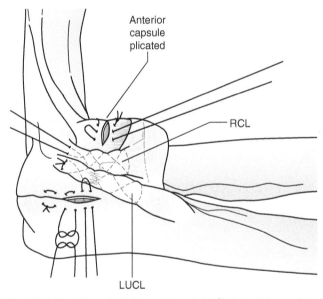

• **Fig. 40.10** Illustration of plication and repair. *LUCL*, lateral ulnar collateral ligament; *RCL*, radial collateral ligament.

Open Technique

In cases where ligament quality is uncertain or in cases where the normal anatomy is distorted (trauma, congenital deformity), the open approach may be preferable. When performing an open repair of the LUCL, a diagnostic arthroscopy may be performed to confirm the presence of instability and the absence of associated pathology, such as loose osteochondral fragments. A posterolateral approach is used, and the anconeus muscle split is retracted anteriorly to access the LUCL complex. The lateral pivot-shift examination maneuver can be used to identify loose areas of the capsule and LUCL. Plication sutures are placed in the redundant areas of the capsule and left untied. The LUCL is then examined, and if found to be detached or stretched, can be repaired using a suture anchor at the LUCL origin on the posterior inferior portion of the lateral epicondyle (Fig. 40.10). We usually place the forearm in pronation and hold the elbow flexed at 30–45 degrees for suture

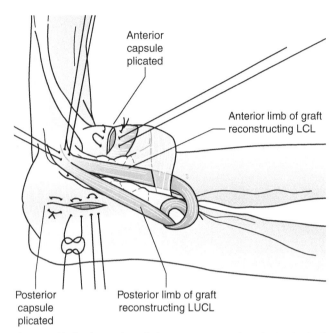

• **Fig. 40.11** If plication and repair does not restore adequate tension to the lateral collateral ligament *(LCL)* complex, open anatomic ligament reconstruction can be performed, as illustrated here. *LUCL*, lateral ulnar collateral ligament.

tightening. We then flex the elbow to 90 degrees while observing the repair to ensure we can regain full motion postoperatively. Capsular plication sutures are then tied down after the repair is complete, tensioning as necessary.

In revision surgery, or in patients with inadequate tissue for repair, a palmaris autograft or gracilis allograft may be used to reconstruct the lateral ligament complex. The supinator crest of the ulna, just posterior to the radial neck, is dissected free and the insertion site identified. A 4-mm bone tunnel is created at the supinator crest, at the ulnar attachment of the LUCL, and the midportion of the graft is secured into the ulna using an interference screw technique. Alternatively, two 4-mm tunnels can be created, leaving a minimum 1 cm of bony bridge in between the tunnels, and one limb of the graft can be passed through the tunnels. This also allows both limbs of the graft to be brought proximally. The two free graft limbs are then brought proximally, pulling one under the annular ligament and one over the ligament, and attached to the isometric point on the posterior aspect of the lateral epicondyle (Fig. 40.11). There are many techniques to fix the graft to the humerus. This may include a blind-ended socket with exit holes to allow the sutures for each end of the graft to be tied over a bone bridge, a single socket with a hole in the posterolateral humerus to allow passage of the sutures that can be tied over a button on the posterior humerus, and so on. Bringing one limb of the graft under the annular ligament creates a more anatomic reconstruction, with the added benefit of increasing stability of the proximal radioulnar joint. The graft should be slightly lax in extension and tighten with flexion.[5]

Postoperative Management

Following repair, patients are immediately placed into a splint or hinged brace with the elbow in approximately 30 degrees of extension to relax tension on the repair. Fluoroscopy or radiographs should be obtained to check the reduction after the splint or brace is applied, as additional flexion may be necessary to tighten the reconstruction and keep the joint reduced. The first postoperative visit usually takes place within 3–5 days of the surgery, and the patient is placed into a hinged elbow brace that allows comfortable movement, usually 0–45 degrees. Motion with the elbow at the side is permitted while the patient is instructed not to lift the arm away from the body (shoulder abduction) as this can place stress on the repair in the acute setting. Shoulder, periscapular, wrist, and hand exercises are allowed as long as they do not produce pain in the elbow.

The patient is then seen at 2-week intervals and motion slowly increased 10–20 degrees per week as pain and swelling allow. Physical therapy is initiated at 6–8 weeks postoperatively to include upper extremity and core strengthening exercises with the elbow brace in place. Full range of motion of the elbow should be obtained by 8 weeks, if not sooner. Depending on individual progression, patients are allowed to start strengthening exercises out of the brace at 10–12 weeks. They must be able to perform all strengthening exercises pain-free in the brace, before progression out of the brace.

PEARLS AND PITFALLS

- Arthroscopic repair allows for direct visualization of the LCL complex, articular surface, and more precise anchor placement.
- Early surgical repair may allow for a faster return to play when compared with conservative treatment for high-level athletes.
- A concrete preoperative plan allows for speed and precision when performing arthroscopic repair.
- Unnecessary steps and wasted time during arthroscopic repair can lead to fluid extravasation and swelling, making the procedure more challenging.
- Ensure posterior central portal and proximal posterior lateral portal are at least 3 cm proximal to the olecranon tip to allow for repair.
- Arthroscopic repair of the LUCL should have the effect of pushing the arthroscope out of the lateral gutter as the repair is tensioned.
- Elimination of the laxity that allows for the "drive-through sign of the elbow" is one of the key aspects of confirming an adequate arthroscopic repair in patients with PLRI.
- Open ligament plication and repair can be performed using a posterolateral approach through the anconeus.
- In revision cases or patients with inadequate tissue for repair, open reconstruction can be performed using a palmaris autograft or gracilis allograft.

References

1. Mehlhoff TL, Noble PC, Bennett JB, Tullos HS. Simple dislocation of the elbow in the adult. Results after closed treatment. *J Bone Jt Surgery Am*. 1988;70(2):244–249. https://www.ncbi.nlm.nih.gov/pubmed/3343270.
2. Stoneback JW, Owens BD, Sykes J, Athwal GS, Pointer L, Wolf JM. Incidence of elbow dislocations in the United States population. *J Bone Jt Surgery Am*. 2012;94(3):240–245. https://doi.org/10.2106/JBJS.J.01663.
3. Smith JP, Savoie FH, Field LD. Posterolateral rotatory instability of the elbow. *Clin Sports Med*. 2001;20(1):47–58. https://www.ncbi.nlm.nih.gov/pubmed/11227708.
4. Savoie FH, Field LD, Gurley DJ. Arthroscopic and open radial ulnohumeral ligament reconstruction for posterolateral rotatory instability of the elbow. *Hand Clin*. 2009;25(3):323–329. https://doi.org/10.1016/j.hcl.2009.05.010.
5. O'Brien MJ, Savoie FH. Arthroscopic and open management of posterolateral rotatory instability of the elbow. *Sports Med Arthrosc Rev*. 2014;22(3):194–200. https://doi.org/10.1097/JSA.0000000000000029.

41

Technique Spotlight: Reconstruction of the Lateral Ulnar Collateral Ligament

ANTONIO M. FORURIA AND BELÉN PARDOS MAYO

Indications

The most common indication for lateral ulnar collateral ligament (LUCL) reconstruction is a chronic posttraumatic posterolateral rotatory instability of the elbow resulting in mechanical symptoms, pain, and disability. While prior trauma is the most common etiology of LUCL insufficiency, other causes of chronic LUCL instability include the following:

- Severe lateral epicondylitis, particularly if several corticosteroid injections were used for treatment, or an aggressive surgical debridement has been performed.
- After lateral elbow or distal humeral surgery for other reasons apart from epicondylitis resulting in iatrogenic injury.
- Cubitus varus deformity resulting in tardy posterolateral rotatory instability.

Preoperative Evaluation

The diagnosis of this pathology is based on history and clinical examination. Patients will typically present with complaints of lateral elbow pain and clicking or locking of the elbow. On examination, a posterior drawer test is typically painful and shows posterior displacement of the radial head with respect to the capitellum. Pivot-shift testing is also positive in these patients.

Imaging is typically not very useful for confirming the posterolateral rotatory instability of the elbow, unless acute rupture or avulsion lesions can be seen. It is important to remember that chronic insufficiency of the LUCL is a dynamic condition. In some cases, the lateral ligaments may appear present and intact on advanced imaging but are clinically incompetent.

If a posterolateral rotatory instability of the elbow is highly suspected but clinical examination is not clear enough or difficult to perform due to pain or poor patient collaboration, an exploration under anesthesia is recommended. Sometimes, an elbow arthroscopy is necessary to reveal the subluxation of the articular surfaces under direct vision.

Positioning

The patient is typically placed in the supine position with the arm extended onto an arm board. The arm is positioned with the shoulder in internal rotation. A towel bump can be placed under the medial elbow to allow for the lateral and dorsal sides to be more accessible. Normally a brachial plexus block is performed and a brachial tourniquet is used.

Procedural Equipment and Material

- Tendon Allograft: this is preferred over autograft to decrease morbidity and expedite the procedure. The allograft must be at least 15 cm in length and 4 mm wide. Round and compact forearm flexor tendons are preferred.
- 2- and 4-mm burr.
- Sutures:
  - Absorbable braided #0 suture → capsule and native ligament tagging.
  - Absorbable braided suture 2/0 (×3) → passing-through tunnel sutures.
  - Nonabsorbable braided #2 suture → for the graft, in a Krackow fashion, native ligament repair, and anterolateral and posterolateral transosseous musculocapsular repair.
  - Absorbable braided 3/0 suture → subcutaneous tissue repair.

Surgical Technique

A 7-cm skin incision is performed over the humeral lateral column, passing over the lateral epicondyle prominence toward the *crista supinatoris* of the ulna. A Kocher interval is developed after dissecting the subcutaneous tissue, between the anconeus and the extensor carpi ulnaris (ECU) muscles. This interval is better identified by a fine adipose stripe between the muscles, where the deep vascular perforating branches pierce the fascial plane to reach the subcutaneous tissue (Fig. 41.1). The anconeus is retracted posteriorly, exposing the lateral collateral ligament and the lateral cortex of the ulnar metaphysis. It is useful to elevate the tendon of the ECU off the anterolateral capsule. By detaching it along with the other extensor muscles from the humerus, greater access is achieved of the anterior and lateral aspect of the proximal LUCL as well as the posterolateral capsuloligamentous unit of the elbow.

The capsule is incised laterally in a plane anterior to the anterior border of the native LUCL, in the area exposed after elevating

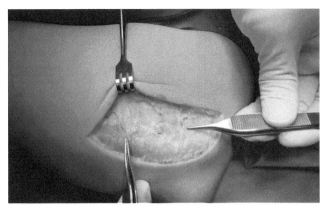

• **Fig. 41.1** Perforating branches that pierce the fascial plane to the subcutaneous tissue are used as a guide to identify the Kocher's interval.

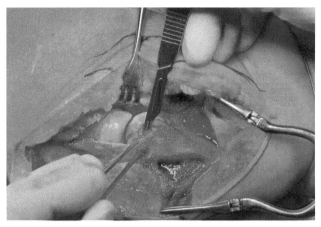

• **Fig. 41.3** The native lateral collateral ligament is elevated off the humerus, in continuity with the posterolateral capsule.

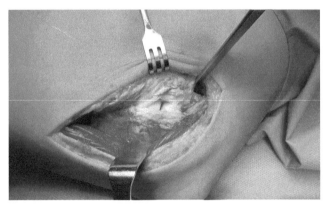

• **Fig. 41.2** The capsule is incised laterally in a plane anterior to the anterior border of the native lateral ulnar collateral ligament.

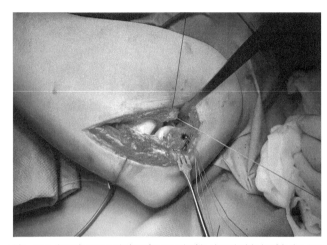

• **Fig. 41.4** Anterior capsule is referenced with absorbable braided suture.

the ECU off the capsule, from the lateral epicondyle to a point distal and anterior to the crista supinatoris tubercle of the ulna (Fig. 41.2). The native LCL is elevated off the humerus, in continuity with the posterolateral capsule (Fig. 41.3). Both capsule and native LUCL are then tagged with absorbable braided #0 sutures (Fig. 41.4).

The lateral cortex of the ulnar metaphysis is then exposed elevating the anconeus. The deep vessels perforating the interosseous membrane and coming into the field are meticulously cauterized. The first ulnar tunnel is located at the crista supinatoris tubercle of the ulna, easily located by palpation distally to the edge of the lesser sigmoid notch, at the level of the radial neck. The hole is created with a 4-mm burr, avoiding damaging the LCL insertion. The second hole is located at least 2 cm proximal and posterior in the lateral ulnar metaphyseal cortex. Both holes are intercommunicated with the burr to ensure a smooth graft passage. A 2/0 stay suture is placed provisionally for humeral isometric point location and graft suture passing.

Attention is turned to the lateral humerus. The stay suture passed through the ulnar tunnel is tensioned, and both strands are fixed by hand at the estimated isometric point (Fig. 41.5). The forearm is fully pronated, and the ulnohumeral joint is tested in flexion and extension correcting and maintaining the isometric point position until a smooth movement not modifying this position is achieved, even when the forearm is supinated. A hole is created with the 4-mm burr so that the isometric point is located in the most anterior and distal margin

of the hole (as it will be the exact point where the allograft will change its direction once under tension through elbow motion) (Fig. 41.6). The tunnel is then developed inside the lateral column directed medially and superiorly. A 2-mm burr is then used to create two smaller tunnels communicating the bigger tunnel with the anterior and posterior humeral cortex. The anterior smaller tunnel is located proximal to the radial fossa, and the posterior tunnel, at the same height as the latter, in the posterior column cortex. A stay 2/0 suture is passed through each tunnel.

A nonabsorbable #2 suture is passed through the extensor tendons and the anterolateral capsule at the same level of the anterior humeral small tunnel. The suture needle is then passed through this anterior hole and the lateral column exiting into the posterior cortex of the lateral column. Perforating the posterior cortex in a virgin location is usually easy, as this is a much softer bone, so the trajectory of our needle does not interfere with the humeral tunnels (Fig. 41.7). Repair the native LUCL to the anterolateral capsule with a nonabsorbable braided suture #2 in a Krackow fashion (Fig. 41.8).

The allograft is typically prepared with nonabsorbable braided #2 suture at the most compact end using a Krackow fashion running locking technique. Pass the allograft through the ulnar tunnel using the previously passed sutures by pulling the suture end of the allograft first, from posterior to anterior, and then

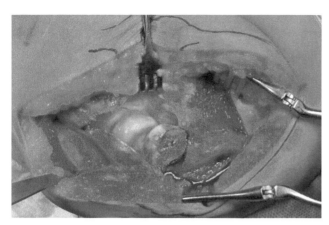

• **Fig. 41.5** The isometric point is located.

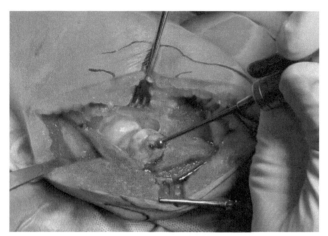

• **Fig. 41.6** The isometric point must be located in the most anterior and distal margin of the humeral tunnel.

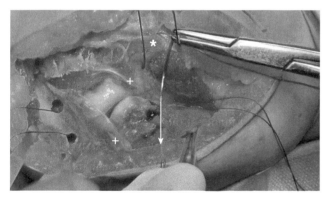

• **Fig. 41.7** A nonabsorbable #2 suture is passed through the extensor tendons and the anterolateral capsule *(asterisk)*. The needle is then passed through the anterior humeral tunnel, exiting into the posterior cortex of the lateral column, where the bone is softer. Native ligament indicated by *crosses (+)*.

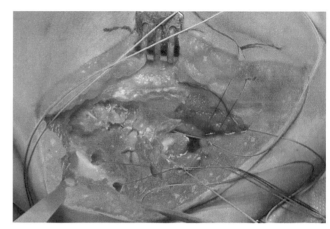

• **Fig. 41.8** Repair the native lateral ulnar collateral ligament to the anterolateral capsule in a Krakow fashion.

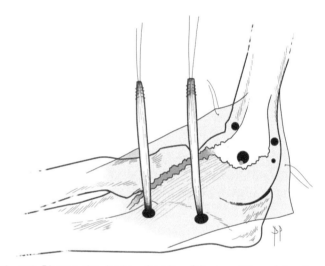

• **Fig. 41.9** Diagram showing how the allograft is passed through the ulnar tunnel.

ligament is removed. The created free end is secured with a nonabsorbable suture in Krackow fashion similar to the other end of the tendon. The anterior native ligament suture and the anterior allograft suture are then passed through the humeral tunnel exiting through the anterior hole of the humerus. The posterior native ligament sutures and the posterior ligament sutures are passed through the humeral tunnel exiting through the posterior hole (Figs. 41.11 and 41.12).

The sequence of tensioning and suture is as follows: the elbow is reduced in flexion and full pronation ensuring a perfect ulnohumeral apposition and a correct radial head reduction to the capitellum. The native ligament is tensioned and tied first. Then, the allograft is fully tensioned, their ends pulled inside the humeral tunnel, and the sutures tied. Finally, the anterolateral and posterolateral capsule-muscular walls (previously transosseous-sutured from the anterior humeral hole to the posterior humeral cortex) are tied over the reconstructed ligament covering the lateral humerus (Fig. 41.13).

The wound is cleaned with saline, the tourniquet is released, and an intensive hemostasis is performed before wound closing. A long arm splint is applied in the operating room in 90-degree flexion and neutral pronosupination.

the ligament, with the aid of the stay sutures (Figs. 41.9 and 41.10). Tension the graft, reduce the elbow in flexion and full pronation, and place and maintain tight the end with the sutures in the humeral hole. The length of the posterior branch of the allograft will be determined under tension at the entrance of the humeral hole. The length is marked with a pen, and the excess

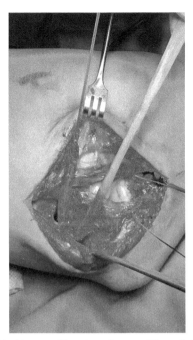

• **Fig. 41.10** Clinical image of the allograft passed through the ulnar tunnel.

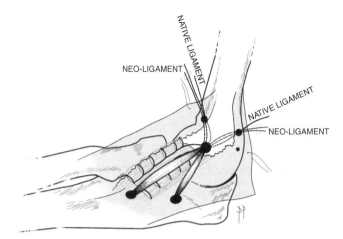

• **Fig. 41.12** The anterior native ligament suture and the anterior allograft suture are passed through the humeral tunnel exiting through the anterior hole of the humerus. The posterior native ligament sutures and the posterior ligament sutures are passed through the humeral tunnel exiting through the posterior hole.

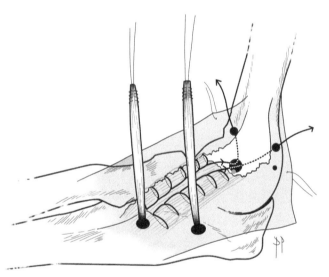

• **Fig. 41.11** Repair the native lateral ulnar collateral ligament to the anterolateral capsule with a nonabsorbable braided suture #2 in a Krakow fashion.

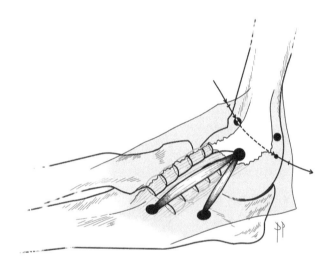

• **Fig. 41.13** The anterolateral and posterolateral capsule-muscular walls are sutured over the reconstructed ligament, using the previous passed transosseous sutures from the anterior humeral tunnel to the posterior humeral cortex. Then, the Kocher's interval is sutured.

Postoperative Care

Based on our experience, patients with posttraumatic unstable elbows, especially those in which the initial injury was treated appropriately, do not develop competent scar tissue, and that is the reason for persistent instability. Furthermore, in our experience, postoperative stiffness is an uncommon complication.

Typically the patient will be immobilized with a long arm splint in 90-degree flexion and neutral pronosupination during 3 weeks. At the third week, the splint is removed and the elbow tested with passive range of motion (ROM). If full or nearly full ROM is demonstrated, the splint is placed back for another week, and the same examination repeated, to continue with splinting either up to 6–8 weeks or until some decrease of ROM is observed, demonstrating some scar tissue formation.

An elbow articulated brace is useful in trustworthy patients after the third week to further protect the repair while scar formation is still occurring. ROM is limited and modified on a weekly basis as follows:
• The first week after splint removing: full flexion, maximum extension of 70 degrees.
• The second week: full flexion, maximum extension of 50 degrees.
• The third week: full flexion, maximum extension of 30 degrees.
• The fourth week: full flexion, maximum extension of 10 degrees.
• After this period, the ROM will be free.

After splint removal, the patient must also perform protected pronosupination exercises in full elbow flexion and extension exercises maintaining the forearm pronated.

PEARLS AND PITFALLS

- Lateral joint opening has to be performed anterior to the body of the ulnar collateral lateral ligament, to avoid further damage to the native ligament. Elevating the ECU off the ligament is advised to achieve this goal.
- Ensure the best reconstruction possible by passing the graft inside the ulnar tunnel from the posterior-proximal hole to the anterior-distal hole, and then secure it inside the humeral tunnel. The posterior allograft branch can be tied to the anterior branch if it does not reach the humeral tunnel.
- Tensioning the native ligament should be performed prior to graft measuring and tensioning.
- Measure the real length of the graft when it is passed through the ulnar tunnel and the anterior allograft branch pulled inside the humeral tunnel.
- The anconeus humeral attachment can be incorporated in the native ligament posterior suture to strengthen the repair.
- Tension and tie the native ligament and the allograft sequentially, with the forearm in full pronation, the elbow flexed, and pressing the proximal ulna toward the humerus. This can be performed with the patient forearm across his chest, so the forearm weight reduces the ulnohumeral joint.
- Additional graft tensioning can be achieved by suturing both branches together with a running suture.
- Protect your reconstruction by suturing the common extensor group to the triceps, covering completely the lateral humerus.
- A wide and strong enough ulnar bony bridge is critical. Not elevating enough the anconeus off the lateral aspect of the ulna may decrease the space to create the ulnar holes, increasing the chance of a short ulnar tunnel and frail bone bridge.
- Choose a compact round graft and completely open the ulnar tunnel to allow smooth passage of the graft passes and avoid fraying.
- When a suture is used to calculate the graft length, it is common to underestimate the needed length.

References

1. Morrey B. *Morrey's the Elbow and its Disorders*. Philadelphia, PA: Elsevier; 2018:670–678.
2. Camp CL, Sanchez-Sotelo J, Shields MN, O'Driscoll SW. Lateral ulnar collateral ligament reconstruction for posterolateral rotatory instability of the elbow. *Arthrosc Tech*. 2017;6(4):e1101–e1105.
3. Sanchez-Sotelo J, Morrey BF, O'Driscoll SW. Ligamentous repair and reconstruction for posterolateral rotatory instability of the elbow. *J Bone Joint Surg Br*. 2005;87(1):54–61.
4. Anakwenze OA, Khanna K, Levine WN, Ahmad CS. Lateral ulnar collateral ligament reconstruction: an analysis of ulnar tunnel locations. *Am J Orthop*. 2016;45(2):53–57.
5. Jones KJ, Dodson CC, Osbahr DC, et al. The docking technique for lateral ulnar collateral ligament reconstruction: surgical technique and clinical outcomes. *J Shoulder Elbow Surg*. 2012;21(3):389–395.
6. Vernet E, Bacle G, Marteau E, Favard L, Laulan J. Lateral elbow ligamentoplasty by autologous tendon graft in posterolateral rotatory instability: results in 18 cases at a mean 5 years' follow-up. *Orthop Traumatol Surg Res*. 2015;101(4 Suppl):S199–S202.
7. Ahmad CS, ElAttrache NS. Elbow valgus instability in the throwing athlete. *J Am Acad Orthop Surg*. 2006;14(12):693–700.

42

Technique Spotlight: Ulnar Collateral Ligament Reconstruction

THEODORE S. WOLFSON, BHARGAVI MAHESHWER, BRADY T. WILLIAMS, AND NIKHIL N. VERMA

Introduction

Ulnar collateral ligament (UCL) reconstruction has grown dramatically in popularity and utilization since the time of Frank Jobe and Tommy John.[1-4] Over this period, UCL reconstruction constructs have evolved significantly from the original Jobe technique. Modifications have included refinements in approach, ulnar nerve (UN) management, tunnel positioning, and graft fixation.[5] Today, "docking" techniques offer the benefit of sparing the common flexor tendon (CFT) origin, standardizing tunnel placement, facilitating graft passage and tensioning, and optimizing biomechanical construct strength.[6-11] Modern studies consistently demonstrate return to play at the same level or higher in 85%–90% of patients with the use of current docking techniques.[12-16] Despite these advancements, complications and failures continue to occur. To achieve optimal outcomes while minimizing complications, it is critical to adhere to strict indications, meticulous surgical technique, and structured rehabilitation. This chapter is designed to provide a concise summary and description of a modified docking technique with a focus on key surgical pearls and pitfalls.

Surgically Relevant Anatomy and Biomechanics

As with all surgical reconstructions, successful UCL reconstruction relies on a complete understanding of the anatomy, biomechanics, and material properties of the native ligament. The UCL is composed of three separate bundles: the anterior, posterior, and transverse bundles. The anterior bundle is comprised of two distinct bands: the anterior band and the posterior band. The anterior bundle originates on the humerus from a flat surface, 11.7–13.4 mm anterior (lateral) and inferior (distal) to the medial epicondyle (ME).[17,18] It traverses the joint and inserts over a broad attachment centered over the sublime tubercle (ST), tapering along the ulnar ridge with a total footprint length of almost 3 cm.[17,19,20] Between footprints it has a total reported length of just over 5 cm.[17,19-21]

Biomechanically, the stability of medial elbow can be broadly categorized into dynamic and static stabilizers. Dynamic stability is provided by the flexor-pronator mass (FPM), while static stability is primarily conferred by the UCL and medial joint capsule. Of the dynamic stabilizers, there are significant contributions from the flexor carpi ulnaris (FCU), flexor digitorum superficialis (FDS), and flexor carpi radialis (FCR), with the FCU being the most significant stabilizer of the FPM.[22,23] Statically, the UCL provides the majority of stability to valgus stress of the elbow. The anterior bundle is the primary restraint to valgus stress, and as a consequence, is the most frequently injured and the focus of surgical reconstruction. The anterior bundle has the highest strength and stiffness of the stabilizers with a mean load to failure of 260.9 N. However, this is regularly exceeded by the valgus torques imposed during overhead throwing leading to repetitive trauma and eventual tearing.[24,25] The consequences of UCL injury have been quantified in cadaveric models demonstrating increased valgus instability of 3.2–11.8 degrees depending on the degree of elbow flexion.[26-31] As our understanding of the anatomy and biomechanics have evolved, so too have reconstruction techniques in an effort to more accurately restore the function of the UCL.

Surgical Indications

The primary surgical indication for UCL reconstruction is persistent medial elbow pain and dysfunction despite a trial of nonoperative treatment, or acute full-thickness UCL tear, coupled with the desire to return to competition at the same level or higher. Nonoperative management should include a structured rehabilitation program with at least 3 months of rest and gradual return to throwing. Surgery may be considered earlier in patients with evidence of complete UCL rupture on examination and imaging. Contraindications to surgery include significant concomitant ulnotrochlear or radiocapitellar arthrosis and inability or unwillingness to participate in the rigorous postoperative rehabilitation program. UCL reconstruction should never be offered to improve performance including pitching velocity, accuracy, or stamina.

Technique

Preoperative Planning

The patient is examined preoperatively for the presence of a palmaris longus (PL) tendon. If the PL tendon is present, we prefer to use a PL tendon autograft for UCL reconstruction. If the PL tendon is absent, a gracilis tendon autograft or allograft can be utilized. On examination of the elbow, the UN is also palpated and assessed for subluxation.

Appropriate preoperative imaging generally includes standard plain radiographs including anteroposterior (AP) and lateral projections to assess for bony anatomy, and osteophyte formation, as well as magnetic resonance imaging (MRI) to assess for ligament tear and other associated pathology. When necessary, computed tomography (CT) should be used to better evaluate for bony abnormality.

Preoperative planning also includes the consideration of additional pathology that may need to be concurrently addressed. For example, the presence of posteromedial osteophytes is common in throwing athletes, particularly baseball pitchers undergoing surgery of the elbow.[32–36] These are thought to be the result of repetitive valgus overload. The osteophytes themselves can cause flexion contractures, posteromedial impingement, pain at terminal extension, and can be excised at the time of surgery.

Essential equipment utilized during UCL reconstruction is detailed in Table 42.1.

Positioning and Anesthesia

The patient is positioned supine with the operative extremity on a hand table. The arm is prepped and draped in the usual fashion and a sterile high arm tourniquet is placed. The limb is exsanguinated and the tourniquet is inflated for the duration of the procedure. Regional nerve blockade in combination with general anesthesia is utilized for appropriate postoperative pain control and minimizes narcotic consumption.

Graft Harvest

The location of the PL is confirmed with Schaeffer's test (the patient actively opposes the thumb and little finger while flexing the wrist, resulting in prominence of the PL and marked preoperatively. A 1-cm transverse incision is made centered over the tendon at the proximal volar wrist crease. The tendon is identified, isolated, and lifted from the incision with a curved hemostat. Elevation of the skin along the correct anatomic course confirms the identity of the PL. A running whipstitch is placed in the distal tendon and it is released from its fascial insertion. Counterincisions more proximally can be used to clearly identify the PL and minimize the risk of neurologic injury. A closed tendon stripper is then used to release the tendon proximally. The harvested PL tendon is measured to confirm adequate length and stored until needed.

In instances where the palmaris longus is insufficient or not present, a hamstring tendon, typically gracilis, can be used. Either autograft or allograft options can be utilized based on graft availability, donor site morbidity, and surgeon and patient preference. Other graft choices do exist; however, the PL and gracilis autografts are among the most common, particularly in high-level throwing athletes.[34] If the decision is made to utilize gracilis autograft, harvest can be performed with the patient supine with a high-thigh tourniquet in place, by bending the knee and externally rotating the hip for access to the medial side of the knee and thigh.

TABLE 42.1	Standardized Postoperative Rehabilitation Protocol After UCL Reconstruction
Postoperative Timepoint	**Guidelines**
Phase I: Weeks 0–4	Weeks 0–1: Immobilization in posterior mold splint and sling
	Weeks 2–4: Conversion to hinged elbow brace, unlocked ROM from 15-degree extension to full flexion
Phase II: Weeks 4–16	Initiate physical therapy, discontinue brace
	Progressively advance from passive ROM, to active assist ROM, to active ROM. Gradually begin wrist, forearm, elbow, and shoulder strengthening as tolerated
Phase III: Months 4–9	Begin interval-throwing program progressing from 45 to 180 ft
	May progress from one distance level to next when the following criteria are met:
	1. No pain/stiffness during or after throwing
	2. Strength is sufficient throughout with minimal fatigue
	3. Accuracy of throws is consistent and throws are on line
Phase IV: Months 9–12	Return to competition is permitted once the following criteria are met:
	1. No pain while throwing
	2. Reestablishment of throwing balance, rhythm, and coordination
	3. Strength/balance of trunk, scapula, shoulder, and arm have normalized

ROM, range of motion; *UCL,* ulnar collateral ligament.

Operative Step	Special Equipment
1. Positioning and setup	• Hand table, pneumatic tourniquet
2. Graft harvest	• Closed tendon stripper
3. Graft preparation	• #2 nonabsorbable UHMWPE suture
4. Approach and exposure	• Penrose drain or vessel loop
5. Tunnel preparation	• Ulnar collateral ligament reconstruction instruments or set
	• Drill guides
	• 2.0-, 3.5-, 4.0-mm drill bits
	• Suture passage devices: nitinol loop, microlasso, skid
	• Small-angle curettes, rasp
6. Graft passage and fixation	• Mineral oil
	• #2 nonabsorbable UHMWPE suture

UHMWPE, ultra high-molecular weight polyethylene suture.

Approach and Exposure

The shoulder is externally rotated, the elbow is flexed 30 degrees, and a small bump is placed under the elbow for optimal exposure of the posteromedial elbow. An 8-cm curvilinear incision is made, centered just posterior to the ME. The incision extends proximally along the medial condylar ridge of the humerus and

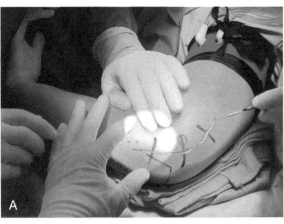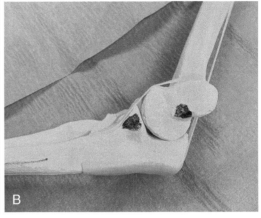

• **Fig. 42.1** Medial view of a right elbow (A) demonstrating patient positioning for ulnar collateral ligament (UCL) reconstruction. Note the sterile high arm tourniquet and bump placed under the elbow. Surface anatomy is marked, indicating the palpated and approximate locations of the medial epicondyle and sublime tubercle (A). The bone model (B) indicates the ulnar and humeral attachments of the UCL.

distally toward the ST of the ulna (Fig. 42.1). Subcutaneous tissue is divided with care to identify and protect branches of the medial antebrachial cutaneous (MABC) nerve, particularly in the distal aspect of the incision.

Ulnar Nerve Decompression

The UN is identified in the cubital tunnel and carefully dissected proximally through the arcade of Struthers and distally between the two heads of the FCU. It is critical to adequately release the UN from the distal FCU fascia to allow its posterior retraction for exposure of the proximal ulna (Fig. 42.2). Care should be taken to identify, protect, and mobilize motor branches to the FCU. Once the decompression is complete, a wide Penrose drain is loosely placed around the nerve.

Ulnar Tunnel Preparation

With the UN identified and protected, the FPM is retracted anteriorly with care to avoid detaching the CFT from the ME. This is done by beginning mobilization posteriorly along the floor of the cubital tunnel. Once the nerve is mobilized, sharp dissection is carried out elevating the FPM directly off the UCL. Once the proximal ulna and ST are exposed, a valgus stress is applied to the elbow to tension the UCL. The ulnar ridge can help identify the center of the UCL insertion on the ST. The anterior bundle of the native UCL is identified and incised longitudinally in line with its fibers (Fig. 42.3). The ulnohumeral (UH) joint is exposed through the split in the UCL to further delineate the ST and subsequent tunnel location. In some cases, medial bone exostosis associated with chronic stress reaction may need to be excised.

The bony prominence of the ST is identified and exposed 7–10 mm distal to the UH joint. Two 3.5-mm converging tunnels are drilled anterior and posterior to the ST spaced approximately 1–2 cm apart (Figs. 42.4 and 42.5). A 55-degree V-shaped drill guide (Arthrex Inc., Naples, FL, USA) can be utilized to ensure an adequate bone bridge. Angled curettes are used to remove bony debris and confirm tunnel convergence. The tunnel apertures are overdrilled and a rasp is used to chamfer and smooth tunnel edges to facilitate graft passage and minimize abrasion. A curved nitinol wire loop is used to shuttle a suture loop for later graft passage.

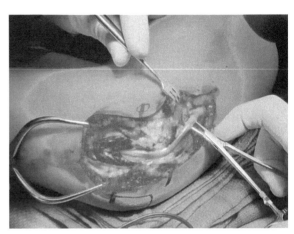

• **Fig. 42.2** Medial view of a right elbow demonstrating the identification and release of the ulnar nerve.

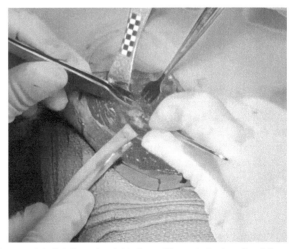

• **Fig. 42.3** Medial view of a right elbow. The anterior bundle of the native ulnar collateral ligament is incised longitudinally in line with its fibers. The flexor-pronator mass is retracted anteriorly, while the ulnar nerve is protected posteriorly.

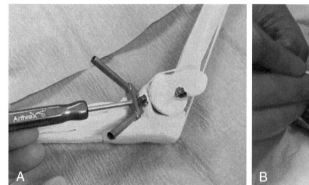
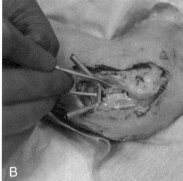
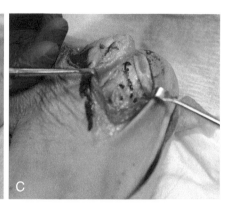

• **Fig. 42.4** Medial view of a right elbow bone model (A) and cadaveric elbow (B) demonstrating the tunnel placement over the sublime tubercle. (B) The native ulnar collateral ligament is split longitudinally to identify the sublime tubercle and facilitate placement of the V-shaped drill guide. Two converging tunnels are subsequently drilled, anterior and posterior to the sublime tubercle, ensuring an adequate bone bridge (C).

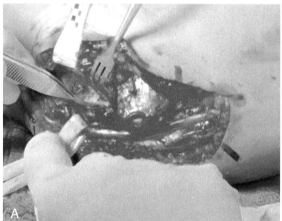
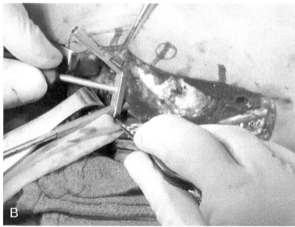

• **Fig. 42.5** Medial view of a right elbow demonstrating the (A) identification of the sublime tubercle followed by (B) the drilling of two converging tunnels anterior and posterior to the sublime tubercle to facilitate graft passage and reconstruction of the ulnar attachment of the ulnar collateral ligament (UCL).

Humeral Tunnel Preparation

Attention is turned to the ME where the origin of the anterior bundle of the UCL is located distal and anterior to the origin of the CFT (Fig. 42.6). The primary "docking" tunnel is centered at the isometric point of the UCL aimed in line with the UCL fibers toward the medial intermuscular septum (Fig. 42.7). A 4.5-mm drill hole is made to a depth of 15 mm using a humeral drill guide with depth stop (Arthrex Inc.). Tunnel containment without cortical breach is confirmed after drilling.

Two small proximal converging tunnels are then connected to the primary docking tunnel. An adjustable guide (Arthrex Inc.) is inserted into the 4.5-mm tunnel and two 2.0-mm tunnels are drilled anterior and posterior spaced at least 1 cm apart for a sufficient bone bridge (Fig. 42.8). The location of the tunnels should be planned such that the knot for graft fixation is positioned away from the native UN or desired transposition site. After drilling, it is helpful to mark the aperture of the proximal tunnels as they are often obscured by soft tissue. A microlasso and skid (Arthrex Inc.) can be used to shuttle a passing suture loop into each 2.0-mm tunnel and out of the primary 4.5-mm tunnel (Fig. 42.9).

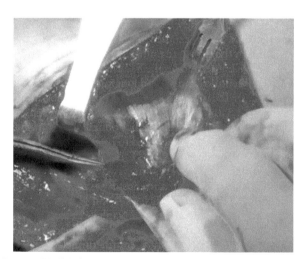

• **Fig. 42.6** Medial view of a right elbow demonstrating palpation of the medial epicondyle. This landmark is used to identify the humeral origin of the anterior band of the ulnar collateral ligament, which is anterior and distal to the epicondyle and origin of the common flexor tendon.

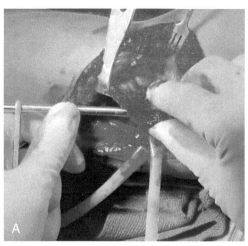
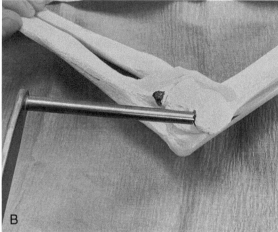

• **Fig. 42.7** (A) Medial view of a right elbow demonstrating the drilling of the primary docking tunnel to recreate the humeral attachment of the ulnar collateral ligament and (B) bone model of same.

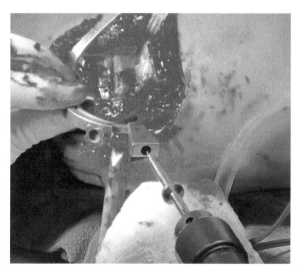

• **Fig. 42.8** Medial view of a right elbow demonstrating the first of two 2.0-mm tunnels drilled into the primary docking tunnel. These tunnels accommodate passing sutures that will be used to dock and secure the graft in the primary docking tunnel.

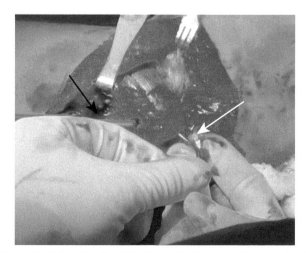

• **Fig. 42.9** Medial view of a right elbow, demonstrating the use of a skid (*left, black arrow*) and microlasso (*right, white arrow*) (Arthrex Inc., Naples, FL, USA) to facilitate introduction of a passing suture loop into the humeral reconstruction tunnels.

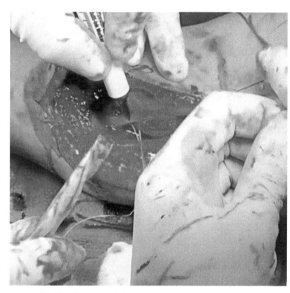

• **Fig. 42.10** Medial view of a right elbow demonstrating the measuring and marking of the graft. The anterior limb is tensioned in the docking tunnel, and the posterior limb is held taught to the aperture of the docking tunnel. A length of 12–13 mm is marked and whipstitched, while the excess remainder is sharply excised.

Graft Passage and Fixation

The graft is first passed through the ulnar tunnel using the previously placed suture loop, resulting in an anterior and posterior limb of the graft. To facilitate passage, the graft should be tapered on one end. Mineral oil can also be used to help provide additional lubrication. The anterior limb is shuttled into the docking tunnel using the anterior tunnel suture loop until it bottoms out. With the anterior limb tensioned, the posterior limb of the graft is held taut to the docking tunnel aperture and marked at this location. A second mark is placed 12–13 mm proximally. The region of the graft between the marks is whipstitched and remaining tendon is sharply removed (Fig. 42.10). It is critical to cut the tendon slightly shorter than 15 mm to prevent it from bottoming out in the tunnel resulting in construct laxity. Loop-type suture devices can be used, which allows for the distal loop to be removed in the event that the graft needs to be shortened.

The joint is then irrigated and the native UCL is closed using interrupted sutures. In cases where proximal or distal avulsion of the native UCL has occurred, sutures can be placed in the graft and shuttled through the reconstruction tunnels. Sutures are shuttled through the ulnar tunnels for distal avulsions, or the humeral tunnels for proximal avulsions to provide primary repair as an augment to reconstruction. The posterior graft limb is then shuttled into the docking tunnel using the posterior tunnel suture loop. With the elbow held in 30 degrees of flexion and a varus force applied, the anterior and posterior suture limbs are tensioned and tied securely over the bone bridge. The knots are intentionally positioned posterior to avoid irritation of the nerve following transposition (Fig. 42.11). The two limbs of the graft are subsequently sutured together to create the final construct (Figs. 42.12 and 42.13). The native UCL can also be incorporated into the body of the graft to reinforce the reconstruction.

Ulnar Nerve Transposition

If indicated, UN transposition can be performed using the surgeon's preferred technique (Fig. 42.14). We routinely perform an anterior transposition by suturing the CFT fascia to the subcutaneous tissue (Fig. 42.15). Mobility and stability of the UN are confirmed by ranging the elbow after transposition. Wounds are thoroughly irrigated, and a standard layered closure is performed.

Postoperative Rehabilitation

Immediately after surgery, the patient is placed in a posterior splint with immobilization of the elbow in 90 degrees of flexion for the first 7–10 days postoperatively.[37] This is done to minimize swelling and pain, facilitate initial healing, and protect the UCL graft and soft tissue slings for the UN transposition.[38] A standardized rehabilitative approach is utilized as detailed in Table 42.1.

Outcomes and Return to Play

There have been multiple studies reporting outcomes after UCL reconstruction. In a systematic review by Ahmad and Vitale, 83% of all patients in the included studies had an excellent result. Several factors were identified as predictors of postoperative outcomes. Transition to the muscle-splitting approach was associated with better outcomes versus detachment of the FPM. Additionally, patients who did not have UN transposition had superior outcomes compared with patients who had obligatory UN transposition. Furthermore, the modified docking technique was associated with superior outcomes, with 95% of patients reporting excellent results compared with 76% of patients treated with a figure-of-eight technique.[39]

With regard to return to play, a systematic review by Romeo et al. found that the docking and modified docking technique had significantly higher rates of return to play compared with the Jobe technique, with rates of 97% and 66.7%, respectively.[40] Specifically, 2-year follow-up of elite throwers who underwent modified docking procedure for UCL reconstruction demonstrated a 92% rate of return to play at preinjury levels of competition.[15]

Failure and revision rates for the modified docking technique are rare in the current literature. A systematic review of UCL reconstruction techniques demonstrated lower rates of complications in modified docking techniques compared with other techniques including Jobe, modified Jobe, interference screw, and docking. Specifically, two studies utilized the modified docking technique on a total of 46 patients, with only two complications reported (UN neuropraxia

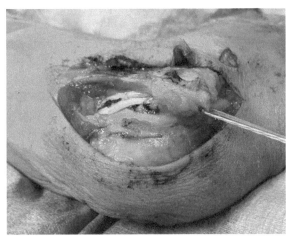

• **Fig. 42.11** Medial view of a right cadaveric elbow. The anterior and posterior graft limbs are docked and the suture limbs are tied over the bone bridge, carefully placing the knots away from the subsequent ulnar nerve transposition.

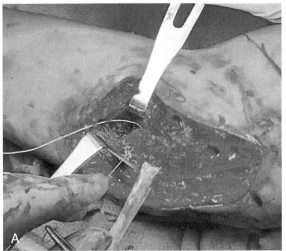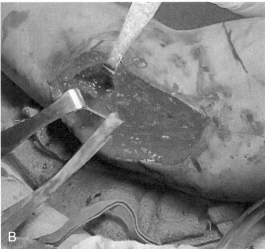

• **Fig. 42.12** Medial view of a right elbow demonstrating the suturing together of the anterior and posterior limbs of the graft (A) to create the final construct (B).

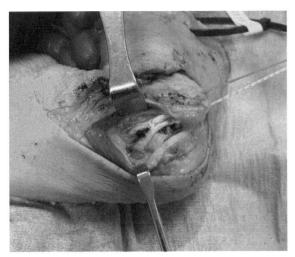

• **Fig. 42.13** Medial view of a right cadaveric elbow. The anterior and posterior limbs of the graft are sutured together to complete the final construct.

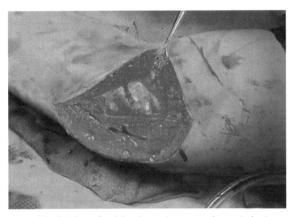

• **Fig. 42.14** Medial view of a right elbow demonstrating anterior transposition of the ulnar nerve.

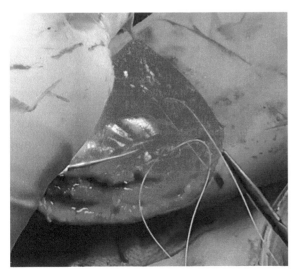

• **Fig. 42.15** Medial view of a right elbow demonstrating the completion of the ulnar nerve anterior transposition by suturing the common flexor tendon fascia to the subcutaneous tissue.

PEARLS AND PITFALLS

Pearls

Palmaris longus harvest: Identify and mark preoperatively and elevate from wound to confirm identity. More proximal incisions can be made to confirm the identity of the palmaris and minimize the risk of neurologic injury.

Graft preparation: Tubularize graft to consistent diameter of 2.5 mm with at least 15 cm of length, whipstitch one end.

Approach: Avoid detachment of FPM from ME, identify and protect MABC nerve.

Ulnar Nerve: Extend decompression distal to FCU, protect with wide Penrose drain, and use judicious indications for UN transposition. Identify and protect motor branches to the FCU.

Ulnar tunnels: Identify ST 7–10 mm distal to the UH joint, drill tunnels at 55-degree angle, smooth tunnels with curette and rasp to facilitate graft passage.

Humeral tunnels: Confirm isometric point on ME prior to drilling, mark proximal tunnels to prevent soft tissue from obscuring passage of passing sutures.

Graft passage and fixation: While tensioning, mark posterior limb of graft <15 mm proximal to docking tunnel to prevent graft from "bottoming out." Suture limbs together after passage to minimize residual laxity and reinforce with native UCL.

Pitfalls

Palmaris longus harvest: Incorrect or inadvertent flexor tendon harvest, or injury to the median nerve.

Graft preparation: Bulky graft interferes with graft passage, inadequate length precludes complete docking and tensioning.

Approach: Trauma to or excessive release of FPM can prolong or compromise recovery.

Ulnar nerve: Obligatory transposition and excessive manipulation can result in high rates of postoperative neuropraxia.

Ulnar tunnels: Maintain sufficient (≥1 cm) bone bridge to minimize fracture, smooth tunnels to avoid graft incarceration.

Humeral tunnels: Cortical breach can occur if tunnel trajectory is too medial or posterior, confirm tunnel containment with curette or probe.

Graft passage and fixation: Avoid graft "bottoming out" in docking tunnel, remove any excess laxity prior to tying limbs over humeral bone bridge.

and ulnar tunnel fracture).[41] In a systematic review examining prevalence and type of UN complications after UCL reconstruction, a 2.5% rate of ulnar neuropathy was found in all-comers (with and without UN transposition) who underwent the modified docking technique, compared to 12.0% overall rate in patients undergoing any UCL reconstruction procedure.[12,14,42]

References

1. Jobe FW, Stark H, Lombardo SJ. Reconstruction of the ulnar collateral ligament in athletes. *J Bone Joint Surg Am*. 1986;68(8):1158–1163.
2. Camp CL, Conte S, D'Angelo J, Fealy SA. Epidemiology of ulnar collateral ligament reconstruction in Major and Minor League Baseball pitchers: comprehensive report of 1429 cases. *J Shoulder Elbow Surg*. 2018;27(5):871–878.
3. DeFroda SF, Goodman AD, Gil JA, Owens BD. Epidemiology of elbow ulnar collateral ligament injuries among baseball players: National Collegiate Athletic Association Injury Surveillance Program, 2009-2010 through 2013-2014. *Am J Sports Med*. 2018;46(9):2142–2147.

4. Hodgins JL, Vitale M, Arons RR, Ahmad CS. Epidemiology of medial ulnar collateral ligament reconstruction: a 10-year study in New York state. *Am J Sports Med.* 2016;44(3):729–734.

5. Chang ES, Dodson CC, Ciccotti MG. Comparison of surgical techniques for ulnar collateral ligament reconstruction in overhead athletes. *J Am Acad Orthopaedic Surg.* 2016;24(3):135–149.

6. Armstrong AD, Dunning CE, Ferreira LM, et al. A biomechanical comparison of four reconstruction techniques for the medial collateral ligament-deficient elbow. *J Shoulder Elbow Surg.* 2005;14(2):207–215.

7. Ciccotti MG, Siegler S, Kuri 2nd JA, Thinnes JH, Murphy DJT. Comparison of the biomechanical profile of the intact ulnar collateral ligament with the modified Jobe and the Docking reconstructed elbow: an in vitro study. *Am J Sports Med.* 2009;37(5):974–981.

8. Jackson TJ, Adamson GJ, Peterson A, et al. Ulnar collateral ligament reconstruction using bisuspensory fixation: a biomechanical comparison with the docking technique. *Am J Sports Med.* 2013;41(5):1158–1164.

9. Leasure J, Reynolds K, Thorne M, Escamilla R, Akizuki K. Biomechanical comparison of ulnar collateral ligament reconstruction with a modified docking technique with and without suture augmentation. *Am J Sports Med.* 2019;47(4):928–932.

10. McGraw MA, Kremchek TE, Hooks TR, Papangelou C. Biomechanical evaluation of the docking plus ulnar collateral ligament reconstruction technique compared with the docking technique. *Am J Sports Med.* 2013;41(2):313–320.

11. Paletta Jr GA, Klepps SJ, Difelice GS, et al. Biomechanical evaluation of 2 techniques for ulnar collateral ligament reconstruction of the elbow. *Am J Sports Med.* 2006;34(10):1599–1603.

12. Bowers AL, Dines JS, Dines DM, Altchek DW. Elbow medial ulnar collateral ligament reconstruction: clinical relevance and the docking technique. *J Shoulder Elbow Surg.* 2010;19(2 Suppl):110–117.

13. Dodson CC, Thomas A, Dines JS, et al. Medial ulnar collateral ligament reconstruction of the elbow in throwing athletes. *Am J Sports Med.* 2006;34(12):1926–1932.

14. Koh JL, Schafer MF, Keuter G, Hsu JE. Ulnar collateral ligament reconstruction in elite throwing athletes. *Arthroscopy.* 2006;22(11):1187–1191.

15. Paletta Jr GA, Wright RW. The modified docking procedure for elbow ulnar collateral ligament reconstruction: 2-year follow-up in elite throwers. *Am J Sports Med.* 2006;34(10):1594–1598.

16. Rohrbough JT, Altchek DW, Hyman J, Williams 3rd RJ, Botts JD. Medial collateral ligament reconstruction of the elbow using the docking technique. *Am J Sports Med.* 2002;30(4):541–548.

17. Camp CL, Jahandar H, Sinatro AM, et al. Quantitative anatomic analysis of the medial ulnar collateral ligament complex of the elbow. *Orthopaed J Sports Med.* 2018;6(3). 2325967118762751.

18. Frangiamore SJ, Moatshe G, Kruckeberg BM, et al. Qualitative and quantitative analyses of the dynamic and static stabilizers of the medial elbow: an anatomic study. *Am J Sports Med.* 2018;46(3):687–694.

19. Dugas JR, Ostrander RV, Cain EL, Kingsley D, Andrews JR. Anatomy of the anterior bundle of the ulnar collateral ligament. *J Shoulder Elbow Surg.* 2007;16(5):657–660.

20. Farrow LD, Mahoney AP, Sheppard JE, Schickendantz MS, Taljanovic MS. Sonographic assessment of the medial ulnar collateral ligament distal ulnar attachment. *J Ultrasound Med.* 2014;33(8):1485–1490.

21. Farrow LD, Mahoney AJ, Stefancin JJ, et al. Quantitative analysis of the medial ulnar collateral ligament ulnar footprint and its relationship to the ulnar sublime tubercle. *Am J Sports Med.* 2011;39(9):1936–1941.

22. Lin F, Kohli N, Perlmutter S, et al. Muscle contribution to elbow joint valgus stability. *J Shoulder Elbow Surg.* 2007;16(6):795–802.

23. Park MC, Ahmad CS. Dynamic contributions of the flexor-pronator mass to elbow valgus stability. *J Bone Joint Surg Am.* 2004;86(10):2268–2274.

24. Fleisig GS, Andrews JR, Dillman CJ, Escamilla RF. Kinetics of baseball pitching with implications about injury mechanisms. *Am J Sports Med.* 1995;23(2):233–239.

25. Werner SL, Fleisig GS, Dillman CJ, Andrews JR. Biomechanics of the elbow during baseball pitching. *J Orthopaedic Sports Physical Therap.* 1993;17(6):274–278.

26. Ahmad CS, Park MC, Elattrache NS. Elbow medial ulnar collateral ligament insufficiency alters posteromedial olecranon contact. *Am J Sports Med.* 2004;32(7):1607–1612.

27. Callaway GH, Field LD, Deng XH, et al. Biomechanical evaluation of the medial collateral ligament of the elbow. *J Bone Joint Surg Am.* 1997;79(8):1223–1231.

28. Floris S, Olsen BS, Dalstra M, Søjbjerg JO, Sneppen O. The medial collateral ligament of the elbow joint: anatomy and kinematics. *J Shoulder Elbow Surg.* 1998;7(4):345–351.

29. Morrey BF, Tanaka S, An KN. Valgus stability of the elbow. A definition of primary and secondary constraints. *Clin Orthop Related Res.* 1991;(265):187–195.

30. Safran M, Ahmad CS, Elattrache NS. Ulnar collateral ligament of the elbow. *Arthroscopy.* 2005;21(11):1381–1395.

31. Søjbjerg JO, Ovesen J, Nielsen S. Experimental elbow instability after transection of the medial collateral ligament. *Clin Orthop Related Res.* 1987;218:186–190.

32. Andrews JR, Timmerman LA. Outcome of elbow surgery in professional baseball players. *Am J Sports Med.* 1995;23(4):407–413.

33. Garcia GH, Gowd AK, Cabarcas BC, et al. Magnetic resonance imaging findings of the asymptomatic elbow predict injuries and surgery in Major League Baseball pitchers. *Orthop J Sports Med.* 2019;7(1). 2325967118818413.

34. Griffith TB, Ahmad CS, Gorroochurn P, et al. Comparison of outcomes based on graft type and tunnel configuration for primary ulnar collateral ligament reconstruction in professional baseball pitchers. *Am J Sports Med.* 2019;47(5):1103–1110.

35. Gutierrez NM, Granville C, Kaplan L, Baraga M, Jose J. Elbow MRI findings do not correlate with future placement on the disabled list in asymptomatic professional baseball pitchers. *Sports Health.* 2017;9(3):222–229.

36. Saper M, Shung J, Pearce S, Bompadre V, Andrews JR. Outcomes and return to sport after ulnar collateral ligament reconstruction in adolescent baseball players. *Orthop J Sports Med.* 2018;6(4). 2325967118769328.

37. Ellenbecker TS, Wilk KE, Altchek DW, Andrews JR. Current concepts in rehabilitation following ulnar collateral ligament reconstruction. *Sports Health.* 2009;1(4):301–313.

38. Wilk KE, Arrigo C, Andrews JR. Rehabilitation of the elbow in the throwing athlete. *J Orthop Sports Physical Therap.* 1993;17(6):305–317.

39. Vitale MA, Ahmad CS. The outcome of elbow ulnar collateral ligament reconstruction in overhead athletes: a systematic review. *Am J Sports Med.* 2008;36(6):1193–1205.

40. Erickson BJ, Chalmers PN, Bush-Joseph CA, Verma NN, Romeo AA. Ulnar collateral ligament reconstruction of the elbow: a systematic review of the literature. *Orthopaed J Sports Med.* 2015;3(12). 2325967115618914.

41. Watson JN, McQueen P, Hutchinson MR. A systematic review of ulnar collateral ligament reconstruction techniques. *Am J Sports Med.* 2014;42(10):2510–2516.

42. Clain JB, Vitale MA, Ahmad CS, Ruchelsman DE. Ulnar nerve complications after ulnar collateral ligament reconstruction of the elbow: a systematic review. *Am J Sports Med.* 2019;47(5):1263–1269.

43

Technique Spotlight: Static, Hinged, and Internal Elbow Joint Fixators

JORGE L. ORBAY

Indications

Damage to bony, muscular, and ligamentous structures from injuries such as simple but unstable elbow dislocations or fracture-dislocations may result in elbow instability. Attempts to repair these structures may not address the resultant elbow instability. When instability persists, the use of an elbow fixator may be necessary to maintain ulnohumeral joint reduction and/or protect the repaired structures. Elbow fixators may also be indicated for instability compounded by delayed treatment. When dislocated elbows remain unreduced for >2 weeks, elastic forces (laxity) from fibrosing soft tissues must be overcome and the joint often requires supplemental stabilization to maintain reduction.[1] Patients undergoing surgery for elbow contracture or heterotopic ossification may require extensive soft tissue release or excision resulting in instability. Therefore the use of an elbow fixation device may be necessary.

Static elbow fixation methods include transarticular pinning and static external fixators. These stabilize but also completely immobilize the elbow joint. Static fixation is simple to apply but has considerable potential drawbacks such as cartilage necrosis, poor soft tissue maturation, and joint stiffness. Therefore they are best indicated for shorter periods of immobilization or when other methods are not available. Hinged external fixators and internal joint stabilizers are indicated when early motion is particularly desired or longer fixation times are needed.[2,3] Early joint motion has been documented to preserve cartilage integrity, improve the maturation and remodeling of healing ligaments, and prevent joint contracture. Hinged external fixators are indicated for distraction interposition arthroplasty, in which the joint is distracted and stabilized to minimize shear forces on the biological resurfacing.

Generally, all elbow fixation devices are relatively contraindicated in the presence of poor bone quality. Bone loss in the humerus or ulna may not allow the use of these devices. The use of transarticular pinning in pediatric patients should be avoided to avoid disturbing growth plates.

Preoperative Evaluation

The nature of elbow instability should be determined by evaluating the patient's history, including the mechanism of injury and the magnitude of energy involved. Also, mechanical symptoms, prior elbow surgery, and peripheral nerve deficits must be investigated and documented. Understanding normal elbow stability is essential for formulating an effective treatment plan. The ulnohumeral articulation, medial collateral ligament (MCL), and lateral collateral ligament (LCL) are considered the primary static elbow joint constraints. The radiocapitellar articulation, joint capsule, and the common flexor and extensor tendon origins are considered secondary static constraints.[4] Diagnostic maneuvers can help elucidate subtle instability patterns. Valgus instability, from injury to the MCL, can be identified through a valgus stress test. Posterolateral rotatory instability, resulting from injuries to the LCL, can be identified through the lateral pivot-shift test or posterolateral rotatory drawer test. Varus posteromedial rotatory instability can be identified through the gravity-assisted varus stress test.[4] Instability can be acute, recurrent, chronic, or surgically induced.

Preoperative planning is enhanced by imaging. Radiographs in multiple views should be acquired to examine fracture pattern, bone defects, or joint malalignment. Computed tomography may also be used for high-resolution characterization of bony structures. Magnetic resonance imaging can be used to assess soft tissue and osteochondral structures. Ultrasonography can also be a valuable tool for identifying concomitant ligamentous damage.[4]

Positioning and Equipment

The patient is typically positioned supine with the arm supported on a hand table or in the lateral decubitus position. A sterile bolster over the chest or a positioning device can facilitate surgery. The arm is prepped from hand to shoulder and the use of a sterile tourniquet is helpful (Fig. 43.1). The surgeon must assure that the necessary instrumentation and equipment are available and ready as these cases are complex and often require alternative procedural plans. Manufacturers of these devices generally provide system-specific instrumentation and system-specific surgical technique guides; a general list of the instrumentation and implant components is available in Table 43.1.

Specific Fixator Techniques

Transarticular or Cross-Pinning

Transarticular or cross-pinning is a time-tested method for static elbow fixation. Stability is provided by one or two Steinmann pins driven across the ulna and into the humerus usually in a position of elbow flexion (Fig. 43.2). It is a low-cost, simple, readily available technique but unfortunately can produce articular surface damage and risk deep joint infection from exposed pins. It is a practical technique for short-term stabilization in cases compounded by vascular injury and often exchanged for other methods of elbow stabilization once the vascular status has stabilized. Transarticular pinning of the elbow joint is done with one or two Steinmann pins of at least 2.0 mm diameter. The joint must be anatomically reduced after all other related procedures have been completed. Pins are inserted through

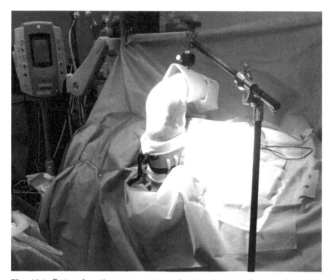

• **Fig. 43.1** Setup for elbow surgery: patient supine, sterile tourniquet, and arm holder.

the proximal ulna into the humerus and through the articular surface. One axial pin or two crossed for more stability can be utilized. They can be cut below the skin or left out for ease of removal. The elbow joint must be additionally supported by a cast or splint as stability is always limited and stress on the pins can cause increased damage to the joint surface. Pins should not be retained for longer than 6 weeks.

Static External Fixation

Static external fixation is a simple and powerful technique. The humerus, ulna, and, at times, the radius are connected with a modular, commonly available external fixator. Frames are usually placed on the lateral or posterior aspect of the arm and half pins used to avoid the medial neurovascular structures. At least two fixation pins must be placed in the humerus and in the ulna to provide sufficient stability. These are fastened to bars which themselves are fastened together by clamps and bars, allowing for positional adjustment (Fig. 43.3). After completing the surgical repair procedure and determining the need for elbow fixation, the surgeon first applies two half pins on the posterior or lateral aspect of the humerus and two half pins on the ulna. Pin insertion must be done with exacting technique and the location of the radial nerve considered. The radial nerve can be injured by humeral pin application but this is less likely if pins are applied using open technique as opposed to blind technique. Open technique requires either extending an existing incision or creating a small one to dissect down to the humeral surface and avoid the nerve. The ulna is more forgiving and pins can be placed medial, posterior, or lateral but the location of the ulnar nerve should be minded when applying pins on its proximal aspect. In general, bone pins should be applied in line with a bone as this facilitates clamping them to a bar. One bar is used for the humeral pins and another one for the ulna and a third bar is then positioned connecting the first two bars together but left loosely attached. The elbow joint is then reduced concentrically and the entire device is rigidly locked. The elbow is usually immobilized in some degree of flexion. Stability is usually adequate but decreases with pin

TABLE 43.1	**Procedural Equipment: A General List of the Instrumentation and Implant Components**	
Fixator Technique	**Instrumentation**	**Implant Components**
Transarticular or cross-pinning	Tissue protector Pin driver	Steinmann pins (≥2.0 mm) Cast/splint
Static external fixator	Pin drivers Tissue protectors/ drill sleeve Drill bit Driver/wrenches	Full pins/half pins Frame - Connectors/clamps - Bars
Hinged or dynamic external fixator	Guidewire Pin drivers Tissue protectors/drill sleeve Drill bit Driver/wrenches	Axis pin Hinge mechanism Full pins/half pins Frame - Connectors/clamps - Bars
Internal joint stabilizer	Guidewire Axis trajectory guide Drills/depth gauges/drivers Cutting pliers	Axis pin Baseplate/bone screws/connecting arm

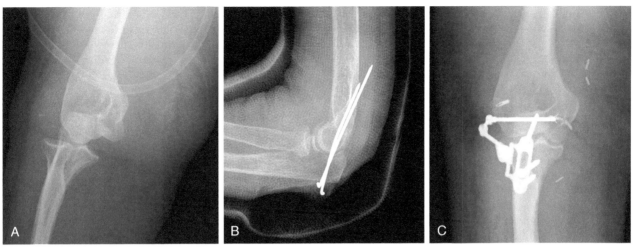

• **Fig. 43.2** Transarticular pinning. (A) A 48-year-old female with a lateral elbow dislocation and brachial artery rupture. (B) Immediate vascular repair with vein graft and temporary cross-pinning stabilization with 2-mm Steinmann pins. (C) One week later, ligaments were repaired and the elbow fixator converted to internal joint stabilizer.

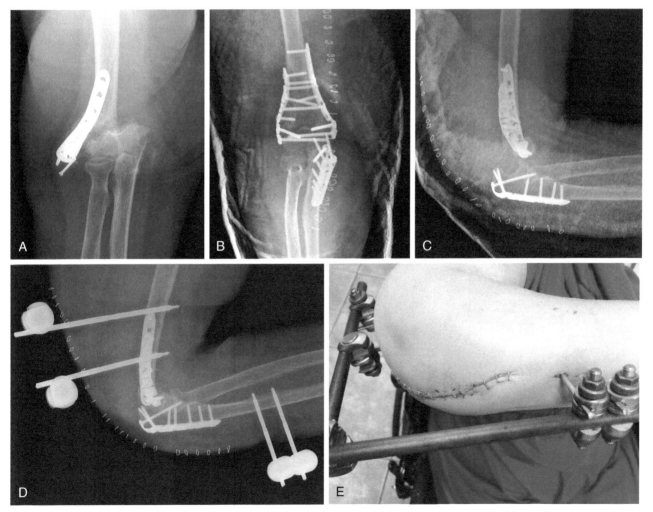

• **Fig. 43.3** Static external fixation. (A) A 56-year-old female with a 9-month-old nonunion of a right low supracondylar fracture. (B) and (C) Anteroposterior and lateral views of the elbow dislocated after osteosynthesis. (D) and (E) After ligament reconstruction, repairs were protected with a posterior static external fixator.

length which can be problematic when treating obese patients. Most complications are associated with pin use. Pin tract infections are frequent but are usually easily treated. Fractures can occur at pin sites and prolonged joint immobilization can promote stiffness. The fixators can be removed following soft tissue healing after about 4–6 weeks.

Hinged or Dynamic External Fixators

Hinged or dynamic external fixators provide stability while allowing elbow motion. They are fixed to the ulna and humerus by means of pins like static external fixators. Some hinged fixators have a unilateral configuration for simplicity and only use half pins. Others have a bilateral or semicircular configuration and can use transfixation pins. Some have worm gears for managing joint contracture. Many have joint distraction features and

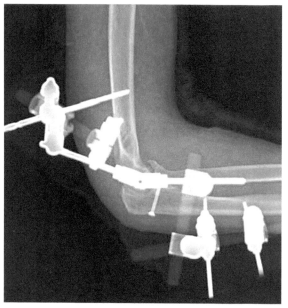

• **Fig. 43.4** Hinged external fixator. The hinge's axis must be aligned coaxially with the axis of ulnohumeral rotation.

are indicated for interposition arthroplasty. Dynamic fixators function as hinge or pivot joint whose axis of rotation must be coaxially aligned with that of the ulnohumeral articulation to permit physiologic elbow motion (Fig. 43.4). Determining the correct axis of rotation is achieved by either open or fluoroscopic technique and is the key step in their application. A guidewire is inserted along the ulnohumeral axis of rotation and the fixator's cannulated hinge mechanism is inserted over it; this assures that the fixator axis is aligned to that of the elbow. The guidewire may function as a temporary alignment tool or remain inserted with the application of the device. The fixator is now completed by either building it around the aligned hinge and finally fixing it to the bony structures or attaching a partially completed fixator to the aligned hinge using adjustable connectors or clamps. Finally, the surgeon must radiographically and visually verify proper reduction through the intended range of motion. Complications of hinged fixators include those related to the use of percutaneous pins or to poor technique. Determining the correct axis of ulnohumeral rotation is a key step (Fig. 43.5) and can be technically difficult; open technique requires a medial and lateral open joint exposure with visual identification of the surface points through which the axis courses. Cues to this are the centers of curvature of the capitellum and trochlea and the origin of the medial and LCLs. An anterior cruciate ligament (ACL)-type guide can be used to insert the guidewire between these two points. Radiographic technique requires percutaneously drilling the guidewire along the direction of the axis of rotation. This is achieved by driving it concentrically through circles seen under fluoroscopy in the coronal plane where the trochlea and capitellum are superimposed. Do not compromise on this step. Malalignment of the fixator axis results in abnormal tracking, nonphysiologic joint compression, and distraction during the arc of motion, which strains repaired ligaments and limits elbow motion. The fixators can usually be removed after 6–12 weeks.

Internal Joint Stabilizers

Internal joint stabilizers are dynamic fixators that provide stability, allow motion, and are placed subcutaneously to avoid pin tract problems.[3] They are located close to the bone surface, therefore have a short working length, and are made smaller

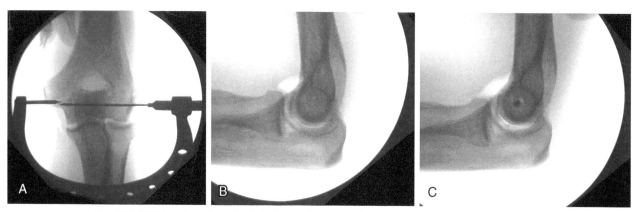

• **Fig. 43.5** (A) Determining the axis of ulnohumeral rotation using an anterior cruciate ligament–type wire guide. The isometric points, revealed by the origin of both collateral ligaments, are identified under direct vision and the guidewire placed between them. (B) and (C) Radiographic technique: the medical trochlea, center trochlea, and capitellum are seen as concentric circles in a lateral fluoroscopic view, and a guidewire is freehand inserted along their centers.

than external fixators. Internal stabilizers allow elbow motion by means of a rotating cobalt-chrome pin (axis pin) inserted into the distal humerus along the axis of ulnohumeral rotation. They function as a hinge and resist abnormal joint movements. The axis pin is connected to a base plate on the ulna via an articulated arm with two joints. These are securely locked after achieving joint reduction. The ulnar base plate is fixed with bone screws. With more complicated injury patterns (Fig. 43.6), multiple repairs may take place during fixator application. The device is usually placed on the lateral side of the elbow and the connecting arm overlies the anconeus muscle and LCL (Fig. 43.7). Internal joint stabilizers can be applied

medially for elbows with disorders of the coronoid or medial side instability. When applied medially, the ulnar nerve must be transposed and the medial epicondyle trimmed to avoid impingement. Collateral ligaments are repaired by tacking them to the humerus slightly proximal to their original position, as the axis pin is located at the isometric point. These ligaments scar back into their original location after fixator removal. Coronoid fractures can also be repaired through the lateral incision in cases where the radial head is removed for repair or replacement (Fig. 43.8). Identify the ulnohumeral joint axis prior to the intended reconstructive procedure when the elbow is maximally unstable and no repairs have yet been made; this

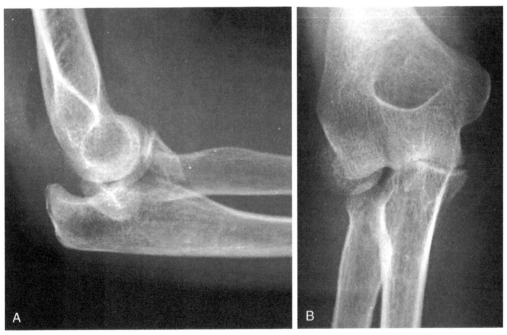

• **Fig. 43.6** (A) Lateral and (B) anteroposterior views of the right elbow of a 38-year-old female presenting with a terrible triad injury and Type III coronoid and Type III radial head fractures.

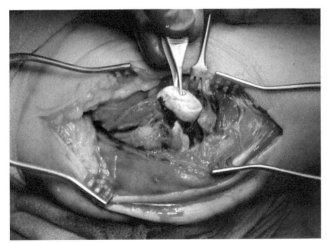

• **Fig. 43.7** Surgical exposure should allow access to the lateral aspect of the elbow joint and olecranon.

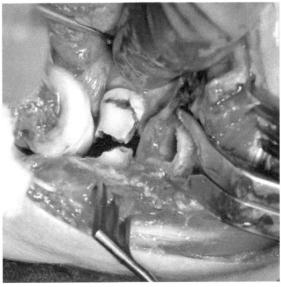

• **Fig. 43.8** Access to a Type III comminuted coronoid fracture after radial head excision.

will facilitate axis guide introduction. The ulnohumeral joint axis is found by determining two points along its axis. The first point is located by identifying the center of curvature on the surface of the lateral capitellum (Fig. 43.9). The second point is located by using a self-centering guide to predictably define the correct trajectory relative to the medial trochlear expansion (Fig. 43.10). The axis guide works best on the lateral side and precludes the need for exposing the opposite side of the joint. A guidewire is inserted across both points defining the axis and fluoroscopy is used to confirm proper guide pin placement: It should be concentric on the lateral view, should bisect the trochlear spool on the frontal view, and should point to the distal aspect of the medial epicondyle where the MCL originates. A cannulated drill is inserted over the guidewire to create a pilot hole for the axis pin. The axis pin length is measured with a depth gauge and the longest pin not traversing the medial cortex is selected. Insert the axis pin into the pilot hole to maintain the axis of rotation. Once the axis is identified, any associated fractures can be addressed starting with the coronoid (Fig. 43.11) and then the radial head (Fig. 43.12). If the surgical repair provides sufficient stability, the stabilizer is

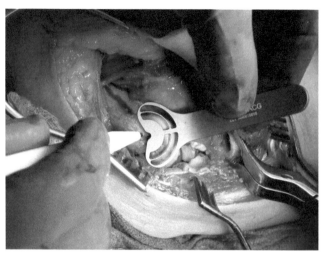

• **Fig. 43.9** Identifying the axis of rotation. The first step when using an internal stabilizer is to find the axis of ulnohumeral rotation. The center of curvature of the capitellum, which is identified using a concentric circle guide, is one of the two points used to determine the axis.

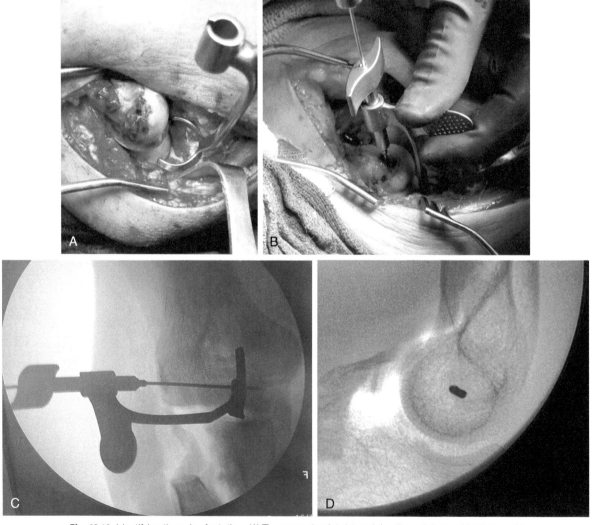

• **Fig. 43.10** Identifying the axis of rotation. (A) The second point determining the axis is provided by a guide that self-centers on the medial trochlea. (B) A guidewire is introduced along the axis. (C, D) Placement confirmed fluoroscopically.

not used and the axis pin is removed and the pilot hole is used to reattach the lateral ligament at its isometric point. If the stabilizer is needed, the surgeon now places the base plate on the posterior ulna immediately distal to the triceps insertion (Fig. 43.13); he should utilize two or three bone screws while assuring all screws are extra-articular as the ulnohumeral joint is at risk. The axis pin is removed from the pilot hole and threaded securely into the connecting arm. The axis pin is inserted into the humeral axis drill hole and simultaneously the connecting arm is inserted into the locking joint on the base plate assembly. The joint at the midpoint of the connecting arm must be kept loose during this step. The pin and connecting arm are fully seated, the elbow joint is concentrically reduced, and the

connecting arm joints are then locked securely. A maneuver to facilitate joint reduction is to position the humerus vertically, flex the elbow, push the ulnar notch against the trochlea, and rotate the shoulder until the patient's hand lies over the patient's face as this eliminates torsional stress (Fig. 43.14). Fixator joints are locked sequentially, starting with the one at the midpoint of the connecting arm and followed by the joint at the baseplate assembly (Fig. 43.15). The connecting arm is finally cut short where it exits the base plate joint to avoid soft tissue irritation (Fig. 43.16). Final repairs are confirmed fluoroscopically (Fig. 43.17). Internal joint stabilizers are usually removed between 12 and 16 weeks after surgery and usually through small new incisions.

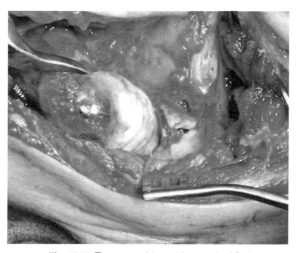

• **Fig. 43.11** The coronoid must be repaired first.

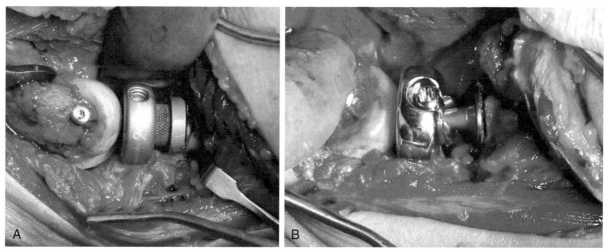

• **Fig. 43.12** (A) Once the coronoid is repaired, the radial head is trialed. (B) The replaced head should have the correct length to prevent overstuffing.

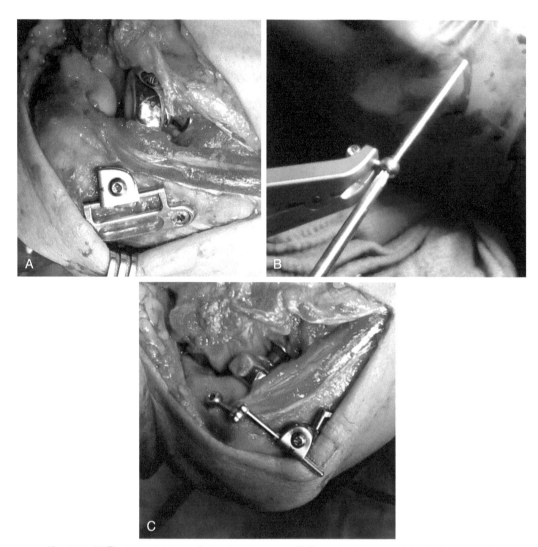

• **Fig. 43.13** (A) The baseplate is applied to the olecranon. (B) The axis pin is assembled to the connecting arm. (C) The internal joint stabilizer is assembled.

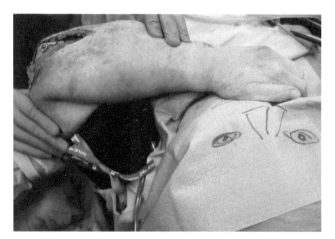

• **Fig. 43.14** The joint is reduced by pressing the ulnar notch down into the trochlea and eliminating torsional stress by placing the hand over the patient's mouth.

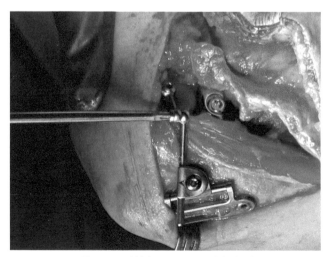

• **Fig. 43.15** All joints are securely locked.

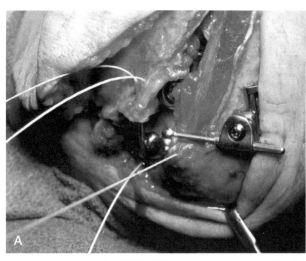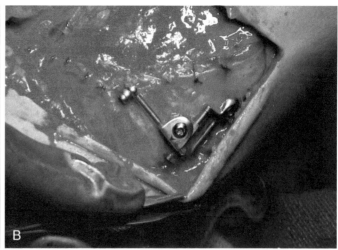

• **Fig. 43.16** (A) Soft tissues are repaired back to the lateral epicondyle just proximal to the axis pin. (B) Finally, the connecting arm is trimmed.

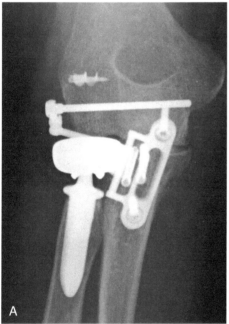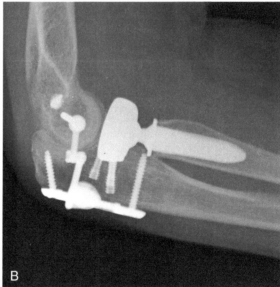

• **Fig. 43.17** (A) Anteroposterior and (B) lateral views of the elbow after repair and fixation with the internal stabilizer.

PEARLS AND PITFALLS

- Transarticular pinning is simple, readily available, and works well for short fixation times but requires additional external support and risks damage to articular surfaces, particularly in osteopenic and noncooperative patients.
- Static external fixators are readily available, are easy to apply, and provide good stability. Injury to peripheral nerves should be avoided by exposing key insertion sites. Excessively long pins may compromise stability, particularly in obese patients.
- Static external fixators carry the risk of limiting joint motion; this should be considered when treating high-demand patients.[5]
- Hinged external fixators permit early motion to address the risk of postoperative joint contracture but can be challenging in application. Precise technique is necessary when determining the axis of rotation.[2] Pain and motion restriction can occur from pin tract irritation.
- Hinged external fixator devices offer unilateral, bilateral, and multiplanar frames to accommodate different stability needs and can be used to provide joint distraction in interposition arthroplasty.

- Internal joint stabilizers also allow elbow motion. They are better tolerated by patients, avoid pin tract issues, and more reliably achieve early postoperative motion. Precise placement of the axis pin is necessary and a special guide facilitates this step through a single exposure.
- The incision utilized for internal stabilizers should expose the olecranon where the base plate will be placed.
- When applying the internal stabilizer, determining the axis of rotation should be performed before repairs are performed.
- Patients requiring fixation and bone or soft tissue repair or reconstruction should be given special attention when placing elbow fixators as device components may interfere with hardware or soft tissue structures.
- Device prominence, patient compliance, potential adverse events, and expected functional outcomes should be analyzed when choosing a fixator.

References

1. Chen N, Jupiter J, Steinmann S, Ring D. Nonacute treatment of elbow fracture with persistent ulnohumeral dislocation or subluxation. *J Bone Joint Surg Am*. 2014;96:1308–1316.
2. Iordens G, Den Hartog D, Van Lieshout E, et al. Good functional recovery of complex elbow dislocations treated with hinged external fixation: a multicenter prospective study. *Clin Orthop Relat Res*. 2015;473:1451–1461.
3. Orbay J, Ring D, Kachooei A, et al. Multicenter trial of an internal joint stabilizer for the elbow. *J Shoulder Elbow Surg*. 2017;26:125–132.
4. Karbach L, Elfar J. Elbow instability: anatomy, biomechanics, diagnostic maneuvers, and testing. *J Hand Surg Am*. 2017;42(2):118–126.
5. Rao A, Cohen M. The use of static external fixation for chronic instability of the elbow. *J Shoulder Elbow Surg*. 2019;28:255–264.

44

Isolated Radial Head/Neck Fractures

ROBERT A. KAUFMANN AND LEIGH-ANNE TU

Introduction

Fractures of the radial head are the most common elbow injuries, accounting for approximately 30% of all elbow fractures in adult patients. The majority of patients are between 20 and 64 years of age with no gender predominance.[1,2] The mechanism of injury is typically a fall on an outstretched arm with the elbow extended and the forearm pronated.

Radial head fractures occur with associated lesions in one-third of cases with coronoid fractures being the most commonly implicated.[3] These injuries can range from simple nondisplaced fractures to those associated with complex elbow instability. Because the radial head is an important stabilizer of the elbow, displaced fractures, particularly when associated with ligamentous injuries, may lead to elbow dysfunction. Management of these injuries, whether nonoperative or operative, is aimed at maintaining radial head alignment while elbow joint motion is encouraged as rapidly as the stability of the fracture affords.

Anatomy and Biomechanics

The radial head is entirely intra-articular and ensures smooth rotation between the radius and ulna while facilitating elbow flexion and extension. It does this through two articulations at the radio-capitellar (RC) and the proximal radioulnar joints (PRUJs). The radial head has a concave surface that articulates with the convex surface of the capitellum and this provides stability through a concavity/compression mechanism as well as through tensioning of the lateral collateral ligament (LCL) complex.[4] Its elliptical shape produces a cam effect at the PRUJ and the proximal radius of curvature is slightly greater when compared to the capitellum, which limits its constraint. These complexities in the radial head as well as a variable neck-shaft angle can make repair and replacement efforts challenging.[5,6] This variability mandates that plates are intraoperatively bent to match the uninjured proximal radius.[7]

When surgically approaching the radial head, there exists a safe zone that does not articulate with the PRUJ, which can be easily located between the palpable radial styloid and Lister's tubercle. These landmarks are then transferred to the proximal radius and represent a safe zone for hardware placement in the nonarticular portion of the radial head. The mean safe zone is an arc of 133 degrees.[8] The posterior interosseous nerve (PIN) winds around the radial neck within the supinator muscle to enter the posterior compartment of the forearm and is located 5–6 cm from the RC joint (Fig. 44.1).

The radial head acts as the main stabilizer of longitudinal forearm stability because it resists proximal axial migration of the radius.[9] On the lateral side of the elbow, the major ligamentous contributors to varus elbow stability are the lateral ulnar collateral ligament (LUCL), the radial collateral ligament (RCL), and the annular ligament. The LUCL courses from the lateral epicondyle to the supinator crest of the ulna and prevents the radial head from subluxating posteriorly, and when injured, plays a crucial role in the development of posterolateral rotatory instability.[10,11] Therefore when approaching a radial head injury with an intact LUCL, it is imperative to stay above the "equator" of the lateral epicondyle to avoid inadvertently detaching the LUCL (Fig. 44.1). The annular ligament wraps around the radial head and stabilizes the head in the lesser sigmoid notch. Elbow fractures are often associated with injuries to the annular ligament; however, the clinical relevance has not been clarified.[12] The RCL originates from the lateral epicondyle and inserts on the annular ligament.

The radial head acts in concert with the bony and static stabilizers to impart elbow stability.[13] Upon application of a valgus load, the radial head experiences a compressive force making it a secondary contributor to valgus elbow stability.[14] Thus the medial collateral ligament (MCL) and radial head integrity influence each other. This should be acknowledged when dealing with radial head fractures, which are often accompanied by lesions of the collateral ligaments.

The primary biomechanical role of the radial head is to transmit forces across the RC joint and tension the LUCL. At the elbow, approximately 60% of the mechanical load is transmitted through the radial column.[15,16] This load transmission has been shown to be altered with lengthening and shortening of the radial head as little as 2.5 mm, which affects ulnohumeral kinematics and RC pressures (Fig. 44.2).[17]

Radial head resection shifts 100% of the loading onto the ulnar column, which is discouraged in unreconstructable fractures, particularly in an acute setting. Without the radial head, proximal migration of the radius is likely, which reliably leads to instability, pain, and limited function.[18] A cadaveric study demonstrated increased varus-valgus laxity and altered elbow kinematics after

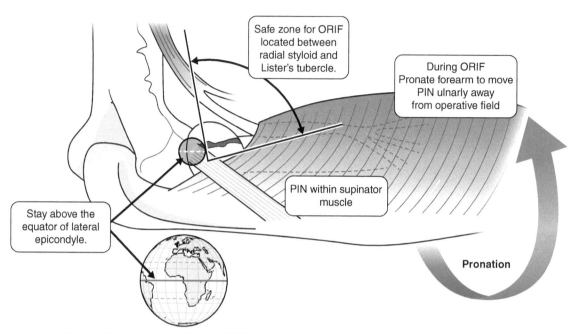

Safe zone for ORIF located between radial styloid and Lister's tubercle.

During ORIF Pronate forearm to move PIN ulnarly away from operative field

PIN within supinator muscle

Stay above the equator of lateral epicondyle.

Pronation

• **Fig. 44.1** The radial head safe zone. *ORIF*, Open reduction internal fixation; *PIN*, posterior interosseous nerve.

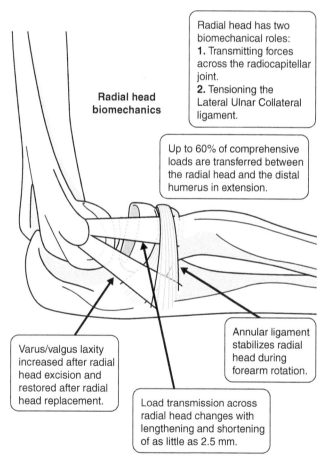

Radial head biomechanics

Radial head has two biomechanical roles:
1. Transmitting forces across the radiocapitellar joint.
2. Tensioning the Lateral Ulnar Collateral ligament.

Up to 60% of comprehensive loads are transferred between the radial head and the distal humerus in extension.

Varus/valgus laxity increased after radial head excision and restored after radial head replacement.

Annular ligament stabilizes radial head during forearm rotation.

Load transmission across radial head changes with lengthening and shortening of as little as 2.5 mm.

• **Fig. 44.2** Radial head biomechanics.

radial head excision and both were corrected after radial head arthroplasty.[19] In the face of biomechanical compromise to the interosseous membrane (IOM), such as in an Essex-Lopresti lesion, disastrous complications may ensue.

Pathoanatomy

Radial head fractures often occur due to a fall onto an outstretched hand where the elbow is extended and the forearm pronated. Because pronation decreases the distance between the radial head and capitellum, substantial force is transmitted in this position. A comminuted radial head or neck fracture is most likely the result of failure in compression due to an axial and valgus load. More substantial radial head fractures are believed to have likely occurred in association with a brief but complete dislocation of the elbow.[19] Concomitant lesions were found in 39% of a study population suggesting that radial head fractures rarely occur in isolation and tend to be a marker of complex elbow trauma.[20] Ligament rupture or avulsion fractures from the coronoid process are, therefore, to be expected.[21] A magnetic resonance imaging (MRI) study of 24 subjects with Mason type II and III fractures demonstrated 54% MCL and 80% LUCL injuries with associated capitellar chondral defects and loose bodies occurring in 30% and 91% of cases, respectively.[5] Frequent lateral ligamentous injuries have been noted even in a Mason type I fracture.[22] These studies emphasize the need to appreciate ligamentous and osseous lesions and how it is to be expected that the elbow's healing response may be a vigorous one that has the potential to lead to stiffness if early motion is not achieved.

Accompanying injuries of the IOM have also been reported with incidence increasing proportionally with the severity of fracture.[23] A complete tear of the IOM was noted in all Mason type III fractures. Even with Mason type I fractures, a partial lesion of the IOM was identified in 9 of 14 individuals.[23] With the increasing severity of the causal injury, the likelihood of wrist or shoulder injuries rises requiring an appropriate emphasis on evaluating these regions as well.[24]

Physical Examination

Elbow swelling, hematoma, and, occasionally, deformity will accompany these proximal radius injuries. Palpation will elicit a point of maximum tenderness, which should correlate with this injury. Palpation along the IOM and distal radioulnar joint stability assessment will identify associated lesions of the forearm and wrist. Active and passive range of motion (ROM) must be documented with attention given to joint crepitus when moving the extremity and, particularly, when rotating the forearm. Varus and valgus stability should be investigated in full extension and 30 degrees of flexion, and, if possible, documented under fluoroscopy.

Imaging

The most basic imaging begins with radiographs, including anteroposterior (AP) and lateral projections of the elbow. The oblique lateral (Greenspan) view of the elbow can also be helpful to evaluate the RC joint and radial head without overlap of the coronoid. Subtle fractures are often difficult to see on radiographs. Soft tissue findings that are typical of occult fractures include the presence of an anterior or a posterior fat pad sign. In addition, a slight irregularity of the transition of the radial head to the neck may be visible on radiographic studies, even in low-grade fractures with minimal displacement.

Adequate articulation of the joint must also be determined, including the presence of free bony fragments or posterolateral subluxation of the radial head suspicious for posterolateral rotatory instability (PLRI). The complete loss of cortical contact of at least one radial head fracture fragment is strongly correlated with a complex injury pattern.[25]

Moreover, the degree of displacement of fracture fragments (>2 mm) can be judged, although the reliability of such predictions is better with a computed tomography (CT) scan. Two-dimensional and three-dimensional reconstructions of the radial head are possible but do not reduce interobserver variation.[26] Small free intra-articular fragments or impacted fractures can be judged best on CT scans.[27]

MRI scans allow the clinician to assess the state of the soft tissues, visualizing even the slightest fracture line within bone and detecting intraosseous edema.[28] An MRI can be useful to evaluate associated collateral ligament or IOM injury.[29] However, the routine use of MRI scans is not necessary because it rarely affects management.[30]

Classification

The Mason classification system is the most widely used classification system for fractures of the radial head.[31] The classification distinguishes nondisplaced fractures (type I), displaced fractures (type II), and fractures that are displaced with comminution (type III). A fourth type was added by Johnston in 1962, describing a fracture of the radial head accompanied by elbow dislocation (Fig. 44.3). In 1987, a metric definition of displacement (<2 or >2 mm) and an area of involvement of the articular surface (>30%) was included to differentiate between Mason types I and II. The Mason classification, however, has shown low interobserver and intraobserver reliability; hence, it is difficult to derive conclusive treatment algorithms.[32]

Type I Fractures

Hotchkiss later modified the Mason type I classification to include nondisplaced or minimally displaced (<2 mm) fractures with no mechanical block to rotation.[33] These are generally small cracks and may not be visible on initial X-rays and yet can usually be seen if the X-ray is taken 3 weeks after the injury. Nonsurgical treatment involves using a splint or a sling for a few days, followed

by an early increase in elbow movement. Many studies have demonstrated good results with most patients achieving full function and recovery of ROM after type I fractures.[34–36]

Assessing elbow joint ROM can be difficult at first due to pain. Therefore reevaluation in a few days is advised. However, if there is suspicion of a mechanical block to rotation, the diagnosis can also be facilitated via the aspiration of trauma hematoma and injection of local anesthetics. Surgery is indicated if substantial loss of motion or clicking and crepitus occurs with forearm rotation despite lidocaine-induced pain relief, which is suggestive of a mechanical block or articular incongruity.

Type II Fractures

Type II fractures are displaced >2 mm or angulated and may result in a mechanical block to forearm rotation. If no mechanical block is identified, a sling or splint may be used for 1–2 weeks, followed by ROM exercises. The amount of radial head fracture displacement that is acceptable for nonoperative treatment remains largely unknown.

Good long-term results of nonsurgically treated 2–5-mm displaced Mason type II fractures have further clouded indications for surgery.[37] Here, 40 of 49 subjects declared that they had no symptoms after a mean follow-up of 19 years and only minimal differences between the injured and uninjured elbow were noted. Subsequent studies confirm these results and call into question whether surgery is indicated for partially displaced fractures.[38,39]

Surgery to restore articular congruence may be preventative for the development of posttraumatic arthritis. In a retrospective comparison of 10 surgically and 16 nonsurgically treated Mason type II fractures, a higher incidence of degenerative changes in the nonoperative group was noted. Overall, 90% of the surgically treated subjects versus only 44% of the nonoperatively treated subjects reached a good outcome.[40] Conversely, Akesson and colleagues reported that most of the degenerative changes resulting after nonoperative treatment of partially displaced fractures remained asymptomatic, an observation that has been confirmed by similar studies.[35,37,39] At present, no randomized controlled trials exist to guide treatment, and it remains unclear how to best manage displaced partial articular fractures of the radial head.

Ultimately, management decisions for these fractures should take into account patient factors including age and activity level as well as bone quality and any associated injuries. Also, given their high association with soft tissue trauma, surgical intervention to address bony pathology affords an opportunity to repair the soft tissue damage.

Type III Fractures

Type III fractures are comminuted and substantially displaced resulting in a mechanical block to forearm rotation. In most type III radial head fractures, substantial damage to the surrounding ligaments is encountered. The surgical treatment of multifragmentary radial head fractures is technically challenging and optimal treatment decisions remain controversial. Injuries that are amenable to anatomic and stable open reduction internal fixation (ORIF) should be fixed as restoration of the lateral column enables physiologic load transmission. Arthroplasty is indicated for comminuted unreconstructable fractures with concomitant ligamentous injuries. Resection of the radial head without prosthetic replacement should only be considered in the case of a stable elbow and, even then, probably not in a younger person. Elbow stability must be examined after resection of the radial head to exclude valgus instability and longitudinal instability of the forearm. Varus,

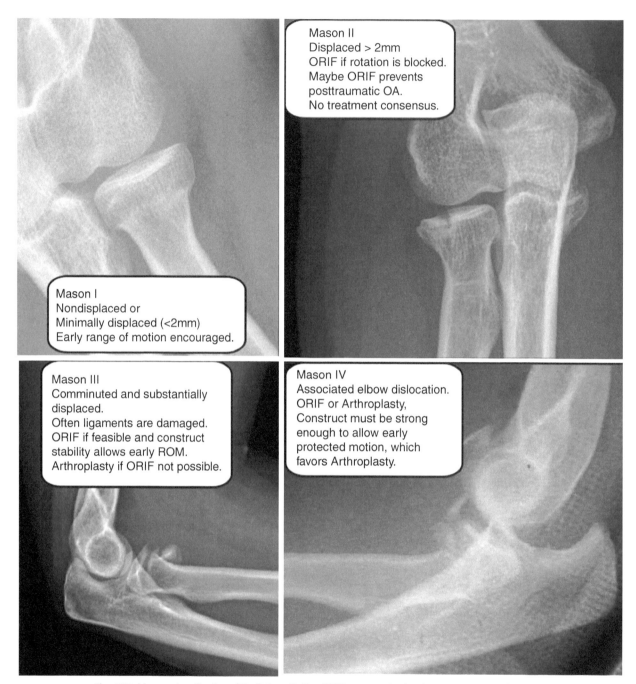

• **Fig. 44.3** Mason classification. *OA*, Osteoarthritis; *ORIF*, open reduction internal fixation; *ROM*, range of motion.

valgus, posterolateral rotatory, and axial stress examination should be carefully performed under fluoroscopic control. Significant instability is often found because unreconstructable Mason type III fractures are accompanied by a high percentage of associated ligament tears. Therefore radial head resection is rarely indicated because it does not sufficiently accommodate these capsuloligamentous injuries. If instability is a concern, radial head replacement should be performed.

Type IV Fractures

Type IV fractures involve an associated elbow dislocation and require surgical intervention. No different than with other complex elbow dislocations, the goal is to convert a complex (associated fracture) to a simple (no bony injury) dislocation, which is then treated with protected early motion within a protected arc. The decision to treat with an ORIF or a replacement is at the discretion of the surgeon with the overriding principle being the creation of adequate construct stability that can withstand the mechanical requirements of early ROM.

Treatment Options

Nonoperative

Nondisplaced and isolated or minimally displaced radial head fractures that do not exhibit a mechanical block to rotation benefit from early ROM at 1 week. Additionally, isolated minimally displaced or impacted radial neck fractures can also be safely treated with a brief period of immobilization and then ROM. It must be emphasized to work on ensuring full extension so as to prevent elbow stiffness. The frequent correlation between collateral ligament injury and displaced radial head and neck fractures has been established. However, regardless of soft tissue trauma, conservative management is the best treatment for an elbow with a firm end point under valgus stress testing.[41] Patients are asked to particularly focus on terminal elbow extension as elbow flexion and forearm rotation improvement is more reliably recovered. Generally, formal physical therapy (PT) is not typically necessary. A prospective randomized controlled trial demonstrated that patients who followed a home exercise program after sustaining a nondisplaced or minimally displaced radial head or neck fracture had a better early function at 6 weeks compared with patients undergoing formal PT and there was no significant difference in outcomes after 6 weeks.[42]

Operative

Surgery is recommended for significantly displaced or comminuted fractures that mechanically limit rotation or if they are associated with complex elbow injuries. The radial head should be preserved or replaced if there is an associated ligamentous or articular injury involving the elbow or the distal radioulnar joint.[43] When possible, ORIF should be chosen over prosthetic replacement. Broadly there are three options. The radial head can be removed, it can be repaired, and it can be replaced.

Radial Head Excision

Although biomechanical data predict that radial head excision significantly alters elbow kinematics even in a stable elbow, good long-term clinical results of primary radial excision have been published. Twenty-six subjects treated with primary radial head excision for isolated Mason type II and III fractures achieved good results in 24 subjects, with a mean Mayo Elbow Performance Score (MEPS) of 95 and a follow-up of 15 years. No correlation between a high rate of degenerative changes and subject disorders was found.[44]

In young patients, higher activity demand is associated with a greater need to preserve the biomechanics of the radial head. Comparing acute radial head excision with ORIF, a better DASH (the Disabilities of the Arm, Shoulder and Hand) score and a lower rate of subsequent elbow dislocation and posttraumatic arthritis for the ORIF group were found.[45] Superior results for ORIF were identified in a retrospective comparison of ORIF and acute radial head resection for comminuted radial head fractures.[46]

The clinical benefit of restoring the radial column is in line with biomechanical findings. Sixty percent of the axial loads are normally transmitted through the humeroradial column. When this relationship is compromised, the ulnohumeral joint must bear the vast majority of axial forces after radial head excision. Therefore the rate of radiographic osteoarthritis progression is high in these circumstances.[47] These findings are in agreement with in vitro biomechanical studies that indicate changes in kinematics and greater laxity after radial head resection compared with the intact, repaired, and replaced radial head.[48–50] Based on these findings, radial head replacement is considered the treatment of choice for the unreconstructable radial head fracture. Excision of the radial head may be considered in acute situations but should be limited to low-demand or elderly patients.[51,52]

ORIF

Fracture reconstruction is recommended for Mason type II fractures with a mechanical block and Mason type III fractures where ORIF is feasible. Furthermore, if elbow instability is noted on examination, a soft tissue repair at the same time as the ORIF or radial head arthroplasty is indicated.

When addressing these fractures, it is important to determine key fracture characteristics. If only a portion of the articular surface is injured and, importantly, the neck is in continuity with the articular surface, simple screw fixation of loose parts to the stable parts of the articular surface may be sufficient.[53] In cases where the whole articular surface is separated from the radial shaft, the free-floating fracture fragments of the head must be pieced together.[54] Subsequently, the restored radial head may be secured to the radial neck within the safe zone. When reconstructing the radial head, typically only unicortical screws can be placed to avoid penetration and impingement of the PRUJ. Due to these limitations, a plate with locking screw options is recommended to maximize construct stability. Radial head–specific plates with locking screws may provide enhanced primary stability with results of ORIF for comminuted radial head fractures demonstrating mostly good outcomes.[46,55,56] When radial head fractures involve more than three fragments, the risk of complications is high and replacement should be considered.[57]

Ultimately, the ability to repair the radial head may only be reliably determined intraoperatively and preparation for both treatments is encouraged. The primary goal of surgical management is to ensure an early advancement in ROM. If adequate construct stability is achieved with ORIF, this approach is advocated. If this cannot be reliably achieved, then an arthroplasty must be considered.

Radial Head Arthroplasty

The decision to replace the radial head can be multifactorial and dependent on patient age and bone quality as well as concomitant bony or ligamentous injuries. Generally, radial head arthroplasty is indicated for displaced and comminuted fractures that are not amenable to achieving an anatomic reduction with a strong internal fixation construct. Many types of metallic radial head prostheses are commercially available. Different head geometries (round vs. elliptical), stem types (smooth vs. ingrowth), methods of head to shaft fixation (monopolar vs. bipolar), and cemented versus cementless fixation exist. Regardless of design, radial head implants have proven to restore elbow stability, even in unstable elbow fracture-dislocations.[58–60] There are currently no studies comparing the clinical outcomes of different radial head implants.

Promising short-term and midterm results have been reported; however, only a few long-term studies exist.[50,61–64] Good results with a bipolar metallic radial head implant after 10-year follow-up with no report of elbow instability were noted.[62] Nevertheless, there certainly are disadvantages to radial head arthroplasty that often relate to the difficulty in replicating the radial head's anatomy. As long as the RC joint is accurately restored, the functional results of radial head arthroplasty exceed those that have undergone radial head excision in the setting of unreconstructable radial head fractures.

Surgical Approaches

Several approaches exist for the surgical management of radial head fractures. The most common incision is centered laterally

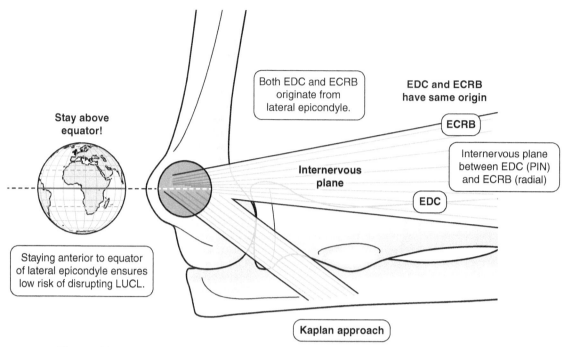

Stay above equator!

Staying anterior to equator of lateral epicondyle ensures low risk of disrupting LUCL.

Both EDC and ECRB originate from lateral epicondyle.

EDC and ECRB have same origin

Internervous plane

ECRB

Internervous plane between EDC (PIN) and ECRB (radial)

EDC

Kaplan approach

• **Fig. 44.4** Kaplan approach. *ECRB,* Extensor carpi radialis brevis; *EDC,* extensor digitorum communis; *LUCL,* lateral ulnar collateral ligament; *PIN,* posterior interosseous nerve.

over the lateral epicondyle and radial head. A posterior incision is employed when a concomitant olecranon fracture requires fixation; however, we would not recommend routine use of a posterior incision for isolated radial head fractures. This approach requires large skin flaps to be mobilized which could increase the risk of hematoma formation and wound complications.

Upon making a lateral incision, a few surgical approaches can be chosen. The most commonly described approaches include the Kaplan, the Kocher, and the extensor splitting approaches. The PIN crosses the proximal radius from anterior to posterior within the supinator muscle 5 cm distal to the RC joint. In all approaches, the forearm should be pronated to protect the PIN. Pronation positions the nerve away from the surgical field to minimize the risk of injury. Try to limit anterior retraction over the radial neck as this could put undue pressure on the PIN. If more visualization is needed, all approaches can be extended proximally and distally.

Kaplan Approach

This muscle-tendon splitting approach lies between the extensor digitorum communis (EDC) (PIN) and extensor carpi radialis brevis (ECRB) (radial n.).[65] Dissection occurs anterior to the equator of the capitellum ensuring a much lower risk of disrupting the LUCL and destabilizing the elbow (Fig. 44.4). This approach allows the best exposure to the anterior aspect of the radial head for ORIF of anterior radial head fragments. If there is a LUCL injury, this approach may make it more difficult to repair the ligament and may require more dissection posteriorly to do so.

Extensor Splitting Approach

This muscle-tendon splitting approach lies between the EDC (Fig. 44.5). As with all approaches, dissection occurs anterior to the equator of the capitellum, which ensures a much lower risk of disrupting the LUCL. This approach is in many respects a compromise between the Kaplan, which is a more anteriorly based interval and has an increased risk of PIN injury, versus the Kocher, which is posterior and has a risk of LUCL injury. The extensor

split reduces the risk of nerve injury and iatrogenic lateral elbow instability making this approach the preferred method by the authors.

Kocher Approach

This approach lies between the extensor carpi ulnaris (ECU) (PIN) and anconeus (radial n.) muscles (Fig. 44.6). It is imperative to dissect anterior to the crista supinatoris, which is where the LUCL inserts so as to avoid damaging this very important elbow stabilizer. Although there is less risk of PIN injury than the Kaplan approach, the risk of destabilizing the LUCL complex makes this approach less desirable. However, if there is a known LUCL injury, as is identified on the preoperative stress examination or with elbow dislocation, then the Kocher approach may be chosen for direct visualization of the ligament. It is also advocated when visualization of the posterior radial head and the PRUJ is paramount and is recommended for multifragmentary radial head fractures.

Relevant Complications

Regardless of whether operative or nonoperative treatment is chosen, restricted elbow motion is common. It is important to begin elbow motion as soon as possible to minimize this risk. Conversely, elbow instability is associated with these injuries and may warrant a period of immobilization to avoid loss of fixation, recurrent instability, and joint malalignment. PIN injury may occur with operative management. ORIF carries a risk of malunion, nonunion, and arthritis. At long-term follow-up from ORIF, patients with a type II radial head fracture had satisfactory results; however, those with a type III fracture were more likely to go on to nonunion (8.3%).[57] While outcomes are generally favorable after radial head replacement, 38% of patients had ulnohumeral arthritis, and 36% developed heterotopic ossification; however, none of these patients required implant removal or revision.[61]

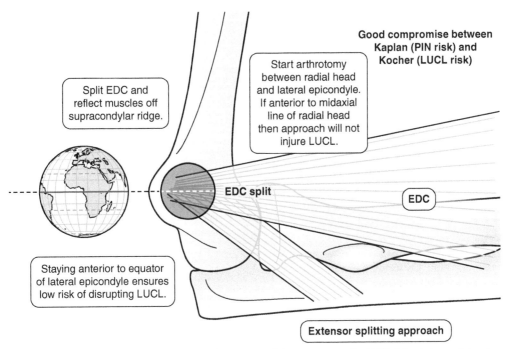

Split EDC and reflect muscles off supracondylar ridge.

Good compromise between Kaplan (PIN risk) and Kocher (LUCL risk)

Start arthrotomy between radial head and lateral epicondyle. If anterior to midaxial line of radial head then approach will not injure LUCL.

EDC split

EDC

Staying anterior to equator of lateral epicondyle ensures low risk of disrupting LUCL.

Extensor splitting approach

• **Fig. 44.5** Extensor splitting approach. *EDC*, Extensor digitorum communis; *LUCL*, lateral ulnar collateral ligament; *PIN*, posterior interosseous nerve.

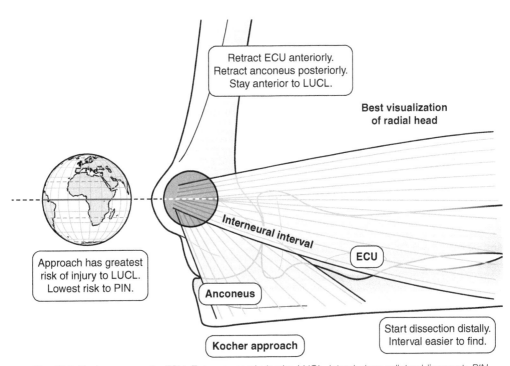

Retract ECU anteriorly. Retract anconeus posteriorly. Stay anterior to LUCL.

Best visualization of radial head

Interneural interval

ECU

Approach has greatest risk of injury to LUCL. Lowest risk to PIN.

Anconeus

Start dissection distally. Interval easier to find.

Kocher approach

• **Fig. 44.6** Kocher approach. *ECU*, Extensor carpi ulnaris; *LUCL*, lateral ulnar collateral ligament; *PIN*, posterior interosseous nerve.

Review of Treatment Outcomes

The outcome of these fractures depends largely on the severity of the injury. A key management component is achieving early ROM. Though nondisplaced, stable fractures have a good prognosis with nonoperative treatment, it is necessary to identify the displaced unstable fractures that may benefit from surgery and then identify whether reduction and fixation is possible, or whether replacement must be performed.

Simple fractures displaced <2 mm can, quite reliably, be treated nonoperatively. The treatment of choice for 2–5 mm displaced partial articular fractures remains without consensus and yet the rate of osteoarthritis seems to be higher with nonoperative treatment. ORIF is preferred whenever an anatomic and stable reduction can be achieved that allows early ROM, and radial head arthroplasty is considered when this cannot be achieved. Radial head arthroplasty is the treatment of choice for those fractures that do not allow anatomic and stable fixation. Patients with fractures involving less of the articular surface, such as those with Mason type II fractures, have good to excellent results following an ORIF. These patients can expect an average arc of motion of 144 degrees of flexion and extension, with an average range of 72 degrees of both pronation and supination. However, patients with Mason type III fractures had much lower patient satisfaction scores and much less ROM following their ORIF.[57]

Though most of the degenerative changes reported in outcome studies after radial head arthroplasty are asymptomatic, they might become symptomatic within the course of time because most patients suffering a radial head fracture are young and may have to cope with fracture sequelae for 30–50 years. A few long-term follow-up studies have found that patients with a radial head arthroplasty have good to excellent functional outcomes and are generally satisfied with their clinical results after 8–12 years.[63,64] However, there is a continued need for long-term follow-up data in the younger population to determine the superiority between ORIF and replacement in the surgically indicated radial head fracture.

References

1. Van Riet RP, Glabbek F, Morrey BF. Radial head fracture. *Elb Its Disord*. 2009:359–389.
2. Duckworth AD, Clement ND, Jenkins PJ, Aitken SA, Court-Brown CM, McQueen MM. The epidemiology of radial head and neck fractures. *J Hand Surg*. 2012;37:112–119.
3. van Riet RP, Morrey BF, O'Driscoll SW, Van Glabbeek F. Associated injuries complicating radial head fractures: a demographic study. *Clin Orthop*. 2005;441:351–355.
4. Jensen SL, Olsen BS, Søjbjerg JO. Elbow joint kinematics after excision of the radial head. *J Shoulder Elbow Surg*. 1999;8:238–241.
5. Itamura JM, Roidis NT, Chong AK, Vaishnav S, Papadakis SA, Zalavras C. Computed tomography study of radial head morphology. *J Shoulder Elbow Surg*. 2008;17:347–354.
6. Kuhn S, Burkhart KJ, Schneider J, et al. The anatomy of the proximal radius: implications on fracture implant design. *J Shoulder Elbow Surg*. 2012;21:1247–1254.
7. Giannicola G, Manauzzi E, Sacchetti FM, et al. Anatomical variations of the proximal radius and their effects on osteosynthesis. *J Hand Surg*. 2012;37:1015–1023.
8. Ries C, Müller M, Wegmann K, Pfau DB, Müller LP, Burkhart KJ. Is an extension of the safe zone possible without jeopardizing the proximal radioulnar joint when performing a radial head plate osteosynthesis? *J Shoulder Elbow Surg*. 2015;24:1627–1634.
9. Wegmann K, Dargel J, Burkhart KJ, Brüggemann GP, Müller LP. The Essex-Lopresti lesion. *Strateg Trauma Limb Reconstr*. 2012;7:131–139.
10. O'Driscoll SW. Classification and evaluation of recurrent instability of the elbow. *Clin Orthop*. 2000:34–43. https://doi.org/10.1097/00003086-200001000-00005.
11. Reichel LM, Milam GS, Sitton SE, Curry MC, Mehlhoff TL. Elbow lateral collateral ligament injuries. *J Hand Surg*. 2013;38:184–201. quiz 201.
12. Mak S, Beltran LS, Bencardino J, et al. MRI of the annular ligament of the elbow: review of anatomic considerations and pathologic findings in patients with posterolateral elbow instability. *AJR Am J Roentgenol*. 2014;203:1272–1279.
13. Hassan SE, Parks BG, Douoguih WA, Osbahr DC. Effect of distal ulnar collateral ligament tear pattern on contact forces and valgus stability in the posteromedial compartment of the elbow. *Am J Sports Med*. 2015;43:447–452.
14. Morrey BF, Tanaka S, An KN. Valgus stability of the elbow. A definition of primary and secondary constraints. *Clin Orthop*. 1991:187–195.
15. Morrey BF, An K-N. Stability of the elbow: osseous constraints. *J Shoulder Elbow Surg*. 2005;14:174S–178S.
16. Morrey BF, An KN, Stormont TJ. Force transmission through the radial head. *J Bone Joint Surg Am*. 1988;70:250–256.
17. Van Glabbeek F, Van Riet RP, Baumfeld JA, et al. Detrimental effects of overstuffing or understuffing with a radial head replacement in the medial collateral-ligament deficient elbow. *J Bone Joint Surg Am*. 2004;86:2629–2635.
18. Loeffler BJ, Green JB, Zelouf DS. Forearm instability. *J Hand Surg*. 2014;39:156–167.
19. Burkhart KJ, Franke S, Wegmann K, et al. [Mason I fracture - a simple injury?]. *Unfallchirurg*. 2015;118:9–17.
20. Gruszka D, Nowak TE, Tkacz T, Wagner D, Rommens PM. Complex radial head and neck fractures treated with modern locking plate fixation. *J Shoulder Elbow Surg*. 2019;28:1130–1138.
21. Duckworth AD, McQueen MM, Ring D. Fractures of the radial head. *Bone Jt J*. 2013;95-B:151–159.
22. Kaas L, van Riet RP, Vroemen JPAM, Eygendaal D. The incidence of associated fractures of the upper limb in fractures of the radial head. *Strateg Trauma Limb Reconstr*. 2008;3:71–74.
23. Itamura J, Roidis N, Mirzayan R, Vaishnav S, Learch T, Shean C. Radial head fractures: MRI evaluation of associated injuries. *J Shoulder Elbow Surg*. 2005;14:421–424.
24. Hausmann J-T, Vekszler G, Breitenseher M, Braunsteiner T, Vécsei V, Gäbler C. Mason type-I radial head fractures and interosseous membrane lesions—a prospective study. *J Trauma*. 2009;66:457–461.
25. Rineer CA, Guitton TG, Ring D. Radial head fractures: loss of cortical contact is associated with concomitant fracture or dislocation. *J Shoulder Elbow Surg*. 2010;19:21–25.
26. Guitton TG. Ring, D, Science of Variation Group: interobserver reliability of radial head fracture classification: two-dimensional compared with three-dimensional CT. *J Bone Joint Surg Am*. 2011;93:2015–2021.
27. Sormaala MJ, Sormaala A, Mattila VM, Koskinen SK. MDCT findings after elbow dislocation: a retrospective study of 140 patients. *Skeletal Radiol*. 2014;43:507–512.
28. Kaas L, Turkenburg JL, van Riet RP, Vroemen JPAM, Eygendaal D. Magnetic resonance imaging findings in 46 elbows with a radial head fracture. *Acta Orthop*. 2010;81:373–376.
29. Timmerman LA, Schwartz ML, Andrews JR. Preoperative evaluation of the ulnar collateral ligament by magnetic resonance imaging and computed tomography arthrography. Evaluation in 25 baseball players with surgical confirmation. *Am J Sports Med*. 1994;22:26–31. discussion 32.
30. Kaas L, van Riet RP, Turkenburg JL, Vroemen JPAM, van Dijk CN, Eygendaal D. Magnetic resonance imaging in radial head fractures: most associated injuries are not clinically relevant. *J Shoulder Elbow Surg*. 2011;20:1282–1288.
31. Mason ML. Some observations on fractures of the head of the radius with a review of one hundred cases. *Br J Surg*. 1954;42:123–132.
32. Sheps DM, Kiefer KRL, Boorman RS, et al. The interobserver reliability of classification systems for radial head fractures: the Hotchkiss modification of the Mason classification and the AO classification systems. *Can J Surg J Can Chir*. 2009;52:277–282.
33. Hotchkiss RN. Displaced fractures of the radial head: internal fixation or excision? *J Am Acad Orthop Surg*. 1997;5:1–10.
34. Duckworth AD, Watson BS, Will EM, et al. Radial head and neck fractures: functional results and predictors of outcome. *J Trauma*. 2011;71:643–648.
35. Duckworth AD, Wickramasinghe NR, Clement ND, Court-Brown CM, McQueen MM. Long-term outcomes of isolated stable radial head fractures. *J Bone Joint Surg Am*. 2014;96:1716–1723.
36. Herbertsson P, Josefsson PO, Hasserius R, Karlsson C, Besjakov J, Karlsson MK. Displaced Mason type I fractures of the radial head and neck in adults: a fifteen- to thirty-three-year follow-up study. *J Shoulder Elbow Surg*. 2005;14:73–77.

37. Akesson T, Herbertsson P, Josefsson P-O, Hasserius R, Besjakov J, Karlsson MK. Primary nonoperative treatment of moderately displaced two-part fractures of the radial head. *J Bone Joint Surg Am.* 2006;88:1909–1914.

38. Lindenhovius ALC, Felsch Q, Ring D, Kloen P. The long-term outcome of open reduction and internal fixation of stable displaced isolated partial articular fractures of the radial head. *J Trauma.* 2009;67:143–146.

39. Yoon A, King GJW, Grewal R. Is ORIF superior to nonoperative treatment in isolated displaced partial articular fractures of the radial head? *Clin Orthop.* 2014;472:2105–2112.

40. Khalfayan EE, Culp RW, Alexander AH. Mason type II radial head fractures: operative versus nonoperative treatment. *J Orthop Trauma.* 1992;6:283–289.

41. Rhyou IH, Kim KC, Kim KW, Lee J-H, Kim SY. Collateral ligament injury in the displaced radial head and neck fracture: correlation with fracture morphology and management strategy to the torn ulnar collateral ligament. *J Shoulder Elbow Surg.* 2013;22:261–267.

42. Egol KA, Haglin JM, Lott A, Fisher N, Konda SR. Minimally displaced, isolated radial head and neck fractures do not require formal physical therapy: results of a prospective randomized trial. *J Bone Joint Surg Am.* 2018;100:648–655.

43. van Riet RP, Morrey BF. Documentation of associated injuries occurring with radial head fracture. *Clin Orthop.* 2008;466:130–134.

44. Antuña SA, Sánchez-Márquez JM, Barco R. Long-term results of radial head resection following isolated radial head fractures in patients younger than forty years old. *J Bone Joint Surg Am.* 2010;92:558–566.

45. Lindenhovius ALC, Felsch Q, Doornberg JN, Ring D, Kloen P. Open reduction and internal fixation compared with excision for unstable displaced fractures of the radial head. *J Hand Surg.* 2007;32:630–636.

46. Ikeda M, Sugiyama K, Kang C, Takagaki T, Oka Y. Comminuted fractures of the radial head. Comparison of resection and internal fixation. *J Bone Joint Surg Am.* 2005;87:76–84.

47. Mikíc ZD, Vukadinovíc SM. Late results in fractures of the radial head treated by excision. *Clin Orthop.* 1983;220–228.

48. Beingessner DM, Dunning CE, Gordon KD, Johnson JA, King GJW. The effect of radial head excision and arthroplasty on elbow kinematics and stability. *J Bone Joint Surg Am.* 2004;86:1730–1739.

49. Johnson JA, Beingessner DM, Gordon KD, Dunning CE, Stacpoole RA, King GJW. Kinematics and stability of the fractured and implant-reconstructed radial head. *J Shoulder Elbow Surg.* 2005;14:195S–201S.

50. King GJ, Zarzour ZD, Rath DA, Dunning CE, Patterson SD, Johnson JA. Metallic radial head arthroplasty improves valgus stability of the elbow. *Clin Orthop.* 1999:114–125.

51. Charalambous CP, Stanley JK, Mills SP, et al. Comminuted radial head fractures: aspects of current management. *J Shoulder Elbow Surg.* 2011;20:996–1007.

52. Solarino G, Vicenti G, Abate A, Carrozzo M, Picca G, Moretti B. Mason type II and III radial head fracture in patients older than 65: is there still a place for radial head resection? *Aging Clin Exp Res.* 2015;27(suppl 1):S77–S83.

53. Burkhart KJ, Wegmann K, Müller LP, Gohlke FE. Fractures of the radial head. *Hand Clin.* 2015;31:533–546.

54. Businger A, Ruedi TP, Sommer C. On-table reconstruction of comminuted fractures of the radial head. *Injury.* 2010;41:583–588.

55. Burkhart KJ, Mueller LP, Krezdorn D, et al. Stability of radial head and neck fractures: a biomechanical study of six fixation constructs with consideration of three locking plates. *J Hand Surg.* 2007;32:1569–1575.

56. Koslowsky TC, Mader K, Dargel J, Koebke J, Hellmich M, Pennig D. Reconstruction of a Mason type-III fracture of the radial head using four different fixation techniques. An experimental study. *J Bone Joint Surg Br.* 2007;89:1545–1550.

57. Ring D, Quintero J, Jupiter JB. Open reduction and internal fixation of fractures of the radial head. *J Bone Joint Surg Am.* 2002;84:1811–1815.

58. Pomianowski S, O'Driscoll SW, Neale PG, Park MJ, Morrey BF, An KN. The effect of forearm rotation on laxity and stability of the elbow. *Clin Biomech Bristol Avon.* 2001;16:401–407.

59. King GJ, Patterson SD. Metallic radial head arthroplasty. *Tech Hand Up Extrem Surg.* 2001;5:196–203.

60. Yian E, Steens W, Lingenfelter E, Schneeberger AG. Malpositioning of radial head prostheses: an in vitro study. *J Shoulder Elbow Surg.* 2008;17:663–670.

61. Marsh JP, Grewal R, Faber KJ, Drosdowech DS, Athwal GS, King GJW. Radial head fractures treated with modular metallic radial head replacement: outcomes at a mean follow-up of eight years. *J Bone Joint Surg Am.* 2016;98:527–535.

62. Sershon RA, Luchetti TJ, Cohen MS, Wysocki RW. Radial head replacement with a bipolar system: an average 10-year follow-up. *J Shoulder Elbow Surg.* 2018;27:e38–e44.

63. Harrington IJ, Sekyi-Otu A, Barrington TW, Evans DC, Tuli V. The functional outcome with metallic radial head implants in the treatment of unstable elbow fractures: a long-term review. *J Trauma.* 2001;50:46–52.

64. Burkhart KJ, Mattyasovszky SG, Runkel M, et al. Mid- to long-term results after bipolar radial head arthroplasty. *J Shoulder Elbow Surg.* 2010;19:965–972.

65. Kaplan EB. Surgical approach to the proximal end of the radius and its use in fractures of the head and neck of the radius. *JBJS.* 1941;23:86–92.

45

Technique Spotlight: ORIF Radial Head and Neck

ROBERT A. KAUFMANN AND LEIGH-ANNE TU

Indications

Open reduction internal fixation (ORIF) is recommended for Mason Type II fractures with a mechanical block and Mason Type III fractures where stable fracture fixation is feasible. Radial head fractures with concomitant injuries (e.g., coronoid, olecranon, and/or capitellum fractures) or substantial elbow instability that requires a soft tissue repair provide an opportunity for an ORIF to be performed.

There is no clear consensus on the optimal treatment of radial head fractures with >2 mm displacement and no mechanical block to rotation. Good results have been shown with nonoperative treatment of these injuries.[1,2] Ultimately, this decision should be made after a thorough discussion with the patient regarding the risks and benefits.

For more comminuted radial head fractures, it is still a matter of debate regarding which ones can be fixed versus replaced. Often, this decision is made intraoperatively after inspecting the fracture fragments. High complication rates and poor clinical results after ORIF of radial head fractures with more than three fragments have been noted prompting recommendation that the radial head be replaced in these cases.[3] However, new techniques and implants, such as radial head–specific plates, have been developed, which have expanded the surgeon's ability to fix more comminuted radial head fractures.

Preoperative Evaluation

The preoperative examination of the patient with a radial head fracture begins with a neurovascular examination and inspection of the soft tissue to rule out open injuries. Palpation along the interosseous membrane and distal radioulnar joint (DRUJ) as well as stability assessment will identify associated injuries of the forearm and wrist. Active and passive elbow motion and any block must be determined and documented. Attention must be given to joint crepitus when moving the extremity and, particularly, when rotating the forearm. Varus and valgus stability should be investigated in full extension and 30 degrees of flexion, and, if possible, documented under fluoroscopy.

Elbow radiographs, including anteroposterior (AP) and lateral projections as well as an oblique lateral view of the elbow, can be helpful. If an Essex-Lopresti injury is suspected, then radiographs of the forearm and wrist should also be taken. Ultimately, the

intraoperative determination of DRUJ stability after radial head fixation is most important to identify an Essex-Lopresti injury. A computed tomography (CT) scan can be used for more comminuted radial head fractures.

Positioning and Equipment: Fixation Options and Plate Options

The ideal approach to the radial head occurs with the patient supine and the arm placed on a hand table. Internal and external rotation of the shoulder provides access to the lateral and the medial sides of the elbow. A nonsterile tourniquet placed on the upper arm usually allows adequate exposure. After anesthesia is induced, and prior to prepping, elbow stability should be assessed with fluoroscopy.

Fracture morphology and bone quality ultimately influence the fixation strategy. Fixation options include using headless screws, 1.5- or 2.0-mm screws, and 2.5- or 3.0-mm cannulated screws. Plate fixation can also be useful for obtaining fixation of radial neck fractures. Plate options include standard small-fixation systems or precontoured locking systems that accommodate screws between 2 and 3 mm in diameter size. Smooth K-wires can be used to reduce fragments and provide provisional fixation but are not used as definitive fixation.

After fixing the radial head, you should be prepared to repair the lateral ulnar collateral ligament (LUCL) if necessary. To do this, we recommend repairing with a heavy nonabsorbable suture over a bone tunnel created in the lateral epicondyle.

Remember that the decision to either fix or replace the radial head can sometimes only be made intraoperatively after evaluating the degree of fracture comminution. Therefore it is prudent to have radial head implants available if needed.

Technique in Detail

The lateral epicondyle and radial head are palpated and the skin incision is usually made to include these landmarks. A curvilinear incision is made 3 cm proximal to the lateral epicondyle along the supracondylar ridge and 4 cm distal to the radial head. Thick skin flaps are created. During the surgical approach, it is often difficult to discern the separate fascial planes of the extensor intervals, especially soon after a trauma when hematoma and tissue destruction can obscure normal anatomy. Often with radial head fractures, the lateral collateral complex and extensor origin is avulsed, making exposure relatively straightforward. In this case, the traumatic avulsion creates the approach interval. When no avulsion has occurred, radial head exposure occurs with an extensor splitting, Kaplan or Kocher approach. If more visualization is needed, all approaches can be extended proximally and distally.

As described previously in Chapter 44, the Kaplan approach is more useful for anterior radial head fractures and the Kocher approach allows for better visualization of the LUCL and ability to repair the ligament (Fig. 45.1A–B).

If the ligament is intact, then the Kaplan and extensor splitting approaches can avoid potential iatrogenic injury to the ligament by staying anterior to the equator of the lateral epicondyle (Fig. 45.1C). If more exposure is needed, all approaches can be extended proximally and distally. The annular ligament is preserved and sharply incised so that it can be repaired at the end of the case (Fig. 45.2). Hohmann retractors around the radial neck can be used to aid exposure; however, we would caution against prolonged retraction around the anterior radial neck because of the pressure placed on the posterior interosseous nerve (PIN). Remember to keep the forearm pronated and avoid any

dissection distal to the bicipital tuberosity to protect the PIN. If the fracture extends distally and mandates greater visualization, then the PIN needs to be formally dissected and protected throughout the case.

After opening the joint, the extent of the fragmentation is inspected and any interposing tissue is cleaned out. For partial articular fractures, the fragments can be reduced back to the intact portion of the radial head's articular surface.

K-wires can be used as joysticks to elevate any depressed fragments and the reduction can be provisionally held with these K-wires, which are then exchanged with 1.5- to 2.5-mm cortical screws according to the sizes of the fracture fragments. Alternatively, cannulated headless compression screws can be used. Screws should be countersunk to prevent impingement with the radial notch and annular ligament even if placed on the nonarticular margin. Also, it is important to avoid perforation of the far cortex while drilling to allow for more accurate length measurements with a depth gauge. Screw penetration of the far cortex could interfere with forearm rotation as well.

In complete articular fractures, the head should be first anatomically reconstructed with free screws. Again, provisional

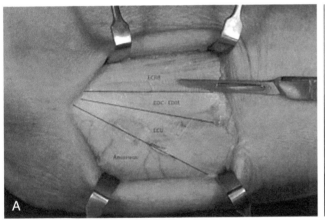
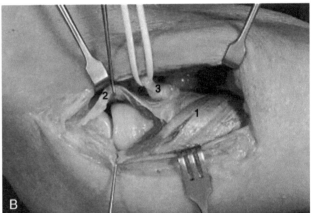
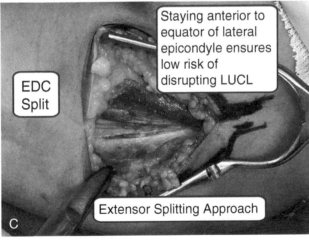

• **Fig. 45.1** Kaplan approach. (A) An interval is developed between the extensor carpi radialis brevis (ECRB) muscle and the extensor digitorum muscle (extensor digitorum communis-extensor digiti minimi [EDC–EDM]). (B) After entering this interval, the supinator muscle (1) and underlying capsule (2) should be longitudinally incised, allowing access to the most anterior part of the radial head. Note the close location of the posterior interosseous nerve (3). (C) If the ligament is intact, then the Kaplan and extensor splitting approaches can avoid potential iatrogenic injury to the ligament by staying anterior to the equator of the lateral epicondyle. *ECU*, Extensor carpi ulnaris; *LUCL*, lateral ulnar collateral ligament. (From Laakso RB, Forcada-Calvet P, Ballesteros-Betancourt JR, Llusa-Pérez M, Antuña SA. Surgical approaches to the elbow. In: Stanley D, Trail I, eds. *Operative Elbow Surgery*. Philadelphia: Elsevier; 2012:91-106.)

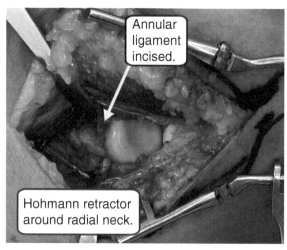

• **Fig. 45.2** The annular ligament is preserved and sharply incised so that it can be repaired at the end of the case. Hohmann retractors around the radial neck can be used to aid exposure.

fixation can be achieved with K-wires. Then, the reconstructed head can be fixed to the neck using divergent cannulated 2.5-mm screws if the neck is not comminuted.

A plate can also be used if there is radial neck comminution. Fixed-angle, precontoured plates are preferred and should be placed in the safe zone to avoid restricting forearm rotation (Fig. 45.3A–B). The fracture morphology may occasionally necessitate placing the plate outside the safe zone. In these cases, the plate should be removed as soon as healing has occurred and a surgical release of the proximal radioulnar joint (PRUJ) is also recommended during the time of hardware removal. If bone graft is needed for defects, cancellous bone from the lateral epicondyle, the proximal ulna, or the distal radius can be obtained.

If ruptured, the LUCL is repaired anatomically with transosseous sutures or suture anchors. The author's preferred method of LUCL repair employs nonabsorbable sutures such as a 5-0 Ticron that is tied over a bone bridge. The center of the capitellum can be used for identifying the placement of the drill hole that represents an isometric location for graft placement. The drill is directed in a

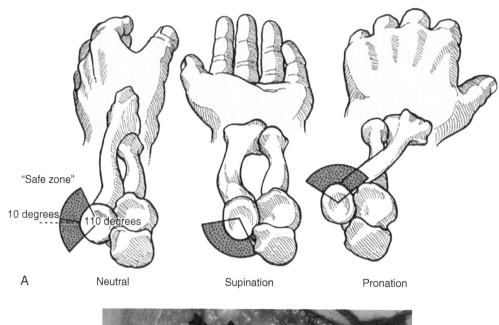

A   Neutral   Supination   Pronation

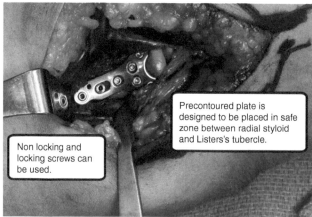

B

• **Fig. 45.3** A. Nonarticular portion of the radial head. The nonarticular portion "safe zone" of the radial head can be identified as a 110-degree arc centered on a point 10 degrees anterior to the midpoint of the lateral side of the radial head with the forearm in neutral rotation. (B) A plate can be placed in the safe zone of the radial head. (From King GJW. Fractures of the radial head. In: Green DP, ed. *Green's Operative Hand Surgery*. Philadelphia: Elsevier; 2017:734-769.)

divergent manner to create two posterior openings. A 5-0 Ticron suture with two needles is passed through the LUCL in a Bunnell fashion. The two needles are both passed through the point of isometry and then posteriorly through the divergent holes. Once the suture is passed, tension both limbs for 2 minutes to remove the viscous properties and then tie the sutures directly over the bone bridge created by the two posterior drill holes in the capitellum. Stability is then checked again after the LUCL is repaired and, if there is still significant medial instability leading to subluxation of the elbow, the medial collateral ligament should be repaired. If repair of the medial collateral ligament does not restore adequate stability, we will place an external static or dynamic elbow fixator or an Internal Joint Stabilizer (Skeletal Dynamics, Miami, FL).

The lateral wound is closed by suturing the anterior limb of the split extensor origin to the posterior limb. The previously incised annular ligament may be repaired with an absorbable suture. If the LUCL is intact at the time of surgery or the repair of the LUCL is stout, the elbow is splinted in 90 degrees of flexion with the forearm in supination. Forearm supination helps close the medial joint space, allowing an injured ulnar collateral ligament to heal in an anatomic position.

Postoperative Rehabilitation

The postoperative regimen is tailored to the individual patient depending on stability and associated injuries. The goal of all rehabilitation protocols is early, safe mobilization (Fig. 45.4). Postoperatively, the elbow is splinted in 90 degrees of flexion for 10 days and then the skin sutures removed. If the LUCL was not injured, then elbow range of motion is initiated. A Munster splint can be used to avoid forearm rotation but still allow for elbow motion. There is a 5-pound lifting restriction until 8 weeks after surgery. If the LUCL was injured and repaired, then a hinged brace is placed and for the first week 90 to full elbow flexion is allowed. The hinged brace can be periodically removed to allow the achievement of full flexion, which may be limited by the brace itself. Forearm rotation is generally restricted until evidence of fracture healing is appreciated radiographically, which is often not until 4 weeks status post radial head fixation. Unlimited forearm rotation is allowed in partial articular fractures where the biomechanical construct will tolerate rotational forces. At 17 days, the hinged brace is adjusted to allow 60 to full flexion. At 24 days, 30 degrees to full flexion is encouraged. The ability to achieve terminal extension is assessed at 31 days. Usually at 31 days, the patient has difficulty extending beyond 30 and the hinged brace is unlocked. However, if terminal extension is easily achieved at this time, then an arc of 30 degrees to full flexion is maintained for another week to protect the soft tissues. At 38 days, the hinged brace is unlocked and at 42 days it is discontinued. Formal physical therapy is used if at any time motion within the prescribed arc is not achieved by the patient. Varus and valgus stresses as well as resistive exercises are not started until 8 weeks after surgery.

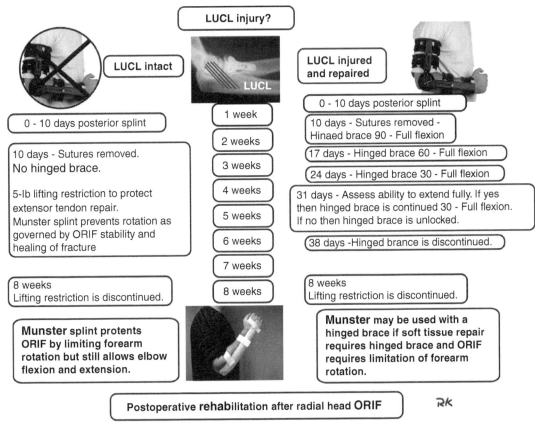

• **Fig. 45.4** Rehabilitation protocols for intact or injured lateral ulnar collateral ligament (*LUCL*).

Procedural Equipment and Material

Positioning	• Hand table
Exposure	• Weitlaner retractors
	• Small Hohmann retractor
Fracture reduction and fixation	• Dental pick
	• Bone clamps
	• 0.35-mm or 0.45-mm K-wires
	• Headless screws: 1.5- or 2.0-mm screws and 2.5- or 3.0-mm cannulated screws
	• Fixed-angle precontoured radial neck/head plates
Lateral ulnar collateral ligament repair	• Nonabsorbable suture: 5-0 Ticron with double-ended needles
	• Drill equipped with 2.0 drill bit
Imaging	• Fluoroscope

PEARLS AND PITFALLS

- We recommend staying anterior to the midpoint of the lateral epicondyle to avoid injury to a potentially intact LUCL.
  - The Kaplan and extensor splitting approaches may be best at avoiding injury to the LUCL.
  - The Kocher interval may be used but the capsular incision must be made anteriorly so as to avoid injury to the LUCL.
- The competency of the lateral ligament complex may be difficult to assess. Gross instability is noted when the lateral complex and the common extensor mechanism are both stripped leaving the lateral epicondyle bare. In other cases, the injury can be more subtle mandating intraoperative assessment of dynamic and static stabilizers.
- The biggest pitfall in dealing with an elbow fracture-dislocation is the inability to maintain elbow stability.
  - A concomitant LUCL injury is common with radial head fractures and should be routinely repaired.
  - An ulnar collateral ligament injury can be managed with protected mobilization, as long as elbow stability is restored with the radial head ORIF, and the LUCL repair.
- Beware of hardware impingement limiting forearm rotation. To avoid this, ensure that there is no screw penetration through the opposite cortex and that the plate and screw construct does not impinge upon the PRUJ. After obtaining fixation and prior to closing the wound, gently pronate and supinate the forearm to ensure that there is no crepitus and no prominent hardware within the PRUJ.

References

1. Akesson T, Herbertsson P, Josefsson P-O, Hasserius R, Besjakov J, Karlsson MK. Primary nonoperative treatment of moderately displaced two-part fractures of the radial head. *J Bone Joint Surg Am.* 2006;88:1909–1914.
2. Yoon A, King GJW, Grewal R. Is ORIF superior to nonoperative treatment in isolated displaced partial articular fractures of the radial head? *Clin Orthop Relat Res.* 2014;472:2105–2112.
3. Ring D, Quintero J, Jupiter JB. Open reduction and internal fixation of fractures of the radial head. *J Bone Joint Surg Am.* 2002;84:1811–1815.

46

Technique Spotlight: Radial Head Arthroplasty

ROBERT A. KAUFMANN AND LEIGH-ANNE TU

Indications

Radial head arthroplasty (RHA) is a valuable surgical option for complex, comminuted radial head fractures with associated elbow instability. An RHA is recommended when anatomic repair and fixation of a radial head fracture is not possible and removal of the radial head alone may not be advantageous due to instability. Injury to the lateral ulnar collateral ligament (LUCL) complex and the medial collateral ligament (MCL) will lead to greater elbow instability if the radial head is simply excised and the ligaments are not repaired. Similarly, injury to the interosseous membrane will lead to longitudinal forearm instability if the radial head is not restored. The majority of these associated ligamentous injuries occur with Mason type III radial head fractures.[1] Furthermore, the elbow that requires a soft tissue repair is also one that benefits from early range of motion so as to prevent stiffness. A radial head replacement can, at times, allow for a more rapid advancement in range of motion than an open reduction internal fixation (ORIF).

Preoperative Evaluation

The key aspects to the preoperative examination of the patient with a radial head fracture are detailed in Chapter 44. Preoperative imaging typically starts with plain radiographs including anteroposterior, lateral, and Greenspan (radial head) views. In most cases, this is sufficient for preoperative planning; however, computed tomography (CT) scan is considered if there are concomitant bony injuries or to further delineate articular fragments when also considering ORIF.

Positioning and Equipment

The patient is supine with the arm placed on a radiolucent hand table. Internal and external rotation of the shoulder provide access to the lateral and the medial sides of the elbow. A nonsterile tourniquet placed on the upper arm usually allows adequate exposure. After anesthesia is induced, and prior to prepping, elbow stability should be assessed with fluoroscopy. If there is an associated olecranon fracture, then it may be more advantageous to make one single posterior incision to access the olecranon and radial head. In this case, it is easier to place the patient lateral with the arm draped over an arm holder.

A variety of radial head replacements are available and have in common their ability to act as a force transmitter between the radius and the distal humerus as well as a tensioner of the LUCL (Fig. 46.1). They are substantially equivalent and differentiate themselves through their stem type (smooth vs. ingrowth), head appearance (round vs. elliptical), and head to shaft connection (rigid vs. flexible). Longer stems for fractures with more distal extension are also available.

Technique in Detail

The approach to the radial head is described in detail in the previous chapter. If choosing a Kaplan or extensor splitting approach, it is important to stay above the "equator" of the lateral epicondyle to avoid injury to an intact LUCL. The annular ligament should be incised sharply and preserved for repair at the end. Remember to keep the forearm pronated and avoid any dissection distal to the radial tuberosity to protect the posterior interosseous nerve.

Once the joint is exposed, the fracture fragments should be examined to ensure that an ORIF is not possible. If it is determined that ORIF is not feasible and radial head replacement is indicated, it is important to inspect the fracture site and remove all bony fragments, many of which can be found in locations far removed from the radiocapitellar (RC) joint. Using a microsagittal saw, the neck is cut perpendicular to the shaft at the metaphyseal-diaphyseal junction. This cut will usually be just distal to the distal margin of the lesser sigmoid notch of the ulna. It is advantageous to preserve as much shaft as possible as this region provides fixation for the radial head implant

After the fragments are removed, the stability of the LUCL, MCL, and the interosseous membrane is assessed. When examining the LUCL, it is important to remember that sometimes LUCL injury may not always be apparent on first glance if the common extensor origin is still intact. In this case, to assess the LUCL, extend the elbow and retract the posterior limb of the extensor origin. The capsule and associated LUCL origin are normally adjacent to the articular cartilage. If the lateral wall of the capitellum is "naked," devoid of any soft tissue or ligamentous attachment, the LUCL origin is ruptured and the elbow is in the early stages of posterolateral rotatory instability (PLRI).[2] The interosseous membrane integrity is determined by pulling on the exposed radial neck and observing proximal migration. With fluoroscopy at the wrist, proximal migration of the radius is estimated using "feel" and the change in ulnar variance at the wrist. A change in variance >3 mm suggests rupture of the interosseous membrane. If the variance changes >6 mm, it is likely that both the triangular

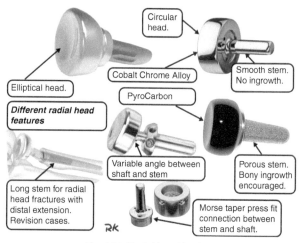

• **Fig. 46.1** Radial head implants.

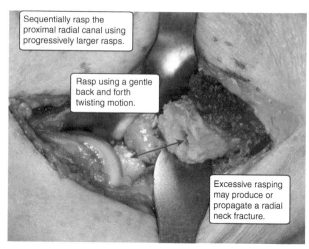

• **Fig. 46.2** Preparation of the proximal radius canal.

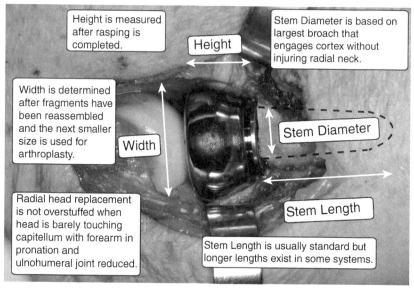

• **Fig. 46.3** Radial head sizing.

fibrocartilage complex (TFCC) and interosseous membrane are disrupted.[3] In this case, the distal radioulnar joint (DRUJ) needs to be inspected and the forearm pinned and the pins cut beneath the skin so that they can be left in place for 8–10 weeks, which should allow the interosseous membrane to heal. An arthroplasty is indicated in this scenario to restore length.

The fractured pieces of the radial head are reassembled typically the back table and the radial head implant size is chosen based on the measured diameter of the native radial head. If between sizes, choose the next smaller size.

The implant stem diameter is assessed through the successive use of trial broaches after a canal finder has been employed to locate the intramedullary canal (Fig. 46.2). Be careful not to be too aggressive with the rasping effort so as to avoid hoop stresses that may fracture bone that has already been traumatized and may be of poor structural integrity.

The height of the radial head is the distance between the articular surface and the remaining bone (Fig. 46.3). This parameter is influenced by the amount of bone left remaining after the comminuted

fragments have been removed. Placement of a radial head implant that is too thick could cause over lengthening of the radius and lead to capitellar wear and pain.[4] This is referred to as "overstuffing" of the RC joint and is a feared complication. Studies have shown that we cannot solely rely on the anteroposterior radiograph of the ulnohumeral joint as a guide to radial head size.[5,6] Although radial height is judged by the dimensions of the resected head and neck, comminution of the radial head may prohibit its accurate measurement. Generally, the implant should articulate at the height of the proximal radioulnar joint, about 2 mm distal to the coronoid.[7]

During radial head implant trialing, the soft tissue trauma has often rendered the elbow unstable and the olecranon may easily subluxate. With the elbow at 90 degrees of flexion, a proximally directed force is applied to the olecranon that seats the trochlea securely into the distal humerus (Fig. 46.4). If ulnohumeral joint subluxation is noted during implant trialing, this may indicate that the implant is "overstuffed" in the RC joint.

After insertion of the trial implants, range of motion is examined and stability is checked through stress testing. Remember

CHAPTER 46 Technique Spotlight: Radial Head Arthroplasty

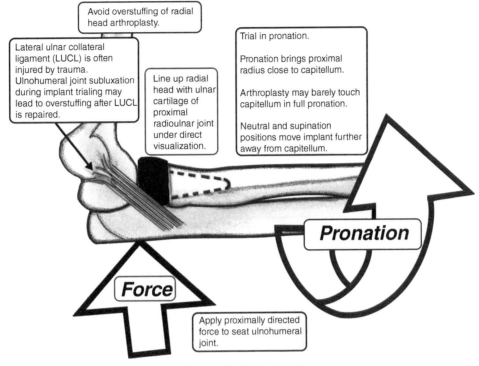

Avoid overstuffing of radial head arthroplasty.

Lateral ulnar collateral ligament (LUCL) is often injured by trauma. Ulnohumeral joint subluxation during implant trialing may lead to overstuffing after LUCL is repaired.

Line up radial head with ulnar cartilage of proximal radioulnar joint under direct visualization.

Trial in pronation.

Pronation brings proximal radius close to capitellum.

Arthroplasty may barely touch capitellum in full pronation.

Neutral and supination positions move implant further away from capitellum.

Pronation

Force

Apply proximally directed force to seat ulnohumeral joint.

• **Fig. 46.4** Radial head trialing.

that the LUCL is often injured leading to lateral elbow instability, which makes trialing of the implant difficult. Seating the ulnohumeral joint with a proximally directed force as shown in Fig. 46.4 makes it less likely for the joint to be overstuffed when trialing implants of different neck heights. Without this proximal force, the ulnohumeral joint may be subtly widened on the lateral side when the radial head is trialed and, once definitively implanted and the ligaments repaired, the implant height is too great and the joint is now overstuffed.

After the implant is placed, the LUCL is repaired anatomically with either transosseous sutures or suture anchors. Our preferred method of LUCL repair employs nonabsorbable sutures such as a 5-0 Ticron that is tied over a bone bridge. The center of the capitellum can be used for identifying the placement of the drill hole that represents an isometric location for graft placement. The drill is directed in a divergent manner to create two posterior openings. A 5-0 Ticron suture with two needles is passed through the LUCL in a Bunnell fashion. The two needles are both passed through the point of isometry and then posteriorly through the divergent holes. Once the suture is passed, both limbs are tensioned for 2 minutes to remove the viscous properties and then tie the sutures directly over the bone bridge created by the two posterior drill holes in the capitellum. Stability is then checked again after the LUCL is repaired and, if substantial medial instability exists, the MCL should be repaired. If repair of the MCL does not restore adequate stability, we will place an external static or dynamic elbow fixator or an Internal Joint Stabilizer (Skeletal Dynamics, Miami, FL, USA).

Once the final implants are seated and any collateral ligament injuries are addressed, fluoroscopic images should be taken with the elbow flexed and extended in both forearm pronation and supination. Radiographically, the ulnohumeral joint space is

assessed for parallelism and ulnar variance is assessed at the wrist. Direct visualization of the implant is very important to avoid overstuffing as the lateral ulnohumeral joint space may radiographically appear wider than the medial ulnohumeral joint even when the joint is not overstuffed[5] (Fig. 46.5). Another way to judge restoration of radial head size radiographically is to compare to the contralateral side.

Postoperative Rehabilitation

Assuming that the head replacement is seated within the proximal radius securely and no other fractures (olecranon, distal humerus) are present, the arthroplasty is not a limiting factor in motion advancement. After surgery, elbow motion is advanced as governed by the soft tissue injury and repair (Fig. 46.6).

Postoperatively, the elbow is splinted in 90 degrees of flexion for 10 days and then the skin sutures are removed. A hinged brace is placed and for the first week, 90 degrees to full elbow flexion is allowed. There are no restrictions placed on forearm rotation. The hinged brace can be periodically removed to allow the achievement of full flexion, which may be limited by the brace itself. At 17 days, the hinged brace is adjusted to allow 60 degrees to full flexion. At 24 days, 30 degrees to full flexion is encouraged. The ability to achieve terminal extension is assessed at 31 days. Usually at 31 days, the patient has difficulty extending beyond 30 degrees and the hinged brace is unlocked. However, if terminal extension is easily achieved during this time, then an arc of 30 degrees to full flexion is maintained for another week to protect the soft tissues. At 38 days, the hinged brace is unlocked and at 42 days it is discontinued. Formal physical therapy is used if at any time motion within the prescribed arc is not achieved by the patient.

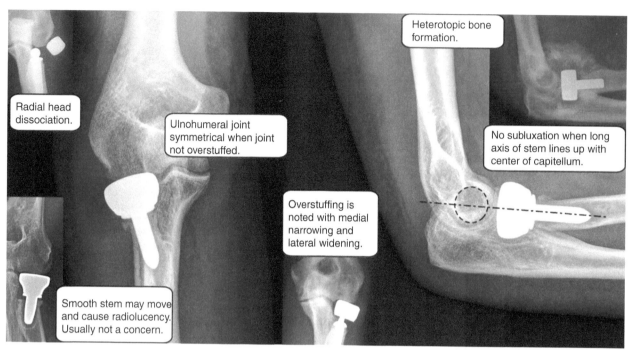

• **Fig. 46.5** Radiographic evaluation.

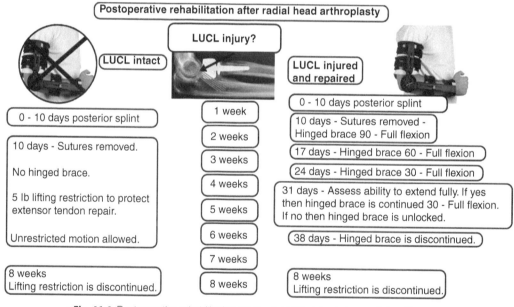

• **Fig. 46.6** Postoperative rehabilitation protocol. *LUCL*, lateral ulnar collateral ligament.

PEARLS AND PITFALLS

- Identify underlying elbow instability if present. Remember a significant portion of radial head fractures will have injuries to the LUCL.
- LUCL injury should be repaired and is often present even when the common extensor origin is intact.
- An MCL injury can be managed with protected mobilization, as long as elbow stability is restored with the combination of the radial head implant and the LUCL repair.
- Forearm supination helps close the medial joint space, allowing an injured ulnar collateral ligament to heal without substantial force to the medial soft tissue structures.
- Avoid overstuffing of the RC joint:
  - ○ Use the reconstructed excised radial head as a template.
  - ○ Select an implant height that is never greater than what was removed.
  - ○ Choose a head diameter that is one size smaller than the native radial head.
  - ○ Use intraoperative fluoroscopy to confirm appropriate implant size.
    - ■ Medial ulnohumeral joint space is parallel.
    - ■ Implant should be at the level of the proximal radial ulnar joint.
    - ■ The ulnar variance should be restored at the wrist compared to the contralateral side.

References

1. van Riet RP, Morrey BF, O'Driscoll SW, Van Glabbeek F. Associated injuries complicating radial head fractures: a demographic study. *Clin Orthop Relat Res.* 2005;441:351–355. https://doi.org/10.1097/01.blo.0000180606.30981.78.
2. Guss MS, Hess LK, Baratz ME. The naked capitellum: a surgeon's guide to intraoperative identification of posterolateral rotatory instability. *J Shoulder Elbow Surg.* 2019;28(5):e150–e155. https://doi.org/10.1016/j.jse.2018.10.028.
3. Smith AM, Urbanosky LR, Castle JA, Rushing JT, Ruch DS. Radius pull test: predictor of longitudinal forearm instability. *J Bone Joint Surg Am.* 2002;84(11):1970–1976.
4. Van Glabbeek F, Van Riet RP, Baumfeld JA, et al. Detrimental effects of overstuffing or understuffing with a radial head replacement in the medial collateral-ligament deficient elbow. *J Bone Joint Surg Am.* 2004;86(12):2629–2635. https://doi.org/10.2106/00004623-200412000-00007.
5. Rowland AS, Athwal GS, MacDermid JC, King GJW. Lateral ulnohumeral joint space widening is not diagnostic of radial head arthroplasty overstuffing. *J Hand Surg Am.* 2007;32(5):637–641. https://doi.org/10.1016/j.jhsa.2007.02.024.
6. Shors HC, Gannon C, Miller MC, Schmidt CC, Baratz ME. Plain radiographs are inadequate to identify overlengthening with a radial head prosthesis. *J Hand Surg Am.* 2008;33(3):335–339. https://doi.org/10.1016/j.jhsa.2007.12.004.
7. Doornberg JN, Linzel DS, Zurakowski D, Ring D. Reference points for radial head prosthesis size. *J Hand Surg Am.* 2006;31(1):53–57. https://doi.org/10.1016/j.jhsa.2005.06.012.

47

Coronoid Fractures and the Terrible Triad: An Algorithm for Successful Management

J. BROCK WALKER AND MICHAEL McKEE

Relevant Anatomy

The elbow is a complex hinge joint connecting the distal end of the humerus with the proximal ends of the radius and ulna, forming three articulations: the ulnohumeral, radiocapitellar, and proximal radioulnar joints (Fig. 47.1). The primary degrees of freedom allowed by the elbow are flexion/extension and pronation/supination. Flexion/extension is accomplished through the ulnohumeral and radiocapitellar joints, while pronation/supination involves the radiocapitellar and proximal radioulnar joints of the elbow as well as the distal radioulnar joint of the wrist.

The elbow is an inherently stable joint due to a combination of bony congruity and dynamic and static stabilizers. The ulnohumeral articulation is a highly congruous joint with the coronoid process serving as a block to posterior translation of the ulna and the olecranon serving as a block to anterior translation (Fig. 47.2). The muscles crossing the elbow (triceps, anconeus, biceps, brachialis, flexor/pronator mass, common extensor origin) serve as dynamic stabilizers at the elbow. Their tone (either resting tone or active tone when bracing for an impact) holds the bony articulations of the elbow tight and congruous by resisting distraction at the joint, similar in function to the rotator cuff of the shoulder. The collateral ligaments, acting together, also resist distractive forces placed on the elbow.

Varus/valgus stability is imparted to the elbow primarily from bony congruity and static stabilizers. The width of the elbow joint in the coronal plane, comprised of the ulnohumeral and radiocapitellar joints, provides inherent stability. The medial collateral ligament (MCL), comprised of anterior, posterior, and transverse bundles, serves to resist valgus stress, with the anterior bundle being the primary constraint (Fig. 47.3). The secondary constraint to valgus stress is the radial head, which becomes the primary constraint in the setting of an MCL injury.

The lateral collateral ligament (LCL) complex consists of the radial collateral ligament, the lateral ulnar collateral ligament (LUCL), the accessory collateral ligament, and the annular ligament. The LUCL serves as the primary constraint against varus stress at the elbow, with the anteromedial facet of the coronoid process providing secondary constraint (Fig. 47.4).

Coronoid Fractures

Pathoanatomy

Anteroposterior (AP) translation of the ulna is resisted by the highly congruous nature of the ulnohumeral joint. The olecranon fossa and the coronoid fossa of the distal humerus accommodate the proximal ulna to allow a nearly 180-degree capture of the distal humerus by the ulna. Simple elbow dislocations, defined as an elbow dislocation without associated fracture, typically occur as the result of a fall onto an outstretched arm. Axial compression, along with a posterolateral rotatory force, causes disruption of the LCL followed by the anterior capsule and lastly the MCL.[1] Disruption of these static structures then allows unopposed distraction, valgus, and rotation of the elbow joint, leading to dislocation.

Coronoid fractures occur in 2%–15% of elbow dislocations as a result of the humerus coming into contact with the coronoid process during an instability event.[2] This contact produces a shear force across the coronoid process leading to fracture. The significance of this fracture on elbow stability depends on both the size of the fracture and the associated injuries to the collateral ligaments and the radial head and will be discussed in subsequent sections.

Fracture of the coronoid can also occur through a primarily varus moment on the elbow which drives the medial aspect of the trochlea into the anteromedial facet of the coronoid. This injury mechanism is best demonstrated in comparing the intraoperative resting AP and stress views shown in Fig. 47.5. This varus moment results in disruption of the LCL (usually through avulsion off the lateral epicondyle of the humerus) as well as a shear-type fracture of the anteromedial facet of the coronoid.[3] While these two injuries can occur in isolation, Klug et al. found 15 of 24 patients with a fracture of the anteromedial facet of the coronoid also had a concomitant avulsion of the LCL.[4] Ring found 15 of 18 patients had an LCL injury.[5]

Classification

Coronoid fractures are classified according to the Regan and Morrey classification (Fig. 47.6).[6] Type I injuries were described as an avulsion of the tip of the coronoid process. Type II injuries involved 50% or less of the coronoid process, while Type III

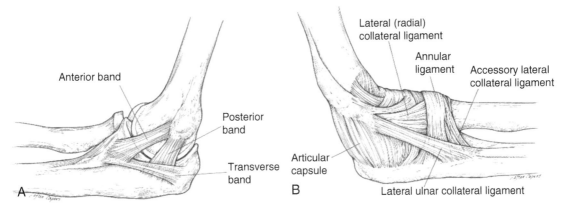

• **Fig. 47.1** (A) Medial side of the elbow depicting the medial collateral ligament which consists of anterior, posterior, and transverse bands. (B) Lateral side of the elbow depicting the lateral collateral ligament complex which primarily includes the lateral radial collateral ligament, lateral ulnar collateral ligament, and annular ligament. (From Dodds SD, Fishler T. Terrible triad of the elbow. *Orthop Clin N Am.* 2013;44:47-58; Fig. 2.)

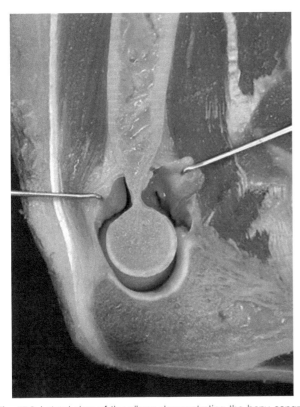

• **Fig. 47.2** Lateral view of the elbow demonstrating the bony congruity. The coronoid process prevents posterior translation of the ulna, especially in flexion, while the olecranon process prevents anterior translation of the ulna, especially in extension. (Morrey's The Elbow and Its Disorders 5th Edition, Morrey, Bernard; Llusa Perez, Manuel. 2018 Elsevier, figue 2-11.)

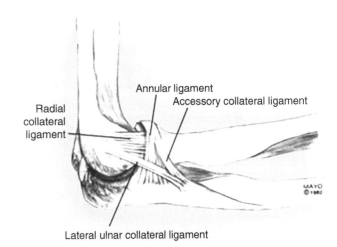

• **Fig. 47.3** Elbow stability to valgus force. A valgus moment placed on the elbow is resisted on the tension side by the medial collateral ligamentous complex, and on the compression side by the articulation of the capitellum with the radial head. The medial collateral ligamentous complex is composed of the anterior and posterior bundles as well as the transverse ligament. The anterior and posterior bundles are the primary contributors to valgus stability. (Morrey's The Elbow and Its Disorders 5th Edition, Morrey, Bernard; Llusa Perez, Manuel. 2018 Elsevier, figure 2-21.)

injuries include fractures of >50% of the height of the coronoid process. Since the adoption of this classification, it has become evident that Type I injuries are usually the result of a shear force imparted by the distal humerus, as opposed to a capsular avulsion, as anatomic studies have demonstrated that the capsule inserts, on average, 6.4 mm distal to the tip of the coronoid.[7]

O'Driscoll popularized a more comprehensive classification of coronoid fractures. In this classification, Type I injuries also represent injuries to the tip of the coronoid process and are subdivided based on the size of less than or greater than 2 mm, but still <50%

of coronoid height. Type II fractures involve the anteromedial facet and are subdivided into three subtypes: anteromedial facet rim, anteromedial facet rim and tip of the coronoid process, and anteromedial facet rim and sublime tubercle (which is the insertion of the anterior bundle of the MCL) with or without fractures of the tip of the coronoid. Type III fractures involve the base of the coronoid and are subdivided into isolated base fractures and those associated with transolecranon fracture-dislocations of the elbow (Fig. 47.7).[3]

Treatment Options

Simple elbow dislocations are typically treated with closed reduction and a brief period (7–10 days) of immobilization followed by early rehabilitation to avoid stiffness. This is typically successful at producing a stable elbow with excellent range of motion, occasionally with negligible limitations at the extremes of motion.

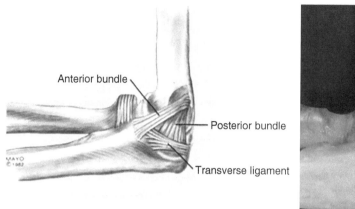
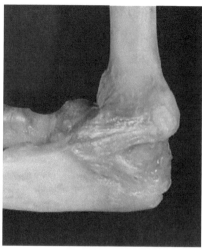

• **Fig. 47.4** Elbow stability to varus force. A varus force placed on the elbow is resisted on the tension side by the lateral collateral ligamentous complex, and on the compression side by the articulation of the trochlea of the distal humerus with the anteromedial facet of the coronoid process. The anatomic image highlights the "Y-shaped" distribution of the lateral ligamentous complex for varus stability. (Morrey's The Elbow and Its Disorders 5th Edition, Morrey, Bernard; Llusa Perez, Manuel. 2018 Elsevier, figue 2-24.)

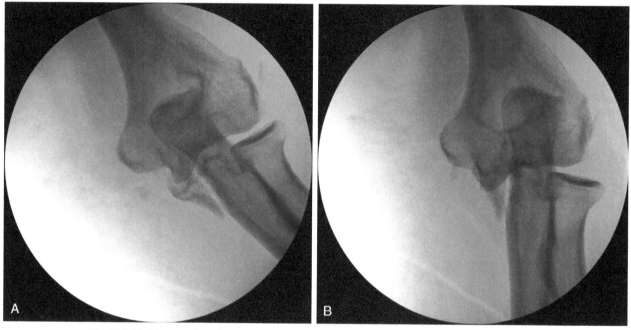

• **Fig. 47.5** (A) Intraoperative, slightly oblique, anteroposterior view of an elbow demonstrating an antero-medial facet coronoid fracture. (B) Intraoperative varus stress applied to the elbow demonstrates significant displacement of the fracture and incongruity of the radiocapitellar and ulnohumeral joints, illustrating the significant instability imparted by anteromedial facet coronoid fractures.

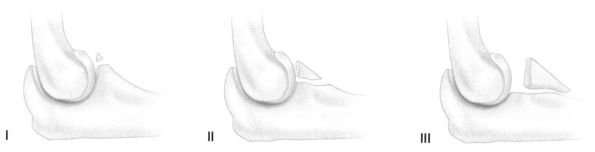

• **Fig. 47.6** Reagan and Morrey classification of fractures of the coronoid process. Type I injuries are fractures of the coronoid tip. Type II fractures involve <50% of the coronoid height. Type III fractures involve >50% of the coronoid height. (Campbell's Orthopedics Fractures and dislocations in Children, Sawyer, Jeffrey; Spence, David Elsevier 2017 fig 36-53.)

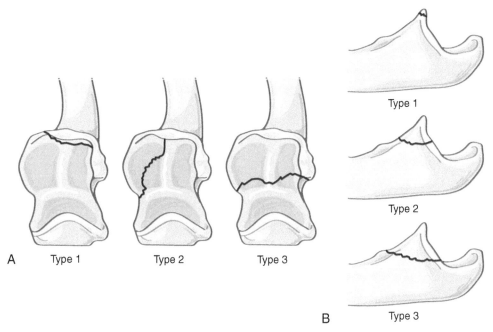

• **Fig. 47.7** (A) O'Driscoll and (B) Regan-Morrey classifications of fracture of the coronoid process. (From Xavier O, Sibont R. Surgical treatment of the terrible triad of the elbow. *Orthop Traumatol Surg Res.* 2021;107(1S):102784.)

Early surgical intervention, when indicated by early recurrent instability, typically consists of collateral ligament repair. Other techniques including external fixation, internal fixation hinge systems, transarticular fixation, or bridge plating are less commonly employed.[8]

Missed or neglected injuries, or failure of closed or open treatment, can result in residual instability, contractures, or a combination thereof which is referred to as the "stiff, unstable elbow" wherein the arc of motion is severely limited, but within the retained arc of motion, significant AP instability exists. In these chronic settings, treatment options depend on specific deficits and goals and include contracture release, transhumeral debridement,[9] collateral ligament reconstruction, transarticular fixation, hinged external fixation, coronoid process reconstruction, radial head replacement, fascial arthroplasty, total elbow arthroplasty, and elbow arthrodesis. In these complex clinical scenarios, often a combination of these treatment options is utilized in an attempt to minimize pain and maximize function. It is crucial that both the clinician and the patient have realistic expectations and thoroughly discuss the functional goals of the patient to select the best treatment options.

Indications for Surgical Treatment

Absolute indications for operative management in the acute setting include inability to obtain a concentric reduction, open injuries, and vascular injuries. A relative indication for operative management following an elbow dislocation includes a greater than normal degree of instability of the elbow after reduction, usually in the setting of a high-energy injury. This can be assessed with the patient still sedated after the elbow has been reduced. Residual AP instability is expected within 30 degrees of full extension after an elbow dislocation. However, if there is instability with >30 degrees of flexion, some authors advocate for early intervention as prolonged immobilization required to stabilize the elbow in this setting would lead to stiffness.

In the setting of elbow dislocation with an associated coronoid shear fracture, the size of the coronoid fragment dictates the effect on elbow stability. Biomechanical studies suggest that resection of 50% of the coronoid, with intact collateral ligaments, leads to increased AP instability of the elbow.[10] From this study, fractures >50% of the height of the coronoid have become a relative indication for operative treatment of a coronoid shear fracture in the setting of elbow dislocation, for fear of residual instability even after the collateral ligaments have healed with nonoperative management and rehabilitation.

Displaced fractures of the anteromedial facet of the coronoid also represent an indication for surgical management. These injuries are caused by a varus moment placed on the elbow and are typically accompanied by an avulsion of the LCL from the lateral epicondyle of the humerus.[4,5] If missed or treated nonoperatively, these elbows can subluxate into varus with resultant posteromedial varus rotatory instability, which is associated with rapid degenerative changes and a poor outcome.[5]

Surgical Approaches

There are two surgical approaches most commonly used to access the coronoid process of the ulna: the anteromedial approach and Hotchkiss "over-the-top" approach.

In the anteromedial approach, a longitudinal, curvilinear incision is made over the anteromedial elbow, approximately 1 cm anterior to the medial epicondyle. The medial antebrachial cutaneous nerve is identified and protected. The ulnar nerve is identified, either through palpation or by performing neurolysis for direct visualization of the nerve, and is protected throughout the operation. The flexor-pronator mass originating from the medial epicondyle is identified and its overlying fascia is exposed. A longitudinal split is performed through this musculature, usually through the flexor carpi ulnaris muscle ("FCU split"), and through this the coronoid process is able to be visualized and exposed (Fig. 47.8).

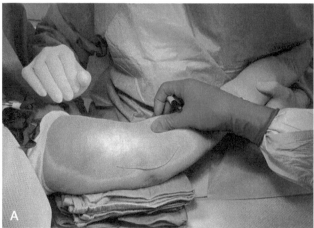

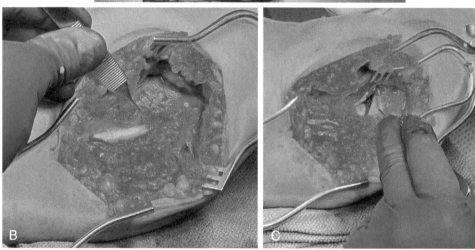

• **Fig. 47.8** Intraoperative pictures of the "FCU split" anteromedial approach to the coronoid. (A) Demonstrates the planned skin incision, (B) shows identification and decompression of the ulnar nerve, (C) shows exposure of the anteromedial facet fracture fragment with the medial collateral ligament attaching to the sublime tubercle.

In the Hotchkiss "over-the-top" approach,[11] neurolysis of the ulnar nerve in the cubital tunnel is performed. The nerve is then mobilized and protected. Through the floor of the cubital tunnel, the proximal ulna is identified. Subperiosteal dissection under the flexor-pronator mass, "over the top" of the anterior proximal ulna is performed to expose the coronoid process. Often, the posterior aspect of the flexor-pronator mass must be elevated from the medial epicondyle for exposure and is repaired during closure.

Huh et al. compared the osseous exposure of the anteromedial FCU split approach and the Hotchkiss "over-the-top" approach to the coronoid process. This study found that the anteromedial FCU split approach provided nearly three times more osseous exposure of the proximal ulna than the Hotchkiss approach; however, they noted that the majority of the increased exposure gained by the FCU split approach was better visualization of the proximal ulnar shaft. Both approaches have been utilized by several authors with good clinical results and clinical comparisons of the two approaches are lacking.[4,5,12]

Once exposed, the coronoid fracture is exposed from distal to proximal, with care being taken to not disrupt soft tissue attachments from the fracture fragment. Doing so would not only devascularize the fragment, but could also destabilize the elbow if the anterior bundle of the MCL is removed from the sublime tubercle of the coronoid. The fracture site is debrided, irrigated, and reduced. The reduction is typically held in place with K-wire fixation. Definitive fixation options include screws, minifragment plates, or precontoured olecranon-specific plates (Fig. 47.9). For large, isolated fractures of the coronoid tip, any of these fixation options can be used with success. For fractures of the anteromedial facet associated with a varus moment placed on the elbow, buttress plating is the preferred method of fixation to resist shear forces across the fracture.[4,12–14]

Once stabilization of the coronoid fracture is achieved, the elbow should again be examined for stability. In the setting of an isolated coronoid tip fracture, typically no further treatment is necessary. In the setting of concomitant radial head and collateral ligament injuries, these are addressed in a stepwise fashion which will be further discussed in the subsequent section. As previously discussed, anteromedial facet fractures of the coronoid usually have a concomitant avulsion of the LCL complex of the lateral epicondyle of the distal humerus. Good clinical outcomes have been obtained with isolated coronoid fixation,[4,13] as well as with coronoid fixation combined with LCL repair,[15] with some authors recommending fixation of the coronoid fracture followed by stress examination to determine the need for LCL repair.[16]

Relevant Complications

With regard to fractures of the coronoid tip, complications of surgical management include infection, heterotopic ossification, ulnar

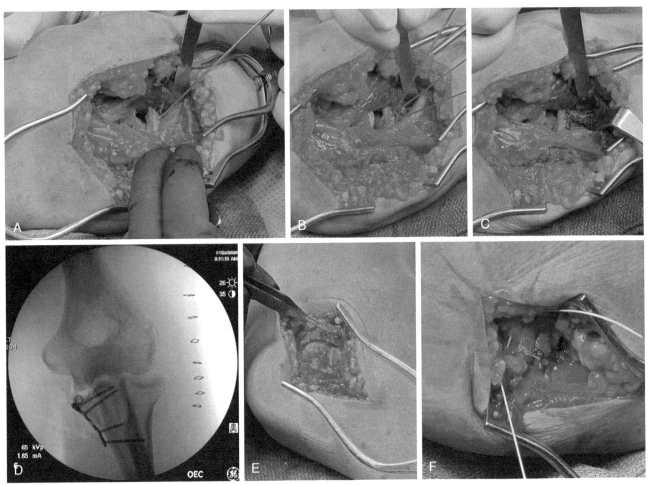

• **Fig. 47.9** Intraoperative pictures of coronoid fracture fixation. (A) The fracture is reduced and provisionally held with K-wire fixation, (B) a minifragment plate is applied and held in place while position is confirmed clinically and radiographically, (C) screws are placed through the plate which is being utilized in buttress mode, and (D) the plate and screw positions are again confirmed clinically and radiographically. Attention is then turned to the lateral side, and (E) the lateral collateral ligamentous complex is found to be avulsed off the lateral epicondyle of the distal humerus. (F) This is repaired through transosseous drill holes through the lateral epicondyle of the distal humerus.

nerve injury, and intra-articular placement of hardware, though these complications are rare. Persistent instability is the most relevant and feared complication and can be the result of either nonoperative management or operative management. With operative management of coronoid tip fractures, persistent instability is typically the result of inadequate stabilization of the other stabilizers of the elbow including the collateral ligaments and radial head, which puts undue stress on the coronoid fixation leading to loss of fixation and persistent instability. In the setting of a chronically unstable elbow with a history of coronoid tip fracture, often there is coronoid bone loss/resorption. In the absence of arthritic symptoms, coronoid reconstruction can be accomplished via olecranon tip autograft from either the ipsilateral or contralateral olecranon.[17] As coronoid deficiency is rarely an isolated cause of elbow instability, this procedure is typically performed with other procedures aimed at improving elbow stability including collateral ligament or radial head reconstructions.

Persistent instability resulting from fractures of the anteromedial facet of the coronoid is usually varus posteromedial rotatory instability (PMRI) of the elbow. This can be the result of missed or neglected injuries, injuries treated nonoperatively with interval displacement of the anteromedial facet of the coronoid, or those treated operatively with loss of fixation of the coronoid fracture. The result

is an elbow that is unstable with varus stress, with resultant subluxation in a posterior medial direction with rotation around the intact lateral column.[18] If identified acutely or subacutely, PMRI can be treated with fixation (or revision fixation) of the coronoid fracture in combination with LCL repair. In the chronic setting, treatment typically involves olecranon and LCL reconstructions.[18,19]

Review of Treatment Outcomes

Isolated fractures of the coronoid in association with an elbow dislocation are typically Type I in nature and do not, in isolation, require surgery.[20] However, when the fracture fragment is large enough to impart significant instability to the elbow joint, or a block to motion, surgical reduction and fixation are indicated. In this setting, surgical stabilization is typically met with good outcomes as the elbow is now stabilized to allow early range of motion and avoid stiffness, and the remainder of the stabilizers of the elbow are intact.[21] More typically, fractures of the coronoid tip are associated with injuries to the collateral ligaments and/or the radial head and will be discussed further in the following section of the text.

Fractures of the anteromedial facet, when recognized early and treated appropriately, are associated with good functional

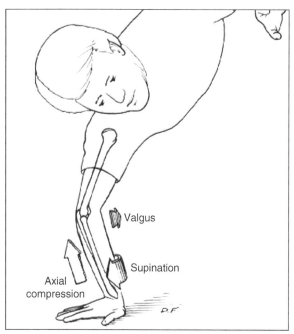

• **Fig. 47.10** Typical mechanism of terrible triad injuries of the elbow consists of a fall onto an outstretched hand. The hand, forearm, and elbow are held fixed while the falling body provides a valgus, rotatory, and axial force on the elbow. (Orthopedic Clinics of America, Terrible Triad of the Elbow Dodds, Seth; Fischler, thomas 2013 Elsevier.)

outcomes. In a report of 12 cases by Lor, all patients treated with buttress fixation of an anteromedial facet coronoid fracture had functional elbow range of motion (at least 30–130 degrees). There were no cases of persistent instability or reoperation, and mean DASH (The Disabilities of the Arm, Shoulder and Hand) scores at 16-month follow-up were 16 points.[13] Similarly, Klug found no cases of persistent instability in 24 patients treated with buttress fixation, with a mean DASH score of 7 points at 2-year follow-up. Five patients in this study required revision surgery for stiffness.[4]

The importance of early recognition of elbow instability in association with anteromedial facet coronoid fractures is highlighted by the poor results associated with late reconstruction. Papandrea found that in 27 patients who underwent reconstruction for chronic elbow instability following coronoid fracture, only 62% had a successful outcome, which was based on the Mayo Elbow Performance score (MEPS) and the patient's willingness to repeat the operation. The duration of treatment delay was significantly associated with outcome, as the treatment of only one of seven elbows with a delay >7 weeks was successful.[22]

Terrible Triad Injuries

Pathoanatomy

The terrible triad injury is defined as an elbow dislocation with fractures of the coronoid and the radial head or neck. There is also typically an associated lateral collateral ligamentous complex disruption, along with variable degree of injury to the medial collateral ligamentous complex.[8]

Terrible triad injuries are typically the result of a fall onto an outstretched arm. In this position, the hand and palm are fixed on the ground, and the elbow is held in space (Fig. 47.10). The falling body then provides a valgus moment to the elbow which, along with rotational and axial forces, leads to disruption of the capsuloligamentous structures of the elbow from lateral to medial.

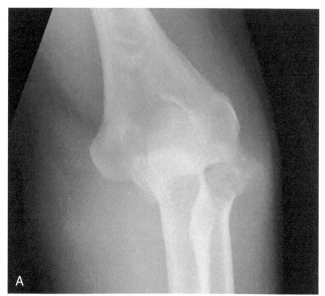

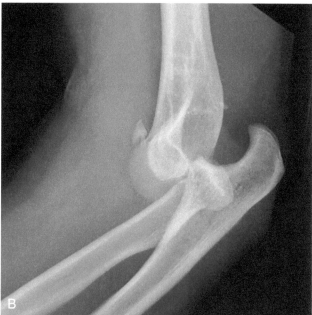

• **Fig. 47.11** Anteroposterior (A) and lateral (B) radiographs of a terrible triad injury of the elbow demonstrating an elbow dislocation with fractures of the coronoid and radial neck.

The valgus moment placed on the elbow drives the capitellum into the radial head, causing a radial head or neck fracture. Disruption of this lateral strut allows posterolateral subluxation of the ulna as it levers out of the trochlea. As the ulna dislocates posteriorly, the lateral collateral ligamentous complex is typically avulsed from the lateral humeral epicondyle. In addition, the anterior coronoid tip abuts the distal humerus, causing a shear-type fracture of the coronoid. The medial collateral ligamentous complex can remain uninjured or can have a variable degree of disruption which is proportional to the energy imparted to the elbow at the time of injury.[1,23–25] The radiographs of a typical terrible triad injury are illustrated in Fig. 47.11.

Classification

While there is no well-adopted classification for terrible triad injuries as a whole, classification systems have been developed to describe the fractures involved.

Coronoid fractures are classified according to the Regan and Morrey system[6] or the O'Driscoll system.[3] These two classifications were delineated in the previous section, but in general classification depends on the size of the coronoid fragment and whether the fracture destabilizes the coronoid tip or the anteromedial facet. Disruption of the anteromedial facet is typically observed in varus-moment injuries to the elbow, which were discussed in the previous section. Terrible triad injuries, as the result of a posterolateral dislocation event, are typically accompanied by fractures of the coronoid tip which are typically described with the Regan and Morrey classification system.

Fractures of the radial head are classified according to the Mason classification system.[26] In this classification, Type 1 fractures are nondisplaced fractures. Type 2 fractures are partial articular injuries with or without comminution. Type 3 fractures are complete articular injuries with comminution of the radial head.

This classification was modified by Hotchkiss in 1997 in an attempt to match the classification to treatment options and to deter surgeons from excising the radial head when fixation is possible.[27] According to the Hotchkiss modification, Type 1 injuries are displaced <2 mm without block to rotation and are typically treated nonoperatively. Type 2 injuries represent radial head fractures that are displaced >2 mm or radial neck fractures that are angulated. These fractures, according to Hotchkiss, should be considered for internal fixation. Type 3 injuries represent fractures that are comminuted to the point that fixation is not feasible, and for which

Hotchkiss recommended excision at the time of original publication of the article. Type 4 injuries represent those with an associated, recognized, elbow dislocation event (Fig. 47.12). Since then, it has been recognized that Type 2 fractures that do not block rotation can be treated nonoperatively.[28] In addition, as radial head replacement implants have evolved, they have largely replaced radial head excision in the treatment of Type 3 injuries due to the improved functional outcomes with radial head replacement.[29]

Treatment Options

The majority of terrible triad injuries are treated surgically. Nonoperative management is an option in a very select subset of terrible triad injuries, and criteria for nonoperative management are reviewed in the following section.

Treatment options for the coronoid fracture include fragment excision, open reduction and internal fixation, and anterior capsular repair. Type I coronoid fractures only involving the tip of the coronoid are typically excised. In this setting, some authors have advocated for anterior capsular repair, in which a posterior-to-anterior drill hole is placed through the proximal ulna, and suture is passed through the capsule to tighten the anterior capsule against the anterior ulna. However, King et al. found no increase in posterolateral laxity with complete transection of the anterior capsule in a cadaveric study, which calls into question the need for anterior capsular repair.[30] Antoni et al. evaluated anterior capsular

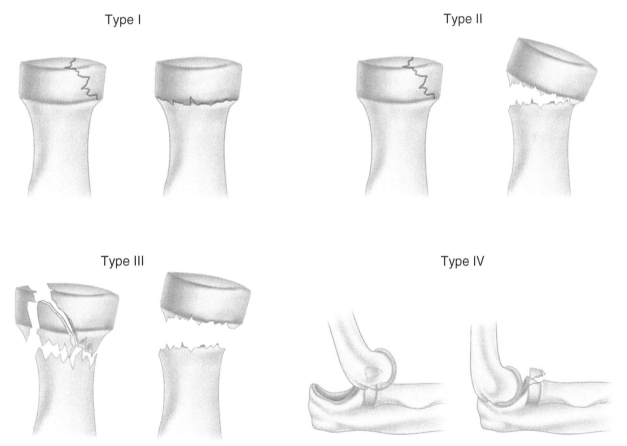

Type I

Type II

Type III

Type IV

• **Fig. 47.12** The modified Mason classification of radial head fractures. Type I fractures are displaced <2 mm. Type II fractures are displaced >2 mm and may or may not cause a block to motion. Type III fractures are comminuted and displaced fractures. Type IV fractures are those with an associated elbow dislocation. (From Perez EA. Fractures of the shoulder, arm, and forearm. In: *Campbell's Operative Orthopaedics.* 2017:2927–3016.)

repair in this setting and found no difference in functional or clinical outcomes in their small, retrospective review.[31]

Type II and III fractures of the coronoid are typically treated with open reduction and internal fixation. Reduction and provisional fixation can be done through the lateral approach. Fixation can be accomplished with minifragment screws placed through the lateral approach, or posterior-to-anterior screws that are placed under fluoroscopic guidance from the subcutaneous border of the posterior border of the ulna into the coronoid tip. In the rare setting of anteromedial facet coronoid fracture in the setting of a terrible triad injury, the coronoid fracture should be approached and buttressed through a medial approach as described in the previous section focused on coronoid fractures.

Radial head and neck fractures are treated with fragment excision, open reduction and internal fixation, or radial head replacement. Historically, irreparable radial head fractures were treated with radial head excision; however, this resulted in recurrent instability with poor functional and clinical outcomes.[29] Fragment excision is an acceptable treatment option for small, peripheral fragments that on examination do not provide significant stability to the radiocapitellar joint. Fragment excision of a small, peripheral fragment can also be used in conjunction with operative fixation of two large, articular fragments.

The decision between radial head fixation and radial head replacement is controversial. Age, activity level, and bone quality are all subjective measures that influence this decision-making but thresholds are poorly defined in the literature. In general, open reduction and internal fixation of the radial head is the preferred treatment in young, active patients when possible. The number of fracture fragments is the most objective measure influencing the decision to fix or replace the radial head. Ring et al. found that most patients who underwent fixation of radial head fractures with more than three articular fragments had a poor result and thus recommended against operative fixation if more than three articular fragments are encountered. In addition, radial head fixation in the setting of concomitant elbow instability had significantly worse outcomes.[32]

The medial side of the elbow is the last to be injured in the terrible triad injury pattern and has a variable injury pattern depending on the severity of the injury.[23] In lower energy injuries, the medial-sided structures may remain completely intact. In higher energy injuries, disruption of the medial collateral ligamentous complex and/or the flexor-pronator mass may be present. Once the injuries on the lateral side of the elbow have been addressed, the elbow is examined intraoperatively for instability. Persistent instability due to injury to the medial-sided structures of the elbow is uncommon, but does occur. Options for this include open repair of the medial collateral ligamentous complex and/or open repair of the flexor-pronator mass. Indirect options for dealing with persistent instability due to incompetency of the medial-sided structures include static external fixation, hinged external fixation, and transarticular pinning or screw fixation. All of these methods are aimed at minimizing stress to the elbow and allowing the medial-sided structures to heal without open intervention. The benefit of hinged external fixation in this setting is the allowance of early motion, though the technical difficulties of pin placement in hinged external fixation of the elbow can be a challenge.

Indications for Surgical Treatment

Terrible triad injuries typically require surgery due to the instability imparted to the elbow from the injury. Outside of the rare instance

of a patient who is moribund or otherwise unfit for surgery, several criteria must all be met for nonoperative management to be considered. First, after reduction the radiocapitellar and ulnohumeral joints must be concentrically reduced radiographically. The coronoid fracture should be small fracture of the coronoid tip which does not involve the anteromedial facet. The radial head/neck fracture should be minimally displaced or angulated, such that there is no block to pronation or supination of the forearm. This can be addressed on examination while the patient is sedated after reduction. Lastly, the elbow should remain stable through a functional arc of motion of 30–130 degrees. This is a good marker that the elbow will be stable with early range of motion, following a brief period of immobilization, with nonoperative management.[24] If nonoperative management is attempted, the patient should be followed closely with serial radiographs and examinations to assess stability with progressive motion of the elbow. If the above criteria are not met or are lost with serial follow-up, then operative management is indicated.

Surgical Approaches

When surgical treatment is selected, treatment should be performed according to the standardized protocol published by Pugh et al.[33] in 2004. The elbow should be approached laterally through a radiocapitellar or Kaplan approach. Typically, after skin incision and subcutaneous dissection, the elbow joint and articular cartilage of the radiocapitellar joint can be visualized through a traumatic defect in the deeper soft tissue structures. At this stage, the lateral collateral ligamentous complex and common extensor origin are typically found to be avulsed off the lateral epicondyle of the humerus, with a corresponding "bare spot" representing their anatomic origin on the epicondyle. When present, the defect in the lateral capsule should be utilized and extended to enter the elbow joint. From there, one should work from deep to superficial, addressing damaged structures sequentially.

The deepest structures that can be reached from the lateral approach include the coronoid fracture and the anterior capsule. If the radial head is to be replaced, the radial head should be excised early in the procedure as this significantly improves coronoid exposure. The coronoid fracture should be exposed and examined. If the anterior capsule is attached to the fragment, this should be left attached. In Type I coronoid tip fractures, these are usually too small for fixation, do not provide significant stability to the elbow joint, and are typically treated with excision. As mentioned earlier, some authors in this setting recommend imbrication of the anterior joint capsule, though this has debatable clinical benefit, with the only available study showing no benefit in a small, retrospective series.[31] Type II or Type III fractures of the coronoid, in the setting of terrible triad injuries, are typically treated with open reduction and internal fixation. Reduction and provisional fixation can be obtained through the lateral approach. Fixation can be achieved through the lateral approach with minifragment screw fixation or through posterior-to-anterior screw fixation starting from the subcutaneous border of the posterior ulna and ending in the coronoid tip, with intraoperative fluoroscopy confirming screw position. In the rare instance of a large coronoid fracture involving the anteromedial facet of the coronoid, a medial approach can be utilized for buttress fixation as outlined in the prior section.

Next, the radial head is addressed. Treatment options include fragment excision, fixation, and radial head replacement. Historically, radial head excision was the treatment of choice for irreparable radial head fractures; however, this has been fraught with poor outcomes.[29] Small, peripheral fragments may be excised if deemed to not contribute significantly to radiocapitellar stability. Caution should be exercised prior to excision of posterior rim fragments of the radial head, as these often contribute significant stability to the elbow. Operative fixation is the treatment of choice for radial head fractures with three or fewer fragments, presuming the bone quality is strong enough to support fixation.[32] In fractures with more than three articular fragments or those with poor bone quality, radial head replacement is the treatment of choice.

Most superficially, on the lateral side, the lateral collateral ligamentous complex and the common extensor origin are addressed. In the rare instance, they were not disrupted by the injury, but were opened longitudinally in the approach, then this longitudinal opening is closed in layers. More commonly, both structures are avulsed off a "bare spot" on the lateral epicondyle of the humerus. Repair of these structures should be performed with a large, nonabsorbable suture either through bone tunnels in the distal humerus or with suture anchors (Fig. 47.13A). If a large bony avulsion fragment is present, this can also be addressed with screw fixation with a soft tissue washer (Fig. 47.13B–C). This repair should be done with the elbow held in flexion and the forearm held pronated to minimize tension of the lateral-sided structures.

Once repair of the lateral-sided structures is completed, the elbow is assessed clinically and radiographically. As with simple elbow dislocations, it is anticipated that the elbow will have some instability at full extension. However, if the elbow remains stable clinically and concentrically reduced radiographically between full flexion and 30 degrees of flexion, then the elbow is splinted in flexion and forearm pronation for 2 weeks, followed by progressive motion of the elbow. Stability up to 30 degrees of flexion serves as a consistent marker of good results without further intervention.[3,8,24] Of note, mildly increased ulnohumeral joint space

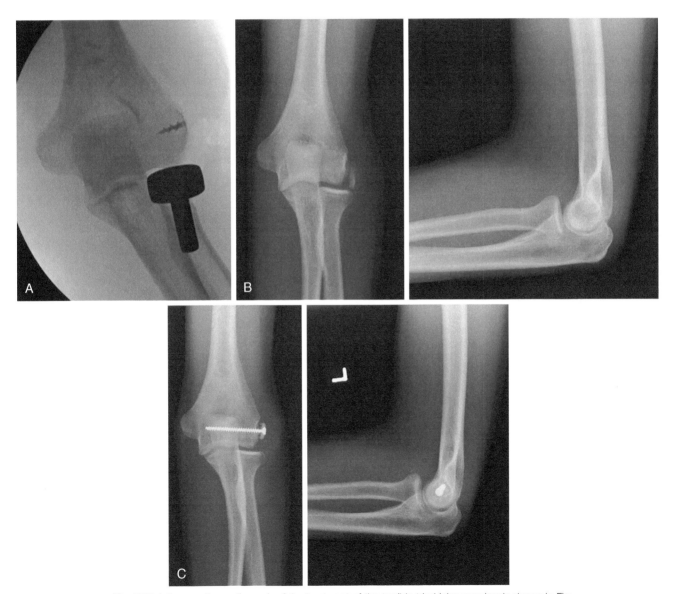

• **Fig. 47.13** Intraoperative radiograph of the treatment of the terrible triad injury previously shown in Fig. 47.10. (A) Treatment consisted of coronoid fragment excision, radial head replacement, and lateral collateral ligamentous complex repair to the lateral epicondyle of the distal humerus with suture anchor fixation. (B and C) In the presence of a large bony avulsion fragment, the lateral ligamentous complex can also be fixed with a screw and soft tissue washer .

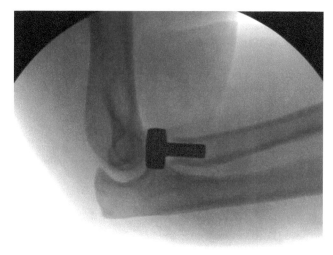

• **Fig. 47.14** Intraoperative lateral radiograph demonstrating mildly increased ulnohumeral joint space, or "drop sign."

Review of Treatment Outcomes

Pugh et al. found an average arc of flexion of 20–135 degrees at final follow-up in their series of 36 patients. As mentioned in the prior section, 22% of patients required revision surgery. At final follow-up, 15 patients had an excellent result, 13 good, 7 fair, and 1 poor as defined by the MEPS. They found patients who were treated acutely had significantly better motion than those in whom treatment was delayed. In addition, they found patients who underwent prolonged immobilization tended to have a poorer result and thus their postoperative rehabilitation protocol evolved to allow earlier range of motion.[33] This finding was also identified in a study by Broberg, who found that immobilization past 4 weeks was associated with poor function.[35]

on the lateral radiograph is common and has been termed the "drop sign" (Fig. 47.14). This represents mild medial-sided laxity that is expected to resolve with time and does not represent an indication for further intervention.[34] This is treated with early active exercises and avoidance of varus stress.

If clinical instability or significant joint incongruity is present with >30 degrees of flexion after repair of the lateral-sided structures, further steps must be taken to stabilize the elbow. In the presence of gapping of the medial side of the ulnohumeral joint, one should consider that the medial soft tissue damage is severe including the MCL and the flexor-pronator mass. This would represent a relative indication for a medial-sided approach with repair of the MCL and flexor-pronator mass. Other treatment options for persistent instability after lateral-sided repair include static external fixation, hinged external fixation, and transarticular pin or screw fixation.[24] These options have not been directly compared in the literature due to the rarity in which their utilization is required. Pugh et al., in their series of 36 terrible triad injuries, had six patients who remained unstable after addressing the lateral-sided structures. After open repair of the medial-sided structures, four were found to be stable and the other two patients were placed in hinged external fixators.

Relevant Complications

Complications following terrible triad injuries are common, especially in injuries that are the result of high-energy mechanisms. Common complications include persistent instability, stiffness, loss of fixation, and heterotopic ossification. Less common complications include wound complications, infection, malunion, nonunion, and ulnar neuropathy. Long-term, radiographic posttraumatic arthrosis of the elbow is common; however, clinical symptoms vary widely and are typically not severe.

In the study by Pugh et al., 22% of patients had a complication requiring reoperation; one patient with persistent instability required hinged external fixation placement, two patients developed radioulnar synostosis, one wound infection, and four patients required hardware removal and elbow contracture release and/or heterotopic bone resection. One more patients in their series had clinical evidence of mild persistent posterolateral rotatory instability but declined further intervention given that they were minimally symptomatic.

References

1. O'Driscoll SW, Morrey BF, Korinek S, An KN. Elbow subluxation and dislocation. A spectrum of instability. *Clin Orthop*. 1992;280:186–197.
2. Wells J, Ablove RH. Coronoid fractures of the elbow. *Clin Med Res*. 2008;6(1):40–44. https://doi.org/10.3121/cmr.2008.753.
3. O'Driscoll SW, Jupiter JB, Cohen MS, Ring D, McKee MD. Difficult elbow fractures: pearls and pitfalls. *Instr Course Lect*. 2003;52:113–134.
4. Klug A, Buschbeck S, Gramlich Y, Buckup J, Hoffmann R, Schmidt-Horlohé K. Good outcome using anatomically pre-formed buttress plates for anteromedial facet fractures of the coronoid-a retrospective study of twenty-four patients. *Int Orthop*. 2019;43(12):2817–2824. https://doi.org/10.1007/s00264-019-04354-6.
5. Ring D, Doornberg JN. Fracture of the anteromedial facet of the coronoid process. Surgical technique. *J Bone Joint Surg Am*. 2007;89(suppl 2 Pt.2):267–283. https://doi.org/10.2106/JBJS.G.00059.
6. Regan W, Morrey B. Fractures of the coronoid process of the ulna. *J Bone Joint Surg Am*. 1989;71(9):1348–1354.
7. Cage DJ, Abrams RA, Callahan JJ, Botte MJ. Soft tissue attachments of the ulnar coronoid process. An anatomic study with radiographic correlation. *Clin Orthop*. 1995;320:154–158.
8. Rockwood Jr CA, Green DP. In: *Rockwood and Green's Fractures in Adults*. 8th ed. Philadelphia, PA: Lippincott; 2015:1179–1227.
9. Kashiwagi D. Osteoarthritis of the elbow joint. Intra-articular changes and the special operative procedure, Outerbridge-Kashiwagi method. *Elbow Joint*. 1985:177–178.
10. Closkey RF, Goode JR, Kirschenbaum D, Cody RP. The role of the coronoid process in elbow stability. A biomechanical analysis of axial loading. *J Bone Joint Surg Am*. 2000;82(12):1749–1753. https://doi.org/10.2106/00004623-200012000-00009.
11. Hotchkiss, RN, Kasparyan, NG. The medial "Over the top" approach to the elbow. *Tech Orthopaedics*. 15(2):105–112.
12. Rausch V, Hackl M, Seybold D, Wegmann K, Müller LP. [Plate osteosynthesis of the coronoid process of the ulna]. *Oper Orthopadie Traumatol*. 2020;32(1):35–46. https://doi.org/10.1007/s00064-019-00647-6.
13. Lor KKH, Toon DH, Wee ATH. Buttress plate fixation of coronoid process fractures via a medial approach. *Chin J Traumatol Zhonghua Chuang Shang Za Zhi*. 2019;22(5):255–260. https://doi.org/10.1016/j.cjtee.2019.05.005.
14. Morellato J, Louati H, Desloges W, Papp S, Pollock JW. Fixation of anteromedial coronoid facet fractures: a biomechanical evaluation of plated versus screw constructs. *J Orthop Trauma*. 2018;32(11):e451–e456. https://doi.org/10.1097/BOT.0000000000001266.
15. Park S-M, Lee JS, Jung JY, Kim JY, Song K-S. How should anteromedial coronoid facet fracture be managed? A surgical strategy based on O'Driscoll classification and ligament injury. *J Shoulder Elbow Surg*. 2015;24(1):74–82. https://doi.org/10.1016/j.jse.2014.07.010.

16. Rhyou IH, Kim KC, Lee J-H, Kim SY. Strategic approach to O'Driscoll type 2 anteromedial coronoid facet fracture. *J Shoulder Elbow Surg.* 2014;23(7):924–932. https://doi.org/10.1016/j.jse.2014.02.016.

17. Wegmann K, Knowles NK, Lalone EE, et al. The shape match of the olecranon tip for reconstruction of the coronoid process: influence of side and osteotomy angle. *J Shoulder Elbow Surg.* 2019;28(4):e117–e124. https://doi.org/10.1016/j.jse.2018.10.022.

18. McLean J, Kempston MP, Pike JM, Goetz TJ, Daneshvar P. Varus posteromedial rotatory instability of the elbow: injury pattern and surgical experience of 27 acute consecutive surgical patients. *J Orthop Trauma.* 2018;32(12):e469–e474. https://doi.org/10.1097/BOT.0000000000001313.

19. Bellato E, Kim Y, Fitzsimmons JS, et al. Role of the lateral collateral ligament in posteromedial rotatory instability of the elbow. *J Shoulder Elbow Surg.* 2017;26(9):1636–1643. https://doi.org/10.1016/j.jse.2017.04.011.

20. Foruria AM, Gutiérrez B, Cobos J, Haeni DL, Valencia M, Calvo E. Most coronoid fractures and fracture-dislocations with no radial head involvement can be treated nonsurgically with elbow immobilization. *J Shoulder Elbow Surg.* 2019;28(7):1395–1405. https://doi.org/10.1016/j.jse.2019.01.005.

21. Kow RY, Mustapha Zakaria Z, Khan ESKM, Low C. Isolated Regan-Morrey type III fracture of the ulnar coronoid process: a report of two cases. *J Orthop Case Rep.* 2018;8(6):65–67. https://doi.org/10.13107/jocr.2250-0685.1262.

22. Papandrea RF, Morrey BF, O'Driscoll SW. Reconstruction for persistent instability of the elbow after coronoid fracture-dislocation. *J Shoulder Elbow Surg.* 2007;16(1):68–77. https://doi.org/10.1016/j.jse.2006.03.011.

23. O'Driscoll SW, Bell DF, Morrey BF. Posterolateral rotatory instability of the elbow. *J Bone Joint Surg Am.* 1991;73(3):440–446.

24. Mathew PK, Athwal GS, King GJW. Terrible triad injury of the elbow: current concepts. *J Am Acad Orthop Surg.* 2009;17(3):137–151. https://doi.org/10.5435/00124635-200903000-00003.

25. Pugh DMW, McKee MD. The "terrible triad" of the elbow. *Tech Hand Up Extrem Surg.* 2002;6(1):21–29. https://doi.org/10.1097/00130911-200203000-00005.

26. Mason ML. Some observations on fractures of the head of the radius with a review of one hundred cases. *Br J Surg.* 1954;42(172):123–132. https://doi.org/10.1002/bjs.18004217203.

27. Hotchkiss RN. Displaced fractures of the radial head: internal fixation or excision? *J Am Acad Orthop Surg.* 1997;5(1):1–10. https://doi.org/10.5435/00124635-199701000-00001.

28. Burkhart KJ, Wegmann K, Müller LP, Gohlke FE. Fractures of the radial head. *Hand Clin.* 2015;31(4):533–546. https://doi.org/10.1016/j.hcl.2015.06.003.

29. Beingessner DM, Dunning CE, Gordon KD, Johnson JA, King GJW. The effect of radial head excision and arthroplasty on elbow kinematics and stability. *J Bone Joint Surg Am.* 2004;86(8):1730–1739. https://doi.org/10.2106/00004623-200408000-00018.

30. Dunning CE, Zarzour ZD, Patterson SD, Johnson JA, King GJ. Ligamentous stabilizers against posterolateral rotatory instability of the elbow. *J Bone Joint Surg Am.* 2001;83(12):1823–1828. https://doi.org/10.2106/00004623-200112000-00009.

31. Antoni M, Eichler D, Kempf J-F, Clavert P. Anterior capsule reattachment in terrible triad elbow injury with coronoid tip fracture. *Orthop Traumatol Surg Res OTSR.* 2019;105(8):1575–1583. https://doi.org/10.1016/j.otsr.2019.09.024.

32. Ring D, Quintero J, Jupiter JB. Open reduction and internal fixation of fractures of the radial head. *J Bone Joint Surg Am.* 2002;84(10):1811–1815. https://doi.org/10.2106/00004623-200210000-00011.

33. Pugh DMW, Wild LM, Schemitsch EH, King GJW, McKee MD. Standard surgical protocol to treat elbow dislocations with radial head and coronoid fractures. *J Bone Joint Surg Am.* 2004;86(6):1122–1130. https://doi.org/10.2106/00004623-200406000-00002.

34. Duckworth AD, Kulijdian A, McKee MD, Ring D. Residual subluxation of the elbow after dislocation or fracture-dislocation: treatment with active elbow exercises and avoidance of varus stress. *J Shoulder Elbow Surg.* 2008;17(2):276–280. https://doi.org/10.1016/j.jse.2007.06.006.

35. Broberg MA, Morrey BF. Results of treatment of fracture-dislocations of the elbow. *Clin Orthop.* 1987;(216):109–119.

48

Technique Spotlight: Terrible Triad Injuries

J. BROCK WALKER AND MICHAEL McKEE

Terrible triad injuries represent a spectrum of complex elbow dislocations that result from a posterolateral rotatory force combined with axial compression, typically on an outstretched arm. This typically results in fractures of the radial head and coronoid, ligamentous disruption of the lateral collateral ligament complex, and variable injury to the medial collateral ligamentous complex. Following the treatment algorithms laid out in Chapter 47, the vast majority of patients will have a good outcome with a pain-free, stable, functional elbow, typically with an asymptomatic limitation in range of motion compared to the uninjured side.

Preoperative Evaluation

A thorough history and physical examination are key to the diagnosis of terrible triad injuries. History should focus on the details of injury as the mechanism and the position of the arm can help inform the surgeon which structures may be injured. Higher energy mechanisms, such as falls from height, are associated with a higher degree of bony and soft tissue injury.

Physical examination should begin with inspection, as any degree of deformity can represent a subluxated or dislocated elbow. At times, terrible triad injuries spontaneously reduce prior to presentation. In this setting, patients typically have tenderness and ecchymosis about the lateral elbow, pain with range of motion, and apprehension with extension of the elbow. Tenderness or ecchymosis to the medial elbow can indicate injury to the medial collateral ligament (MCL), but is not necessarily an indication for medial-sided repair. A careful neurovascular examination should also be performed. If there is any concern for vascular injury based on physical examination, computed tomography arthrography (CTA) and/or vascular consultation should be obtained immediately. In addition to examination of the entire injured extremity, special attention should be given to the examination of the wrist. Tenderness or pain with range of motion of the wrist can indicate a concomitant Essex-Lopresti injury, which is a disruption of the interosseous membrane and distal radioulnar joint (DRUJ).

Anteroposterior (AP) and lateral radiographs are obtained on presentation and after reduction and splinting. The radiographs should be critically examined to determine the severity of injury as well as identification of injured structures. The radial head should be assessed for the size and location of fracture fragments, as well as degree of comminution. If the coronoid is fractured, the size and orientation of the fracture should be evaluated as this dictates

fixation strategy. A CT scan is not typically necessary unless a coronal shear fracture of the capitellum is suspected, or radiographs are of poor quality and further delineation of fracture patterns is required for preoperative planning.

Positioning and Equipment

Terrible triad elbow injuries are typically treated surgically in the supine position, with the arm at the side on a hand table. This allows access to the medial and lateral sides of the elbow, but requires a second incision if medial-sided repair is performed. In high-energy injuries, where there is a high probability that medial-sided repair will be necessary to restore stability to the elbow, or if there is associated ulnar nerve pathology, a posterior incision can also be utilized. The patient is placed in the lateral position with the affected side up and the arm draped over a bolster, and the medial and lateral sides of the elbow can be accessed through a single, posterior incision.

Although preoperative planning is of paramount importance in the treatment of terrible triad injuries, there is some requirement for intraoperative decision-making. As such, it is the responsibility of the treating surgeon to ensure all possible required equipment is available including instrumentation for coronoid fixation, anterior capsular repair, radial head fixation, radial head replacement, medial/lateral collateral ligament repairs, medial/lateral ligament reconstructions, and common flexor/extensor mass repairs, and external fixation.

Surgical Technique

Fig. 48.1 demonstrates the presenting radiographs of a healthy 50-year-old man who fell from a bicycle onto an outstretched arm. Radiographs demonstrate a fracture of the coronoid tip, a posteriorly subluxated ulnohumeral joint, and a dislocated radiocapitellar joint with a fracture of the radial head and neck. These findings were confirmed with a CT scan, shown in Fig. 48.2, which better delineated the size of the coronoid fracture that did not involve the anteromedial facet, and was deemed small enough to not require fixation. A CT scan also better demonstrated the radial neck fracture and exposed two additional fracture lines within the radial head. While surgeons should always have a radial head replacement set available when planning fixation of a radial head or neck, these CT findings raised concern that radial head fixation may not be a good option for this patient.

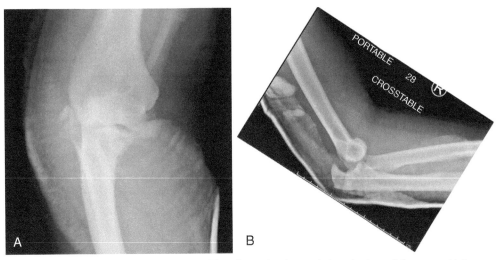

• **Fig. 48.1** Anteroposterior (A) and lateral (B) radiographs demonstrate a fracture of the coronoid tip, a posteriorly subluxated ulnohumeral joint, and a dislocated radiocapitellar joint with a fracture of the radial head and neck.

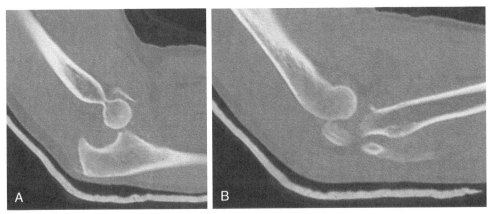

• **Fig. 48.2** Representative sagittal cut through the ulnohumeral joint (A) better delineated the size of the coronoid fracture that did not involve the anteromedial facet and therefore did not require fixation. Representative sagittal cut through the radiocapitellar joint (B) demonstrates a comminuted radial head and neck fracture dislocation.

Patients are typically placed supine on an operating room table with the head of the bed elevated approximately 30 degrees with the injured extremity at the side on a hand table. A lateral radiocapitellar (Kocher) approach is utilized (Fig. 48.3). In this case, fragments of the fractured and posteriorly dislocated radial head were encountered. Dissection was performed to identify the extent of lateral collateral ligament injury. This is most often found to be avulsed from the lateral epicondyle of the humerus and is illustrated by the Adson forceps in Fig. 48.3B. A matching bare spot on the humeral epicondyle is commonly present, representing the avulsed lateral collateral ligamentous complex as well as the common extensor origin.

There is often a lateral capsular defect in terrible triad injuries which can be utilized when approaching the elbow joint. In this case, the radial head and neck fragments were then exposed, found to be free of any soft tissue attachments and were thus brought out of the wound (Fig. 48.4A). The coronoid fragment was also identified, brought out of the wound, and deemed too small to warrant fixation (Fig. 48.4B). In this setting, or in the absence of a coronoid fracture, one can consider anterior capsular repair as further means for stabilizing the elbow. This is typically performed by making a small incision over the subcutaneous border of the ulna and creating two drill holes through the base of the coronoid. A suture is then passed through

one drill hole, through the anterior capsule in a "lasso" fashion with multiple passes, back through the other drill hole and tied over the ulna. Since the need for anterior capsular repair is controversial, is case dependent, and may lead to further limitations in extension, the authors prefer to pass this suture early in the case, while the coronoid is easily exposed either through the defect in the radial head or by gently subluxating the elbow. Once the other structures of the injured elbow are repaired, the decision can be made at the end of the case whether to tie down or remove the anterior capsular suture based on the stability of the elbow and the quality of the repairs.

Given the comminution of the radial head fracture, two small peripheral rim fragments, and the patient's age, the decision was made to proceed with radial head replacement. The native radial head was sized (Fig. 48.4C), and the proximal radius was prepared (Fig. 48.5). Overstuffing of the radiocapitellar joint by implantation of a radial head which is too large should be avoided. Overstuffing leads to increased force across the radiocapitellar joint, limitations of motion, and altered elbow mechanics. Intraoperatively, overstuffing can be assessed radiographically by the incongruity of the ulnohumeral joint with widening of the lateral side during trialing (Fig. 48.6). To avoid overstuffing, the radial head is typically downsized one size relative to the native head

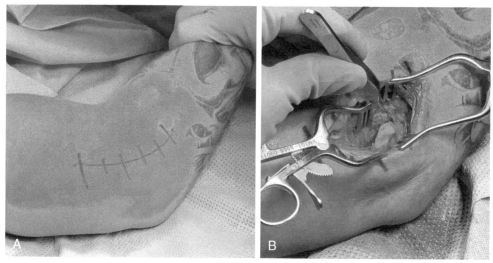

• **Fig. 48.3** (A) A lateral radiocapitellar (Kocher) approach is utilized. (B) A matching bare spot on the humeral epicondyle is commonly present, representing the avulsed lateral collateral ligamentous complex as well as the common extensor origin.

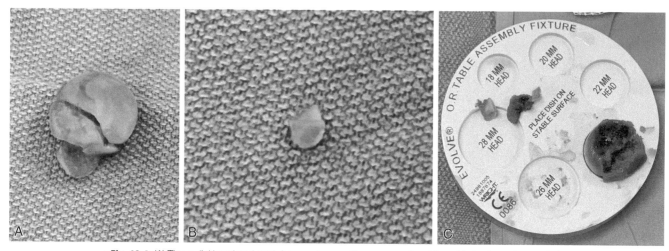

• **Fig. 48.4** (A) The radial head and neck fragments were then exposed and found to be free of any soft tissue attachments and were thus brought out of the wound. (B) The coronoid fragment was also identified, brought out of the wound, and deemed too small to warrant fixation. (C) The native radial head was sized.

measurement. In this case, the native head measured 24 mm in diameter, and thus a 22-mm smooth metal implant was trialed (Fig. 48.7A), selected (Fig. 48.7B), and implanted without cementation. Intraoperative fluoroscopy demonstrated concentrically reduced ulnohumeral and radiocapitellar joints with symmetric medial and lateral joint spaces of the ulnohumeral joint on the AP radiograph (Fig. 48.8A). The intraoperative lateral radiograph (Fig. 48.8B) demonstrates mildly increased ulnohumeral joint space, termed the "drop sign." This common finding represents mild laxity of the medial-sided structures and is not an indication for medial-sided intervention. It is treated with early active motion and avoidance of varus stress to the elbow.

After addressing the radial head fracture, attention is typically turned to the lateral ligamentous complex. In this case, the lateral ligamentous complex and the common extensor origin had torn off the lateral epicondyle in a large, confluent sheet of tissue, as is often seen with this injury pattern. This left a bare spot on the lateral epicondyle from where these structures had originated. This bare spot was roughened up with a curette to encourage healing. A size #1 nonabsorbable suture was passed multiple times, in

Krackow fashion, through the proximal aspect of the ligament. The isometric point of the ligament origin is determined by holding tension on the suture and ranging the elbow from full flexion to 30 degrees of flexion, determining the orientation of the ligament which obtained optimal stability of the elbow throughout motion. A drill hole was then placed from anterior to posterior, centered on this isometric point, and one end of the suture was then passed through this transosseous tunnel. A second suture was similarly passed through the common extensor tendon, and passed through a drill tunnel placed on the lateral epicondyle, just proximal to the lateral collateral ligament tunnel. Suture anchors can also be utilized instead of drill tunnels at the discretion of the treating surgeon. The elbow was then gently examined both clinically and radiographically at full flexion, and again at 30 degrees of flexion. If any instability persists, medial-sided repair is indicated. This is performed with a separate medial incision, identification and protection of the ulnar nerve, and repair of the MCL and common flexor tendon in a similar fashion to the lateral side. In this case, stability to the elbow was restored from full extension to 30 degrees of flexion, and thus medial-sided intervention was not

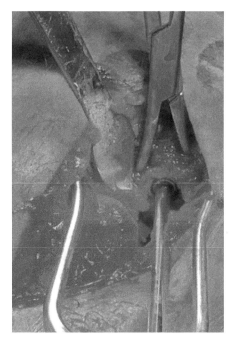

• **Fig. 48.5** The proximal radius was then prepared with sequential broaching up the appropriate size.

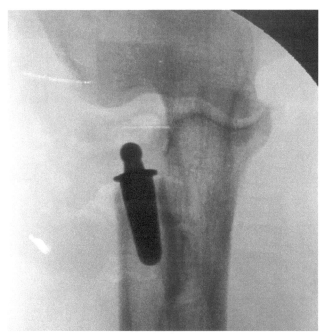

• **Fig. 48.6** Intraoperatively, overstuffing can be assessed radiographically by the incongruity of the ulnohumeral joint with widening of the lateral side during trialing.

indicated. For the remainder of the case until application of the splint, the forearm was held in 90 degrees of elbow flexion and pronation to minimize tension on the lateral ligamentous complex, and the sutures were then tied over the top of the lateral humeral epicondyle (Fig. 48.9). After closure, the arm is splinted in 90 degrees of elbow flexion and maximal forearm pronation, and a sling is applied.

Postoperatively, the patient is held in the sling for 2 weeks. The sling is removed at the 2-week postoperative visit and the wound examined. Postoperative radiographs are obtained to confirm reduction. At this point, if the elbow is found on examination to be stable throughout a passive arc of motion, the patient will be allowed to actively and passively range their elbow as tolerated. Over the next 6 weeks, patients are instructed to avoid weight-bearing or shoulder abduction (which puts a varus moment on the elbow, stressing the collateral ligament repair). After that time, they will be able to advance activity gradually as tolerated. If, at the 2-week postoperative visit, instability is found with extension of the elbow, a hinged elbow brace will be prescribed to block full extension to ensure a stable arc of motion. This block to extension will be minimized in subsequent weeks with close follow-up and serial examinations of the patient.

PEARLS AND PITFALLS

- Careful attention should be given to the mechanism of injury, as this provides important clues to which structures may be injured and to what extent.
- Any concern for a vascular injury requires further evaluation immediately, either with CTA or vascular surgery consultation.
- Ensure all possible necessary equipment is available, including instrumentation for coronoid fixation, anterior capsular repair, radial head fixation, radial head replacement, medial/lateral collateral ligament repairs, medial/lateral ligament reconstructions, and common flexor/extensor tendon repairs, and external fixation.
- Repair of injured structures should proceed in a stepwise fashion from deep to superficial starting with the coronoid/anterior capsule, then the radial head, then the lateral collateral ligament and common extensor origin, followed by the medial side stabilization if necessary.
- Once a collateral ligament repair has been performed, careful attention should be given to avoid undue stress on the repair throughout the remainder of the procedure including closure and splinting.
- At the conclusion of the procedure, ensure the elbow has adequate stability between full flexion and 30 degrees of flexion. If achieved, the patient may reliably return to early (<3 weeks postoperatively) range-of-motion exercises, which is associated with improved outcomes.

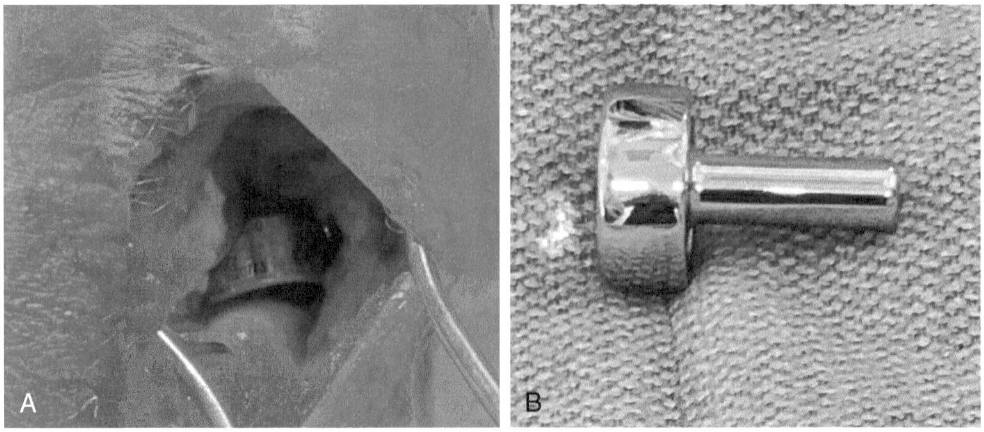

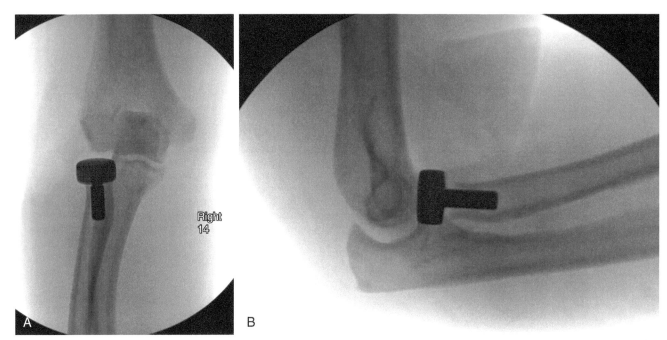

• **Fig. 48.7** The native head measured 24 mm in diameter, and thus a 22-mm smooth metal implant was trialed (A), selected (B), and implanted without cementation.

• **Fig. 48.8** (A) Intraoperative fluoroscopy demonstrated concentrically reduced ulnohumeral and radiocapitellar joints with symmetric medial and lateral joint spaces of the ulnohumeral joint on the anteroposterior radiograph. (B) The intraoperative lateral radiograph demonstrates mildly increased ulnohumeral joint space, termed the "drop sign."

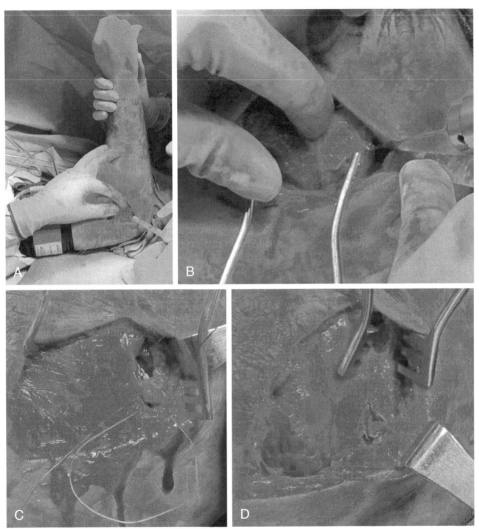

• **Fig. 48.9** For the remainder of the case until application of the splint, the forearm was held in 90 degrees of elbow flexion and pronation (A) to minimize tension on the lateral ligamentous complex. Drill tunnels are placed through the lateral epicondyle (B) and passed through the lateral ligamentous complex to secure it to the lateral epicondyle (C). The interval through the extensor mass is then oversewn (D).

49

Technique Spotlight: ORIF Medial Coronoid Fracture

JULIE ADAMS AND SCOTT STEINMANN

Indications

Indications for open reduction internal fixation of a medial coronoid fracture include a large medial coronoid fracture in the setting of an unstable elbow. Regan and Morrey[1] described coronoid fractures based upon the lateral plain film radiographs (Fig. 49.1), but the advent and widespread use of computed tomography (CT) scan with two- and three-dimensional reconstructions expanded our understanding of coronoid fracture anatomy and biomechanics (Table 49.1; Fig. 49.2). We now know that the anteromedial facet of the coronoid is especially important to buttress and stabilize the elbow particularly against varus posteromedial rotatory forces. Varus posteromedial rotatory forces may act to avulse the lateral ulnar collateral ligament (LUCL) and impact the medial coronoid against the medial aspect of the trochlea, resulting in a fracture of the anteromedial coronoid. Large fragments include the sublime tubercle and, therefore, the medial collateral ligament (MCL) becomes incompetent. Surgical fixation for these large fragments is generally recommended to restore stability to the elbow, as unrecognized instability will lead to medial joint narrowing and wear, and rapid onset of arthrosis.[2]

Preoperative Evaluation (Imaging, Examination, etc.)

Preoperative evaluation includes plain film radiographs of the elbow and most commonly a CT scan with two- and three-dimensional reconstructions. CT scan is ideally obtained after a closed reduction for elbow dislocations, with the elbow splinted in as much extension as possible. The elbow is ideally centered in the scanner, usually with the arm elevated above the patient's head rather than resting at the patient's side. This will allow for the most useful images. Reconstructions including three-dimensional studies and joint subtraction views are helpful to determine fracture size and location and presence of additional injuries.

Physical examination documents the status of the radial, median, and, particularly, the ulnar nerve function and excludes concomitant injuries to the limb by palpating for tenderness, to determine if additional radiographs are needed, and documenting stability or lack of stability of the elbow. Typically, an examination under anesthesia and fluoroscopy may be performed to evaluate stability of the elbow, but is usually done in the operating room.

To assess for posteromedial instability in clinic, a stress examination that is reasonably well tolerated by patients is to have the patient abduct his arm to 90 degrees, then have him actively flex and extend the elbow. Gravity acts to create instability, crepitus, and apprehension in those with medial coronoid fractures associated with posteromedial instability (Fig. 49.3A–B). It is important to understand that in the setting of posteromedial instability, in which the patient is treated operatively, typically we first address the large medial coronoid fragment with fixation. Subsequently, one may reassess stability intraoperatively with examination under

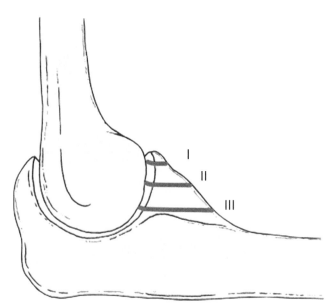

• **Fig. 49.1** Regan-Morrey classification of coronoid fractures is based upon the lateral radiograph of the elbow. Type I fractures represent the tip of the coronoid, type II are those that represent <50% of the coronoid on the lateral film, and type III are those that comprise >50% of the coronoid on the lateral film. (From Browner B, Jupiter J. Skeletal Trauma, 5th edition 2014.)

anesthesia and fluoroscopy. If lateral-sided instability is problematic, one can address it by repair of the LUCL.[3-5] One should also recognize that if medial stability is restored, even if LUCL instability is present at terminal extension, in some cases the LUCL may be left alone if the elbow can be immobilized in a position of congruency and stability. In many cases, fixation of the coronoid may not be robust enough to allow early unrestricted motion; therefore the patient may be immobilized for a few weeks anyway, and provided that the patient is monitored closely with weekly radiographs to ensure the joint remains congruently located, it may be acceptable and even desirable to avoid the trauma of a second lateral incision and fixation of the LUCL, and rather to allow it to heal on its own. Small coronoid fractures, in contrast to larger fragments, may be indicative of posterolateral instability,

which should be distinguished from posteromedial rotatory instability (PMRI).

Positioning and Equipment

The patient is positioned usually supine and one may use an arm board or arm table. A sterile tourniquet may be used. In terms of fixation of coronoid fractures, if the patient has a concomitant radial head fracture that is replaced, the laterally based approach through window afforded by the excised radial head is used.

TABLE 49.1 Coronoid Fractures Classification (O'Driscoll)

Fracture	Subtype	Description
Tip	1	≤2 mm of coronoid bony height (i.e., "Flake" fracture)
	2	<2 mm of coronoid height
Anteromedial	1	Anteromedial rim
	2	Anteromedial rim + tip
	3	Anteromedial rim + sublime tubercle (±tip)
Base	1	Coronoid body and base
	2	Transolecranon basal coronoid fractures

From O'Driscoll SW, Jupiter JB, Cohen MS, Ring D, McKee MD. Difficult elbow fractures: pearls and pitfalls. *Instr Course Lect* . 2003;52:113-134.

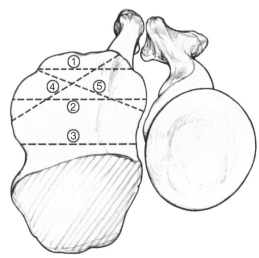

• **Fig. 49.2** A revision of the Regan-Morrey classification includes the original types I, II, and III, but also accounts for the anteromedial *(line 4)* and anterolateral *(line 5)* fracture types and is based upon a review of computed tomography scans. (From Browner B, Jupiter J. Skeletal Trauma, 5th edition 2014.)

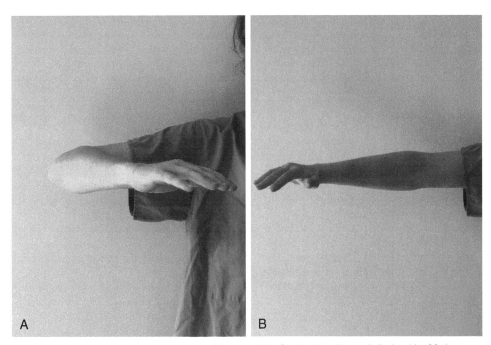

• **Fig. 49.3** To assess for subtle medial instability, the patient is asked to abduct their shoulder 90 degrees, and to (A) flex and (B) extend the elbow. Gravity exerts a stress across the elbow and presence of apprehension or crepitus indicates instability of the elbow.

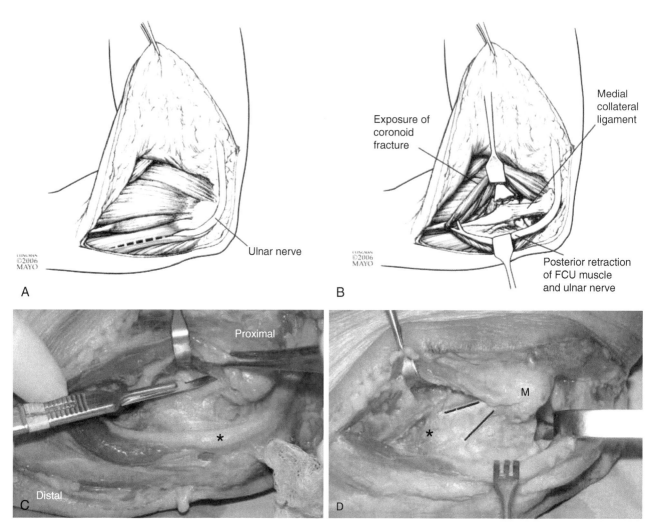

A

B

Exposure of
coronoid
fracture

Medial
collateral
ligament

Ulnar nerve

Posterior retraction
of FCU muscle
and ulnar nerve

Proximal

Distal

C

D

M

*

*

• **Fig. 49.4** Medial approach to the coronoid process on a right elbow. (A) Illustration demonstrating how the flexor carpi ulnaris *(FCU)* is split between the two heads *(dashed line)* to enable in situ release of the ulnar nerve. (B) Illustration demonstrating the cubital tunnel retinaculum following the release of the ulnar nerve. The floor of the cubital tunnel is exposed as the ulnar nerve is gently retracted posteriorly. (C) Intraoperative photograph showing the ulnar nerve *(asterisk)* after it has been carefully dissected off of the anterior band of the medial collateral ligament (MCL). (D) Intraoperative photograph. The anterior band of the MCL lies between the lines. The base of the coronoid process *(asterisk)* is exposed. The posterior and transverse bands of the MCL have been excised for the purpose of illustration. Reflection of the humeral head of the FCU laterally and superiorly allows nearly full visualization of the anterior bundle of the MCL. This exposure affords complete access to the coronoid process and the MCL as well as limited access to the posterior fossa. *M,* medial epicondyle. (From Cheung EV, Steinmann SP. Surgical approaches to the elbow. *J Am Acad Orthop Surg.* 2009;17(5):325-333.)

However, in most cases of large medial coronoid fractures, a separate medially based incision is used to expose and fixate the fracture. Of note, an anterior incision has been described,[6] although for substantial medial fracture fragments, these authors prefer a medial incision. Although sizes vary among manufacturers, typically plate and screw systems for fixation of the coronoid range between 2.0 and 2.7 mm, with most around 2.5 mm in size. Purpose-made contoured plates are now available from a number of manufacturers, although one may alternatively bend appropriately sized plates intraoperatively.

Surgical Technique

An incision is made, similar to the one preferred for a cubital tunnel decompression (Fig. 49.4A). A longitudinal incision is made just posterior to the medial epicondyle. Dissection proceeds, identifying and preserving (if possible) branches of the medial antebrachial cutaneous nerve. The ulnar nerve is identified, and distally over the proximal forearm, it is mobilized such that it may be retracted anteriorly, as the dissection proceeds at the distal aspect of the cubital tunnel region. Care is taken to avoid excessive disruption of the nerve or mobilization more proximally.

Thus the so-called floor of the cubital tunnel is exposed, and the surgeon works distally to proximally, palpating the sublime tubercle as a landmark, as he or she works from distal to proximal (Fig. 49.4B). With careful palpation and by working from distal to proximal, the surgeon can readily identify the sublime tubercle as a clue to the insertion site of the MCL (Fig. 49.4C). By doing so, the surgeon can avoid iatrogenic injury to

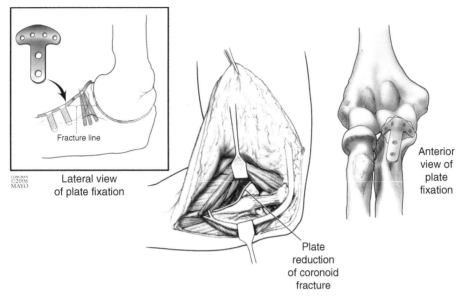

CLINGMAN
©2006
MAYO

Lateral view
of plate fixation

Fracture line

Plate
reduction
of coronoid
fracture

Anterior
view of
plate
fixation

• **Fig. 49.5** The coronoid fracture has been reduced from a medial approach and plate fixation utilized. Care is taken to protect the ulnar nerve.(from the Mayo Clinic.)

the MCL (Fig. 49.4D). The fracture site is exposed (Fig. 49.5), the surgeon reduces the fracture, and determines if plate versus screw fixation is appropriate. It is often helpful to provisionally place the plate over the fracture site, which may be temporarily fixated with K-wires through the plate. The plate position may be checked under fluoroscopy and adjusted, or the plate retrieved and bent to contour to the bone to serve as a buttress. A variety of purpose-made precontoured plating systems are available for fixation of coronoid fractures. Some plates are designed to allow in situ bending, while others should be removed for additional contouring. Fixation is applied and fluoroscopy confirms appropriate fixation and stability of the elbow.

The ulnar nerve is allowed to fall back into place, and care is taken to assure there has not been an area of potential compression or tethering of the nerve created. The nerve is assessed for subluxation, which is generally not a problem unless there has been excessive mobilization more proximally. The elbow is checked for range of motion to ensure it is full and that there is no crepitus. Stability is gently assessed. If the elbow is stable, the tourniquet is released, and the wound is closed, and the elbow is typically splinted in about 90 degrees of flexion and supination. If there is

concern about lateral-sided elbow instability, the LUCL may be repaired, and then the forearm is immobilized in 90 degrees of flexion and neutral forearm rotation.

References

1. Regan W, Morrey B. Fractures of the coronoid process of the ulna. *J Bone Joint Surg Am*. 1989;71(9):1348–1354.
2. Steinmann SP. Coronoid process fracture. *J Am Acad Orthop Surg*. 2008;16(9):519–529.
3. Ramirez MA, Stein JA, Murthi AM. Varus posteromedial instability. *Hand Clin*. 2015;31(4):557–563.
4. Doornberg JN, Ring DC. Fracture of the anteromedial facet of the coronoid process. *J Bone Joint Surg Am*. 2006;88(10):2216–2224. https://doi.org/10.2106/JBJS.E.01127.
5. Adams JE, Hoskin TL, Morrey BF, Steinmann SP. Management and outcome of 103 acute fractures of the coronoid process of the ulna. *J Bone Joint Surg Br*. 2009;91(5):632–635. https://doi.org/10.1302/0301-620X.91B5.21755.
6. Reichel LM, Milam GS, Reitman CA. Anterior approach for operative fixation of coronoid fractures in complex elbow instability. *Tech Hand Up Extrem Surg*. 2012;16(2):98–104. https://doi.org/10.1097/BTH.0b013e31824e6a74.

PEARLS AND PITFALLS

- Special attention is required for coronoid fractures and their impact on elbow stability. Failure to recognize these patterns can have a significant impact upon stability and lead to rapid and inevitable onset of arthritis of the elbow.
- The ulnar nerve may be irritated or injured with this approach. Most commonly, such cases represent a neurapraxia which is temporary, likely due to traction, although permanent injury may occur. It is important to counsel the patient about this preoperatively.
- Work from distal to proximal in order to avoid iatrogenic injury to the MCL; the surgeon is constantly palpating for the sublime tubercle as a landmark. Working from proximal to distal or with a direct medial approach is likely to result in exposure of the coronoid and injury to the MCL which often "appears before you know it."

50

Technique Spotlight: Approach to Chronic Elbow Instability

AUSTIN A. PITCHER AND PETER J. EVANS

The elbow is a complex joint comprising three distinct articulations and stabilized by multiple osseous and ligamentous structures. As a result, elbow instability can be a challenging problem to successfully treat.[1] Elbow instability can present on a spectrum of severity, ranging from subtle ligamentous laxity to severe multidirectional instability with bony changes.

Indications

Patients with subtle instability often present with complaints of pain, mechanical symptoms, or a sense of instability with certain activities. In contrast, patients with more severe injuries present with a stiff, painful elbow with little functional use. Elbow instability is classified as either posteromedial or posterolateral instability. Posteromedial instability is due primarily to insufficiency of the medial structures including the anterior band of the ulnar collateral ligament (UCL), whereas posterolateral instability stems from insufficiency of the lateral ligamentous complex and the lateral ulnar collateral ligament (LUCL).[2–5]

Patients with more severe injuries may present with chronic dislocation of the ulnohumeral and radiocapitellar joints and may have multiple associated bony injuries including distal humeral, radial head, and coronoid fractures. Associated fractures may be nonunited or malunited and there can be significant bone loss that needs to be addressed to restore stability. In the chronic setting, it is common to have extensive heterotopic ossification and scarring which may need to be resected before a congruent articulation is achieved.[6,7]

In all cases of elbow instability, a careful clinical assessment with appropriate imaging and careful preoperative planning is essential for success. In cases of isolated posterolateral rotatory instability (PLRI) or posteromedial rotatory instability (PMRI) without bony injury, appropriate ligament reconstruction may be all that is necessary to restore stability. However, in cases of chronic instability with bony abnormalities, liberal resection of scar tissue, reconstruction of bony defects, and multiple ligament reconstruction may be necessary.

Coronoid fractures except small avulsions (O'Driscoll type I) should be repaired or reconstructed as this is a primary stabilizer of the ulnohumeral joint. In cases where the bony fragment is not amenable to fixation, it may be reconstructed from an excised radial head if available, the tip of the ipsilateral olecranon, the distal clavicle, or a costochondral autograft.[8–14] The literature supporting different coronoid graft options does not support making strong conclusions regarding donor selection, and thus the choice is primarily a matter of surgical convenience and the surgeon's preference.[14]

Radial head deficiency should also be addressed. While radial head resection remains an option for comminuted radial head fractures, surgeons must assure that the collateral ligaments, forearm longitudinal ligaments, and the triangular fibrocartilage complex (TFCC) in the wrist are stable.[15] Although the radial head is not considered a primary stabilizer of the elbow joint, its role in stabilizing the traumatized elbow has been well established. Small fractures of the radial head may be amenable to fixation, but chronic bone loss or comminuted fracture patterns are best addressed with radial head arthroplasty.[16]

Preoperative Evaluation

Evaluation should begin with a detailed history including mechanism of injury along with initial management including any prior surgical treatment. Examination should include a careful neurovascular examination, range of motion of the elbow including pronation and supination of the forearm, and careful palpation of the bony and ligamentous structures about the elbow. The shoulder and wrist should also be evaluated as they may be concurrently injured. Provocative maneuvers including push-up from chair, moving valgus stress, lateral pivot shift, and stability to varus and valgus stress can be included to test for more subtle signs of instability.

Plain radiographs should be obtained in all patients, and care should be taken to obtain high-quality lateral views of the elbow. Computed tomography (CT) should be obtained in most patients with chronic instability to evaluate for bone loss of the coronoid process, radial head, or distal humerus, and to evaluate for potential sites of bony impingement. The CT should be obtained with thin cuts through the elbow with three-dimensional reconstructions to aid in visualization of bony abnormalities and for preoperative planning. Stress examination under fluoroscopy in the clinic setting can add valuable information utilizing all of the above-listed provocative maneuvers and can yield additional information. This is useful to strategically plan medial, lateral, or combined bony and ligamentous reconstruction. If this cannot be performed in the clinical setting, it is routinely obtained in the operating room prior to starting the procedure. Magnetic resonance imaging (MRI) plays a limited role in evaluation of chronic instability.

Positioning and Equipment

The elbow can be approached in the supine, lateral, or prone positions and is largely a matter of the surgeon's preference. We prefer to position the patient in the supine position with the arm on a radiolucent hand table, as this provides ready access to both the medial and lateral sides of the elbow, allows for facile imaging, and allows for convenient examination of the elbow including performance of the hanging arm test to assess gross collateral ligament laxity. Equipment includes fluoroscopy via a mini or large C-arm, suture anchors, tendon allograft, drill, and splint material. In cases with bony abnormalities, the surgeon should have available a sagittal saw, radial head arthroplasty components, minifragmentation set, headless compression screws (2.4 and 3.0 mm), and any instruments necessary for coronoid reconstruction. An external fixator or internal joint stabilizer should be available as a backup option in case a stable ulnohumeral joint cannot be obtained following appropriate bony and soft tissue reconstruction or to protect the reconstruction.

Technique

A tourniquet is applied to the upper arm. In cases where both the lateral and medial sides will need to be addressed, we prefer to use two incisions as this prevents having to raise large skin flaps which can create wound issues and maximizes each exposure. The elbow joint should be reconstructed systematically, first addressing bony defects from medial to lateral, and then ligamentous structures starting with the LUCL, moving on to the UCL only if there is persistent instability (Fig. 50.1).

The lateral exposure can be done through the interval between the extensor carpi radialis brevis (ECRB) and the extensor digitorum communis (EDC, Kaplan's interval), or through the interval between the anconeus and the extensor carpi ulnaris (ECU, Kocher's interval). The skin incision for both approaches is the same, starting over the lateral elbow just proximal to the lateral epicondyle, continued distally over the epicondyle, and ending over the proximal ulna. The chosen interval is identified and bluntly dissected to expose the joint capsule. The joint capsule should be incised just anterior to the midpoint of the radial head, taking care to avoid unnecessary injury to the LUCL or annular ligaments (Fig. 50.2).

In cases of chronic instability, significant scar tissue or heterotopic ossification may be preventing normal elbow range of motion or even prevent reduction of the elbow joint. Contracture release should be performed at this stage and continued until the elbow can be reduced and reduction can be maintained throughout full range of motion.[17] A column approach is useful here and provides good access to the anterior and posterior capsules as well as the olecranon fossa and lateral side of the olecranon.[18] A medial approach is often necessary, particularly in cases with limited

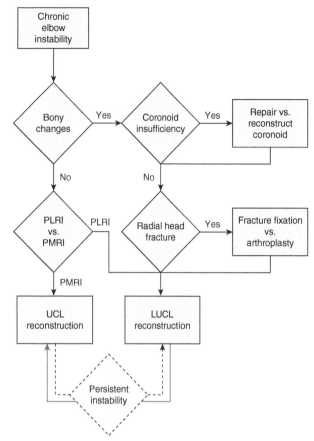

• **Fig. 50.1** Algorithmic approach for reconstruction in elbow instability. *LUCL*, Lateral ulnar collateral ligament; *PLRI*, posterolateral rotatory instability; *PMRI*, posteromedial rotatory instability; *UCL*, ulnar collateral ligament.

flexion as it allows for ulnar nerve decompression and release of the posterior band of the UCL (Fig. 50.3).

Following contracture release, the first decision to be made is determining if the radial head is able to be salvaged or if an arthroplasty is necessary. In cases where arthroplasty is determined to be appropriate, excision of remaining radial head often significantly improves exposure to the coronoid process. Fixation or reconstruction of the coronoid process is the first structure that should be addressed to restore elbow stability. Capsular avulsion or Type I coronoid fractures may at times require capsular reapproximation to the remaining coronoid by either a trans-ulna suture loop or bone anchor placed in the coronoid stump. Some coronoid fractures may be able to be fixed from the lateral approach, but larger, more complex, or predominantly anteromedial facet fractures are best addressed through a medial approach. Subsequently, if the radial head has been excised, arthroplasty can be performed at this time. Alternatively, fracture fixation can be performed if amenable.

The LUCL is one of the key structures required to restore elbow stability. There are numerous techniques described in the literature including bone tunnels, button fixation, and interference screw fixation. We prefer a docking technique, and the graft is first anchored to the ulna at the LUCL insertion at the supinator crest. The graft is then tensioned with the elbow held reduced and the forearm in supination. It is essential that the humeral insertion of the graft be just superior to the center of rotation of the capitellum (allowing for the size of the docking hole) to ensure constant tension throughout elbow range of motion.[19] The anchor site can

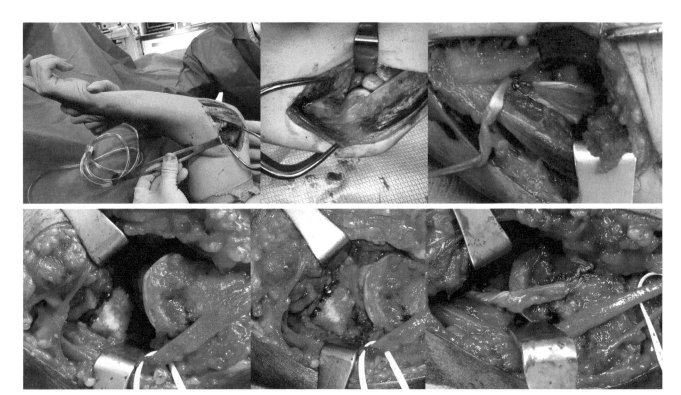

• **Fig. 50.2** The patient is placed in the supine position. The elbow is first approached laterally *(top left)* allowing for contracture release *(top center)*, fixation or replacement of the radial head, and lateral ulnar collateral ligament reconstruction *(top right)*. If there is persistent instability, extension contracture, or coronoid fracture, the elbow is then approached medially *(bottom)*. The ulnar nerve is decompressed *(bottom left)*, the coronoid reconstructed *(bottom center)*, and the ulnar collateral ligament is reconstructed *(bottom right)*.

also be confirmed by holding the graft with a clamp and ranging the elbow to ensure constant tension throughout the range. On closure, reefing up slack posterior capsule first and then anterior capsule to the ligament reconstruction can add additional stability (Fig. 50.4).

The elbow should be carefully tested clinically and radiographically for signs of instability following LUCL reconstruction. The hanging arm test can be utilized here. The arm is placed in the supinated position and supported at the humerus. The elbow is then extended and the forearm allowed to hang while obtaining a lateral fluoroscopic view of the elbow. Maintenance of concentric reduction of the ulnohumeral joint confirms adequate reconstruction of the elbow stability. A minimal amount of radiocapitellar sag is common and acceptable. If instability persists at this point, assess medially and UCL reconstruction should be performed through the medial approach. Similar to the LUCL reconstruction, the graft is first anchored at the ulnar insertion on the sublime tubercle. The graft is then tensioned and anchored into the humeral origin of the UCL via a docking technique. Holding the graft with a clamp at the planned insertion site while ranging the elbow to ensure constant tension throughout the arc is again useful (Fig. 50.5). Following UCL reconstruction the elbow should again be critically evaluated for instability. If there is persistent instability, ligament reconstruction should be critically evaluated for proper graft tensioning and anchor placement in the humerus.

If instability still persists, then a hinged external fixator or an internal joint stabilizer should be placed.

PEARLS AND PITFALLS

- Although medial and lateral reconstruction can be performed through a single posterior incision, we recommend separate medial and lateral incisions to maximize exposure and avoid creating large skin flaps.
- Contracture release should be performed prior to any reconstructive procedures and should be performed algorithmically until adequate flexion and extension are obtained.
- Bony issues should be carefully evaluated preoperatively as they can require significant preoperative planning should defects need to be reconstructed. Having a primary and secondary plan for bony procedures will ensure that all necessary equipment is available.
- If radial head arthroplasty is performed, care should be taken to avoid overstuffing the radiocapitellar joint by aligning the proximal aspect of the prosthesis with sigmoid notch on the ulna.
- Appropriate placement of the humeral docking sites for LUCL and UCL reconstruction is key to restoring stability throughout range of motion, and extra care should be taken to ensure appropriate placement as this can be a challenging error to fix should an anchor or tunnel be placed in an incorrect position.
- The ulnar nerve should be decompressed in any cases with flexion limited to <90 degrees.

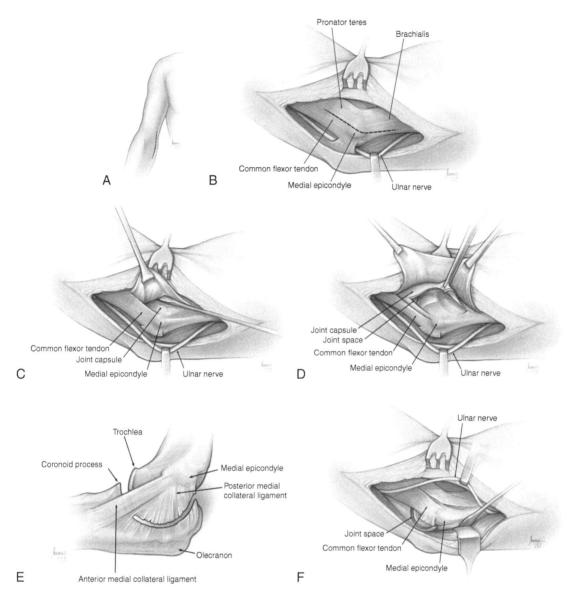

• **Fig. 50.3** Illustration demonstrating the medial approach for elbow instability. In patients with limited elbow flexion, ulnar nerve decompression and posterior band of the ulnar collateral ligament (UCL) should be released. (A) Location of the medial incision, (B) superficial dissection, (C) deep dissection, (D) anterior capsular release, (E) release of posterior band of the UCL, and (F) completion of release with intact common flexor tendon and anterior band of the UCL. (Reprinted with permission, Cleveland Clinic Center for Medical Art & Photography ©2021. All Rights Reserved.)

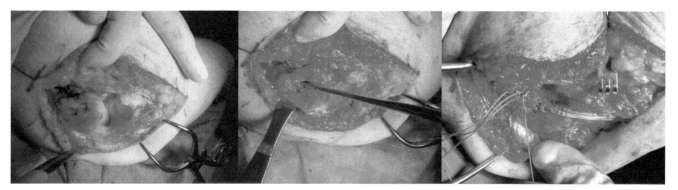

• **Fig. 50.4** The docking technique for lateral ulnar collateral ligament (LUCL) reconstruction. The graft is first placed through bone tunnels in the ulna at the LUCL insertion at the supinator crest *(not shown)*. The center of rotation of the capitellum is determined clinically and fluoroscopically by identifying the center-center position on a perfect lateral fluoroscopic view. The tunnel is placed just superior to the center of rotation to allow for the size of the drill *(left)*. The tunnel is then widened using curettes *(middle)*. Finally, the graft is docked into the humeral tunnel and tensioned with the forearm held in supination and a valgus stress applied across the elbow *(right)*.

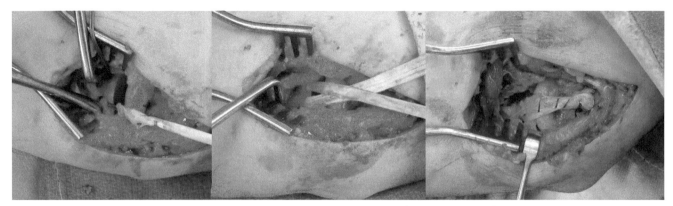

• **Fig. 50.5** The docking technique for ulnar collateral ligament (UCL) reconstruction. Bone tunnels are made through ulna at the UCL insertion at the supinator crest and the graft is passed *(left)*. The humeral tunnel is made at the UCL origin at the intersection of the medial condyle and epicondyle. The graft is tensioned with the forearm held in pronation. If lateral ulnar collateral ligament (LUCL) reconstruction has already been performed, care is taken to not apply excessive varus force across the elbow when tensioning the UCL graft to avoid injury to the LUCL reconstruction *(middle)*. The graft is then secured in the humeral tunnel. Suturing limbs of the graft together can allow fine-tuning of graft tensioning and can more accurately reconstruct the normal UCL anatomy *(right)*.

References

1. Morrey BF, An KN. Articular and ligamentous contributions to the stability of the elbow joint. *Am J Sport Med*. 1983;11(5):315–319.
2. Oka K, Murase T, Moritomo H, et al. Accuracy of corrective osteotomy using a custom-designed device based on a novel computer simulation system. *J Orthop Sci*. 2011;16(1):85–92. https://doi.org/10.1007/s00776-010-0020-4.
3. Grace SP, Field LD. Chronic medial elbow instability. *Orthop Clin N Am*. 2008;39:213–219. https://doi.org/10.1016/j.ocl.2007.12.003.
4. Charalambous CP, Stanley JK. Posterolateral rotatory instability of the elbow. *J Bone Jt Surg Br*. 2008;90B:272–279. https://doi.org/10.1302/0301-620X.90B3.19868.
5. Lee JH, Lee JH, Kim KC, Ahn KB, Rhyou IH. Treatment of posteromedial and posterolateral dislocation of the acute unstable elbow joint: a strategic approach. *J Shoulder Elb Surg*. 2019;28(10):2007–2016. https://doi.org/10.1016/j.jse.2019.05.029.
6. Lee ML, Rosenwasser MP. Chronic elbow instability. *Orthop Clin North Am*. 1999;30(1):81–89.
7. Tashjian RZ, Katarincic JA. Complex elbow instability. *J Am Acad Orthop Surg*. 2006;14:278–286.
8. Garrigues GE, Wray WH, Lindenhovius ALC, Ring DC, Ruch DS. Fixation of the coronoid process in elbow fracture-dislocations. *J Bone Jt Surg Am*. 2011;93:1873–1881.
9. Ramirez MA, Ramirez JM, Parks BG, Tsai MA, Murthi AM. Olecranon tip osteoarticular autograft transfer for irreparable coronoid process fracture: a biomechanical study. *Hand*. 2015;10:695–700. https://doi.org/10.1007/s11552-015-9776-5.
10. Silveira GH, Eng K. Reconstruction of coronoid process using costochondral graft in a case of chronic posteromedial rotatory instability of the elbow. *J Shoulder Elb Surg*. 2013;22:e14–e18. https://doi.org/10.1016/j.jse.2013.01.015.
11. Yasui Y, Uesugi A, Kataoka T, Kuriyama K, Hamada M. Reconstruction of the coronoid process using a costal osteochondral autograft for acute comminuted coronoid fracture : a case report. *J Shoulder Elb Surg*. 2018;27:e167–e171. https://doi.org/10.1016/j.jse.2018.01.019.
12. Papandrea RF, Morrey BF, O'Driscoll SW. Reconstruction for persistent instability of the elbow after coronoid fracture-dislocation. *J Shoulder Elb Surg*. 2007;16:68–77. https://doi.org/10.1016/j.jse.2006.03.011.
13. Ring D, Guss D, Jupiter JB. Reconstruction of the coronoid process using a fragment of discarded radial head. *J Hand Surg Am*. 2012;37A(3):570–574. https://doi.org/10.1016/j.jhsa.2011.12.016.
14. Bellato E, O'Driscoll SW. Management of the posttraumatic coronoid-deficient elbow. *J Hand Surg Am*. 2019;44:400–410. https://doi.org/10.1016/j.jhsa.2018.08.001.
15. Aburto Bernardo M, Arnal Burró J, López Mombielo F, Pérez Martín A, López Torres I, Álvarez González C. A retrospective comparative cohort study of radial head arthroplasty versus resection in complex elbow dislocations. *Injury*. 2020 Apr;51(suppl 1):S89–S93. https://doi.org/10.1016/j.injury.2020.02.028.
16. Leigh WB, Ball CM. Radial head reconstruction versus replacement in the treatment of terrible triad injuries of the elbow. *J Shoulder Elb Surg*. 2012;21:1336–1341. https://doi.org/10.1016/j.jse.2012.03.005.
17. Haglin JM, Kugelman DN, Christiano A, Konda SR, Paksima N, Egol KA. Open surgical elbow contracture release after trauma: results and recommendations. *J Shoulder Elb Surg*. 2018;27:418–426. https://doi.org/10.1016/j.jse.2017.10.023.
18. Nandi S, Maschke S, Evans PJ, Lawton JN. The stiff elbow. *Hand*. 2009;4(4):368–379. https://doi.org/10.1007/s11552-009-9181-z.
19. Moritomo H, Murase T, Arimitsu S, Oka K, Yoshikawa H, Sugamoto K. The in vivo isometric point of the lateral ligament of the elbow. *J Bone Jt Surg - Ser A*. 2007;89(9):2011–2017. https://doi.org/10.2106/JBJS.F.00868.

51

Proximal Ulna Fractures and Fracture-Dislocations— Monteggia and Beyond

DAVID R. VELTRE AND HARRY A. HOYEN

Introduction

Proximal ulna fractures and fracture-dislocations present a unique challenge to the orthopedic surgeon. It is one of the few joints with multiple articulations and degrees of freedom. Due to these intricate relationships, the disruption of the elbow's complex osseous and ligamentous anatomy can have profound effects on the ability to perform activities of daily living. Recognition of the patterns of injury and timely treatment are critical to getting patients back to full function as soon as possible.

Relevant Osseous Anatomy

The elbow provides flexion, extension, and rotation around the central axis of the forearm. The ability of the elbow joint to perform these movements is due to its unique anatomy including its three articulations: the proximal radioulnar, the radiocapitellar, and the ulnotrochlear joints. The congruity that these joints provide and the soft tissue surrounding the elbow provide its stability.

The ulnotrochlear joint is primarily stabilized by the trochlear notch of the ulna. The trochlear notch consists of a nearly 190-degree articulation from the coronoid distally to the olecranon process proximally.[1] The trochlear notch is not hemispherical, but rather ellipsoid, which explains the articular gap in the midportion. This gap, which appears as a transverse nonarticular groove that cuts across the trochlear notch, separates the coronoid and olecranon articular areas of the notch (Fig. 51.1). When reconstructing an olecranon fracture, it is important to reestablish the anatomic relationship between these two main articular regions.

The angle between the tip of the olecranon and the coronoid processes, when viewed in the sagittal plane, is approximately 30 degrees posteriorly tilted in respect to the long axis of the ulna.[2] This angle corresponds to the 30 degrees of anterior angulation of the articular condyles of the distal humerus. This synergistic anatomy provides the stability of the elbow joint and allows the elbow to obtain full extension.

The olecranon process is the most posterior aspect of the trochlear notch and the location of the triceps insertion. At full extension of the elbow, the olecranon tip rests in the olecranon fossa of the distal humerus. There are three distinct insertional areas of the triceps on the olecranon corresponding to the posterior capsular insertion, the deep muscular portion, and the superficial tendinous portion of the triceps. The triceps insertion is 2.6-cm wide and attaches approximately 1 cm from the tip of the olecranon.[3]

The coronoid process consists of the coronoid tip, base, lesser sigmoid notch, and the anteromedial facet. The anteromedial facet, in particular, is essential for elbow stability under posterior and varus stress. Understanding the soft tissue attachments to the coronoid area is critical to understanding the stability of the elbow joint. The anterior band of the medial collateral ligament attaches

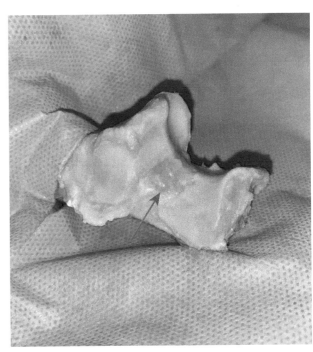

• **Fig. 51.1** View from the lateral aspect of the olecranon of a cadaveric specimen indicated the bare spot (arrow) between the coronoid and olecranon articular areas.

to the base of the coronoid at the sublime tubercle and provides stability in valgus stress while remaining isometric during elbow range of motion (ROM).[4–6] On the lateral side of the elbow, the lateral ulnar collateral ligament (LUCL) attaches to the tubercle of the supinator crest of the ulna and is the primary stabilizer to varus and external rotation stress of the elbow. The anterior capsule inserts on average 6 mm distal to the coronoid tip and injury to the capsule should be suspected in any coronoid tip fracture.

Pathoanatomy

A firm understanding of the pathoanatomy of the elbow allows the surgeon to anticipate and identify associated injuries after an injury, which is essential to timely and appropriate treatment.

When a proximal ulna fracture is first identified, it is important to recognize whether there is a dislocation component in relation to the ulnohumeral or proximal radioulnar articulations. A fracture of the proximal ulna and a disruption of the proximal radioulnar joint is known as a Monteggia fracture. Initially described by Giovanni Battista Monteggia in 1814,[7] it was further expanded upon by Jose Luis Bado in 1958.[8] Today, we reserve the label of a Monteggia to apply to a dislocation of the proximal radioulnar joint in association with a fracture of the ulna. Monteggia fractures should be distinguished from transolecranon fracture-dislocations. In Monteggia fractures, the fracture of the ulna is generally distal to the coronoid and there is a dislocation of the radiocapitellar and proximal radioulnar joints. In a transolecranon fracture-dislocation, the fracture is in the region of the coronoid and there is radiocapitellar joint dislocation with preserved radioulnar articulation.[9,10]

Monteggia fractures and transolecranon fracture-dislocations of the elbow are often associated with injuries including radial head fractures, capitellum fractures, coronoid fractures, and injuries to the lateral ligamentous complex of the elbow, particularly the LUCL. A surgical plan should be developed to address the other concomitant injuries. While Monteggia fractures are less common in adults than in children, all patients with a proximal ulna fracture should be evaluated for these associated injuries and treated accordingly. Standard radiographic analysis should include anteroposterior (AP), lateral, and radial head views. Traction radiographs obtained at the time of reduction can be very useful in identifying the fracture patterns. Ancillary studies such as a computed tomography (CT) scan or magnetic resonance imaging (MRI) should be obtained after fracture or joint reduction.

Classification

The purpose of a classification system is to aid the surgeon in understanding the prognosis of an injury and help guide in deciding the appropriate treatment. An understanding of the classification systems below is essential in maximizing the outcomes in patients with proximal ulna and Monteggia fractures.

Olecranon Fractures

The treatment-driven classification system used for olecranon fractures is the Mayo classification system.[2] The Mayo classification system describes proximal ulna fractures on the basis of displacement, then stability, and comminution. There are three fracture types and each type is then subdivided into comminuted (A) or noncomminuted (B) fractures (Fig. 51.2). Type I proximal ulna fractures are nondisplaced. These fractures are the least common type of olecranon fracture, occurring only 5% of the time.

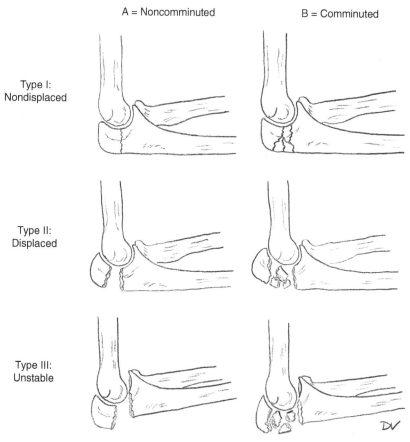

A = Noncomminuted   B = Comminuted

Type I:
Nondisplaced

Type II:
Displaced

Type III:
Unstable

• **Fig. 51.2** Mayo classification of olecranon fractures.

Whether these fractures are comminuted or not, these fractures are typically treated nonoperatively. Type II fractures are displaced but stable. Eighty to eighty-five percent of all olecranon fractures are Mayo Type II.[11,12] The collateral ligament and fracture fragments are intact in Type II fractures and, therefore, the elbow is typically stable. Type III fractures are displaced and unstable. These fractures are the most unstable of the olecranon fracture types and represent transolecranon fracture-dislocations.

While not a formal classification system, we have developed a treatment algorithm based on the fracture patterns and extensions. Fractures of the olecranon process (A type) are mainly due to an avulsion mechanism and are proximal to the nonarticular portion of the proximal ulna. The elbow articulations are stable in these situations. Overcoming the proximal pull of the triceps is important in planning fracture reconstruction. Fractures involving the coronoid region (B type) are often a result of higher energy mechanisms and result in more instability patterns. As the fractures extend and displace the ligament insertion areas, the ulnohumeral and proximal radioulnar joints are rendered unstable. Fracture fixation of the critical coronoid ligament insertion fragments is essential. Because these are also articular injuries around the nonarticular (bare area) of the proximal ulna, it is also important to concentrate on the fixation of the olecranon process into the coronoid. Fractures more distal to the coronoid (C type) are largely nonarticular or minimally articular. These fractures are more similar to forearm shaft fractures sharing similar fixation principles and are more likely to result in radial head instability. Proximal ulna fractures can certainly involve multiple zones. The surgeon should be prepared to gain stability across the different regions. Fracture plating systems have been designed to best capture and gain stability in each of these different zones.

Monteggia Fractures

The Bado description of Monteggia fractures is most commonly used (Fig. 51.3, Table 51.1).[8] It involves four types based on the direction of the dislocation of the radial head and the apex of the ulnar fracture, which are always in the same direction. Type I fractures are dislocated anteriorly, Type II fractures are displaced posteriorly, Type III fractures are displaced laterally, and Type IV fractures can be displaced in any direction but are characterized by a diaphyseal fracture of the radius.

Type I fractures are the most common among all patients (55%–80%) but occur more commonly in children.[13,14] These injuries typically occur following a direct blow to the ulna or a hyperextension injury during a fall on an outstretched hand. Type II fractures are less common. They occur in 10%–15% of patients and are more likely to be in adults (particularly osteoporotic adults) rather than in children. These fractures were further subclassified by Jupiter and colleagues to highlight the spectrum of injury within this subgroup. It is subdivided based on the location of the ulna fracture relative to the coronoid. Type IIA fractures involve the coronoid, Type IIB are distal to the coronoid, Type IIC represent a diaphyseal fracture, and Type IID include comminuted fractures extending from the proximal portion of the ulna, including the coronoid, to the proximal half of the ulna.[15] Type III fractures occur primarily in children and represent 7%–20% of Monteggia fractures.[8] Type IV are the least common (<5%) and the least well-understood Monteggia fractures. These injuries could be due to an injury to a pronated forearm.

Treatment Options

The treatment options for olecranon, proximal ulna, and Monteggia fractures range from nonoperative to open reduction and internal fixation. Nonoperative treatment consists of immobilization at 45–90 degrees of flexion for 3–4 weeks, at which point gentle ROM exercises can begin. Nonoperative treatment is reserved for nondisplaced fractures or low-demand, elderly patients. Nonoperative treatment, however, does not necessarily mean poor outcomes. A recent prospective study by Duckworth et al. found satisfactory short-term and long-term outcomes with the nonoperative management of isolated displaced olecranon fractures in older, lower demand patients.[16] In a subsequent prospective randomized trial of

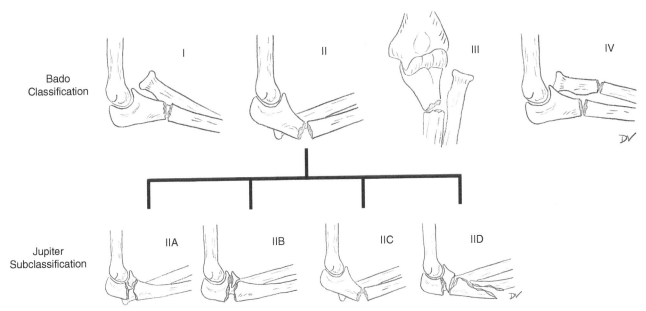

• **Fig. 51.3** Bado classification of Monteggia fractures with Jupiter subclassification of posterior Monteggia fractures.

TABLE 51.1	Bado Classification of Monteggia With Jupiter Subclassification of Type II Fractures	
	Description	Incidence
Type I	Anterior dislocation of radial head and apex anterior ulna fracture	55%–80%
Type II	Posterior dislocation of radial head and apex anterior ulna fracture	10%–15%
Type IIA	Type II with fracture involving the olecranon and coronoid processes	
Type IIB	Type II with fracture just distal to the trochlear notch	
Type IIC	Type II with fracture in the ulna diaphysis	
Type IID	Type II with comminuted fracture in multiple locations	
Type III	Lateral dislocation of radial head and apex anterior ulna fracture	7%–20%
Type IV	Involve diaphyseal fracture of radius	<5%

acute isolated displaced fractures of the olecranon in patients aged ≥75 years comparing nonoperative versus operative (primarily tension band wiring [TBW]), the same group found no difference in the Disabilities of the Arm, Shoulder and Hand (DASH) score and higher complications in patients being treated operatively at 1 year.[17]

Surgical Treatment

Most patients with displaced fractures will require operative fixation to maximize their functional outcomes and return to regular activities as soon as possible. Excision of the proximal olecranon fragment and advancement of the triceps tendon can be an effective technique in the treatment of nonunions, severely comminuted fractures, or in acute fractures in elderly, osteoporotic patients as long as >50% of the olecranon joint intact. This technique is particularly useful if the posterior elbow skin is at risk but the patient is not a candidate for operative fixation.

Fixation Options and Indications

For stable, noncomminuted fractures, intramedullary screw fixation or tension band construct provide appropriate stability. Fixation with intramedullary cancellous screws has also had good historical results[18] when properly placed along the intramedullary shaft axis. A smaller screw (3.5 mm) can be used with a washer to accommodate the bow of the proximal ulna. Alternatively, a larger screw (4.5–6.5 mm) can be used for more stability. Care should be taken that the fracture is not tipped or angulated as the larger screw engages the cortex distal to the ulnar bow. A tension band wire fixation converts the extensor force of the triceps to a dynamic compressive force across the articular surface.[19] Tension band wire and screw fixation is contraindicated if the fracture is unstable (comminuted or long oblique), involves the coronoid region, or is associated with any instability patterns.

The preferred treatment option for most displaced olecranon fractures is open reduction and plate fixation. More simple oblique fractures can be provisionally stabilized with a single lag screw with a posterior plate applied for neutralization and rotational stability. One-third tubular and reconstruction plates have historically been used; however they may not be strong enough for fracture-dislocations.[20] Precontoured locked olecranon plates have gained popularity due to ease of use and superior biomechanical strength.[21,22] Details of these fixation strategies will be described further in technique chapters (see Chapters 52–55).

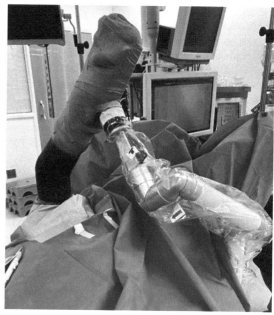

• **Fig. 51.4** Supine positioning using a surgical arm holder to position the arm in an adducted and partially extended position. Full or mini-fluoroscopy can be brought in from the contralateral side to facilitate imaging.

Surgical Approach

The patient may be positioned supine with the arm draped across the chest and supported with either a padded Mayo stand, arm holder, stack of sterile towels above the drapes, or nonsterile folded blankets on the chest underneath the drapes. The goal of positioning the arm this way is to allow the forearm to rest comfortably across the body with the elbow at approximately 90 degrees of flexion. This positioning typically requires one assistant to support the arm during the operation. However, if no assistant is available or if placing the arm on the chest is contraindicated (such as a polytrauma patient with a chest wound), a surgical arm holder (e.g., Trimano Fortis by Arthrex, Naples, FL or Spider by Smith & Nephew, Memphis, TN) can be used to hold the arm across the body above the chest (Fig. 51.4).

The more common method is the lateral decubitus position with their arm over a padded support with their forearm hanging down (Fig. 51.5). This does not require an assistant to hold the

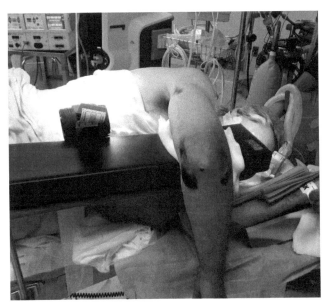

• **Fig. 51.5** Lateral decubitus positioning with arm over a padded radiolucent support.

arm and, if positioned correctly, allows the fluoroscopic machine to take orthogonal views without moving the arm. The ability of the fluoroscopic machine to obtain the appropriate views should be confirmed after the patient is positioned but prior to draping to ensure all adjustments are made prior to the initial incision. Traction radiographs are often obtained at this juncture. These may aid to fracture pattern extension and overall joint alignment. The lateral position is the senior author's preferred positioning. A nonsterile tourniquet is placed on the upper arm and the patient is draped in the standard fashion.

The posterior approach extends proximal to the triceps insertion and then longitudinally to the ulnar shaft. The incision is curved laterally around the tip of the olecranon to avoid a painful scar on pressure points on the medial aspect of the elbow or over the olecranon. Sharp dissection is carried through the subcutaneous tissue to the musculature fascia (Fig. 51.6). Care is taken to find the intramuscular raphe between the volar and dorsal compartments of the forearm and splitting the raphe with electrocautery down to the crest of the ulna (Fig. 51.7). Typically, this raphe is slightly dorsal to the ulnar shaft since the volar musculature typically wraps slightly dorsal around the ulna. On the medial (volar) side, the muscular origins of the flexor digitorum profundus, flexor digitorum superficialis, and the deep head of the pronator teres may be elevated. On the lateral (dorsal) side, the insertion of the anconeus may need to be elevated as well. In our experience, the ulnar nerve does not typically need to be exposed unless there is more extensive involvement of the medial column. If plate fixation requires a triceps split, a definitive and sharp split is made in the triceps insertion for the proximal aspect of the plate to lay flush on the proximal olecranon. This incision in the triceps insertion should go completely through the triceps tendon to allow for appropriate visualization and later repair. The olecranon fossa of the distal humerus should be palpable.

Once the fracture is visualized, it is debrided of any soft tissue or clot that could impede anatomic reduction of the fracture. If the fracture involves the articular surface, inspection of the joint should be made to identify marginal impaction. If there are impacted articular fragments, they should be reduced and elevated

to its anatomic location. K-wires can be placed in subchondral position within the fracture or from outside the fracture to support the articular fragments. The void behind it can be filled with a bone substitute that provides structural support such as impacted cancellous allograft chips. After the articular fragments are supported, the main fracture is reduced and typically maintained with provisional K-wire fixation. Clamps can also be placed along the medial or lateral columns because direct posterior placement often interferes with posterior plate application. Pilot holes may need to be drilled to allow the clamps to be stabilized in the distal segments.

Postoperative Management

Postoperative rehabilitation depends partly on the extent of the injury and the associated injured or repaired structures. For simple proximal ulna and olecranon fractures, gentle ROM exercises can be initiated approximately 1 week after surgery to allow for soft tissue rest and decrease in swelling. Strengthening and more aggressive ROM and weight-bearing activities can be initiated once evidence of radiographic union is seen. Some period of immobilization is often necessary for the soft tissue in more high-energy injuries. Immobilization should not exceed 3 weeks. Swelling reduction is an essential facet of the early rehabilitation process.

Relevant Complications

The most common complications seen after treatment of a proximal ulna fracture and fracture-dislocations are joint stiffness due to heterotopic ossification (HO) and capsular contracture, wound dehiscence with infection, elbow instability, and symptomatic hardware. Less common complications include malunion, nonunion, and nerve injury.

Joint Stiffness and Heterotopic Ossification

Loss of flexion or extension of the elbow after an elbow injury, including an olecranon fracture, is very common. The most common complication is lack of full extension with an average of 10–15 degrees in most patients compared to the contralateral limb[23–26] but has been reported to be up to 30 degrees or more.[12] Typically, joint stiffness that is not associated with a mechanical block to motion, such as HO, typically responds well to occupational therapy and dynamic or static progressive splints. If those nonoperative measures are unsuccessful, surgery can be performed to excise the scarred and contracted capsule.

HO can contribute to the joint stiffness found in patients with elbow trauma with an overall incidence of approximately 7%.[27] A delay in treatment is associated with a higher risk of HO. Isolated olecranon fractures are less likely to develop HO and, therefore, prophylaxis should be reserved for injuries with a high risk of HO, such as patients with head injuries or severe soft tissue damage. If symptomatic heterotopic bone develops, it can be removed after radiographic maturation, or once the patient is beyond the inflammatory phase of the injury and surgery.

Symptomatic Hardware

Symptomatic hardware can be the cause of significant pain and can ultimately lead to additional surgical procedures to remove hardware. Symptomatic hardware can be due to loosening hardware,

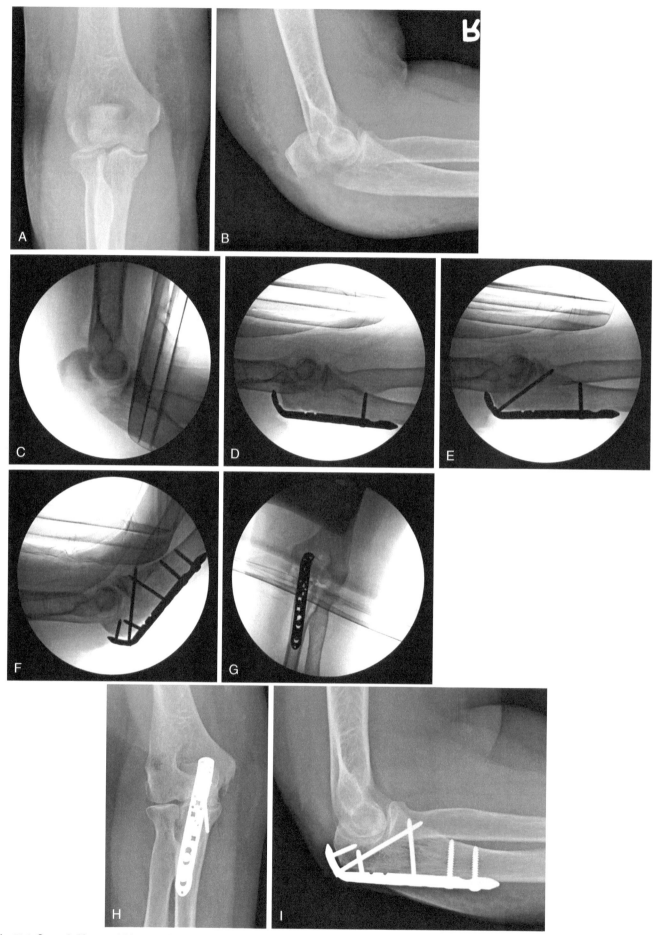

• **Fig. 51.6** Case: A 56-year-old female with an olecranon fracture (Mayo IIA) after a fall from standing. (A) Anteroposterior (AP) and (B) lateral images at the time of injury. Intraoperative fluoroscopy images demonstrating (C) displacement at the time of surgery, (D) placement of plate with shaft screw, (E) metaphyseal screw placement below articular surface compressing the fracture, (F) additional locking screws placed proximally and bicortical nonlocking screws placed distally along the shaft. (G) AP fluoroscopy demonstrating appropriate placement of plate and screws. (H and I) 3-month follow-up imaging demonstrating healed fracture and maintained alignment.

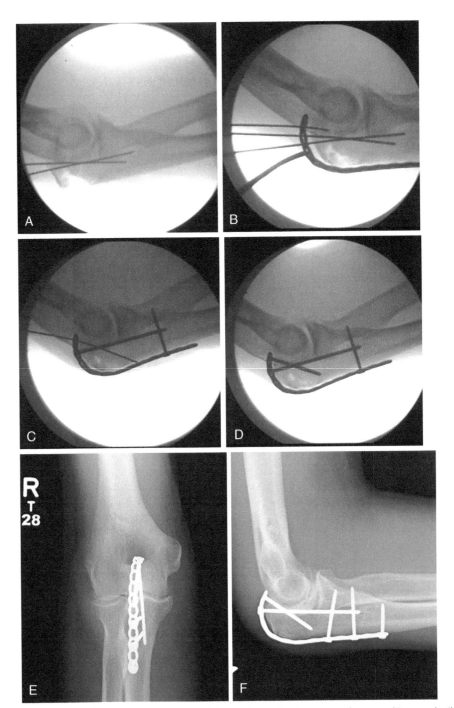

• **Fig. 51.7** Case: An 80-year-old man who sustained this proximal olecranon fracture with comminution (Mayo IIB) after a fall on his elbow. (A) The proximal fracture was reduced and held in position with K-wires. (B) The triceps was split and a locking compression plate was curved to provide maximal proximal fixation and placed on the proximal ulna. (C and D) The plate was held in place with a K-wire and a shaft screw was drilled eccentrically to provide compression across the joint. Locking screws were placed as proximal as possible to stabilize fracture and avoid hardware prominence. Not shown, heavy nonabsorbable suture was placed between the triceps and the olecranon proximally, crossed the construct posteriorly, and wrapped around a cortical screw underneath the plate to function as a tension band construct due to the very proximal nature of the fracture. (E and F) Final follow-up imaging demonstrating healed fracture and maintained alignment. At 4 months, patient reports he has returned to his baseline two sets of 100 push-ups in a row.

or placement of hardware in subcutaneous locations. The patient is likely to rest their arm such as the medial side or over the corner of the olecranon. In tension band fixation, the end of the twisted wires, a new break in the wire, or proximal migration of the K-wires can irritate local soft tissue and become painful requiring

removal.[28] Avoiding placing hardware at the bend of the olecranon plate may prevent irritation with certain plate designs.[23] Rates of hardware removal vary widely in the literature ranging from 0% to 49%[23,24,26,29] in plates but rates of removal are universally higher in tension band constructs.[12,30–33]

Wound Breakdown and Infection

Wound breakdown and subsequent infection typically occur in situations of compromised soft tissues associated with open fractures. However, due to the necessary subcutaneous placement of the implant around the proximal ulna, excessive pressure over prominent hardware can also cause wound breakdown in an olecranon fracture or fracture-dislocation.[28] Any potential wound complication should be treated urgently to avoid contamination of the metallic implants and hardware removal should be considered whenever hardware is exposed. Local skin flaps, such as a bipedicle flap,[34] can be used to cover hardware if the wound is not able to cover primarily.

Nonunions and Malunions

Nonunion after an olecranon fracture is rare and more likely to occur with fracture-dislocations or higher energy injuries. Nonunion can be treated with revision open reduction and internal fixation with autogenous bone graft, but may require olecranon fragment excision or joint replacement.[35–37]

Malunions are more likely to occur in segmental, multifragment articular, and comminuted fracture. Fracture subsidence results in articular incongruity or main fracture malalignment. Overcompression of a comminuted fracture at the joint can decrease the distance between the coronoid and the olecranon tip resulting in increased stress across the joint, decreased ROM, and early arthrosis. Extra-articular malreduction along the shaft or shortening of the ulna can result in instability of the elbow or radial head. Malunion should always be suspected in cases of radial head subluxation or instability postoperatively. Malunions can be treated with revision open reduction and internal fixation, but may require arthroplasty in cases where significant damage to the joint has already occurred. In cases where ulnar malreduction causes persistent radial head subluxation or dislocation, an ulnar osteotomy with revision fixation, along with open reduction of the radial head, should be performed.

Ulnar and Anterior Interosseous Nerve Injury

Direct injury to the ulnar nerve is uncommon in proximal ulna fractures and fracture-dislocations, but irritation to the nerve can occur in up to 12% of cases.[28,38–40] The ulnar nerve does not typically need to be identified and released during operative fixation unless the patient has definitive preoperative symptoms or the fracture pattern necessitates more medial column exposure. Ulnar neuritis postoperatively can occur due to swelling and irritation of the nerve, but can also be due to small fracture fragments or osteophyte formation postoperatively. Intraoperative and postoperative imaging can identify potential hardware of osseous causes of compression.[38] If there is no mechanical compression of the ulnar nerve, observation typically results in a return to baseline. Alternatively, postoperative patients who struggle with stiffness in flexion and have complaints of hypersensitivity or signs of ulnar neuropathy can benefit from ulnar nerve release postoperatively.

Injury to the anterior interosseous nerve (AIN) during tension wire fixation has been reported.[41] To avoid iatrogenic neurovascular injury during tension band wiring of the olecranon, the wire tips should not extend beyond the anterior ulnar cortex by more than 1 cm at a distance of 1.5 cm distal to the coronoid.[42] The AIN is also at risk during plate fixation as well, particularly during placement of the subchondral metaphyseal screws. Care should be taken when drilling and placing screws that exit distal to the coronoid.

Instability

Residual instability can occur after proximal ulna fractures or Monteggia fractures. Often, instability is due to inadequate reduction of the ulna fracture, typically in the form of persistent posterior angulation of the proximal ulna and posterior subluxation of the radial head. Inadequate identification or treatment such as injury to the radial head, coronoid, or lateral/medial collateral ligament fracture zones can also be a source of instability. Instability should be assessed intraoperatively and any associated injuries should be treated at the initial surgery. Postoperatively, persistent instability can be treated with secondary surgery, prolonged immobilization, or temporary hinged devices.

Treatment Outcomes

Proximal ulna fractures and fracture-dislocations typically result in good functional outcomes. In order to assess the functional outcomes of these fractures, two commonly used assessments are used: the Broberg and Morrey rating system[43] and the Disability of the Arm, Shoulder and Hand (DASH) Questionnaire.[44] Most studies of proximal ulna fractures treated with plate fixation have shown average DASH scores between 10 and 13.[23,26,29] Most olecranon and proximal ulna injuries result in some residual loss of elbow flexion and extension with preservation of forearm rotation except in fractures associated with a radial head injury.

Most recent investigations have centered on comparing types of fixation. Hume and Wiss[30] performed the first prospective and randomized trial comparing TBW to plate fixation using a one-third tubular plate for these displaced simple olecranon fractures. They found postoperative loss of reduction to be more common in TBW (53%) than after plate fixation (5%). There were better clinical and radiographic results with plate fixation, as compared with TBW. In a prospective randomized trial comparing TBW against plating for displaced proximal ulna fractures, Duckworth et al.[32] found equivalent functional outcomes scores between plating and TBW at 1 year. Patients with TBW had higher complication rates (63% vs. 38%, P = .042) primarily due to the increased rate of removal of metalwork in symptomatic patients (50% vs. 22%, P = .021). Loss of reduction was more common in TBW patients (27% vs. 13%). However, there were more infections in the plate group (n = 4, 13% in plate fixation vs. 0% in TBW) and four revision surgeries in the plating group for nonhardware irritation issues. A similar study by Powell et al.[33] comparing TBW with locking plate fixation found equivalent QuickDASH scores in both groups. However, 40% of the tension band wire patients had complications including a 33% chance of reoperations and a 27% chance of removal of metalwork for hardware irritation. There were no complications and had no reoperations in the 16 patients who received locking plate fixation. Radiographic signs of arthrosis in transolecranon fractures occur up to 30% of the time.[20,45,46]

While the Monteggia fracture-dislocation involves greater injury to the surrounding structures including the coronoid, radial head, coronoid, and collateral ligamentous complexes, most will have good outcomes when treated appropriately. In a long-term retrospective review, Konrad et al.[13] evaluated 47 patients at an average of 8.4 years and found a mean Broberg and Morrey score of 87.2 with 72% good or excellent results (>80) and a mean

DASH score of 17.4. A recent retrospective review on Monteggia-like lesions by Jungbluth et al.[47] evaluating a total of 46 patients at an average of 65 months found a mean Broberg and Morrey score of 86.6 with 83% good or excellent results. They also found a mean DASH score of 15. Bado II Monteggia fractures (posterior dislocations), Jupiter Type IIA fractures (fractures involving the coronoid), radial head fractures, coronoid fractures, and reoperations are associated with worse clinical outcomes.[13,47]

References

1. Sorbie C, Shiba R, Siu D, Saunders G, Wevers H. The development of a surface arthroplasty for the elbow. *Clin Orthop.* 1986;208:100–103.

2. Morrey BF. Current concepts in the treatment of fractures of the radial head, the olecranon, and the coronoid. *Instr Course Lect.* 1995;44:175–185.

3. Barco R, Sánchez P, Morrey ME, Morrey BF, Sánchez-Sotelo J. The distal triceps tendon insertional anatomy-implications for surgery. *JSES Open Access.* 2017;1(2):98–103. https://doi.org/10.1016/j.jses.2017.05.002.

4. Callaway GH, Field LD, Deng XH, et al. Biomechanical evaluation of the medial collateral ligament of the elbow. *J Bone Joint Surg Am.* 1997;79(8):1223–1231. https://doi.org/10.2106/00004623-199708000-00015.

5. Jackson TJ, Jarrell SE, Adamson GJ, Chung KC, Lee TQ. Biomechanical differences of the anterior and posterior bands of the ulnar collateral ligament of the elbow. *Knee Surg Sports Traumatol Arthrosc Off J ESSKA.* 2016;24(7):2319–2323. https://doi.org/10.1007/s00167-014-3482-7.

6. Morrey BF. Applied anatomy and biomechanics of the elbow joint. *Instr Course Lect.* 1986;35:59–68.

7. Monteggia GB. Lussazioni delle ossa delle estremita superiori. [Dislocations of the bones of the upper extremities.] In: 2nd ed. Monteggia GB, ed. *Instituzioni Chirurgiches [Surgical Institutions].* Vol. 5. Milan: Maspero; 1814:131–133. [In Italian].

8. Bado JL. The Monteggia lesion. *Clin Orthop.* 1967;50:71–86.

9. Ring D, Jupiter JB, Waters PM. Monteggia fractures in children and adults. *J Am Acad Orthop Surg.* 1998;6(4):215–224. https://doi.org/10.5435/00124635-199807000-00003.

10. Biga N, Thomine JM. [Trans-olecranal dislocations of the elbow]. *Rev Chir Orthop Reparatrice Appar Mot.* 1974;60(7):557–567.

11. McKay PL, Katarincic JA. Fractures of the proximal ulna olecranon and coronoid fractures. *Hand Clin.* 2002;18(1):43–53. https://doi.org/10.1016/s0749-0712(02)00013-6.

12. Rommens PM, Schneider RU, Reuter M. Functional results after operative treatment of olecranon fractures. *Acta Chir Belg.* 2004;104(2):191–197. https://doi.org/10.1080/00015458.2004.11679535.

13. Konrad GG, Kundel K, Kreuz PC, Oberst M, Sudkamp NP. Monteggia fractures in adults: long-term results and prognostic factors. *J Bone Joint Surg Br.* 2007;89(3):354–360. https://doi.org/10.1302/0301-620X.89B3.18199.

14. Tompkins DG. The anterior Monteggia fracture: observations on etiology and treatment. *J Bone Joint Surg Am.* 1971;53(6):1109–1114.

15. Jupiter JB, Leibovic SJ, Ribbans W, Wilk RM. The posterior Monteggia lesion. *J Orthop Trauma.* 1991;5(4):395–402. https://doi.org/10.1097/00005131-199112000-00003.

16. Duckworth AD, Bugler KE, Clement ND, Court-Brown CM, McQueen MM. Nonoperative management of displaced olecranon fractures in low-demand elderly patients. *J Bone Joint Surg Am.* 2014;96(1):67–72. https://doi.org/10.2106/JBJS.L.01137.

17. Duckworth AD, Clement ND, McEachan JE, White TO, Court-Brown CM, McQueen MM. Prospective randomised trial of non-operative versus operative management of olecranon fractures in the elderly. *Bone Jt J.* 2017;99-B(7):964–972. https://doi.org/10.1302/0301-620X.99B7.BJJ-2016-1112.R2.

18. Johnson RP, Roetker A, Schwab JP. Olecranon fractures treated with AO screw and tension bands. *Orthopedics.* 1986;9(1):66–68.

19. Müller ME, Allgöwer M, Schneider R, Willenegger H. *Manual of Internal Fixation: Techniques Recommended by the AO-ASIF Group.* 3rd ed. In: Allgöwer M, ed. Berlin, Heidelberg: Springer-Verlag; 1991: 978-3-662-02695-3.

20. Ring D, Jupiter JB, Sanders RW, Mast J, Simpson NS. Trans-olecranon fracture-dislocation of the elbow. *J Orthop Trauma.* 1997;11(8):545–550. https://doi.org/10.1097/00005131-199711000-00001.

21. Wilson J, Bajwa A, Kamath V, Rangan A. Biomechanical comparison of interfragmentary compression in transverse fractures of the olecranon. *J Bone Joint Surg Br.* 2011;93(2):245–250. https://doi.org/10.1302/0301-620X.93B2.24613.

22. Wegmann K, Engel K, Skouras E, et al. Reconstruction of Monteggia-like proximal ulna fractures using different fixation devices: a biomechanical study. *Injury.* 2016;47(8):1636–1641. https://doi.org/10.1016/j.injury.2016.05.010.

23. De Giacomo AF, Tornetta P, Sinicrope BJ, et al. Outcomes after plating of olecranon fractures: a multicenter evaluation. *Injury.* 2016;47(7):1466–1471. https://doi.org/10.1016/j.injury.2016.04.015.

24. Anderson ML, Larson AN, Merten SM, Steinmann SP. Congruent elbow plate fixation of olecranon fractures. *J Orthop Trauma.* 2007;21(6):386–393. https://doi.org/10.1097/BOT.0b013e3180ce831e.

25. Siebenlist S, Torsiglieri T, Kraus T, Burghardt RD, Stöckle U, Lucke M. Comminuted fractures of the proximal ulna—preliminary results with an anatomically preshaped locking compression plate (LCP) system. *Injury.* 2010;41(12):1306–1311. https://doi.org/10.1016/j.injury.2010.08.008.

26. Buijze G, Kloen P. Clinical evaluation of locking compression plate fixation for comminuted olecranon fractures. *J Bone Joint Surg Am.* 2009;91(10):2416–2420. https://doi.org/10.2106/JBJS.H.01419.

27. Bauer AS, Lawson BK, Bliss RL, Dyer GSM. Risk factors for post-traumatic heterotopic ossification of the elbow: case-control study. *J Hand Surg.* 2012;37(7):1422–1429. https://doi.org/10.1016/j.jhsa.2012.03.013. e1-6.

28. Macko D, Szabo RM. Complications of tension-band wiring of olecranon fractures. *J Bone Joint Surg Am.* 1985;67(9):1396–1401.

29. Bailey CS, MacDermid J, Patterson SD, King GJ. Outcome of plate fixation of olecranon fractures. *J Orthop Trauma.* 2001;15(8):542–548. https://doi.org/10.1097/00005131-200111000-00002.

30. Hume MC, Wiss DA. Olecranon fractures. A clinical and radiographic comparison of tension band wiring and plate fixation. *Clin Orthop.* 1992;(285):229–235.

31. Wolfgang G, Burke F, Bush D, et al. Surgical treatment of displaced olecranon fractures by tension band wiring technique. *Clin Orthop.* 1987;(224):192–204.

32. Duckworth AD, Clement ND, White TO, Court-Brown CM, McQueen MM. Plate versus tension-band wire fixation for olecranon fractures: a prospective randomized trial. *J Bone Joint Surg Am.* 2017;99(15):1261–1273. https://doi.org/10.2106/JBJS.16.00773.

33. Powell AJ, Farhan-Alanie OM, McGraw IWW. Tension band wiring versus locking plate fixation for simple, two-part Mayo 2A olecranon fractures: a comparison of post-operative outcomes, complications, reoperations and economics. *Musculoskelet Surg.* 2019;103(2):155–160. https://doi.org/10.1007/s12306-018-0556-6.

34. Chepla KJ, Shue S, Kafuman BR. Bipedicle flaps for posterior elbow reconstruction. *Tech Hand Up Extrem Surg.* 2017;21(4):161–163. https://doi.org/10.1097/BTH.0000000000000174.

35. Papagelopoulos PJ, Morrey BF. Treatment of nonunion of olecranon fractures. *J Bone Joint Surg Br.* 1994;76(4):627–635.

36. Ring D, Jupiter JB, Gulotta L. Atrophic nonunions of the proximal ulna. *Clin Orthop.* 2003;409:268–274. https://doi.org/10.1097/01.blo.0000052936.71325.eb.

37. Rotini R, Antonioli D, Marinelli A, Katušić D. Surgical treatment of proximal ulna nonunion. *Chir Organi Mov.* 2008;91(2):65–70. https://doi.org/10.1007/s12306-007-0011-6.

38. Ishigaki N, Uchiyama S, Nakagawa H, Kamimura M, Miyasaka T. Ulnar nerve palsy at the elbow after surgical treatment for fractures of the olecranon. *J Shoulder Elbow Surg.* 2004;13(1):60–65. https://doi.org/10.1016/s1058-2746(03)00220-9.

39. Shin R, Ring D. The ulnar nerve in elbow trauma. *JBJS.* 2007;89(5):1108–1116. https://doi.org/10.2106/JBJS.F.00594.

40. Claessen FMAP, Braun Y, Peters RM, Dyer G, Doornberg JN, Ring D. Factors associated with reoperation after fixation of displaced olecranon fractures. *Clin Orthop.* 2016;474(1):193–200. https://doi.org/10.1007/s11999-015-4488-2.

41. Parker JR, Conroy J, Campbell DA. Anterior interosseus nerve injury following tension band wiring of the olecranon. *Injury.* 2005;36(10):1252–1253. https://doi.org/10.1016/j.injury.2004.12.028.

42. Prayson MJ, Iossi MF, Buchalter D, Vogt M, Towers J. Safe zone for anterior cortical perforation of the ulna during tension-band wire fixation: a magnetic resonance imaging analysis. *J Shoulder Elbow Surg.* 2008;17(1):121–125. https://doi.org/10.1016/j.jse.2007.04.010.

43. Broberg MA, Morrey BF. Results of delayed excision of the radial head after fracture. *JBJS.* 1986;68(5):669–674.

44. Jester A, Harth A, Germann G. Measuring levels of upper-extremity disability in employed adults using the DASH Questionnaire. *J Hand Surg.* 2005;30(5):1074.e1–1074.e10. https://doi.org/10.1016/j.jhsa.2005.04.009.

45. Mouhsine E, Akiki A, Castagna A, et al. Transolecranon anterior fracture dislocation. *J Shoulder Elbow Surg.* 2007;16(3):352–357. https://doi.org/10.1016/j.jse.2006.07.005.

46. Mortazavi SMJ, Asadollahi S, Tahririan MA. Functional outcome following treatment of transolecranon fracture-dislocation of the elbow. *Injury.* 2006;37(3):284–288. https://doi.org/10.1016/j.injury.2005.10.028.

47. Jungbluth P, Tanner S, Schneppendahl J, et al. The challenge of Monteggia-like lesions of the elbow. *Bone Jt J.* 2018;100-B(2):212–218. https://doi.org/10.1302/0301-620X.100B2.BJJ-2017-0398.R2.

52

Technique Spotlight: Parallel Plating of Olecranon Fractures

WILLIAM B. GEISSLER

Fractures of the proximal ulna may severely compromise function of the elbow both in flexion/extension and forearm rotation (Figs. 52.1 and 52.2). The anatomy of the olecranon is quite complex. The junction of the olecranon process with the metaphysis of the proximal ulna is a nonarticulate area with less subchondral bone. This area is relatively narrow in the sagittal plane and increases the risk of fracture. The trochlear notch of the ulna has a circumference of nearly 180 degrees, making this an inherently constrained joint. The articular surface of the trochlear notch has a separate coronoid and olecranon areas, separated by a small nonarticulate transverse groove previously mentioned. The coronoid process has the anteromedial facet, which is a critical stabilizer of the elbow in varus stress. In addition, it is composed of the lesser sigmoid notch region, the tip and the base.

Indications

The Mayo classification of olecranon fractures is frequently used to describe the fracture pattern. It is based on three factors that have a direct influence on operative management, that being fracture displacement, comminution, and elbow instability. Type 1 fractures are nondisplaced or minimally displaced and can be either minimally comminuted (Type 1A) or comminuted (Type 1B). These fractures being nondisplaced are frequently treated nonoperatively. Type 2 fractures have displacement of the proximal fragment without elbow instability. These fractures will require operative fixation. Type 2A fractures are without comminution and can usually be treated with tension band or intramedullary screw fixation. Type 2B fractures are comminuted and traditionally have been treated with plate fixation. Type 3 fractures present with elbow instability. Type 3A fractures are noncomminuted, and Type 3B are comminuted. Traditionally, these fractures are treated with plate fixation. Tension band wiring has typically been reserved for relatively simple fractures at the level of the transverse groove of the trochlear notch without any associated ligamentous injuries or fractures of the coronoid or radial head. These would involve <50% of the articular surface. If the fracture is more comminuted or more distal, tension band techniques will generally fail. Plate and screw fixation is recommended for fractures involving >50%

articular surface and for all Type 3 fractures. Traditionally, when plate fixation has been recommended, the plate is placed straight dorsal. The problem with the elbow is that it is quite subcutaneous with minimal muscle coverage. Both tension band fixation and dorsal plates frequently are systematic and require removal (Fig. 52.3). Also in more frail patients with thin skin, the concern with a dorsal plate is soft tissue breakdown and the plate penetrating through the skin (Fig. 52.1).

Recently, parallel plating of olecranon fractures has been introduced (Fig. 52.4). Parallel plating has several advantages compared with the previously described techniques. By placing the plates on the radial and ulnar side of the olecranon, rather than straight dorsal, there is significantly decreased hardware irritation with the chance of skin breakdown and hardware removal. In addition, if the olecranon fracture is quite comminuted with a small proximal fragment, parallel plating potentially allows for increased screw placement in the small proximal fragment compared with traditional posterior plating (Fig. 52.5). Lastly, parallel plating can make the reduction of the fracture much easier (Fig. 52.6). A bone tenaculum can be placed through a drill hole on the distal olecranon and used to help compress and provisionally reduce the proximal olecranon fragments. The parallel plates can then be placed both on the radial and ulnar side of the olecranon while the provisional fixation is held by the bone tenaculum compressing the fracture.

Positioning and Equipment

The patient is placed in the lateral decubitus position. The nonoperative upper extremity and lower extremities are well padded with foam and pillows. A triangle foam support braces the operative extremity in slight flexion for the posterior approach.

Surgical Technique

A curved incision is made radial to the tip of the olecranon to preserve sensation to the back of the elbow. Sharp dissection is carried down to the level of the fascia where thick skin flaps are elevated. In most instances it is not necessary to dissect out the ulnar nerve.

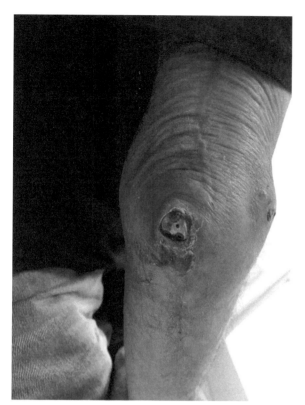

• **Fig. 52.1** Photograph of a posterior olecranon plate with soft tissue breakdown exposing the plate.

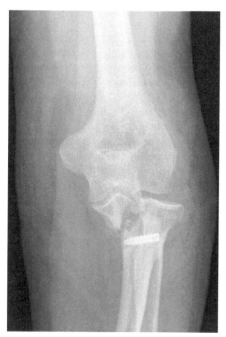

• **Fig. 52.2** Anteroposterior radiograph of a transverse olecranon fracture. The patient had a previous ulnar collateral ligament reconstruction with a screw which acted as a stress riser.

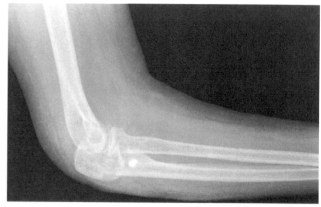

• **Fig. 52.3** Lateral radiograph showing the proximal olecranon fracture.

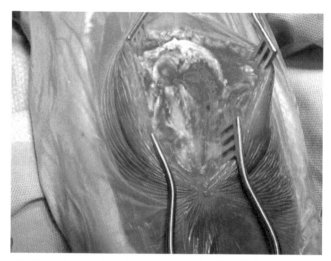

• **Fig. 52.4** Intraoperative photograph showing the displaced transverse fracture of the olecranon.

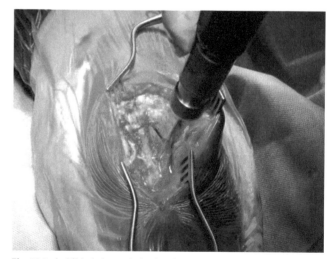

• **Fig. 52.5** A drill hole is made in the distal olecranon starting perpendicularly then angling at approximately 45-degrees for the bone tenaculum.

The interval between the flexor carpi ulnaris and extensor carpi ulnaris is subperiosteally elevated, exposing the fracture to the olecranon (Figs. 52.2–52.4). A drill hole is made at a 45-degree angle in the distal portion of the olecranon for the bone tenaculum (Fig. 52.5). The fracture is anatomically reduced and provisionally stabilized with bone tenaculum straight posteriorly (Fig. 52.6).

This technique provides excellent stability and reduction to the fracture while the two are being applied compared to a dorsal plate, in which case the bone tenaculum would prevent placement of the plate. Fixation utilized for this technique involves radial- and ulnar-sided plates. These plates are typically 2.7–3.5 mm in size and stock. Straight plates can be contoured to the patient's

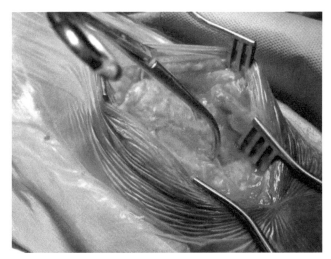

• **Fig. 52.6** A bone tenaculum provides excellent provisional stability in compression to the olecranon fracture.

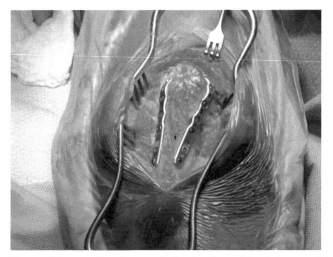

• **Fig. 52.7** Intraoperative photograph showing the radial and ulnar parallel plates stabilizing the fracture.

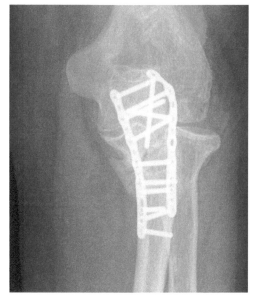

• **Fig. 52.8** Anteroposterior radiograph demonstrating the parallel plates in fixation of the olecranon fracture.

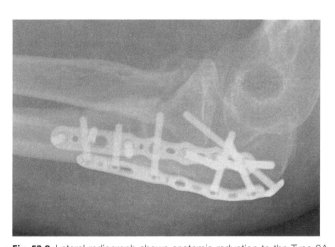

• **Fig. 52.9** Lateral radiograph shows anatomic reduction to the Type 2A olecranon fracture.

anatomy intraoperatively. Several manufacturers provide plating systems that will accommodate cortical and locking screws for this application. Alternatively, the author prefers the Medartis (Basel, Switzerland) parallel olecranon plate system, which is composed of short and long radial and ulnar plates, and short and long straight plates. These can be used in whatever combination necessary to achieve stability to the fracture. In less comminuted Type 2 fractures, usually the short radial and ulnar plates will be utilized. With both the radial and ulnar plates applied, the first screw is placed in a nonlocking screw hole to compress the plate down to bone. The screws in the oblong holes are placed first and are nonlocking. These screws are inserted just until they touch the plate but, are not tightened at this time. This allows the plate to slide for positioning or compression during the placement of the "home run" screws. The home run screws are placed second and are also nonlocking. The home run screw is the most proximal screw on the plate. The screw hole position and a standard nonlocking screw allows for compression of the soft tissues and the fracture or osteotomy site. The remaining round holes are locking.

After compression by the home run screw the screws in the oblong holes are tightened and the remaining locking screws are placed. Both the medial and lateral plates are applied simultaneously on the ulna. Alternating tightening of the home run screw allows for uniform compression of the osteotomy or fracture (Figs. 52.7–52.9).

Suture augmentation can be used for small fractures of the olecranon (less than 1cm). A 1.5-mm labral tape or #2 nonabsorbable suture can be placed 2-3 cm proximal to the fracture. A Bunnell weave is used, and the ends are brought out just proximal to the tip of the olecranon. The fracture is reduced, and the plate is applied. The suture or tape is passed through the most proximal small oblong holes. The clamp is compressed, and the screws are tightened. The sutures are then tied, and the remainder of the screws are inserted. This augments the fixation and stability of the construct when screw fixation alone may be insufficient.

- In more comminuted Type 3 fractures, traditionally the longer radial plates are placed or they overlap with a straight plate. In this manner, the plates are offset distally to help decrease the chance of a stress riser (Figs. 52.10–52.13).

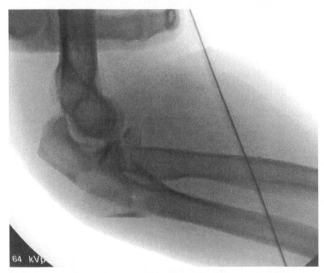

• **Fig. 52.10** Lateral radiograph of the Type 3B olecranon fracture.

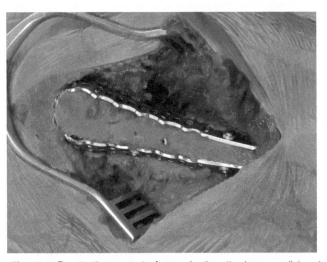

• **Fig. 52.11** Due to the amount of comminution, the longer radial and ulnar olecranon plates were placed to bridge across the comminution.

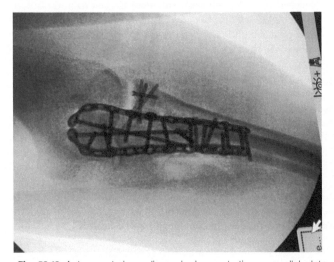

• **Fig. 52.12** Anteroposterior radiograph demonstrating a parallel plate fixation.

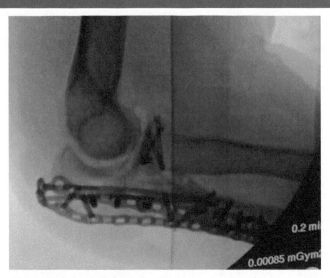

• **Fig. 52.13** Lateral radiograph with longer parallel olecranon plates shows anatomic reduction to the comminuted Type 3B olecranon fracture. Once the fracture was reduced, this restored stability back to the elbow.

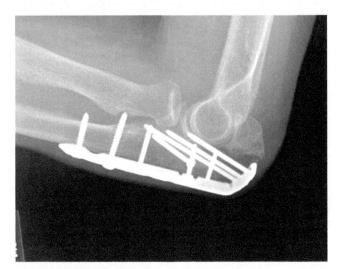

• **Fig. 52.14** Lateral radiograph of previously applied posterior plate with displacement of the proximal olecranon fragment.

- Parallel plate fixation is ideal for small proximal olecranon fractures compared with standard posterior plate fixation.
- Technical pearl: We will often use two tenaculums to hold provisional fixation of the fracture or osteotomy. The 2.8mm drill is used to make a bicortical hole that is 1-2 cm distal to the anticipated ends of the olecranon double plates. One end of the tenaculums is placed in this hole and the other is placed through the most proximal holes of the plates. Drill holes are placed distally in the oblong holes and the screws are inserted until they just touch the plate. One clamp is left on and the other hole for the home run screw is drilled and placed until it just touches the plate. The remaining tenaculums is removed and the second home run screw is inserted. These screws are then alternately tightened.
- Dual plate fixation allows for a greater number of proximal screws to stabilize the fragment compared with posterior plates (Figs. 52.14–18).

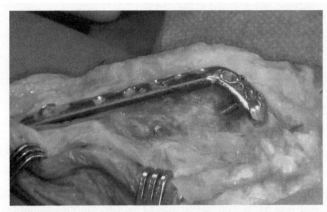

• **Fig. 52.15** Intraoperative photograph showing the previously applied posterior plate with displacement of the proximal fragment.

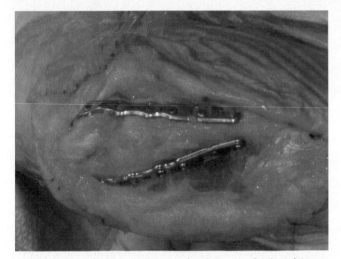

• **Fig. 52.16** Intraoperative photograph showing an application of the parallel olecranon plates to the small proximal fragment. The use of parallel plates allowed multiple screw fixation into the small olecranon fragment, compared with a straight posterior plate.

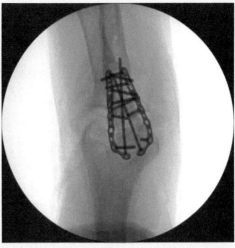

• **Fig. 52.17** Anteroposterior radiograph shows anatomic reduction from revision of a previous applied posterior plate.

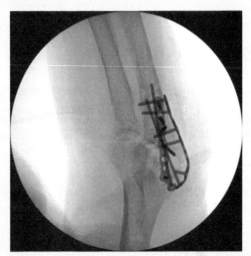

• **Fig. 52.18** Lateral radiograph shows anatomic reduction to the small proximal olecranon fragment.

• Parallel fixation potentially is easier technically for the surgeon by allowing a bone tenaculum placed straight posteriorly to provisionally hold the fracture reduced and compressed while the parallel plates are applied.

53

Technique Spotlight: ORIF with Intramedullary Screw Fixation

ANDY EGLSEDER JR. AND DAVID POTTER

Olecranon fractures have historically been treated with tension band wires and recently plates. Plate and tension band hardware have been associated with soft tissue irritation from hardware prominence and migration due to improper seating at the time of surgery. Another treatment option is intramedullary (IM) screws. The goals of proximal ulna fracture fixation are joint reduction, rigid fixation, and early range of motion. IM screw fixation for proximal ulna or olecranon fractures provides rigid fixation, excellent compression, and minimal soft tissue irritation. The IM screw provides excellent compression perpendicular to the typical fracture lines of the proximal ulna. It also has a long working length that increases stability and allows for early range of motion. Additionally, the cost of an IM screw is 20 times lower than that of a proximal ulnar plate system.

Indications

Operative indications for fixation with an IM screw are based on the proximal fragment size. If the fragment size is large enough to accept a 6.5- or 7.3-mm partially threaded screw, the fixation can be performed. Comminution is not a contraindication for IM screw usage. Augmenting the IM screw fixation with miniplates using both bicortical and unicortical locking screws allows for fracture-specific fixation around the IM screw in setting of comminution. Fractures occurring at the coronoid flair can still be treated with the IM screw as long as there is enough cortical contact of the proximal and distal fragments to provide length stability. Proximal shaft screws are also feasible as the length of fixation and compressive effect by the IM screw is limited by the screw length and purchase distal to the shaft fracture.

Contraindications for surgical management by the IM screw involve any fractures in which there is a coronal or sagittal split in the proximal fragment. Further, small-comminuted subchondral bone fragments with articular cartilage attached will not be secured by the IM screw and would be an indication for fragment-specific minifragment plate fixation or rafting K-wires to augment the length stabilizing effect of the IM screw.

Preoperative Evaluation

Initial physical examination typically demonstrates a significant soft tissue swelling and pain, mostly localized posteriorly over the olecranon. A palpable defect is often encountered where the olecranon fracture has occurred. The patient may have loss of active elbow extension depending on the location and displacement of fracture relative to the triceps insertion. Range-of-motion examination of the elbow joint is often not well tolerated.

Standard anteroposterior (AP) and lateral X-rays of the elbow are typical for primary assessment. Computed tomography (CT) is typically not indicated in isolated olecranon process fractures; however, it may be helpful if there is a concern for fracture extension into the coronoid or concomitant humeral articular injury.

Positioning and Equipment

Patient can be positioned supine. The patient's arm is at their side on a bump during exposure, allowing for direct joint visualization at the time of reduction (Fig. 53.1). An abducted arm on an arm board may provide easier visualization while incorporating intraoperative fluoroscopy (Fig. 53.2). Once reduction is achieved and provisional fixation is applied, it is easier to drill and place the IM screw with the arm laid over the chest/abdomen on a bump (Fig. 53.3). An alternative positioning option in the setting of multiple injuries is to position the patient laterally. The arm is extended out over a Mayo stand or similar arm holder. In the supine position, the patient's body should be positioned so the medial edge of the scapular body is hanging over the edge of the operating room table. This allows for maximum motion/movement for intraoperative fluoroscopy. If lateral, ensure the positioning of the supportive device is placed where maximum flexion and extension can be completed. Surgical skin preparation and drapes should include the entire arm to the axilla. A sterile tourniquet can be applied if needed. The pneumatic tourniquet can limit the triceps distal excursion and hamper reduction. See Table 53.1 for associated equipment and material.

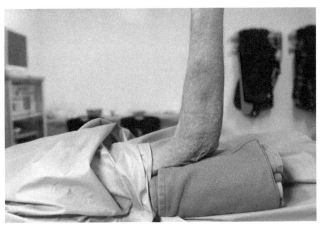

• **Fig. 53.1** Patient is supine with a small bump at the patient's side to allow for joint visualization during exposure and reduction.

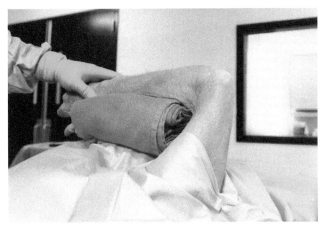

• **Fig. 53.3** Patient is supine with a bump on the abdomen. This position is helpful for drilling and screw placement after reduction has been performed.

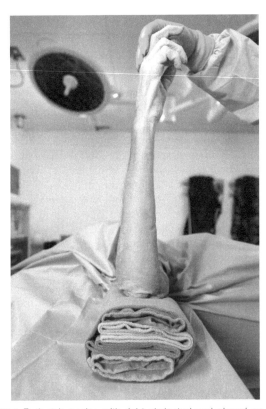

• **Fig. 53.2** Patient is supine with right abducted and placed on a small radiolucent arm board.

TABLE 53.1	**Procedural Equipment and Material**
Positioning	Regular operating room table with towel bump and radiolucent arm board. Alternatively, if positioned laterally, a Mayo stand or elbow arm holder.
Fracture reduction	Medium serrated reduction forceps that function as "goal post" Two large pointed reduction clamps.
Fracture fixation	3.2-mm solid drill bit 4.5-mm solid drill bit 6.5-mm calibrated tap 2.0-mm minifragment plating system and/or 24- or 26-gauge dental wire if needing augmented fixation 6.5-mm partially threaded, 32-mm length thread solid core screw 7.3-mm partially threaded, 32-mm length thread screw (will need a 7.3 tap if upsizing diameter of screw)
Imaging	Fluoroscope

Detailed Technique Description

A posterolateral approach is used to address the proximal ulnar fracture (Fig. 53.4). The ulna is a subcutaneous bone and palpation of landmarks is easily identified. Mark out the shaft distally. Your incision should cheat just lateral, off the boney edge of the ulnar shaft to avoid placement of the scar directly over the subcutaneous border of the ulna. Proximally, the incision should extend approximately 3–5 cm; this allows for soft tissue excursion and proper exposure for accessing the IM canal. Carry the incision down sharply to the fascial tissue covering the anconeus and triceps. Unless concerned, you do not need to dissect down medially to look for the ulnar nerve.

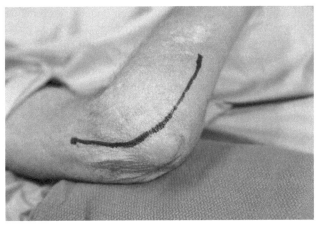

• **Fig. 53.4** Posterolateral incision is made on the right elbow.

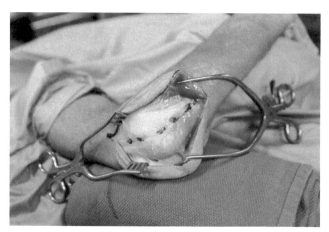

• **Fig. 53.5** Fascial incision along interval of the anconeus and soft tissue lateral border of the ulna.

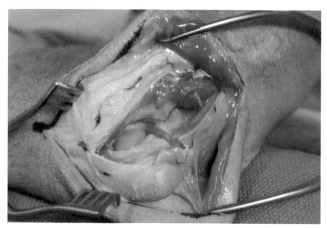

• **Fig. 53.6** Posterolateral exposure to the joint allows you to visualize the fracture lines and joint surface, and provide exposure for synovectomy and fixation.

Once the anconeus is identified, incise along the edge of the ulnar shaft (Fig. 53.5). If the quality of the soft tissue allows, you may be able to create a fascial cuff to repair at the time of closure. Often, the tissue is too thin or traumatized to have any integrity to hold a suture. Sharply elevate the proximal attachment of muscle off the bone and carry this down to the anterior edge of the ulna. A posterolateral capsulotomy and synovectomy is performed in order to directly visualize the joint. Care should be taken during joint exposure to protect and preserve the annular ligament. Full-thickness elevation of the joint capsule allows the identification of the intra-articular extension of the fracture and allows for direct visualization for reduction at the articular surface (Fig. 53.6). Distally, approximately 4–5 cm from the fracture, elevate down the medial and lateral sides of the ulna with a freer or small periosteal elevator. This will allow for the placement of a clamp to counteract the torque applied with performing fixation.

Tease out any intra-articular fragments that may have migrated anterior or posteriorly. Extending the elbow will provide joint soft tissue laxity to allow for easy irrigation and fragment removal. Once the fracture has been debrided and the pattern discovered, proceed with direct reduction. Initial reduction is easier to achieve with the arm fully extended. If the proximal fragment will not migrate distally, consider releasing the tourniquet if insufflated. Additionally, relaxing the lateral soft tissue by supinating in extended position can also help in this aspect. Utilization of a dental pic and large point-to-point reduction clamps will assist in mobilizing and performing reduction with provisional fixation. Fracture-specific fixation of small-comminuted fragments and subchondral bone with articular cartilage should be performed during provisional fixation. A variation of miniplate fixation and 24- or 26-gauge wire can capture and hold fragments in anatomic position (Fig. 53.7A–D). The placement of these implants should be on the lateral edge of the ulna, deep to the soft tissue of the anconeus, thus reducing prominence.

Direct visualization of joint reduction is achieved through the anconeus-triceps interval and allows for palpation of the articular surface with a blunt probe. Once clamped, the fixation should be sufficient to withstand the forces of semiflexed elbow to allow for easier technique of fixation (Fig. 53.8). After the reduction and provisional fixation is achieved, find the center-center of the posterior aspect of the proximal olecranon fragment. Identify the medial and lateral borders of the olecranon with direct palpation. The proximal tip of the olecranon should be easily palpated

through the tendinous insertion of the triceps fibers. The subcutaneous border of the ulna provides the last point of defining reference. Once the center-center starting point is located, look along the lateral border through the anconeus interval and ensure the trajectory would be extra-articular. Using electrocautery or knife, make a 3- to 4-cm longitudinal incision at the location of the starting point. Undermine and elevate triceps fibers medial and laterally to allow for the washer to subside under the soft tissue and rest directly on the bone (Fig. 53.9). Prior to drilling, confirm the reduction is maintained. Use a soft tissue guide to protect the triceps fibers and assist with maintaining an accurate trajectory. Begin drilling with a long 3.2-mm drill. The drill's trajectory should split the "goalpost" of the bone clamp applied to the ulnar shaft that is used to prevent torque. Pass the drill at full speed, typically to a depth of 150–180 mm (Fig. 53.10A–B). Be sure to reduce torque by applying counterforce to the direction of rotation to prevent displacement of provisional fixation. A key is to not force the 3.2-mm drill bit. If it is not a smooth pass and without resistance, stop drilling and remove the drill bit. Forcing the drill can cause a perforation or a "shoulder" within the IM canal by partially drilling the inner cortical wall. In order to prevent fracture or penetration when having difficulty passing the 3.2-mm bit, proceed to the next step with the 4.5-mm drill bit. Use a 4.5-mm drill bit to drill a "glide hole" in the proximal fragment only. Do not cross the fracture line with the 4.5-mm drill bit. Next, use the calibrated 6.5-mm tap to "sound" and find the natural progression of the canal. If you maintain the soft tissue guide in place when changing drill bits, you will see it is easier to find the starting hole and prior trajectory.

A calibrated 6.5-mm tap is used to find the appropriate length of screw (Fig. 53.11). It is important to provide counter-torque to the proximal fragment through the reduction clamps and distally through the "goalpost" clamp when passing the screw tap as it imparts large amounts of torque. The tap should encounter significant endosteal contact as demonstrated by torquing of the distal shaft and likely a cracking sensation or disconcerting creak. This typically is around 120 mm. Do not stop. Continue the tap past this finding until there is excellent purchase with the tap, thus indicating the anticipated screw's significant IM endosteal purchase. Once satisfied with the purchase, measure the length of the screw. It is recommended to subtract 5–10 mm to ensure there is a portion of intramedullary bone that has been tapped and will provide endosteal contact to allow for compression.

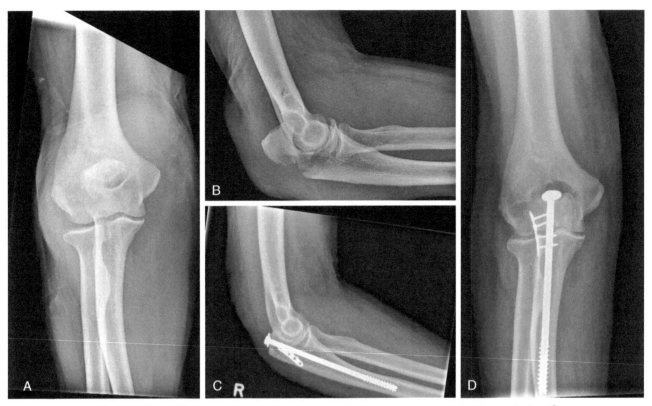

• **Fig. 53.7** (A) and (B) demonstrate a displaced olecranon fracture with lateral cortical wall comminution. (C) and (D) demonstrate minifragment plate augmentation to the intramedullary screw. The plate is placed to aid in joint support and reduction. It is placed deep within the elevated anconeus interval to avoid prominence.

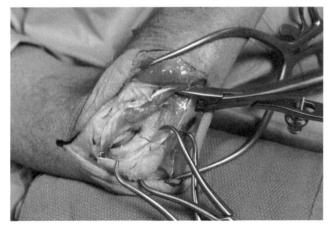

• **Fig. 53.8** Direct visualization is best performed with arm at the side of the patient's body on a bump. Provisional fixation with two point-to-point reduction clamps adequately will hold reduction. It helps to cross the clamp's points to avoid blocking the starting point and give equal compression.

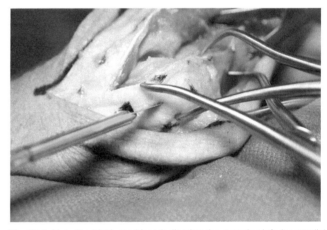

• **Fig. 53.9** Note the black markings indicating the superior, inferior, medial, and lateral borders of the proximal ulnar olecranon fragment. The knife blade is marking the "center-center" starting point.

The 6.5-mm solid core screw should be used with 32-mm threads. Placing the screw with power and finishing with hand allows for better control and ability to apply counterforce with the "goalpost" clamp on the distal shaft. The screw will naturally conform and bend to follow the IM canal and provide three points of fixation with the screw threads, the varus bend of the ulna, and the screw head. As the screw head approaches the soft tissue, use a blunt tip tissue elevator to mobilize the soft tissue around the washer and screw head (Fig. 53.12A–B). When seating the screw, your screw purchase should improve. The washer will tilt to match

the inherent angle built into the posterior cortex of the olecranon. Intraoperative fluoroscopy will demonstrate this tilt and indicates the washer is fully seated without soft tissue entrapment. It should be a significant bite that provides reassuring compression and have an assertive endpoint.

If you did not achieve significant fixation with appreciable compression, consider either exchanging for a longer screw or increasing the diameter to a 7.3-mm partially threaded screw. You should utilize a tap for a 7.3-mm screw prior to upsizing the screw. Reexamine the joint to ensure congruence with this final fixation complete (Fig. 53.13). Remove the provisional clamps and irrigate

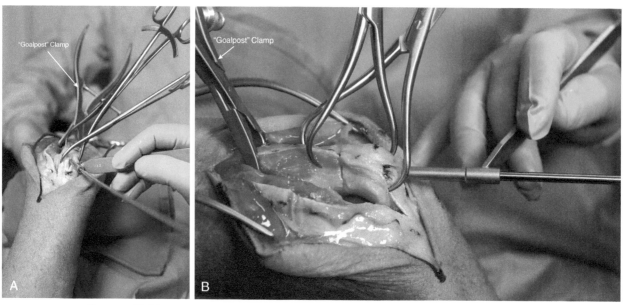

• **Fig. 53.10** (A) When drilling with a 3.2-mm bit, the trajectory should be through the "goalpost" clamp distally. (B) On the lateral view, the drill bit trajectory is confirmed to be extra-articular.

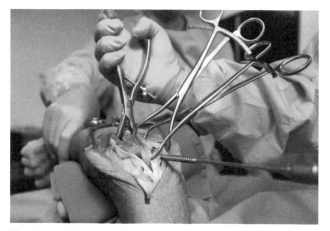

• **Fig. 53.11** A 6.5-mm tap is used to find the appropriate screw length. Note the surgeon's right hand is applying counter-torque to the tap by holding the "goalpost" clamp.

the joint again. Test range of motion to ensure appropriate alignment. The patient's elbow should tolerate near-normal range of motion with gentle passive motion to test for congruence and ease of tracking. Once satisfied, proceed with closure. Soft tissue repair of the joint capsule to the remaining cuff will allow for near anatomic soft tissue approximation and closure. The cuff of the anconeus is typically not robust enough to hold a suture. The most reliable closure is reapproximating the extensor carpi ulnaris/anconeus soft tissue sleeve to the flexor carpi ulnaris. Suture the triceps split to cover the screw head and washer (Fig. 53.14). Final X-rays are obtained with a true lateral of the elbow and fully extended AP of the elbow (Fig. 53.15).

Postoperatively, the patient should be splinted in a semiextended position, just shy of 90 degrees. The patient remains immobilized for soft tissue rest and healing for 2 weeks and then begins active-assisted range of motion. If the patient has no significant soft tissue trauma or concerns and achieved excellent fixation, one can forego the splint and start range of motion at 3–5 days postoperatively. Six weeks postoperatively, the patient may begin using for activities of daily living with a 1-pound weight limit. Around the 10- to 12-week postoperative mark and based on radiographic confirmation of healing, the patient may progress to weight-bearing and activity.

PEARLS AND PITFALLS

- Utilize minifragment fixation and small gauge wire to capture and hold fragments in anatomic position.
- Place a clamp on the ulna distal to fracture to serve as "goalposts" when preparing for IM fixation. This clamp is also used to counteract torque forces when applying screw.
- 3.2-mm drill should advance smoothly. Stop when meeting resistance to avoid a false passage and risk of fracture.
- A 6.5-mm tap should impart a large amount of torque. This typically is encountered around 120 mm. Continue to advance until excellent purchase and subtract 5–10 mm from tap length for screw selection.
- Screw should have significant purchase with an assertive endpoint.
- If you did not achieve significant compression, consider exchanging for longer screw or increasing to larger diameter screw.

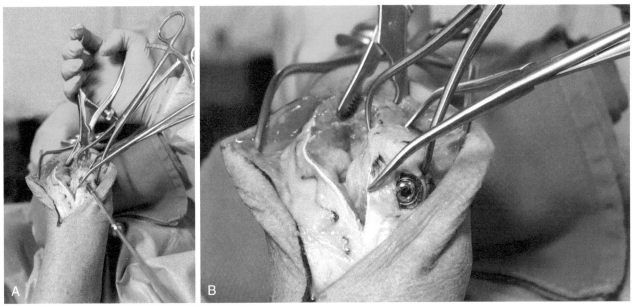

• **Fig. 53.12** (A) Screw is placed on power and finished by hand. Remember to apply counter-torque when applying intramedullary screw with the "goalpost" clamp. (B) Ensure the triceps split is elevated so soft tissue sits over the washer and screw head. This helps minimize prominence and allows for full compression without soft tissue entrapment.

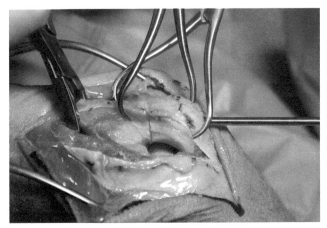

• **Fig. 53.13** Note the maintenance of reduction and congruence achieved after compressive fixation with the intramedullary screw.

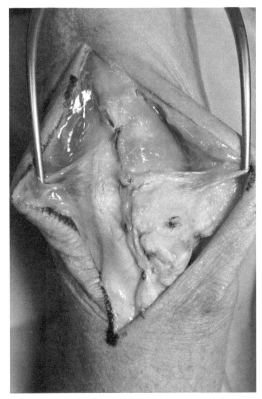

• **Fig. 53.14** The extensor carpi ulnaris/anconeus tissue sleeve may be reapproximated to the flexor carpi ulnaris with absorbable suture. It is possible there will not be a soft tissue cuff to repair. The triceps split is closed with absorbable suture over the screw head.

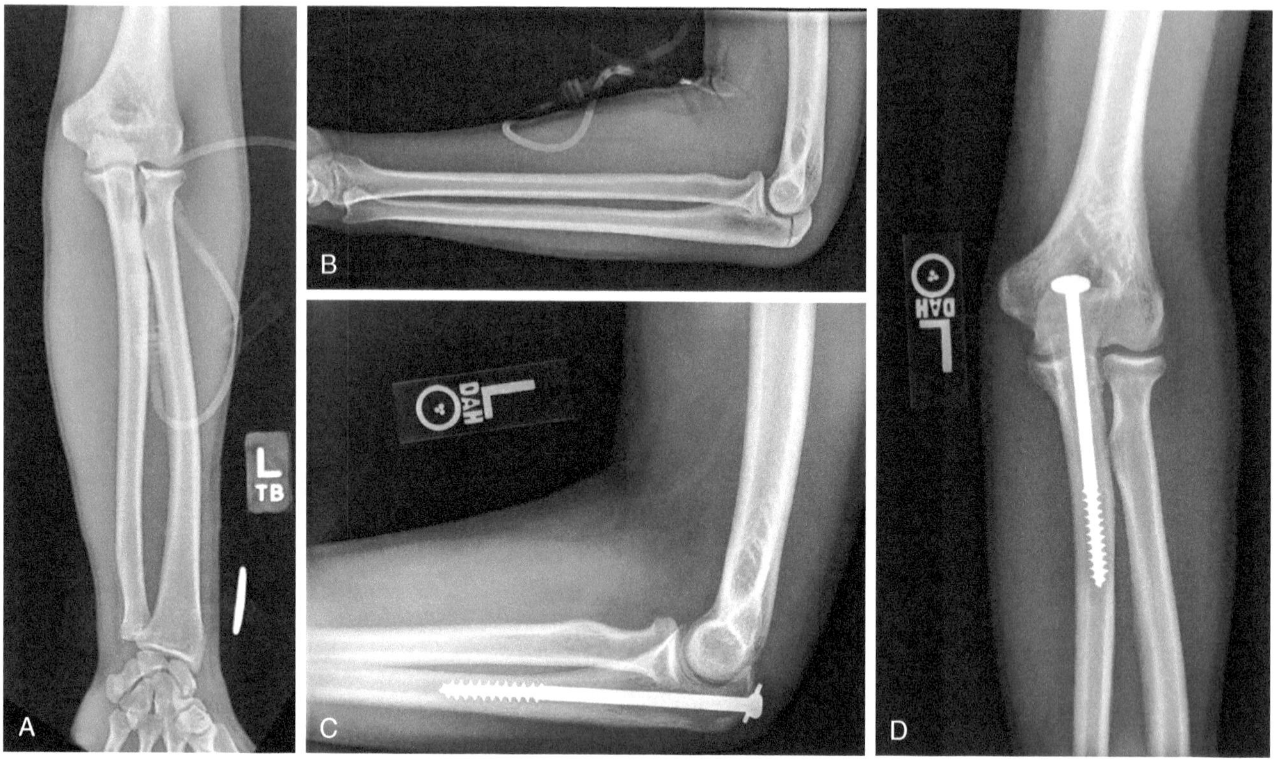

• **Fig. 53.15** (A–D) Injury films of a simple olecranon fracture with single intramedullary screw fixation.

54

Technique Spotlight: Anterior (Trans-olecranon) Olecranon Fracture-Dislocation

DAVID F. BRUNI, LEE M. REICHEL, AND DAVID RING

Indications

Anterior olecranon fracture-dislocation of the elbow (also referred to as transolecranon fracture-dislocation) is characterized by disruption of the trochlear notch, loss of radiocapitellar alignment, maintenance of some apposition of the articular surfaces, intact collateral ligaments, and a normal radioulnar relationship (Fig. 54.1).[1,2] The loss of the elbow congruity is due to fracture of the olecranon and coronoid rather than ligament injury. The proximal radioulnar joint can be affected by the coronoid fracture, but the radial head is not fractured. The goal of treatment is stable restoration of concentric elbow joint alignment.[3] The olecranon and coronoid fragments are realigned and secured to the ulnar shaft.

It is important to distinguish this injury from a forearm fracture-dislocation or anterolateral Monteggia injury.[4] In a transolecranon fracture-dislocation, the radioulnar relationship remains intact (Fig. 54.1A). The primary surgical aim is to restore the trochlear notch and proximal ulna. In contrast, anterolateral Monteggia forearm fracture-dislocations feature dislocation of the proximal radioulnar joint and fracture of the ulna diaphysis (Fig. 54.1B).[5] For forearm fracture-dislocations, the key is anatomical alignment of the ulnar shaft, which restores alignment of the radiocapitellar joint and the proximal radioulnar joint.

Preoperative Evaluation

The entire extremity from the cervical spine to the fingertip can be visualized, palpated, and imaged if helpful, to identify any injury. A documented neurovascular examination is standard. Specifically, the soft tissue envelope is assessed at the proximal forearm and elbow to evaluate for open fracture and to anticipate planned skin incisions.[6]

Anterior olecranon fracture-dislocation is usually apparent on radiographs. The radial head is positioned anteriorly, and the olecranon is fractured (Fig. 54.1A). Computed tomography can help identify the shape and complexity of the coronoid or olecranon fracture.[7] The coronoid is usually a single large fragment in this injury pattern, which makes it relatively easy to realign and secure.[8] Subluxation is usually a result of fragmentation in the center of the trochlear notch, which can be identified and planned for on computed tomography (Fig. 54.2A). Residual subluxation is often due to inadequate realignment of impaction at the depths of the trochlear notch (Fig. 54.2B).

Positioning and Equipment

Supine positioning with the injured arm over the body or lateral decubitus positioning with the arm on a holder or bump are both acceptable. With lateral positioning, gravity may assist in restoring ulnar length. If there is difficulty achieving ulnar length, occasionally an external distractor can be helpful (Fig. 54.3). Supine positioning may be advantageous for visualization and ease of hardware placement if a medial approach to the coronoid is needed. Although the medial approach for a large fragment is accomplished by elevating the entire flexor-pronator mass, which is relatively easy in a lateral decubitus position. A nonsterile pneumatic tourniquet is placed on the upper arm.

Technique

The dorsal incision can be straight or curved radially around the olecranon. If there is a soft tissue injury or skin defect in this area, the incision can be adjusted to optimize wound healing (Fig. 54.4A). Open fractures are debrided of devitalized tissue. The need for specific procedures for soft tissue coverage is unusual. The skin incision is deepened to the proximal ulna proximally and the fascia distally. The skin is mobilized medially and laterally as full-thickness flaps (Fig. 54.4B).

The distal humerus and radial head can be visualized through the olecranon fracture once it is mobilized as with olecranon

423

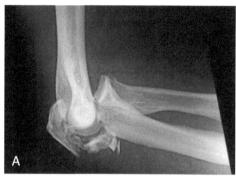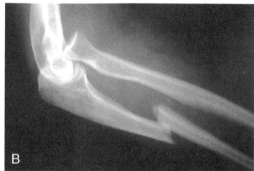

• **Fig. 54.1** (A) Lateral radiograph of an anterior (transolecranon) olecranon fracture-dislocation. The radio-ulnar relationship is intact and the entire forearm is subluxated anteriorly. There is impaction in the depths of the trochlear notch. (B) Lateral radiograph of an anterolateral Monteggia injury: diaphyseal fracture of the ulna with anterolateral dislocation of the radial head from the proximal radioulnar and radiocapitellar joints.

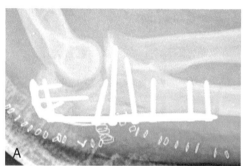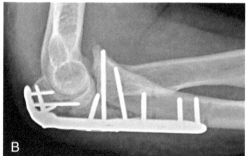

• **Fig. 54.2** (A) Inadequate support is noted at the transverse ridge of the olecranon. (B) As a result, settling of the distal humerus into the trochlear groove is demonstrated.

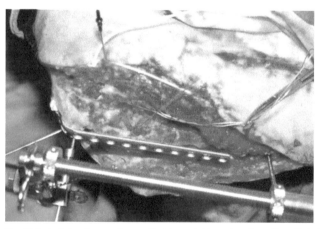

• **Fig. 54.3** A distractor can be applied to assist in restoration of length but is rarely required.

osteotomy (Fig. 54.5). If the distal humerus is also fractured, it can be repaired through this exposure.

Restoration of the proximal ulna (olecranon, transverse ridge of the olecranon, and coronoid) is the most important and difficult portion of the procedure. Coronoid fractures tend to be large basal fractures, typically a single fragment. This allows for reduction and stabilization of coronoid fragments through the olecranon fracture in most cases (Fig. 54.5). Often the coronoid fragment can be reduced and stabilized through the posterior approach. The coronoid can be secured with screws either through the plate or independently. We have found it easier and more secure to elevate the flexor-pronator mass off the medial ulna until the coronoid

fracture is encountered and place a medial plate to secure the coronoid (Fig. 54.6A–B). Unroof the ulnar nerve, protect it, and consider transposing it subcutaneously. Connect the proximal ulnar fragments to the ulnar shaft with plate and screw fixation.

Realign the proximal olecranon fragment to the distal humerus using the trochlea as a "template" (Fig. 54.5). Using the trochlea as a "template" restores the articular relationship between the distal humerus, olecranon, and radial head. More specifically, use of the trochlear template restores the greater sigmoid notch to its appropriate dimensions and congruency, thus restoring ulnohumeral stability. If the olecranon is fragmented, 0.045- and 0.062-inch K-wires can be used for provisional fixation. Additional fixation with suture, wire, screws, or a small plate can be considered as needed. The olecranon fragment can be pinned to the distal humerus if needed to help stabilize its position for reduction of other fragments.

Residual subluxation is usually due to impaction at the center of the trochlear notch. Make sure where the coronoid and olecranon fragments meet that the articular surface is properly contoured. Small wires may be placed to raft beneath or maintain the impacted segments in the elevated anatomic position. These wires can be cut and retained to maintain stability as further olecranon reconstruction is performed (Figs. 54.7 and 54.8). If you need to elevate in this area, you might need to move some cancellous bone from the proximal ulna dorsal to the coronoid process, under the articular fragments to support them.

Plate and screw fixation is recommended. These include 3.5-mm dynamic compression or similar strength precontoured plates (Fig. 54.7). Avoid one-third tubular plates and tension band constructs in this injury pattern. A straight plate may be contoured

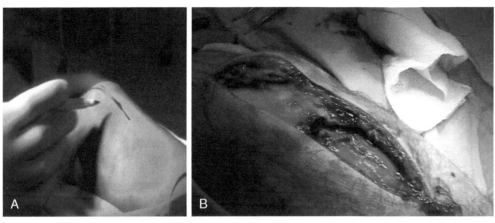

• **Fig. 54.4** (A) A dorsal incision can be made straight or curved radially around the olecranon. (B) Skin is mobilized medially and laterally as full-thickness flaps.

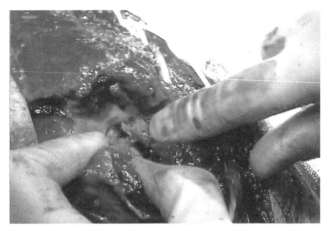

• **Fig. 54.5** Coronoid fragment exposure. The coronoid is exposed through the fracture site similar to an olecranon osteotomy. Bony fragments are templated to the distal humerus.

with "cross-table" lateral view to prevent torsional stress on the elbow joint after fixation of the fracture and reduction of the joint to evaluate reduction of the ulnohumeral and radiocapitellar joints.

Postoperatively, the elbow is placed in a posterior splint at 90 degrees of flexion. This can be removed the next day when fixation is secure, and the patient is ready to start using and moving the arm. It is also reasonable to delay motion a week or so for comfort. It is important to use the hand and make a tight fist repeatedly to work out the swelling and ecchymosis in the fingers.

At the first postoperative visit, elbow radiographs are obtained to confirm elbow alignment, and active and active self-assisted stretching exercises are initiated. Supervised therapy with emphasis on elbow stability may be helpful in some patients who might benefit from additional coaching, supervision, and encouragement.[11] If you refer the patient to a therapist, make sure the therapist understands the importance of cognitive bias and psychological distress in recovery. The dynamic relationship between a therapist and a patient is

to the patient's anatomy. Alternatively, precontoured olecranon plates may offer ease of fit. These precontoured plates also offer clustered and variable angle locking screws that may help secure coronoid fragments and position screws in the subchondral bone[9] (Fig. 54.8A–F). It can be helpful to add a wire or suture that incorporates the triceps insertion into the construct and reinforce the olecranon process fixation. This is particularly useful in an older patient with lower quality bone[10] (Fig. 54.9A and B).

Indirect reduction techniques may be helpful in minimizing soft tissue stripping although generally not utilized. Ulnar length is maintained by the intact radius. When using indirect reduction techniques, a 2.5- or 4.0-mm Schanz pin in the distal fragments connected to a K-wire in the proximal fragment by a distraction device can be used as an indirect reduction technique. Fluoroscopy is used for intraoperative imaging.

If there is bone loss from an open fracture, fill it with autograft (e.g., iliac crest bone graft). Typically, the fragments are viable in this injury and are not debrided, so use of bone graft is typically not needed. The objective of the completed construct is to provide stability to the ulnohumeral joint by providing sound fixation of the fracture fragments and articular congruency of the semilunar notch. (Fig. 54.10 A and B)

After anatomical restoration of bony anatomy, stability should be evaluated. The elbow is taken through full range of motion

PEARLS AND PITFALLS

The primary goal of surgery is to restore the trochlear notch. Surgical technique is aimed at restoring the anatomic relationship between the proximal ulna, distal humerus, and radial head.

- Conceptualize surgical stabilization in four components:
  1. olecranon
  2. transverse ridge of the olecranon (area between the olecranon and coronoid)
  3. coronoid
  4. ulnar shaft
- Stable restoration of the trochlear groove (olecranon, transverse ridge of the olecranon, and coronoid) is the most difficult and critical step to achieving elbow stability.[12]
- Use the olecranon fracture for exposure. Mobilize it like an olecranon osteotomy.
- Use the trochlea as a template for anatomic restoration of the coronoid and olecranon fragments.
- Restore the coronoid to the trochlea and secure it to the ulna shaft as a first step in fracture reduction and fixation.
- Plate and screw fixation is performed with 3.5-mm plates. Avoid one-third tubular plates and tension band constructs.
- Impaction at the greater sigmoid notch is the most common reason for residual radiocapitellar subluxation. Look carefully for this and consider bone grafting when disimpacted fragments are unstable.

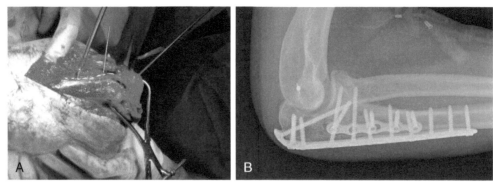

• **Fig. 54.6** (A) A medial approach, elevating the flexor-pronator mass of the medial ulna allowing for reduction and fixation of the coronoid fragment is demonstrated. It is important to unroof the ulnar nerve, protect it, and consider transposing it subcutaneously. (B) Coronoid fragments are connected to the ulnar shaft with plate and screw fixation.

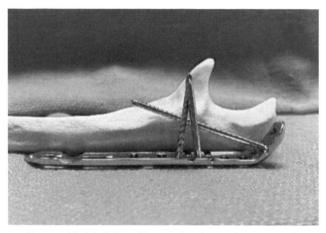

• **Fig. 54.7** Model of ulna with posterior plate and screws overlay.

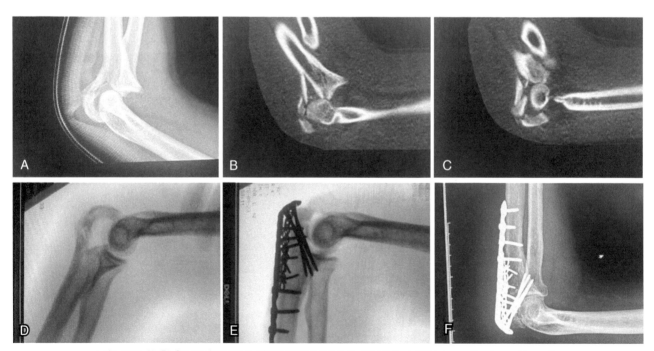

• **Fig. 54.8** (A–D) Severe impaction of the trochlear notch. (E) Here, a locking construct provides subchondral support to help prevent subsidence of articular fragments at the olecranon and transverse ridge. A supplemental lateral plate also is utilized to stabilize the olecranon and transverse ridge segments. (F) Healed fracture at 3 months.

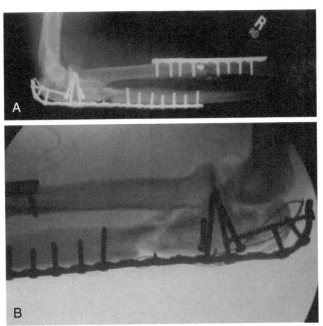

• **Fig. 54.9** (A, B) Photograph of plate options. Locking or nonlocking plates can provide adequate stabilization of bony fragments at the trochlear notch. Locking plates may provide subchondral support to the olecranon, transverse ridge, and coronoid fragments.

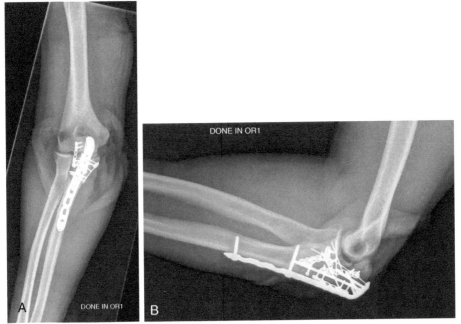

• **Fig. 54.10** Plate application. (A) In this case, a nonlocking plate is fashioned with supplemental olecranon wire fixation to stabilize the comminuted olecranon fragment. (B) Fluoroscopic lateral demonstrating posterior plating, wire stabilization of the olecranon fragment and outside the plate stabilization of the coronoid fragment. (From David Ring, MD, PhD, operative photos.)

often overlooked in fracture care and can have profound impact on patient-reported outcomes. While therapy can have a profound positive impact, a potential for a negative effect exists. Therapists might inadvertently reinforce unhelpful cognitive biases such as "hurt equals harm" through common recommendations such as "work to pain and not beyond," which evidence would suggest is not helpful.

References

1. Biga N, Thomine JM. [Trans-olecranal dislocations of the elbow]. *Rev Chir Orthop Reparatrice Appar Mot*. 1974;60(7):557–567.
2. Ring D, Jupiter JB, Sanders RW, Mast J, Simpson NS. Transolecranon fracture-dislocation of the elbow. *J Orthop Trauma*. 1997;11(8):545–550.
3. Doornberg J, Ring D, Jupiter JB. Effective treatment of fracture-dislocations of the olecranon requires a stable trochlear notch. *Clin Orthop Relat Res*. 2004;429:292–300.
4. Ring D, Jupiter JB, Waters PM. Monteggia fractures in children and adults. *J Am Acad Orthop Surg*. 1998;6(4):215–224.
5. Scolaro JA, Beingessner D. Treatment of Monteggia and transolecranon fracture-dislocations of the elbow: a critical analysis review. *JBJS Rev*. 2014;2(1):2–3.
6. Biberthaler P. Acute elbow trauma fractures and dislocation injuries. In: Beberthaler P, Siebenlist S, Waddell J, eds. *Acute Elbow Trauma*. New York: Springer International Publishing; 2019:219–226.
7. Lubberts B, Janssen S, Mellema J, Ring D. Quantitative 3-dimensional computed tomography analysis of olecranon fractures. *J Shoulder Elbow Surg*. 2016;25(5):831–836.
8. Doornberg JN, Ring D. Coronoid fracture patterns. *J Hand Surg Am*. 2006;31(1):45–52.
9. Mofidi A, Tiessen L, Maripuri N, Mohanty K. Comminuted proximal ulna fractures: injury pattern surgical techniques and outcome. *Eur J Orthop Surg Traumatol*. 2010:545.
10. Izzi J, Athwal GS. An off-loading triceps suture for augmentation of plate fixation in comminuted osteoporotic fractures of the olecranon. *J Orthop Trauma*. 2012;26(1):59–61.
11. Duckworth AD, Kulijdian A, McKee MD, Ring D. Residual subluxation of the elbow after dislocation or fracture-dislocation: treatment with active elbow exercises and avoidance of varus stress. *J Shoulder Elbow Surg*. 2008;17(2):276–280.
12. Lindenhovius AL, Brouwer KM, Doornberg JN, Ring DC, Kloen P. Long-term outcome of operatively treated fracture-dislocations of the olecranon. *J Orthop Trauma*. 2008;22(5):325–331.

55

Technique Spotlight: ORIF Monteggia Fractures

EMILIE J. AMARO AND MIHIR J. DESAI

Introduction

A Monteggia fracture-dislocation, defined as a proximal ulna fracture with a concurrent proximal radioulnar joint dislocation, is a rare but complex injury of the forearm and elbow.[1] Monteggia fracture-dislocations account for 1%–2% of forearm fractures and are commonly secondary to a direct force to the forearm while the elbow is extended and the forearm is pronated.[2] Several classification systems have been proposed to describe these injuries based on both the direction of radial head dislocation and the osseous structures involved. Stability of the elbow is conferred by the ulnar collateral ligament, the coronoid, the radial head, the radial collateral ligament, and the annular ligament.[3] Concurrent injury to these structures can destabilize the elbow and should be carefully evaluated prior to surgical management, as the goal of treatment is to restore elbow stability and facilitate early range of motion.[4]

Indications

The vast majority of Monteggia fractures in adults require operative management to ensure reduction of the ulna and radial head. Loss of alignment and reduction is common in adults treated with closed management and the morbidity of persistent elbow dislocation is high.[5] Furthermore, operative fixation allows for early range of motion, preventing the development of arthrofibrosis and loss of elbow motion.

Preoperative Evaluation

Patient evaluation begins with a detailed history and examination. Examination should include a thorough secondary examination to rule out any associated injuries. A neurovascular examination should be performed to rule out a concomitant neurovascular injury. The posterior interosseous nerve (PIN) is the most commonly associated neurovascular structure injured with Monteggia fracture-dislocations and therefore a careful evaluation of wrist, thumb, and metacarpophalangeal (MCP) extension should be performed.[6] Furthermore, the ulnar nerve should be carefully examined if the fracture pattern involves the olecranon process.[7]

Diagnostic imaging begins with plain radiographs of the elbow involving anteroposterior (AP), lateral, and oblique views. Radial head dislocation or subluxation is a frequently missed injury that carries high morbidity.[8,9] Therefore any patient with a proximal or ulnar shaft fracture should have dedicated elbow radiographs with the radiocapitellar joint scrutinized on the lateral view. Furthermore, approximately 70%–80% of posterior radial head dislocations also involve a fracture of the radial head.[1] A dedicated Greenspan view or radial head view can also be obtained to rule out an associated radial head fracture. If plain radiographs of a Monteggia fracture-dislocation demonstrate a complex pattern involving a fracture of either the radial head or coronoid, computed tomography (CT) imaging is helpful in preoperative planning.[1,10]

Positioning and Equipment

The patient is positioned supine using a radiolucent arm board (Fig. 55.1; Table 55.1). A nonsterile tourniquet is placed on the upper arm proximal to the level of the sterile field. If there is a complex fracture-dislocation or a fracture involving the olecranon, the patient can be placed in the lateral decubitus position with the arm draped over a radiolucent arm post or bolster (Fig. 55.2; Table 55.2). The hand table and/or post should be radiolucent to allow for intraoperative fluoroscopy.

Surgical Technique

The operative management of simple Monteggia fracture-dislocations should first focus on anatomic reduction of the ulna.[9–11] The accurate restoration of length, rotation, and alignment of the ulnar shaft typically leads to spontaneous reduction of the radial head without further operative intervention.[11] Intraoperative fluoroscopy evaluating the radial head following fixation of the ulna is essential as soft tissue structures of the elbow can become entrapped in the radiocapetellar joint, preventing reduction of the radial head even with anatomic alignment of the ulnar shaft.[12]

Simple Monteggia fracture-dislocations including Bado Types I, IIC, and III fractures are often treated with contoured ulnar shaft locking compression plating systems or with bridge plating systems[6,9] (see Chapter 51 for Bado classification details). The subcutaneous approach to the ulnar shaft using the internervous plane between flexor carpi ulnaris (FCU) and extensor carpi ulnaris (ECU) is used to locate and reduce the fracture (Figs. 55.3 and 55.4). Compression, lag, or bridging constructs may be utilized depending on the morphology of the fracture. For example, in patients with comminuted Bado Type I Monteggia

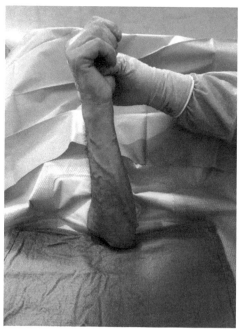

• **Fig. 55.1** Patient is positioned supine with the arm on a radiolucent arm board. A nonsterile tourniquet can be placed on the upper arm, away from the surgical field.

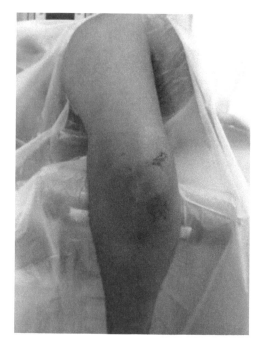

• **Fig. 55.2** Patient is positioned in the lateral decubitus position with the arm draped over a radiolucent arm post.

TABLE 55.1	Procedural Equipment for Simple Bado Types I, IIC, and III Fractures	
Positioning	•	Supine with arm on a radiolucent table
	•	Nonsterile tourniquet proximal to sterile field
Approach	•	Subcutaneous approach to the ulna between flexor carpi ulnaris and extensor carpi ulnaris
Reduction	•	Direct anatomic reduction of ulna using pointed reduction clamps which leads to indirect reduction of the radial head
Plating systems	•	Lag screw fixation with neutralization plate OR
	•	Compression plating system OR
	•	Bridging system in comminuted fractures
Imaging	•	Fluoroscopy

TABLE 55.2	Procedural Equipment for Monteggia Variants Involving the Olecranon	
Positioning	•	Lateral on a bean bag with the arm over a radiolucent post
	•	Nonsterile tourniquet proximal to sterile field
Approach	•	Posterior approach to the elbow
Reduction	•	Direct anatomic reduction of the olecranon using pointed reduction clamps
	•	Indirect reduction of the olecranon by extending the elbow and placing the elbow in extension on a well-padded Mayo stand
Plating systems	•	Precontoured olecranon plating systems
	•	Plate benders can be used to contour plates to the olecranon
Imaging	•	Fluoroscopy

fracture-dislocations, a bridge plate can be used for fracture fixation (Fig. 55.5). With appropriate restoration of length and alignment, the radial head often spontaneously reduces. The surgical goal of ulnar shaft fractures is anatomic reduction and/or restoration of length as this often leads to spontaneous and stable reduction of the radial head.[9] In the event that the radiocapitellar joint does not reduce, the first step is to reassess your ulna reduction. Once confirmed that the reduction is appropriate, explore the radiocapitellar joint. In some cases, the annular ligament is torn and incarcerated within the joint preventing reduction of the radial head. This should be reduced and the ligament repaired primarily.

There is a subset of Monteggia fractures that involve the olecranon (Fig. 55.6).[13] Similar to ulnar shaft fractures, the surgical goal should be anatomic reduction of the proximal ulna.[5] The posterior approach to the elbow is commonly used in the fixation of olecranon fractures. The patient is placed in a lateral decubitus position with the operative extremity positioned over a post (Fig. 55.2). A longitudinal incision is made extending just proximal to the tip of the olecranon, curving laterally around the tip of olecranon, and continuing along the subcutaneous border of the ulna.[14] The ulnar nerve should be located and protected medially. The medial border of the triceps is identified and the triceps is incised allowing for exposure of the olecranon. Oftentimes, direct visualization of the ulnohumeral joint is not needed for reduction of an olecranon fracture. Extending the arm frequently leads to indirect reduction, which can be provisionally held with pointed reduction clamps and K-wires (Fig. 55.7). Throughout the surgery, the

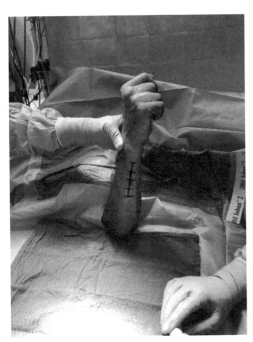

• **Fig. 55.3** The subcutaneous approach to the ulna involves an incision directly centered over the palpable surface of the ulna.

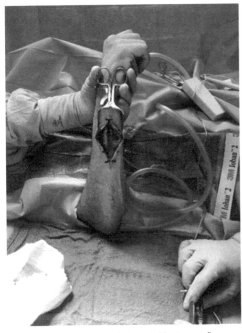

• **Fig. 55.4** The internervous plane is located between flexor carpi ulnaris and extensor carpi ulnaris. This allows direct access to the ulnar shaft.

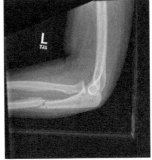
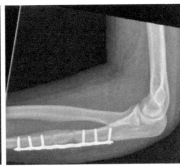

• **Fig. 55.5** Anteroposterior and lateral radiographs demonstrating a left Bado I fracture-dislocation. There is a comminuted ulnar shaft fracture with anterior radial head subluxation. This was treated using a bridge plating construct with spontaneous reduction of the radial head.

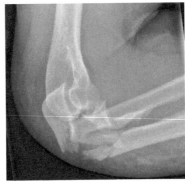
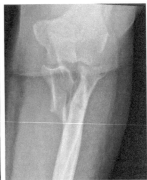

• **Fig. 55.6** Anteroposterior and lateral radiographs demonstrating a right Jupiter IIA fracture-dislocation. There is a comminuted proximal ulna shaft fracture with posterior radial head dislocation.

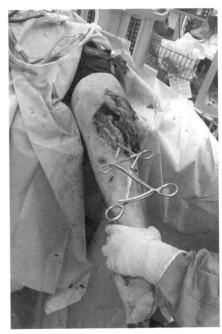

• **Fig. 55.7** The ulnar nerve should be located and protected medially. Extending the arm often assists with reduction.

arm can be held in extension using a padded Mayo stand to assist with maintaining anatomic reduction. In comminuted and/or displaced olecranon fractures, the fracture itself allows for direct visualization of the ulnohumeral joint line. Articular fragments can be tamped, reduced, and provisionally held using the direct visualization the fracture naturally provides.

The orientation of the olecranon fracture and the degree of comminution should guide the method of fixation. Although tension banding can be used in transversely oriented fractures, olecranon fractures with an associated radial head dislocation should be treated with plate fixation (Fig. 55.8).[15,16] Either a precontoured

plate can be utilized or an existing plate can be contoured to the olecranon. The olecranon plate can be placed directly over the triceps insertion; however, the triceps is often incised longitudinally to allow the plate to contact the bone directly.[5] Olecranon plates can be placed laterally or posteriorly. Posterior plates may increase

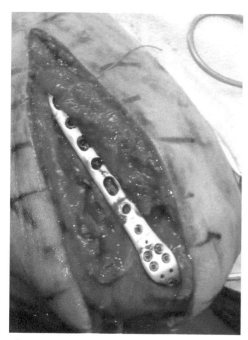

• **Fig. 55.8** Olecranon fracture fixed with a plate leading to spontaneous reduction of the radial head.

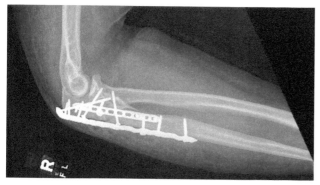

• **Fig. 55.9** A medial and posterior plate was used in conjunction with several lag screws to achieve anatomic reduction of the ulnohumeral joint and coronoid. The radial head spontaneously reduced with fixation of the proximal ulna.

skin irritation, but they allow for placement of lag screws, an intermedullary screw, and fixation that captures the coronoid.[17,18] While lateral plates are associated with less plate prominence, they often limit the screw fixation options available.[17,18] Significantly comminuted and unstable fractures of the olecranon may require a combination of techniques including lag screws, neutralization plating, and contoured plating (Fig. 55.9).

In addition to olecranon involvement, there can also be associated injury to the coronoid (Figs. 55.10 and 55.11). These would be classified as Bado Type II and Jupiter Type IIA fractures. These fractures are critical to both recognize and treat. The lateral ulnar collateral ligament inserts at the base of the coronoid and can be involved in Regan and Morrey Type III coronoid fractures.[19] Furthermore, the anteromedial facet of the coronoid confers significant stability to the elbow and it is imperative that these fractures are identified and treated with fixation.[20,21] Further details on approaches and fixation strategies of coronoid fractures are detailed separately in other dedicated technique chapters.

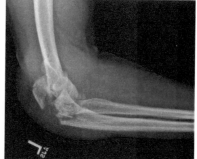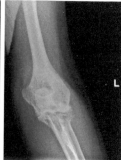

• **Fig. 55.10** Anteroposterior and lateral radiographs demonstrating a complex Monteggia variant fracture-dislocation involving a comminuted olecranon fracture, a large displaced coronoid fracture, and a comminuted radial head fracture-dislocation.

Lastly, concomitant radial head fracture is also a concern with Monteggia injuries (Figs. 55.10 and 55.12). The radial head is an important lateral stabilizer of the elbow. In simple Monteggia fracture-dislocations involving an ulnar shaft fracture and a simple radial head dislocation, anatomic fixation of the ulnar shaft will often lead to reduction of the radial head. In this scenario, no further management of the radial head is needed. However, in Bado Type II or Jupiter Type IIA injuries, the radial head can often be fractured as well as dislocated.[22] The techniques for addressing these fractures are detailed separately in a dedicated chapter to these injuries.

Postoperative Care and Management

The postoperative management of Monteggia fractures involves early mobilization, particularly in a stable construct.[5] The elbow joint has a predilection to develop postoperative stiffness and therefore early exercise and rehabilitation are instrumental in facilitating a full recovery.[23–25] Postoperatively, patients are placed in a well-padded posterior long arm splint for 2 weeks. At the 2-week visit, a wound check is performed and sutures are removed. Patients are then started on a regimen of gentle passive range of motion as tolerated as well as active range of motion guided by physical and occupational therapists. Patients are also given posterior long arm orthosis to wear for comfort when not performing exercises.

PEARLS AND PITFALLS

Pearls
- Achieve anatomic reduction of the ulna when possible as this will often lead to spontaneous reduction of the radial head.
- Surgical priority is fixation of the ulna.

Pitfalls
- Inadequate preoperative imaging.
- When in doubt obtain advanced imaging as elbow injuries can be associated with injury to the coronoid, ligamentous structures, and radial head.
- Appropriate stabilization of all injured structures is paramount to a functional and stable elbow.

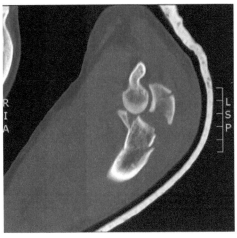
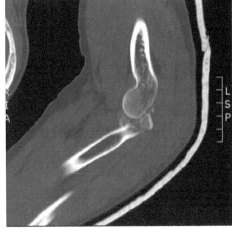

• **Fig. 55.11** Computed tomography scans were obtained in the emergency department for further characterization of the radial head fracture-dislocation as well as the coronoid fracture.

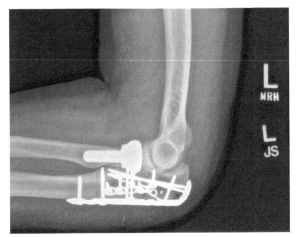

• **Fig. 55.12** A dual plating system of the olecranon was utilized along with lag screws for anatomic fixation of the coronoid. The radial head was excised and replaced due to significant comminution.

References

1. Eathiraju S, Mudgal CS, Jupiter JB. Monteggia fracture-dislocations. *Hand Clin.* 2007;23:165–177.
2. Reckling F. Unstable and Galeazzi of the forearm lesions. *J Bone Jt Surg.* 1982;64A:857–863.
3. Aquilina AL, Grazette AJ. Clinical anatomy and assessment of the elbow. *Open Orthop J.* 2017;11:1347–1352.
4. Matar HE, Akimau PI, Stanley D, Ali AA. Surgical treatment of Monteggia variant fracture dislocations of the elbow in adults: surgical technique and clinical outcomes. *Eur J Orthop Surg Traumatol.* 2017;27:599–605.
5. Siebenlist S, Buchholz A, Braun KF. Fractures of the proximal ulna: current concepts in surgical management. *EFORT Open Rev.* 2019;4:1–9.
6. Josten C, Freitag S. Monteggia and Monteggia-like-lesions: classification, indication, and techniques in operative treatment. *Eur J Trauma Emerg Surg.* 2009;35:296–304.
7. Shin R, Ring D. The ulnar nerve in elbow trauma. *J Bone J Surg Ser* 2007;A89:1108–1116.
8. Mathur N, Lau KK. Monteggia fracture: an easy fracture to miss. *Emerg Radiol.* 2020;10. https://doi.org/10.1007/s10140-020-01763-8.
9. Delpont M, Louahem D, Cottalorda J. Monteggia injuries. *Orthop Traumatol Surg Res.* 2018;104:S113–S120.
10. Calderazzi F, Galavotti C, Nosenzo A, Menozzi M, Ceccarelli F. How to approach Monteggia-like lesions in adults: a review. *Ann Med Surg.* 2018;35:108–116.
11. Ring D, Jupier J, Simpson S. Monteggia fractures in adults. *J Bone Jt Surg.* 1998;80A:1733–1744.
12. Tanner C, Johnson T, Kolahi K, Husak L, Hoekzema N. Irreducible Monteggia fracture: interposed radial nerve and capsule. *JSES Open Access.* 2017;1:85–89.
13. Jupiter JB, Leibovic SJ, Ribbans W, Wilk RM. The posterior Monteggia lesion. *J Orthop Trauma.* 1991;5:395–402.
14. Gartsman G, Sculco T, Otis J. Operative treatment of olecranon fracture. *J Bone Jt Surg.* 1981;63A:718–721.
15. Ring D, Jupiter JB, Sanders R, Mast J, Simpson N. Transolecranon fracture dislocation of the elbow. *J Orthop Trauma.* 1997;11:545–550.
16. Doornberg J, Ring D, Jupiter JB. Effective treatment of fracture-dislocations of the olecranon requires a stable trochlear notch. *Clin Orthop Relat Res.* 2004:292–300. https://doi.org/10.1097/01.blo.0000142627.28396.cb.
17. Niglis L, Bonnomet F, Schenck B, et al. Critical analysis of olecranon fracture management by pre-contoured locking plates. *Orthop Traumatol Surg Res.* 2015;101:201–207.
18. Rochet S, Obert L, Lepage D, et al. Proximal ulna comminuted fractures: fixation using a double-plating technique. *Orthop Traumatol Surg Res.* 2010;96:734–740.
19. Rhyou IH, Lee JH, Kim KC, et al. What injury mechanism and patterns of ligament status are associated with isolated coronoid, isolated radial head, and combined fractures? *Clin Orthop Relat Res.* 2017;475:2308–2315.
20. Chen ACY, Weng CJ, Chou YC, Cheng CY. Anteromedial fractures of the ulnar coronoid process: correlation between surgical outcomes and radiographic findings. *BMC Musculoskelet Disord.* 2018;19:248.
21. Pollock JC, Brownhill J, Ferreira L, et al. The effect of anteromedial facet fractures of the coronoid and lateral collateral ligament injury on elbow stability and kinematics. *J Bone Jt Surg Ser.* 2009;A91:1448–1458.
22. Ring D, Jupiter J, Zilberfarb J. Posterior dislocation of the elbow with fractures of the radial head and coronoid. *J Bone Jt Surg Am.* 2002;84:547–551.
23. Marti RK, Kerkhoffs GMMJ, Maas M, Blankevoort L. Progressive surgical release of a posttraumatic stiff elbow: technique and outcome after 2-18 years in 46 patients. *Acta Orthop Scand.* 2002;73:144–150.
24. Dávila SA, Johnston-Jones K. Managing the stiff elbow: operative, nonoperative, and postoperative techniques. *J Hand Ther.* 2006;19:268–281.
25. Lindenhovius A, Doornberg JN, Brouwer JM, et al. A prospective randomized controlled trial of dynamic versus static progressive elbow splinting for posttraumatic elbow stiffness. *J Bone Jt Surg Ser.* 2012;A94:694–700.

56

Essex-Lopresti—When Do All Three Levels Require Attention?

A. LEE OSTERMAN, RICK TOSTI, AND RYAN TARR

History

Although the eponym for forearm longitudinal instability is known as Essex-Lopresti, Dr. Peter Essex-Lopresti was not the first person who reported the injury. It was first described by Brockman in 1931.[1] Curr and Coe later reported on a case of a dislocation "on both ends of the radius" 15 years later in 1946.[2] However, in a case report by Dr. Essex-Lopresti in 1951, he correctly identified forearm instability as part of the injury constellation after his first patient had severe radial impingement following a radial head excision. It was his observation that expanded the diagnosis from a proximal radius injury and distal radioulnar joint (DRUJ) dislocation to include the disruption of the interosseous membrane (IOM). He predicted that preventing proximal migration by maintaining radial length was paramount for healing of the IOM and DRUJ, and therefore a successful recovery.[3]

Anatomy and Biomechanics

In one sense, the forearm can be visualized as a bicondylar joint with the proximal radioulnar joint and DRUJ as the condyles and the IOM as the cruciate ligament. The three levels are interdependent. Thus an injury at one level has a high likelihood of a reciprocal injury at the other two levels. The radius travels like a bucket handle around the ulna in pronation and supination.

Hennequin, a French anatomist, first characterized the IOM as a ligament in 1894. Subsequently, more detailed histologic studies have confirmed that the structural arrangement of the collagen and its biomechanical behavior is that of a ligament and not just a membrane that separates the flexor and extensor compartments.[4,5] Microscopically, the IOM can be divided into three sections: (1) proximally with the proximal oblique cord (known as the ligament of Weitbrecht) and the dorsal oblique accessory cord[6]; (2) centrally, the major central band and variable accessory bands; and (3) distally, the distal oblique bundle (DOB) as seen in Fig. 56.1.

The central band is the largest component and the major IOM stabilizer to axial stability. It is stout with an average width of 1.1 cm. Its origin begins at 7.7 cm from the radial head and spans obliquely at an angle of 21 degrees to the ulna axis to insert on the ulna 13.7 mm from the olecranon tip. Noda localized the origin of the central band to 60% of the radial length and 33% of the ulnar length (Fig. 56.2).[7] In a biomechanical study, Pfaeffle confirmed that the modulus of elasticity and the ultimate tensile strength was similar to that of the patellar tendon.[8] The central band plays a major role in the longitudinal load transfer of the wrist to the elbow and of the radius to the ulna. It also helps to maintain transverse forearm stability.

The DOB is a short ligament that runs from the proximal ulnar border of the pronator quadratus distally toward the sigmoid notch on the radius.[7] It is a major stabilizer of the DRUJ and adds support to axial and transverse stability. The role of the proximal IOM ligaments is yet to be fully defined; currently, they are felt to play a role in stabilizing the proximal radioulnar joint similar to the role of the DOB distally. Werner and colleagues calculated the contributions of the various portions of IOM to transverse stability: proximal 18%, central band 25%, and DOB 31%.[9]

The IOM has four primary functions: (1) transmit load from the wrist to the elbow, (2) transfer load from the radius to the ulna, (3) maintain forearm stability, and (4) help maintain DRUJ stability.[10] In a cadaveric study by Birkbeck et al., axial forces in supination through the distal radius and distal ulna are 68% and 32%, respectively. The force is then translated through the IOM to equilibrate, resulting in 51% at the proximal radius and 49% at the proximal ulna. However, when the IOM was divided, there was no load transfer within the forearm, and the proximal radiocapitellar joint experienced significantly larger amount of force than the proximal ulna (Fig. 56.3).[11]

Pathomechanics

Essex-Lopresti injuries result from an axial force to the upper extremity. Reports in the literature range from high-energy motor vehicle accidents to low-energy falls from height.[10,12–15] The differing amount of force required to create this injury leads to varying severities and presentations. The position of the forearm influences the injury pattern as well. In a cadaveric study by McGinley, the authors noted that Essex-Lopresti injuries occurred more frequently when the forearm was pronated at an average 70 ± 25 degrees, while isolated radial head fractures and both bone forearm fractures occurred in less pronation.[16]

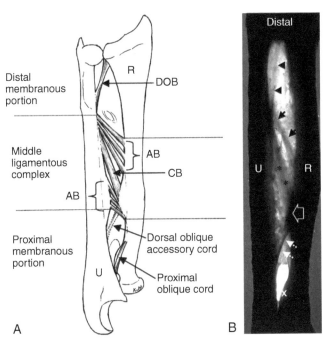

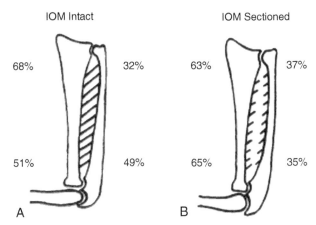

• **Fig. 56.3** (A) Artistic depiction of the transfer of force from the distal radius and ulna to the elbow, with equilibrium of force. (B) Demonstrates that no force is transferred through the interosseous membrane *(IOM)* after injury and the radiocapitellar joint experiences increased pressure. (Recreated with permission from Pfaeffle HJ, Tomaino MM, Grewal R, et al. Tensile properties of the interosseous membrane of the human forearm. *J Orthop Res.* 1996;14(5):842-845. https://doi.org/10.1002/jor.1100140525.)

• **Fig. 56.1** (A) Schematic of the interosseous membrane (IOM) viewed from the anterior aspect. The IOM consists of three main portions: distal, middle, and proximal. The proximal oblique cord is present on the anterior side of the forearm and the dorsal oblique accessory cord on the posterior side in the proximal membranous portion. The middle portion is a ligamentous complex (middle ligamentous complex) that is further divisible into the central band *(CB)* and the accessory band *(AB)*. The distal oblique bundle *(DOB)* is present within the distal membranous portion. (B) Backlit photograph of IOM ligaments. *Asterisks* indicate the CB as part of the middle ligamentous complex, which originates from the radial crest *(white arrow)*, runs distally and ulnarly, and inserts into the interosseous border of the ulna. (B, Courtesy Noda et al. The interosseous membrane of the forearm: an anatomical study of ligament attachment locations. *J Hand Surg.* 2009; 34A: 415-422.)

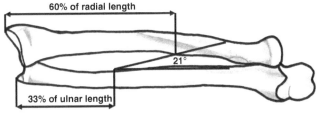

• **Fig. 56.2** Schematic of the suggested location of central band reconstruction.

Many studies have evaluated the strength of the central band to identify the force needed to disrupt it.[4,8,17,18] Wegmann applied 210 J to cadaveric specimen forearms while filming with a high-speed video. He reported that with increasing longitudinal force, the central band failed first, followed by radial head fracture and then the triangular fibrocartilage complex (TFCC).[19] However, these in vitro models neither evaluate the role of the accessory structures (such as the TFCC and the distal oblique ligament) nor explain the incompetence of the central band that can occur after radial head excision. In one cadaver study, the strength of the central and accessory bands was tested with a slow force application and revealed a biphasic failure.[17]

The two common scenarios are the acute presentation recognized at the time of initial injury and the chronic presentation, which occurs over time and only after the radial head is excised.

The primary stabilizer to axial instability is the radial head and thus preservation of the radial head is the first line of treatment. When the radial head is not salvageable and removed, the secondary restraints, that is, the central band and the DRUJ stabilizers, become critical. The early literature debated the relative contributions of these secondary restraints. Hotchkiss showed that with radial head excision, the IOM contributes to 71% of axial load stability compared to only 8% in the TFCC.[20] He also noted that for the radius to migrate proximally >2 mm, the TFCC must also be disrupted. Other studies emphasized the role of the DRUJ stabilizers. Skahen, using a three-space tracking system and a differential variable reluctance transducer (DVRT) strain gauge attached to the central band, concluded that the central band and the distal DRUJ stabilizers were of equal importance in preventing axial migration of the radius.[21]

Diagnosis

Essex-Lopresti injuries are rare. Most textbooks report an incidence of 1% though Duckworth, in a review of forearm and elbow injuries, felt the incidence was closer to 11%.[22] Given its relative rarity, the injury is often underrecognized. Trousdale showed that only 5 out of 20 patients with Essex-Lopresti injuries had an accurate diagnosis at the time of referral.[14] Our more recent data suggest that in only 38% of 106 proven cases was the diagnosis initially made.[23]

An accurate diagnosis is critical in obtaining a successful outcome after a longitudinal radioulnar dissociation; chronic injuries require more surgery and portend an inferior outcome. Trousdale et al. reported that only 20% of patients with a delayed diagnosis had a satisfactory result after treatment.[14] Jupiter had good to excellent outcomes in 78%–88% when the diagnosis was recognized and treated acutely.[24] Schnetzke showed that although range of motion between the two groups showed no difference, the acutely treated group scored better in every objective outcome measure and had significantly fewer complications (38% vs. 93%) at a 5-year follow-up.[25]

A history of a high-energy fall on the outstretched hand should raise the examiner's suspicion. While more commonly associated

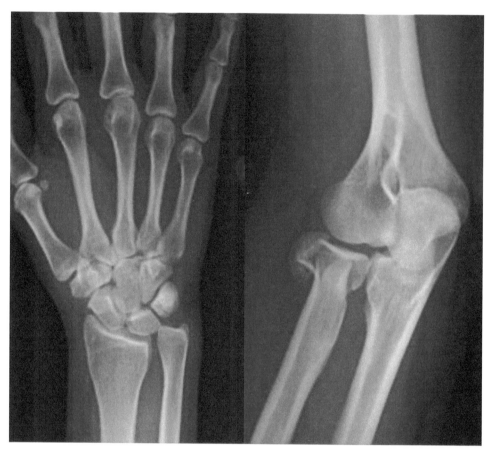

• **Fig. 56.4** Radiographs of a 49-year-old female bicyclist who was involved in a bicyclist versus motor vehicle accident. She sustained a distal radioulnar joint dislocation and a comminuted radial head fracture.

with a Type III comminuted radial head fracture, any radial head fracture or significant elbow injury can be associated with an Essex-Lopresti injury. Hausmann studied 14 patients with a non-displaced Type I radial head fracture and noted that using forearm magnetic resonance imaging (MRI), 64% showed evidence of central band injury. Since the radial head was intact, treatment required only symptomatic elbow support and elbow range of motion.[26]

The clinical workup of a potential Essex-Lopresti injury should include a DRUJ examination for tenderness and instability. Palpation for tenderness over the central band in the forearm is another clue. In the chronic setting after radial head resection, patients may complain of ulnar wrist pain, limited forearm rotation, and a prominent ulnar head. At the elbow, there may be signs of radiocapitellar impingement with worsening elbow pain and decreased motion. Grip strength as measured by a Jamar dynamometer will be reduced.

Besides images of the elbow, the standard radiographic examination in a suspected Essex-Lopresti injury should include the forearm and wrist with particular attention paid to ulnar variance, widening of the DRUJ, or ulnar styloid fracture (Fig. 56.4). In one series, such standard initial injury films were positive for axial instability in only 12%.[27] Specialty views can include a grip-loaded, pronated posteroanterior (PA) to demonstrate any dynamic instability as well as contralateral wrist films for comparison.

Other advanced imaging techniques have been studied. A triple-phase bone scan may show increased uptake at the elbow and wrist but is relatively silent for IOM injury. In forearm cadaver

specimens, Failla demonstrated that ultrasound could readily distinguish an intact from a disrupted central band and was useful as well in the acute clinical setting.[28] Dynamic ultrasonography may better identify membrane disruption than static testing. A "muscular hernia sign" (Fig. 56.5) may be visible by ultrasound when the ultrasound probe was placed dorsally, and a volar counterforce is applied from anterior to posterior across the forearm.[29] Multiple researchers have applied MRI scanning and shown that a consistent image of the central band is seen on an axial T2, fast spin-echo, fat-suppressed sequence (Fig. 56.6).[30–32] While results have been encouraging in cadavers, it has not demonstrated comparable accuracy in diagnosing the acutely torn central band in the clinical situation.

The more common need for definitive diagnosis of an Essex-Lopresti instability occurs at the primary surgery and when the radial head is not reconstructable and a decision on excision versus prosthetic replacement is required. A number of intraoperative tests exist. Smith and Ruch described the radius pull test.[33] Traction is applied to the proximal radial stump and the ulnar variance is observed fluoroscopically at the wrist. Greater than 3 mm of positive variance is a concern for instability and >6 mm is diagnostic. To refine this fluoroscopic test further, Rynning and Osterman developed the RIST (radioulnar instability stress test), which uses both axial compression and axial distraction. If the combined variance change is >6 mm, then axial instability is present. The lateral pull test or "joystick" test is performed by pulling the radial neck laterally while the forearm is pronated. A positive test is observing lateral dissociation of the forearm, which was noted to be 100%

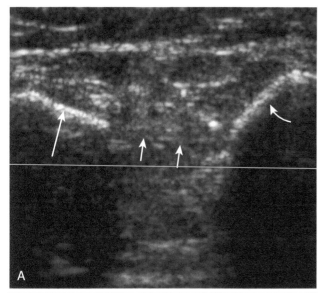

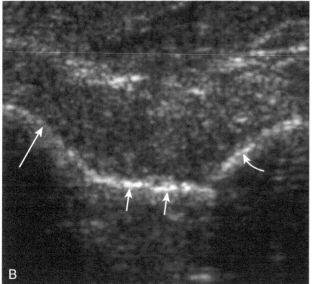

• **Fig. 56.5** (A) A dynamic ultrasound revealing disruption of the interosseous membrane (IOM) with interposed muscle termed "muscular hernia sign" by Soubeyrand et al. (B) Central *arrows* represent intact IOM.

sensitive in the cadaver model.[34] Finally, the RAIL (radial axial interosseous load) test uses the simple fact that if on axial compression the radial stump abuts against the capitellum, then axial instability is present (Fig. 56.7).

Classification

Edwards and Jupiter developed a classification system based on the status of the radial head. They defined Type 1 injuries as an acute radial head fracture with large pieces that were amenable to open reduction internal fixation (ORIF). Type 2 represented a nonreconstructable radial head fracture with instability and best treated with a prosthetic implant. Type 3 represented a chronic longitudinal injury with irreducible proximal radial migration.[24] Limitations of this classification system are that it does not address the status of the secondary stabilizers and thus does not provide guidance for treatment at the forearm or wrist. Our group defines an acute injury as axial instability identified at the time of injury.

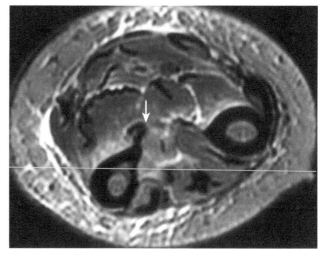

• **Fig. 56.6** T2 axial view demonstrates central band disruption as a wavy, bowed, and discontinuous ligament with interposed muscle.

Subacute injury is defined within 3 months of radial head excision. With the exception of needing a radial head replacement in the subacute group, such injuries are treated similarly to the acute category at the wrist and forearm. Chronic injuries are those identified after 3 months that require attention to all three levels of the injury (Table 56.1).

Treatment

Acute and Subacute Essex-Lopresti

Once axial instability has been identified, a three-pronged strategy of treatment is planned for each level of injury: the elbow, the DRUJ, and the forearm central band. The treatment algorithm starts at the elbow, followed by the wrist, and then the IOM.

At the elbow, the concept is to preserve the radial head whenever possible. It is the primary restraint against axial migration. If the radial head can be fixed, the development of late axial instability is uncommon. Geel and Palmer showed that preserving the radial head resulted in no symptomatic cases of late wrist pain.[35] Ikeda compared a series of Type III comminuted radial head fractures of which half were treated by internal fixation and the other half by excision. In the ORIF group, there was improved grip strength and function and no axial instability.[36]

Karlstad examined the use of radial head allografts in both acute and chronic Essex-Lopresti injuries.[37] The case series had four patients undergoing a total of five procedures which resulted in a failure rate of 80% with only one of the radial heads uniting. The technique was abandoned.

If radial head preservation is not possible, then a radial head prosthesis is indicated. A variety of implants have been introduced in the past decade; these differ in metallic composition, design, and method of fixation. Our studies have not shown an advantage of a particular type with the exception of a silastic prosthesis. A silastic implant is not load bearing and thus is not indicated—especially in the Essex-Lopresti injury. In the Essex-Lopresti setting, the prosthesis is required to withstand greater loads. Gong reported a patient treated with radial head replacement and DRUJ pinning in supination still resulted in migration and lateral arm pain.[38] We have concerns for this and hence, in most acute cases, will address the more distal levels as well to further neutralize the axial forces.

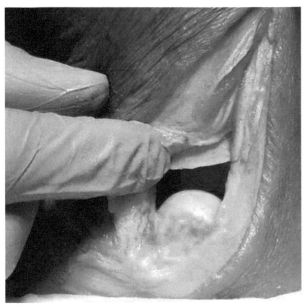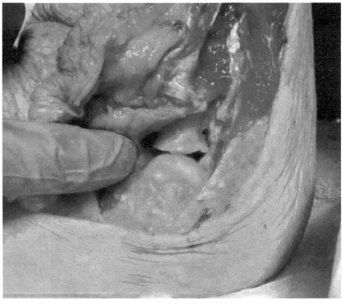

• **Fig. 56.7** Clinical photographs demonstrating the radial axial interosseous load (RAIL) test. With axial pressure applied to the distal radius, there will be complete collapse of the radial capitellar space with interosseous injury.

TABLE 56.1	Reconstruction Techniques by Location	
	Acute Reconstruction	**Chronic Reconstruction**
Elbow	ORIF radial head vs. radial head replacement	± Radial head replacement
Forearm	Primary central band repair Pronator rerouting Suture button construct	Bone-patella tendon-bone graft Suture button construct
DRUJ	Foveal TFC repair Distal oblique bundle reconstruction	Ulnar shortening osteotomy ± Wrist arthroscopy to debride TFC and assess LT ligament

DRUJ, distal radioulnar joint; *LT*, lunatotriquetral ligament; *ORIF*, open reduction internal fixation; *TFC*, triangular fibrocartilage.

The strategy at the wrist level is a foveal TFC repair either by an arthroscopically assisted or open method. If such a repair is not feasible or is insufficient, our new approach is to add a reconstruction of the distal oblique band. We prefer the technique described by Wright over that by Brink, but both are straightforward and add stability both to the DRUJ and axially to the forearm.[39,40] Wright's technique is a dorsal exposure of the distal radius and ulna. A tendon graft is passed through drill holes, from the lateral aspect of the ulna obliquely to the sigmoid notch of the radius and tensioned in supination as depicted in Fig. 56.8.

At the forearm, the goal is to restore the central band function. In acute injuries, the torn central band can easily be exposed through a dorsal incision at the level of the distal third of the ulna and in line with the extensor digiti minimi tendon. The problem arises that in 80% of these cases, the ligament is disrupted centrally and is not amenable to repair. In the other 20% it has sheared off the ulna attachment and can be reattached using suture anchors.

In the more common central disruption, there is a valid concern as to whether the membrane can heal. There are a number of reasons for this observation. The edges of the torn ligament do not align in any forearm position and muscle tissue herniates between the torn edges. Finally, the loss of transverse stability allows for gapping between the radius and ulna. Werner has calculated this divergence to be significant going from 13 mm in an intact ligament to 23 mm when the ligament is torn.[41] This may explain why earlier prolonged immobilization or transient fixation with pins or syndesmotic screws across both bones yielded unpredictable results. This has directed our forearm strategy toward augmentation in the acute injury and reconstruction in the chronic type.

For augmentation we use a rerouted slip of the pronator teres or a suture button construct. The pronator teres rerouting was described by Kuzma and Ruch.[42] The fascia of the pronator teres is harvested in a proximal to distal direction to its radial insertion which is kept intact and reinforced with an anchor. The fascia is then rotated distally at a 20-degree angle and tunneled at the central band level to the distal ulna where it is attached via a drill hole with the tension set in mid-supination. A second and simpler option that we are using more frequently is to pass one or two suture buttons from the ulna to the radius. In passing either of these augments, care should be taken not to go too proximally and thus avoid the terminal branch of the posterior interosseous nerve. It is important to expose and protect the dorsal radial sensory nerve because the exit point of the suture button is most commonly between the radial wrist extensors and the brachioradialis.

In the chronic presentation status post radial head excision, the more symptomatic area is usually the ulnar impaction syndrome at the wrist. Here, the strategy is an ulnar shortening osteotomy, as long as the DRUJ is not arthritic. The desired amount of final variance is 2 mm negative, as our studies show the reconstruction subsides about 1 mm over 10 years.[13] Often the required amount of ulnar shortening is >5 mm, so it is helpful to use a jigged osteotomy system that can accommodate that degree of shortening. To allow for attachment of the central band construct, the plate is

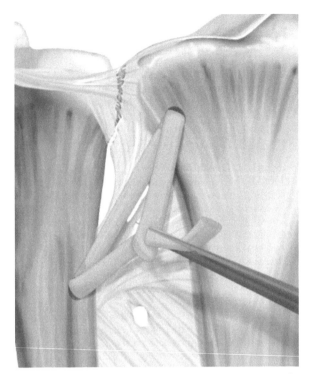

• **Fig. 56.8** Depiction of the distal oblique bundle reconstruction as described by Wright. The graft has been passed through the radius and ulna through a dorsal approach and will be weaved to itself for tensioning.

usually applied volarly or ulnarly. Such a joint leveling procedure has complications such as delayed and nonunion. Risk factors for these complications include smoking, poor bone quality, poor wrist motion, and the use of a double-blade saw.[43] If the joint is arthritic, we have recently been using a constrained DRUJ prosthesis.

To address the ulnar impaction lesion, a concomitant wrist arthroscopy is done to assess the degree of ulnar impaction and the state of the TFCC, lunatotriquetral ligament, and lunate and ulna articular surfaces. Arthroscopic debridement is usually performed.

To reconstruct the central band, a number of grafts have been evaluated both in vitro and in vivo.[12,42,44–49] Most tendon grafts have been unsuccessful, reflecting the inadequacy of replacing a ligament with a tendon. Laboratory studies have demonstrated that no graft substitute is as good as the native central band, but the patellar bone-ligament-bone graft was the closest equivalent.[47,50] We have used patellar bone-ligament-bone grafts exclusively for over 20 years. The initial study involved autografts, but over the last 10 years we have used allografts to reduce knee pain and have not noted any deterioration of results.[13,51]

At the elbow level, we will use a radial head implant if there is valgus instability but not routinely. Our initial 10-year follow-up study did not include replacement and in that series no evidence of recurrent proximal radiocapitellar impingement occurred.[13] Ouellette and Latta's cadaver study showed that normal forearm loading was best approximated by both radial head replacement and bone-ligament-bone reconstruction.[50] A future development that may prove very useful is a constrained proximal radioulnar joint replacement.

Outcomes

Early diagnosis and reparative treatment lead to an improved outcome in both acute and subacute cases. Jupiter had good to excellent outcomes in 78%–88% when the diagnosis was recognized and treated acutely.[24] Schnetzke confirmed that early recognition and treatment led to better DASH (The Disabilities of the Arm, Shoulder and Hand), Mayo Elbow and Wrist, and pain scores. However, in their acute series, despite an appropriate radial head strategy and immobilization, many patients had >2 mm of proximal migration likely because they did not have any DRUJ or central band augmentation. Even though patients with this subsidence had good clinical outcomes at 5 years, their grip strength was reduced and their clinical scores were inferior to those of patients with <2 mm of axial migration.[25] Gaspar and Osterman analyzed a series of acute and subacute cases where, besides stabilizing the elbow and DRUJ areas, a suture button was used to augment the central band. They concluded that this construct was effective with good patient outcomes in the short to midterm follow-up.[12] Similar results have been demonstrated by other authors.[52,53]

In chronic cases, historic treatment strategies often yielded poor results. Sowa reported on eight cases where proximal migration occurred after excision of the radial head. Although patients underwent a combination of silicone radial head replacement, DRUJ pinning, and an ulnar shortening procedure, all techniques failed to provide longitudinal stability.[27] Sotereanos et al. reported results in seven patients treated with radial head replacement and ulnar shortening osteotomy. At 33-month follow-up, there was significant improvement in elbow arc of motion (79–120 degrees), forearm rotation (76–112 degrees), and wrist motion (94–119 degrees). However, patients maintained an average of 3.5 mm of ulnar positive variance.[54]

Marcotte and Osterman described a surgical technique of IOM reconstruction using bone-patellar tendon-bone graft. At an average of 78 months, 15 of 16 patients reported improved wrist pain, grip strength improved from 59% to 86% of the unaffected arm, and no patients needed secondary surgery to address instability. However, 25% of patients reported knee pain, and thus the authors suggested considering an allograft.[51]

Gaspar and Osterman published a series of 33 patients who presented at an average of 10 months post radial head excision.[13] All were treated with ulnar shortening osteotomy and bone-patella-bone graft for IOM reconstruction. The series included both autograft and allograft reconstructions. Radial head replacement was rare, only performed in two patients. Patients were seen at a mean follow-up of 10.9 years. They reported significant improvements in range of motion of the elbow, wrist, and forearm, decreased pain, increased grip strength, and a high rate of good to excellent functional scores. Correction of ulnar variance improved from +3.9 mm preoperatively to −1.1 mm variance at final follow-up. No significant differences in performance were noted between autograft and allograft, and no cases of graft rejection were recorded. The most common complications were symptomatic hardware or nonunion from ulnar shortening osteotomy and residual knee pain in autograft patients.

Salvage

Despite encouraging results with reconstruction, not all patients with chronic Essex-Lopresti injuries are candidates. For those patients with severely limited forearm motion, excessive resections of the proximal radius or distal ulna, or where the reconstructive techniques are not applicable or have failed, then the creation of a one bone forearm is considered for definitive management.

References

1. Brockman EP. Two cases of disability at the wrist-joint following excision of the head of the radius. *Proc R Soc Med.* 1931;24(7):904–905.
2. Curr JF, Coe WA. Dislocation of the inferior radio-ulnar joint. *Br J Surg.* 1946;34:74–77. https://doi.org/10.1002/bjs.18003413312.
3. Essex-Lopresti P. Fractures of the radial head with distal radio-ulnar dislocation; report of two cases. *J Bone Joint Surg Br.* 1951;33B(2):244–247.
4. McGinley JC, Kozin SH. Interosseous membrane anatomy and functional mechanics. *Clin Orthop Relat Res.* 2001;383:108–122.
5. McGinley JC, Heller JE, Fertala A, Gaughan JP, Kozin SH. Biochemical composition and histologic structure of the forearm interosseous membrane. *J Hand Surg Am.* 2003;28(3):503–510. https://doi.org/10.1053/jhsu.2003.50059.
6. Hollister AM, Gellman H, Waters RL. The relationship of the interosseous membrane to the axis of rotation of the forearm. *Clin Orthop Relat Res.* 1994;298:272–276.
7. Noda K, Goto A, Murase T, Sugamoto K, Yoshikawa H, Moritomo H. Interosseous membrane of the forearm: an anatomical study of ligament attachment locations. *J Hand Surg Am.* 2009;34(3):415–422. https://doi.org/10.1016/j.jhsa.2008.10.025.
8. Pfaeffle HJ, Tomaino MM, Grewal R, et al. Tensile properties of the interosseous membrane of the human forearm. *J Orthop Res.* 1996;14(5):842–845. https://doi.org/10.1002/jor.1100140525.
9. Anderson A, Werner FW, Tucci ER, Harley BJ. Role of the interosseous membrane and annular ligament in stabilizing the proximal radial head. *J Shoulder Elbow Surg.* 2015;24(12):1926–1933. https://doi.org/10.1016/j.jse.2015.05.030.
10. Matthias R, Wright TW. Interosseous membrane of the forearm. *J Wrist Surg.* 2016;5(3):188–193. https://doi.org/10.1055/s-0036-1584326.
11. Birkbeck DP, Failla JM, Hoshaw SJ, Fyhrie DP, Schaffler M. The interosseous membrane affects load distribution in the forearm. *J Hand Surg Am.* 1997;22(6):975–980. https://doi.org/10.1016/S0363-5023(97)80035-4.
12. Gaspar MP, Kane PM, Pflug EM, Jacoby SM, Osterman AL, Culp RW. Interosseous membrane reconstruction with a suture-button construct for treatment of chronic forearm instability. *J Shoulder Elbow Surg.* 2016;25(9):1491–1500. https://doi.org/10.1016/j.jse.2016.04.018.
13. Gaspar MP, Adams JE, Zohn RC, et al. Late reconstruction of the interosseous membrane with bone-patellar tendon-bone graft for chronic Essex-Lopresti injuries: outcomes with a mean follow-up of over 10 years. *J Bone Joint Surg Am.* 2018;100(5):416–427. https://doi.org/10.2106/JBJS.17.00820.
14. Trousdale RT, Amadio PC, Cooney WP, Morrey BF. Radio-ulnar dissociation. A review of twenty cases. *J Bone Joint Surg Am.* 1992;74(10):1486–1497.
15. Hey HW, Chong AKS, Peng LL. Atypical Essex-Lopresti injury of the forearm: a case report. *J Orthop Surg.* 2011;19(3):373–375. https://doi.org/10.1177/230949901101900324.
16. McGinley JC, Hopgood BC, Gaughan JP, Sadeghipour K, Kozin SH. Forearm and elbow injury: the influence of rotational position. *J Bone Joint Surg Am.* 2003;85(12):2403–2409.
17. McGinley JC, D'addessi L, Sadeghipour K, Kozin SH. Mechanics of the antebrachial interosseous membrane: response to shearing forces. *J Hand Surg Am.* 2001;26(4):733–741. https://doi.org/10.1053/jhsu.2001.24961.
18. Wallace AL, Walsh WR, van Rooijen M, Hughes JS, Sonnabend DH. The interosseous membrane in radio-ulnar dissociation. *J Bone Joint Surg Br.* 1997;79(3):422–427. https://doi.org/10.1302/0301-620x.79b3.7142.
19. Wegmann K, Engel K, Burkhart KJ, et al. Sequence of the Essex-Lopresti lesion—a high-speed video documentation and kinematic analysis. *Acta Orthop.* 2014;85(2):177–180. https://doi.org/10.3109/17453674.2014.887952.
20. Hotchkiss RN, An KN, Sowa DT, Basta S, Weiland AJ. An anatomic and mechanical study of the interosseous membrane of the forearm: pathomechanics of proximal migration of the radius. *J Hand Surg Am.* 1989;14(2 Pt 1):256–261. https://doi.org/10.1016/0363-5023(89)90017-8.
21. Skahen JR, Palmer AK, Werner FW, Fortino MD. The interosseous membrane of the forearm: anatomy and function. *J Hand Surg Am.* 1997;22(6):981–985. https://doi.org/10.1016/S0363-5023(97)80036-6.
22. Duckworth AD, McQueen MM, Ring D. Fractures of the radial head. *Bone Joint Lett J.* 2013;95-B(2):151–159. https://doi.org/10.1302/0301-620X.95B2.29877.
23. Trousdale R, Osterman AL, Warhold L, Culp R, Bednar J. Reconstruction of the interosseous membrane using a bone-ligament-bone graft. In: *Presented at the American Society for Surgery of the Hand 52nd Annual Meeting, September 11.* Denver, CO; 1997.
24. Edwards GS, Jupiter JB. Radial head fractures with acute distal radioulnar dislocation. Essex-Lopresti revisited. *Clin Orthop Relat Res.* 1988;234:61–69.
25. Schnetzke M, Porschke F, Hoppe K, Studier-Fischer S, Gruetzner P-A, Guehring T. Outcome of early and late diagnosed Essex-Lopresti injury. *J Bone Joint Surg Am.* 2017;99(12):1043–1050. https://doi.org/10.2106/JBJS.16.01203.
26. Hausmann J-T, Vekszler G, Breitenseher M, Braunsteiner T, Vécsei V, Gäbler C. Mason type-I radial head fractures and interosseous membrane lesions—a prospective study. *J Trauma.* 2009;66(2):457–461. https://doi.org/10.1097/TA.0b013e31817fdedd.
27. Sowa DT, Hotchkiss RN, Weiland AJ. Symptomatic proximal translation of the radius following radial head resection. *Clin Orthop Relat Res.* 1995;317:106–113.
28. Failla JM, Jacobson J, van Holsbeeck M. Ultrasound diagnosis and surgical pathology of the torn interosseous membrane in forearm fractures/dislocations. *J Hand Surg Am.* 1999;24(2):257–266. https://doi.org/10.1053/jhsu.1999.0257.
29. Soubeyrand M, Lafont C, Oberlin C, France W, Maulat I, Degeorges R. The "muscular hernia sign": an original ultrasonographic sign to detect lesions of the forearm's interosseous membrane. *Surg Radiol Anat.* 2006;28(4):372–378. https://doi.org/10.1007/s00276-006-0100-5.
30. Starch DW, Dabezies EJ. Magnetic resonance imaging of the interosseous membrane of the forearm. *J Bone Joint Surg Am.* 2001;83(2):235–238. https://doi.org/10.2106/00004623-200102000-00011.
31. Fester EW, Murray PM, Sanders TG, Ingari JV, Leyendecker J, Leis HL. The efficacy of magnetic resonance imaging and ultrasound in detecting disruptions of the forearm interosseous membrane: a cadaver study. *J Hand Surg Am.* 2002;27(3):418–424. https://doi.org/10.1053/jhsu.2002.32961.
32. McGinley JC, Roach N, Hopgood BC, Limmer K, Kozin SH. Forearm interosseous membrane trauma: MRI diagnostic criteria and injury patterns. *Skeletal Radiol.* 2006;35(5):275–281. https://doi.org/10.1007/s00256-005-0069-x.
33. Smith AM, Urbanosky LR, Castle JA, Rushing JT, Ruch DS. Radius pull test: predictor of longitudinal forearm instability. *J Bone Joint Surg Am.* 2002;84(11):1970–1976.
34. Soubeyrand M, Ciais G, Wassermann V, et al. The intra-operative radius joystick test to diagnose complete disruption of the interosseous membrane. *J Bone Joint Surg Br.* 2011;93(10):1389–1394. https://doi.org/10.1302/0301-620X.93B10.26590.
35. Geel CW, Palmer AK. Radial head fractures and their effect on the distal radioulnar joint. A rationale for treatment. *Clin Orthop Relat Res.* 1992;275:79–84.
36. Ikeda M, Sugiyama K, Kang C, Takagaki T, Oka Y. Comminuted fractures of the radial head. Comparison of resection and internal fixation. *J Bone Joint Surg Am.* 2005;87(1):76–84. https://doi.org/10.2106/JBJS.C.01323.
37. Karlstad R, Morrey BF, Cooney WP. Failure of fresh-frozen radial head allografts in the treatment of Essex-Lopresti injury. A report of four cases. *J Bone Joint Surg Am.* 2005;87(8):1828–1833. https://doi.org/10.2106/JBJS.D.02351.

38. Gong HS, Chung MS, Oh JH, Lee YH, Kim SH, Baek GH. Failure of the interosseous membrane to heal with immobilization, pinning of the distal radioulnar joint, and bipolar radial head replacement in a case of Essex-Lopresti injury: case report. *J Hand Surg Am.* 2010;35(6):976–980. https://doi.org/10.1016/j.jhsa.2010.03.004.

39. Brink PRG, Hannemann PFW. Distal oblique bundle reinforcement for treatment of DRUJ instability. *J Wrist Surg.* 2015;4(3):221–228. https://doi.org/10.1055/s-0035-1556856.

40. Riggenbach MD, Conrad BP, Wright TW, Dell PC. Distal oblique bundle reconstruction and distal radioulnar joint instability. *J Wrist Surg.* 2013;2(4):330–336. https://doi.org/10.1055/s-0033-1358546.

41. Skahen JR, Palmer AK, Werner FW, Fortino MD. Reconstruction of the interosseous membrane of the forearm in cadavers. *J Hand Surg Am.* 1997;22(6):986–994. https://doi.org/10.1016/S0363-5023(97)80037-8.

42. Chloros GD, Wiesler ER, Stabile KJ, Papadonikolakis A, Ruch DS, Kuzma GR. Reconstruction of Essex-Lopresti injury of the forearm: technical note. *J Hand Surg Am.* 2008;33(1):124–130. https://doi.org/10.1016/j.jhsa.2007.09.008.

43. Cha SM, Shin HD, Ahn KJ. Prognostic factors affecting union after ulnar shortening osteotomy in ulnar impaction syndrome: a retrospective case-control study. *J Bone Joint Surg Am.* 2017;99(8):638–647. https://doi.org/10.2106/JBJS.16.00366.

44. Miller AJ, Naik TU, Seigerman DA, Ilyas AM. Anatomic interosseus membrane reconstruction utilizing the biceps button and screw tenodesis for Essex-Lopresti injuries. *Tech Hand Up Extrem Surg.* 2016;20(1):6–13. https://doi.org/10.1097/BTH.0000000000000107.

45. Tomaino MM, Pfaeffle J, Stabile K, Li Z-M. Reconstruction of the interosseous ligament of the forearm reduces load on the radial head in cadavers. *J Hand Surg Br.* 2003;28(3):267–270. https://doi.org/10.1016/s0266-7681(03)00012-3.

46. Gaspar MP, Kearns KA, Culp RW, Osterman AL, Kane PM. Single- versus double-bundle suture button reconstruction of the forearm interosseous membrane for the chronic Essex-Lopresti lesion. *Eur J Orthop Surg Traumatol.* 2018;28(3):409–413. https://doi.org/10.1007/s00590-017-2051-4.

47. Tejwani SG, Markolf KL, Benhaim P. Graft reconstruction of the interosseous membrane in conjunction with metallic radial head replacement: a cadaveric study. *J Hand Surg Am.* 2005;30(2):335–342. https://doi.org/10.1016/j.jhsa.2004.07.022.

48. Bigazzi P, Marenghi L, Biondi M, Zucchini M, Ceruso M. Surgical treatment of chronic Essex-Lopresti lesion: interosseous membrane reconstruction and radial head prosthesis. *Tech Hand Up Extrem Surg.* 2017;21(1):2–7. https://doi.org/10.1097/BTH.0000000000000143.

49. Adams JE, Osterman MN, Osterman AL. Interosseous membrane reconstruction for forearm longitudinal instability. *Tech Hand Up Extrem Surg.* 2010;14(4):222–225. https://doi.org/10.1097/BTH.0b013e3181e2457d.

50. Jones CM, Kam CC, Ouellette EA, Milne EL, Kaimrajh D, Latta LL. Comparison of 2 forearm reconstructions for longitudinal radioulnar dissociation: a cadaver study. *J Hand Surg Am.* 2012;37(4):741–747. https://doi.org/10.1016/j.jhsa.2012.01.025.

51. Marcotte AL, Osterman AL. Longitudinal radioulnar dissociation: identification and treatment of acute and chronic injuries. *Hand Clin.* 2007;23(2):195–208. https://doi.org/10.1016/j.hcl.2007.01.005.vi.

52. Drake ML, Farber GL, White KL, Parks BG, Segalman KA. Restoration of longitudinal forearm stability using a suture button construct. *J Hand Surg Am.* 2010;35(12):1981–1985. https://doi.org/10.1016/j.jhsa.2010.09.009.

53. Meals CG, Forthman CL, Segalman KA. Suture-button reconstruction of the interosseous membrane. *J Wrist Surg.* 2016;5(3):179–183. https://doi.org/10.1055/s-0036-1584547.

54. Venouziou AI, Papatheodorou LK, Weiser RW, Sotereanos DG. Chronic Essex-Lopresti injuries: an alternative treatment method. *J Shoulder Elbow Surg.* 2014;23(6):861–866. https://doi.org/10.1016/j.jse.2014.01.043.

57

Technique Spotlight: Interosseous Membrane Reconstruction

RYAN TARR, RICK TOSTI, AND A. LEE OSTERMAN

Indications

The primary indication to reconstruct the interosseous membrane (IOM) is a longitudinal radioulnar dissociation also known as an Essex-Lopresti injury (ELI). An ELI is an injury triad involving fracture of the radial head, rupture of the interosseous ligaments, and instability of the distal radioulnar joint (DRUJ). Early diagnosis is paramount for a favorable outcome, as timing affects the strategy of treatment.[1]

In the acute setting, the surgeon will repair or replace the radial head, repair the triangular fibrocartilage complex (TFCC), and stabilize the interosseous interval with a tendon graft or a suture-button device. Acutely diagnosed injuries with proper stabilization may yield a good result in 80% of cases. However, unrecognized injury and poor stabilization lead to an 80% failure rate.[2,3]

In the chronic setting, the radius has migrated proximally, and the IOM has no potential for healing. Radiocapitellar impingement and instability at the DRUJ are often identified. To address the pathology at the elbow, the radial head may be excised as long as axial stability has been reestablished, or it may be replaced with implant arthroplasty. Proximal radial migration also causes a relative shortening at the DRUJ with symptomatic ulnar impaction. Wrist arthroscopy is valuable to evaluate the lunate articular cartilage and the TFCC. Then, ulnar shortening osteotomy is utilized to correct the ulnar variance at the wrist. Finally, IOM reconstruction of the central band imparts additional stability to the forearm for force transmission and prevents further radial migration.

Preoperative Evaluation

A thorough history should focus on the mechanism of action and location of pain. An axial load injury should clue the physician to evaluate not only the elbow, but also the forearm and wrist. The elbow flexion-extension arc, as well as varus/valgus stability, should be scrutinized for a deficit compared to the contralateral extremity. Similarly, the wrist is examined to identify signs of ulna impaction. Examination should include evaluation for TFCC mechanical symptoms, foveal tenderness, and lunotriquetral (LT)

ballottement. The DRUJ is assessed in both supination and pronation to identify loss of motion or joint laxity.

Imaging of both the elbow and wrist should be obtained. Grip-loaded view or axial loading under fluoroscopy can be acquired to look for dynamic instability at the wrist. Greater than 6 mm of proximal migration is indicative of forearm dissociation. In the acute setting, advanced imaging can be used to assess the IOM. Magnetic resonance imaging (MRI) has been shown to identify IOM disruption; herniation of musculature through the IOM is pathognomonic. However, edematous or attenuated ligaments may be difficult to correlate with clinical stability. Ultrasound has also been used acutely albeit less commonly than MRI.

Equipment

- Wrist arthroscopy tower and instruments
- Radiolucent hand table
- Sagittal saw
- Mini C-arm fluoroscopy
- Ulna shortening osteotomy set versus 3.5-mm dynamic compression plate
- IOM reconstruction graft of choice (autograft, allograft, suture-button device)
- Radial head fixation and/or arthroplasty set

Positioning

The patient is positioned supine with the operative extremity on a hand table. A well-padded tourniquet is placed on the upper arm. Care is taken to make sure both the wrist and elbow are easily visualized with the mini C-arm. If not, a standard C-arm fluoroscopy unit is used.

After the arm is prepped and draped, the extremity is positioned in the arthroscopy tower with 10–15 pounds of traction applied. This is helpful regardless of whether wrist arthroscopy is planned or not as the axial traction helps to correct the radial proximal migration.

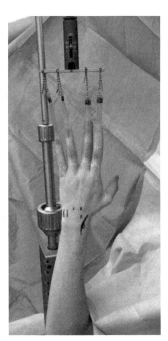

• **Fig. 57.1** Clinical photograph of wrist in skeletal traction with standard portals illustrated.

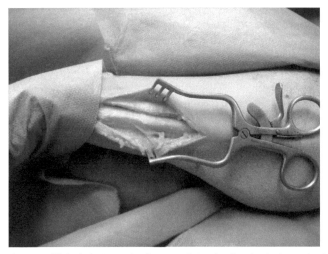

• **Fig. 57.2** Clinical photograph of approach to ulna for shortening osteotomy. Care is taken to stay 2 cm proximal to ulnar head to avoid iatrogenic injury to dorsal ulnar cutaneous nerve.

Detailed Technique Description of Treatment of Chronic ELI

Step 1: Wrist Arthroscopy

1. Using standard 3-4 and 6R portals, diagnostic wrist arthroscopy is performed (Fig. 57.1). Examination of the intrinsic and extrinsic ligaments, articular surface, and TFCC is performed. Synovectomy and debridement are performed as needed until a stable cartilage edge is achieved.
2. A half-filled syringe is then used to inject air into the midcarpal space to evaluate the integrity of the scapholunate (SL) and LT ligaments. Intact ligaments will cause distention, whereas torn ligaments will result in bubbles within the radiocarpal joint.

3. The midcarpal joint is then visualized through standard midcarpal radial and ulnar portals. The chondral surfaces are inspected paying close attention to the capitohamate region for signs of ulnar impaction and hamate arthrosis lunate triquetral (HALT) lesions. If identified, 2–3 mm of the proximal hamate are removed utilizing the arthroscopic shaver. The LT and SL are inspected from this perspective as well.

Step 2: Ulna Shortening Osteotomy

1. The arm is exsanguinated with an Esmarch and the tourniquet is elevated to 250 mm Hg.
2. Make a longitudinal incision in line with the subcutaneous border of the ulna approximately 10 cm long with the center approximately over the distal third of the ulna (near the insertion for the central band of the interosseous ligament).
3. Elevate the periosteum off of the ulna, but do not release extensor carpi ulnaris (ECU) from its subsheath. To protect the dorsal ulnar sensory branch, the surgeon should remain at least 2 cm from the articular surface of the distal ulna (Fig. 57.2).
4. Score the ulna longitudinally approximately 6–7 cm from the ulna styloid to mark the site for the IOM graft. This will also facilitate normalizing rotational alignment once the osteotomy is performed.
5. Perform the shortening osteotomy with either a commercial system or a 3.5-mm limited contact dynamic compression plate. The magnitude of the shortening osteotomy should be based on preoperative planning with a goal of 1–2 mm ulnar negative variance.
   a. We prefer an oblique osteotomy due to the increased surface contact area of the osteotomy. We also place the plate along the volar or subcutaneous border of the ulna as it allows for ease of graft placement along the dorsal surface for IOM reconstruction. If utilizing a suture-button reconstruction, place the plate on the volar or dorsal surface of the ulna.

Step 3: IOM Reconstruction

1. Ensure maximal tension is still applied using the wrist traction tower. Prior to placement of the IOM graft, confirm an ulnar negative variance using fluoroscopy. Next, pass a Kelly clamp proximally and radially along the dorsal aspect of the forearm between the IOM and extensor tendons (Fig. 57.3). This point of entry should intersect the radius at a 21-degree angle to recreate the central band.[4]
2. Make a 5-cm incision along the radius centered over the Kelly clamp. Identify interval between brachioradialis and extensor carpi radial longus (Fig. 57.4). Find and protect the superficial branch of the radial nerve. The interval is then extended revealing the dorsal aspect of the radius and pronator insertion.
3. In our technique, we utilize a bone-patellar-tendon allograft (Fig. 57.5). A trough is measured and created in the dorsal ulna approximately the same size as the bone graft. The graft is secured to the ulna with a 3.5-mm screw. The graft is then passed under the extensor tendons to the radial side and tensioned while supinating the wrist. The insertion site of the radius is marked, a trough is made, and the graft is secured to the radius with a 3.5-mm screw (Fig. 57.6).
4. The hand is removed from the traction tower and examined with axial loading under fluoroscopy. The surgeon should note the absence of axial instability and a functional range of pronation and supination at the forearm as well as flexion and extension at the elbow (Fig. 57.7).

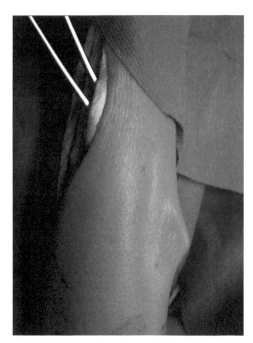

• **Fig. 57.3** Depiction of Kelly clamps passed distal to proximal along the dorsal aspect of the interosseous membrane at an approximate angle of 21 degrees.

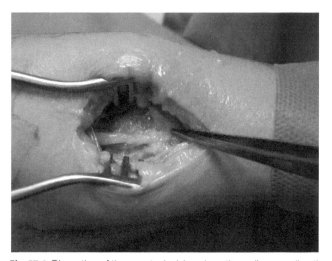

• **Fig. 57.4** Dissection of the counter incision along the radius revealing the place between the brachioradialis and the extensor carpi radialis longus.

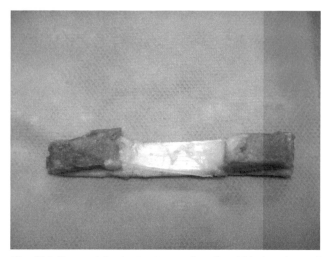

• **Fig. 57.5** Bone-patellar-tendon-bone allograft, which has been the authors' preferred graft.

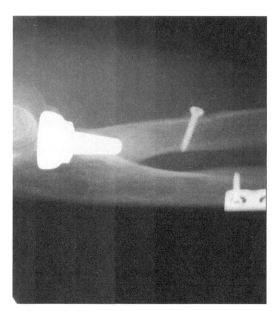

• **Fig. 57.6** Radiograph demonstrating fixation of bone-tendon-bone plug into radial trough using 3.5-mm screw.

5. We prefer to perform a radial head excision if one exists. If the radial head had already been previously removed, then the radiocapitellar joint is not addressed. The senior author has observed that the radius tends to settle 1–2 mm, which can lead to radiocapitellar impingement and decreased flexion-extension arc within an intact radial head.[1]

Step 4: Closure

1. The tourniquet is released, and hemostasis is obtained. The skin is closed in a layered fashion.
2. Final radiographs of the wrist, forearm, and elbow are obtained.
3. A sterile dressing and long arm plaster splint are placed.

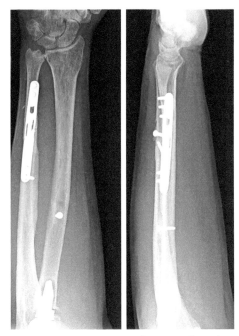

• **Fig. 57.7** Anteroposterior and lateral radiographs of a patient who underwent radial head replacement, ulna shortening osteotomy, and interosseous membrane reconstruction 11 years prior. Radiographs reveal no recurrent radial migration or radiocapitellar impingement.

PEARLS AND PITFALLS

Pearls

- A complete physical examination is paramount. There are multiple variants to the typical ELI. Case reports have reported ELIs in radial head dislocations and Monteggia fracture-dislocations. It is imperative to examine the elbow, forearm, and wrist in the setting of an axial load injury to the wrist.
- The ulnar insertion of the IOM is one-third the length of the ulna from the ulnar styloid. The radial insertion is approximately 60% of the radial length from the radial styloid.[5]
- Take care to protect the dorsal ulnar sensory branch as well as the anterior and posterior interosseous nerve.
- The central band is shortest in supination, so tensioning should be done in this position to prevent laxity during forearm rotation.
- Although the central band only measures 4 cm, a soft tissue graft needs to be at least 11 cm for appropriate tensioning during reconstruction.[6] Bone-tendon-bone (BTB) graft lengths are not adjustable and therefore can lead to variation in graft placement and trajectory.

Pitfalls

- A radial head excision in isolation is never indicated acutely, and only in chronic cases where there is preexisting radiocapitellar arthritis.
- A transosseous tunnel technique can compromise cortical integrity of bone as fractures have been reported in the postoperative period. Some authors prophylactically plate in this setting.[7]

References

1. Marcotte AL, Osterman AL. Longitudinal radioulnar dissociation: identification and treatment of acute and chronic injuries. *Hand Clin.* 2007;23(2):195–208. https://doi.org/10.1016/j.hcl.2007.01.005. vi.
2. Trousdale RT, Amadio PC, Cooney WP, Morrey BF. Radioulnar dissociation. A review of twenty cases. *J Bone Joint Surg Am.* 1992;74(10):1486–1497.
3. Edwards GS, Jupiter JB. Radial head fractures with acute distal radioulnar dislocation. Essex-Lopresti revisited. *Clin Orthop Relat Res.* 1988;234:61–69.
4. Skahen JR, Palmer AK, Werner FW, Fortino MD. The interosseous membrane of the forearm: anatomy and function. *J Hand Surg Am.* 1997;22(6):981–985. https://doi.org/10.1016/S0363-5023(97)80036-6.
5. Noda K, Goto A, Murase T, Sugamoto K, Yoshikawa H, Moritomo H. Interosseous membrane of the forearm: an anatomical study of ligament attachment locations. *J Hand Surg Am.* 2009;34(3):415–422. https://doi.org/10.1016/j.jhsa.2008.10.025.
6. Chandler JW, Stabile KJ, Pfaeffle HJ, Li Z-M, Woo SL-Y, Tomaino MM. Anatomic parameters for planning of interosseous ligament reconstruction using computer-assisted techniques. *J Hand Surg Am.* 2003;28(1):111–116. https://doi.org/10.1053/jhsu.2003.50033.
7. Miller AJ, Naik TU, Seigerman DA, Ilyas AM. Anatomic interosseous membrane reconstruction utilizing the biceps button and screw tenodesis for Essex-Lopresti injuries. *Tech Hand Up Extrem Surg.* 2016;20(1):6–13. https://doi.org/10.1097/BTH.0000000000000107.

58

Radial and Ulnar Shaft Fractures: Choice of Approach, Nails vs. Plates, Compression Tips and Tricks

ROBIN KAMAL AND NATHANIEL FOGEL

Relevant Anatomy

The diaphyseal forearm functions to provide a stable platform upon which the hand can be positioned in space, as well as to facilitate forearm rotation. The ulna functions as the dominant load-bearing structure, with the radius rotating about it in pronation and supination. The soft tissue envelope about the diaphysis of the forearm is composed of the superficial and deep volar compartments, the extensor compartment, and the mobile wad. Transiting neurovascular structures are at risk both at the time of injury and during the surgical approach. Proximally, the median nerve enters the mid-forearm between the heads of pronator teres and runs between flexor digitorum superficialis (FDS) and flexor digitorum profundus (FDP). The anterior interosseous nerve branches from the proper median nerve at the proximal aspect of FDS and courses between the two heads of FDS. More distally, the palmar cutaneous nerve comes off the median nerve 8.5 cm from the volar wrist crease, putting it at risk during the surgical approach for distal-third fractures. The ulnar nerve exits the cubital tunnel between the heads of flexor carpi ulnaris (FCU) and travels between FDP and FCU as it traverses the mid-forearm.[1] The radial nerve divides in the proximal forearm into the posterior interosseous nerve (PIN) and the superficial sensory branch. The course of the PIN is particularly important in considering the treatment of radial shaft fractures, as it runs in close proximity to the proximal third of the radial shaft and pierces through the supinator, placing it at risk from traumatic injury as well as from iatrogenic injury during a surgical exposure. The superficial radial nerve is also at risk as it travels deep to brachioradialis throughout the entirety of the mid-forearm before exiting dorsally 8 cm proximal to the radial styloid. The nerve travels with the radial artery beneath brachioradialis, with the radial artery coming off the brachial artery as it passes beneath the bicipital aponeurosis.[2]

At the diaphysis, the structures of the interosseous membrane (IOM) are the primary stabilizers of the radius in axial load and pronosupination. The IOM also contributes to the stability of the proximal radioulnar joint (PRUJ) as well as resists proximal migration of the ulna relative to the radius.[3] The distal radioulnar joint (DRUJ) and the PRUJ play important roles in stability proximally and distally and are often injured in the setting of shaft fractures. Radiographic fracture displacement is itself a marker of potential significant disruption of the IOM, and subsequent instability.[4] The IOM is divided into distal and proximal membranous portions, with a middle ligamentous portion providing stability in the mid-diaphysis (Fig. 58.1). The complex mechanism

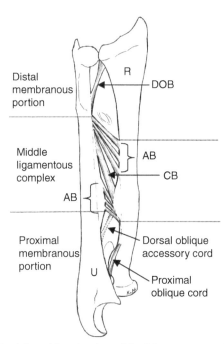

• **Fig. 58.1** Depiction of the structure of the interosseus membrane anatomy. *AB*, Accessory band; *CB*, central band; *DOB*, distal oblique bundle; *R*, radius; *U*, ulna. (With permission from Noda K, Goto A, Murase T, Sugamoto K, Yoshikawa H, Moritomo H. Interosseous membrane of the forearm: an anatomical study of ligament attachment locations. *J Hand Surg.* 2009;34A:415-422.)

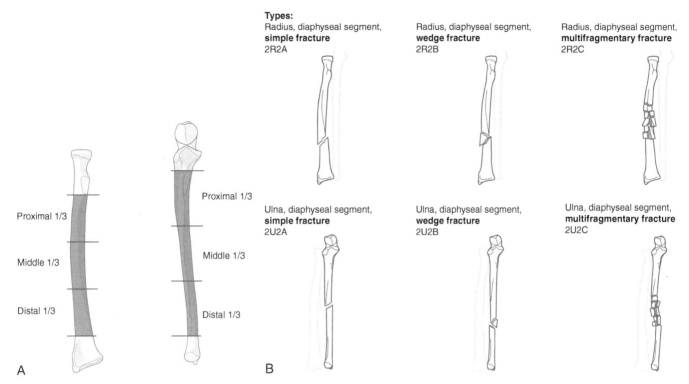

Types:
Radius, diaphyseal segment, **simple fracture** 2R2A

Radius, diaphyseal segment, **wedge fracture** 2R2B

Radius, diaphyseal segment, **multifragmentary fracture** 2R2C

Proximal 1/3

Middle 1/3

Distal 1/3

Proximal 1/3

Middle 1/3

Distal 1/3

Ulna, diaphyseal segment, **simple fracture** 2U2A

Ulna, diaphyseal segment, **wedge fracture** 2U2B

Ulna, diaphyseal segment, **multifragmentary fracture** 2U2C

A

B

• **Fig. 58.2** (A) The diaphysis of the radius and ulna is divided into the proximal 1/3, middle 1/3, and distal 1/3. *There is no uniformly agreed-upon classification for fractures* of the diaphysis of the radius and ulna. (B) AO classification fractures of the diaphysis of the ulna and radius. (With permission from Meinberg EG, Agel J, Roberts CS, Karam MD, Kellam JF. Fracture and dislocation classification and compendium. *J Orthop Trauma.* 2018;32(1):S24.)

of forearm rotation is predicated upon the anatomic relationship between the bowed radius and the relatively straight ulna. The bow of the radius is directed radially and dorsally and establishes a spatial relationship between the radius, ulna, and IOM.[3] Disruption of this relationship leads to functional deficit, primarily in pronosupination, often necessitating surgical intervention to restore the native anatomy.[2] In addition to establishing length, alignment, and rotation, recreating the radial bow is essential in the treatment of forearm fractures.

Pathoanatomy

Fractures of the diaphyseal radius and ulna are typically the result of a high-energy trauma or fall. Both bone forearm fractures often result from an axial load through the hand and wrist, or in the case of isolated ulnar shaft fractures, a direct blow to the medial forearm.[2,5] It is important in the initial evaluation of these injuries to rule out associated injuries at the wrist and elbow. Radial and ulnar shaft fractures as discussed in this chapter are distinct from related injuries such as Galeazzi and Monteggia fractures and are isolated from the wrist joint distally and the elbow joint proximally.

Classification

There is no universally accepted classification method for diaphyseal forearm fractures.[6] For the purposes of surgical intervention, the radial and ulnar shafts are divided into thirds (Fig. 58.2A). The proximal third is demarcated by the radial tuberosity and the beginning of the radial bow, with the middle third encompassing the bow to the point where the diaphysis begins to straighten distally,

and the distal third ending at the metaphyseal flare. The AO classification is most useful in aiding decision-making on direct versus indirect reduction, approach, and implant choice (Fig. 58.2B).

Isolated ulnar shaft fractures are classified as either "stable" or "unstable." Stable fractures are considered those in the mid-third or distal third of the diaphysis with <50% displacement or 10 degrees of angulation. Fractures with >50% displacement, >10 degrees of angulation, and those involving the proximal third are generally more unstable. Those associated with instability at the PRUJ and DRUJ are inherently unstable and represent a distinct entity from isolated shaft fractures.[4]

Treatment Options

Given the importance of anatomic reduction of radial shaft in maintaining range of motion in pronation and supination, nearly all radial shaft fractures in adults are treated with operative intervention. Only in the setting of limited baseline function or specific patient goals of care would nonoperative management be considered. Isolated ulnar shaft fractures, however, are often amenable to nonoperative measures and there remains no absolute indication for surgical intervention.[4] The primary distinction in the management of isolated ulnar shaft fractures is dictated by whether the fracture is deemed stable or unstable, as discussed above. Functional bracing provides stability while allowing for range of motion at the elbow and is preferred for nonoperative management over long arm cast immobilization. Completely nondisplaced fractures of the radius may also be treated with a period of cast immobilization, but these are rare.

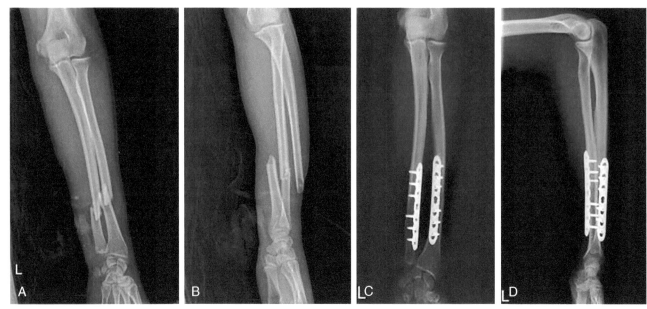

• **Fig. 58.3** Radiographs (A) and (B) are of a 26-year-old male with a diaphyseal both bone forearm fracture. (C) and (D) demonstrate union following open reduction internal fixation after compression plating. (With permission from Lee S, Kim K, Choy W. Plate osteosynthesis versus intramedullary nailing for both forearm bones fractures. *Eur J Orthop Surg Traumatol.* 2014;24:769-776.)

Plate fixation is the mainstay of surgical treatment for fractures of the radial and ulnar diaphysis (Fig. 58.3). Open reduction and fixation allows for anatomic reduction of the radial bow, provides the surgeon with the option to bone graft primarily should there be extensive bone loss, and has a proven track record in the literature with a high rate of union.[7–9] Plate fixation can provide a rigid construct, theoretically allowing for primary bone healing and minimal callus formation. In the setting of the complex anatomic relationship of the radius and ulna with respect to forearm rotation, this is a potential benefit over a relative stability construct generating robust callus in close proximity to the IOM. In the setting of extensive comminution, bridge plate constructs are optimal to help maintain length and rotation. Postoperative immobilization can be minimal, and patients are able to begin early range of motion at the wrist and elbow. However, open reduction internal fixation (ORIF) of the forearm comes with well-documented challenges related to management of soft tissues, as well as the neurovascular structures in close proximity to the radial and ulnar diaphysis. Plating of the radius often necessitates attempting to fit a straight plate at the apex of the radial bow, which can lead to malreduction if not appropriately contoured or positioned.[10] The recommended approaches, potential pitfalls, and outcomes related to plate fixation are detailed in the remainder of this chapter.

Intramedullary (IM) fixation is a frequently used technique for stabilization of long bones in both upper and lower extremities (Fig. 58.4). However, while the IM constructs for the forearm have been frequently employed in the pediatric population, nailing of diaphyseal radius and ulna fractures in adults remains relatively rare in comparison. The first IM devices used for forearm fixation were a series of unlocked implants, including K-wires and Rush rods.[11,12] Historically, IM implants were problematic for a number of reasons. While the length, alignment, and rotation of the relatively straight ulna seemed amenable to IM fixation, it was difficult to restore the natural anatomic bow of the radius. Unlocked nailing constructs were prone to rotational deformity. Biomechanical studies of unlocked nails demonstrate less stiffness

to torsion, with increased distraction at the fracture site compared to plate constructs.[13] With the advent of interlocked and precontoured implants, modern IM devices are potential options for the treatment of isolated shaft and both bone forearm fractures. IM implants offer the benefit of respecting a soft tissue envelope in the acute setting, often are associated with shorter operative times and lead to less periosteal stripping.[14] Furthermore, they can easily span the entire length of the radius or ulna, offering stabilization to the entirety of the bone in the setting of a pathologic fracture.[11] Contraindications to nailing include active osseous infection, canal diameter too small to accommodate implants (generally 3 mm), and intra-articular fractures requiring reduction and subsequent fixation.[12] Despite design advances, IM fixation still has limitations—it requires longer postoperative immobilization compared to ORIF, has lower torsional stiffness compared to plate constructs, is suboptimal for maintaining length and rotation in the setting of extensive comminution, and can be associated with distraction at fracture site when compared to compression plating.[11]

Indications for Surgical Treatment

In the case of isolated fractures of the ulna, surgical treatment is indicated in the case of an unstable fracture of the distal or middle third. As previously discussed, radiographic parameters of 50% displacement and 10 degrees of angulation are generally accepted cutoffs for surgical intervention. Isolated fractures of the proximal third are typically more unstable and have been shown historically to be associated with decreased range of motion with nonoperative management compared with operative fixation.[15] Other indications include open fracture and neurovascular compromise, though injury to the ulnar neurovascular bundle in the case of an isolated, closed ulnar shaft fracture is rare.[4] Fixation in the polytraumatized patient is a weak relative indication, but should be considered if lengthy immobilization in a fracture brace or long arm cast will limit their ability to participate in therapy.

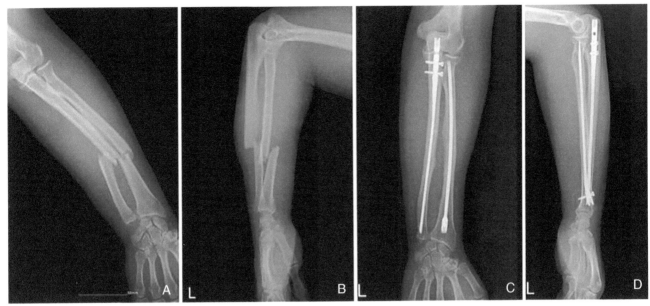

• **Fig. 58.4** Radiographs (A) and (B) are of a 56-year-old female with a diaphyseal both bone forearm fracture. (C) and (D) demonstrate union following intramedullary nailing. (With permission from Lee S, Kim K, Choy W. Plate osteosynthesis versus intramedullary nailing for both forearm bones fractures. *Eur J Orthop Surg Traumatol*. 2014;24:769-776.)

Given the importance of anatomic reduction of the radial bow to forearm rotation, essentially all radial shaft and both bone forearm fractures should be treated with operative intervention except in rare cases where the patient is unable to tolerate surgery.

Surgical Approaches and Techniques

Approaches for ORIF

The anterior or volar approach of Henry provides an extensile approach to the forearm, allowing for access from the radial head to the radial styloid through a single incision. This utilitarian approach is amenable to fracture fixation for all diaphyseal fractures of the radius and can be extended to access additional pathology both proximally and distally. Ample overlying flexor musculature provides for volar instrumentation to be placed without concern for irritation of the subcutaneous tissues.[2]

The skin is incised along a line from the insertion of the distal biceps to the radial styloid (Fig. 58.5). For diaphyseal fractures such as those addressed in this chapter, the fascia of the volar compartment is incised in longitudinal fashion off the ulnar edge of the brachioradialis. The radial artery is then identified and protected as the interval between brachioradialis and the proper radial artery is further developed. At the level of the mid-forearm, the radial artery may be deep to the brachioradialis muscle belly prior to emerging as it travels into the distal third. As the relationship between the brachioradialis and the radial artery is defined, the superficial sensory branch of the radial nerve will also be encountered. More proximally, the lateral antebrachial cutaneous nerve transits between the brachioradialis and the distal biceps and should be protected. The superficial dissection of this approach is relatively constant, while the deep dissection interval differs depending on whether exposure is needed proximally or distally.

Distally, the radial shaft is accessed between the radial artery and flexor carpi radialis (FCR; Fig. 58.6A–B). The underlying flexor pollicis longus and pronator quadratus (PQ) are released

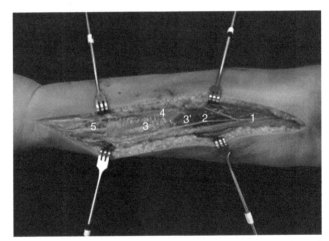

• **Fig. 58.5** Superficial exposure for the volar (Henry) approach to the radius. The skin incision is made in a straight line from the radial aspect of the flexor carpi radialis (FCR) tendon to the insertion of the distal biceps tendon. *(1)* cephalic vein; *(2)* lateral antebrachial cutaneous nerve; *(3)* brachioradialis tendon; *(3')* brachioradialis muscle belly; *(4)* FCR; and *(5)* radial artery. (With permission from Ballesteros-Betancourt J, Llusa-Perez M, Sanchez-Sotelo J. Surgical exposures of the forearm. In: Morrey BF, Sanchez-Sotelo J, Morrey ME, eds. *Morrey's The Elbow and Its Disorders*. 5th ed. Philadelphia, PA: Elsevier; 2018.)

from the radial border of the shaft and elevated ulnarly to allow for fracture reduction and instrumentation. Proximally, the insertion of the distal biceps provides a point of orientation for the interval of deep dissection. The bursa lying lateral to the biceps tendon is entered and dissected. The radial artery remains medial to the distal biceps and should remain medial to the tendon as the approach is carried deep. The recurrent branch of the radial artery is encountered off the ulnar edge of the brachioradialis. It can be ligated if its course interferes with further dissection. Supination of the forearm brings the supinator muscle belly into view. The forearm should remain supinated as the supinator is subperiosteally elevated off

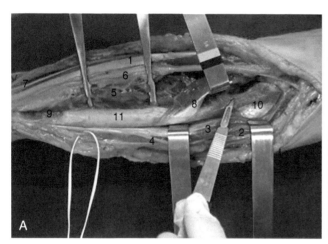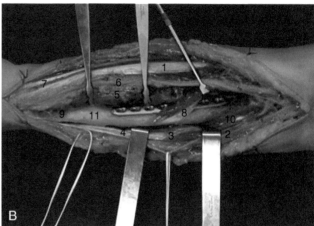

• **Fig. 58.6** (A) and (B) Deep exposure for the volar (Henry) approach to the radius. Pronator teres may be released if necessary, though its attachment can be left intact with instrumentation placed via tunneling under the muscle belly. *(1)* Flexor carpi radialis; *(2)* brachioradialis; *(3)* extensor carpi radialis longus; *(4)* superficial radial nerve; *(5)* flexor pollicis longus; *(6)* radial artery; *(7)* palmaris longus; *(8)* pronator teres; *(9)* pronator quadratus; *(10)* supinator; and *(11)* radial shaft. (With permission from Ballesteros-Betancourt J, Llusa-Perez M, Sanchez-Sotelo J. Surgical exposures of the forearm. In: Morrey BF, Sanchez-Sotelo J, Morrey ME, eds. *Morrey's The Elbow and Its Disorders*. 5th ed. Philadelphia, PA: Elsevier; 2018.)

the ulnar aspect of the radius to protect the PIN. Care should be taken to avoid placing retractors around the posterior aspect of the proximal radial shaft. Pronator teres is divided and elevated off its insertion onto the radius to provide exposure for plate fixation of the diaphysis and proximal third of the radius if needed.

The dorsal approach to the forearm, or Thompson approach, allows access to the entire length of the forearm (Fig. 58.7A–B).[16] Surface landmarks of the exposure are the lateral epicondyle of the humerus and Lister's tubercle, with a skin incision being a straight line between these points. The proximal interval utilizes the plane between extensor carpi radialis brevis (ECRB) and the extensor digitorum communis (EDC). Abductor pollicis longus (APL) and extensor pollicis brevis (EPB) come through this interval more distally in the mid-forearm and are useful in identifying the proper intermuscular plane before. Proximal dissection can work proximally from this point. The supinator lies deep to this interval, with the PIN piercing the muscle approximately 3 cm distal to the radiocapitellar joint.[17] The forearm is supinated to move the PIN out of the way prior to elevation of the muscle belly from the radius to allow for access to the diaphysis of the radius. The course of the PIN proximally as it crosses the radial neck limits the Thompson from being a true extensile approach proximally. Distally, the interval between ECRB and extensor pollicis longus (EPL) is exploited to expose the distal third of the radial shaft.

Advantages to the dorsal approach include access to fractures of the proximal third of the radius without the extensive dissection required in the volar proximal third. This negates the need for dissection of the recurrent radial vessels and allows access to the radial neck if fixation needs to be extended proximally.[18] More distally, the radius is relatively subcutaneous in the dorsal interval, again limiting soft tissue manipulation. Further, dorsal plating allows for positioning the implant on the tension side of the diaphysis, which is optimal from the perspective of AO principles. For middle-third diaphyseal fractures without proximal extension, the volar approach remains the mainstay surgical approach.

In the setting of an isolated ulnar shaft fracture or in both bone forearm fractures, the ulna is traditionally accessed via the approach to the subcutaneous border of the ulna. The interval

between FCU and extensor carpi ulnaris (ECU) is developed in longitudinal fashion centered over the fracture. If the fracture is in the distal third, the dorsal ulnar sensory nerve can be found in the subcutaneous tissues at the distal aspect of the incision and should be protected. Implants should be placed on the volar or dorsal aspect. Plates can be placed on the subcutaneous border of the ulna, though this subcutaneous location can result in prominent hardware that may necessitate removal at a later date.[4]

While the volar and dorsal approaches have traditionally been the workhorse approaches for ORIF of radial and ulnar shaft fracture, alternative surgical approaches have been described. A single incision volar approach utilizes a radial window and ulnar window for access to distal-third both bone forearm fractures through a single incision. A skin incision is made over palmaris longus (PL), and the superficial interval between FCR and PL is utilized. The radial window is accessed through the FCR sheath, with FCR being taken radially, and FPL and FDS retracted ulnar. PQ is released in its radial insertion. The ulnar window utilizes the interval between FCU and FDS. FDS and FDP are released at their ulnar border and the ulnar neurovascular bundle is identified, protected, and taken ulnarly.[1] The risks associated with this approach are similar to the volar Henry with regard to the radial window, along with relative increased risk to the ulnar neurovascular bundle.

For diaphyseal fractures of the radius, a direct lateral approach has also been described. The incision is made in line from the radial styloid to the lateral epicondyle of the humerus at the level of the fracture. The interval between brachioradialis and ECRL is utilized to access the fracture site. The attachment of the pronator teres at the lateral aspect of the radius is released while maintaining the dorsal attachment to create space for a plate.[19] The proposed benefit of this approach is that it eliminates the risk of injury to the PIN that comes with the dorsal approach, as well as the potential insult to the radial artery and its branches that comes with a volar approach. In the lateral approach, the superficial radial nerve may be encountered more distally, as it traverses from under brachioradialis through the fascia approximately 8 cm proximal to the radial styloid.[2]

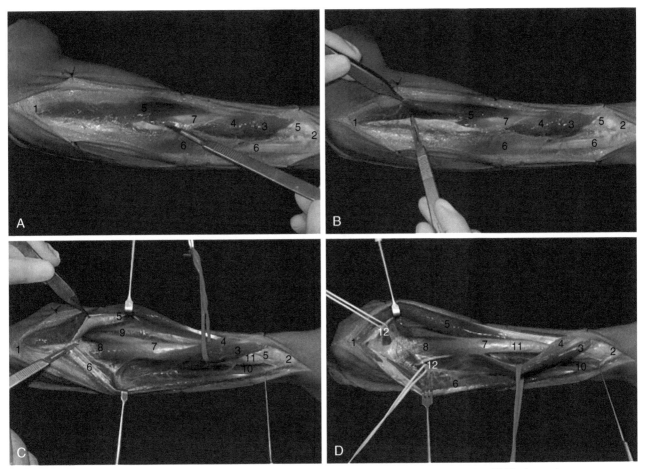

• **Fig. 58.7** (A) The superficial exposure of the dorsal (Thompson) approach to the radius. (B) The interval between extensor digitorum communis (EDC) and extensor carpi radialis brevis (ECRB) is developed. (C) Supinator is exposed beneath EDC and ECRB. (D) Posterior interosseous nerve and its relationship to supinator can be seen. *(1)* Lateral epicondyle; *(2)* Lister's tubercle; *(3)* extensor pollicis brevis; *(4)* abductor pollicis longus; *(5)* ECRB; *(6)* EDC; *(7)* pronator teres; *(8)* supinator; *(9)* superficial radial nerve; *(10)* extensor pollicis longus; *(11)* radial shaft; and *(12)* radial nerve. (With permission from Ballesteros-Betancourt J, Llusa-Perez M, Sanchez-Sotelo J. Surgical exposures of the forearm. In: Morrey BF, Sanchez-Sotelo J, Morrey ME, eds. *Morrey's The Elbow and Its Disorders*. 5th ed. Philadelphia, PA: Elsevier; 2018.)

Approaches for IM Nailing

Proper approach and surgical technique are crucial to successful treatment of radial and ulnar shaft fractures with IM devices. The patient is positioned in either the supine or lateral position with the elbow flexed at 90 degrees about a post or arm holder allowing sustained axial traction of the forearm to be applied.[20] When addressing the ulna, the procedure is typically performed with the identification of the proximal start point at the olecranon tip under fluoroscopic guidance (Fig. 58.8). A 10-mm incision is made just radial to the center of the olecranon to allow for passage of the awl and reamers. Care should be taken to avoid drifting ulnar off the tip of the olecranon to protect the ulnar nerve.[21] The triceps is split longitudinally to facilitate the entry of the opening awl and any subsequent reamers.[12] In the setting of both bone forearm fractures, it is recommended that the ulna be nailed first in part to provide stability for the subsequent retrograde nailing of the radius. Traction and manual manipulation of the fracture is required and necessitates the use of a surgical assistant. A limited open reduction can be utilized if soft tissues allow (Fig. 58.9). Nail sizing should be approximated during preoperative planning with the use of injury radiographs or contralateral films if available.

While the specifics can vary based on implant model and manufacturer, the length of the ulnar implant is typically measured from the tip of the olecranon to 1 cm proximal to the ulnar head.

Nailing of the radius is achieved via either radial styloid or second dorsal compartment entry site. For second dorsal compartment entry, a small incision is made just radial to Lister's and the EPL is protected and typically mobilized ulnar. The start point is typically 5 mm to 1 cm proximal to the articular surface of the dorsal aspect of the distal radius, though it can vary slightly depending on implant specifications (Fig. 58.10). Care must be taken to ensure that any interlocking screw in the proximal radius must be at least 3 cm distal to the radial head, and placed radial to ulnar, in order to avoid iatrogenic injury to the PIN. Postoperative care typically includes 10–14 days in a long arm splint or cast given the inferior rotational control with an IM implant (Fig. 58.11).

Relevant Complications

Complications related to treatment of diaphyseal radius and ulna fracture are not an infrequent occurrence. A recent meta-analysis

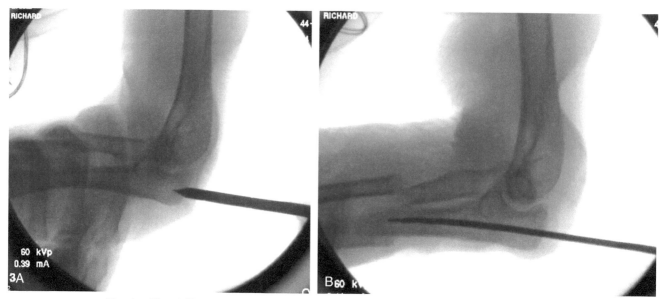

• **Fig. 58.8** (A) and (B) Lateral fluoroscopic imaging demonstrating appropriate start point (A) and passage (B) of the nail for antegrade nailing of the ulna.

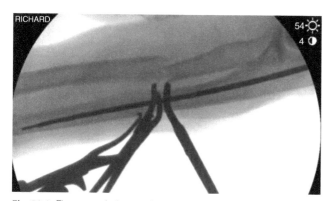

• **Fig. 58.9** Fluoroscopic image demonstrating clamp application to hold alignment after a limited open reduction was performed.

of plate fixation versus IM nailing for both bone forearm fractures reported an overall complication rate of 21.6% and 13.7%, respectively.[22]

Nonunion and delayed union of the radius and ulna are relatively uncommon. Historically, nonunion rates were reported as high as 10%, but recent studies with modern compression plating and IM fixation report rates between 2% and 5%.[4,7,23,24] Malunion represents a unique complication in the treatment of radial shaft fractures, as failure to restore the anatomic relationship of the radius and ulna, as well as the native radial bow, has been shown to lead to disability and loss of forearm pronosupination.[5] Cadaveric studies suggest that malunion resulting in <10 degrees of deformity of the radius or ulna is likely to be tolerated.[9] Even with anatomic reduction and union, loss of motion in the pronosupination arc is a known complication of the treatment of both bone forearm fractures, with small but statistically significant limitations in motion present even in long-term follow-up.[8] The majority of forearm malunions are the result of nonoperative management of pediatric fractures with a loss of reduction.

Postoperative radioulnar synostosis or robust callous formation can occur whether operative or nonoperative treatment is pursued. The incidence of postoperative synostosis is low in the setting of appropriate surgical technique (1.2%–6%) and early range

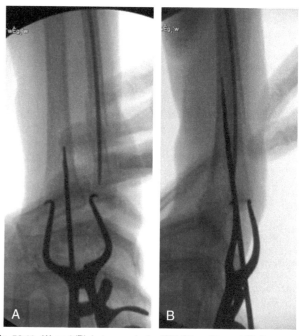

• **Fig. 58.10** (A) and (B) Anteroposterior (AP) (A) and lateral (B) fluoroscopic images demonstrating appropriate start point and initial passage of the intramedullary implant after successful instrumentation of the ulna.

of motion postoperative protocols.[2,6] Thought to be associated with soft tissue trauma and injury to the IOM, the incidence of synostosis is increased in the setting of concomitant head injury. Radioulnar synostosis is classified on its given location, with type I involving the DRUJ, type II involving the middle third of the forearm, and type III involving the proximal third. Surgical resection should be deferred until there is no radiographic evidence of expanding heterotopic bone formation. Recurrence of heterotopic ossification after excision is highest in type I and type III.[25] Postoperative heterotopic ossification prophylaxis with perioperative radiation or nonsteroidal anti-inflammatory medication is not routinely recommended as there is no consensus on the efficacy of

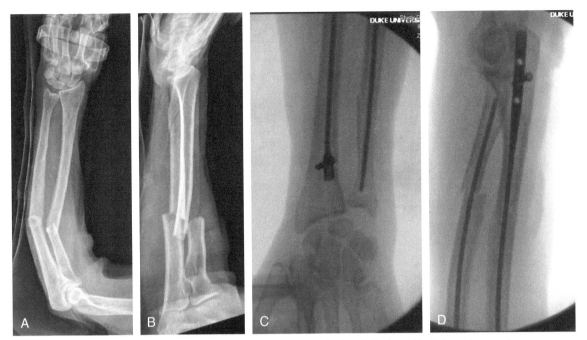

• **Fig. 58.11** (A) and (B) Injury radiographs demonstrating displaced diaphyseal both bone forearm fractures. (C) and (D) Fluoroscopic images demonstrating final alignment and construct after intramedullary fixation for both bone forearm fractures.

these modalities. However, small cohort studies have shown good results with resection and irradiation, as well as with resection and placement of interposition material.[26]

A high rate of hardware removal after ORIF has been documented in numerous studies. Refracture after plate represents a nontrivial complication of ORIF.[27] Yao et al. published on 122 patients with history of diaphyseal forearm fractures who underwent ORIF and reported at 12.9% refracture rate in patients who underwent hardware removal compared with 2.8% in those who retained their implants. Further, all refractures in the retained hardware group were as a result of high-energy trauma, whereas those who underwent implant removal sustained refracture related to lower energy mechanisms.[28] They reported no significant difference in mean time to implant removal between those who went on to refracture and those who did not (14.8 and 19 months, respectively). Hidaka et al. reported an increased risk of refracture when implant removal occurred prior to 1 year postoperatively, as four of the seven refractures in their study occurred when removal took place prior to 12 months from the index procedure.[29] Other studies published in the literature recommend waiting at least 18 months prior to removal if possible.[27,28,30]

Compartment syndrome represents a rare but potentially devastating consequence of radial and ulnar shaft fractures. A systematic review by Kalyani et al. found the overall complication rate of forearm compartment syndrome to be 42%, with neurologic deficit and contracture being the two most common etiologies.[31] In the same review, radial shaft or both bone fractures accounted for 25% of fracture-associated compartment syndromes. Isolated ulnar shaft–associated compartment syndrome was not reported. Fractures associated with high-energy injuries require close clinical observation in the immediate postinjury and postoperative periods. Should there be clinical suspicion for a developing compartment syndrome at the time of planned definitive fixation, compartment releases can be performed volarly through

a modified Henry approach in addition to releases of the dorsal compartments and mobile wad.

Intraoperative neurovascular injury has also been reported in both ORIF and IM fixation techniques. The volar approach to the radius requires manipulation of the radial artery both distally and proximally, with recurrent branches in the proximal forearm requiring meticulous dissection. The superficial radial nerve and PIN are also at risk of injury during ORIF. IM techniques place the patient at risk of PIN injury if the proximal radial interlock screws are used,[12] as well as superficial radial nerve injury related to the radial start point for retrograde nailing.

Review of Treatment Outcomes for ORIF Versus IM Nailing

ORIF

There are extensive data on plate fixation over the past 50 years. In 1975 Anderson reported a series of 244 patients with radius and ulna fractures fixed with compression plate constructs. They reported 95% and 98% union rate of the radius and ulna, respectively.[7] In 1989 Chapman et al. reported 98% fracture union with 91% of patients reporting satisfactory or excellent outcomes in 127 diaphyseal forearm fractures treated with 4.5- and 3.5-mm dynamic compression plate (DCP) fixation. Thirty-eighty percent represented open fracture, with 68 undergoing primary autografting at the time of fixation. Infection rate was 2.3%, with two refractures reported after removal of hardware.[32] This replicated similar findings to a prior study by Hadden et al. with 177 forearm fractures treated with plate fixation where they reported 97% union rate with 80% of patients reporting good or excellent outcomes.[33]

In the setting of robust literature detailing the efficacy of compression plate fixation for the treatment of diaphyseal radius and ulna fractures, Droll et al. investigated patient-based functional measures following fixation. They reported on 30 patients with

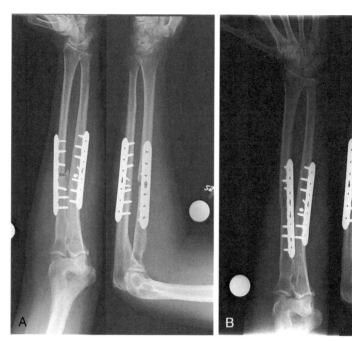

• **Fig. 58.12** (A) Radiographs demonstrating nonunion of the radius following open reduction internal fixation of left both bone forearm fracture. (B) Healed nonunion following revision compression plating with bone grafting. (With permission from Regan D, Crespo A, Konda S, Egol K. Functional outcomes of compression plating and bone grafting for operative treatment of nonunions about the forearm. *J Hand Surg.* 2018;43(6):564.e1-564.e9.)

mean follow-up of over 5 years and concluded that despite a high rate of union, patients were found to have decreased strength in the affected arm compared to the contralateral side at end follow-up (70% strength in forearm pronation, 67% strength in forearm supination, 84% in wrist flexion, 63% in wrist extension, and 75% in grip strength).[24] There were statistically significant lasting range-of-motion deficits in pronosupination and wrist flexion. Mean DASH (The Disabilities of the Arm, Shoulder and Hand) scores demonstrated ongoing functional disability in many patients even after surgical intervention resulting in bony union and restoration of radial bow. They concluded that while motion and bony anatomy were consistently restored, strength deficits persist in long-term follow-up. Bot et al. reported a mean 21-year follow-up on 71 patients who underwent ORIF for both bone forearm fractures, and their group reported similar objective measures to Droll's study (flexion/extension arc 91%, grip strength 94% of contralateral side). Twenty-eight percent of patients still reported some residual pain.[8] While the conclusion of both studies was ultimately that patients report overwhelmingly good outcomes with plate fixation, it is still important to counsel patients that both bone forearm fractures have the potential to have lasting effects regardless of the method of treatment pursued.

While beyond the scope of this chapter, it is important to note that plate fixation remains the standard for treatment of nonunion. Recent case series investigating surgical intervention with ORIF and bone grafting report upwards of 90% union rate (Fig. 58.12).[23,34,35]

IM Nailing

While there are few studies detailing outcomes related to IM fixation, there is still a significant body of literature reporting excellent outcomes in the treatment of isolated shaft fractures and both bone forearm fractures. Lil et al. reported a series of 34 adult patients with both bone forearm fractures treated with Talwalkar

square nails in which 31 patients went on to union of both fractures with 27 patients reporting good or excellent Grace and Eversmann ratings. Complications included two superficial infections, one olecranon bursitis and one case of radioulnar synostosis.[21] Lee et al. reported on 38 interlocking IM nails in 27 patients for a variety of diaphyseal forearm fractures. Their implant of choice is precontoured to accommodate the anatomy of the radius and ulna. They selectively chose fractures they considered to be amenable to IM fixation—simple fracture pattern, fractures with poor overlying soft tissue envelope, segmental fractures, and floating elbow. Contraindications to nailing in their study included osteopenic bone, comminution, and segmental fractures with significant comminution, where the authors felt that preservation of length would be difficult. Thirty-seven of 38 fractures went on to union with a mean time to union of 14 weeks. Twenty-five of 27 patients had either excellent or good results according to the Grace and Eversmann rating system, with average DASH scores of 15. Their study suggests that interlocking IM fixation is a safe and effective alternative to plate fixation in properly selected patients.[36]

Saka et al. reported a series of locked IM nails for radius, ulna, and both bone forearm fractures with 1-year follow-up in which 59 fractures (43 patients) went onto union with no episodes of nonunion, deep infection, or radioulnar synostosis.[37] The average DASH score was 6.5, and 42 of the 43 patients reported good or excellent Grace and Eversmann ratings.

With regard to the treatment of nonunion with IM devices, Hong et al. reported 96% radiographic union with locked interlocking nails with iliac crest bone grafting. However, there was a significant loss of arc of range of motion, and only 53% of patients reported excellent or satisfactory outcomes, with mean DASH scores of 35. Hong and colleagues concluded that interlocked nailing should not be seen as a viable alternative to plate fixation for nonunion of the ulnar or radial diaphysis.[38] However, a more recent study by Vitis et al. reported 93% union in 49 patients with radial, ulnar, or both bone nonunions with unlocked Rush rods. The use of autologous bone graft was used at the discretion of the surgeon when deemed appropriate.[39]

Plate Versus IM Nail

There are limited head-to-head prospective data comparing plate versus nail for diaphyseal forearm fractures in any population. In a meta-analysis of the pediatric literature, where IM fixation is more commonly used, no level I or level II studies were reported.[40] Of note, four adult randomized controlled trials (RCTs) were reviewed in meta-analysis that concluded there were no significant differences in postoperative forearm rotation, restoration of radial bow, time to union, and overall union rate.[22] Further, it is difficult to compare the techniques given the wide range of associated factors in many studies that complicate direct comparison, namely the presence of open fracture, degree of comminution, and presence or lack of bone loss. Most studies looking at IM implants address closed fractures without bone loss, as compared with those more complex fractures that would necessitate a formal debridement and ORIF.[41]

Lee et al. reported outcomes on 67 patients randomized to nail versus plate fixation for both bone forearm fractures. All injuries were closed and treated with closed reduction and nailing, followed by immobilization in a long arm cast before transition into a hinged elbow brace.[42] Those treated with plate osteosynthesis were found to have faster time to union (10 vs. 14 weeks, respectively) and decreased fluoroscopy time compared to the IM nailing group. At final follow-up, function, range of pronosupination, Grace and Eversmann rating, and DASH were all found to have no statistical difference between treatment groups. One patient in the IM nailing group went on to nonunion, while one patient in the plate fixation sustained refracture after removal of hardware.

Ozkaya et al. reported on the retrospective review of 42 patients treated with either locked IM nailing (20 patients) or dual plating (22 patients) for both bone forearm fractures. Those in the nailing group were found to have significantly less blood loss and a shorter time to union (10 vs. 14 weeks). There was no significant difference in DASH or Grace and Eversmann scores, or in postoperative complications between groups. Hardware was removed in 12 of 22 of the ORIF group, with 7 of 20 of the nailing group subsequently undergoing removal of either the nail or interlocking screws.[43]

Hybrid plate and nail constructs have also been reported in the literature. Behnke et al. conducted a retrospective review of dual plating (27 patients) versus hybrid fixation with IM nailing of the ulna and plate fixation of the radius (29 patients) for both bone forearm fractures.[44] They reported no significant difference in range of motion through the pronosupination arc, Grace and Eversmann scores (>70% excellent or good in both groups), or complication rate. There was one nonunion in each group. However, a series by Kim et al. reported inferior time to union, pronosupination arc, Grace and Eversmann ratings, and DASH scores in hybrid fixation as compared to dual plating in a retrospective series of 47 patients with 1-year follow-up.[45] It is important to note that in Kim's series, fractures of the radius were treated with IM nailing in the hybrid fixation group (with plate fixation of the ulna) as well as with combination of plate fixation for the radius and IM nailing for the ulna, as opposed to Behnke's study where only the ulna was treated with IM nailing and all fractures of the radius were treated with plate fixation.

References

1. Procaccini R, Martiniani M, Farinelli L, Luciani P, Specchia N, Gigante A. A new single volar approach for the both-bone fractures of the forearm: the mediolateral windows approach extended. *Tech Hand Up Extrem Surg.* 2020;24(3):114–118.
2. Baratz M. Disorders of the forearm axis. In: Wolfe S, Hotchkiss R, Pederson W, Kozin S, Cohen M, eds. *Green's Operative Hand Surgery.* 7th ed. Philadelphia, PA: Elsevier; 2017:786–809.
3. Stutz C, Waters P. Fractures and dislocations of the forearm, wrist and hand. In: Mencio G, Swiontkowski M, eds. *Green's Skeletal Trauma in Children.* 5th ed. Philadelphia, PA: Elsevier; 2014:142–181.
4. Sauder D, Athwal G. Management of isolated ulnar shaft fractures. *Hand Clin.* 2007;23(2):179–184.
5. Schulte L, Meals C, Neviaser R. Management of adult diaphyseal both-bone forearm fractures. *J Am Acad Orthop Surg.* 2014;22(7):437–446.
6. Jupiter J, Kellam J. Diaphyseal fractures of the forearm. In: Browner B, Levine A, Jupiter J, Trafton P, Krettek C, eds. *Skeletal Trauma.* 4th ed. Philadelphia, PA: Saunders; 2008:1459–1502.
7. Anderson L, Sisk D, Tooms R, Park W. Compression-plate fixation in acute diaphyseal fractures of the radius and ulna. *J Bone Joint Surg Am.* 1975;57(3):287–297.
8. Bot A, Doornberg J, Lindenhovius A, Ring D, Goslings C, van Dijk N. Long-term outcomes of fractures of both bones of the forearm. *J Bone Joint Surg Am.* 2011;93(6):527–532.
9. Matthews L, Kaufer H, Garver D, Sonstegard D. The effect on supination-pronation of angular malalignment of fractures of both bones of the forearm. *J Bone Joint Surg Am.* 1982;64(1):14–17.
10. Adams MR, Domes C, Githens MF, Sirkin MS, Sullivan MP, Taitsman LA, Wright RD. Forearm fractures. In: *Harborview Illustrated Tips and Tricks in Fracture Surgery.* 2nd ed. Philadelphia, PA: Wolters Kluwer; 2019:199–221.
11. Dehghan N, Schemitsch E. Intramedullary nail fixation of non-traditional fractures: clavicle, forearm, fibula. *Injury.* 2017;48(S):S41-S46.
12. Rehman S, Sokunbi G. Intramedullary fixation of forearm fractures. *Hand Clin.* 2010;26(3):391–401.
13. Jones D, Henley M, Schemitsch E, Tencer A. A biomechanical comparison of two methods of fixation of fractures of the forearm. *J Orthop Trauma.* 1995;9(3):198–206.
14. Eglseder W. Shaft fractures of the radius and ulna. In: Eglseder W, ed. *Atlas of Upper Extremity Trauma, A Clinical Perspective.* Philadelphia, PA: Springer; 2018:585–642.
15. Sarmiento A, Latta L, Zych G. Isolated ulnar shaft fractures treated with functional braces. *J Orthop Trauma.* 1998;12(6):420–424.
16. Thompson J. Anatomical methods of approach in operations on the long bones of the extremities. *Ann Surg.* 1918;68(3):309–329.
17. Moss J, Bynum D. Diaphyseal fractures of the radius and ulna in adults. *Hand Clin.* 2007;23(2):143–151.
18. Catalano L, Zlotolow D, Hitchcock P, Shah S, Barron O. Surgical exposures of the radius and ulna. *J Am Acad Orthop Surg.* 2011;19(7):430–438.
19. Haseeb M, Muzafar K, Ghani A, Bhat K, Butt M. A fresh look at radial shaft fixation: the lateral approach to the radius. *J Orthop Surg.* 2018;26(2):1–8.
20. Cossio A, Cazzaniga C, Gaddi D, Zatti G. Treatment of diaphyseal forearm fractures with intramedullary nailing. *Tech Orthop.* 2014;29(3):140–144.
21. Lil N, Makkar D, Aleem A. Results of closed intramedullary nailing using Talwarkar square nail in adult forearm fractures. *Malays Orthop J.* 2012;6(3):7–12.
22. Zhao L, Wang B, Bai X, Liu Z, Gao H, Li Y. Plate fixation versus intramedullary nailing for both-bone forearm fractures: a meta-analysis of randomized controlled trials and cohort studies. *World J Surg.* 2017;41(3):722–733.
23. Boussakri H, Elibrahimi A, Bachiri M, Elidrissi M, Shimi M, Elmrini A. Nonunion of fractures of the ulna and radius diaphyses: clinical and radiological results of surgical treatment. *Malays Orthop J.* 2016;10(2):27–34.

24. Droll K, Perna P, Potter J, Harniman E, Schemitsch E, McKee M. Outcomes following plate fixation of fractures of both bones of the forearm in adults. *J Bone Joint Surg Am.* 2007;89(12):2619–2624.

25. Vince KG, Miller JE. Cross-union complicating fracture of the forearm Part I: adults. *J Bone Joint Surg Am.* 1987;69(5):640–653.

26. Hanel D, Pfaeffle H, Ayalla A. Management of posttraumatic metadiaphyseal radioulnar synostosis. *Hand Clin.* 2007;23(2):227–234.

27. Rosson J, Petley G, Shearer J. Bone structure removal of internal fixation plates. *J Bone Jt Surg Br.* 1991;73:65–67.

28. Yao CK, Lin KC, Tarng YW, Chang WN, Renn JH. Removal of forearm plate leads to a high risk of refracture: decision regarding implant removal after fixation of the forearm and analysis of risk factors of refracture. *Arch Orthop Trauma Surg.* 2014;134:1691–1697.

29. Hidaka S, Gustilo R. Refracture of bones of the forearm after plate removal. *J Bone Joint Surg Am.* 1984;66(8):1241–2143.

30. Muller M, Allgower M, Schneider R, Willenegger H. In: *Manual of Internal Fixation: Techniques Recommended by the AO-ASIF Group.* 3rd ed. New York, NY: Springer; 1991.

31. Kalyani B, Fisher B, Roberts C, Giannoudis P. Compartment syndrome of the forearm: a systematic review. *J Hand Surg Am.* 2011;36(3):535–543.

32. Chapman M, Gordon J, Zissimos A. Compression-plate fixation of acute fractures of the diaphyses of the radius and ulna. *J Bone Joint Surg Am.* 1989;71(2):159–169.

33. Hadden W, Reschauer R, Seggl W. Results of AO plate fixation of forearm shaft fractures in adults. *Injury.* 1983;15(1):44–52.

34. Kloen P, Wiggers J, Buijze G. Treatment of diaphyseal non-unions of the ulna and radius. *Arch Orthop Trauma Surg.* 2010;130(12):1439–1445.

35. Regan D, Crespo A, Konda S, Egol K. Functional outcomes of compression plating and bone grafting for operative treatment of nonunions about the forearm. *J Hand Surg Am.* 2018;43(6):564.e1–564.e9.

36. Lee Y, Lee S, Chung M, Baek G, Gong H, Kim K. Interlocking contoured intramedullary nail fixation for selected diaphyseal fractures of the forearm in adults. *J Bone Joint Surg Am.* 2008;90(9):1891–1898.

37. Saka G, Saglam N, Kurtulmus T, et al. New interlocking intramedullary radius and ulna nails for treating forearm diaphyseal fractures in adults: a retrospective study. *Injury.* 2013;45(S1):S16-S23.

38. Hong G, Cong-Feng L, Hui-Peng S, Cun-Yi F, Bing-Fang Z. Treatment of diaphyseal forearm nonunions with interlocking intramedullary nails. *Clin Orthop Relat Res.* 2006;450:186–192.

39. De Vitis R, Passiatore M, Cilli V, Maffeis J, Milano G, Taccardo G. Intramedullary nailing for treatment of forearm non-union: is it useful – a case series. *J Orthop.* 2020;20:97–104.

40. Baldwin K, Morrison M, Tomlinson L, Ramirez R, Flynn J. Both bone forearm fractures in children and adolescents, which fixation strategy is superior – plates or nails? A systematic review and meta-analysis of observational studies. *J Orthop Trauma.* 2014;28(1):e8–e14.

41. Jones D, Kakar S. Adult diaphyseal forearm fractures: intramedullary nail versus plate fixation. *J Hand Surg Am.* 2011;36(7):1216–1219.

42. Lee S, Kim K, Lee J, Choy W. Plate osteosynthesis versus intramedullary nailing for both forearm bones fractures. *Eur J Orthop Surg Traumatol.* 2014;24(5):769–776.

43. Ozkaya U, Kilic A, Ozdogan U, Beng K, Kabukcuoglu Y. Comparison between locked intramedullary nailing and plate osteosynthesis in the management of adult forearm fractures. *Acta Orthop Traumatol Turc.* 2009;43(1):14–20.

44. Behnke N, Redjal H, Nguyen V, Zinar D. Internal fixation of diaphyseal fractures of the forearm: a retrospective comparison of hybrid fixation versus dual plating. *J Orthop Trauma.* 2012;26(11):611–616.

45. Kim S, Heo Y, Yi J, Lee J, Lim B. Shaft fractures of both forearm bones: the outcomes of surgical treatment with plating only and combined plating and intramedullary nailing. *Clin Orthop Surg.* 2015;7(3):282–290.

59

Technique Spotlight: ORIF of Both Bones Forearm Fractures—Approaches

RAMESH C. SRINIVASAN

Indications

Surgical indications for both bones forearm fractures include the following: (1) nondisplaced or minimally displaced both bones forearm fractures with a propensity for instability (comminution, initial displacement prior to reduction, and polytrauma patients) and (2) significantly displaced or angulated radius or ulna or both bones forearm fractures.

Preoperative Evaluation (Imaging, Examination, Etc.)

Preoperative evaluation includes standard anteroposterior (AP), lateral, and oblique X-rays of the entire injured forearm. Because of the risk of concomitant injury to the wrist or elbow, dedicated wrist and elbow X-rays should also be obtained. The patient should be carefully examined for wrist and/or elbow joint pain or physical examination findings consistent with distal radioulnar joint (DRUJ) or proximal radioulnar joint (PRUJ) instability concerning Galeazzi, Monteggia, or Essex-Lopresti injuries.

In the setting of significant loss of length, comminution, or segmental bone loss, X-rays of the contralateral side can be helpful as a template for restoring normal anatomy on the injured side intraoperatively.

Adjunctive testing includes computed tomography (CT) scan and laboratory testing (vitamin D, calcium, thyroid labs, erythrocyte sedimentation rate, C-reactive protein). Rarely is a CT scan indicated, although it is useful in the setting of concomitant wrist and/or elbow joint injury or nonunion. In the setting of nonunion, laboratory testing to optimize the patient's biology is paramount for successful subsequent surgery. For elderly patients or patients with known systemic disorders, vitamin D, calcium, and thyroid labs should be checked and normalized immediately after surgery to optimize bony healing.

Positioning and Equipment

Supine positioning is ideal for standard forearm fractures because it allows for standard AP, oblique, and lateral X-rays. A nonsterile tourniquet is applied to the upper arm. General anesthesia is used with or without a regional block (typically axillary block). If there is any concern for compartment syndrome (swelling or severe injury), a regional block should be avoided to allow for regular postoperative examination. Alternatively, intraoperative prophylactic forearm fasciotomies may be considered.

A roll-in hand table (Fig. 59.1) can be used in order to leave the patient on the stretcher and to avoid moving the patient to an operating room bed. Over the course of a busy elective day, avoidance of this transfer can save 5–10 minutes per case which can result in an hour or more saved throughout the course of a day.

The author prefers the use of a large C-arm fluoroscopy unit rather than the mini C-arm for more accurate assessment of forearm length and radial bow.[1] The author of this chapter has a low threshold for obtaining X-rays of the contralateral side preoperatively or intraoperatively if there is any question with regard to anatomic restoration of length or radial bow during the operation.

Surgical Technique Description

Two different surgical approaches for the radius may be considered: (1) the volar Henry approach or (2) the dorsal Thompson approach. Classically, the volar Henry approach is used for midshaft or more distal fractures. It is more cosmetic than a dorsal approach for distal fractures and offers the benefit of avoidance of extensor tendon irritation. Although the volar approach may be used for proximal one-third fractures of the radius, this approach becomes more challenging due to the insertion of the supinator and pronator, the girth of the extensor and flexor wads, as well as the proximity of the posterior interosseous nerve. For these reasons, the author of this chapter prefers the dorsal Thompson approach for proximal one-third fractures.

Prophylactic antibiotics are administered prior to surgical incision.[2] The volar Henry approach begins with a skin incision marked out directly over a palpable flexor carpi radialis (FCR) tendon which heads towards the distal pole of the scaphoid and inserts on the base of the second metacarpal (Fig. 59.2A–I). Proximally, this line can be carried to where the distal biceps tendon is palpated at the elbow flexion crease. The skin is incised sharply with a #15 scalpel and careful sharp dissection is carried down to the FCR tendon. The superficial sheath of the FCR tendon is incised.

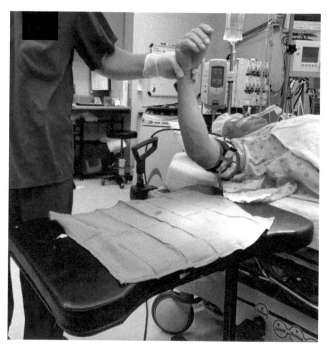

• **Fig. 59.1** Roll-in hand table setup.

Distally, the FCR tendon is retracted in an ulnar direction protecting the palmar cutaneous branch of the median nerve. The deep FCR sheath is incised while protecting the radial artery which is identified and retracted radially for the remainder of the case. The FCR sheath is released proximally. The flexor pollicis longus muscle belly is bluntly dissected off of the radial septum and retracted in an ulnar direction, protecting the median nerve. Depending on the site of the fracture, the pronator quadratus is released as needed to facilitate fracture reduction and/or plate placement. As the dissection continues more proximally, the interval is opened between the FCR and brachioradialis (BR). The radial artery, which courses between these muscles, is retracted ulnarly with the FCR as there tend to be more vascular connections to the FCR than the BR. For more proximal fractures, the pronator teres and supinator are released as needed in a limited fashion to facilitate fracture reduction and/or plate placement (Fig. 59.3A–E). This is best done by performing the action of the muscle to be released. For example, to release the pronator teres muscle, the forearm is placed in maximal pronation and the terminal fibers of the insertion of the tendon are identified and released. Similarly, to release the supinator, placing the forearm in maximal supination exposes the attachment of the supinator tendon and facilitates release.

The dorsal Thompson approach involves a skin incision extending in line from the lateral epicondyle to Lister's tubercle (Fig. 59.4A–I). Proximally, the dissection occurs between extensor carpi radialis brevis (ECRB) and extensor digitorum communis (EDC). Distally, the dissection plane is in between ECRB and extensor pollicis longus (EPL). This author prefers to start distally, finding the dissection plane between EPL and ECRB, and then bluntly carry the dissection proximally between ECRB and EDC after completely releasing the dorsal forearm fascia. Proximally, the posterior interosseous nerve is palpated running perpendicular to the fibers of the supinator muscle. Careful blunt dissection allows for exposure of this nerve and subsequent protection for the remainder of the surgical procedure. The fracture site is exposed with careful subperiosteal dissection, minimizing muscular stripping to preserve blood supply to the fracture. Soft tissue attachments are preserved for separate comminuted fragments. The fracture site is cleaned of fracture hematoma and early adhesions. The fracture is anatomically reduced and held with a reduction clamp. A 3.5-mm limited contact dynamic compression (LCDC) plate between six and eight holes is placed for simple fracture patterns. A minimum of six cortices of bicortical fixation is achieved on both sides of the fracture with compression at the fracture site.

For transverse fractures, anatomic reduction and compression are achieved through the use of a compression plate. For short or long oblique fractures, the fracture is anatomically reduced and provisionally stabilized with one or more lag screws. After compression is achieved, the fracture is stabilized with a neutralization plate with a minimum of six cortices of fixation on both sides of the fracture.[3,4] Care is taken to apply the lag screws perpendicular to the fracture line and outside of the position planned for plate placement (Fig. 59.3A–E). Alternatively, if the orientation of the fracture is amenable, lag screws can be placed through the plate. Two published reports have demonstrated a high union rate (>90%) with only four cortices of fixation proximal and distal to the fracture site when supplemental lag screw fixation is used.[5,6]

Fractures of the ulna are approached through a skin incision directly over the subcutaneous border of the ulna (Fig. 59.5A–G). The intermuscular interval is between the extensor carpi ulnaris (ECU) dorsally and the flexor carpi ulnaris (FCU) volarly. The fracture site is exposed with careful subperiosteal dissection. It is anatomically reduced and fixed with a 3.5-mm LCDC plate with or without lag screws according to the principles described above. Fractures of the distal ulna may be treated with contoured distal ulna plating, hook plating, or headless compression screws. Care must be taken to identify and protect dorsal cutaneous branches of the ulnar nerve when treating distal ulna fractures.

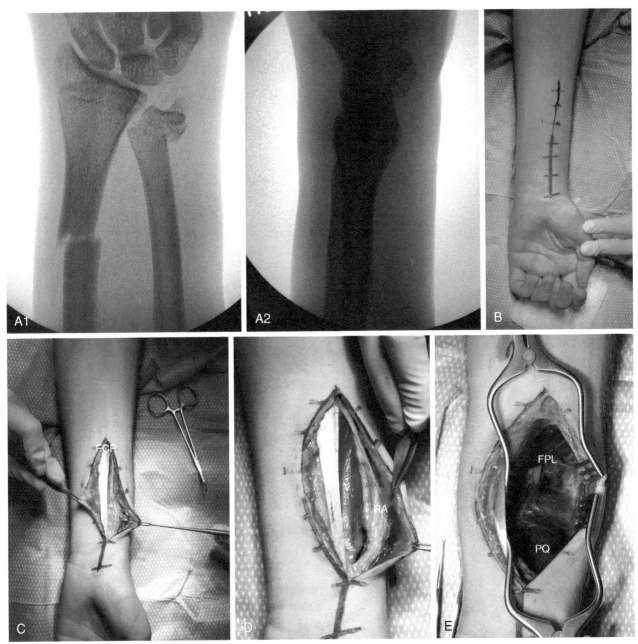

• **Fig. 59.2** (A) 20-year-old male status post fall off of skateboard with these injury films demonstrating radial shaft fracture and ulnar neck fracture. (B) Volar Henry approach marked out with incision over the palpable flexor carpi radialis (FCR) tendon. If the FCR is difficult to palpate due to body habitus or swelling, wrist extension will make the tendon more prominent and taut against the volar skin. (C) *FCR* tendon exposed. (D) Radial artery is identified and protected for the remainder of the procedure. (E) The flexor pollicis longus muscle belly is bluntly dissected off of the radial septum and retracted in an ulnar direction to expose the pronator quadratus.

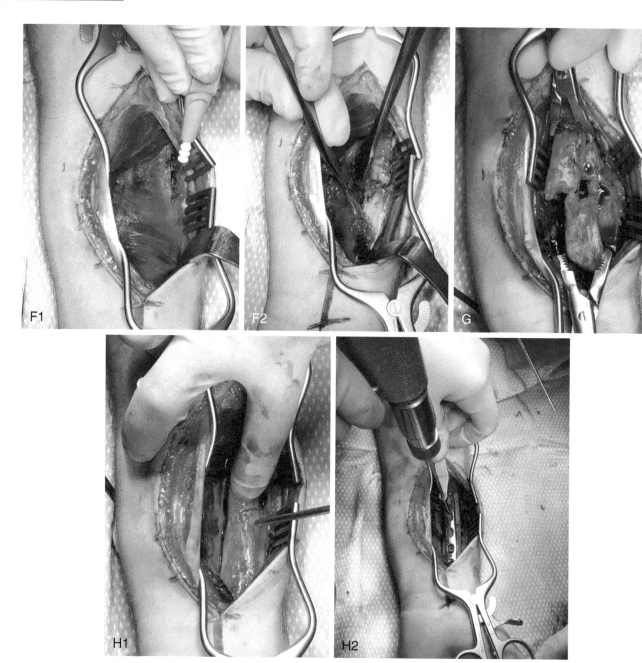

• **Fig. 59.2, cont'd** (F) The pronator quadratus is released and the fracture site is exposed. (G) The fracture site is distracted with the assistance of serrated bone clamps and cleaned of hematoma and early adhesions. (H) Once the fracture edges are accurately identified, the fracture is anatomically reduced and a 3.5-mm limited contact dynamic compression plate is placed with a minimum of six cortices of fixation on each side of the fracture.

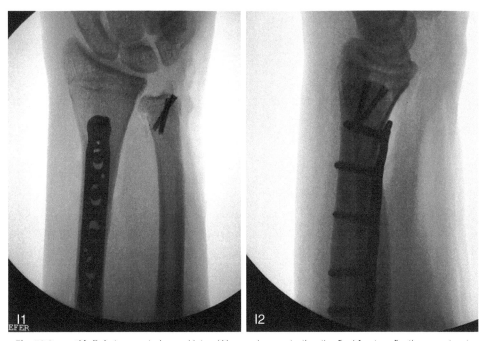

• **Fig. 59.2, cont'd** (I) Anteroposterior and lateral X-rays demonstrating the final fracture fixation construct.

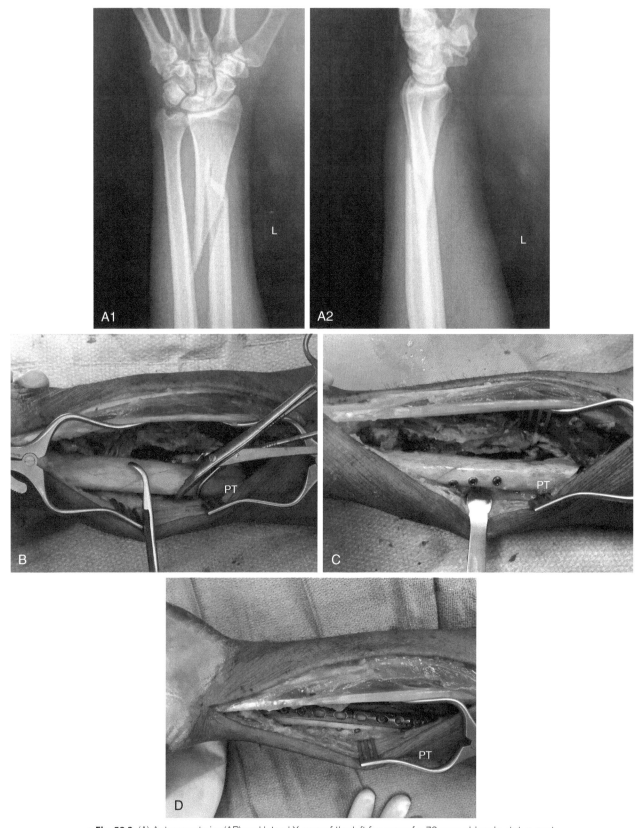

• **Fig. 59.3** (A) Anteroposterior (AP) and lateral X-rays of the left forearm of a 73-year-old male status post fall onto an outstretched arm demonstrating a displaced long oblique radial shaft fracture. (B) Anatomic reduction requires release and retraction of the pronator teres *(PT)* insertion off of the dorsolateral aspect of the radial shaft. (C) After anatomic reduction, three lag screws are placed across this long oblique fracture to achieve compression. (D) A 3.5-mm limited contact dynamic compression plate is placed in neutralization mode with six cortices of fixation on each side of the fracture.

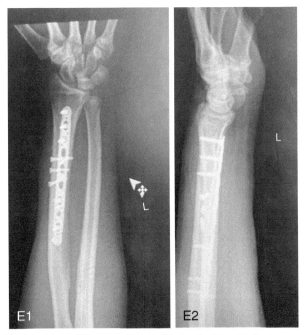

• **Fig. 59.3, cont'd** (E) AP and lateral X-rays demonstrating the final fracture fixation.

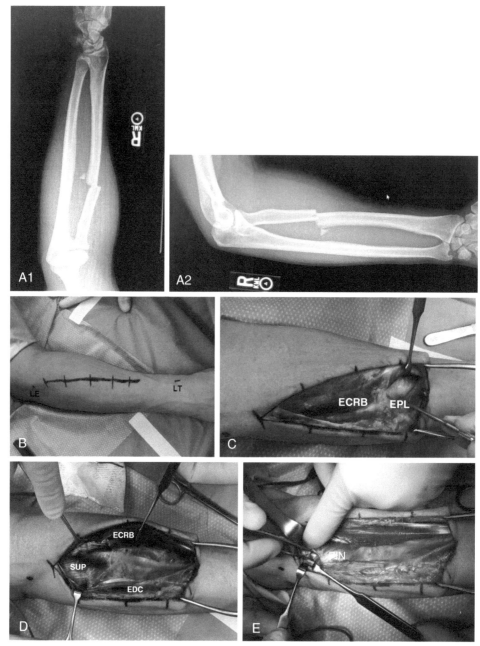

• **Fig. 59.4** (A) Anteroposterior (AP) and lateral X-rays of 35-year-old male who presented with a displaced proximal one-third radial shaft fracture after fall from a mountain bike. (B) Dorsal Thompson skin incision extending in line with the lateral epicondyle and Lister's tubercle. (C) The surgical interval is identified proximally between extensor carpi radialis brevis *(ECRB)* and extensor digitorum communis (EDC) and distally between ECRB and extensor pollicis longus *(EPL)*. (D) With *ECRB* and *EDC* retracted, the supinator *(SUP)* muscle is exposed proximally. (E) The SUP muscle can be bluntly split perpendicular to its fibers in order to find and protect the posterior interosseous nerve *(PIN)*.

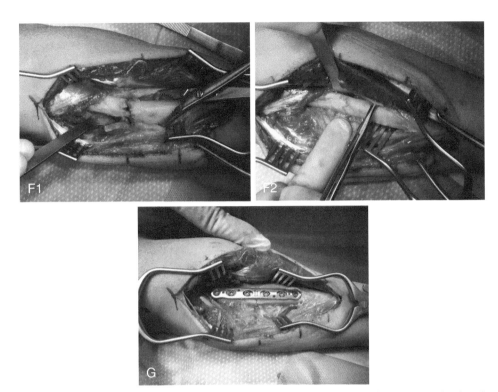

• **Fig. 59.4, cont'd** (F) Once the PIN is identified and protected, the fracture site is exposed and reduced. (G) Clinical photo of fracture reduction and plate placement.

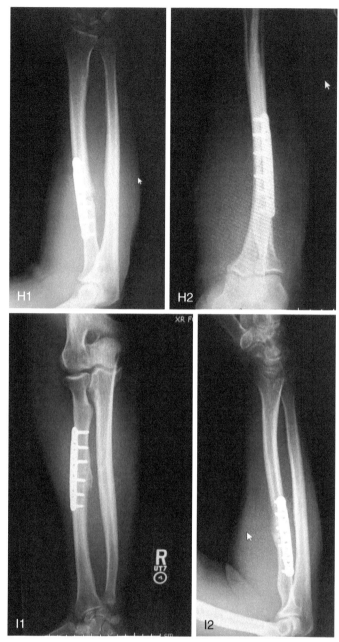

• **Fig. 59.4, cont'd** (H) AP and lateral X-rays of the reduced and fixed fracture. (I) Final X-rays (AP and lateral) demonstrating a healed fracture.

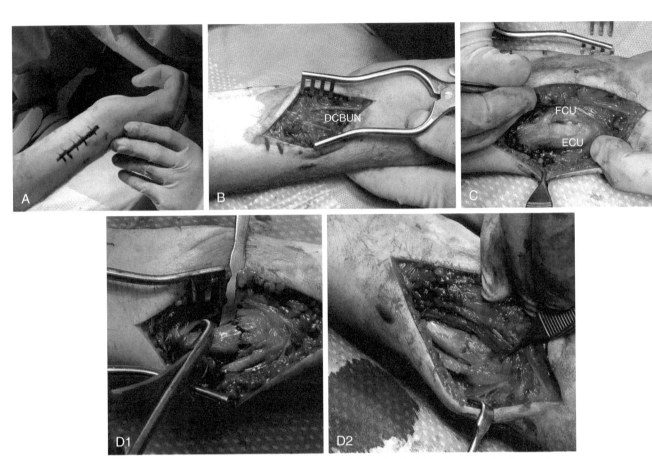

• **Fig. 59.5** (A) Fractures of the ulna can be approached through an incision along the subcutaneous border of the ulna. (B) For distal ulna fractures, dorsal cutaneous branches of the ulnar nerve *(DCBUN)* should be identified and protected for the remainder of the procedure. (C) The muscular interval is between the flexor carpi ulnaris *(FCU)* and the extensor carpi ulnaris *(ECU)*. (D) The fracture site is exposed and anatomically reduced. Fixation depends on the fracture pattern and location. In this case, headless compression screws were used.

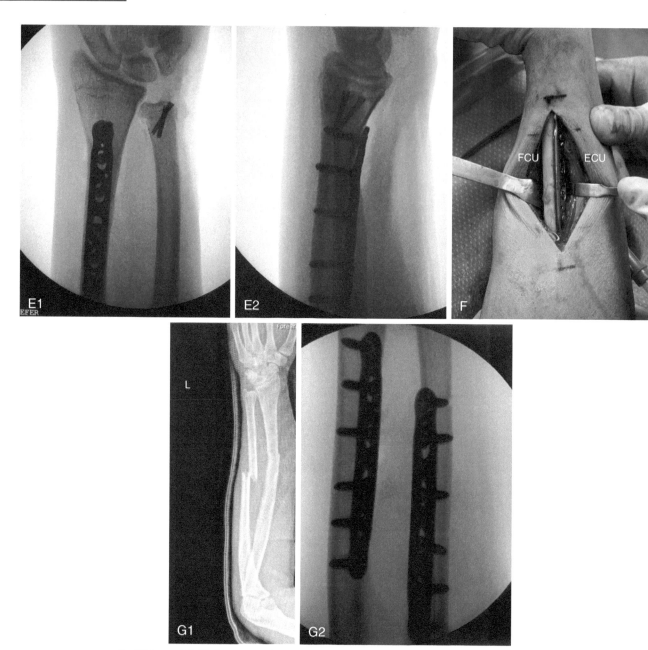

• **Fig. 59.5, cont'd** (E) Anteroposterior and lateral X-rays demonstrating the final fixation construct. (F) For midshaft ulna fractures, the surgical approach is the same, between *FCU* and *ECU*. The fracture is anatomically reduced and a 3.5-mm plate with a minimum of six cortices of fixation on each side of the fracture is achieved. (G) Preoperative and postoperative X-rays of displaced both bones forearm fractures anatomically fixed with 3.5-mm plates.

PEARLS AND PITFALLS

- For proximal one-third fractures of the radius the author prefers a dorsal approach with formal protection and identification of the posterior interosseous nerve.
- A minimum of six cortices of fixation should be achieved on each side of the fracture.
- 3.5-mm LCDC plates are typically used in the adult population.
- Short and long oblique fractures can be treated with lag screw fixation prior to plate neutralization; lag screws should be placed orthogonal to the fracture and placed outside of the plane of planned plate placement. Alternatively, lag screws may be placed through the plate across the fracture site.

References

1. Schemitsch EH, Richards RR. The effect of malunion on functional outcomes after plate fixation of fractures of both bones of the forearm in adults. *J Bone Joint Surg Am.* 1992;74(7):1068–1078.
2. Rizvi M, Bille B, Holtom P, Schnall SB. The role of prophylactic antibiotics in elective hand surgery. *J Hand Surg.* 2008;33:413–420.
3. Chapman MW, Gordon JE, Zissimos AG. Compression-plate fixation of acute fractures of the diaphysis of the radius and ulna. *J Bone Joint Surg Am.* 1989;71:159–169.
4. Stern PJ, Drury WJ. Complications of plate fixation of forearm fractures. *Clin Orthop Relat Res.* 1983;175:25–29.
5. Crow BD, Mundis G, Anglen JO. Clinical results of minimal screw plate fixation of forearm fractures. *Am J Orthop.* 2007;36:477–480.
6. Lindvall EM, Sagi HC. Selective screw placement in forearm compression plating: results of 75 consecutive fractures stabilized with 4 cortices of screw fixation on either side of the fracture. *J Orthop Trauma.* 2006;20:157–162. discussion 162–163.

60

Distal Radius Fractures

DANIEL A. LONDON AND RYAN P. CALFEE

Introduction

Distal radius fractures are the most common upper extremity fracture in patients in the United States,[1] accounting for 0.7%–2.5% of emergency department visits.[2,3] Worldwide, the incidence of distal radius fractures has increased over the past 40–50 years, almost doubling in certain populations.[4,5]

Distal radius fractures occur in a bimodal distribution with the highest frequency in youths under the age of 18 years and a secondary peak in adults over 50 years old.[1] In the older adults, osteoporosis and poor postural stability are associated with these fractures after falls onto an outstretched hand.[1,6–9] Increasing age and obesity levels are risk factors for more complex injury patterns.[10] Distal radius fractures in young patients usually occur in the setting of play or sports and account for 23% of all sports-related fractures in adolescents.[11]

Regardless of patient age, comorbidity burden, or fracture pattern, the overall principles in management remain the same. First, the fracture must be stabilized and any secondary injuries evaluated. Next, the determination of operative versus nonoperative treatment must be made. Currently, the most common surgical procedure for distal radius fractures in adults is open reduction and internal fixation with a volar plate, but the specific procedure should be tailored to individual patients and their injuries.

Relevant Anatomy

The distal radius has three articular surfaces: the scaphoid facet, the lunate facet, and the sigmoid notch, which articulate with the scaphoid, lunate, and distal ulna, respectively. Several measurements describe the normal distal radius: height (radial styloid 12 mm longer than the ulnar corner of the lunate facet), lateral tilt (11 degrees volar), radial inclination (22 degrees), and ulnar variance (the length of the radius relative to the ulna, with neutral to ulnar negative being normal) (Fig. 60.1). After a fracture, changes from these normative values or changes compared to the contralateral, uninjured radius are assessed and often guide the decision to pursue operative versus nonoperative management. Decreased radial height and inclination result in a hand that appears radially deviated with increased prominence of the ulnar head. Altered lateral tilt of the articular surface may produce visible deformity, but this alteration of the normal anatomy is more important as a cause of adaptive midcarpal instability, which is one cause of long-term wrist pain secondary to the malalignment between the lunate and capitate. When clinically relevant changes in lateral tilt or radial length occur, patients may also experience

restricted forearm rotation secondary to altered distal radioulnar joint (DRUJ) mechanics. Finally, loss of radial length producing an ulnar positive wrist increases the chances of patients developing symptomatic ulnar impaction syndrome.

The median nerve and flexor tendons for the fingers course volar to the distal radius. Distal radius fractures increase the pressure within the carpal tunnel, a finding potentiated by immobilization in a position of wrist flexion.[12] Excessive pressure may produce symptomatic carpal tunnel syndrome that may necessitate emergent release or contribute to the development of complex regional pain syndrome (CRPS).

In the setting of a distal radius fracture, soft tissue injuries to nearby structures are common. Most frequently occurring is an injury to the triangular fibrocartilage complex (TFCC), which comprises the meniscal homolog triangular fibrocartilage, the dorsal and volar radioulnar ligaments, the ulnar collateral ligament, the extensor carpi ulnaris (ECU) subsheath, and the origins of the ulnolunate and ulnotriquetral ligaments. The second most frequent is injury to the scapholunate (SL) ligament, which is a C-shaped structure that consists of dorsal, volar, and proximal portions, and is essential to providing intracarpal stability and preventing dorsal intercalated segmental instability. Lunotriquetral (LT) ligament injuries are also possible. This is also a ligament that has dorsal, volar, and proximal components, and injury to this ligament can result in volar intercalated segmental instability. Hanker et al. reviewed the cases of 173 athletes presenting with distal radius fractures. The most common soft tissue injury was TFCC tears in 61% of patients, followed by carpal instability in 20%, and DRUJ instability in 9%.[13] Studies performed to document the incidence of associated carpal pathology consistently report a high incidence from 68% to 98%.[14–16] Although these associated injuries are often partial or low-grade injuries that do not require dedicated treatment, surgeons should remain aware of the potential of clinically relevant associated injuries when screening for these associated injuries on physical and radiographic examination.

Evaluation

Initial assessment begins with assessing the skin about the wrist to confirm that it is a closed injury. This should be followed by a thorough neurovascular assessment with evaluation of the radial and ulnar arteries, as well as the median, radial, and ulnar nerves. After assessing for neurovascular injury, distal radius fractures require lateral and posteroanterior (PA) radiographs. A standard PA radiograph should profile the ECU tendon groove, which should be at the level of or radial to the base of the ulnar styloid (Fig. 60.2).[17] A true lateral radiograph is defined by the relationship of the scaphoid,

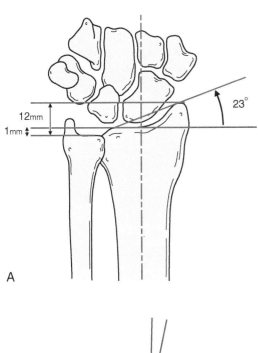

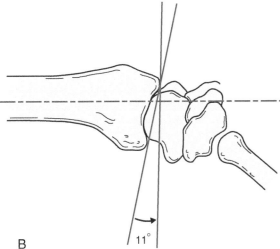

• **Fig. 60.1** Diagram of normal bony anatomy of the distal radius. (A) Normal 23 degrees of radial inclination, 12 mm of radial height, and 1mm of negative ulnar variance. (B) Normal 11 degress of palmar tilt. (Reprinted from *Skeletal Trauma.* 4th ed., Fig. 40.2.)

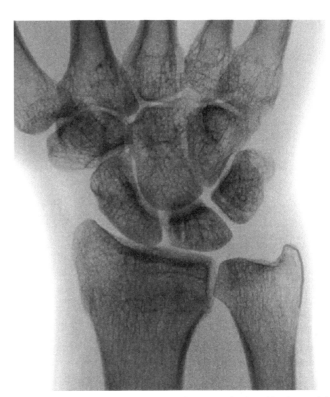

• **Fig. 60.2** Neutral rotation posteroanterior X-ray of wrist with ulnar styloid *(blue outline)* at ulnar border of ulna.

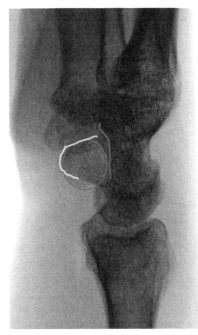

• **Fig. 60.3** True lateral X-ray of wrist with distal pole of scaphoid *(yellow outline)* just volar to pisiform *(blue outline)* which is volar to the capitate *(orange outline)*.

the pisiform, and the capitate. An acceptable position is when the volar cortex of the pisiform lies between the volar cortex of the distal pole of the scaphoid and the volar margin of the capitate head (Fig. 60.3).[18] If the pisiform is dorsal to the distal scaphoid pole, then the arm is overly pronated, and if the pisiform is volar to the distal scaphoid pole, then the arm is excessively supinated. Additionally, because of the normal 11 degrees of volar tilt, a true lateral X-ray does not allow for assessment of the articular surface. To account for this, Medoff suggested a 10-degree lateral X-ray.[19] This positioning profiles the distal radius' articular surface and allows the surgeon to assess the dorsal and volar rims.

For complex distal radius fractures with a high degree of comminution and/or intra-articular extension, computed tomography (CT) can allow for a detailed understanding of the fracture fragments (Fig. 60.4). This advanced imaging can provide assistance in surgical planning with regard to fixation method and surgical approach.

Fractures are examined for displacement according to the normative values for radial height, length, inclination, and lateral tilt. The articular surfaces of the radiocarpal joint and the DRUJ are assessed

for step-off and gapping. Loss of normal alignment with articular incongruity over 2 mm, radial shortening over 3 mm, or dorsal tilt over 10 degrees generally requires reduction. Failure to obtain or maintain reduction better than these parameters is an accepted indication for operative treatment. Obviously, patient-specific needs and comorbidities influence the ultimate treatment decision and the standard parameters may provide less guidance in the older adult.[20]

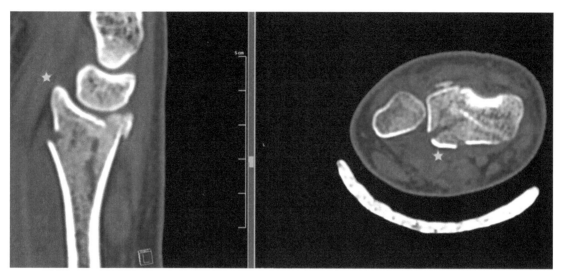

• **Fig. 60.4** Sagittal and axial computed tomography cuts of distal radius fracture demonstrating the exact size of volar lunate facet fracture *(star)*.

As of 2016, there were at least 15 fracture classification systems for distal radius fractures. Several recent studies have found that not one of them provides enough reliability, reproducibility, or clinical usefulness to become the dominant method for describing distal radius fractures.[21,22] Still, for completeness sake, we will succinctly describe several of the more common classification systems.

Eponyms

Historically, certain common fracture patterns were described by surgeons, whose names then became eponyms for those patterns, all of which are still used today. Most common is the Colles' fracture which was described by Dr. Abraham Colles in 1814 and refers to an extra-articular, dorsally displaced metaphyseal fracture with radial shortening.[23] Then, in 1838, Dr. John Rhea Barton described an intra-articular distal radius fracture with either volar or dorsal displacement of the respective lip, now referred to as a volar or dorsal Barton's fracture.[24] Finally, in 1847, Dr. Robert William Smith classified extra-articular volarly displaced distal radius fractures, which are now called Smith's fractures.[25]

Frykman

The Frykman system is based on whether or not the fracture lines extend into the radiocarpal and radioulnar joints, as well as the presence of an associated ulnar styloid fracture. Emphasis on this system was based on the presence of intra-articular extension to the DRUJ portending a poor outcome.[26]

Melone

The Melone classification focuses on intra-articular distal radius fractures and highlights the importance of four fragments in these fractures: the radial shaft, the radial styloid, the dorsal ulnar fragment, and the volar ulnar fragment.[27] Particular emphasis is placed on the volar ulnar fragment and its significance in achieving an anatomic reduction. This classification system is also the basis for fragment-specific fixation of distal radius fractures.

AO Foundation/Orthopaedic Trauma Association (AO/OTA)

The AO/OTA classification offers a simple descriptive classification system which may imperfectly predict treatment, but facilitates communication about the injury and is readily understood (Fig. 60.5). A-type fractures are extra-articular injuries typically in the metaphysis of the radius. B-type fractures are partial articular injuries that are frequently associated with abnormal carpal translation in the direction of the displaced fragment. Partial articular fractures of the dorsal and volar rim of the lunate facet are notoriously unstable and are routinely stabilized operatively. C-type fractures are complete articular injuries where the metaphyseal fracture completely separates each of the articular fragments from the diaphysis. This classification is also the basis for the American Academy of Orthopaedic Surgeons' (AAOS) Appropriate Use Criteria on distal radius fractures.

Fernandez

The Fernandez classification is unique in that it is based on the mechanism of injury and includes mechanisms of bending, shear, compression, avulsion, and high energy. In doing so, this system attempts to take into account the level of bony and soft tissue injury. Its usefulness includes its focus on practical aspects of patient care, provides information on the stability of the fracture, and suggests treatment algorithms based on the severity of the injury.[28]

Nonoperative Treatment

Nonoperative treatment is recommended for the nondisplaced, extra-articular fracture or the stable, reduced fracture. However, predicting fracture stability is challenging. Lafontaine's criteria of stability was one of the first scores used to predict secondary displacement after reduction. They determined if three or more of the following criteria are met, then a fracture is at increased risk of displacement if managed nonoperatively: age >60 years, dorsal comminution, extension of the fracture through the radiocarpal articulation, an associated ulnar fracture, and dorsal angulation >20 degrees.[29]

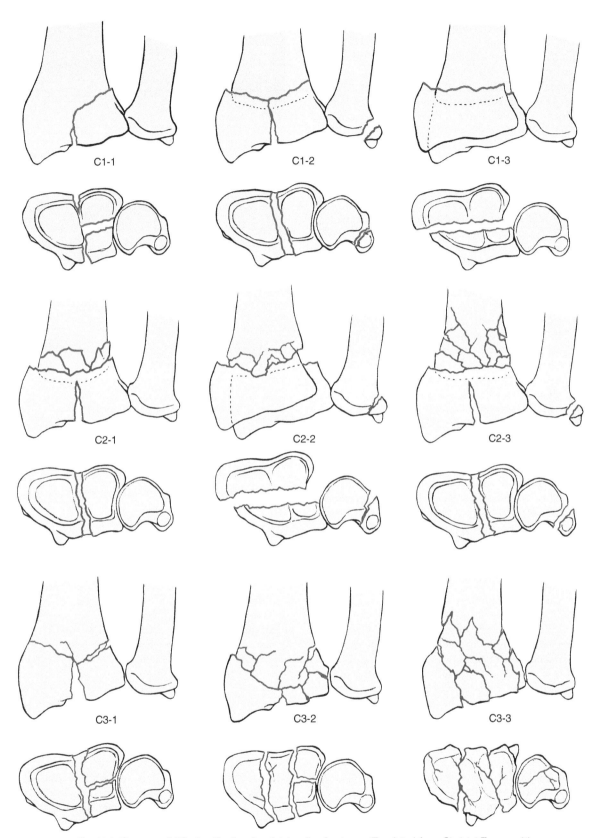

• **Fig. 60.5** Diagram of AO classification for distal radius fractures. (Reprinted from *Skeletal Trauma*. 4th ed., Fig. 40.3.)

Meanwhile, Nesbitt et al. showed that age >60 years was the only significant predictor of instability, even when accounting for all the other variables considered by Lafontaine. Following an acceptable reduction at the time of injury, they found that a 40-year-old patient has a 27% risk of displacement, and this increases to 50% for a 58-year-old patient and 77% for an 80-year-old patient. All these risks decrease if the patient's reduction is maintained 1 week later (10%, 25%, and 57%, respectively).[30] Similarly, Mackenney et al. created calculations to predict the risk of early (2 weeks) and late (time of union) instability based on a patient's age, the presence of comminution, the dorsal angle at presentation, and the ulnar variance at presentation.[31] However, the resultant Edinburgh Wrist Calculator may require validation to individual patient populations.[32]

The importance of age was confirmed by LaMartina et al., as they showed it to be predictive of changes in radial height and radial inclination, as well as the final ulnar variance, radial height, and radial inclination in a multivariable analysis. Additionally, they demonstrated the importance of reestablishing the volar cortical integrity with a closed reduction in regard to maintaining dorsal/volar tilt.[33] Finally, in a systematic review and meta-analysis, Walenkamp et al. demonstrated that dorsal comminution and age >60 years were the only variables that held as being significant predictors of eventual fracture displacement.[32] Regardless of how fracture stability is assessed, it is important to remember that even if no instability criteria are met, there is still the chance of secondary displacement in a reduced fracture. Therefore we recommend that nonoperative treatment includes follow-up in the first 3 weeks after injury to monitor radiographic alignment.

Displaced fractures have historically been indicated for closed reduction and initial immobilization. There is no consensus on the ideal splint/cast design (bivalved short arm cast vs. sugar tong splint vs. reverse sugar tong splint) and positioning to maintain a reduction. It is best to avoid extreme flexion and ulnar deviation to lower the risk of acute carpal tunnel syndrome and to possibly decrease pressure on the volar lunate facet (Fig. 60.6). It has been demonstrated that patients requiring multiple reductions in the emergency department rarely achieve an alignment that is good enough to avoid surgical fixation.[34] Similarly, for patients whose fracture demonstrates initial instability and a likely need for surgery, it has been shown that there is no clear additional benefit to preoperative reduction in the absence of nerve compromise or gross malignment.[35] Furthermore, the closed reduction process is associated with increased pain when just intravenous pain medication is given.[36] Instead, a closed reduction is more commonly done after the administration of a hematoma block, which was recently shown in a meta-analysis to provide adequate pain relief for patients.[37]

For patients treated nonoperatively, we recommend clinical and radiographic evaluation two to three times over the first 3 weeks after the injury so that any displacement will be detected and can be corrected prior to bony malunion. A recent randomized controlled trial demonstrated that there is no clinical benefit for obtaining X-rays after the initial 2 weeks of follow-up, as this treatment plan did not impact patient-rated outcomes or the risk of complications.[38] Once the fracture has solidified in position—typically within 2–3 weeks—these patients can be changed from their initial immobilization into a short arm cast.

These patients—with either nondisplaced fractures or displaced fractures that have since been reduced and are stable—can be treated conservatively with 6 weeks of a short arm cast followed by use of an orthosis as needed for comfort. Christersson et al. showed that there is no clinical benefit to immobilization for <4 weeks, as range of motion is not significantly improved and the risk of displacement is too great.[39] Any significant displacement during healing prompts indication for surgical fixation and a discussion with the patient regarding the risks and benefits.

Range-of-motion exercises for the fingers, elbow, and shoulder should be started immediately (Fig. 60.7). These are performed without resistance and can include gentle active and passive motions. Forearm rotation is often possible as the fracture begins to consolidate by 3 weeks and can be performed within

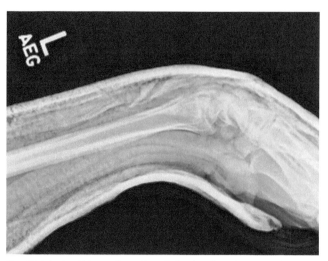

• **Fig. 60.6** Lateral X-ray of a reduced distal radius demonstrating excessive flexion through the carpus which increases the risk of carpal tunnel compression.

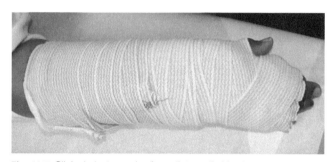

• **Fig. 60.7** Clinical photograph of a splint applied in the emergency room for a distal radius fracture that inappropriately immobilizes the fingers.

the confines of a short arm cast. Casts are removed only when radiographs demonstrate fracture healing (disappearance of fracture line, presence of callus formation). Wrist range of motion commences once the cast is removed but is often associated with soreness following weeks of immobilization. Strengthening exercises should be delayed until there is radiographic evidence of union accompanied by a resolution of fracture tenderness. Both of these activities can be performed at home once patients are properly instructed. Routine formal physical therapy referrals for all patients have shown to not provide clinical benefit.[40] However, specific patients with aversions to stretching or difficulty with rehabilitation will benefit from one-on-one sessions with a therapist. Resuming activity after immobilization is important, as a recent study suggests that patients who are immediately active have a reduced tendency to have disproportionate pain.[41] After cast removal, patients are transitioned to a removable brace or orthosis to be used for comfort over the first week. In the case of a nondisplaced, simple fracture, we may discontinue the cast at 4 weeks and start active range of motion (wrist and forearm rotation) earlier, but still delay strengthening until 6 weeks.

One of the primary potential complications with a nondisplaced distal radius fracture is rupture of the extensor pollicis longus (EPL). It is estimated that this complication impacts ~5% of nondisplaced distal radius fractures, and, on average, occurs 6.5 weeks after the injury.[42] If such an injury occurs, it is recommended to be treated surgically with a tendon transfer of either extensor indicis proprius (EIP) or extensor carpi radialis brevis (ECRB).[43] It has been hypothesized that the attritional rupture of the EPL is due to the combination of poor vascularity at the level of Lister's tubercle, as well as the maintenance of the extensor retinaculum despite the injury, which with the addition of fracture hematoma creates a constrictive space that even further limits blood flow to the tendon.[44] EPL rupture is best detected by the loss of active thumb retropulsion, as well as the loss of active hyperextension at the thumb interphalangeal joint.

Operative Treatment

There are several surgical options for patients with unstable fractures or for those patients who value a more rapid rehabilitation and desire anatomic restoration. However, it should be noted that most studies show equivalent results at 1–2 years after adequate fracture reduction regardless of fixation choice, leaving the specific treatment dependent on fracture characteristics.[45,46]

Internal fixation will generally provide an earlier return to function in the first 6–12 weeks compared with pin fixation or wrist spanning fixation. The most commonly used method is open reduction and internal fixation with volar plating. While some earlier studies showed no difference, more recent studies have demonstrated both improved functional outcomes and fewer complications with the use of volar plates relative to both external fixation and dorsal plating, especially in the first months after surgery.[47–50] Along with the ease of the volar approach, the advent of precontoured volar locking plates has made the technical aspect of the procedure simpler as well. The volar aspect of the radius is frequently less comminuted, allowing for easier assessment of reduction (Fig. 60.8).

Although volar would be our routine approach for most displaced fractures, an exception should be made for the displaced intra-articular fracture that requires reduction under direct visualization. In this situation, dorsal plating would be recommended in order to clearly visualize the articular surface. Alternatively, a volar approach can be supplemented with wrist arthroscopy to facilitate articular reduction.

Dorsal spanning plates have largely replaced the use of external fixation, but should be reserved as a last resort to avoid loss of motion at the wrist. However, it may be required in the setting of a highly comminuted articular surface to maintain reduction and restore radial length.

The open distal radius physis in the child or adolescent requires alternative operative approaches to preserve future growth. Closed reduction with K-wires is typically sufficient for patients with open physes and extra-articular fractures, with open reduction performed only if required.[51] However, these patients should be monitored closely for subsequent displacement, as this technique provides only relative fracture stability.

Surgical Approach for Volar Fixation

Several anatomic features of the wrist are relevant to operative management of the distal radius. During a volar approach to the radius through the flexor carpi radialis (FCR) sheath, surgeons must be aware of the palmar cutaneous branch of the median nerve. Although most commonly located between the FCR and the palmaris longus, this causalgic nerve is located within the FCR sheath in up to 6% of individuals (Fig. 60.9).[52] The watershed line, a prominent transverse ridge on the volar aspect of the distal radius, is the most volar prominence of the distal radius. Volar plates placed on the distal radius are ideally positioned against the bone proximal to this ridge to prevent the flexor tendons from contacting the plate (Fig. 60.10). Plate prominence otherwise risks tenosynovitis of the flexor tendons and potential tendon ruptures,

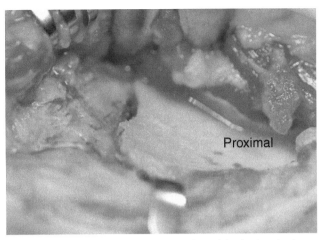

• **Fig. 60.8** Clinical image of intraoperative view of the fractured volar cortex of the distal radius that can be readily reduced.

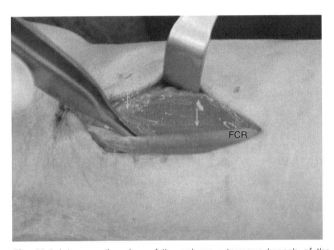

• **Fig. 60.9** Intraoperative view of the palmar cutaneous branch of the median nerve adjacent to the flexor carpi radialis tendon.

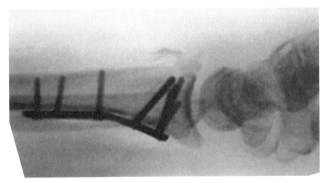

• **Fig. 60.10** Lateral X-ray demonstrating a volar plate tightly applied to the distal radius and positioned proximal to the volar lip of the distal radius to protect the flexor tendons.

most commonly affecting the flexor pollicis longus (FPL) and index finger flexor digitorum profundus.[53] During volar plate fixation, direct visualization of the radiocarpal articular reduction is not possible secondary to the radioscaphocapitate and radiolunate ligaments, which originate from the volar articular margin of the distal radius. These must be noted and preserved during a volar approach to prevent an iatrogenic ulnar carpal translation.

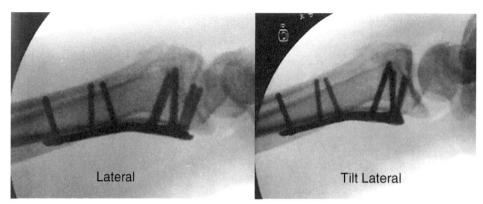

• **Fig. 60.11** Lateral X-ray and lateral tilt X-rays demonstrating how the tilt image clarifies the extra-articular position of the screws.

After appropriately prepping and draping the injured limb on a hand table, the limb is exsanguinated with an Esmarch and an upper arm tourniquet is inflated. A volar longitudinal incision through the skin and subcutaneous tissue is made along the FCR tendon. The FCR tendon sheath is then opened, with care to avoid injury to the palmar cutaneous branch of the median nerve (Fig. 60.1). The tendon is retracted and the floor of the sheath is incised and blunt dissection can proceed radial to the FPL muscle to allow identification of the pronator quadratus (PQ), which is then released distally and radially. If radial length and inclination are not readily restored, the brachioradialis tendon fibers are released from the radial styloid. The fracture is manually reduced and the volar plate is positioned on the distal radius just proximal to the watershed line. We typically stabilize the plate in position with a screw through the oblong hole proximal to the fracture and a K-wire through a wire hole in the distal plate, followed by fluoroscopic confirmation of adequate reduction and plate placement. Second and third screws are then placed into the radial diaphysis. This is followed by drilling and insertion of distal locking screws. For metaphyseal fractures, we utilize only unicortical distal screws to minimize the risk of either rupturing the extensor tendons or placing intra-articular hardware. As long as screws are 75% the length of the measured bicortical distance, then the resultant construct stiffness is comparable to bicortical screw fixation.[54] This surgical choice has also clinically demonstrated the ability to maintain reductions in almost all cases.[55]

After fixation, clinical evaluation of the distal radius alignment, DRUJ stability, and forearm range of motion is performed. Fluoroscopic confirmation of appropriate alignment, plate placement, and screw length is confirmed. This is best achieved with a combination of several fluoroscopic views beyond the standard PA and lateral images. Tweet et al. demonstrated the value of rotational fluoroscopy,[56] and Pace and Cresswell demonstrated that images with the arm held 11 degrees above the table for PA views and 23 degrees above the table for lateral views, to best assess intra-articular penetration (Fig. 60.11).[57] Additionally, a Skyline view was first described in 2010 by Jacob and Clay[58] and allows for easy assessment of dorsal cortical perforation (Fig. 60.12). This intraoperative image has been found to be more sensitive than a lateral fluoroscopic view in assessing this.[59] Notably, no study has identified an imaging modality or specialized view that is 100% sensitive for detecting intra-articular screw penetration. Therefore surgeons must remain vigilant when assessing for intra-articular crepitus when examining wrists after fixation.

Some surgeons advocate repair of the PQ. A systematic review published in 2017 demonstrated no significant differences in the Disabilities of the Arm, Shoulder and Hand (DASH) scores, range

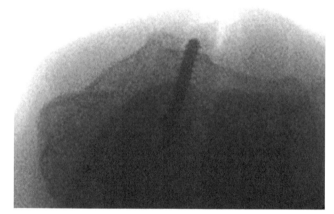

• **Fig. 60.12** Skyline X-ray demonstrating the dorsal profile of the distal radius allowing for assessment of dorsal cortex screw penetration. Screw in this image just ulnar to Lister's tubercle.

of motion, postoperative pain, and complication rates between patients who underwent a repair and those who did not.[60] Furthermore, a recent randomized controlled trial by Sonntag et al. demonstrated no significant differences in patient-rated wrist evaluation scores at 12 months regardless of PQ repair status.[61] Surprisingly, patients who did not have a repair had a significantly higher rating of pronation strength. They did find that in patients who did not undergo a repair of PQ, that at 3 months their PQ was significantly shortened with increased retractions, but that this finding did not correlate with functional scores or complication rates.[62] Although not evidence based, we prefer to repair the pronator over the distal plate when possible (Fig. 60.13).

Irrigation is then used to clean the surgical wound. It is then up to the operating surgeon whether to proceed with closure or to deflate the tourniquet and obtain hemostasis. We prefer tourniquet deflation prior to wound closure due to the proximity of the radial artery to the surgical field. We also prefer closing the subcutaneous layer with a monofilament, absorbable deep dermal suture, and then closure of the skin with a running subcuticular stitch, followed by application of Steri-Strips. A soft dressing is then applied, and a short arm, volar, plaster splint is placed prior to leaving the operating room.

Risks of Volar Plate Fixation

Although any surgical procedure carries inherent risk, the incidence of complications after volar plating for a distal radius

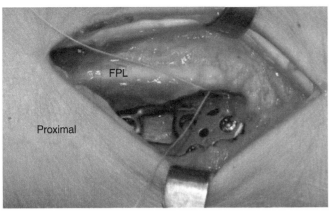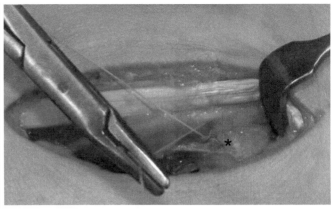

• **Fig. 60.13** Intraoperative view of the pronator quadratus being repaired over the distal plate to protect the flexor pollicis longus *(FPL)* tendon.

fracture repair is low. Overall, minor complications (transient paresthesias, DeQuervain's tenosynovitis, ulnar-sided wrist pain, tendon irritation, delayed union, prolonged stiffness) were recently reported to be at 13.8% and major complications (painful/intra-articular hardware, flexor/extensor tendon rupture, return to the operating room for tendon repair/transfer, carpal/intercarpal ligament injury, carpal tunnel syndrome within 3 months of surgery, compartment syndrome, malunion, DRUJ instability requiring surgery, posttraumatic arthritis requiring additional procedures, nonunion, radial artery injuries requiring repair, and major medical complications) were reported in 17.5% of cases.[63] There is an increased risk of median nerve dysfunction after volar approaches to the distal radius with reported incidence from 0% to 10.2%.[64–69] However, most of these median nerve symptoms are mild and self-limited, resolving in the first few months after surgery.

Although the flexor tendons do not contact the radius as intimately as the extensor tendons, even low-profile volar plates may irritate the flexor tendons if the tendons glide repetitively over the distal edge of the plate. Rates of postoperative flexor tendon rupture are reported from 0% to 1.8%.[53,64,66–69] This risk can be reduced by ensuring the entirety of the plate remains proximal to the transverse ridge at the distal aspect of the radius, keeping the distal plate tightly applied to the bone, and restoring the volar tilt of the radius.[53,70,71] We also attempt to center the plate in the coronal plane so as not to impinge on the DRUJ ulnarly or create a symptomatic radial prominence.

Extensor tendon ruptures, especially the EPL, certainly occur after volar plate fixation. Although this can occur following non-operatively treated fractures, prominent screws placed from volar plates have been implicated in postoperative ruptures. Extensor tendon ruptures complicate up to 6.5% of distal radius fractures treated with a volar locking plate.[64,66–69]

Additionally, generalized risk factors for complications in operative management of distal radius fractures include obesity, diabetes, and smoking, with the latter leading to higher rates of tenderness, stiffness, nonunion, as well as need for hardware removal and revision procedures.[63,72,73]

Surgical Approach for Dorsal Fixation

The utilization of a dorsal approach for distal radius fractures depends on the surgeon's preference, fracture configuration, or the need to directly visualize the radiocarpal articular reduction

(Fig. 60.14). This approach requires the dissection and exposure of the extensor compartments. A longitudinal dorsal incision is made just ulnar to the palpable Lister's tubercle. When dissecting the subcutaneous tissues off the extensor retinaculum, branches of the superficial radial nerve and dorsal cutaneous branch of the ulnar nerve are visualized and kept superficial with the subcutaneous fat.

At the wrist, the extensor tendons run under the extensor retinaculum in six separate fibro-osseous sheaths. The EPL is the only extensor tendon that deviates substantially from a longitudinal course. As such, care must be taken to identify and protect the EPL during a dorsal approach to the distal radius. The extensor digitorum communis (EDC) tendons should be visible proximally, and once these are identified, the extensor retinaculum above them can be incised. When planning to plate the radius dorsally, we prefer to make a step cut in the retinacular tissue. This approach guards against difficulty closing the retinaculum over the fourth compartment and frequently produces one limb of tissue that can be interposed between the plates and tendons (Fig. 60.15). Once the retinaculum is dissected free, the interval between the tendons within the third and fourth compartments is developed to allow access to the dorsal distal radius as well as any free, impacted, articular fragments (Fig. 60.16).

The fourth extensor compartment also contains the posterior interosseous nerve, which is commonly excised as a partial wrist denervation for pain relief during dorsal approaches. Furthermore, careful elevation of the fourth extensor compartment near the DRUJ is essential to preservation of the dorsal radioulnar ligament. The extensor digiti minimi located in the fifth extensor compartment is a commonly used landmark for operative exposure of the DRUJ and the TFCC. Additionally, an interval between the fourth and fifth compartments can be developed to allow access to the dorsal ulnar corner fragment. Deep to the extensor tendons, the dorsal intercarpal and radiocarpal ligaments stabilize the carpus. The primary intrinsic carpal ligaments of the proximal carpal row are the SL and LT ligaments, which are strongest dorsally and volarly, respectively. Care is taken during all dorsal exposures of the wrist to avoid iatrogenic injury to the SL ligament which is located just distal to Lister's tubercle of the distal radius.

Small dorsal fracture fragments are routinely ignored except when encountering dorsal subluxation of the carpus resulting from partial articular fracture of the dorsal lunate facet. In these situations, dorsal fixation can be achieved with a dorsal plate, or in

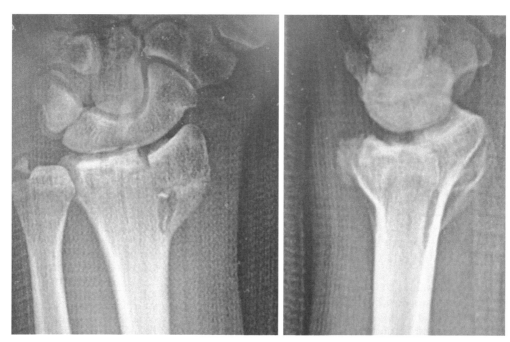

• **Fig. 60.14** X-rays of a comminuted intra-articular fracture felt to be best served with a dorsal approach to ensure articular reduction.

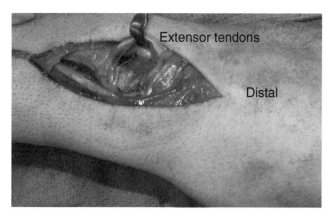

Extensor tendons

Distal

• **Fig. 60.15** Intraoperative image after application of dorsal plates on the radius with half of the extensor retinaculum repaired under the extensor digitorum communis tendons to prevent direct contact with plates.

the case of more comminuted fractures, fragment-specific fixation implants can be used such as pin plates and hook plates.

In the setting of high-energy trauma, the possibility exists that the distal radius fracture is too comminuted in the metaphysis for the typical volar plate or fragment-specific fixation. Under these circumstances, along with carpal instability, dorsal bridge plating serves as a viable treatment alternative. Of note, some surgeons are also utilizing this fixation method in low-demand patients who rely on weight-bearing through assistive devices.[74]

Two surgical approaches are possible.[75,76] First is the use of the fourth dorsal compartment floor to span a plate from the radial diaphysis to the third metacarpal. The approach to the floor of the fourth compartment is the same as previously described. Second is the utilization of the second dorsal compartment to span a plate from the radial aspect of the radial diaphysis to the second metacarpal (Fig. 60.17). There are no clinical data comparing the two constructs. Biomechanical studies have demonstrated

that dorsal bridge plating is stiffer than external fixation,[77] and that third metacarpal fixation is stiffer than second metacarpal fixation.[78,79]

For both approaches, traction is applied to establish radial length. For the second metacarpal approach, an incision is identified with the use of fluoroscopy to mark the proximal and distal extents based on the need for three to four screw holes in both the second metacarpal and the radial shaft. An incision should then be made at the base of the second metacarpal and the insertions of the ECRB and extensor carpi radialis longus (ECRL) should be identified. The proximal incision is then made along the radial shaft in the interval between the ECRB and the ECRL. The plate can then be passed minimally invasively above the periosteum in the proximal to distal direction.

Regardless of approach, the plate should be first fixed distally with a nonlocking screw. The plate can then be used as an adjunct to help restore adequate radial length. Once this is achieved, and proper plate alignment is confirmed via fluoroscopy, the plate can be fixed proximally. We recommend then placing an additional three screws both proximally and distally to complete the fixation. The incisions are then irrigated and closed in a similar fashion as previously described. Patients should be placed into a plaster volar splint for immobilization. A complete detailed description of the technique is outlined in Chapter 64.

One advantage of the dorsal bridge plate is that patients are allowed to weight bear through the forearm and elbow immediately after surgery. Lifting and carrying is still typically limited to less than five pounds until the fracture has healed. This is particularly helpful in the polytrauma setting. However, this tenet has recently come into question, with biomechanical data demonstrating that fixation along the second metacarpal fails in wrist flexion—a typical position associated with weight-bearing.[80] Once the fracture has healed, a second surgery can be performed to remove the plates and screws, typically no earlier than 12 weeks after the original fixation, and usually between 3 and 6 months.

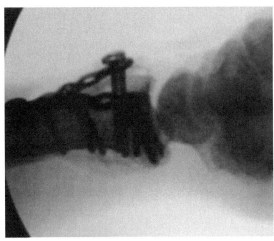
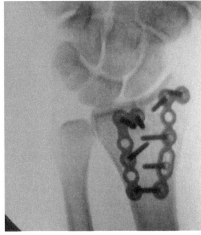

• **Fig. 60.16** X-rays after fixation of the intra-articular fracture confirming reduction of joint congruity and alignment with dorsal plates.

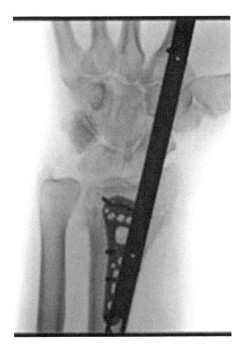

• **Fig. 60.17** X-ray of a distal radius fracture treated with a volar plate and supplemented with a spanning plate to the second metacarpal due to excessive comminution.

Risks of Dorsal Bridge Plate Fixation

Overall, complication rates are low in dorsal bridge plating. Pooled data from eight clinical studies show complication rates ranging from 0.3% to 3.3% with the most frequent issues being finger stiffness and implant failures.[81] Despite the plate's placement extraperiosteally along the extensor compartments, extensor tendon complications including adhesions, finger extension lag, and tendon rupture are all quite rare (0.7%–1.0%).[81] From biomechanical data, differences have been noted between the two described approaches. Placement of the plate along the second metacarpal is associated with increased ECRL and ECRB plate/tendon contact but no tendinous entrapment, while the third metacarpal approach is associated with entrapment of the EPL, abductor pollicis longus, and abductor pollicis brevis, along with

contact of the EIP and EDC tendons.[82,83] Additionally, the second metacarpal approach puts branches of the radial sensory nerve at risk, while the third metacarpal approach has the risk of splitting or entrapping the extensor retinaculum with the plate.[82,83]

Role of Arthroscopy

Distal radius fractures are frequently accompanied by soft tissue injuries, particularly in high-energy injuries.[13,14,84,85] Despite the high frequency of these associated injuries, a routine arthroscopic examination has not been shown to routinely improve outcomes. A postoperative retrospective study analyzed CT scans at the 3-month postoperative time point and found no significant differences in articular step-offs or articular gaps between surgical fixation with fluoroscopy only versus fluoroscopy and arthroscopy.[86] Similar findings have been observed by other researchers.[87] In contrast, others have found that arthroscopy allowed the identification of articular reductions achieved via fluoroscopy alone with up to 3 mm of step-off[88] and helped achieve significantly better articular reductions as measured by the intra-articular reduction index.[89]

We do not routinely incorporate arthroscopy in the treatment of distal radius fractures but believe there are several settings in which arthroscopy can be a useful adjunct. Arthroscopy offers a unique ability to provide assurance that screws do not penetrate the radiocarpal joint and is invaluable when assessing for suspected SL ligament injury while treating a distal radius fracture with a volar approach. It can also assist in the reduction of small displaced articular fractures, such as in a die punch impaction, by providing better visualization of the articular surface. Furthermore, in the setting of persistent DRUJ instability after volar plate fixation, arthroscopy can facilitate TFCC repair in a minimally invasive fashion.

Postoperative Rehabilitation

Following rigid internal fixation, patients are immobilized in a nonremovable, volar, plaster splint for 10–14 days. Such action may decrease patients' postoperative pain and need for analgesic medication.[90] When sutures are removed at 10–14 days, a removable orthosis is fashioned (Fig. 60.4). Active wrist motion and forearm rotation are initiated between 2 and 6 weeks depending on fracture severity and presumed construct rigidity. Although earlier range-of-motion exercises typically speed early recovery, it is not anticipated to change the ultimate outcome.[91] We routinely follow patients every 2 weeks until healing. At 6 weeks, or when healing is demonstrated radiographically, we then introduce passive range of motion while also discontinuing orthotic use and allowing gradual strengthening. Similar to patients treated nonoperatively, there does not appear to be any clinical benefit to universally requiring formal physical/occupational therapy sessions.[92]

Although the majority of motion and function is regained within 3 months of treatment, gradual improvements in motion, strength, endurance, and patient-reported function continue for at least 1 year after distal radius fracture.[93–95]

In the AAOS' 2010 Clinical Practice Guideline, it was recommended to treat patients postoperatively with 500 mg vitamin C daily for 50 days to reduce the incidence of CRPS. This was based on a randomized clinical trial performed by Zollinger et al. who demonstrated a 7.7% reduction in the incidence of CRPS.[96] However, a more recent randomized, placebo-controlled trial examining the effect of daily vitamin C postoperatively showed no differences in range of motion, function, or pain scores at either 6 weeks or 6 months postoperatively.[97] Currently, the AAOS' Appropriate Use Criteria does not comment on the use of vitamin C.[98] As it is unclear in our minds if vitamin C is beneficial, but as we are not aware of the risk associated with taking a vitamin C supplement, we recommend it in patients anticipated to be at higher risk for disproportionate pain following fracture.

Finger Motion

For both nonoperatively and operatively treated distal radius fractures, achieving full finger motion is stressed as a primary goal beginning at the initial evaluation. Patients are recommended to work toward making a full fist without any resistance and to fully extend their digits. This is explained to patients with the common "six-pack" of exercises. These include (1) fully extending the fingers at the metacarpophalangeal (MCP), proximal interphalangeal (PIP), and distal interphalangeal (DIP) joints; (2) keeping the fingers extended at the PIP and DIP joints while flexing at the MCP joints to 90 degrees; (3) keeping the MCP joints extended, while flexing at the PIP and DIP joints; (4) making a complete fist by flexing at the MCP, PIP, and DIP joints; (5) full finger spread via abduction; and (6) touching each fingertip to the thumb one at a time. A common misperception among patients is that squeezing a ball helps achieve full finger motion. We explain that squeezing a ball only adds resistance and actually blocks fingers from making a full fist. In our experience, prolonged finger stiffness after distal radius fracture is difficult to treat and imparts greater impairment than wrist stiffness. Regaining finger motion is stressed at every office visit.

Outcomes

When the distal radius heals in reasonable alignment, regardless of the modality of treatment employed, most patients ultimately do well.[45,46,99,100] Nonunion of the distal radius is rare following both nonoperative and operative treatment as these fractures routinely heal in 6–8 weeks.[101,102] Return of range of motion occurs primarily within the first 3 months, with pronation/supination reaching 92% of the uninjured wrist by this time. Flexion and extension are slower to return, but on average regain 87% and 90% of the contralateral wrist's motion by 1 year.[95] Return of strength progresses more slowly, and patients often experience a

return of grip strength to approximately 81%–94% of the contralateral wrist.[95,102] Most importantly, patients tend to demonstrate excellent functional outcomes.[95,101–103] Rozental and Blazar reviewed 41 patients treated with volar locking plates at an average follow-up of 17 months.[68] These patients reported exceptional return to function, with an average DASH Questionnaire scores of 14/100 (lower scores indicate less disability). Higher energy trauma is associated with worse wrist range of motion, grip strength, and functional scores at 3 and 6 months, but this difference may diminish by 9 months.[104]

Better short-term outcomes can be achieved with early surgical rather than delayed surgical fixation. At 12 weeks, patients surgically treated within the first few days of injury have shown significantly improved range of motion, strength, and functional outcome scores compared with patients treated one or more weeks after their injury.[105,106] These differences disappear by 1 year, suggesting that while earlier surgery may lead to earlier mobilization, long-term outcomes are the same whether or not surgery is delayed.

Radiocarpal arthritic changes are frequently noted on long-term follow-up after intra-articular distal radius fractures. Goldfarb et al. found radiocarpal arthrosis in 13 out of 16 patients 15 years after surgery.[107] However, these changes had no effect on the patients' self-evaluation of function or their clinical examination. Knirk and Jupiter found that this delayed arthritis was best correlated with the accuracy of articular reduction, where 91% of patients with incongruous joint surfaces after surgery developed arthritis versus only 11% of those with congruent articular surfaces.[108] An increased articular gap and postoperative displacement of articular fragments have also been associated with higher stages of arthritis at long-term follow-up.[103,109]

Moving forward, the Distal Radius Outcomes Consortium has proposed a systematic approach to documenting outcomes after distal radius fractures are treated both operatively and nonoperatively.[110] They focus on five domains: performance, patient-rated outcomes, pain, complications, and radiographs, and they provide recommendations for assessment metrics and time points to collect data.

The Older Patient

Bone density is frequently compromised with distal radius fractures in older adults. Regardless of the mechanism, sustaining a distal radius fracture as an older adult is associated with both osteoporosis and subsequent risk of hip fracture in men and women. Unfortunately, orthopedists historically are not adept at facilitating the proper evaluation and management of the underlying endocrine abnormalities that can place patients at risk for these and subsequent bony injuries, including hip and vertebral body fractures, both of which carry significant mortality and morbidity burdens.[111–116] It is now recommended that older patients who experience distal radius fractures from a low-energy injury should undergo bone mineral density testing, assessment of vitamin D and calcium levels, and screening for potential causes of secondary osteoporosis.[117] Because orthopedists are not always comfortable with ordering and/or interpreting these tests, it has been demonstrated that fracture liaison services can be instrumental in implementing this level of care, with significant clinical benefit for patients as seen by higher levels of screening and treatment, along with reduced rates of subsequent fracture and 2-year mortality.[118–122] Remarkably, among patients over the age of 60 years, distal radius fracture portends an 8.7 times increased risk of subsequent hip fracture compared with controls without distal radius fracture.[114]

Advanced age also predicts lost alignment after reduction and casting of distal radius fractures. In this age group, final radiographic appearance of the distal radius most often mirrors the appearance at the time of injury as opposed to postreduction images. Although this would seemingly suggest that surgical intervention is preferred, the impact of distal radius malunion in the older adult is controversial. Grewal and MacDermid found that the number needed to harm from malunion was greater in older adults compared with young adults.[20] Furthermore, a retrospective analysis has shown that surgical treatment is associated with great complications in patients older than 65.[123] Randomized trials have not consistently demonstrated superior objective or patient-reported outcomes with operative treatment for displaced distal radius fractures in older adults and a cross-sectional evaluation was unable to demonstrate any significant negative impact of distal radius malunion in older adults stratified by activity level.[64,124] In one recent randomized trial of patients over 70 years of age, volar plating improved patient-reported outcomes without increasing complications when treating dorsally displaced distal radius fractures.[125] Outside of randomized trials, investigators acknowledge that they have little to no experience treating particular fracture patterns (e.g., partial articular fractures associated with carpal subluxation) or fractures with more extreme displacement nonoperatively. In our practice, we explain to the older patient that operative treatment for mildly displaced fractures (even those somewhat exceeding those values for an acceptable reduction detailed earlier) may not change the ultimate functional outcome. The risks of surgery are, therefore, weighed against the advantages of earlier rehabilitation and a more normal appearance of the wrist.

The Wrist and Radius Injury Surgical Trial (WRIST) is a recently completed, multicenter, randomized clinical trial that evaluated patients >60 years of age with displaced, extra-articular, and intra-articular distal radius fractures.[126] Patients were enrolled at one of 24 clinical sites in the United States, Canada, and Singapore, and patients were randomized to volar locking plate fixation, percutaneous pinning, or external fixation with or without supplemental pinning. Patients treated nonoperatively were also followed as an observation group. Evidence from the study demonstrated that older patients (age >60 years) focus more on the recovery process and differences in this process between operative and nonoperative management once they are informed of the clinically equivalent outcomes.[127] Discussions between older patients and their surgeons should place more emphasis on this topic to allow patients to make an informed decision in a shared decision-making process.[128]

This study also found that older adult function, as measured by patient-rated outcomes, is not associated with the degree of anatomic restoration achieved 1 year after surgery or the type of treatment patients received (open reduction internal fixation vs. external fixation vs. closed reduction and percutaneous pinning vs. casting).[129] Furthermore, in this population, it appears that patients obtain satisfaction with their results if they have achieved 59% of their contralateral hand's grip strength and 79% of their contralateral hand's wrist motion by 1 year after surgery.[130] Predictors of poor patient-rated outcomes included patients with severe baseline pain (Michigan Hand Questionnaire Pain score ≥93/100), more than two comorbidities, and less than a high school education.[131] The presence of any complication after patients undergo open reduction internal fixation with a volar locked plate, external fixation, or closed reduction and percutaneous pinning is not significantly different.[132]

Summary

Distal radius fractures commonly affect patients of all ages. General treatment principles are similar for all patients. Decisions regarding operative versus nonoperative management are complex and are based on fracture morphology and a shared decision-making process between a surgeon and a patient taking into account a patient's goals and risk tolerance in relation to the timeline for recovery. If operative management is chosen, multiple fixation constructs exist, which can achieve favorable outcomes. Ultimately, patients should anticipate a near-full recovery by 1–2 years after their injury.

References

1. Karl JW, Olson PR, Rosenwasser MP. The epidemiology of upper extremity fractures in the United States, 2009. *J Orthop Trauma.* 2015;29(8):E242–E244.
2. Chung KC, Spilson SV. The frequency and epidemiology of hand and forearm fractures in the United States. *J Hand Surg-Am.* 2001;26A(5):908–915.
3. Larsen CF, Lauritsen J. Epidemiology of acute wrist trauma. *Int J Epidemiol.* 1993;22(5):911–916.
4. Bengner U, Johnell O. Increasing incidence of forearm fractures - a comparison of epidemiologic patterns 25 years apart. *Acta Orthop Scand.* 1985;56(2):158–160.
5. Nellans KW, Kowalski E, Chung KC. The epidemiology of distal radius fractures. *Hand Clinics.* 2012;28(2):113.
6. Curtis EM, van der Velde R, Moon RJ, et al. Epidemiology of fractures in the United Kingdom 1988-2012: variation with age, sex, geography, ethnicity and socioeconomic status. *Bone.* 2016;87:19–26.
7. Ismail AA, Pye SR, Cockerill WC, et al. Incidence of limb fracture across Europe: results from the European Prospective Osteoporosis Study (EPOS). *Osteoporosis International.* 2002;13(7):565–571.
8. Louer CR, Boone SL, Guthrie AK, Motley JR, Calfee RP, Wall LB. Postural stability in older adults with a distal radial fracture. *J Bone Joint Surg-Am.* 2016;98(14):1176–1182.
9. Sakai A, Oshige T, Zenke Y, Suzuki M, Yamanaka Y, Nakamura T. Association of bone mineral density with deformity of the distal radius in low-energy Colles' fractures in Japanese women above 50 years of age. *J Hand Surg-Am.* 2008;33A(6):820–826.
10. Ebinger T, Koehler DM, Dolan LA, McDonald K, Shah AS. Obesity increases complexity of distal radius fracture in fall from standing height. *J Orthop Trauma.* 2016;30(8):450–455.
11. Wood AM, Robertson GA, Rennie L, Caesar BC, Court-Brown CM. The epidemiology of sports-related fractures in adolescents. *Injury-Int J Care Inj.* 2010;41(8):834–838.
12. Gelberman RH, Szabo RM, Mortensen WW. Carpal tunnel pressures and wrist position in patients with Colles' fractures. *J Trauma-Injury Infect Crit Care.* 1984;24(8):747–749.
13. Hanker GJ. Radius fractures in the athlete. *Clin Sports Med.* 2001;20(1):189–201.
14. Geissler WB, Freeland AE, Savoie FH, McIntyre LW, Whipple TL. Intracarpal soft-tissue lesions associated with an intra-articular fracture of the distal end of the radius. *J Bone Joint Surg-Am.* 1996;78A(3):357–365.
15. Lindau T, Arner M, Hagberg L. Intraarticular lesions in distal fractures of the radius in young adults. A descriptive arthroscopic study in 50 patients. *J Hand Surg (Edinburgh, Scotland).* 1997;22(5):638–643.

16. Forward DP, Lindau TR, Melsom DS. Intercarpal ligament injuries associated with fractures of the distal part of the radius. *J Bone Joint Surg Am.* 2007;89(11):2334–2340.

17. Jedlinski A, Kauer JMG, Jonsson K. X-ray evaluation of the true neutral position of the wrist: the groove for extensor carpi ulnaris as a landmark. *J Hand Surg.* 1995;20(3):511–512.

18. Yang Z, Mann F, Gilula L, Haerr C, Larsen C. Scaphopisocapitate alignment: criterion to establish a neutral lateral view of the wrist. *Radiol.* 1997;205(3):865–869.

19. Medoff RJ. Essential radiographic evaluation for distal radius fractures. *Hand Clin.* 2005;21(3):279–288.

20. Grewal R, MacDermid JC. The risk of adverse outcomes in extra-articular distal radius fractures is increased with malalignment in patients of all ages but mitigated in older patients. *J Hand Surg-Am.* 2007;32A(7):962–970.

21. Shehovych A, Salar O, Meyer C, Ford D. Adult distal radius fractures classification systems: essential clinical knowledge or abstract memory testing? *Annals Royal Coll Surg Eng.* 2016;98(8):525–531.

22. Wæver D, Madsen ML, Rölfing JHD, et al. Distal radius fractures are difficult to classify. *Injury.* 2018;49:S29–S32.

23. Colles A. On the fracture of the carpal extremity of the radius. *N Eng J Med, Surg Collateral Branches Sci.* 1814;3(4):368–372.

24. Barton JR. Views and treatment of an important injury of the wrist. *The Medical Examiner.* 1838;1:365–368.

25. Smith RW. *A Treatise on Fractures in the Vicinity of Joints, and on Certain Forms of Accidental and Congenital Dislocations.* Dublin: Hodges & Smith; 1847.

26. Frykman G. Fracture of the distal radius including sequelae—shoulder-hand-finger syndrome, disturbance in the distal radio-ulnar joint and impairment of nerve function. A clinical and experimental study. *Acta Orthop Scand.* 1967;Suppl 108:103+.

27. Melone Jr CP. Distal radius fractures: patterns of articular fragmentation. *Orthoped Clin Nor Am.* 1993;24(2):239–253.

28. Fernandez DL. Fractures of the distal radius: operative treatment. *Instructional Course Lectures.* 1993;42:73–88.

29. Lafontaine M, Hardy D, Delince P. Stability assessment of distal radius fractures. *Injury-Int J Care Inj.* 1989;20(4):208–210.

30. Nesbitt KS, Failla JM, Les C. Assessment of instability factors in adult distal radius fractures. *J Hand Surg Am.* 2004;29(6):1128–1138.

31. Mackenney PJ, McQueen MM, Elton R. Prediction of instability in distal radial fractures. *J Bone Joint Surg Am.* 2006;88(9):1944–1951.

32. Walenkamp MM, Aydin S, Mulders MA, Goslings JC, Schep NW. Predictors of unstable distal radius fractures: a systematic review and meta-analysis. *J Hand Surg, Eur.* 2016;41(5):501–515.

33. LaMartina J, Jawa A, Stucken C, Merlin G, Tornetta 3rd P. Predicting alignment after closed reduction and casting of distal radius fractures. *J Hand Surg Am.* 2015;40(5):934–939.

34. Schermann H, Kadar A, Dolkart O, Atlan F, Rosenblatt Y, Pritsch T. Repeated closed reduction attempts of distal radius fractures in the emergency department. *Arch Orthop Trauma Surg.* 2018;138(4):591–596.

35. Teunis T, Mulder F, Nota SP, Milne LW, Dyer GSM, Ring D. No difference in adverse events between surgically treated reduced and unreduced distal radius fractures. *J Orthop Trauma.* 2015;29(11):521–525.

36. Low S, Papay M, Eingartner C. Pain perception following initial closed reduction in the preoperative care of unstable, dorsally displaced distal radius fractures. *J Hand Microsurg.* 2019;11(2):111–116.

37. Tseng P-T, Leu T-H, Chen Y-W, Chen Y-P. Hematoma block or procedural sedation and analgesia, which is the most effective method of anesthesia in reduction of displaced distal radius fracture? *J Orthopaed Surg Res.* 2018;13(1):62.

38. van Gerven P, El Moumni M, Zuidema WP, et al. Omitting routine radiography of traumatic distal radial fractures after initial 2-week follow-up does not affect outcomes. *JBJS.* 2019;101(15):1342–1350.

39. Christersson A, Larsson S, Sanden B. Clinical outcome after plaster cast fixation for 10 days versus 1 month in reduced distal radius fractures: a prospective randomized study. *Scand J Surg: SJS: Official Organ for the Finnish Surgical Society and the Scandinavian Surgical Society.* 2018;107(1):82–90.

40. Wakefield AE, McQueen MM. The role of physiotherapy and clinical predictors of outcome after fracture of the distal radius. *J Bone Joint Surg Br.* 2000;82(7):972–976.

41. Boersma EZ, Meent H Vd, Klomp FP, Frölke JM, Nijhuis-van der Sanden MWG, Edwards MJR. Treatment of distal radius fracture: does early activity postinjury lead to a lower incidence of complex regional pain syndrome? *Hand.* January: 2020. 1558944719895782. https://doi.org/10.1177/1558944719895782.

42. Roth KM, Blazar PE, Earp BE, Han R, Leung A. Incidence of extensor pollicis longus tendon rupture after nondisplaced distal radius fractures. *J Hand Surg Am.* 2012;37(5):942–947.

43. Yu W, Yang G, Li Q, Zhang J, Wu Z, Wang Z. Long-term functional evaluation on tendon transfer to restore extension of the thumb using extensor carpi radialis brevis. *Int J Surg Res Pract.* 2015;2(2):1–2.

44. Engkvist O, Lundborg G. Rupture of the extensor pollicis longus tendon after fracture of the lower end of the radius—a clinical and microangiographic study. *Hand.* 1979;11(1):76–86.

45. Gartland JJ, Werley CW. Evaluation of healed Colles fractures. *J Bone Joint Surg-Am.* 1951;33(4):895–907.

46. Karnezis IA, Fragkiadakis EG. Association between objective clinical variables and patient-rated disability of the wrist. *J Bone Joint Surg-Br.* 2002;84B(7):967–970.

47. Chappuis J, Boute P, Putz P. Dorsally displaced extra-articular distal radius fractures fixation: dorsal IM nailing versus volar plating. A randomized controlled trial. *Orthop Traumatol-Surg Res.* 2011;97(5):471–478.

48. Grewal R, Perey B, Wilmink M, Stothers K. A randomized prospective study on the treatment of intra-articular distal radius fractures: open reduction and internal fixation with dorsal plating versus mini open reduction, percutaneous fixation, and external fixation. *J Hand Surg-Am.* 2005;30A(4):764–772.

49. Ruch DS, Papadonikolakis A. Volar versus dorsal plating in the management of intra-articular distal radius fractures. *J Hand Surg-Am.* 2006;31A(1):9–16.

50. Wei DH, Poolman RW, Bhandari M, Wolfe VM, Rosenwasser MP. External fixation versus internal fixation for unstable distal radius fractures: a systematic review and meta-analysis of comparative clinical trials. *J Orthop Trauma.* 2012;26(7):386–394.

51. Clancey GJ. Percutaneous Kirschner-wire fixation of Colles fractures - a prospective-study of 30 cases. *J Bone Joint Surg-Am.* 1984;66A(7):1008–1014.

52. Jones C, Beredjiklian P, Matzon JL, Kim N, Lutsky K. Incidence of an anomalous course of the palmar cutaneous branch of the median nerve during volar plate fixation of distal radius fractures. *J Hand Surg-Am.* 2016;41(8):841–844.

53. Soong M, Earp BE, Bishop G, Leung A, Blazar P. Volar locking plate implant prominence and flexor tendon rupture. *J Bone Joint Surg-Am.* 2011;93A(4):328–335.

54. Wall LB, Brodt MD, Silva MJ, Boyer MI, Calfee RP. The effects of screw length on stability of simulated osteoporotic distal radius fractures fixed with volar locking plates. *J Hand Surg Am.* 2012;37(3):446–453.

55. Dardas AZ, Goldfarb CA, Boyer MI, Osei DA, Dy CJ, Calfee RP. A prospective observational assessment of unicortical distal screw placement during volar plate fixation of distal radius fractures. *J Hand Surg Am.* 2018;43(5):448–454.

56. Tweet ML, Calfee RP, Stern PJ. Rotational fluoroscopy assists in detection of intra-articular screw penetration during volar plating of the distal radius. *J Hand Surg Am.* 2010;35(4):619–627.

57. Pace A, Cresswell T. Use of articular wrist views to assess intra-articular screw penetration in surgical fixation of distal radius fractures. *J Hand Surg Am.* 2010;35(6):1015–1018.

58. Jacob J, Clay NR. Re: Pichler et al. Computer tomography aided 3D analysis of the distal dorsal radius surface and the effects on volar plate osteosynthesis. *J Hand Surg Eur*. 2009;34: 598–602. J Hand Surg, Eur Vol. 2010;35(4):335–336.

59. Vaiss L, Ichihara S, Hendriks S, Taleb C, Liverneaux P, Facca S. The utility of the fluoroscopic skyline view during volar locking plate fixation of distal radius fractures. *J Wrist Surg*. 2014;3(4):245–249.

60. Mulders MAM, Walenkamp MMJ, Bos F, Schep NWL, Goslings JC. Repair of the pronator quadratus after volar plate fixation in distal radius fractures: a systematic review. *Strateg Trauma Limb Reconstruction*. 2017;12(3):181–188.

61. Sonntag J, Woythal L, Rasmussen P, et al. No effect on functional outcome after repair of pronator quadratus in volar plating of distal radial fractures: a randomized clinical trial. *Bone Jt J*. 2019;101-B(12):1498–1505.

62. Sonntag J, Hern J, Woythal L, Branner U, Lange KHW, Brorson S. The pronator quadratus muscle after volar plating: ultrasound evaluation of anatomical changes correlated to patient-reported clinical outcome. *Hand (New York, NY)*. 2021;16(1):32–37.

63. DeGeorge Jr BR, Brogan DM, Becker HA, Shin AY. Incidence of complications following volar locking plate fixation of distal radius fractures: an analysis of 647 cases. *Plast Reconstruct Surg*. 2020;145(4):969–976.

64. Arora R, Lutz M, Hennerbichler A, Krappinger D, Espen D, Gabl M. Complications following internal fixation of unstable distal radius fracture with a palmar locking-plate. *J Orthop Trauma*. 2007;21(5):316–322.

65. Ho AWH, Ho ST, Koo SC, Wong KH. Hand numbness and carpal tunnel syndrome after volar plating of distal radius fracture. *Hand*. 2010;6(1):34–38.

66. Hove LM, Nilsen PT, Furnes O, Oulie HE, Solheim E, Molster AO. Open reduction and internal fixation of displaced intraarticular fractures of the distal radius - 31 patients followed for 3-7 years. *Acta Orthop Scand*. 1997;68(1):59–63.

67. Musgrave DS, Idler RS. Volar fixation of dorsally displaced distal radius fractures using the 2.4-mm locking compression plates. *J Hand Surg-Am*. 2005;30A(4):743–749.

68. Rozental TD, Blazar PE. Functional outcome and complications after volar plating for dorsally displaced, unstable fractures of the distal radius. *J Hand Surg-Am*. 2006;31A(3):359–365.

69. Ward CM, Kuhl TL, Adams BD. Early complications of volar plating of distal radius fractures and their relationship to surgeon experience. *Hand*. 2010;6(2):185–189.

70. Kitay A, Swanstrom M, Schreiber JJ, et al. Volar plate position and flexor tendon rupture following distal radius fracture fixation. *J Hand Surg-Am*. 2013;38A(6):1091–1096.

71. Tanaka Y, Aoki M, Izumi T, Fujimiya M, Yamashita T, Imai T. Effect of distal radius volar plate position on contact pressure between the flexor pollicis longus tendon and the distal plate edge. *J Hand Surg-Am*. 2011;36A(11):1790–1797.

72. Hess DE, Carstensen SE, Moore S, Dacus AR. Smoking increases postoperative complications after distal radius fracture fixation: a review of 417 patients from a level 1 trauma center. *Hand (New York, NY)*. 2018;15:686–691. https://doi.org/10.1177/1558944718810882.

73. London DA, Stepan JG, Lalchandani GR, Okoroafor UC, Wildes TS, Calfee RP. The impact of obesity on complications of elbow, forearm, and hand surgeries. *J Hand Surg Am*. 2014;39(8):1578–1584.

74. Hyatt BT, Hanel DP, Saucedo JM. Bridge plating for distal radius fractures in low-demand patients with assist devices. *J Hand Surg*. 2019;44(6):507–513.

75. Hanel DP, Lu TS, Weil WM. Bridge plating of distal radius fractures: the Harborview method. *Clin Orthopaed Related Res*. 2006;445:91–99.

76. Ruch DS, Ginn TA, Yang CC, Smith BP, Rushing J, Hanel DP. Use of a distraction plate for distal radial fractures with metaphyseal and diaphyseal comminution. *J Bone Joint Surg Am*. 2005;87(5):945–954.

77. Wolf JC, Weil WM, Hanel DP, Trumble TE. A biomechanic comparison of an internal radiocarpal-spanning 2.4-mm locking plate and external fixation in a model of distal radius fractures. *J Hand Surg Am*. 2006;31(10):1578–1586.

78. Alluri RK, Bougioukli S, Stevanovic M, Ghiassi A. A biomechanical comparison of distal fixation for bridge plating in a distal radius fracture model. *J Hand Surg*. 2017;42(9):748. e741–e748.

79. Guerrero EM, Lauder A, Federer AE, Glisson R, Richard MJ, Ruch DS. Metacarpal position and lunate facet screw fixation in dorsal wrist-spanning bridge plates for intra-articular distal radial fracture: a biomechanical analysis. *J Bone Joint Surg Am*. 2020;102(5):397–403.

80. Huang JI, Peterson B, Bellevue K, Lee N, Smith S, Herfat S. Biomechanical assessment of the dorsal spanning bridge plate in distal radius fracture fixation: implications for immediate weight-bearing. *Hand*. 2018;13(3):336–340.

81. Lauder A, Hanel DP. Spanning bridge plate fixation of distal radial fractures. *JBJS Reviews*. 2017;5(2): e2. 01874474-201702000-00002. https://doi.org/10.2106/JBJS.RVW.16.00044.

82. Lewis S, Mostofi A, Stevanovic M, Ghiassi A. Risk of tendon entrapment under a dorsal bridge plate in a distal radius fracture model. *J Hand Surg Am*. 2015;40(3):500–504.

83. Dahl J, Lee DJ, Elfar JC. Anatomic relationships in distal radius bridge plating: a cadaveric study. *Hand (New York, NY)*. 2015;10(4):657–662.

84. Carlsen BT, Rizzo M, Moran SL. Soft-tissue injuries associated with distal radius fractures. *Operative Tech Orthopaed*. 2009;19(2):107–118.

85. Ogawa T, Tanaka T, Yanai T, Kumagai H, Ochiai N. Analysis of soft tissue injuries associated with distal radius fractures. *Sports Med, Arthroscopy, Rehabilitation, Ther Technol*. 2013;5(1):19.

86. Saab M, Wunenburger PE, Guerre E, et al. Does arthroscopic assistance improve reduction in distal articular radius fracture? A retrospective comparative study using a blind CT assessment. *Eur J Orthopaed Surg Traumatol: Orthopedie Traumatologie*. 2019;29(2):405–411.

87. Ruch DS, Vallee J, Poehling GG, Smith BP, Kuzma GR. Arthroscopic reduction versus fluoroscopic reduction in the management of intra-articular distal radius fractures. *Arthroscopy*. 2004;20(3):225–230.

88. Lutsky K, Boyer MI, Steffen JA, Goldfarb CA. Arthroscopic assessment of intra-articular distal radius fractures after open reduction and internal fixation from a volar approach. *J Hand Surg Am*. 2008;33(4):476–484.

89. Burnier M, Le Chatelier Riquier M, Herzberg G. Treatment of intra-articular fracture of distal radius fractures with fluoroscopic only or combined with arthroscopic control: a prospective tomodensitometric comparative study of 40 patients. *Orthopaed Traumatol, Surg Res: OTSR*. 2018;104(1):89–93.

90. Andrade-Silva FB, Rocha JP, Carvalho A, Kojima KE, Silva JS. Influence of postoperative immobilization on pain control of patients with distal radius fracture treated with volar locked plating: a prospective, randomized clinical trial. *Injury*. 2019;50(2):386–391.

91. Lozano-Calderon SA, Souer S, Mudgal C, Jupiter JB, Ring D. Wrist mobilization following volar plate fixation of fractures of the distal part of the radius. *J Bone Joint Surg-Am*. 2008;90A(6):1297–1304.

92. Chung KC, Malay S, Shauver MJ. The relationship between hand therapy and long-term outcomes after distal radius fracture in older adults: evidence from the randomized Wrist and Radius Injury Surgical Trial. *Plastic Reconstructive Surg*. 2019;144(2):230e–237e.

93. Bobos P, Nazari G, Lalone EA, Grewal R, MacDermid JC. Recovery of grip strength and hand dexterity after distal radius fracture: a two-year prospective cohort study. *Hand Therap*. 2017;23(1):28–37.

94. Abramo A, Kopylov P, Tagil M. Evaluation of a treatment protocol in distal radius fractures. *Acta Orthop*. 2008;79(3):376–385.

95. Dillingham C, Horodyski M, Struk AM, Wright T. Rate of improvement following volar plate open reduction and internal fixation of distal radius fractures. *Adv Orthop*. 2011;2011. 565642-565642.

96. Zollinger PE, Tuinebreijer WE, Breederveld RS, Kreis RW. Can vitamin C prevent complex regional pain syndrome in patients with wrist fractures? A randomized, controlled, multicenter dose-response study. *J Bone Joint Surg Am.* 2007;89(7):1424–1431.

97. Özkan S, Teunis T, Ring DC, Chen NC. What is the effect of vitamin C on finger stiffness after distal radius fracture? A double-blind, placebo-controlled randomized trial. *Clin Orthopaed Related Res.* 2019;477(10):2278–2286.

98. American Academy of Orthopaedic Surgeons. *Appropriate Use Criteria for Treatment of Distal Radius Fractures.* Rosemont, IL: American Academy of Orthipaedic Surgeons; 2013.

99. McQueen M, Caspers J. Colles fracture - does the anatomical result affect the final function. *J Bone Joint Surg-Br.* 1988;70(4):649–651.

100. Wilcke MKT, Abbaszadegan H, Adolphson PY. Patient-perceived outcome after displaced distal radius fractures - A comparison between radiological parameters, objective physical variables, and the DASH score. *J Hand Ther.* 2007;20(4):290–298.

101. Fok MWM, Klausmeyer MA, Fernandez DL, Orbay JL, Bergada AL. Volar plate fixation of intra-articular distal radius fractures: a retrospective study. *J Wrist Surg.* 2013;2(3):247–254.

102. MacFarlane RJ, Miller D, Wilson L, et al. Functional outcome and complications at 2.5 years following volar locking plate fixation of distal radius fractures. *J Hand Microsurg.* 2015;7(1):18–24.

103. Catalano LW, Cole RJ, Gelberman RH, Evanoff BA, Gilula LA, Borrelli J. Displaced intra-articular fractures of the distal aspect of the radius - long-term results in young adults after open reduction and internal fixation. *J Bone Joint Surg-Am.* 1997;79A(9):1290–1302.

104. Roh YH, Lee BK, Noh JH, Oh JH, Gong HS, Baek GH. Factors delaying recovery after volar plate fixation of distal radius fractures. *J Hand Surg-Am.* 2014;39(8):1465–1470.

105. Weil YA, Mosheiff R, Firman S, Liebergall M, Khoury A. Outcome of delayed primary internal fixation of distal radius fractures: a comparative study. *Injury-Int J Care Inj.* 2014;45(6):960–964.

106. Yamashita K, Zenke Y, Sakai A, Oshige T, Moritani S, Maehara T. Comparison of functional outcome between early and delayed internal fixation using volar locking plate for distal radius fractures. *J UOEH.* 2015;37(2):111–119.

107. Goldfarb CA, Rudzki JR, Catalano LW, Hughes M, Borrelli J. Fifteen-year outcome of displaced intra-articular fractures of the distal radius. *J Hand Surg-Am.* 2006;31A(4):633–639.

108. Knirk JL, Jupiter JB. Intra-articular fractures of the distal end of the radius in young adults. *JBJS.* 1986;68(5):647–659.

109. Lutz M, Arora R, Krappinger D, Wambacher M, Rieger M, Pechlaner S. Arthritis predicting factors in distal intraarticular radius fractures. *Arch Orthop Trauma Surg.* 2011;131(8):1121–1126.

110. Waljee JF, Ladd A, MacDermid JC, Rozental TD, Wolfe SW. A unified approach to outcomes assessment for distal radius fractures. *J Hand Surg Am.* 2016;41(4):565–573.

111. Cuddihy MT, Gabriel SE, Crowson CS, O'Fallon WM, Melton 3rd LJ. Forearm fractures as predictors of subsequent osteoporotic fractures. *Osteoporosis International.* 1999;9(6):469–475.

112. Gupta MJ, Shah S, Peterson S, Baim S. Rush fracture liaison service for capturing "missed opportunities" to treat osteoporosis in patients with fragility fractures. *Osteoporosis International.* 2018;29(8):1861–1874.

113. Haentjens P, Autier P, Collins J, Velkeniers B, Vanderschueren D, Boonen S. Colles fracture, spine fracture, and subsequent risk of hip fracture in men and women. A meta-analysis. *J Bone Joint Surg Am.* 2003;85(10):1936–1943.

114. Chen CW, Huang TL, Su LT, et al. Incidence of subsequent hip fractures is significantly increased within the first month after distal radius fracture in patients older than 60 years. *J Trauma Acute Care Surg.* 2013;74(1):317–321.

115. Freedman KB, Kaplan FS, Bilker WB, Strom BL, Lowe RA. Treatment of osteoporosis: are physicians missing an opportunity? *J Bone Joint Surg Am.* 2000;82(8):1063–1070.

116. Robin BN, Ellington MD, Jupiter DC, Brennan ML. Relationship of bone mineral density of spine and femoral neck to distal radius fracture stability in patients over 65. *J Hand Surg Am.* 2014;39(5):861–866. e863.

117. Ostergaard PJ, Hall MJ, Rozental TD. Considerations in the treatment of osteoporotic distal radius fractures in elderly patients. *Curr Rev Musculoskelet Med.* 2019;12(1):50–56.

118. Huntjens KM, van Geel TA, van den Bergh JP, et al. Fracture liaison service: impact on subsequent nonvertebral fracture incidence and mortality. *J Bone Joint Surg Am.* 2014;96(4):e29.

119. Nakayama A, Major G, Holliday E, Attia J, Bogduk N. Evidence of effectiveness of a fracture liaison service to reduce the re-fracture rate. *Osteoporosis International.* 2016;27(3):873–879.

120. Walters S, Khan T, Ong T, Sahota O. Fracture liaison services: improving outcomes for patients with osteoporosis. *Clin Interventions in Aging.* 2017;12:117–127.

121. Curtis JR, Silverman SL. Commentary: the five Ws of a Fracture Liaison Service: why, who, what, where, and how? In osteoporosis, we reap what we sow. *Curr Osteoporosis Rep.* 2013;11(4):365–368.

122. Dell R. Fracture prevention in Kaiser Permanente Southern California. *Osteoporosis International.* 2011;22(Suppl 3):457–460.

123. DeGeorge Jr BR, Van Houten HK, Mwangi R, Sangaralingham LR, Larson AN, Kakar S. Outcomes and complications in the management of distal radial fractures in the elderly. *J Bone Joint Surg Am.* 2020;102(1):37–44.

124. Nelson GN, Stepan JG, Osei DA, Calfee RP. The impact of patient activity level on wrist disability after distal radius malunion in older adults. *J Orthop Trauma.* 2015;29(4):195–200.

125. Saving J, Severin Wahlgren S, Olsson K, et al. Nonoperative treatment compared with volar locking plate fixation for dorsally displaced distal radial fractures in the elderly: a randomized controlled trial. *J Bone Joint Surg Am.* 2019;101(11):961–969.

126. Wrist, Radius Injury Surgical Trial (WRIST) Study Group. Reflections 1 year into the 21-Center National Institutes of Health—funded WRIST study: a primer on conducting a multicenter clinical trial. *J Hand Surg Am.* 2013;38(6):1194–1201.

127. Nasser JS, Huetteman HE, Shauver MJ, Chung KC. Older patient preferences for internal fixation after a distal radius fracture: a qualitative study from the Wrist and Radius Injury Surgical Trial. *Plast Reconstruct Surg.* 2018;142(1):34e–41e.

128. Huetteman HE, Shauver MJ, Nasser JS, Chung KC. The desired role of health care providers in guiding older patients with distal radius fractures: a qualitative analysis. *J Hand Surg.* 2018;43(4):312–320. e314.

129. Chung KC, Cho HE, Kim Y, Kim HM, Shauver MJ, WRIST Group. Assessment of anatomic restoration of distal radius fractures among older adults: a secondary analysis of a randomized clinical trial. *JAMA Network Open.* 2020;3(1). e1919433-e1919433.

130. Chung KC, Sasor SE, Speth KA, Wang L, Shauver MJ. Patient satisfaction after treatment of distal radial fractures in older adults. *J Hand Surg, Eur.* 2020;45(1):77–84.

131. Chung KC, Kim HM, Malay S, et al. Predicting outcomes after distal radius fracture: a 24-center international clinical trial of older adults. *J Hand Surg.* 2019;44(9):762–771.

132. Chung KC, Malay S, Shauver MJ, Kim HM, WRIST Group. Assessment of distal radius fracture complications among adults 60 years or older: a secondary analysis of the WRIST randomized clinical trial. *JAMA Network Open.* 2019;2(1). e187053-e187053.

61

Technique Spotlight: ORIF of Intra-Articular Distal Radius Fractures—Volar Approach

JOSHUA A. GILLIS AND SANJEEV KAKAR

Introduction

It is important to try and achieve as close as an anatomic reduction of the articular surface as possible, especially in a young patient, in the management of intra-articular distal radius fractures to reduce the chance of posttraumatic radiocarpal arthritis.[1,2] Visualization of the radiocarpal articular surface was historically performed through a dorsal approach to the distal radius fracture via a dorsal capsulotomy.[1] With the advent of volar locking plates, many surgeons now prefer to fix an intra-articular fracture through a volar approach.[1,2]

Confirmation of the reduction of the articular surface is typically performed using fluoroscopy. This is an indirect assessment of the articular cartilage reduction and can underestimate the step-offs or gaps of the articular surface.[1,3,4] Wrist arthroscopy can be used to confirm, measure, and assist in articular reduction; assess intercarpal ligaments and the triangular fibrocartilage complex (TFCC); and has been shown to demonstrate significant step-offs and gaps not identified radiographically.[3] Abe et al. evaluated 155 wrists arthroscopically during distal radius fracture fixation after reduction was achieved using fluoroscopy. They found residual intra-articular gaps or step-off >2 mm in 35.2% of patients.[4] In addition, they found scapholunate ligament and TFCC injury in 28.9% and 63.2% of patients, respectively. The use of arthroscopy allows a magnified, high-resolution view of the articular surface to guide reduction compared to the indirect method of fluoroscopy.[1,5,6] The use of arthroscopic-assisted reduction has correlated with improved patient-reported outcomes, wrist and forearm motion, and radiographic alignment compared to fluoroscopy.[2]

Indications

The volar approach to the distal radius with arthroscopic guidance is typically performed for displaced intra-articular distal radius fractures, AO types B and C, that have failed closed management and are amenable to volar plate fixation.[3] It is primarily used to

guide articular reduction but can be used to address other carpal or soft tissue pathology, as indicated. Given the fluid extravasation that can be seen with traditional arthroscopy, we advocate "dry" arthroscopy.[7–9]

Preoperative Evaluation

Preoperative and postreduction radiographs are assessed to determine the displacement of the distal radius fracture and the degree of articular congruity. The radial tilt, inclination, width, and height are measured. Particular attention is paid to assess for articular step-offs and gaps (Fig. 61.1). A computed tomography (CT) scan is helpful to appropriately measure the size of any step-offs and gaps and to determine the size and number of intra-articular fragments (Fig. 61.2). A CT scan can help to plan the proper reduction of these fragments, determine the reference fragment, and determine the appropriate plate placement and need for disimpaction of fracture fragments.[10] A detailed discussion is then had with the patient to determine whether one should proceed with nonsurgical or operative intervention.

Positioning and Equipment

The patient is positioned supine on the operating table with the operative extremity abducted 90 degrees on an arm table. A nonsterile tourniquet is applied to the upper arm. Prior to starting surgery on the affected wrist, we always examine the uninjured contralateral extremity's distal radioulnar joint (DRUJ) in neutral, pronation, and supination to ascertain baseline examination of DRUJ stability.

Technique

The extended flexor carpi radialis (FCR) volar approach to the radius is performed first.[11] A 6- to 8-cm incision is made overlying the FCR tendon proximal to the proximal wrist crease. The

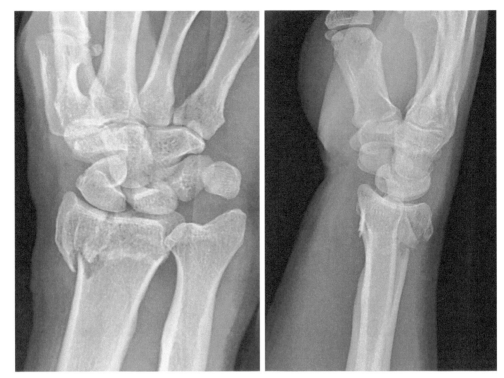

• **Fig. 61.1** Posteroanterior and lateral radiographic views of a comminuted distal radius fracture with intra-articular extension.

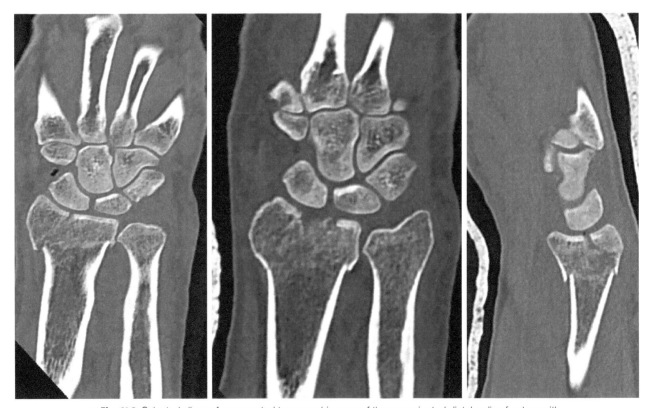

• **Fig. 61.2** Selected slices of a computed tomographic scan of the comminuted distal radius fracture with intra-articular extension demonstrating the articular step-offs and incongruity.

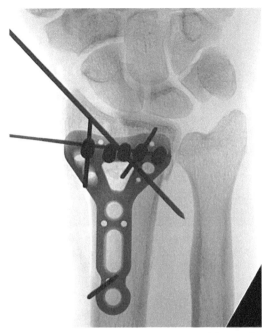

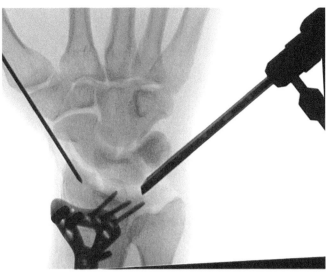

• **Fig. 61.3** Fluoroscopic image of a volar plate provisionally fixed to the comminuted intra-articular distal radius fracture using K-wires with a K-wire placed through the radial styloid to obtain provisional fracture stabilization.

• **Fig. 61.4** Fluoroscopic image of a volar plate fixed to the comminuted intras-articular distal radius fracture with three distal screws, working from ulnar to radial. A K-wire remains through the radial styloid for provisional fracture stabilization as the fragments are fixed to the plate from the ulnar to radial direction, with arthroscopic assisted reduction. The arthroscope can be seen intra-articularly.

skin and subcutaneous tissue are dissected, and care is taken to identify the palmar cutaneous branch of the median nerve and the superficial branch of the radial artery, especially at the distal aspect of the incision, given that we do cross the wrist crease to access the very distal aspect of the radius. The anterior sheath of the FCR is divided and the FCR is retracted ulnarly, with care taken to identify and protect the palmar cutaneous branch of the median nerve. The posterior sheath of the FCR is then opened over the pronator quadratus (PQ). The thick septum between the FCR and flexor pollicis longus (FPL) is divided distally, allowing the tendons and median nerve to be retracted ulnarly.

The PQ fascia is released in an L-shaped manner at its distal and radial insertions, retracting it ulnarly with the FPL. The PQ is then elevated subperiosteally along the volar margin of the radius and fracture site. This is done from the radial border to the volar ulnar corner, which supports the lunate fossa, ensuring not to injure the extrinsic carpal ligaments.[3] The periosteum over the fracture is incised and removed. To facilitate reduction of the fracture, the brachioradialis tendon is divided. The fracture is then cleaned of hematoma and debris volarly, provisionally reduced and stabilized with K-wires, as indicated. A volar locking plate is applied to the distal radius, its position confirmed fluoroscopically, and the nonlocking shaft screw is applied proximally through the oblong hole. K-wires can be applied through the distal aspect of the plate to obtain the best reduction possible using fluoroscopy (Fig. 61.3). It is critical that no screws are placed through the distal screw holes at this time.[7,12–14]

The hand is then placed in a standard arthroscopic tower, with finger traps applied to the index through small fingers. No more than five to seven pounds of traction is used. Given the fracture comminution, typical bony landmarks used to establish the arthroscopy portals such as Lister's tubercle may be lost. As such, we typically start with the 6R portal as the ulnar head is often devoid of injury. Using a 22-gauge needle, the proximal aspect of

the triquetrum is palpated and the 6R portal created. The arthroscope is placed through this portal to evaluate the reduction of the articular surface. Typically the view is obscured with fracture hematoma which can be removed using the "automatic washout technique" in which a 2.5-mm shaver is introduced into the radiocarpal joint through a 3–4 portal and a 10-mL saline-filled syringe is attached to the side port of the arthroscope.[7] The joint is lavaged until the hematoma is evacuated. The valve of the scope's sheath should be kept open at all times to allow air to circulate freely inside the joint.[12] It is important that the arthroscope does not rest on the distal radius as it can lead to fracture displacement. The quality of the articular reduction of the lunate facet is first evaluated. If this is deemed satisfactory, fixation of this fragment can be performed through the plate by placing the distal ulnar screws (Fig. 61.4). If the fracture is malreduced, the K-wires are removed, the articular fragments are reduced under arthroscopic control with a shoulder probe, and the K-wires are reinserted (Fig. 61.5). Once the lunate facet has been reduced and stabilized with screw fixation, attention is directed to the radial column of the distal radius fracture and a similar procedure performed. It is critical that the surgeon alternate the arthroscope between the 6R and 3–4 portals to ensure the adequacy of the reduction is viewed from multiple angles. The remainder of the diaphyseal screws are inserted to create a rigid construct[10] (Fig. 61.6).

The TFCC is examined and DRUJ stability is checked in neutral, pronation, and supination by stabilizing the radius with one hand while the ulna is grasped with the examiner's other hand and translated volarly and dorsally in relation to the radius. If the DRUJ is found to be unstable in ulnar deviation as compared to the contralateral extremity but tightens up in radial deviation, the TFCC is not addressed given that the secondary stabilizers of the DRUJ appear to be intact. If the DRUJ is unstable in both ulnar and radial deviation, the TFCC is arthroscopically repaired.[15,16] Lindau et al. looked retrospectively at 51 patients with displaced

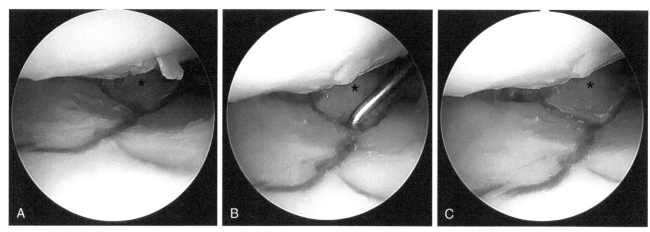

• **Fig. 61.5** Arthroscopic views of the displaced intra-articular distal radius fracture. (A) The radial styloid fragment *(asterisk)* is displaced and (B) reduction is performed using the shoulder probe to achieve (C) adequate reduction of the articular surface, which is then fixated using the radial column screws of the volar plate.

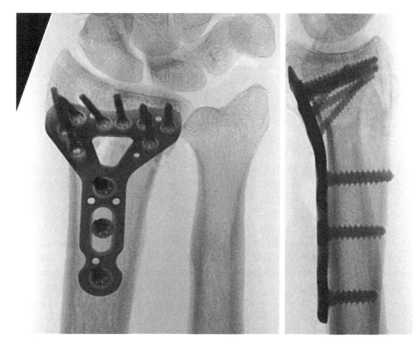

• **Fig. 61.6** Posteroanterior and lateral fluoroscopic views of the intra-articular distal radius fracture post open reduction internal fixation using a volar approach with a volar plate and arthroscopic-guided reduction.

distal radius fractures of which 43 had arthroscopically confirmed TFCC tears.[17] None of these TFCC injuries were treated and the patients were evaluated at a median of 12 months. They found that 19 patients (37%) had instability of the DRUJ, which was painful in 13 patients. Ten of 11 patients with a complete peripheral tear demonstrated DRUJ instability. Those with a partial or no peripheral tear had DRUJ instability in 7 of 32 patients.[17] Instability was not associated with any radiographic features. The same group looked at 38 of these patients 13–15 years post injury, of which 25 had had a partial or central tear and 8 had a complete peripheral tear.[18] Of the original 51 patients, one patient had undergone a repair of their TFCC tear secondary to painful DRUJ instability. They found 17 of the 38 patients to have a lax DRUJ, and those with laxity had worse grip strength. There was a trend towards improved DASH (The Disabilities of the Arm, Shoulder and Hand) and Gartland and Werley scores with a stable DRUJ; however, this did not reach significance. There was no difference

in the presence of DRUJ arthritis between those with a lax or stable DRUJ.[18] Given these findings, the authors suggest that aggressive management of the TFCC may not be necessary; however, any true difference in subjective outcome needs to be delineated with proper randomized trials.[17,18]

PEARLS AND PITFALLS

- Dry arthroscopy can be used to aid in intra-articular distal radius reduction and fixation, which reduces the risk of fluid extravasation, swelling, postoperative pain, and compartment syndrome that may be associated with wet arthroscopy.
- Pitfalls of arthroscopy may include iatrogenic injury of the carpus or distal radius as the bony landmarks can be lost, longer operative times, and a learning curve associated with starting this technique.

References

1. Lutsky K, Boyer MI, Steffen JA, Goldfarb CA. Arthroscopic assessment of intra-articular distal radius fractures after open reduction and internal fixation from a volar approach. *J Hand Surg Am.* 2008;33(4):476–484.
2. Herzberg G. Intra-articular fracture of the distal radius: arthroscopic-assisted reduction. *J Hand Surg Am.* 2010;35(9):1517–1519.
3. Henry MH, Griggs SM, Levaro F, Clifton J, Masson MV. Volar approach to dorsal displaced fractures of the distal radius. *Tech Hand Up Extrem Surg.* 2001;5(1):31–41.
4. Abe Y, Yoshida K, Tominaga Y. Less invasive surgery with wrist arthroscopy for distal radius fracture. *J Orthop Sci.* 2013;18(3):398–404.
5. Edwards 2nd CC, Haraszti CJ, McGillivary GR, Gutow AP. Intra-articular distal radius fractures: arthroscopic assessment of radiographically assisted reduction. *J Hand Surg Am.* 2001;26(6):1036–1041.
6. Auge 2nd WK, Velazquez PA. The application of indirect reduction techniques in the distal radius: the role of adjuvant arthroscopy. *Arthroscopy.* 2000;16(8):830–835.
7. del Pinal F, Garcia-Bernal FJ, Pisani D, Regalado J, Ayala H, Studer A. Dry arthroscopy of the wrist: surgical technique. *J Hand Surg Am.* 2007;32(1):119–123.
8. del Pinal F, Garcia-Bernal FJ, Delgado J, Sanmartin M, Regalado J, Cerezal L. Correction of malunited intra-articular distal radius fractures with an inside-out osteotomy technique. *J Hand Surg Am.* 2006;31(6):1029–1034.
9. Kakar S, Burnier M, Atzei A, Ho PC, Herzberg G, Del Pinal F. Dry wrist arthroscopy for radial-sided wrist disorders. *J Hand Surg Am.* 2020;45(4):341–353.
10. Del Pinal F, Klausmeyer M, Moraleda E, de Piero GH, Ruas JS. Arthroscopic reduction of comminuted intra-articular distal radius fractures with diaphyseal-metaphyseal comminution. *J Hand Surg Am.* 2014;39(5):835–843.
11. Orbay JL, Gray R, Vernon LL, Sandilands SM, Martin AR, Vignolo SM. The EFCR approach and the radial septum-understanding the anatomy and improving volar exposure for distal radius fractures: imagine what you could do with an extra inch. *Tech Hand Up Extrem Surg.* 2016;20(4):155–160.
12. Del Pinal F. Technical tips for (dry) arthroscopic reduction and internal fixation of distal radius fractures. *J Hand Surg Am.* 2011;36(10):1694–1705.
13. Del Pinal F. Arthroscopy: some dos and don'ts. In: Del Pinal F, ed. *Atlas of Distal Radius Fractures.* Stuttgart: Thieme; 2018:51–72.
14. Del Pinal F. Treatment of explosion type distal radius fractures. In: del Piñal FMC, Luchetti C, eds. *Arthroscopic Management of Distal Radius Fractures.* Berlin: Springer Verlag; 2010:41–65.
15. Atzei A, Luchetti R, Braidotti F. Arthroscopic foveal repair of the triangular fibrocartilage complex. *J Wrist Surg.* 2015;4(1):22–30.
16. Atzei A. New trends in arthroscopic management of type 1-B TFCC injuries with DRUJ instability. *J Hand Surg Eur.* 2009;34(5):582–591.
17. Lindau T, Adlercreutz C, Aspenberg P. Peripheral tears of the triangular fibrocartilage complex cause distal radioulnar joint instability after distal radial fractures. *J Hand Surg Am.* 2000;25(3):464–468.
18. Mrkonjic A, Geijer M, Lindau T, Tagil M. The natural course of traumatic triangular fibrocartilage complex tears in distal radial fractures: a 13-15 year follow-up of arthroscopically diagnosed but untreated injuries. *J Hand Surg Am.* 2012;37(8):1555–1560.

62

Technique Spotlight: Dorsal Plating for Distal Radius Fractures

SCOTT G. EDWARDS, NICHOLAS S. ADAMS, AND
PAUL A. TAVAKOLIAN

Indications

Open reduction with internal fixation has become the preferred treatment for most unstable intra-articular and periarticular fractures; however, there is no consensus regarding optimal treatment algorithms and predicted outcomes with various surgical options. Like any fixation technique, each has advantages and disadvantages. Volar locked plating, for example, although popular for most fractures that are dorsally displaced, relies on locking screws to buttress the subchondral bone at the joint. The more the articular surface is compromised, however, the less mechanical advantage these screws have to neutralize the deforming forces. Furthermore, poor bone quality potentially may not allow for enough purchase for screw threads and may allow avulsion of dorsal fragments and consequent loss of reduction. Additionally, the volar approach can lead to greater neuropathic complications or carpal tunnel syndrome from retraction of the median nerve.[1,2] Dorsal plating has an advantage in these fractures by providing buttress support; however, there are potential complications, notably hardware irritation and extensor tendon–related complications.[3]

Biomechanically, dorsal plating has been shown to be at least equivalent and perhaps superior to volar locking plates in previous investigations. Kandemir et al. demonstrated no difference between volar and dorsal plating in an extra-articular fracture model and in a dorsally comminuted model.[4] Trease et al. found dorsal plates to have a greater rigidity than volar plates and Gondusky et al. noted that dorsal plating resulted in less fracture motion.[5,6]

The dorsal approach to the distal radius is a reproducible and straightforward approach with no detachment of muscles or mobilization or retraction of significant neurovascular structures. If intra-articular inspection is desired, the visualization afforded by a dorsal approach via a dorsal arthrotomy does so without the need to violate the critical volar wrist ligaments.[7]

Additional advantages of dorsal plate fixation include the ability of more recent plate designs to address more complex fracture patterns than volar plates in isolation, thus minimizing the need for supplemental fragment–specific fixation. An intra-articular fracture with a displaced, far distally fractured radial styloid fragment, for example, may pose a challenge for the one or two screws of a volar plate to secure adequately in order to allow for early motion. Supplemental fixation may be required in addition to the volar plate. Current dorsal plates, on the other hand, extend to the radial styloid by design in a manner in which volar plates cannot. As another example, fragility fractures predictably fracture close to the joint. These far distal fractures are challenging for any fixation technique, but since dorsal plates have the ability to align along the dorsal rim, these plates have the best opportunity to stabilize these fractures.

In summary, the advantages of the dorsal plating techniques for distal radius fractures include (1) the ability to address complex fracture patterns with little need for supplemental fragment–specific fixation; (2) a better option for far distal, fragility fractures; (3) a relatively easier reduction opportunity and a sound, and perhaps superior biomechanical fixation alternative for severely angulated and dorsally comminuted fractures; (4) the ease of dissection without placing major neurovascular structures at risk; (5) the opportunity for hematoma evacuation of the third dorsal compartment and release of the extensor pollicis longus (EPL) tendon from adjacent fracture lines; (6) a relatively less invasive direct visualization of the articular surfaces, if desired; and (7) ability to perform corrective osteotomies, if needed.

Preoperative Assessment

All patients with fractures of the distal radius should have a comprehensive clinical evaluation in terms of usual activity status, potential comorbidities, associated injuries, and soft tissue concerns. As with any distal radius fracture, preoperative zero rotation posteroanterior, oblique, and lateral radiographs of the affected wrist should be obtained and evaluated for fracture angulation, displacement, radial shortening, comminution, intra-articular extension, any ulnar-sided injury, and stability (Fig. 62.1). Comparison views, traction radiographs, and advanced imaging can be helpful in further characterizing the injury.

Particular attention to identify fracture patterns that may be challenging for volar plating techniques or well suited for dorsal plates should be identified, as discussed in the previous section. In addition, dorsal radiocarpal fracture-dislocation along with dorsally displaced and angulated fracture patterns require dorsal buttress fixation and may be best offered by dorsal plates. The dorsal

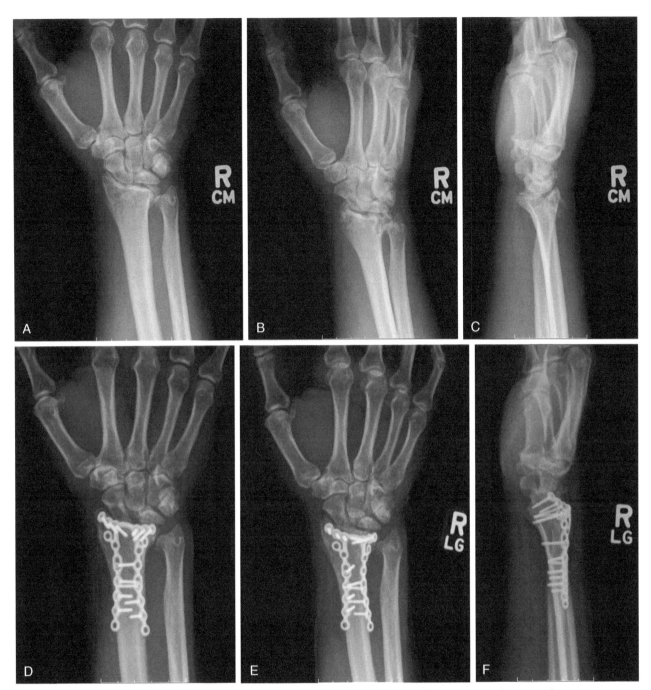

• **Fig. 62.1** Preoperative (A) right wrist posteroanterior (PA), (B) oblique, (C) and lateral radiographs of a 64-year-old female following a ground-level fall. Postoperative (D) PA, (E) oblique, and (F) lateral radiographs taken 4 months following dorsal plate fixation. As with any distal radius fracture, preoperative zero rotation posteroanterior, oblique, and lateral radiographs of the affected wrist should be obtained and evaluated for fracture angulation, displacement, radial shortening, comminution, intra-articular extension, any ulnar-sided injury, and stability.

rim of the distal radius extends more distal than the volar surface given the natural volar tilt and thus allows for a more distal plate placement to capture more distal, comminuted, and articular fragments with (1) dorsal shear fractures, (2) dorsal die-punch fractures or fracture patterns in which an indirect reduction from the volar approach cannot be obtained, and (3) fractures with associated scapholunate ligament injury or other bony and ligamentous lesions requiring operative intervention.

Relative contraindications to the dorsal approach and fixation to the distal radius include patients with poor dorsal soft tissues, volarly displaced and angulated fracture patterns (Smith), volar shear fractures (Barton), and isolated marginal lunate facet fractures. Also, comminuted articular distal radius fractures in which locking screws will not achieve fixation distally may be better addressed using either an external fixator or a dorsal spanning plate.

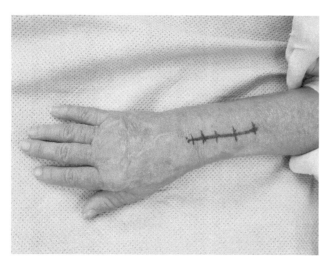

• **Fig. 62.2** The affected limb is prepared and draped under sterile conditions. Using a surgical marker, the longitudinal incision is positioned over the distal forearm just ulnar to Lister's tubercle.

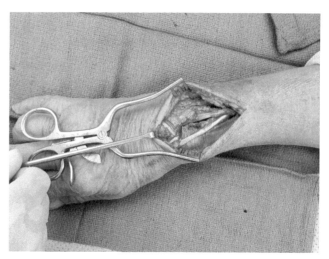

• **Fig. 62.4** Sharp dissection elevates the second and fourth dorsal compartments radially and ulnarly, respectively. This is done in a subperiosteal plane to minimize scarring and adhesion of the extensor tendons and to provide a layer of soft tissue between the tendons and plate during closure.

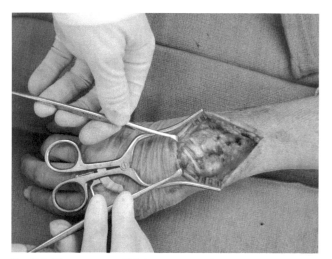

• **Fig. 62.3** The extensor pollicis longus tendon is identified distally, sharply released from the third dorsal compartment and retracted radially.

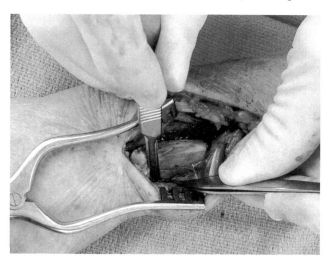

• **Fig. 62.5** Care should be taken to protect the branches of superficial radial nerve and tendons of the first dorsal compartment during this step. Throughout elevation and exposure, care is taken not to disrupt the soft tissue attachments to the distal-most dorsal comminuted fragments.

Positioning and Equipment

Patient positioning for open reduction and internal fixation of distal radius fractures with a dorsal approach should be in the supine position with the affected extremity extended onto a radiolucent table located next to the operating table or patient stretcher. It should be noted that this position may force the fracture into relative pronation inadvertently and care must be taken to neutralize these imposed forces across the wrist when reducing the fracture. Usually being mindful to rotate through the shoulder rather than the wrist can be helpful. A nonsterile, pneumatic, upper arm tourniquet is applied to facilitate hemostasis and visualization throughout the procedure. Intraoperative fluoroscopy is essential to assess reduction, confirm hardware positioning, as well as determine postfixation stability and motion. We prefer regional anesthesia and a single dose of preoperative, prophylactic antibiotics are routinely given.

Detailed Technique Description

The affected limb is prepared and draped under sterile conditions. Using a surgical marker, the longitudinal incision is positioned over the distal forearm just ulnar to Lister's tubercle (Fig. 62.2).

After the affected extremity is exsanguinated and a pneumatic tourniquet is inflated, sharp dissection is used to incise through the skin and down to the extensor retinaculum. Full-thickness flaps are elevated to expose the retinaculum using care to avoid damage to the superficial radial nerve branches (Fig. 62.3). The EPL tendon is identified distally, sharply released from the third dorsal compartment, and retracted radially (Fig. 62.4). Sharp dissection elevates the second and fourth dorsal compartments radially and ulnarly, respectively. This is done in a subperiosteal plane to minimize scarring and adhesion of the extensor tendons and to provide a layer of soft tissue between the tendons and plate during closure. Dissection is carried radially to the brachioradialis tendon and ulnarly to the ulnar border of the radius with careful attention to avoid detaching the dorsal radioulnar ligaments of the triangular fibrocartilage complex. Tenotomy of the brachioradialis tendon can be performed to ease reduction (Fig. 62.5). Care should be taken to protect the branches of superficial radial nerve and tendons of the first dorsal compartment during this step. Throughout elevation and exposure, care is taken not to disrupt the soft tissue attachments to the distal-most dorsal comminuted

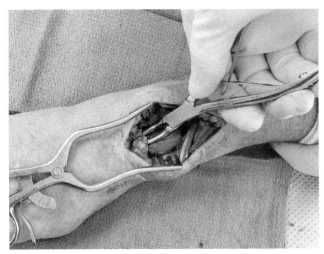

• **Fig. 62.6** The fracture is mobilized and any interposed fibrous tissue is debrided with a rongeur. This should be done cautiously while maintaining the dorsal distal capsular tissues.

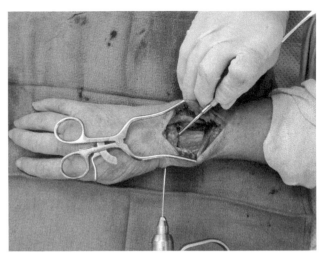

• **Fig. 62.8** Once reduced, one or two transversely directed 0.062-inch Kirschner pins are placed immediately deep to the subchondral bone to support reduced die-punch fragments or articular comminution.

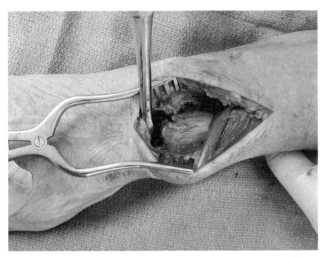

• **Fig. 62.7** While assessment of the reduction may be done with fluoroscopy, there may be times to further critically assess the articular surface directly through a capsulotomy of the radiocarpal joint.

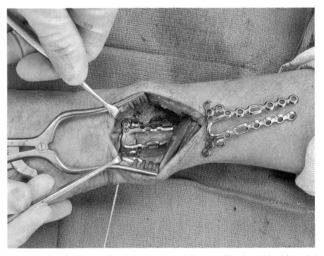

• **Fig. 62.9** Implant selection is important. A low-profile dorsal locking plate must match the width of the radius. Multiple widths are available through most manufacturers.

fragments. Leaving a continuous sleeve of periosteum over these distal fragments will preserve whatever vascularity remains and will allow the fragments to be manipulated while maintaining a "leash" on the fragments to assist in the reduction.

The fracture is mobilized and any interposed fibrous tissue is debrided with a rongeur. This should be done cautiously while maintaining the dorsal distal capsular tissues (Fig. 62.6).

After mobilization of the fracture, reduction is facilitated with a wide elevator placed in the subchondral space (Fig. 62.7). While assessment of the reduction may be done with fluoroscopy, there may be times to further critically assess the articular surface directly through a capsulotomy of the radiocarpal joint. This may be performed through a longitudinal incision while protecting the underlying cartilage and intrinsic ligaments. Once reduced, one or two transversely directed 0.062-inch Kirschner pins are placed immediately deep to the subchondral bone to support reduced die-punch fragments or articular comminution (Fig. 62.8).

Implant selection is important. A low-profile dorsal locking plate must match the width of the radius. Multiple widths are available through most manufacturers (Fig. 62.9). Apply the plate to assess any discrepancies between the plate and the underlying

bone. Contour the plate as necessary to match the profile of the bone. Most dorsal plates are designed to be positioned distal to Lister's tubercle, but if Lister's tubercle prevents the plate from lying close to the bone, it can be removed and used as bone graft. The plate can be provisionally fixed with pins while positioning is assessed. At this point, articular tilt, inclination, and congruity should be adequately reduced. Radial height, however, will be corrected later in the procedure. Once the plate position is confirmed, the distal holes are drilled and locking screws are placed. It is imperative that these be placed immediately below the subchondral bone to support the reduced articular surface. Subchondral screw placement may be assessed with a 20-degree lateral fluoroscopy view (Fig. 62.10). If there is any question of joint penetration with the screws, a small dorsal capsulotomy may be performed for direct visualization. Depending on the specific fracture, nonlocking screws through the dorsal plate may be required to capture and compress volar fragments, such as a volar tear-drop-type fragment or a segment of volar cortical bone from the metaphysis.

With the distal locking screws placed, restoration of radial height and small modifications to volar tilt is done through

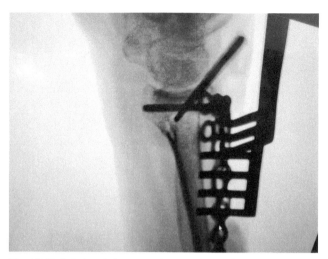

• **Fig. 62.10** Subchondral screw placement may be assessed with a 20-degree lateral fluoroscopy view.

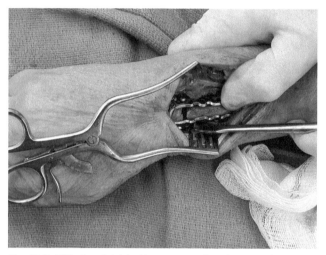

• **Fig. 62.11** With the distal locking screws placed, restoration of radial height and small modifications to volar tilt is done through traction as well as translating the plate distally with the aid of a blunt instrument, such as a Key elevator.

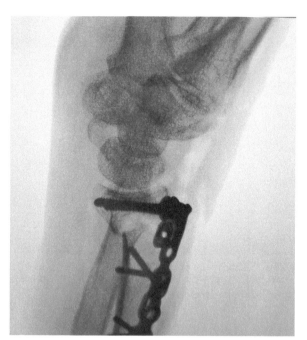

• **Fig. 62.12** A final assessment of screw positioning and lengths is done with fluoroscopy.

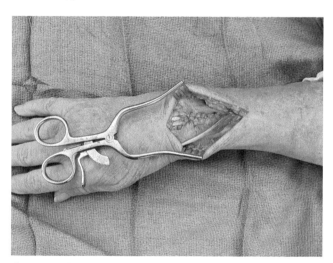

• **Fig. 62.13** It is common not to be able to close the periosteum completely over the plate. The extensor pollicis longus tendon remains radialized in the subcutaneous plane.

traction as well as translating the plate distally with the aid of a blunt instrument, such as a Key elevator (Fig. 62.11). This can be held provisionally with pins through the plate while the oblong hole is drilled and a nonlocking screw is placed. Reduction is again assessed via fluoroscopy. Adjustments are made if needed and the remaining proximal screw holes are drilled and screws are placed. Nonlocking screws should be used to draw the plate close to the bone. Once the bone and plate are in contact, locking screws can be placed. A final assessment of screw positioning and lengths is assessed with fluoroscopy (Fig. 62.12). Although not routinely performed for acute fractures, bone graft can be placed within the metaphysis, if desired.

Prior to closure, motion of the wrist, especially extension, should be assessed for potential screw articular penetration or plate impingement. Stability of the distal radioulnar joint should also be assessed for laxity in all positions of forearm rotation. The operative site is irrigated copiously and closure is begun. If a capsulotomy was performed, this is repaired with 3-0 braided, nonabsorbable suture. The elevated second and fourth compartments, along with their underlying periosteum are reapproximated over

the plate and secured with nonabsorbable 3-0 braided suture. It is common not to be able to close the periosteum completely over the plate. The EPL tendon remains radialized in the subcutaneous plane (Fig. 62.13). The skin is closed as per the surgeon's preference. A well-padded, volar-based splint is applied to immobilize the wrist. Immediate elevation and digital motion is encouraged. Assuming confidence in the fixation, hand therapy is begun within 3–5 days to begin wrist motion, edema control, and fabrication of a custom resting splint. Patients are weaned from the splint over the next 4–6 weeks.

Follow-up with the surgeon occurs at 10–14 days for a wound check and suture removal. Limited weight-bearing to two pounds is allowed for the first 4 weeks and continues until adequate callous formation is demonstrated on radiographs, usually at 6 weeks. There should be a specific discussion with the patient regarding the potential need for dorsal plate removal. Although dorsal plate implant design has evolved substantially over the past two decades, tendon-related complications are still a concern. Failure to progress in rehabilitation, particularly in wrist and/or digital flexion, should raise suspicions that tendon adherence may be an issue and plate removal may be indicated at the appropriate time. Even after union, patients are instructed to report any pain or swelling that may occur over the dorsal wrist. Routine plate removal after 6 months is not unreasonable, though may not be necessary.

PEARLS AND PITFALLS

- Correct identification of fracture patterns that are optimally addressed through a dorsal fixation.
- Subperiosteal elevation of the second and fourth dorsal compartments allows for a soft tissue layer between the implant and extensor tendons.
- It is imperative that the distal screws be placed to support the subchondral bone to prevent subsidence and shortening of the radius. These should be of proper length to avoid irritation of the underlying flexor tendons.
- Contour the plate to match the morphology of the dorsal distal radius to optimize plate mechanics. Lister's tubercle can be excised, if not already fragmented, and used as bone graft to better accommodate the plate.
- Adequately restore radial length through a combination of traction and translation of the plate after distal screw placement (Fig. 62.10).
- Visual assessment of gliding of all tendons should be performed to ensure unrestricted movement over the plate to minimize postoperative tenosynovitis or the risk of attritional tendon ruptures.
- The surgeon should stay vigilant for signs of extensor tenosynovitis postoperatively and maintain a low threshold for hardware removal.
- Early active range of motion should be initiated to prevent tendon adhesions and stiffness.

References

1. Yu YR, Makhni MC, Tabrizi S, Rozental TD, Mundanthanam G, Day CS. Complications of low-profile dorsal versus volar locking plates in the distal radius: a comparative study. *J Hand Surg Am.* 2011;36(7):1135–1141. https://doi.org/10.1016/j.jhsa.2011.04.004.
2. Chou Y-C, Chen AC-Y, Chen C-Y, Hsu Y-H, Wu C-C. Dorsal and volar 2.4-mm titanium locking plate fixation for AO type C3 dorsally comminuted distal radius fractures. *J Hand Surg Am.* 2011;36(6):974–981. https://doi.org/10.1016/j.jhsa.2011.02.024.
3. Azzi AJ, Aldekhayel S, Boehm KS, Zadeh T. Tendon rupture and tenosynovitis following internal fixation of distal radius fractures: a systematic review. *Plast Reconstr Surg.* 2017;139(3):717e–724e. https://doi.org/10.1097/PRS.0000000000003076.
4. Kandemir U, Matityahu A, Desai R, Puttlitz C. Does a volar locking plate provide equivalent stability as a dorsal nonlocking plate in a dorsally comminuted distal radius fracture? A biomechanical study. *J Orthop Trauma.* 2008;22(9):605–610. https://doi.org/10.1097/BOT.0b013e318186006f.
5. Trease C, McIff T, Toby EB. Locking versus nonlocking T-plates for dorsal and volar fixation of dorsally comminuted distal radius fractures: a biomechanical study. *J Hand Surg Am.* 2005;30(4):756–763. https://doi.org/10.1016/j.jhsa.2005.04.017.
6. Gondusky JS, Carney J, Erpenbach J, et al. Biomechanical comparison of locking versus nonlocking volar and dorsal T-plates for fixation of dorsally comminuted distal radius fractures. *J Orthop Trauma.* 2011;25(1):44–50. https://doi.org/10.1097/BOT.0b013e3181d7a3a6.
7. Müller A, Child C, Allemann F, Pape H-C, Breiding P, Hess F. Using mini-arthrotomy for dorsal plating to treat intraarticular distal radius fractures: can it improve radiological and clinical outcomes? *Eur J Trauma Emerg Surg.* March 2020:1-8. https://doi.org/10.1007/s00068-020-01354-9.

63

Technique Spotlight: Fragment Specific Options for Distal Radius Fractures

FRANCIS J. AVERSANO AND DAVID M. BROGAN

Introduction

The last two decades have seen the introduction of new implants and techniques revolutionize the capacity to successfully stabilize displaced and unstable distal radius fractures. The advent and sweeping adoption of volar locked plating in the new millennium quickly broadened indications for surgery.[1,2] The demonstrated success[3] and versatility[4] of volar locked plating have led to its adoption as the most common method of fixation of distal radius fractures.[5] However, while volar locking plates (VLPs) are a crucial tool in a surgeon's armamentarium, they are not the panacea for all distal radius fractures. A subset of fracture patterns will benefit from alternative approaches and implant selection. Fragment-specific fixation[6] utilizes multiple implants, through one or more incisions, each designed to secure an individual fracture fragment. In comminuted intra-articular distal radius fractures, the epiphysis commonly separates into five characteristic fragments with fault lines at the intervals between radiocarpal ligament attachments.[7] The most common fragments include the radial column, dorsal ulnar corner, dorsal wall, volar rim or volar ulnar corner (VUC), and free intra-articular fragments (Fig. 63.1).[8]

Advantages of Fragment-Specific Fixation

Increased articular cavity depth or intra-articular step-off ≥3 mm has been shown to increase radiocarpal contact stress.[9–11] The goals of fragment-specific techniques are to achieve direct open visualization, manipulation, and buttress-style fixation of each fragment to facilitate anatomic reduction and create a load-sharing construct. Buttress-style fixation with low-profile implants eliminates dependency on screw thread purchase of the dorsal ulnar corner, dorsal wall, and radial styloid fracture fragments, as is necessary when relying on isolated fixation with a volar plate. Often these fragments are small, secondary to a shear or avulsion mechanism, and pose a challenge in capturing from the volar side while minimizing dorsal prominence of the screws.[12,13] Distal fractures of the volar surface are also difficult to stabilize with a standard VLP without risking flexor tendon injury.[14–20] Low-profile fragment-specific implants minimize tendon irritation on the dorsal surface[20–22] or when volar fixation is required distal to the watershed line,[20–22] as is often the case with the critical VUC

fragment. Fragment-specific implants can be utilized in isolation, in combination, or as adjunctive fixation[23,24] to other fixation methods to stabilize very distal or highly comminuted distal radius fractures.

Radiographic Considerations

Careful analysis of injury radiographs is crucial when considering or planning fragment-specific fixation techniques.[8] Measurements of radial height, radial inclination, ulnar variance, volar tilt, and articular step-off provide insight into the global displacement of a distal radius fracture; well-described thresholds for each value identify unacceptable deformity and inform indications for operative treatment. Abnormalities in these radiographic parameters act synergistically and should be considered in the context of the total deformity, rather than in isolation (Fig. 63.2).

A systematic and reproducible method for identifying the character and degree of displacement of each fracture fragment is critical for treatment planning. The central reference point (CRP) is an important landmark to identify on the posteroanterior (PA) radiograph (Fig. 63.3). The CRP is the point halfway between the dorsal and volar corners of the sigmoid notch. This point should be used as the more proximal reference point when measuring radial inclination, ulnar variance, and radial height because it remains consistent despite excess dorsal or volar angulation.[25]

On both the PA and lateral radiographs, radiodense lines below the subchondral radius may represent a rotated dorsal wall fragment (Fig. 63.4) or a free intra-articular fragment that has rotated into the metaphyseal cavity. On the lateral radiograph, it is important to identify incongruency of the joint interval, widening of the anteroposterior (AP) distance, depression of the teardrop angle, and carpal malalignment. In the absence of radiocarpal ligament injury or articular step-off, a contiguous and smooth radiocarpal articulation should be noted, from the dorsal to volar margin. Similarly, the arc of curvature of the articular surface of the distal radius should be congruent to the proximal pole of the lunate; incongruency can occur when volar or dorsal ulnar corner fragments separate or rotate in the sagittal plane (Fig. 63.5). A 10-degree lateral view provides a clearer view of the articular surface by positioning the X-ray beam parallel to the radial inclination of the joint.[26]

In extra-articular fractures, a depression of the teardrop angle implies increased dorsal angulation of the epiphyseal fragment. However, in an intra-articular fracture, a depressed teardrop angle of <45 degrees often corresponds to dorsal angulation of the volar portion of the lunate facet, as is seen in a standard Colles' fracture (Fig. 63.6).[27]

Alternatively, a volar shear injury may cause proximal displacement of the VUC and subsequent volar translation of the carpus. In some fractures, a small avulsion fracture of the attachment of the volar carpal ligaments may escape distally with corresponding volar subluxation of the carpus, particularly in the setting of an impacted volar lunate facet. Recognition of this carpal malalignment on injury radiographs is critical to inform surgical planning; distal radius fractures with carpal malalignment are usually treated

operatively. To better evaluate these fractures, computed tomography (CT) scans are often employed. While not critical for every pattern, CT scans can help with preoperative planning for complex intra-articular fractures, particularly if the surgeon has less experience with highly comminuted fractures.[28–32]

Positioning and Operating Room Setup

Generally, we prefer to position the patient supine with the arm outstretched on an arm board. A tourniquet is placed on the upper

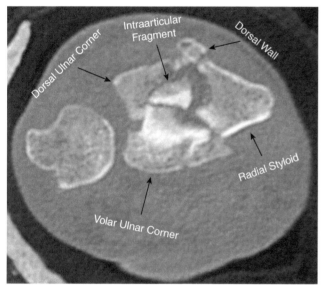

• **Fig. 63.1** Fragment-specific fracture fragments.

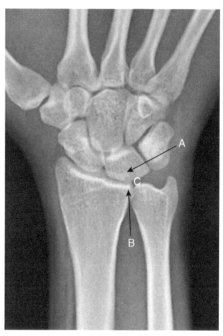

• **Fig. 63.3** Central reference point. The midpoint between the dorsal (A) and volar (B) corners of the sigmoid notch is called the central reference point (C).

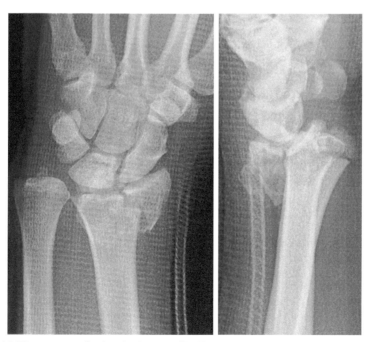

• **Fig. 63.2** Multifragmentary distal radius fracture. Significant loss of radial column height, positive ulnar variance, dorsal and radial translation, and dorsal tilt with depressed teardrop angle.

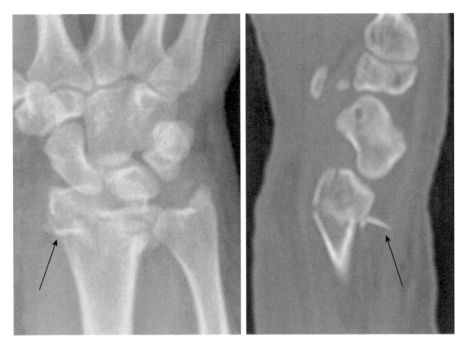

• **Fig. 63.4** Rotated dorsal wall fragment.

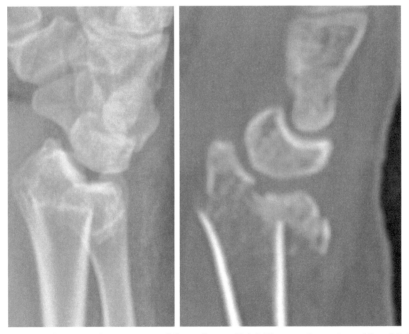

• **Fig. 63.5** Discontinuity and incongruency of the radiocarpal joint. The arc of curvature of the distal radius is in discontinuity and does not match with that of the proximal pole of the lunate.

arm and the arm is prepped to the level of the tourniquet, well above the elbow. The wrist is positioned over a rolled towel and finger traps are applied to the index and long fingers. A Kerlix gauze connects the finger traps with 5–10 lbs of traction hung over the end of the arm table. Our preference is to utilize a large C-arm, brought in 45 degrees from the end of the arm table in order to avoid the traction rope/weights, with the monitor positioned orthogonally to the C-arm to allow visualization by the surgeon and assistant.

General Principles for Fragment-Specific Fixation

In this section, we will present our preferred techniques and sequence to address each fracture fragment that may be present. The ultimate goals are to achieve articular congruency, restore length, and ensure stability of the radiocarpal and distal radioulnar joints (DRUJ). When planning to utilize a fragment-specific technique, our preferred sequence to address each fracture fragment is as follows: (1) reduction of intra-articular fragments, (2) bone grafting of the metaphyseal void, (3) reduction and provisional stabilization of the radial column, (4) fixation of the volar lunate facet, (5) fixation of the dorsal ulnar corner, (6) additional fixation of the radial column as needed, and (7) fixation of the dorsal wall.

Intra-articular Fragments

Prior to reducing and stabilizing any other fracture fragments, depressed intra-articular fragments must be addressed. Implants will later interfere with the ability to access the metaphyseal void, to tamp up depressed intra-articular fragments, and/or to apply bone graft to this area. During the initial reduction, a window for insertion of a tamp, elevator, or bone graft can be created by booking open a dorsal wall, radial styloid, or metaphyseal fracture fragment. Traction, flexing the wrist over a rolled towel bump,

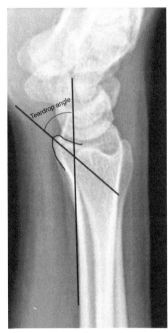

• **Fig. 63.6** Teardrop angle—the angle formed between the radial diaphysis and a line drawn down the center of the volar rim of the distal radius.

and levering with a freer elevator can help to maintain adequate distraction of the fracture fragments during this process. If none of the other fracture fragments will provide an adequate window, a cortical window may be created with an osteotome through the volar or dorsal metaphyseal surface. If a dorsal approach is planned, it will allow direct or indirect assessment of the joint to evaluate congruency of the articular surface. Otherwise, the articular congruity can be assessed with AP and 10-degree lateral radiographs.

Metaphyseal Void

For fractures with segmental articular pieces not attached to the volar or dorsal lunate facet nor scaphoid facet fragments, bone grafting provides an effective method to reduce and temporarily support these chondral pieces. Subsequent reduction and stabilization of the volar and/or dorsal fragments will buttress the reduced intra-articular fragment and keep the bone graft contained. When possible, it may be advantageous to have a fixed-angle volar or dorsal implant supporting the subchondral bone beneath this fragment, particularly if the applied bone graft does not effectively support the articular piece. If the fixation construct will not otherwise include an adequate fixed-angle implant to support the subchondral bone, a buttress-style wire form can also be used for this purpose. Legs of the wire form are cut to end short of the far cortex and are bent to support the articular fragment prior to insertion through a 2 × 5-mm cortical window in the dorsal cortex.[33]

Initial Reduction and Temporary Fixation

The next priority is to restore and stabilize the length of the radial column. This is best achieved with traction and ulnar deviation to restore length and correct radial translation, followed by provisional trans-styloid pin fixation. We employ a 16-gauge needle as a drill guide for two 0.045-inch K-wires if done percutaneously. These wires are placed obliquely and penetrate the ulnar cortex of the metadiaphyseal radius. These wires can later be used as the distal fixation in a radial column pin plate if there is a free radial styloid fragment requiring fixation. Alternatively, a radial buttress plate may be used for provisional stabilization, with placement of subchondral screws deferred until after distal volar and/or dorsal fixation (Fig. 63.7).

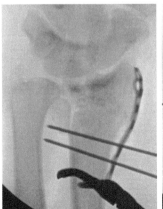 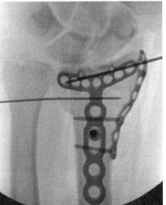 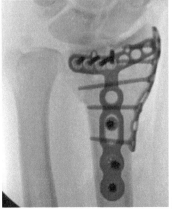 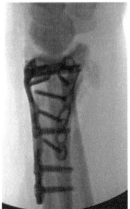

• **Fig. 63.7** Fixation sequence of the fracture in Fig. 63.2. The radial column buttress plate is secured proximally, to buttress and maintain the length of the radial column. Subchondral screws are placed through the dorsal rim plate prior to distal fixation of the radial plate.

Volar Rim or Volar Ulnar Corner

Definitive fixation is first applied to the volar rim or VUC. Stabilization of the radiolunate joint, restoration of the length of the intermediate column, and reduction of the ulnar aspect of the sigmoid notch create a foundation from which to build the remainder of the construct. Critical assessment of the teardrop angle informs the surgeon as to whether the reduction is anatomic. When reducing and fixing the volar and dorsal articular fragments, it is important to avoid over-reduction in the sagittal plane, which leads to an undesirable V-deformity, narrowing the radiocarpal surface. Reducing and stabilizing the radial column prior to this step facilitate appropriate reduction of the sigmoid notch in the axial and coronal planes by seating it against the ulnar head. The anatomy of the VUC makes it particularly vulnerable to injury and challenging to secure with conventional implants. It extends 5 mm distal and 3 mm anterior to the watershed line and the flat volar surface of the distal radius.[14] The smaller this fragment is, the more difficult it is to properly capture, even if utilizing a VLP with ulnar extension.[15] A volar-ulnar approach[34,35] allows the most direct access to this fracture fragment (Fig. 63.8). The approach is made through the internervous plane between palmaris longus and flexor carpi ulnaris (FCU). To improve exposure of the carpus or more radial aspect of the volar distal radius, the incision may be angled obliquely at the wrist flexion crease to include an extended carpal tunnel release. The ulnar neurovascular bundle is retracted ulnarly and contents of the carpal tunnel radially. Specific dissection of the median nerve is not necessary or recommended.[35] Access to the VUC fragment is also possible through a trans-flexor carpi radialis (FCR) or Henry approach, but is more difficult for small ulnar fragments. However, the more radial approaches offer better exposure of the more radial aspect of the volar surface and can also be easily extended to allow access to

the diaphysis or the radial column. The FCR approaches also facilitate easier placement of a standard VLP. In all three approaches, it is important to avoid dissection more than 2 mm past the distal ridge of the radius to avoid violating the volar carpal ligaments. The pronator quadratus can be reflected from its radial attachment in each of these approaches or, alternatively, may be detached from its ulnar attachment in the volar-ulnar approach. We find it helpful to apply a lobster claw forceps to the proximal aspect of the visualized radial diaphysis to control the metaphyseal/diaphyseal segments during manipulation and reduction and provide soft tissue retraction.

VLPs with or without an ulnar extension are useful for stabilizing a larger metaphyseal fragment and can successfully capture some VUC fragments. Smaller, fragment-specific implants, which can extend distal to the watershed line (Fig. 63.8D–F), are recommended for fragments with <15 mm available for fixation in the radial-ulnar dimension or that have subsided more than 5 mm.[15] Hook plates are a type of fragment-specific implant useful for fragments of adequate size: at least 7 mm medial-lateral, 5 mm proximal-distal, and 4 mm in the AP dimensions (Fig. 63.9).[36] These may be placed at or just distal to the watershed line[37] and the fragment should be reduced and provisionally stabilized before predrilling holes for the hooks to be inserted.

For smaller or more distal fractures, a wire form, buttress pin plate, free K-wires bent and secured under a plate, or suture anchors can be used. If planning to use a buttress pin plate, the K-wires stabilizing the distal fragment can be incorporated into the plate with two additional screws placed proximally. When inserting the K-wires, limit penetration of the far cortex to 1–2 mm. When used in pin plates, the K-wire is marked where it interfaces the plate and is then withdrawn 1 cm and cut 1 cm above that mark. A wire bender is used to create a hook with the mark placed between the two lower posts of the bender. The

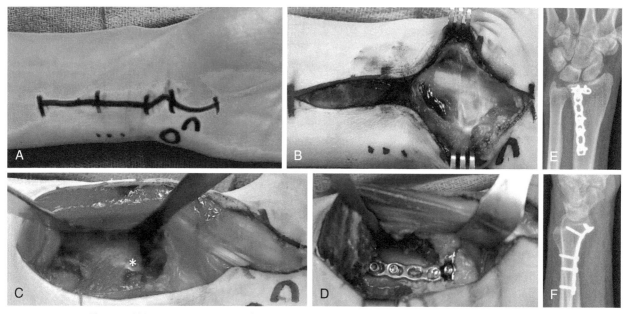

• **Fig. 63.8** Volar-ulnar approach and fragment-specific fixation of volar ulnar corner. (A) Incision angled obliquely at the wrist flexion crease to include an extended carpal tunnel release and improve exposure. (B and C) Internervous plane between palmaris longus and flexor carpi ulnaris is developed, the contents of the carpal tunnel are retracted radially, and pronator quadratus is elevated off the radius. (D–F) Fixation of the volar ulnar corner fragment *(asterisk)* with low-profile implant placement at or just distal to the watershed line. (Copyright Christopher J. Dy, MD.)

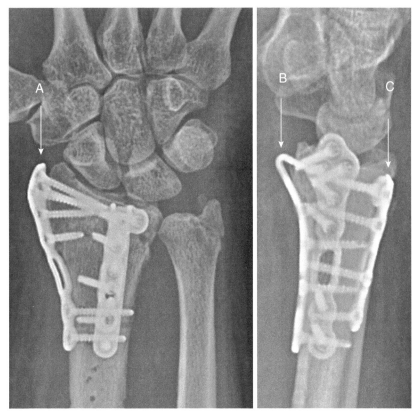

• **Fig. 63.9** Fragment-specific fixation—radial column locking plate *(A)*, volar ulnar corner hook plate *(B)*, and dorsal ulnar corner locking plate *(C)*.

wire is overbent slightly with a pin clamp and impacted into the plate to fully seat the hook in an adjacent pinhole. We find a pin plate to be more useful for fragments that are too narrow in the radial-ulnar dimension to accept two drill holes 5–7 mm apart, as would be required for a hook plate or wire form. Predrilled holes for a buttress wire form should be oriented perpendicular to the long axis of the radius and angled approximately 20 degrees in the sagittal plane away from the articular surface.[33] Before insertion, pre-bend the wire to match the contour of the volar ulnar cortex of the radius and trim the legs to avoid contact with the dorsal cortex. Cutting one leg shorter than the other facilitates insertion of the legs into the predrilled holes. An alternative technique to capture very distal VUC pieces, when pin plates are not available, is to stabilize the fragments with K-wires, then bend and secure them beneath a volar plate (Fig. 63.10).[38] One to three 0.028- or 0.035-inch K-wires are placed through the fracture fragment into the opposite cortex. They are each backed out 1 cm and bent proximally to match the contour of the volar radius. Each K-wire is tamped back into place and a volar plate is secured over them. For fractures too small to be captured with a rigid implant, sutures can be placed into the capsule just distal to the fracture fragment and secured with a suture plate or bone anchors.[39,40] The sutures can be used to de-rotate the fragment under direct visualization, as is often necessary.

Dorsal Ulnar Corner

Next, our attention is turned to the dorsal ulnar corner, which can be accessed through a standard dorsal approach or the more limited dorsal ulnar approach. A standard dorsal approach is centered over the ulnar aspect of Lister's tubercle. Full-thickness skin flaps are created over the extensor retinaculum, preserving the radial sensory and dorsal ulnar sensory nerves and any dorsal veins.

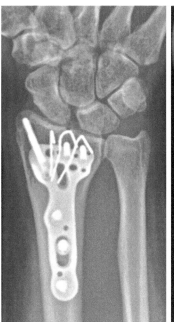
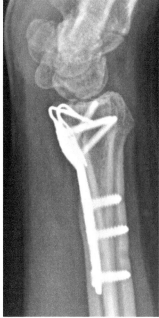

• **Fig. 63.10** K-wires bent under volar locking plate for fixation of volar ulnar corner. (Courtesy Robin Kamal, MD.)

The roof of the extensor pollicis longus (EPL) tendon sheath is incised and the tendon is retracted radially. Subperiosteal elevation of second and fourth extensor compartments is performed, providing access to the entire dorsal surface of the distal radius (Fig. 63.11). The posterior interosseous nerve may be excised,

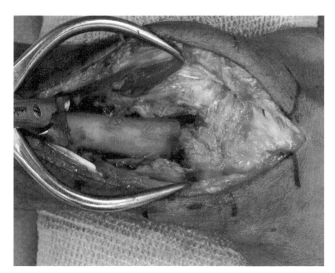

• **Fig. 63.11** Exposure provided by the dorsal approach.

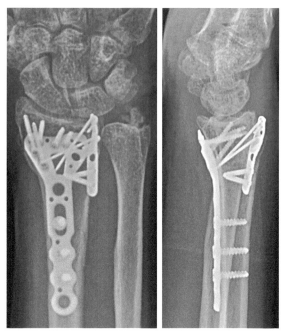

• **Fig. 63.12** Dorsal ulnar corner pin plate and volar locking plate.

and a capsulotomy may be made to access the radiocarpal joint. However, our standard practice is to leave the radiocarpal ligaments intact and perform an indirect reduction of the articular surface, visualizing the subchondral bone through the dorsal wall fragment.

Alternatively, a dorsal ulnar approach centered over the DRUJ may be used. A 3- to 4-cm incision is carried down through the roof of the fifth dorsal compartment and the extensor digiti minimi is transposed; the ligaments of the DRUJ are just deep to this. This approach cannot be easily extended to access other fracture fragments; therefore its utility is limited to fixation of the dorsal ulnar corner. If planning to stabilize the dorsal ulnar corner after applying a VLP, it is important to postpone use of any ulnar-distal holes in the VLP until after the dorsal fixation of the DUC is complete,[41] or intentionally leave these screws short to allow manipulation of the dorsal fragment after the volar fragment is secured. Modern precontoured dorsal ulnar plates are lower profile, with smoother edges, and come in various shapes compared to earlier generations, which were frequently implicated in tendon irritation or rupture.[42] Alternatively, a hook plate, pin plate (Fig. 63.12), or wire forms may be utilized for the dorsal ulnar corner as well. To achieve buttress-style fixation, it is important to precontour the plate to affect a compressive force when it is secured with the proximal cortical screws. Precise contouring is critical given the dorsal slope of the distal radius and the metaphyseal flare leading to the dorsal DRUJ. Pin plates can be twisted to allow adaptation to the dorsal ulnar corner and the proximal dorsal metaphysis with minimal prominence. Contouring should be completed before application of the plate to the cortical bone but after provisional fixation of the articular fragment with an initial K-wire. The plate is then slid over the established K-wire to check the fit of the contouring and adjustments are made prior to drilling cortical screws.

Radial Column

The approach to the radial styloid can be accomplished in several ways, depending on the type of fixation required and the other approaches used. The distal limb of the volar Henry or standard dorsal approach can be used to access the radial column, or a separate incision centered between the first and second dorsal compartments can be used. If an FCR approach is otherwise being utilized, it can be converted to the volar Henry approach through the same

skin incision by elevating a subcutaneous skin flap superficial to the radial artery. After initial skin incision, care must be taken to avoid injury to the radial sensory nerve within the subcutaneous tissue, usually found adjacent to the cephalic vein. The first dorsal compartment sheath is identified, and the subcutaneous tissue is bluntly dissected away from proximal to distal to elevate a skin flap. The forearm is pronated to present the radial column into the wound and the radial styloid exposed between the first and second dorsal compartments by performing subperiosteal elevation of the first and second dorsal compartments. Conversely, the forearm is supinated to present the radial styloid when using a dorsal approach. If more proximal exposure is required to accommodate a plate, the first dorsal compartment is opened proximally, leaving the distal 1 cm intact, allowing retraction of the tendons. The insertion of the brachioradialis is reflected or split longitudinally to complete exposure of the radial column. Implant selection depends largely on the character of the fracture. Simple, isolated radial styloid fractures are well suited for one or two compression screws. This technique does not require an extensive approach and the screws can be cortical, headless, cannulated, or solid.[43,44] Our typical practice, for more complex fractures, is to use a radial column locking plate or pin plate to buttress the fragment (Figs. 63.2, 63.7, and 63.9). The provisional K-wires that were used to stabilize the radial column can be used at this step if in an appropriate position. Alternatively, radial column locking plates are useful to bridge metaphyseal comminution. A plate will sit dorsal to the first dorsal compartment distally and cross under the tendons to sit volar to the tendons proximally. If the brachioradialis tendon was split, it may be closed over the plate.

Dorsal Wall

The dorsal wall fragment can also be accessed through the standard dorsal approach and stabilized in the same manner as the dorsal ulnar corner. This fragment is typically a larger metaphyseal fragment that serves as a buttress to prevent dorsal instability of the carpus. Pin plates, wire forms, or buttress plates may all adequately secure this fragment, although it is generally the last fragment to be fixed, as it does not typically contain articular pieces. Reduction of this piece helps to maintain any bone graft that was placed into the metaphyseal void and provides a strut to buttress any segmental articular pieces or the subchondral bone attached to the scaphoid facet.

Intraoperative Assessment

Intraoperative fluoroscopy is critical to appropriate anatomic fixation of these comminuted fractures, including judicious use of AP, lateral, 10-degree lateral, PA, and dorsal tangential fluoroscopic images to evaluate for radial height, inclination, articular surface congruency, and screw length. Additionally, many of the shear, avulsion, and articular fractures we choose to fix with fragment-specific techniques represent or correspond with significant injury to the DRUJ, and radiocarpal or intracarpal ligaments.[7,8,40,45,46] Final fluoroscopic images should be carefully inspected to ensure that all other aspects of the carpus appear in normal alignment. If fluoroscopic images are satisfactory, assessment of DRUJ stability is performed with ballottement in pronation, supination, and neutral. If there is radiographic evidence of DRUJ instability or a significant difference in ballottement test compared to the contralateral wrist, consideration should be given to open or arthroscopic repair of the triangular fibrocartilage complex (TFCC); the authors do not routinely pin the DRUJ.

Postoperative Protocol

A sugar tong splint is applied at the conclusion of the surgery with the forearm positioned in supination to minimize the risk of pronation contracture and scarring. Patients are encouraged to work on digital range of motion immediately after surgery. The postoperative splint is removed at 10–14 days and the surgical wound is assessed; routine X-rays are not taken at the initial postoperative appointment.[47] The patient is given an off-the-shelf wrist splint and encouraged to begin gentle active forearm rotation immediately and wrist range-of-motion exercises at 4 weeks postoperatively. The patient is seen again at 6 weeks after surgery and radiographs are obtained at this visit. If there are no concerns with healing and motion, the patient may discontinue use of the splint and begin to progress activity.

References

1. Chung KC, Shauver MJ, Birkmeyer JD. Trends in the United States in the treatment of distal radial fractures in the elderly. *J Bone Joint Surg Am*. 2009;91(8):1868–1873.
2. Koval KJ, Harrast JJ, Anglen JO, Weinstein JN. Fractures of the distal part of the radius. The evolution of practice over time. Where's the evidence? *J Bone Joint Surg Am*. 2008;90(9):1855–1861.
3. Sammer DM, Fuller DS, Kim HM, Chung KC. A comparative study of fragment-specific versus volar plate fixation of distal radius fractures. *Plast Reconstr Surg*. 2008;122(5):1441–1450.
4. Chung KC, Squitieri L, Kim HM. Comparative outcomes study using the volar locking plating system for distal radius fractures in both young adults and adults older than 60 years. *J Hand Surg Am*. 2008;33(6):809–819.
5. Salibian AA, Bruckman KC, Bekisz JM, Mirrer J, Thanik VD, Hacquebord JH. Management of unstable distal radius fractures: a survey of hand surgeons. *J Wrist Surg*. 2019;8(4):335–343.
6. Leslie BM, Medoff RJ. Fracture specific fixation of distal radius fractures. *Tech Orthop*. 2000;15:336–352.
7. Mandziak DG, Watts AC, Bain GI. Ligament contribution to patterns of articular fractures of the distal radius. *J Hand Surg Am*. 2011;36(10):1621e–1625.
8. Medoff RJ. Radiographic evaluation and classification of distal radius fractures. In: Slutsky DJ, Osterman AL, eds. *Fractures and Injuries of the Distal Radius and Carpus: The Cutting Edge*. 1st ed. Philadelphia: Elsevier; 2009:17–31.
9. Anderson DD, Bell AL, Gaffney MB, Imbriglia JE. Contact stress distributions in malreduced intraarticular distal radius fractures. *J Orthop Trauma*. 1996;10(5):331–337.
10. Erhart S, Schmoelz W, Lutz M. Clinical and biomechanical investigation of an increased articular cavity depth after distal radius fractures: effect on range of motion, osteoarthrosis and loading patterns. *Arch Orthop Trauma Surg*. 2013;133(9):1249–1255.
11. Baratz ME, Des Jardins J, Anderson DD, Imbriglia JE. Displaced intra-articular fractures of the distal radius: the effect of fracture displacement on contact stresses in a cadaver model. *J Hand Surg Am*. 1996;21(2):183–188.
12. Farhan MF, Wong JH, Sreedharan S, Yong FC, Teoh LC. Combined volar and dorsal plating for complex comminuted distal radial fractures. *D J Orthop Surg (Hong Kong)*. 2015;23(1):19–23.
13. Zimmer J, Atwood DN, Lovy AJ, Bridgeman J, Shin AY, Brogan DM. Characterization of the dorsal ulnar corner in distal radius fractures in postmenopausal females: implications for surgical decision making. *J Hand Surg Am*. 2020;45(6):495–502.
14. Andermahr J, Lozano-Calderon S, Trafton T, Crisco JJ, Ring D. The volar extension of the lunate facet of the distal radius: a quantitative anatomic study. *J Hand Surg Am*. 2006;31(6):892–895.
15. Beck JD, Harness NG, Spencer HT. Volar plate fixation failure for volar shearing distal radius fractures with small lunate facet fragments. *J Hand Surg*. 2014;39(4):670–678.
16. Harness NG, Jupiter JB, Orbay JL, Raskin KB, Fernandez DL. Loss of fixation of the volar lunate facet fragment in fractures of the distal part of the radius. *J Bone Joint Surg Am*. 2004;86(9):1900–1908.

PEARLS AND PITFALLS

Pearls

- Be critical of injury radiographs.
  - All fracture lines will not be visible on radiographs. Look for indirect evidence of displaced intra-articular fragments, articular incongruency, and carpal malalignment.
- Make a preoperative plan. Anticipate what approaches, instruments, and implants you will use. Obtain a CT scan if necessary.
- Insert bone graft before implanting hardware.
- Examine closely for a small VUC fragment and ensure adequate fixation of this critical fragment if present.
- Fractures caused by a shearing or avulsion mechanism frequently coexist with intercarpal, radiocarpal, or DRUJ ligament injuries. It is important to maintain high index of suspicion for these injuries.

Pitfalls

- Plate prominence.
  - Use low-profile plates, avoid prominent screws or pins, and cover dorsal implants with the extensor retinaculum.
- Postoperative stiffness.
  - Create a stable, load-sharing construct to allow early motion; patients should be encouraged to begin wrist range of motion within 4 weeks of surgery.
  - Digital range of motion should begin preoperatively and emphasis should be placed on this at every postoperative visit.
- Loss of fixation.
  - Judicious use of fluoroscopic imaging to evaluate fixation construct; stress testing of fracture fixation during surgery is critical to avoid inadequate fragment capture.

17. Rampoldi M, Marsico S. Complications of volar plating of distal radius fractures. *Acta Orthop Belg.* 2007;73(6):714–719.

18. Soong M, Earp BE, Bishop G, Leung A, Blazar P. Volar locking plate implant prominence and flexor tendon rupture. *J Bone Joint Surg Am.* 2011;93(4):328–335.

19. Monaco NA, Dwyer CL, Ferikes AJ, Lubahn JD. Hand surgeon reporting of tendon rupture following distal radius volar plating. *Hand (NY).* 2016;11(3):278–286.

20. Yu YR, Makhni MC, Tabrizi S, Rozental TD, Mundanthanam G, Day CS. Complications of low-profile dorsal versus volar locking plates in the distal radius: a comparative study. *J Hand Surg Am.* 2011;36(7):1135–1141.

21. Simic PM, Robinson J, Gardner MJ, Gelberman RH, Weiland AJ, Boyer MI. Treatment of distal radius fractures with a low-profile dorsal plating system: an outcomes assessment. *J Hand Surg.* 2006;31A:382–386.

22. Kamath AF, Zurakowski D, Day CS. Low-profile dorsal plating for dorsally angulated distal radius fractures: an outcomes study. *J Hand Surg Am.* 2006;31:1061–1067.

23. Rhee PC, Medoff RJ, Shin AY. Complex distal radius fractures: an anatomic algorithm for surgical management. *J Am Acad Orthop Surg.* 2017;25(2):77–88.

24. Grindel SI, Wang M, Gerlach M, McGrady LM, Brown S. Biomechanical comparison of fixed-angle volar plate versus fixed-angle volar plate plus fragment-specific fixation in a cadaveric distal radius fracture model. *J Hand Surg Am.* 2007;32(2):194–199.

25. Palmer AK, Glisson RR, Werner FW. Ulnar variance determination. *J Hand Surg Am.* 1982;7(4):376–379.

26. Lundy DW, Quisling SG, Lourie GM, Feiner CM, Lins RE. Tilted lateral radiographs in the evaluation of intra-articular distal radius fractures. *J Hand Surg Am.* 1999;24(2):249–256.

27. Fujitani R, Omokawa S, Iida A, Santo S, Tanaka Y. Reliability and clinical importance of teardrop angle measurement in intra-articular distal radius fracture. *J Hand Surg Am.* 2012;37(3):454–459.

28. Pruitt DL, Gilula LA, Manske PR, Vannier MW. Computed tomography scanning with image reconstruction in evaluation of distal radius fractures. *J Hand Surg.* 1994;19A:720–727.

29. Cole RJ, Bindra RR, Evanoff BA, Gilula LA, Yamaguchi K, Gelberman RH. Radiographic evaluation of osseous displacement following intra-articular fractures of the distal radius: reliability of plain radiography versus computed tomography. *J Hand Surg Am.* 1997;22(5):792–800.

30. Katz MA, Beredjiklian PK, Bozentka DJ, Steinberg DR. Computed tomography scanning of intra-articular distal radius fractures: does it influence treatment? *J Hand Surg Am.* 2001;26(3):415–421.

31. Harness NG, Ring D, Zurakowski D, Harris GJ, Jupiter JB. The influence of three-dimensional computed tomography reconstructions on the characterization and treatment of distal radial fractures. *J Bone Joint Surg Am.* 2006;88(6):1315–1323.

32. Tanabe K, Nakajima T, Sogo E, Denno K, Horiki M, Nakagawa R. Intra-articular fractures of the distal radius evaluated by computed tomography. *J Hand Surg Am.* 2011;36(11):1798–1803.

33. Schumer ED, Leslie BM. Fragment-specific fixation of distal radius fractures using the Trimed device. *Tech Hand Up Extrem Surg.* 2005;9(2):74–83.

34. Ilyas AM. Surgical approaches to the distal radius. *Hand (NY).* 2011;6(1):8–17.

35. Tordjman D, Hinds RM, Ayalon O, Yang SS, Capo JT. Volar-ulnar approach for fixation of the volar lunate facet fragment in distal radius fractures: a technical tip. *J Hand Surg Am.* 2016;41(12):e491–e500.

36. O'Shaughnessy MA, Shin AY, Kakar S. Stabilization of volar ulnar rim fractures of the distal radius: current techniques and review of the literature. *J Wrist Surg.* 2016;5(2):113–119.

37. Bakker AJ, Shin AY. Fragment-specific volar hook plate for volar marginal rim fractures. *Tech Hand Up Extrem Surg.* 2014;18(1):56–60.

38. Moore AM, Dennison DG. Distal radius fractures and the volar lunate facet fragment: Kirschner wire fixation in addition to volar-locked plating. *Hand (NY).* 2014;9(2):230–236.

39. Apergis E, Darmanis S, Theodoratos G, Maris J. Beware of the ulno-palmar distal radial fragment. *J Hand Surg.* 2002;27B:139–145.

40. Geissler WB, Clark SM. Fragment-specific fixation for fractures of the distal radius. *J Wrist Surg.* 2016;5(1):22–30.

41. Ikeda K, Osamura N, Tada K. Fixation of an ulnodorsal fragment when treating an intra-articular fracture in the distal radius. *Hand Surg.* 2014;19(1):139–144.

42. Spiteri M, Ng W, Matthews J, Power D, Brewster M. Three year review of dorsal plating for complex intra-articular fractures of the distal radius. *J Hand Surg Asian Pac.* 2018;23(2):221–226.

43. Helm RH, Tonkin MA. The Chauffeur's fracture: simple or complex? *J Hand Surg Br.* 1992;17(2):156–159.

44. Reichel LM, Bell BR, Michnick SM, Reitman C. Radial styloid fractures. *J Hand Surg Am.* 2012;37(8):1726–1741.

45. Yang Y, Yin Q, Li D, et al. A new classification and its value evaluation for intermediate column fractures of the distal radius. *J Orthop Surg Res.* 2018;13(1):221.

46. Thomas BP, Sreekanth R. Distal radioulnar joint injuries. *Indian J Orthop.* 2012;46(5):493–504.

47. Stone JD, Vaccaro LM, Brabender RC, Hess AV. Utility and cost analysis of radiographs taken 2 weeks following plate fixation of distal radius fractures. *J Hand Surg Am.* 2015;40(6):1106–1109.

64

Technique Spotlight: Bridge Plating for Distal Radius Fractures

JORDAN GRIER AND DAVID RUCH

Indications

Initially described by Burke and Singer as an alternative to wrist-spanning external fixation, dorsal bridge plate fixation has proven to be a versatile option for the management of fractures of the distal radius.[1] Bridge plate fixation is most frequently utilized in the treatment of distal radius fractures with significant articular or metadiaphyseal comminution which would be suboptimally treated with a conventional locked volar plate construct.[2,3] Bridge plating has also shown favorable results in patients with osteoporotic bone with comminuted fracture patterns.[4] The use of a bridge plate construct in this scenario, rather than a conventional locked volar plate, may allow for elderly patients reliant on gait aids to mobilize and regain their baseline ambulatory ability more quickly following surgery.[5] The allowance of early weight-bearing through the injured upper extremity following bridge plate fixation has also proven advantageous in the treatment of distal radius fractures in polytraumatized patients who are reliant upon their upper extremities to facilitate rehabilitation of lower extremity injuries.

Preoperative Evaluation

Preoperative evaluation should consist of a thorough history and physical examination, with specific attention paid to the condition of the affected upper extremity. Assessment of injuries to adjacent joints should be considered as these may alter the overall treatment plan related to the fracture of the distal radius. A careful assessment of the soft tissue envelope of the forearm and hand should be performed to ensure no open wounds or soft tissue lesions exist which would preclude bridge plate fixation, and that adequate coverage of the planned fixation construct will be achievable. A detailed evaluation for associated neurovascular or tendinous injuries should be conducted to determine if concomitant, or more acute, procedures are indicated to address these associated injuries. Radiographic assessment of the affected limb should include, at minimum, orthogonal radiographs of the ipsilateral radius and ulna, wrist, and hand to evaluate for associated bony injuries and allow for preoperative planning. The patient's overall bone quality should also be carefully assessed on preoperative radiographs as the presence of osteopenia or osteoporosis (if known) may alter the proposed treatment plan.

Positioning and Equipment

Traditionally, bridge plating of the distal radius is performed with the patient in the supine position with the affected extremity supported on a radiolucent hand table extension. The use of a stretcher-based radiolucent hand table may be utilized if available as this form of positioning obviates the need to transfer the patient to a standard operating table and allows for increased operating room efficiency. Alternatively, the patient may be positioned prone or in the ipsilateral decubitus position with the affected upper extremity on a radiolucent hand table extension if this positioning will allow for other injuries to be addressed concomitantly in the polytrauma setting. The immediate availability of fluoroscopy should be confirmed prior to beginning the procedure. A mini C-arm may provide a sufficient field of view and clarity for the procedure to be performed; however, a traditional C-arm is typically utilized in order to visualize the entire construct in one field of view. The fluoroscopy machine should be positioned either parallel to the patient and operating table coming from the head of the bed, or brought in from the ipsilateral side directly over the hand table extension. If desired, a nonsterile pneumatic tourniquet may be applied high on the ipsilateral arm prior to limb preparation. Alternatively, a sterile tourniquet may be applied after prepping and draping has been completed. The operative extremity should be prepped and draped in accordance with the surgeon's preferences for fracture surgery.

Detailed Technique

Bridge plating can be performed via either a two-incision or three-incision technique (Fig. 64.1). Similarly, the bridge plate can be affixed to either the index or long metacarpal distally. The authors' preferred method is to utilize the long finger metacarpal for bridge plate application. This technique is outlined in this chapter. The technique for application of the bridge plate to the index metacarpal is identical with the exception of not requiring the middle incision at the dorsum of the distal radius.

First, an approximately 3-cm incision is marked over the dorsum of the long finger metacarpal from the proximal diaphysis to the metacarpal base. A second 4-cm incision is marked over the dorsal radial aspect of the radial diaphysis just proximal to the

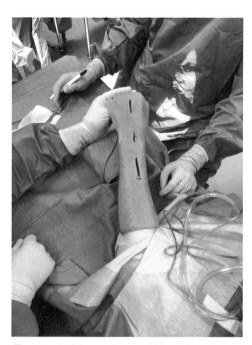

• **Fig. 64.1** The three incisions to be used (dorsal long finger metacarpal, dorsal radiocarpal joint, distal radial diaphysis) are marked with indelible surgical marker prior to beginning the procedure.

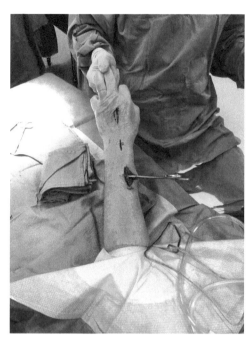

• **Fig. 64.2** A serrated bone holding forceps is used to provisionally affix the plate to radial diaphysis within wound over distal radial diaphysis.

outcropping muscle bellies of the adductor pollicis longus (APL) and extensor pollicis brevis (EPB). This incision should be marked at least 4 cm proximal to the most proximal extent of the fracture comminution observed on the patient's radiographs. If desired, an optional third 3-cm incision can be marked over the dorsal aspect of the radiocarpal joint just ulnar to Lister's tubercle. This incision should also be centered on Lister's tubercle in the proximal-distal orientation. The authors' preferred technique routinely involves the third incision as this window allows for direct visualization and protection of the extensor pollicis longus (EPL) and extensor digitorum communis (EDC) tendons during plate placement. The dorsal radiocarpal incision also allows for placement of bone graft in metaphyseal bone defects if present, as well as direct articular reduction through a dorsal radiocarpal arthrotomy if desired.

The dorsal long finger exposure is made by sharply incising the skin overlying the third metacarpal. Dissection is carried through subcutaneous tissues to the level of the long finger EDC tendon. Care is taken to preserve any traversing branches of the superficial branch of the radial nerve (SBRN) or juncturae tendinum encountered during dissection. The retinacular tissue overlying the long finger EDC tendon is sharply incised, and the tendon is then retracted radially to expose the dorsal aspect of the third metacarpal.

The dorsal radiocarpal incision, if utilized, is exploited first with sharp dissection through skin and subcutaneous tissues to the level of the extensor retinaculum. Care is taken to identify and protect traversing branches of the SBRN throughout the duration of the procedure. The EPL tendon is identified, and its retinaculum is incised proximally and distally in line with the tendon fibers. The EPL tendon is transposed from the third extensor compartment and retracted radially to prevent iatrogenic injury during instrumentation of the radius. The fourth extensor compartment is identified within the ulnar aspect of the wound. The enveloping retinaculum of the EDC and extensor indicis proprius (EIP) tendons is incised in line with the skin incision. Extraperiosteal dissection of the fourth extensor compartment tendons is performed, and the tendons are carefully protected in the ulnar

aspect of the wound throughout instrumentation. The posterior interosseous nerve (PIN) and artery (PIA) should be identified in the floor of the fourth compartment, and if desired a PIN neurectomy may be performed at this time. If a PIN neurectomy is not performed, particular attention should be paid to the terminal radiocarpal branches of the PIN during instrumentation to avoid painful compressive neuropathy symptoms postoperatively.

Exposure of the radial shaft is achieved by sharp dissection through the skin and subcutaneous tissues to the level of the second dorsal compartment. The SBRN may be encountered emerging from deep to the brachioradialis-extensor carpi radialis longus (ECRL) interval at this level. If encountered, branches of the SBRN should be carefully protected throughout the duration of instrumentation. The lateral antebrachial cutaneous nerve (LABCN) may also be encountered in this portion of the forearm traversing longitudinally in close proximity to the cephalic vein. If encountered, the LABCN should also be protected throughout the duration of instrumentation. The ECRL should be taken volarly, and the extensor carpi radialis brevis (ECRB) taken dorsally to expose the radial diaphysis.

A soft tissue corridor for placement of the bridge plate is created by passing a small periosteal elevator from the dorsal long finger incision, through dorsal radiocarpal incision, and ultimately through the floor of the proximal radius incision. The appropriate length bridge plate should next be identified by selecting the shortest plate from the manufacturer's set which allows for a minimum of the three bicortical screws to be placed distally in the metacarpal and three bicortical screws to be placed proximal to the fracture site in the radial diaphysis. The chosen plate is then introduced in a retrograde fashion beginning in the long finger metacarpal wound. Care is taken to avoid iatrogenic injury or entrapment of the SBRN, EPL, EDC, or EIP tendons during plate application. The absence of tendon entrapment should be visually confirmed in the dorsal radiocarpal wound prior to proceeding with instrumentation. The plate is then secured to the proximal radial diaphysis using a small serrated bone holding forceps (Fig. 64.2). Attention is then turned to the long metacarpal. The plate is centered on the metacarpal in the radial-ulnar plane, and a bicortical nonlocking screw is placed in the most central hole which will allow for the placement of two additional bicortical metacarpal screws. If an oblong plate hole is available, this should be utilized first. With distal fixation in the metacarpal achieved, provisional fracture reduction is performed by placing the elbow in 90 degrees of flexion, maximally supinating the forearm, and applying longitudinal traction (Fig. 64.3). The previously applied small serrated bone holding forceps is replaced to maintain the reduction. Fluoroscopy is utilized to confirm a satisfactory reduction has been achieved on orthogonal fluoroscopic views prior to proceeding with instrumentation

(Fig. 64.4A–B). If desired, direct reduction of articular fragments accessible via the dorsal radiocarpal incision may be performed until a satisfactory reduction has been achieved prior to proceeding (Fig. 64.5A–B). With fracture reduction achieved, a bicortical nonlocking screw is placed in the proximal radial diaphysis. Two additional bicortical screws should then be placed in both the proximal and distal-most aspects of the plate to achieve sufficient fixation.

After the completion of instrumentation, fluoroscopic images should be obtained confirming the desired fracture reduction has been achieved and that adequate fixation has been employed to maintain this reduction over the course of fracture healing. The dorsal radiocarpal wound should be inspected once again prior to closure to confirm the absence of tendon entrapment. The EPL tendon is left in a transposed position at the completion of the case. The wounds are thoroughly irrigated before being closed in layers in accordance with the surgeon's preferences. Postoperatively the patient may be immobilized in either a removable volar forearm-based wrist-spanning orthosis or a volar resting plaster splint depending on the surgeon's preference.

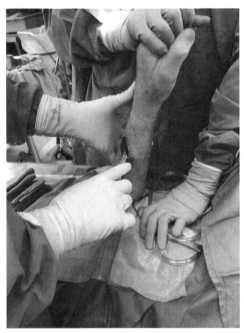

• **Fig. 64.3** The arm is positioned in 90 degrees of elbow flexion, maximal forearm supination, and longitudinal traction is subsequently applied in order to achieve provisional fracture reduction.

PEARLS AND PITFALLS

- Several bridge plate designs offer supplementary screw hole options over the dorsum of the distal radius that can be utilized to provide additional fragment-specific buttress support to the subchondral bone. This may be particularly advantageous in preventing collapse of critical dorsal lunate facet fragments (Fig. 64.6A–B).
- The necessary length and location of the planned incisions can often be estimated by taking a fluoroscopic image of the desired plate applied directly over the dorsal aspect of the radius in line with the desired metacarpal for distal fixation (Fig. 64.7).
- Digital motion should be carefully scrutinized after the completion of instrumentation to ensure that normal tenodesis is maintained, and full passive composite digital flexion can be achieved. Overlengthening of the extrinsic digital extensors has been correlated with decreased postoperative grip strength, inferior functional outcome scores, and worse patient-reported pain scores in spanning external fixation models similar to the described bridge plating technique.

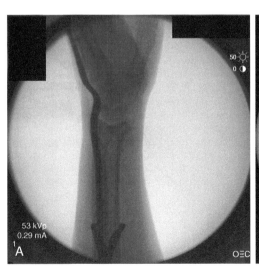
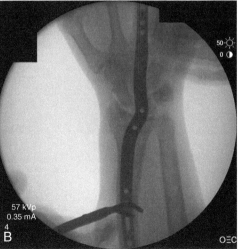

• **Fig. 64.4** (A) Lateral and (B) posteroanterior fluoroscopic views of provisional fracture reduction with dorsal bridge plate applied.

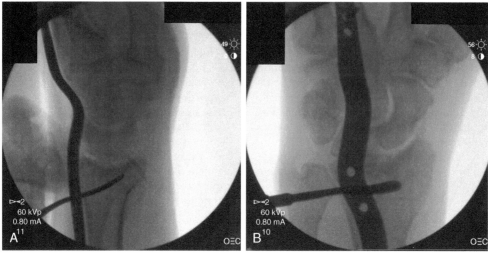

• **Fig. 64.5** (A) Lateral and (B) posteroanterior fluoroscopic views demonstrating direct articular reduction achieved via the dorsal radiocarpal incision.

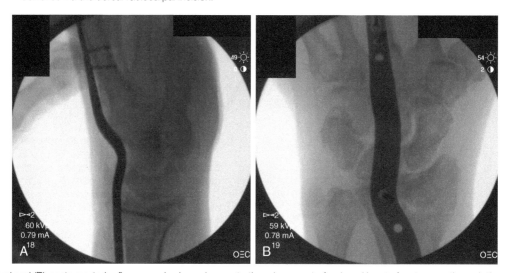

• **Fig. 64.6** (A) Lateral and (B) posteroanterior fluoroscopic views demonstrating placement of a dorsal lunate facet screw through the corresponding plate hole to aid in preventing loss of articular reduction.

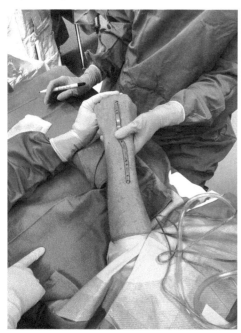

• **Fig. 64.7** The desired dorsal bridge plate selected from the manufacturer's set can be utilized preoperatively to estimate the length and location of planned incisions.

References

1. Burke EF, Singer RM. Treatment of comminuted distal radius with the use of an internal distraction plate. *Tech Hand Up Extrem Surg.* 1998;2(4):248–252.
2. Ruch DS, Ginn TA, Yang CC, Smith BP, Rushing J, Hanel DP. Use of a distraction plate for distal radial fractures with metaphyseal and diaphyseal comminution. *J Bone Joint Surg Am.* 2005;87(5):945–954.
3. Hanel DP, Lu TS, Weil WM. Bridge plating of distal radius fractures: the Harborview method. *Clin Orthop Relat Res.* 2006;445:91–99.
4. Richard MJ, Katolik LI, Hanel DP, Wartinbee DA, Ruch DS. Distraction plating for the treatment of highly comminuted distal radius fractures in elderly patients. *J Hand Surg Am.* 2012;37(5):948–956.
5. Hyatt BT, Hanel DP, Saucedo JM. Bridge plating for distal radius fractures in low-demand patients with assist devices. *J Hand Surg Am.* 2019;44(6):507–513.

65

Distal Radioulnar Joint Instability and Galeazzi Fractures

HASSAN J. AZIMI AND ROBERT W. WYSOCKI

Introduction

The Galeazzi fracture-dislocation is a fracture of the distal one-third of the radial shaft with an associated distal radioulnar joint (DRUJ) dislocation. This injury was described first by Astley Cooper[1] in 1826 and later named after Riccardo Galeazzi who published his series of cases in 1934.[2,3] The Galeazzi fracture has been given the name the "fracture of necessity," referring to its need for anatomic reduction and rigid internal fixation in order to achieve optimal results.[4–7] Galeazzi fracture-dislocations require a high index of suspicion and can frequently go underdiagnosed.

Relevant Anatomy

The forearm rotates about an axis that starts proximally at the center of the radial head and travels through the ulnar fovea distally. The radius, attached carpal bones, and hand rotate around a relatively fixed ulna.[8] The ulna is constrained proximally at the elbow through tight bony and ligamentous constraints, allowing it to function only as a hinge joint. In full supination, the radius and ulna are essentially parallel and in full pronation, the radius rotates across the anterior border of the ulna. To allow rotation of the radius around the straight ulna the radius has a natural bow. This bow is best seen in the sagittal plane on a neutral rotation posteroanterior (PA) radiograph of the forearm.

The radius and ulna have ligamentous connections at the proximal and DRUJs as well as the intervening interosseous membrane. The interosseous membrane is a stout ligamentous complex consisting of proximal, middle, and distal portions. The distal interosseous membrane (DIOM) has been shown by several authors to be a stabilizer of the DRUJ.[9,10] Within the DIOM is the distal oblique bundle (DOB) which is a thickening of the membrane that runs from the proximal attachment of the pronator quadratus at the ulna to the proximal aspect of the sigmoid notch of the radius with some fibers running dorsal and volar to the DRUJ ligaments.[11] Cadaver studies have shown the DOB to be present to a varying degree within the DIOM, being present in 23%–50% of specimens.[11–13] Kitamura et al. showed in a cadaver model that specimens with a DOB had increased stability of the DRUJ in

the neutral position when compared with specimens without a DOB.[14]

The DRUJ is an inherently unstable joint due to the radius of curvature of the sigmoid notch being greater than that of the ulnar head.[15] This radius of curvature mismatch leads to volar/dorsal translation of the ulna in relation to the sigmoid notch of the radius through a full arc of rotation. The limited congruency of the DRUJ necessitates strong soft tissue support, and the triangular fibrocartilage complex (TFCC) serves as the major soft tissue stabilizer of the DRUJ. The TFCC (Fig. 65.1) is a complex structure, composed of the ulnocarpal meniscus (meniscus homolog), the ulnar collateral ligament, the dorsal radioulnar ligament, the palmar radioulnar ligament, and the subsheath of the extensor carpi ulnaris (ECU). The dorsal and palmar distal radioulnar ligaments are thought to provide the majority of the stability to the DRUJ and are subdivided into superficial and deep portions.[16,17] They originate at the sigmoid notch of the radius with the deep portion inserting at the fovea and the superficial portion inserting at the base of the ulnar styloid. In full pronation and supination, the deep portion of the TFCC (ligamentum subcruentum) becomes the primary stabilizer of the DRUJ. In full pronation, the dorsal superficial fibers, the dorsal joint capsule, and the deep palmar fibers tighten for stability and prevent dorsal dislocation of the ulna. The reciprocal occurs in supination.[16]

Pathoanatomy

The deforming forces on a fracture of the distal third of the radial shaft cause a typical deformity of shortening and rotation of the radius (Fig. 65.2). Shortening of the fracture is created by pull from the brachioradialis as well as the wrist and finger flexors and extensors which cross the fracture. The pronator quadratus creates a rotational deformity on the distal fragment and the pronator teres creates a rotational deformity of the proximal fragment of the radius.

The degree of shortening is determined by the severity of the soft tissue injury to the TFCC and DIOM. Cadaver studies in which a radial osteotomy was created have correlated the amount

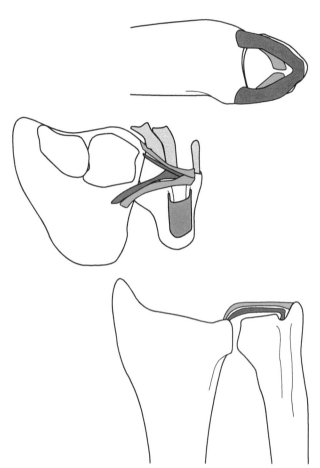

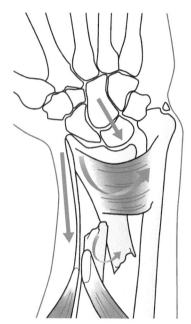

• **Fig. 65.2** Deforming forces are demonstrated with longitudinal shortening from the brachioradialis as well as the extrinsic flexors and extensors of the fingers and wrist. Rotational forces on the proximal and distal fragments are made by the pronator teres and pronator quadratus.

• **Fig. 65.1** The triangular fibrocartilage complex consists of a meniscus homolog *(blue)*, deep dorsal and palmar radioulnar ligaments *(red)* which attach at the ulnar fovea, superficial deep dorsal and palmar radioulnar ligaments *(green)* which attach at the ulnar styloid, extensor carpi ulnaris subsheath *(orange)*, and the ulnocarpal and ulnar collateral ligaments *(pink)*.

of ulnar positive variance to the degree of injury to the TFCC and/or DIOM.[18,19] Moore et al.[19] found that following an isolated radius osteotomy, an average of 4.1 mm of ulnar positive variance was noted with a maximum displacement of 7 mm. With release of the TFCC or the DIOM, an additional 2.9 and 1.3 mm, respectively, of shortening was noted. With subsequent release of both structures, 21 mm of shortening was noted. Schneiderman et al.[18] repeated this study and found similar results with 7.7 mm of shortening with a TFCC release, 6.25 mm of shortening with DIOM release, and 15–40 mm of shortening with both structures released. Both studies concluded that the DIOM and TFCC provide stabilization to the DRUJ in fractures of the radius and >10 mm of shortening is indicative of both structures being disrupted. In a retrospective study of diaphyseal radius fractures, Tsismenakis and Tornetta found that an average of 10.9 mm of ulnar positive variance was associated with persistent intraoperative instability of the DRUJ after open reduction and internal fixation (ORIF) of the radius fracture, in comparison with 3.5 mm of ulnar positive variance in a stable DRUJ.[20]

It has been suggested that an intact DOB after anatomic reduction and stable plate fixation can provide sufficient stability to the DRUJ despite a TFCC tear or ulnar styloid fracture.[21] The mechanism for this is thought to be by restoring tension to the DOB with anatomic and stable fixation of the radius fracture; this

creates a compressive force in the coronal plane from the ulna towards an intact sigmoid notch of the radius through a tensioned DOB (Fig. 65.3). The heterogeneity in the presence and thickness of the DOB in cadaver specimens may account for the variable incidence of DRUJ instability after ORIF of a distal-third radial shaft fracture.[20–23] Furthermore, it is not entirely clear if a dislocation of the DRUJ requires both the palmar and dorsal deep fibers of the foveal attachment of the TFCC to be completely injured. It has been described that with forearm pronation, dorsal dislocation of the ulna occurs with isolated sectioning of the palmar radioulnar ligament, dorsal joint capsule, and dorsal superficial fibers, with the reverse found in palmar dislocations of the ulna.[16] This may indicate that there is a varying degree of injury to the TFCC in the context of an acute DRUJ dislocation. Examination of the DRUJ under anesthesia will demonstrate the degree of injury to the TFCC based upon the direction of instability with forearm rotation.[17]

Classifications

There are several classifications used to described Galeazzi fracture-dislocations. The first was adopted from a series of 41 Galeazzi fracture-dislocations in children.[24] In this series, Walsh et al. categorized the fracture pattern into two groups, palmar or dorsal displacement of the distal radius fragment, and then subdivided these groups into fractures within the distal third of the radial shaft or fractures outside of the distal-third border, creating a total of four groups. Walsh Type 1 fractures demonstrate dorsal displacement of the distal radius fragment and palmar displacement of the distal ulna. Type 2 fractures demonstrate palmar displacement of the distal radius fragment and dorsal displacement of the distal ulna.

Bruckner et al.[25] described complex Galeazzi fracture-dislocations in a series of four cases of an irreducible DRUJ. Simple injury described a DRUJ that was easily reduced and maintained. Complex injuries referred to joints that had recurrent subluxation,

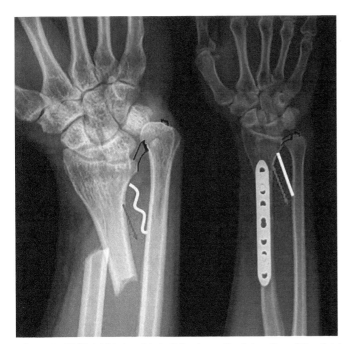

• **Fig. 65.3** (A) Distal-third radial shaft fracture with dislocation of the distal radioulnar joint (DRUJ) and a fractured ulnar styloid with significant shortening of the radial shaft. The torn triangular fibrocartilage complex (TFCC) and a shortened but intact distal oblique bundle (DOB) are demonstrated. (B) After anatomic reduction and plate fixation of the radial shaft fracture, the DOB is brought back to normal tension, restoring a compressive force from the ulna to the stable sigmoid notch. Despite a fractured ulnar styloid and presumed TFCC tear, this patient had a stable DRUJ and did not require additional treatment.

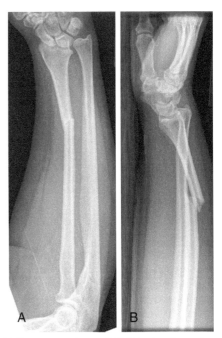

• **Fig. 65.4** (A) Posteroanterior and (B) lateral radiographs of a forearm demonstrating a distal-third radial shaft fracture with volar displacement of the radius, consistent with a Walsh type 2 injury.

dislocation, or were irreducible due to interposed soft tissues. Most commonly, the ECU is displaced palmar to the ulna, preventing a closed reduction of the DRUJ.[26,27] However, the extensor digitorum communis tendons, extensor digiti minimi tendon, dorsal joint capsule, and a displaced ulnar styloid fracture have all been described as structures that can displace palmar to the ulna and become interposed, causing a complex Galeazzi fracture-dislocation.[28–35] Complex dislocations required an open reduction to remove the interposed tissue from the joint.

Rettig and Raskin[36] categorized 40 adult injuries into two groups: Type I, in which the radial shaft fracture was located <7.5 cm from the articular surface of the radius and Type II in which this distance was >7.5 cm. They found that 12 of the 13 cases that required treatment for a persistently unstable DRUJ after ORIF of the radial shaft fracture were Type I injuries. The authors concluded that Type I injuries should have a high index of suspicion for combined TFCC/DIOM disruption that can cause persistent DRUJ instability after ORIF of the radial shaft fracture.

Although fractures in the distal third of the radius are the most likely to cause dislocations of the DRUJ, not all distal-third fractures of the radius are associated with dislocations of the DRUJ. Several studies have found that the location of the fracture alone is insufficient to determine if the DRUJ is stable.[20,23,37] Ring et al.[23] reviewed a series of 36 diaphyseal radius fractures, 8 of which were distal-third diaphyseal fractures. Using 5 mm of ulnar positive variance as a measure of DRUJ dislocation, they found nine DRUJ injuries. Of the nine injuries, five were located in the distal third of the radius. Tsismenakis and Tornetta[20] reviewed a series of 66 isolated diaphyseal radius fractures. Intraoperative assessment of DRUJ stability after radial shaft fixation was used as the

definition for a fracture-dislocation of the DRUJ. Of the 66 radial shaft fractures, 29 were in the distal third of the radial shaft and 7 were fracture-dislocations. Of the 26 fractures occurring within 7.5 cm of the radiolunate joint, only 5 were associated with DRUJ instability. There is a large discrepancy between the incidence of DRUJ instability with distal-third radial shaft fracture between the studies by Ring (63%) and Tsismenakis (19%). Thus the index of suspicion for a combined injury should remain high.

Galeazzi equivalent lesions refer to injuries that occur in children with concomitant fracture of the distal ulna. This can consist most commonly of an ulnar styloid fracture in adults or a transphyseal fracture of the distal ulna in a child with an open distal ulna physis.[38] The latter injury pattern leaves the distal radioulnar ligaments intact, remaining attached to the ulna epiphysis. The ulnar styloid fracture in an adult will have variable amounts of attached soft tissues depending on the size of the fragment.

Presentation and Evaluation

Patients typically present with characteristic swelling and deformity due to prominence of the ulna from a dislocated DRUJ and shortened radius (Fig. 65.3). With less displaced radial shaft fractures, palpation of the DRUJ should be performed to identify tenderness that could indicate DRUJ disruption. A thorough neurovascular examination should be performed as rare injuries to the median and ulnar nerve have been reported.[39,40] Skin should be fully assessed to evaluate for an open fracture. History obtained from the patient typically reveals a high-energy fall or mechanism of injury such as a motor vehicle accident.[41] While a fall onto an outstretched arm with forced pronation or supination of the forearm is the typically described mechanism, the characteristic Galeazzi fracture-dislocation has not been reproduced in a biomechanics laboratory.[7]

Radiographs of the wrist, forearm, and elbow should be obtained and should include PA and lateral views (Fig. 65.4). On the PA

TABLE 65.1	Radiographic Findings That Should Raise Suspicion for a Galeazzi Fracture-Dislocation

Posteroanterior View

Fracture within 7.5 cm of midarticular surface of the radius

Ulnar positive variance of >10 mm

Increased distance between the sigmoid notch of radius and distal ulna

Ulnar styloid fracture

Lateral View

Dorsal or palmar displacement of the distal radius in comparison to the ulnar head

view, characteristic shortening and rotation of the radius is noted (Fig. 65.2) as well as widening of the space between the sigmoid notch of the radius and the distal ulna. A lateral radiograph (Fig. 65.4B) will demonstrate either dorsal or palmar displacement of the radius; this should be noted as it may help the surgeon identify the direction of instability after reduction of the radius. The majority of these injuries will be Walsh Type 2 injuries.[42] While not diagnostic for DRUJ instability, specific attention should be made to the level of the radius fracture and amount of ulnar positive variance due to proximal displacement of the radius, as a radius fracture <7.5 cm away from the articular surface of the radius and with >10 mm ulnar positive variance have been associated with DRUJ instability after radial shaft ORIF (Table 65.1). Radiographs should also be scrutinized for the presence of an ulnar styloid fracture. Contralateral wrist radiographs or a computerized tomography (CT) scan of the wrist and forearm can be performed to assess the DRUJ if radiographs are not clear and suspicion is high for a DRUJ injury, but these are not routinely obtained. The use of magnetic resonance imaging has not been studied in the context of Galeazzi fracture-dislocations and is not a part of routine evaluation.

Treatment Options

Management in Pediatric and Adolescent Patients

Nonoperative management of radial shaft fractures is much more successful in children and adolescents in comparison with adults.[6,24] In children, treatment should begin with attempted closed reduction under sedation. Using fluoroscopic guidance, a closed reduction of the fractured radius is performed. Anatomic reduction of the radius should result in reduction of the DRUJ. Stability of the DRUJ can be assessed at this time.[42] A long arm cast with a good interosseous mold should be placed with the forearm in supination. The cast should be split to allow for swelling that will occur and prevent a potential compartment syndrome. Follow-up evaluation should be performed at 1 week with repeat radiographs, and if reduction is maintained, then the cast is overwrapped. Loose or ill-fitting casts should be replaced during the treatment period to prevent loss of reduction. The patient is immobilized in a long arm cast for 4–6 weeks.[6,24,42] Indications for operative management in pediatric patients include an inability to obtain or maintain a closed reduction of the radius and the DRUJ. The degree of acceptable malalignment will be highly variable depending on the skeletal age of the child.

Eberl et al.[42] reviewed all pediatric radial shaft fractures that were treated at their institution over a 3-year period totaling 198 fractures, 26 of which (13%) were Galeazzi fracture-dislocations. Seventy-nine percent were Walsh Type 2 and the average age was 11 years, consistent with prior reports of a peak incidence of 9–13 years of age.[24] Eighty-five percent of cases were successfully treated with sedation and closed reduction of the radius fracture. Fifty-seven percent of patients were treated in a well-molded short arm cast. Four patients required operative management due to inability to obtain a closed reduction and were treated with either retrograde elastic nailing of the radius or open plate fixation.

Galeazzi equivalent lesions are treated in a similar fashion. Closed reduction of the radius fracture and the displaced ulna epiphysis is attempted. Successful reduction is treated in a similar fashion. Failure of reduction of the distal ulna epiphysis is common due to interposed periosteum, ECU tendon, and/or ECU subsheath.[38] Indications for open reduction of the distal ulna epiphysis include a failed reduction or persistent widening of the physis after reduction, which may indicate interposed tissue. Open reduction and removal of interposed structures followed by pinning of the ulna fracture across the physis is performed. Cha et al.[38] present a series of 10 patients with Galeazzi equivalent lesions with an average follow-up of 6 years. They noted 8 of 10 patients had premature physeal closure at the distal ulna, indicating that long-term follow-up in these patients is required.

Management in Adult Patients

Nonoperative management of adult Galeazzi fracture-dislocations has been less successful with a high incidence of failure. Successful nonoperative management in children may be due to an ability to remodel, a thick periosteum, and a higher incidence of incomplete or greenstick bending fractures that may increase the stability of the radius with closed treatment. Adult diaphyseal radius fractures that are associated with a dislocated DRUJ are highly unstable and prone to displacement and malunion.[7] Fair to poor results with attempted cast immobilization range from 80% to 100% due to radius malunion, DRUJ instability, and pain.[6,43] For this reason, nearly all diaphyseal radius fractures that are associated with DRUJ injuries are treated with open reduction and rigid internal fixation of the radius.

Surgical Options

Pediatric and Adolescent Patients

There are several described techniques for the rare instance in which closed treatment fails. Surgical options include open reduction and casting, open reduction and intramedullary elastic nail fixation, open reduction and pin fixation, and open reduction and plate fixation.[24,42] Plate fixation in pediatric patients is limited by the size of the diaphysis and may require 2.7-mm implants or smaller. Intramedullary elastic nailing has the benefit of percutaneous fixation and smaller incisions. Direct comparisons of these techniques have not been performed in the setting of Galeazzi fracture-dislocations and the decision to use one over the other should be made based upon fracture morphology, location, and ability to obtain an adequate reduction with stable fixation. In Galeazzi equivalent lesions that require surgical management of the distal ulna physeal fracture, fixation should be performed with fine smooth K-wires to limit iatrogenic injury to the physis.

Adult Patients: Radial Shaft Fracture

Open reduction and plate fixation of the radius fracture is the standard treatment for diaphyseal radius fractures in adults. An anatomic reduction is needed to restore the DRUJ relationship.

Fixation with a 3.5-mm dynamic compression plate (DCP) is the most often described method of treatment in these injuries.[20,23,36,37,41] While plating the tension side of fractures is often preferred from a biomechanical standpoint, placing a plate on the radial surface of the radius is fraught with difficulty and is complicated by the insertions of several structures as well as proximity of the superficial branch of the radial nerve. The volar radius is much easier for plating, and Henry approach to the radius provides safe and appropriate exposure for nearly all distal-third radial shaft fractures. Restoration of the radial bow is required to obtain an adequate reduction of the DRUJ and allow full rotation of the forearm. Other methods of fixation have been described, including K-wires, interfragmentary screws, external fixation, and intramedullary pinning. Early reports of these techniques demonstrated poor outcomes due to loss of fixation and displacement of the radius in adults.[43] Intramedullary elastic nailing, similar to that of pediatric forearm fractures, has been reported with good results in adults; however, there are limited data on this technique and it has not gained widespread popularity.[44]

The DRUJ should be scrutinized after initial stable reduction of the radius. This is sometimes achieved with pointed reduction clamps versus preliminary plate fixation. It is helpful to obtain preoperative anteroposterior (AP) and lateral radiographs of the contralateral forearm to determine the normal radial bow, ulnar variance, and DRUJ morphology for a given patient. Fluoroscopic images should be obtained of the injured wrist to confirm an anatomic reduction of the DRUJ prior to placing all of the fixation screws. The ulna should not be forced into the sigmoid notch while obtaining these images as this may mask underlying instability, malreduction, or interposed tissue blocking a concentric reduction. If malreduction of the DRUJ is noted upon initial reduction of the radius, any preliminary hardware should be removed and the reduction of the radius adjusted until the DRUJ easily reduces. Once appropriate reductions of both the radial shaft fracture and the DRUJ dislocation are verified, the provisional fixation can be completed. In the rare instances when an anatomic reduction of the radius is confirmed and the DRUJ remains dislocated, then a complex Galeazzi fracture-dislocation should be suspected and an open reduction of the DRUJ should be performed and interposed tissue removed and repaired.

The reduced DRUJ is now assessed for stability. Objective findings for DRUJ stability often rely on the examining physician's experience and perception of instability. Assessment of palmar and dorsal translation of the radius in relation to the ulna in neutral, pronation, and supination is a well-described examination maneuver.[17] Supination places the dorsal fibers of the ligamentum subcruentum under tension; depending on the severity of the soft tissue injury, the radius will displace dorsal and ulnar head will displace palmar. In pronation, the palmar fibers of the ligamentum subcruentum are under tension; depending on the severity of the soft tissue injury, the radius will displace palmar and ulnar head will displace dorsal. If instability is noted in both directions, then complete avulsion of the fovea has occurred. There is some degree of normal translation of the DRUJ that varies from patient to patient. For this reason, the injured DRUJ should be compared with the contralateral DRUJ with the patient under anesthesia to remove the confounding factor of muscle relaxation. DRUJ instability has been described as the ability to dislocate the ulna out of the sigmoid notch.[36] Another examination maneuver has been described in which the ulna is compressed against the radius while the forearm is rotated. If a clunk is palpated during this maneuver, then instability is confirmed.[21] If stability is confirmed after examination of the DRUJ, then no further treatment is needed. There is no consensus on the position of immobilization in the postoperative period. Our preference is immobilization in neutral forearm rotation, which has been shown to have equivalent outcomes to immobilization in supination and has the added benefit of a more functional position for the patient.[45]

Options for an Unstable DRUJ After ORIF

An unstable DRUJ after ORIF of the radius requires that the DRUJ be treated. There is no comparative data to suggest superiority in any specific treatment. Treatment options that have been described range in complexity from simply splinting in a position of stability,[20,23] K-wire fixation of the radius to the ulna,[20,23,36,41] to more complex procedures such as arthroscopic-assisted DRUJ reduction, ulnar styloid fracture fixation, or repair of the TFCC, and any other associated soft tissue injuries. K-wire stabilization is the most cited treatment and has been described in positions of forearm full supination, partial supination, and neutral rotation.[7,23] The exact position is likely unimportant as long as the ulnar head is reduced within the sigmoid notch. Two 0.062-inch K-wires are passed transversely proximal to DRUJ across both cortices of the ulna and radius while the DRUJ is held reduced. Passing the K-wires through four cortices always allows removal if breakage of the wires were to occur. The pins are removed after 6 weeks, allowing for soft tissue healing.

Open procedures to stabilize the DRUJ include repair of an ulnar styloid fracture and open exploration and foveal repair of the TFCC. Additionally, an open exploration is indicated in cases of complex fracture-dislocations in order to remove interposed soft tissue that is preventing a reduction. In cases of an ulnar styloid fracture that involve the base of the styloid, it is recommended to perform an ORIF of the styloid. Stability of the DRUJ should be assessed after ulnar styloid fixation to confirm adequate stability has been obtained. If the joint is stable, then no further treatment is needed; however, if the DRUJ remains unstable, then K-wire fixation of the ulna to the radius is added. Open foveal repair of the TFCC ensures an anatomic repair of the primary stabilizer of the DRUJ. However, due to the relatively low incidence of true Galeazzi fracture-dislocations, no direct comparisons have been studied to demonstrate that a direct foveal repair adds any additional benefit over K-wire fixation. If an open exploration is indicated, such as in complex fracture-dislocations, then we would recommend a visual inspection of the TFCC fovea and, if torn, an open foveal repair of the TFCC. While arthroscopic and arthroscopic-assisted repairs of the TFCC in the setting of distal radius fractures or isolated DRUJ instability have been well described,[46-50] these techniques are more demanding, require specialized equipment, and have not been shown to have better outcomes in comparison with open TFCC repair techniques.[51,52] For these reasons, we prefer treatment based on the degree of surgeon perceived DRUJ instability. In cases in which a position of stability is found, splinting (sugar tong or above elbow) in the position of stability with or without cross-pinning of the DRUJ is recommended. While open repair of the TFCC is recommended in cases of complex DRUJ dislocation that require open reduction, the indications for TFCC repair in the setting of a reducible DRUJ dislocation have not been established. A decreased threshold for TFCC repair may be warranted with combined dorsal and volar instability.

Relevant Complications

Complications associated with the treatment of these injuries include nonunion, malunion, delayed union, symptomatic hardware, failure of fixation, and injury to neurovascular structures. Loss of a closed reduction in pediatric patients is reported to be 5%–10%.[24,42] Radial shaft malalignment may lead to subluxation of the DRUJ. Unrecognized DRUJ subluxation or dislocation is a devasting complication that can lead to pain, posttraumatic arthritis, and decreased forearm rotation.[5,6,36] Intramedullary elastic nails have reported complications of injury to the superficial sensory branch of the radial nerve and extensor pollicis longus (EPL) tendon rupture.[42]

Review of Treatment Outcomes

Outcomes for management in children were recently reported by Eberl et al.,[42] who reported Gartland-Werley scores for their series of 26 children. The authors reported 23 excellent and 3 good results in this series. There were no cases of ongoing DRUJ instability or malalignment on radiographs at an average follow-up of 22 months. Galeazzi equivalent lesions in children have been reported to have more complications associated with physeal arrest at the distal ulna.[38,53] Cha et al.[38] noted that at an average follow-up of 6 years in 10 patients, premature physeal closure was noted in 8. Other growth abnormalities included bowed distal ulnas, misshaped ulnar heads, and mismatch in DRUJ congruency, indicating that long-term follow-up is required in these injuries to follow and address growth abnormalities.

Mikić[6] reported outcomes for Galeazzi fracture-dislocations with "excellent" defined by near-perfect alignment and length, no subluxation, no limitation in function at the elbow or wrist, and no limitation in pronation or supination. A "fair" result was defined by having at least one abnormal finding including delayed union, subluxation of the ulnar head, limitation of up to 45 degrees in pronation or supination, or restriction of elbow or wrist function. A "poor" result was defined as having at least one of the following: patient dissatisfaction, pain, obvious deformity of the forearm, nonunion, shortening of the radius, >45 degrees of limitation in pronation or supination, or excessive restriction of elbow or wrist function. Using these criteria, Rettig and Raskin[36] reported excellent results from operative management in 95% of their adult patients. Poor outcomes in their series of 40 patients were noted in two cases of persistent DRUJ subluxation. Both patients had persistent dorsal subluxation of the ulnar head despite healing of the radius in adequate alignment. These patients were treated with Darrach resection arthroplasty and ECU tenodesis at 8 and 10 months after initial ORIF.

Ring et al.[23] reported 28% satisfactory and 67% excellent results in their series of 38 adult patients using outcomes described by Anderson et al.,[54] in which an excellent result is defined by a healed fracture with <10-degree loss of elbow or wrist motion and <25% loss of forearm rotation. A satisfactory result is defined by a healed fracture with <20-degree loss of elbow or wrist motion and <50% loss of forearm rotation. An unsatisfactory result is defined by a healed fracture with >30-degree loss of elbow or wrist motion and >50% loss of forearm rotation and a failure is defined as malunion, nonunion, or unresolved chronic osteomyelitis. Two unsatisfactory results were attributed to central nervous system injuries.

They noted no cases of DRUJ subluxation or pain at an average follow-up of 43 months.

Van Duijvenbode et al.[37] compared outcomes of diaphyseal radius fractures with and without DRUJ dislocation with an average follow-up of 19 years and a minimum follow-up of 13 years. They reported no differences in the Disability of Arm, Shoulder, and Hand (DASH) score, Mayo Modified Wrist score, Mayo Clinic Performance Index for the Elbow, forearm rotation, or DRUJ stability. Korompilias et al.[41] reported no DRUJ instability or need for revision surgery with an average follow-up of 6.8 years in a series of 40 radial shaft fractures with concomitant K-wire transfixation for persistent DRUJ instability noted intraoperatively after radial shaft ORIF.

Summary

Galeazzi fracture-dislocations require a high index of suspicion to diagnose correctly. Recognition of the injury and maintenance of an anatomic reduction of the radius and DRUJ are the goals of treatment regardless of nonoperative or operative management. The inherent instability associated with a radial shaft fracture with concomitant DRUJ dislocation makes this injury difficult to treat nonoperatively in adults. Anatomic open reduction and stable internal fixation with intraoperative evaluation of the DRUJ is critical when treating this injury operatively. Outcomes are generally excellent and equivalent to isolated radial shaft fractures when reduction of the DRUJ is maintained. Poor or unsatisfactory outcomes are generally associated with unrecognized and inadequately treated injuries, resulting in loss of reduction of the DRUJ.

References

1. Sebastin SJ, Chung KC. A historical report on Riccardo Galeazzi and the management of Galeazzi fractures. *J Hand Surg Am.* 2010;35(11):1870–1877. https://doi.org/10.1016/j.jhsa.2010.08.032.
2. Galeazzi R. Di una particolare sindrome traumatica dello scheletro dell' avambraccio. *Atti e Mem della Soc Lomb di Chir.* 1934;2:663–666.
3. Galeazzi R. Uber ein besonderes Syndrom bei Verletzungen im Bereich der Unterarmknochen. *Arch Orthop Unfall-Chir.* 1935;35:557–562.
4. Wong PC. Galeazzi fracture-dislocations in Singapore 1960-64; incidence and results of treatment. *Singapore Med J.* 1967;8(3):186–193. http://www.ncbi.nlm.nih.gov/pubmed/5587810.
5. Hughston JC. Fracture of the distal radial shaft; mistakes in management. *J Bone Joint Surg Am.* 1957;39-A(2):249–264. passim http://www.ncbi.nlm.nih.gov/pubmed/13416321.
6. Mikić ZD. Galeazzi fracture-dislocations. *J Bone Joint Surg Am.* 1975;57(8):1071–1080. http://www.ncbi.nlm.nih.gov/pubmed/1201989.
7. Giannoulis FS, Sotereanos DG. Galeazzi fractures and dislocations. *Hand Clin.* 2007;23(2):153–163. https://doi.org/10.1016/j.hcl.2007.03.004.
8. Palmer AK, Werner FW. Biomechanics of the distal radioulnar joint. *Clin Orthop Relat Res.* (187):26-35. http://www.ncbi.nlm.nih.gov/pubmed/6744728.
9. Watanabe H, Berger RA, Berglund LJ, Zobitz ME, An KN. Contribution of the interosseous membrane to distal radioulnar joint constraint. *J Hand Surg Am.* 2005;30(6):1164–1171. https://doi.org/10.1016/j.jhsa.2005.06.013.
10. Kihara H, Short WH, Werner FW, Fortino MD, Palmer AK. The stabilizing mechanism of the distal radioulnar joint during pronation and supination. *J Hand Surg Am.* 1995;20(6):930–936. https://doi.org/10.1016/S0363-5023(05)80139-X.

11. Noda K, Goto A, Murase T, Sugamoto K, Yoshikawa H, Moritomo H. Interosseous membrane of the forearm: an anatomical study of ligament attachment locations. *J Hand Surg Am.* 2009;34(3):415–422. https://doi.org/10.1016/j.jhsa.2008.10.025.

12. Hohenberger GM, Schwarz AM, Weiglein AH, Krassnig R, Kuchling S, Plecko M. Prevalence of the distal oblique bundle of the interosseous membrane of the forearm: an anatomical study. *J Hand Surg Eur.* 2018;43(4):426–430. https://doi.org/10.1177/1753193417727138.

13. Dy CJ, Jang E, Taylor SA, Meyers KN, Wolfe SW. The impact of coronal alignment on distal radioulnar joint stability following distal radius fracture. *J Hand Surg Am.* 2014;39(7):1264–1272. https://doi.org/10.1016/j.jhsa.2014.03.041.

14. Kitamura T, Moritomo H, Arimitsu S, et al. The biomechanical effect of the distal interosseous membrane on distal radioulnar joint stability: a preliminary anatomic study. *J Hand Surg Am.* 2011;36(10):1626–1630. https://doi.org/10.1016/j.jhsa.2011.07.016.

15. af Ekenstam F, Hagert CG. Anatomical studies on the geometry and stability of the distal radio ulnar joint. *Scand J Plast Reconstr Surg.* 1985;19(1):17–25. https://doi.org/10.3109/02844318509052861.

16. Hagert CG. Distal radius fracture and the distal radioulnar joint—anatomical considerations. *Handchir Mikrochir Plast Chir.* 1994;26(1):22–26. http://www.ncbi.nlm.nih.gov/pubmed/8150382.

17. Kleinman WB. Stability of the distal radioulna joint: biomechanics, pathophysiology, physical diagnosis, and restoration of function what we have learned in 25 years. *J Hand Surg Am.* 2007;32(7):1086–1106. https://doi.org/10.1016/j.jhsa.2007.06.014.

18. Schneiderman G, Meldrum RD, Bloebaum RD, Tarr R, Sarmiento A. The interosseous membrane of the forearm: structure and its role in Galeazzi fractures. *J Trauma.* 1993;35(6):879–885. http://www.ncbi.nlm.nih.gov/pubmed/8263987.

19. Moore TM, Lester DK, Sarmiento A. The stabilizing effect of soft-tissue constraints in artificial Galeazzi fractures. *Clin Orthop Relat Res.* 1985;194:189–194. https://doi.org/10.1097/00003086-198504000-00028.

20. Tsismenakis T, Tornetta P. Galeazzi fractures: is DRUJ instability predicted by current guidelines? *Injury.* 2016;47(7):1472–1477. https://doi.org/10.1016/j.injury.2016.04.003.

21. Jupiter JB. Commentary: the effect of ulnar styloid fractures on patient-rated outcomes after volar locking plating of distal radius fractures. *J Hand Surg Am.* 2009;34(9):1603–1604. https://doi.org/10.1016/j.jhsa.2009.06.022.

22. Moritomo H. The distal interosseous membrane: current concepts in wrist anatomy and biomechanics. *J Hand Surg Am.* 2012;37(7):1501–1507. https://doi.org/10.1016/j.jhsa.2012.04.037.

23. Ring D, Rhim R, Carpenter C, Jupiter JB. Isolated radial shaft fractures are more common than Galeazzi fractures. *J Hand Surg Am.* 2006;31(1):17–21. https://doi.org/10.1016/j.jhsa.2005.09.003.

24. Walsh HP, McLaren CA, Owen R. Galeazzi fractures in children. *J Bone Joint Surg Br.* 1987;69(5):730–733. http://www.ncbi.nlm.nih.gov/pubmed/3680332.

25. Bruckner JD, Lichtman DM, Alexander AH. Complex dislocations of the distal radioulnar joint. Recognition and management. *Clin Orthop Relat Res.* 1992;275:90–103. http://www.ncbi.nlm.nih.gov/pubmed/1735239.

26. Lichtman D, Alexander A, Bruckner J. Complex dislocations of the distal radioulnar joint: Recognition and management. *J Orthop Trauma.* 1991;5(2):220. https://doi.org/10.1097/00005131-199105020-00034.

27. Yohe NJ, De Tolla J, Kaye MB, Edelstein DM, Choueka J. Irreducible Galeazzi fracture-dislocations. *Hand (N Y).* 2019;14(2):249–252. https://doi.org/10.1177/1558944717744334.

28. Kikuchi Y, Nakamura T. Irreducible Galeazzi fracture-dislocation due to an avulsion fracture of the fovea of the ulna. *J Hand Surg Br.* 1999;24(3):379–381. https://doi.org/10.1054/jhsb.1998.0007.

29. Alexander AH, Lichtman DM. Irreducible distal radioulnar joint occurring in a Galeazzi fracture - case report. *J Hand Surg Am.* 1981;6(3):258–261. https://doi.org/10.1016/s0363-5023(81)80081-0.

30. Cetti NE. An unusual cause of blocked reduction of the Galeazzi injury. *Injury.* 1977;9(1):59–61. https://doi.org/10.1016/0020-1383(77)90053-5.

31. Budgen A, Lim P, Templeton P, Irwin LR. Irreducible Galeazzi injury. *Arch Orthop Trauma Surg.* 1998;118(3):176–178. https://doi.org/10.1007/s004020050343.

32. Biyani A, Bhan S. Dual extensor tendon entrapment in Galeazzi fracture-dislocation: a case report. *J Trauma.* 1989;29(9):1295–1297. https://doi.org/10.1097/00005373-198909000-00022.

33. Itoh Y, Horiuchi Y, Takahashi M, Uchinishi K, Yabe Y. Extensor tendon involvement in Smith's and Galeazzi's fractures. *J Hand Surg Am.* 1987;12(4):535–540. https://doi.org/10.1016/s0363-5023(87)80203-4.

34. Giangarra CE, Chandler RW. Complex volar distal radioulnar joint dislocation occurring in a Galeazzi fracture. *J Orthop Trauma.* 1989;3(1):76–79. https://doi.org/10.1097/00005131-198903010-00015.

35. Jenkins NH, Mintowt-Czyz WJ, Fairclough JA. Irreducible dislocation of the distal radioulnar joint. *Injury.* 1987;18(1):40–43. https://doi.org/10.1016/0020-1383(87)90384-6.

36. Rettig ME, Raskin KB. Galeazzi fracture-dislocation: a new treatment-oriented classification. *J Hand Surg Am.* 2001;26(2):228–235. https://doi.org/10.1053/jhsu.2001.21523.

37. Van Duijvenbode DC, Guitton TG, Raaymakers EL, Kloen P, Ring D. Long-term outcome of isolated diaphyseal radius fractures with and without dislocation of the distal radioulnar joint. *J Hand Surg Am.* 2012;37(3):523–527. https://doi.org/10.1016/j.jhsa.2011.11.008.

38. Cha SM, Shin HD, Jeon JH. Long-term results of Galeazzi-equivalent injuries in adolescents - open reduction and internal fixation of the ulna. *J Pediatr Orthop Part B.* 2016;25(2):174–182. https://doi.org/10.1097/BPB.0000000000000259.

39. Galanopoulos I, Fogg Q, Ashwood N, Fu K. A widely displaced Galeazzi-equivalent lesion with median nerve compromise. *BMJ Case Rep.* 2012:10–13. https://doi.org/10.1136/bcr-2012-006395.

40. Roettges P, Turker T. Ulnar nerve injury as a result of Galeazzi fracture: a case report and literature review. *Hand.* 2017;12(5):NP162–NP165. https://doi.org/10.1177/1558944717715137.

41. Korompilias AV, Lykissas MG, Kostas-Agnantis IP, Beris AE, Soucacos PN. Distal radioulnar joint instability (Galeazzi type injury) after internal fixation in relation to the radius fracture pattern. *J Hand Surg Am.* 2011;36(5):847–852. https://doi.org/10.1016/j.jhsa.2010.12.020.

42. Eberl R, Singer G, Schalamon J, Petnehazy T, Hoellwarth ME. Galeazzi lesions in children and adolescents: treatment and outcome. *Clin Orthop Relat Res.* 2008;466(7):1705–1709. https://doi.org/10.1007/s11999-008-0268-6.

43. Reckling FW. Unstable fracture-dislocations of the forearm (Monteggia and Galeazzi lesions). *J Bone Jt Surg - Ser A.* 1982;64(6):857–863. https://doi.org/10.2106/00004623-198264060-00007.

44. Gadegone WM, Salphale Y, Magarkar D. Percutaneous osteosynthesis of Galeazzi fracture-dislocation. *Indian J Orthop.* 2010;44(4):448–452. https://doi.org/10.4103/0019-5413.67121.

45. Park MJ, Pappas N, Steinberg DR, Bozentka DJ. Immobilization in supination versus neutral following surgical treatment of Galeazzi fracture-dislocations in adults: case series. *J Hand Surg Am.* 2012;37(3):528–531. https://doi.org/10.1016/j.jhsa.2011.12.021.

46. Iwamae M, Yano K, Kaneshiro Y, Sakanaka H. Arthroscopic reduction of an irreducible distal radioulnar joint in Galeazzi fracture-dislocation due to a fragment of the ulnar styloid: a case report. *BMC Musculoskelet Disord.* 2019;20(1):1–5. https://doi.org/10.1186/s12891-019-2735-5.

47. Iwasaki N, Minami A. Arthroscopically assisted reattachment of avulsed triangular fibrocartilage complex to the fovea of the ulnar head. *J Hand Surg Am.* 2009;34(7):1323–1326. https://doi.org/10.1016/j.jhsa.2009.02.026.

48. Chen WJ. Arthroscopically assisted transosseous foveal repair of triangular fibrocartilage complex. *Arthrosc Tech.* 2017;6(1):e57–e64. https://doi.org/10.1016/j.eats.2016.09.004.

49. Park JH, Kim D, Park JW. Arthroscopic one-tunnel transosseous foveal repair for triangular fibrocartilage complex (TFCC) peripheral tear. *Arch Orthop Trauma Surg.* 2018;138(1):131–138. https://doi.org/10.1007/s00402-017-2835-3.

50. Frank RM, Slikker W, Al-Shihabi L, Wysocki RW. Arthroscopic-assisted outside-in repair of triangular fibrocartilage complex tears. *Arthrosc Tech.* 2015;4(5):e577–e581. https://doi.org/10.1016/j.eats.2015.06.002.

51. Andersson JK, Åhlén M, Andernord D. Open versus arthroscopic repair of the triangular fibrocartilage complex: a systematic review. *J Exp Orthop.* 2018;5(1):1–10. https://doi.org/10.1186/s40634-018-0120-1.

52. Nakamura T, Sato K, Okazaki M, Toyama Y, Ikegami H. Repair of foveal detachment of the triangular fibrocartilage complex: open and arthroscopic transosseous techniques. *Hand Clin.* 2011;27(3):281–290. https://doi.org/10.1016/j.hcl.2011.05.002.

53. Letts M, Rowhani N. Galeazzi-equivalent injuries of the wrist in children. *J Pediatr Orthop.* 13(5):561-566. http://www.ncbi.nlm.nih.gov/pubmed/8376552.

54. Anderson LD, Sisk D, Tooms RE, Park WI. Compression-plate fixation in acute diaphyseal fractures of the radius and ulna. *J Bone Joint Surg Am.* 1975;57(3):287–297. http://www.ncbi.nlm.nih.gov/pubmed/1091653.

66

Technique Spotlight: ORIF of Galeazzi Fracture-Dislocations

HASSAN J. AZIMI AND ROBERT W. WYSOCKI

Indications

The decision between surgical and nonsurgical management is largely guided by patient age. In children, closed reduction and casting is the mainstay of treatment if an adequate reduction of both the radius fracture and the distal radioulnar joint (DRUJ) dislocation can be maintained. In adults, a fracture of the radial shaft with concomitant DRUJ dislocation has been termed "a fracture of necessity," referring to the necessity for surgical treatment of all such fractures in order to obtain adequate outcomes. Multiple series[1,2] have reported on nonoperative treatment with closed reduction and immobilization of Galeazzi fractures in adults with nearly uniform poor results. For this reason, open reduction and internal fixation is the standard of care for adults.[3]

Preoperative Evaluation

Physical examination will demonstrate swelling, deformity, and tenderness at the forearm. The ulnar head may be prominent in the dorsal or volar soft tissues. A detailed neurovascular evaluation should be performed, although neurovascular injuries associated with this fracture are rare.[3–5] Suspicion for DRUJ dislocation should be high with all radial shaft fractures.[6,7] The wrist should be palpated for prominence of the ulnar head and tenderness at the DRUJ. Radiographic evaluation should include posteroanterior (PA) and lateral views of the forearm, wrist, and elbow. The radius may appear shortened and there may be widening of the DRUJ that is best seen on the PA radiograph (Fig. 66.1). The lateral radiograph is best to visualize whether the ulnar head is displaced volarly, or more commonly, dorsally. Radiographs should also be scrutinized for an ulnar styloid fracture. Cross-sectional imaging is typically not necessary but may be used to evaluate fracture comminution or joint incongruity. The utilization of magnetic resonance imaging (MRI) to evaluate the triangular fibrocartilage complex (TFCC) has not been studied in the setting of Galeazzi fracture-dislocations and the authors do not typically obtain an MRI. While radiographic parameters are not diagnostic for DRUJ instability, the following findings should raise suspicion for a Galeazzi injury and prompt further evaluation of the DRUJ at the time of surgery: radial shaft fractures within 7.5 cm of the lunate facet, 5 mm of radial shortening, widening of the DRUJ, concomitant ulnar styloid base fractures, and ulnar head dislocation.[6]

Positioning

The operation can be performed under regional or general anesthesia. The patient is placed supine on an operating table with the arm abducted onto a hand table. A well-padded tourniquet is applied above the elbow. A fluoroscopy unit is typically brought into the surgical field from the head of the table, with the primary surgeon positioned in the patient's axilla and the assistant on the opposite side of the hand table.

Equipment

Equipment List

- 3.5-mm locking compression plate (LCP) system with 3.5-mm screws or similar
- 2.7-mm LCP system with 2.0-, 2.4-, and 2.7-mm screws or similar
- Multiple fracture reduction clamps, pointed and serrated
- K-wire tray with 0.062- and 0.045-inch wires
- Stainless steel surgical wire: 22- or 24-gauge (for ulnar styloid fixation)
- Portable fluoroscopy unit
- Trauma drill

For the average patient, we prefer a 3.5-mm limited-contact dynamic compression plate. It should be noted that a seven-hole plate is typically the ideal length, and this may need to be specially requested as it does not always come standard in the tray (Fig. 66.2). If there is obliquity or comminution at the fracture site, a six-hole plate places the center holes close to the fracture line, which may affect screw purchase. Due to the curvature of the radius in the coronal plane, an eight-hole plate may be prominent off the side of the radius either proximally or distally. If a plate of this length is needed to bridge comminution, then consider the use of precontoured radius plates with scallops that allow for easier bending of the plate to accommodate the radial bow. In smaller patients, it may be necessary to have a 2.7-mm dynamic

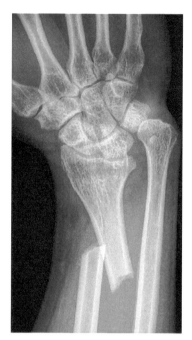

• **Fig. 66.1** Posteroanterior radiograph of the wrist demonstrating a distal-third radial shaft fracture with shortening of the radius, ulnar styloid fracture, ulnar head prominence, and widening of the distal radioulnar joint.

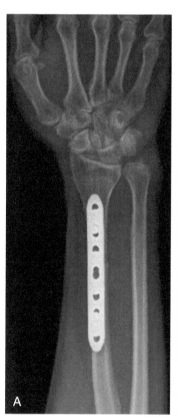 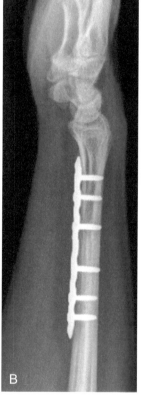

• **Fig. 66.2** Posteroanterior (A) and lateral (B) radiographs status post open reduction and internal fixation with a seven-hole 3.5-mm locking compression plate.

compression plating system available. In our experience, 2.7-mm dynamic compression plates are not rigid enough and are more prone to bending or breaking. If the bone can accommodate a 3.5-mm plate, this is our preference. If the fracture is distal and near the metaphyseal flare, a metadiaphyseal plate with clustered holes distally may be needed to obtain adequate distal fixation.

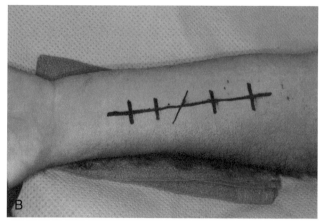

• **Fig. 66.3** The fracture is marked (*oblique hash mark*) to center the incision.

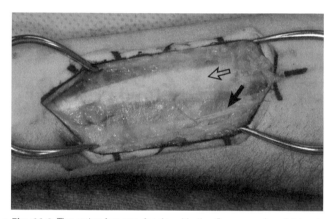

• **Fig. 66.4** The volar forearm fascia with the flexor carpi radial tendon and muscle visible deep (*open arrow*). The lateral antebrachial cutaneous nerve is seen in the radial subcutaneous tissue (*solid arrow*).

Technique

Approach

This technique pertains to distal-third radial shaft fractures that make up the vast majority of Galeazzi injuries. We strongly favor a volar approach given its extensile nature distally with less risk of tendon adhesions and plate prominence. Center the incision on the fracture by using a fluoroscopic image to identify the fracture. Distally, the flexor carpi radial (FCR) tendon and radial artery can be palpated and the incision is drawn longitudinal at the radial edge of the FCR tendon and muscle belly (Fig. 66.3). The radius is approached through a modified Henry approach utilizing the interval between the FCR and the radial artery. Skin is incised and dissection to the volar forearm fascia is performed. Careful dissection is required in the radial subcutaneous tissues as the lateral antebrachial cutaneous (LABC) nerve is present here (Fig. 66.4). The volar forearm fascia is incised along the radial border of the FCR tendon and muscle with identification and protection of the radial artery which runs longitudinally radial to the FCR. The modified Henry interval is between the FCR and the radial artery (Fig. 66.5A). Care should be taken along the radial border of the forearm as the superficial branch of the radial nerve (SBRN) is deep to the brachioradialis (BR) tendon and can be encountered (Fig. 66.5B). Vigorous retraction should be avoided on this sensitive sensory cutaneous nerve. We typically do not identify

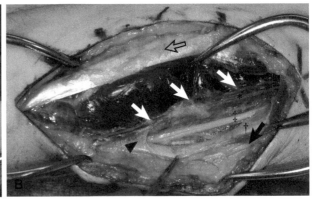

• **Fig. 66.5** Deep interval between the flexor carpi radial *(open arrow)* and the radial artery *(asterisk)* with perforators from the radial artery to the muscle. (A) The brachioradialis tendon *(dagger)* is shown and when reflected (B) the superficial branch of the radial nerve *(double dagger)* is visualized just deep the brachioradialis tendon. The fascia *(arrowhead)* has been incised to expose the superficial branch of the radial nerve (SBRN). The SBRN should not be confused for the lateral antebrachial cutaneous nerve *(solid arrow)* in the subcutaneous tissues.

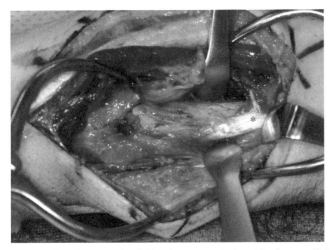

• **Fig. 66.6** The flexor carpi radial has been retracted and the flexor pollicis longus elevated off the radius radially. The pronator teres tendon *(asterisk)* insertion is seen proximally. The radial artery is retracted radially with the brachioradialis tendon and muscle.

the SBRN as it is deep to a fascial layer. Several perforators off of the radial artery to the FCR and underlying flexor pollicis longus (FPL) will need to be ligated with electrocautery, allowing the FCR and FPL to be retracted ulnarly and the radial artery and BR retracted radially (Fig. 66.6), exposing the fracture. With more proximal fractures, the pronator teres (PT) tendon insertion will be encountered (Fig. 66.6) and may need to be elevated. If so, pronate the forearm to sharply elevate the PT off the radial border in a dorsal-radial to volar-ulnar direction. In more distal fractures, the pronator quadratus (PQ) will need to be elevated off the radius from radial to ulnar, ligating perforator vessels. Sufficient PT and PQ must be released to allow fracture visualization and reduction, and sufficient space for placement of the internal fixation plate. In an effort to maximize perfusion to the fracture fragments, extraperiosteal dissection should be performed over the length of the dissection, minimizing subperiosteal dissection to only what is necessary to view and obtain the fracture reduction. Subacute fractures will typically have greater adaptive periosteal thickening and require greater subperiosteal dissection than acute injuries.

Reduction Maneuvers

We prefer the use of serrated blunt reduction clamps to control the fracture fragments (Fig. 66.7A) and perform a manual reduction (Fig. 66.7B). The deforming force on the proximal fragment in these distal-third injuries is the PT, thus a supination force is needed to counteract its pull. The deforming forces on the distal fragment are due to the BR and PQ which cause pronation and shortening of the distal fragment, thus supination and longitudinal traction counteract these forces. Fluoroscopy is used to confirm fracture reduction, radial bow, and the DRUJ reduction. If fracture reduction is anatomic, the DRUJ alignment is restored in the vast majority of cases. Strategies to address the DRUJ in cases of anatomic fracture fixation are addressed elsewhere in this text. An appropriate length plate is applied to the volar cortex. The plate can aid as a reduction tool to control volar-dorsal displacement and the clamps reapplied as the radial and ulnar cortices are aligned. Fluoroscopy is used to confirm the reduction (Fig. 66.8).

Fracture Fixation

Once the fracture alignment is anatomic, the DRUJ is reduced and the radial bow is restored, fixation can be performed (Fig. 66.9). Fractures that allow for compression (simple transverse and short oblique without comminution) are preferably treated with standard AO techniques with pre-bending the plate and utilizing dynamic compression. If comminution is present, a bridge plate construct is utilized. For simple fracture patterns, we prefer to center the plate over the fracture to allow for six cortices of fixation proximal and distal to the fracture (Fig. 66.2).

After fixation is obtained, forearm rotation should be assessed for any blocks to motion and the DRUJ should be stressed in pronation, neutral, and supination. Addressing an unstable DRUJ after radial shaft fixation will be discussed elsewhere in this text. Finally, fluoroscopic images are obtained to confirm reduction of the DRUJ (Fig. 66.10). The tourniquet is released, the radial artery is assessed, and hemostasis is obtained. We do not routinely close the fascia or repair the PQ or PT. The incision is closed with interrupted subcutaneous sutures and interrupted nonabsorbable skin closure.

Postoperative Care

In cases with a stable DRUJ, we prefer a sugar-tong splint in neutral forearm rotation until the first postoperative visit in 10–14

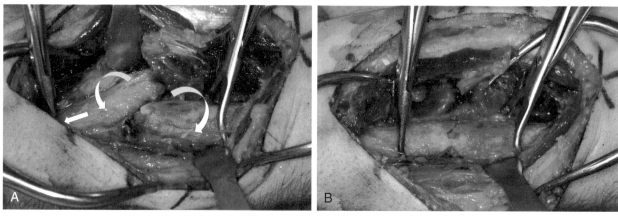

• **Fig. 66.7** (A) Reduction clamps are used to grasp the fragments and perform a reduction maneuver which includes supinating the fragments with longitudinal traction. (B) The reduction is held manually while assessing radiographs.

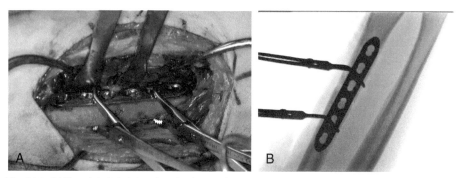

• **Fig. 66.8** (A) The plate is held against the bone with the use of two reduction clamps. (B) Fluoroscopic images of reduction.

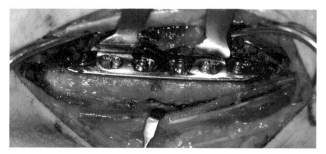

• **Fig. 66.9** Final fixation, note, the two cortical screws near the fracture to allow for dynamic compression through the plate.

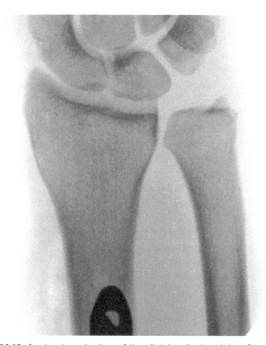

• **Fig. 66.10** Anatomic reduction of the distal radioulnar joint after fracture fixation.

days. At that visit, we place the patient into a removable custom-fabricated long arm or sugar-tong orthosis with the forearm in neutral rotation and begin gentle active and active-assist range-of-motion exercises for the forearm and wrist. Passive range of motion and strengthening begins at 6 weeks. Radiographs are checked at 6 and 12 weeks postoperatively to assess union. Return to full activities is expected by 12–16 weeks.

PEARLS AND PITFALLS

Pearls

- Center the incision using fluoroscopy.
- A 3.5-mm seven-hole LCP is most often used for simple fracture patterns; this may need to be preordered.
- Use the plate to help as a reduction aid.
- Fluoroscopy should be scrutinized to assess the DRUJ and radial bow prior to fixation and after fixation.
- Carefully assess forearm rotation and DRUJ stability after fixation of the radial shaft.

Pitfalls

- Long (eight-hole and greater) straight plates that fit well on the radius may be malreducing the fracture; carefully assess the radial bow with these constructs.
- Overcompression of oblique fractures can shorten the radius and subsequently cause malreduction of the DRUJ.
- Be aware of the location of the dorsal sensory branch of the radial nerve and the LABC nerve to avoid injury.
- Applying compression plating principles without pre-bending the plate can lead to gaping on the far side of the fracture.
- Overzealous subperiosteal dissection can lead to decreased perfusion to the fracture fragments and may impair healing.

References

1. Reckling FW. Unstable fracture-dislocations of the forearm (Monteggia and Galeazzi lesions). *J Bone Jt Surg Ser A*. 1982;64(6):857–863. https://doi.org/10.2106/00004623-198264060-00007.
2. Mikić ZD. Galeazzi fracture-dislocations. *J Bone Joint Surg Am*. 1975;57(8):1071–1080. http://www.ncbi.nlm.nih.gov/pubmed/1201989.
3. Giannoulis FS, Sotereanos DG. Galeazzi fractures and dislocations. *Hand Clin*. 2007;23(2):153–163. https://doi.org/10.1016/j.hcl.2007.03.004.
4. Van Duijvenbode DC, Guitton TG, Raaymakers EL, Kloen P, Ring D. Long-term outcome of isolated diaphyseal radius fractures with and without dislocation of the distal radioulnar joint. *J Hand Surg Am*. 2012;37(3):523–527. https://doi.org/10.1016/j.jhsa.2011.11.008.
5. Atesok KI, Jupiter JB, Weiss APC. Galeazzi fracture. *J Am Acad Orthop Surg*. 2011;19(10):623–633. https://doi.org/10.5435/00124635-201110000-00006.
6. Tsismenakis T, Tornetta P. Galeazzi fractures: is DRUJ instability predicted by current guidelines? *Injury*. 2016;47(7):1472–1477. https://doi.org/10.1016/j.injury.2016.04.003.
7. Ring D, Rhim R, Carpenter C, Jupiter JB. Isolated radial shaft fractures are more common than Galeazzi fractures. *J Hand Surg Am*. 2006;31(1):17–21. https://doi.org/10.1016/j.jhsa.2005.09.003.

67

Technique Spotlight: Tips and Tricks for Predicting Which Radial Shaft Fractures Will Be Unstable; Repair Options for the DRUJ/TFCC After Radial Fixation

HASSAN J. AZIMI, JOHN J. FERNANDEZ, AND ROBERT W. WYSOCKI

Indications

Persistent distal radioulnar joint (DRUJ) instability or an irreducible DRUJ after anatomic fixation of a radial shaft fracture requires further evaluation and management. The following scenarios are typically encountered after radial shaft fixation:

1. Reduced and stable DRUJ
2. Reduced and DRUJ stable only in specific forearm positions (supination or pronation)
3. Reduced but unstable DRUJ with concomitant large ulnar styloid fracture
4. Reduced but unstable DRUJ and intact or small ulnar styloid fracture
5. Irreducible DRUJ

A reduced and stable DRUJ requires no further surgical management. In cases with an ulnar styloid fracture that involves the base or ulnar fovea with concomitant instability of the DRUJ, fixation of the ulnar styloid fracture is recommended to restore the anatomic insertion of the dorsal and palmar ligaments and stabilize the DRUJ.[1] Techniques for fixation of ulnar styloid fractures are discussed in another chapter. An irreducible DRUJ is uncommon, with several case reports describing this clinical scenario.[2] In these cases, an open reduction of the DRUJ should be performed to remove the interposed structures which most commonly includes the extensor carpi ulnaris (ECU) tendon,

but also may include tendons of the extensor digitorum communis (EDC) and extensor digiti minimi (EDM), the dorsal joint capsule, and the fractured ulnar styloid.[2–11] An unstable and reducible DRUJ in a patient with a small ulnar styloid fracture or an intact ulnar styloid should be treated with cast or splint immobilization. In these cases the DRUJ is typically stable and reduced in particular forearm rotations. For example, if the DRUJ is unstable in forearm pronation or neutral but stable in supination, then the patient is immobilized in supination to maintain a reduced position.[12–14] A persistently or globally unstable DRUJ that cannot be held reduced with immobilization alone will typically be treated either with rigid immobilization in a position of stability with K-wire fixation of the radius to ulna or triangular fibrocartilage complex (TFCC) repair to bone depending on surgeon preference and perception of how high-grade the soft tissue disruption is. Many techniques have been described to perform a TFCC repair in this setting, including all-inside arthroscopic, arthroscopic-assisted open, or full open repair.[14–21] Regardless of the technique, it is critical that the repair in the setting of DRUJ instability directly reattaches the TFCC to its insertion on the ulnar fovea. The open transosseous repair of the TFCC to the fovea described here allows for reproducible anatomic reattachment without the need for additional skills in wrist arthroscopy, which have not demonstrated superior outcomes.[19]

Preoperative and Intraoperative Evaluation

The amount of DRUJ translation with loading differs from patient to patient, and thus evaluation of the contralateral wrist should be used for comparison. This examination should be performed prior to beginning the operation. While radiographic parameters are not diagnostic for DRUJ instability,[22–24] the following findings should raise suspicion for a Galeazzi injury in the presence of an isolated radial shaft fracture and prompt further evaluation of the DRUJ after fixation of the radial shaft: radial shaft fractures within 7.5 cm of the lunate facet, 5 mm of radial shortening, widening of the DRUJ, concomitant ulnar styloid base fractures, and ulnar head dislocation.[24] A preoperative lateral radiograph may show dorsal or ulnar dislocation of the ulnar head, with dorsal dislocation being most common.[25] The direction of the dislocation can guide the surgeon on the potential direction of instability after radial shaft fixation. In full pronation, the dorsal superficial fibers, the dorsal joint capsule, and the deep palmar fibers tighten for stability and prevent dorsal dislocation of the ulna, while the reciprocal occurs in supination. As such, the deep palmar ligament is tested in pronation, and the deep dorsal ligament is tested in supination.[26]

Positioning

The operation can be performed under regional or general anesthesia. The patient is placed supine on an operating table with the arm abducted onto a hand table. A well-padded tourniquet is applied above the elbow. A fluoroscopy unit is brought into the surgical field from the head of the table, with the primary surgeon positioned in the patient's axilla and the assistant on the opposite side of the hand table. The hand and wrist are well padded and placed into the traction tower. In open cases when approaching the subcutaneous border of the ulna, the traction tower case is used to hold the hand without applying traction; this frees your assistant from having to hold the forearm in an elevated position throughout the operation.

Equipment List

- 1.1-mm guidewire, 2.0-mm cannulated drill, wire driver, and power drill
- Wrist arthroscopy traction tower
- 2-0 PDS suture
- Suture passer
- Small bone anchor: 2.5 mm × 8 mm, or similar

Surgical Technique

Open Dorsal Approach With Transosseous TFCC Repair for Unstable or Irreducible DRUJ

The DRUJ is approached through the floor of the fifth dorsal wrist compartment. With the forearm pronated, a 5-cm longitudinal incision is made between the EDM and ECU tendons. Care should be taken to identify and protect the dorsal sensory branches of the ulnar nerve. The extensor retinaculum is incised along the radial aspect of the EDM (Fig. 67.1). The DRUJ may be exposed if there is a traumatic capsulotomy, if not an L-shaped capsulotomy is made, starting with a longitudinal limb between the EDM and ECU (Fig. 67.2A), leaving a cuff on both sides for later repair (Fig. 67.2B). The transverse limb of the arthrotomy is made proximal and parallel to the dorsal radioulnar ligament, which allows inspection of the foveal attachment of the TFCC and radioulnar ligaments (Fig. 67.3A). Any interposed tissue within the DRUJ should

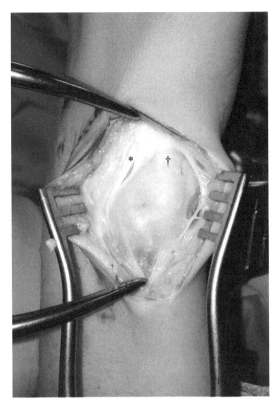

• **Fig. 67.1** The retinaculum over the extensor digiti minimi (EDM) is released. *(Asterisk)* EDM and *(dagger)* extensor carpi ulnaris.

be removed and the joint reduced. Assuming the TFCC is determined to be torn and reparable, a second transverse capsulotomy is made distal to the dorsal radioulnar ligament (Fig. 67.3B) allowing visualization of the TFCC's distal surface and the eventual passing of sutures for a repair.

With the ulnar head exposed, a curette is used to remove any fibrous tissue and prepare the insertion site of the TFCC at the fovea down to healthy bone. A 1.1-mm guidewire is placed at the foveal isometric point (Fig. 67.4A) and passed proximally to exit along the volar and ulnar border of the ulna (Fig. 67.4B). This prevents subcutaneous suture placement which can be symptomatic. A cannulated 2.0-mm drill is passed over the wire and creates the transosseous tunnel. A 2-0 PDS suture is used to create two horizontal mattresses broadly positioned in the body of the TFCC (Fig. 67.5). Direct inspection with tension applied through the sutures should ensure the TFCC is brought evenly down to the foveal insertion site. If needed, adjust the horizontal mattress suture placement to ensure an even repair. A suture passer is passed through the osseous tunnel from the ulnar cortex into the joint and the repair sutures are shuttled out. At least 1 cm proximal to the transosseous tunnel, the drill hole is placed for the first anchor. The second anchor should be drilled at an angle that avoids the first anchor. The sutures are tensioned and the TFCC is brought to the foveal insertion site. With the forearm in neutral rotation, the anchors are placed sequentially (Fig. 67.6) with appropriate suture tension. The sutures are cut after confirmation of secure anchor fixation. The capsule and retinaculum are repaired followed by subcutaneous and skin closure.

Postoperative Rehabilitation

The patient is placed in a long-arm splint in full supination. At 4 weeks, the long-arm splint is removed, and the patient is allowed to move from supination to neutral rotation. At 5 weeks, the

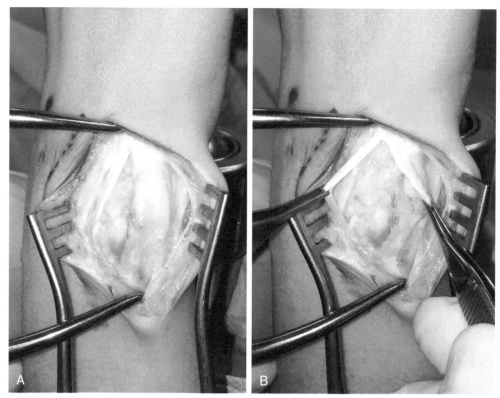

• **Fig. 67.2** (A) The capsule is elevated longitudinally from radial to ulnar. (B) The extensor carpi ulnaris and extensor digiti minimi are retracted to expose the dorsal radioulnar ligament and ulnar head and neck, allowing visualization for the transverse limb of the capsulotomy to be made.

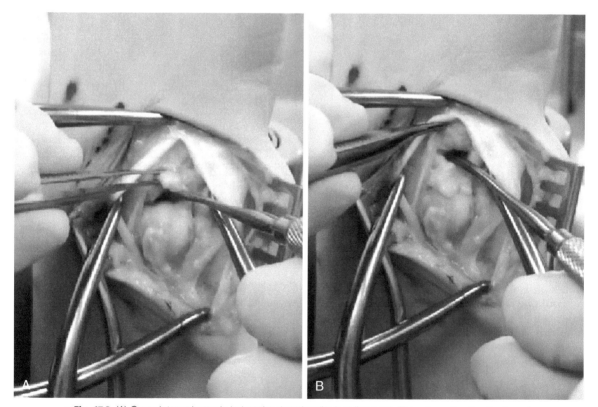

• **Fig. 67.3** (A) Capsulotomy is made below the dorsal radioulnar ligament. This allows for visualization of the triangular fibrocartilage complex (TFCC) fovea and proximal surface. (B) If the TFCC fovea is torn and reparable, then a second transverse capsulotomy is made superior to the dorsal radioulnar ligament and the distal surface is visualized.

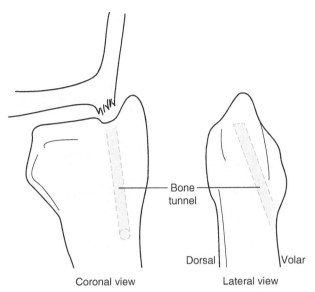

Coronal view   Lateral view

• **Fig. 67.4** A 0.045 K-wire is used to create a transosseous tunnel at the foveal insertion of the triangular fibrocartilage complex. The wire is angled to exit along the volar and ulnar border of the ulna. This prevents subcutaneous knots and sutures that can be symptomatic.

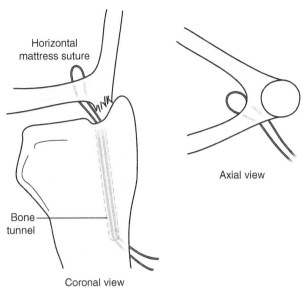

Axial view

Coronal view

• **Fig. 67.5** Correct placement of a horizontal mattress suture at the isometric point of the triangular fibrocartilage complex.

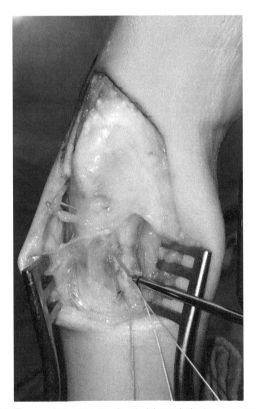

• **Fig. 67.6** The repair sutures are shuttled through the transosseous tunnel and secured to the ulna 1 cm proximal to the transosseous tunnel. The anchors are drilled to avoid each other and with sufficient bridging bone to avoid iatrogenic fracture. Notice the bone anchors are placed along the volar surface to avoid symptomatic sutures.

amount of rotation can be advanced to include up to 60 degrees of pronation. At 6 weeks postoperatively, all splinting is discontinued (except during at-risk activities) and active/passive wrist range of motion is begun with unlimited active and passive forearm rotation. At 10 weeks postoperatively, the patient can begin light strengthening. Return to high-demand activities is restricted until 12 weeks after surgery.

PEARLS AND PITFALLS

Pearls

Fractures in the distal third of the radial shaft should raise suspicion for DRUJ instability.

Exam the contralateral DRUJ under sedation prior to starting the operation.

Use of an arthroscopic traction tower, without traction, is helpful to position and stabilize the forearm, freeing up your assistant.

Drill anchors at different levels or angles to prevent convergence.

Ensure adequate bone bridges between osseous tunnels.

Tension the repair in neutral forearm rotation.

Pitfalls

Failure to examine the DRUJ after radial shaft fixation.

Relying on radiographic findings to diagnose DRUJ stability.

Injury to the dorsal sensory ulnar nerve during the exposure.

Transection of the dorsal radioulnar ligament.

Suboptimal placement of the horizontal mattress sutures into the TFCC, causing asymmetric or inadequate reapproximation of the tissue at the fovea.

References

1. Haugstvedt JR, Berger RA, Nakamura T, Neale P, Berglund L, An KN. Relative contributions of the ulnar attachments of the triangular fibrocartilage complex to the dynamic stability of the distal radioulnar joint. *J Hand Surg Am.* 2006;31(3):445–451. https://doi.org/10.1016/j.jhsa.2005.11.008.
2. Yohe NJ, De Tolla J, Kaye MB, Edelstein DM, Choueka J. Irreducible Galeazzi fracture-dislocations. *Hand (N Y).* 2019;14(2):249–252. https://doi.org/10.1177/1558944717744334.
3. Bruckner JD, Lichtman DM, Alexander AH. Complex dislocations of the distal radioulnar joint. Recognition and management. *Clin Orthop Relat Res.* 1992;275:90–103.
4. Kikuchi Y, Nakamura T. Irreducible Galeazzi fracture-dislocation due to an avulsion fracture of the fovea of the ulna. *J Hand Surg Br.* 1999;24(3):379–381. https://doi.org/10.1054/jhsb.1998.0007.
5. Alexander AH, Lichtman DM. Irreducible distal radioulnar joint occurring in a Galeazzi fracture - case report. *J Hand Surg Am.* 1981;6(3):258–261. https://doi.org/10.1016/s0363-5023(81)80081-0.
6. Cetti NE. An unusual cause of blocked reduction of the Galeazzi injury. *Injury.* 1977;9(1):59–61. https://doi.org/10.1016/0020-1383(77)90053-5.
7. Budgen A, Lim P, Templeton P, Irwin LR. Irreducible Galeazzi injury. *Arch Orthop Trauma Surg.* 1998;118(3):176–178. https://doi.org/10.1007/s004020050343.
8. Biyani A, Bhan S. Dual extensor tendon entrapment in Galeazzi fracture-dislocation: a case report. *J Trauma.* 1989;29(9):1295–1297. https://doi.org/10.1097/00005373-198909000-00022.
9. Itoh Y, Horiuchi Y, Takahashi M, Uchinishi K, Yabe Y. Extensor tendon involvement in Smith's and Galeazzi's fractures. *J Hand Surg Am.* 1987;12(4):535–540. https://doi.org/10.1016/s0363-5023(87)80203-4.
10. Giangarra CE, Chandler RW. Complex volar distal radioulnar joint dislocation occurring in a Galeazzi fracture. *J Orthop Trauma.* 1989;3(1):76–79. https://doi.org/10.1097/00005131-198903010-00015.
11. Jenkins NH, Mintowt-Czyz WJ, Fairclough JA. Irreducible dislocation of the distal radioulnar joint. *Injury.* 1987;18(1):40–43. https://doi.org/10.1016/0020-1383(87)90384-6.
12. Rettig ME, Raskin KB. Galeazzi fracture-dislocation: a new treatment-oriented classification. *J Hand Surg Am.* 2001;26(2):228–235. https://doi.org/10.1053/jhsu.2001.21523.
13. Atesok KI, Jupiter JB, Weiss APC. Galeazzi fracture. *J Am Acad Orthop Surg.* 2011;19(10):623–633. https://doi.org/10.5435/00124635-201110000-00006.
14. Giannoulis FS, Sotereanos DG. Galeazzi fractures and dislocations. *Hand Clin.* 2007;23(2):153–163. https://doi.org/10.1016/j.hcl.2007.03.004.
15. Dunn J, Polmear M, Daniels C, Shin E, Nesti L. Arthroscopically assisted transosseous triangular fibrocartilage complex foveal tear repair in the United States military. *J Hand Surg Glob Online.* 2019;1(2):79–84. https://doi.org/10.1016/j.jhsg.2019.01.006.
16. Chen WJ. Arthroscopically assisted transosseous foveal repair of triangular fibrocartilage complex. *Arthrosc Tech.* 2017;6(1):e57–e64. https://doi.org/10.1016/j.eats.2016.09.004.
17. Frank RM, Slikker W, Al-Shihabi L, Wysocki RW. Arthroscopic-assisted outside-in repair of triangular fibrocartilage complex tears. *Arthrosc Tech.* 2015;4(5):e577–e581. https://doi.org/10.1016/j.eats.2015.06.002.
18. Iwasaki N, Minami A. Arthroscopically assisted reattachment of avulsed triangular fibrocartilage complex to the fovea of the ulnar head. *J Hand Surg Am.* 2009;34(7):1323–1326. https://doi.org/10.1016/j.jhsa.2009.02.026.
19. Andersson JK, Åhlén M, Andernord D. Open versus arthroscopic repair of the triangular fibrocartilage complex: a systematic review. *J Exp Orthop.* 2018;5(1):1–10. https://doi.org/10.1186/s40634-018-0120-1.
20. Park JH, Kim D, Park JW. Arthroscopic one-tunnel transosseous foveal repair for triangular fibrocartilage complex (TFCC) peripheral tear. *Arch Orthop Trauma Surg.* 2018;138(1):131–138. https://doi.org/10.1007/s00402-017-2835-3.
21. Nakamura T, Sato K, Okazaki M, Toyama Y, Ikegami H. Repair of foveal detachment of the triangular fibrocartilage complex: open and arthroscopic transosseous techniques. *Hand Clin.* 2011;27(3):281–290. https://doi.org/10.1016/j.hcl.2011.05.002.
22. Van Duijvenbode DC, Guitton TG, Raaymakers EL, Kloen P, Ring D. Long-term outcome of isolated diaphyseal radius fractures with and without dislocation of the distal radioulnar joint. *J Hand Surg Am.* 2012;37(3):523–527. https://doi.org/10.1016/j.jhsa.2011.11.008.
23. Ring D, Rhim R, Carpenter C, Jupiter JB. Isolated radial shaft fractures are more common than Galeazzi fractures. *J Hand Surg Am.* 2006;31(1):17–21. https://doi.org/10.1016/j.jhsa.2005.09.003.
24. Tsismenakis T, Tornetta P. Galeazzi fractures: is DRUJ instability predicted by current guidelines? *Injury.* 2016;47(7):1472–1477. https://doi.org/10.1016/j.injury.2016.04.003.
25. Eberl R, Singer G, Schalamon J, Petnehazy T, Hoellwarth ME. Galeazzi lesions in children and adolescents: treatment and outcome. *Clin Orthop Relat Res.* 2008;466(7):1705–1709. https://doi.org/10.1007/s11999-008-0268-6.
26. Kleinman WB. Stability of the distal radioulna joint: biomechanics, pathophysiology, physical diagnosis, and restoration of function what we have learned in 25 years. *J Hand Surg Am.* 2007;32(7):1086–1106. https://doi.org/10.1016/j.jhsa.2007.06.014.

68

Radiocarpal Dislocations and Fracture Dislocation

CHELSEA C. BOE AND JERRY I. HUANG

Introduction

Radiocarpal dislocations are rare injuries that occur as a result of a high-energy mechanism. The initial descriptions of this injury were prior to the advent of radiographs, at which time the clinical deformity of a distal radius fracture was presumed to be a dislocation of the joint.[1] The advent of radiography naturally elucidated the bony injuries underlying clinical deformities and allowed better comprehension of the spectrum of distal radial injuries. In fact, true radiocarpal dislocation was not confirmed until the postmortem examinations by Malle in 1838.[1] Subsequent published series have documented these injuries, with a reported incidence of 0.2% of all wrist injuries.[2]

Since the original documentation of these injuries in 1838, we have come to appreciate that radiocarpal dislocations are, in fact, a spectrum of injuries involving the bony and ligamentous structures which allow "internal disarticulation of the wrist joint."[3] This can be associated with intercarpal instability, multiplanar instability of the radiocarpal joint, progressive ulnar translation of the carpus, as well as posttraumatic arthritis.

The most common causes of radiocarpal dislocation include falls from height, motor vehicle collisions, and industrial accidents.[4–7] These are typically polytrauma patients with high-energy mechanisms. In one series, all patients had injury to another organ system, highlighting the importance of looking beyond the distracting extremity injury to focus on the whole patient.[7] Given the energy imparted to create these injuries, associated traumatic neurovascular insults are not uncommon and demand scrutiny in the workup and evaluation of these patients. Arterial occlusion can occur secondary to the deformity of the dislocation and is often remedied with reduction by longitudinal traction.[4,8] Neurologic injuries may occur, especially in open fracture-dislocations, with the median nerve more often affected than the ulnar nerve.[6,7]

The radiographs of these injuries are often dramatic, with obvious dislocation at the radiocarpal joint. In contrast, the appearance postreduction can be deceivingly benign, with limited or even no fractures appreciated. Films should be scrutinized for joint diastasis suggestive of intercarpal ligament injury in addition to radial and ulnar styloid fractures. Gilula's lines may be disrupted in severe carpal instability or fracture to the carpal bones. Evaluation of these lines is an imperative tool in any examination of traumatic wrist films. The films should also be interrogated for dorsal or volar rim fractures. The inclusion of a 10-degree lateral radiograph allows the best appreciation of the volar aspect of the lunate facet to visualize subtle fractures that can be hidden in a standard lateral film. With regard to advanced imaging, computed tomography (CT) is the most sensitive for evaluation of bony injuries. Likewise, magnetic resonance imaging (MRI) is the most sensitive modality for ligamentous injuries, though this is rarely required in the acute setting. These injuries are almost uniformly treated with open reduction, at which point the ligamentous structures are directly identified, obviating the need for advanced imaging. Careful evaluation of plain radiographs with an understanding of the underlying bony and ligamentous anatomy is typically sufficient to identify these injuries and guide appropriate treatment strategies.

Relevant Anatomy

The bony anatomy of the radiocarpal joint is composed of the biconcave articular surface of the radius composed of the lunate and scaphoid facets, as well as the bony buttress of the radial styloid. The extrinsic radiocarpal ligaments, joint capsule, and bony congruity confer stability to the radiocarpal joint.[9]

The volar ligaments take their origin from the volar ridge of the radius. The short radiolunate ligament originates from the most ulnar aspect of the lunate facet and inserts on the volar surface of the lunate. This ligament represents the primary restraint to volar translation of the carpus.[10] The long radiolunate (LRL), radioscaphocapitate (RSC), and radioscapholunate (RSL) ligaments originate more radially along the volar ridge. The RSC is a robust ligamentous structure that is the primary restraint to ulnar translation of the carpus.[11] The radial collateral ligament is an extracapsular ligament that originates from the palmar tip of the radial styloid spanning to the base of the thumb metacarpal and can be confluent with the RSC.[11,12]

The dorsal radiocarpal (DRC) ligaments originate from the most dorsal and distal edge of the radius.[11,13] The DRC ligament originates 15 mm from the tip of the radial styloid, between the scaphoid and lunate facet.[12] Along with the dorsal intercarpal (DIC) ligament, the DRC acts as a dorsal stabilizer for the radioscaphoid joint.

Pathoanatomy

Radiocarpal dislocation is distinct from volar– or dorsal– rim-type fractures of the distal radius in that it contains some element of ligamentous disruption which lends the wrist to the previously

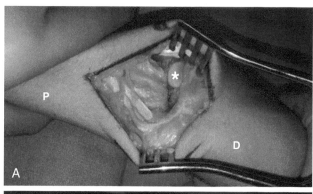

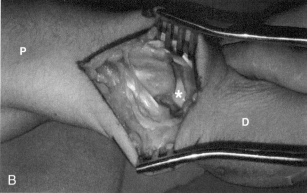

• **Fig. 68.1** Simulated volar dislocation viewed from (A) dorsal/radial approach and (B) volar approach. *D*, Distal; *P*, proximal; (*) scaphoid.

mentioned complications. The mechanism of radiocarpal dislocation is believed to have components of shear and rotation, distinct from the compression force which creates bony rim-type fractures.[3] Bohler et al. in 1930 suggested that the requisite mechanism to create a radiocarpal dislocation mandated a component of compression and rotation applied to a hyperextended and pronated wrist (Fig. 68.1A–B).[3] This rotational component was later designated as an "intercarpal supination" force, which in conjunction with ulnar deviation and wrist extension tensions the volar radiocarpal ligaments and produces the characteristic radial styloid and/or volar radial lip fractures as the carpus is peeled from the pedestal of the radioulnar articulation at the level of the radiocarpal joint.[11,12]

The most common avulsions seen in radiocarpal dislocations include the radial styloid via the RSC ligament,[11,12] the volar rim at the lunate facet via the short radiolunate ligament,[10,14] and ulnar styloid fractures with triangular fibrocartilage complex (TFCC) avulsions. Dorsal dislocations are more commonly reported than volar dislocations[5–7,15] and almost universally include a radial styloid fracture given the triangulation of dorsal, radial, and volar stout ligamentous attachments.[12]

Classification

Radiocarpal dislocations are often described by the direction of dislocation, volar or dorsal. They are often associated with varying degrees of distal radius fractures. While the isolated ligamentous dislocation is described and published in the literature, the vast majority of dislocations include some degree of fracture, ranging from small avulsion fractures to large articular fractures with associated dislocation. Complex intra-articular fracture-dislocations are considered separately on the spectrum of distal radius

fractures and will not be included in the discussion of radiocarpal dislocations.

There are two main classification systems in use to describe radiocarpal dislocations, and an understanding of these systems is imperative to the study and discussion of these injuries. The first was described in 1983 by Moneim et al. and based upon observations of seven patients with radiocarpal dislocation injuries. This classification delineates two groups of radiocarpal dislocation injuries on the basis of intercarpal ligamentous involvement.[8] The first group represents those with no demonstrable intercarpal injury. These are generally more stable post reduction. The second group represents patients with intercarpal injury in addition to radiocarpal dislocation. These patterns tend to have a greater degree of instability, which is less likely to be restored by means of closed reduction and may be at greater risk of long-term instability and the corresponding sequelae. This group and specific injury has been previously described as a perilunate variant injury due to the similarities in the manner by which the force is transmitted around the carpus.[12]

The second classification system commonly used to describe these injuries was presented by Dumontier in 2001 based on his review of 27 patients over 25 years.[5] He defined two groups, based on the involvement of the radial styloid, along with the origin of the injured radiocarpal ligaments. In Group I injuries, the styloid is not fractured, or the avulsion fracture comprises less than one-third of the scaphoid facet of the radius (Fig. 68.2A–B). Group II includes patients in whom the fracture of the radial styloid extends beyond one-third of the scaphoid facet of the radius (Fig. 68.3A–B). The purely ligamentous dislocations or those with small avulsion-type fractures encompassed in the Group I distinction are prone to multidirectional instability, whereas the Group II injuries retain the ligamentous attachments on the radial styloid which can be stabilized with bony fixation. With anatomic fracture reduction and fixation, more radiocarpal anatomy and kinematics are restored.[16,17] Wang et al. proposed addition of a Group III to this classification signified by associated radioulnar injury, but this has not been widely adopted.[18]

Treatment Options/Indications for Surgical Treatment

While reports of successful conservative management with closed reduction and immobilization alone exist in the literature,[4,8,19] the general consensus is that these are unstable injuries that mandate urgent surgical stabilization.[1,4,6,13,19,20] The reported cases of conservative management treated by closed reduction and immobilization for various periods of time ranging from 2 to 9 weeks were associated with ongoing instability.[4,5,13]

General treatment principles in approaching radiocarpal dislocations include recognition of all injured structures based on radiographic evaluation, achieving reduction of the radiocarpal joint, followed by stabilization of fractures and repair of involved radiocarpal ligaments. Associated intercarpal and distal radioulnar joint injuries also need to be addressed. Appropriate comprehensive management includes addressing associated injuries including neurovascular injury and compressive neuropathy as well as soft tissue coverage as needed for open injuries with soft tissue loss.

Method of fixation of the bony injuries is variable and based on the mechanism of injury, size of articular fragment, degree of comminution, as well as proximity to the articular surface. Fixation options include K-wires, compression screws, fragment-specific

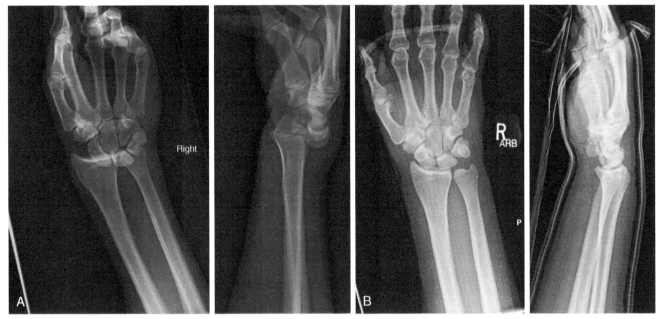

• **Fig. 68.2** Dumontier Type I radiocarpal dislocation without a fracture (A) pre- and (B) postreduction.

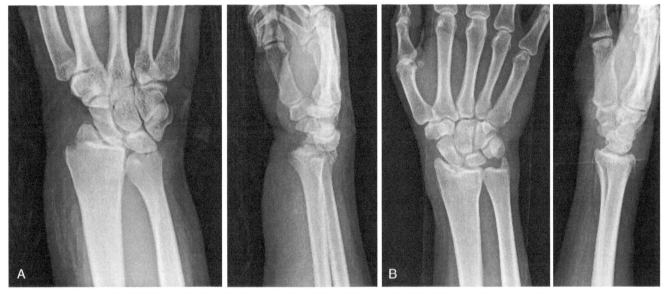

• **Fig. 68.3** Dumontier Type II radiocarpal dislocation with large radial styloid fragment (A) pre- and (B) post closed reduction.

plates such as hook plates, pin plates, radial column plates, as well as suture anchors for relatively small and very distal bony avulsions.[21] Traditionally, Type 1 radiocarpal fracture-dislocations were stabilized with an external fixation in addition to ligament repair.[6] A dorsal spanning plate can also be utilized to hold appropriate ligamentotaxis and offload small avulsion fragments.[22] This has largely supplanted external fixation as internal-external fixators as they serve the similar function of holding ligaments at appropriate tension during healing, without the concerns of pin care and pin tract infections. External fixation may continue to play a role in the setting of severe soft tissue disturbance.[6] Temporary pinning across the radiocarpal joint can also be performed to protect the joint after direct suture repair or suture anchor repair of the injured radiocarpal ligaments (Fig. 68.4).

Repair of ligamentous structures is arguably the most critical component of treatment.[16,23] The ligamentous structures are either repaired directly with sutures or with the use of suture anchors. A variety of 2-0 and 3-0 suture anchor devices are available on the market and the surgeon's comfort and preference often appropriately dictates the specific implant selected.

Arthroscopy

Arthroscopy is helpful in some of these cases, especially those with small articular fragments that are difficult to visualize radiographically. Moreover, in cases where the dorsal or palmar radiocarpal ligaments have been avulsed with small rim fractures, the visualization of the articular surface is blocked following reduction of

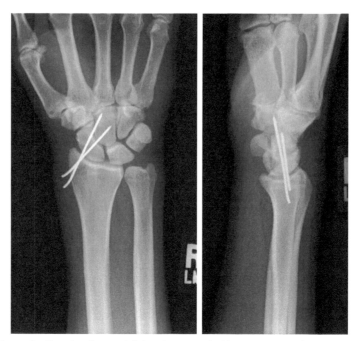

• **Fig. 68.4** Dumontier Type I radiocarpal dislocation treated with temporary radioscaphocapitate pinning as well as repair of the radiocarpal ligaments using suture anchors.

the bony fragment. Arthroscopy can be utilized to allow a direct view of the articular surface to augment surgical reduction. In a fracture setting, this is often performed as dry arthroscopy, a technique well described and published by del Pinal.[24] Arthroscopy additionally allows for visualization and treatment of other carpal injuries which are not infrequently encountered given the high-energy mechanism of these injuries (Fig. 68.5).

Relevant Complications and Review of Treatment Outcomes

Given the rare nature of these injuries, the literature specific to radiocarpal dislocations is somewhat sparse. It mainly comprises case reports and small case series with only a few series containing more than a handful of patients.[5,6,8,25,26] Generally, poor outcomes are predicted by open injury, more severe radiocarpal ligamentous injury, volar dislocation, intercarpal ligament injury, and associated nerve injury.[6,8,16,17,27,28] A recent study also noted that 80% of radiocarpal fracture-dislocations have marginal fractures of the radius and, especially when comminuted, these portend a poor prognosis presumably due to the difficulty in obtaining an anatomic reduction of the articular surface.[26] In a series of 41 patients with 4 Type I and 37 Type II injuries treated with anatomic reduction and stabilization of the radiocarpal joint, Spiry et al. reported good functional outcomes with absence of posttraumatic arthritis.[26] However, others report an "inevitable" degree of impairment or alteration of short- and long-term function of the wrist despite surgical stabilization and fracture healing (Fig. 68.6).[19]

Nerve injuries associated with radiocarpal fracture-dislocations have a somewhat guarded prognosis for recovery. Thankfully, the majority seem to be neurapraxic in nature and recover with reduction, decompression, and time.[6,27] However, in their series of open injuries, Nyquist and Stern noted that all patients who had symptoms of nerve injury at initial presentation had persistent dysfunction at 15-month follow-up (Fig. 68.7).[7]

Permanent loss of motion and strength is frequently reported, as with most major insults to the wrist joint. In one series of eight patients, average motion on clinical examination was 55-degree extension, 35-degree flexion, 88-degree pronation, and 70-degree supination at 4.1-year follow-up.[25] The most recently published study of long-term outcomes in 13 patients suggests similar motion with an average of 55-degree extension, 47-degree flexion, 76-degree pronation, and 70-degree supination.[26] Other large series suggest that 30%–40% loss of motion in the flexion-extension plane is to be anticipated following treatment.[5,7] The loss of strength is reported between 15% and 50% of the contralateral side.[6,7,26,29]

Persistent instability of the radiocarpal joint, most notably progressive ulnar translation of the carpus, can occur following radiocarpal dislocations given the substantial ligament damage necessary to allow the carpus to dislocate (Fig. 68.8). The carpus tends to translate down the radial slope of the radiocarpal articulation in the absence of the strong fibrous volar radiocarpal ligaments that generally prevent such migration. Cadaveric studies have demonstrated that the RSC ligament is the most significant restrictor of this translation. However, RSC sectioning in isolation is not sufficient to allow ulnar translocation. A near global ligamentous disruption is required in order to allow for the carpus to slide towards the ulna.[13,30] Volar translation often accompanies ulnar translation, again suggestive of the significant loss of restraint from the radiocarpal joint stabilizers. This complication tends to be more commonly seen in patients treated by closed means and patients with more significant ligamentous involvement from high-energy injuries.[5,13,16]

Posttraumatic arthritis is a somewhat anticipated long-term complication given the nature of these injuries, though it is by no means universal. In a series of five patients, Schoenecker et al. reported degenerative changes or articular step-off in 60% of their patients; however, Dumontier et al. reported degenerative changes in only 3 of 18 patients in their series followed up for >40 months.[5,19] Other published series report rates of posttraumatic

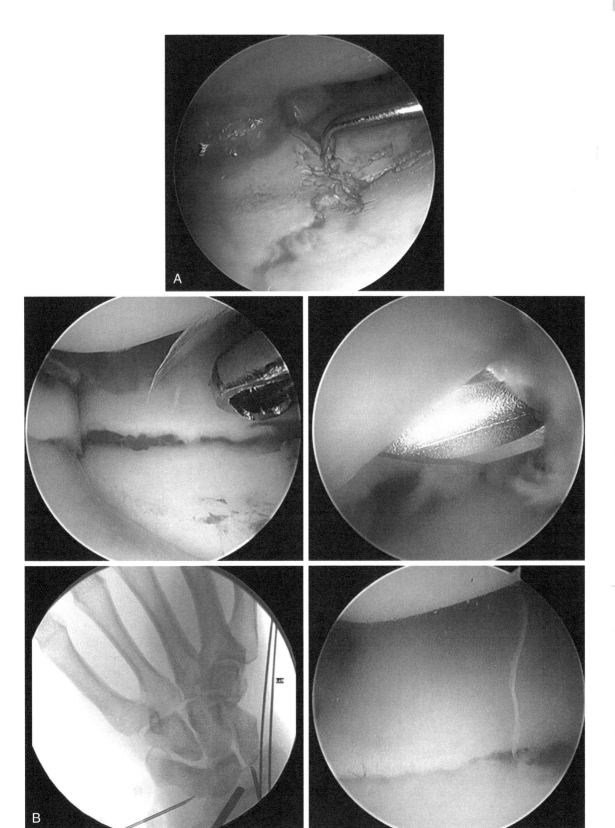

• **Fig. 68.5** Arthroscopic reduction of displaced radial styloid fragment (A). Arthroscopic visualization of scaphoid fracture, with guide pin placement under direct view, complemented by radiographic triangulation and restoration of normal scaphoid contour after fixation (B). (Images courtesy Dr. Sanjeev Kakar, Mayo Clinic, Rochester, MN.)

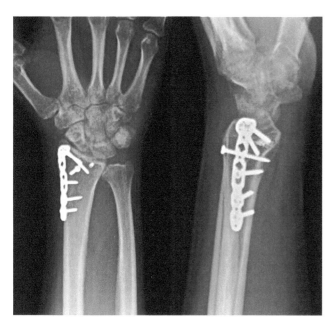

• **Fig. 68.6** Three months following fixation of Dumontier Type II radiocarpal fracture-dislocation, the patient had a 100-degree arc of motion in the flexion/extension plane, full pronation, and 10-degree loss of supination relative to the contralateral side. He was noted to have a chronic extensor pollicis longus rupture which he elected to observe given his overall satisfactory function. He was able to return to unrestricted work as a plumber.

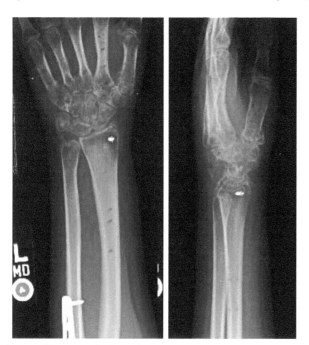

• **Fig. 68.7** Three months following dorsal spanning plate fixation of his Dumontier Type I radiocarpal dislocation and volar ligament repair, the plate was removed. At final follow-up, 6 weeks after hardware removal, the patient had a 90-degree arc of motion in the flexion/extension plane, normal pronation, and 30-degree loss of supination relative to the contralateral side. He also had persistent paresthesias in the superficial radial nerve distribution.

arthritis within this wide range, suggesting that there are other contributing factors to the development of posttraumatic arthritis that are not fully understood or illuminated by these small series.[6,7,25] Recently, it has been presented that anatomic reduction

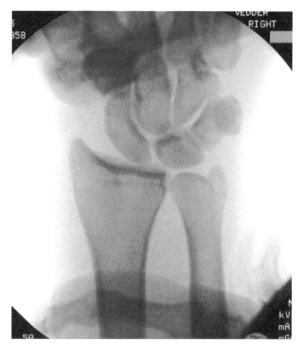

• **Fig. 68.8** Ulnar translation and instability after apparent congruent reduction of Dumontier Type I radiocarpal dislocation demonstrating the extensive ligamentous damage and residual instability in these injuries.

of radial styloid fractures, particularly significant in Dumontier Type II fractures, may be protective against the development of radiocarpal arthritis, though the same is not true of intercarpal lesions.[26]

Patient-reported outcomes including long-term pain and loss of function are variable in these injuries, as would be expected for this spectrum of severe pathology. A series published in 2006 specifically looking at dorsal fracture subluxations and dislocations presented an average Mayo wrist score of 75, which represents a fair result.[29] Another study published in 2018 reported an average quick DASH (The Disabilities of the Arm, Shoulder and Hand) of 23.17 and PRWE (The Patient-Rated Wrist Evaluation) of 27.23 in 13 patients followed up for an average of 14 years.[26] It would seem that reasonable functional outcomes are attainable, and perhaps these patient-reported findings are evidence that the radiographic and clinical results do not always correlate with patient perceptions of function.

Conclusion

Radiocarpal dislocations and fracture-dislocations are rare and devastating injuries to the radiocarpal joint. They occur as a result of high-energy trauma and are often associated with other injuries, both local and systemic. They represent a spectrum of injuries, often with both bony and ligamentous components. Early reduction and aggressive surgical management with the goals of anatomic bony reduction and repair of ligamentous structures is the mainstay of treatment and associated with the best potential for long-term function. However, given the severity of injury to the wrist, even the best outcomes involve stiffness and weakness as well as the propensity for posttraumatic arthritis, a risk of persistent instability, and ulnar translation of the carpus.

References

1. Fernandez DL, Jupiter JB. *Fractures of the Distal Radius: A Practical Approach to Management.* New York: Springer; 1996.
2. Dunn AW. Fractures and dislocations of the carpus. *Surg Clin North Am.* 1972;52(6):1513–1538.
3. Ilyas AM, Mudgal CS. Radiocarpal fracture-dislocations. *J Am Acad Orthop Surg.* 2008;16(11):647–655.
4. Bilos ZJ, Pankovich AM, Yelda S. Fracture-dislocation of the radiocarpal joint. *J Bone Joint Surg Am.* 1977;59(2):198–203.
5. Dumontier C, Meyer zu Reckendorf G, Sautet A, Lenoble E, Saffar P, Allieu Y. Radiocarpal dislocations: classification and proposal for treatment. A review of twenty-seven cases. *J Bone Joint Surg Am.* 2001;83(2):212–218.
6. Mudgal CS, Psenica J, Jupiter JB. Radiocarpal fracture-dislocation. *J Hand Surg Br.* 1999;24(1):92–98.
7. Nyquist SR, Stern PJ. Open radiocarpal fracture-dislocations. *J Hand Surg Am.* 1984;9(5):707–710.
8. Moneim MS, Bolger JT, Omer GE. Radiocarpal dislocation—classification and rationale for management. *Clin Orthop Relat Res.* 1985;(192):199–209.
9. Ritt MJ, Stuart PR, Berglund LJ, Linscheid RL, Cooney 3rd WP, An KN. Rotational stability of the carpus relative to the forearm. *J Hand Surg Am.* 1995;20(2):305–311.
10. Berger RA, Landsmeer JM. The palmar radiocarpal ligaments: a study of adult and fetal human wrist joints. *J Hand Surg Am.* 1990;15(6):847–854.
11. Siegel DB, Gelberman RH. Radial styloidectomy: an anatomical study with special reference to radiocarpal intracapsular ligamentous morphology. *J Hand Surg Am.* 1991;16(1):40–44.
12. Mayfield JK, Johnson RP, Kilcoyne RK. Carpal dislocations: pathomechanics and progressive perilunar instability. *J Hand Surg Am.* 1980;5(3):226–241.
13. Rayhack JM, Linscheid RL, Dobyns JH, Smith JH. Posttraumatic ulnar translation of the carpus. *J Hand Surg Am.* 1987;12(2):180–189.
14. Medoff RJ. Essential radiographic evaluation for distal radius fractures. *Hand Clin.* 2005;21(3):279–288.
15. Obert L, Loisel F, Jardin E, Gasse N, Lepage D. High-energy injuries of the wrist. *Orthop Traumatol Surg Res.* 2016;102(1 Suppl):S81–S93.
16. Penny 3rd WH, Green TL. Volar radiocarpal dislocation with ulnar translocation. *J Orthop Trauma.* 1988;2(4):322–326.
17. Thomsen S, Falstie-Jensen S. Palmar dislocation of the radiocarpal joint. *J Hand Surg Am.* 1989;14(4):627–630.
18. Wang GX, Zhu XJ, Wang ZG, Zhou HD. [Operative treatment for adult patients with simultaneous fracture and dislocation of ipsilateral elbow and radiocarpal joint: 3 cases report]. *Zhong Guo Gu Shang.* 2012;25(4):345–347.
19. Schoenecker PL, Gilula LA, Shively RA, Manske PR. Radiocarpal fracture—dislocation. *Clin Orthop Relat Res.* 1985;197:237–244.
20. Tanzer TL, Horne JG. Dorsal radiocarpal fracture dislocation. *J Trauma.* 1980;20(11):999–1000.
21. Biondi M, Keller M, Merenghi L, Gabl M, Lauri G. Hook plate for volar rim fractures of the distal radius: review of the first 23 cases and focus on dorsal radiocarpal dislocation. *J Wrist Surg.* 2019;8(2):93–99.
22. Wahl EP, Lauder AS, Pidgeon TS, Guerrero EM, Ruch DS, Richard MJ. Dorsal wrist spanning plate fixation for treatment of radiocarpal fracture-dislocations. *Hand (N Y).* 2019. 1558944719893068.
23. Weber O, Muller M, Fischer P, et al. [Diagnosis and treatment of radiocarpal fracture dislocations]. *Unfallchirurg.* 2011;114(7):565–574.
24. del Pinal F, Garcia-Bernal FJ, Pisani D, Regalado J, Ayala H, Studer A. Dry arthroscopy of the wrist: surgical technique. *J Hand Surg Am.* 2007;32(1):119–123.
25. Oberladstatter J, Arora R, Dallapozza C, Smekal V, Rieger M, Lutz M. [Sagittal wrist motion following dorsal radiocarpal fracture dislocations]. *Handchir Mikrochir Plast Chir.* 2007;39(1):49–53.
26. Spiry C, Bacle G, Marteau E, Charruau B, Laulan J. Radiocarpal dislocations and fracture-dislocations: injury types and long-term outcomes. *Orthop Traumatol Surg Res.* 2018;104(2):261–266.
27. Girard J, Cassagnaud X, Maynou C, Bachour F, Prodhomme G, Mestdagh H. [Radiocarpal dislocation: twelve cases and a review of the literature]. *Rev Chir Orthop Reparatrice Appar Mot.* 2004;90(5):426–433.
28. Jardin E, Pechin C, Rey PB, Gasse N, Obert L. Open volar radiocarpal dislocation with extensive dorsal ligament and extensor tendon damage: a case report and review of literature. *Hand Surg Rehabil.* 2016;35(2):127–134.
29. Lozano-Calderon SA, Doornberg J, Ring D. Fractures of the dorsal articular margin of the distal part of the radius with dorsal radiocarpal subluxation. *J Bone Joint Surg Am.* 2006;88(7):1486–1493.
30. Viegas SF, Patterson RM, Ward K. Extrinsic wrist ligaments in the pathomechanics of ulnar translation instability. *J Hand Surg Am.* 1995;20(2):312–318.

69

Technique Spotlight: Dumontier Type 1 vs. Type 2; When and How to Fix the Radial Styloid Fragment; Neutralization Device Options

CHELSEA C. BOE AND JERRY I. HUANG

The surgical approaches for treating radiocarpal dislocations and fracture-dislocations are variable, dependent on the specific injury pattern. It is not unusual for these injuries to require multiple surgical approaches to address all the fracture fragments and achieve ligamentous stability. In a series of patients with dorsal articular rim fractures with radiocarpal fracture-dislocation, 7 of 19 patients required both a dorsal and volar incision to address distal articular fractures dorsally and volarly.[1] Some surgeons feel that the volar approach may not be necessary if the injury can be anatomically reduced and the radiocarpal joint stabilized, with primary healing of the ligament.[2]

Volar Approach

For a volar approach, we favor an extended carpal tunnel approach. This approach provides for excellent visualization of the volar radiocarpal ligaments for direct suture or suture anchor–augmented repair. The extended carpal approach also allows for direct reduction of palmar lip fractures of the radius and application of appropriate fixation. In these injuries, there is often rupture of the ligaments or traumatic avulsion through bony fragments with a traumatic arthrotomy of the joint capsule; thus the dissection is often completed upon exposing the volar wrist. With this incision, carpal tunnel release can be performed which is particularly advantageous in the event of acute median nerve compression or to mitigate the risk of developing acute carpal tunnel in patients with severe swelling.

An incision is planned just ulnar to the thenar crease, in line with radial aspect of the fourth digit with an ulnar-directed Bruner zigzag incision proximally across the wrist crease (Fig. 69.1). A standard carpal tunnel release is performed distally with the release

of the antebrachial fascia proximally. With retraction of the entire contents of the carpal tunnel, there is extensive visualization of the volar wrist capsule and ligamentous structures (Fig. 69.2). From this vantage, the volar radiocarpal ligaments can be assessed and repaired (Fig. 69.3).

A sample case demonstrates the small, comminuted bony fragments more appropriately described as ligamentous avulsions that require open approach for repair (Fig. 69.4). In this case, a 24-year-old male was involved in a high-energy motor vehicle collision resulting in a Dumontier Type I radiocarpal fracture-dislocation in addition to other carpal and metacarpal injuries. His radiocarpal injury was treated with open repair through a volar extended carpal tunnel approach with the addition of a dorsal spanning plate to offload and protect the radiocarpal joint to allow for ligament healing (Fig. 69.5).

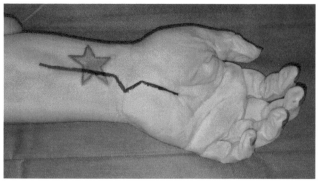

• **Fig. 69.1** Skin marking for extended carpal tunnel incision.

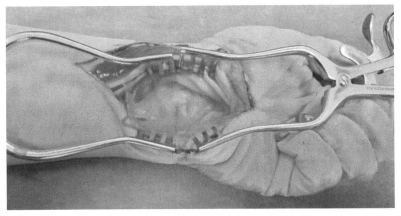

• **Fig. 69.2** After carpal tunnel release and release of the antebrachial fascia, the entire contents of the carpal tunnel are retracted radially, providing excellent visualization of the volar wrist capsule and radiocarpal ligaments.

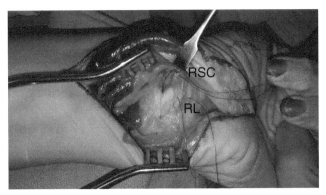

• **Fig. 69.3** Suture tags in the radiolunate *(RL)* and radioscaphocapitate *(RSC)* ligaments demonstrating the ease of visualization and repair from extended carpal tunnel approach.

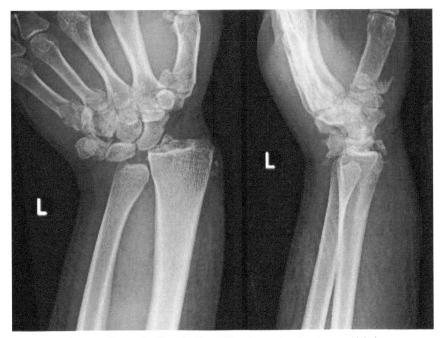

• **Fig. 69.4** Dumontier Type I with additional carpal and metacarpal injuries.

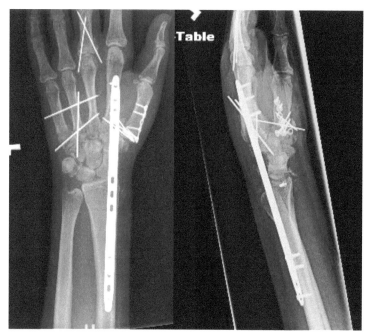

• **Fig. 69.5** Dumontier Type I with dorsal approach for dorsal spanning plate and volar approach to repair the important volar radiocarpal ligaments.

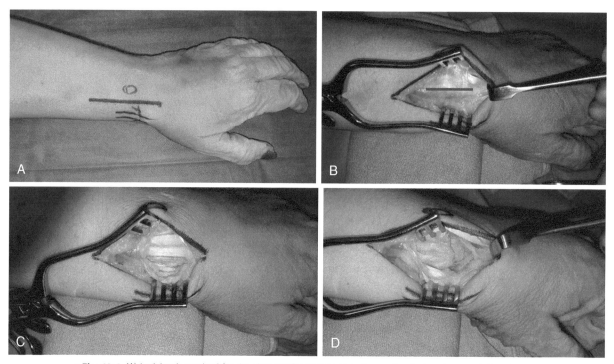

• **Fig. 69.6** (A) Incision is marked for the dorsoradial approach between the first and second dorsal compartments, over the anatomic snuffbox. (B) Following skin incision, the extensor pollicis longus tendon is visualized as well as the sheath overlying the first dorsal extensor compartment. (C) The interval between those structures is split revealing the underlying second dorsal extensor compartment tendons. (D)The radial styloid can be well visualized for reduction and fixation and/or repair of dorsal radiocarpal ligaments.

Dorsal Approach

Dorsally, a standard approach between the third and fourth dorsal compartments can be performed. Like the volar side, there is often traumatic dissection which allows for rapid visualization of ruptured and avulsed ligamentous structures. The standard dorsal approach allows for easy access for reduction and fixation of dorsal lip fractures, as well as extension distally for treatment of intercarpal injuries. Given

the traumatic injury to the ligaments, a ligament-sparing approach is not generally needed or feasible, but can be utilized, if necessary, to expose the carpus for interosseous ligament repair.

For a direct exposure of an isolated large radial styloid fragment, an incision is made over the dorsoradial wrist between the first and second dorsal extensor compartment tendons (Fig. 69.6A). The extensor pollicis longus (EPL) and second dorsal compartment tendons are reflected and retracted dorsal and the

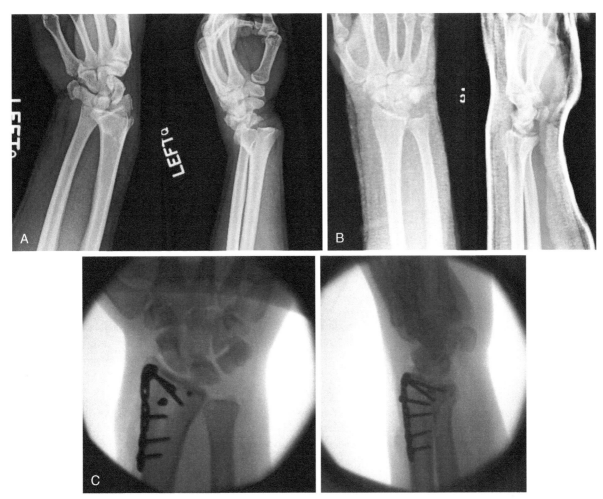

• **Fig. 69.7** (A) Dumontier Type II radiocarpal fracture-dislocation with a large radial styloid fragment. (B) Closed reduction was performed with excellent restoration of gross alignment though with persistent articular step-off between the scaphoid and lunate facets. (C) The large radial styloid fracture fragment was reduced and fixated with a locking plate through a dorsoradial approach with an additional dorsal approach more ulnarly for suture anchor–augmented ligamentous repair.

first dorsal extensor compartment volarly. Incision directly down to bone and subperiosteal reflection of the extensor compartments from bone allows direct visualization of the dorsoradial articular fragment (Fig. 69.6D). In traumatic situations, the capsular ligamentous structures may be torn from the osseous insertions allowing for evaluation of the articular surface.

Case Example

A 41-year-old man fell from a height of 30 ft with numerous injuries, including this Dumontier Type II radiocarpal fracture-dislocation (Fig. 69.7A). After provisional reduction, general alignment was restored though with residual articular step-off and presumed extensive ligamentous injury (Fig. 69.7B). This injury

was approached through a combined dorsal radial approach for radial styloid fracture reduction and fixation and a separate dorsal approach for ligamentous repair, augmented with suture anchor given the limited residual tissue at the radial attachment of the dorsal radiocarpal ligament (Fig. 69.7C).

References

1. Lozano-Calderon SA, Doornberg J, Ring D. Fractures of the dorsal articular margin of the distal part of the radius with dorsal radiocarpal subluxation. *J Bone Joint Surg Am*. 2006;88(7):1486–1493.
2. Spiry C, Bacle G, Marteau E, Charruau B, Laulan J. Radiocarpal dislocations and fracture-dislocations: injury types and long-term outcomes. *Orthop Traumatol Surg Res*. 2018;104(2):261–266.

70

Scaphoid Fractures

MICHAEL N. NAKASHIAN AND THOMAS B. HUGHES

Relevant Anatomy

The scaphoid bone functions as a link between the proximal and the distal carpal rows through ligamentous attachments and articular mechanics. It has a fairly complex and certainly unique anatomy. It is often described as having a peanut shell shape. The scaphoid articulates with the distal radius proximally and the lunate ulnarly. It also articulates with the trapezium, trapezoid, and capitate of the distal carpal row. While it is one of the four bones of the proximal carpal row, it acts as the linkage between the proximal and distal row and is therefore integral to wrist biomechanics in creating motion and stability of the wrist. When this linkage is damaged, as with fracture or scapholunate ligament disruption, carpal instability ensues. One of the fairly unique features of the scaphoid is the relatively large surface area covered by articular cartilage reported to be approximately 80%.[1] This leads to multiple articulating forces being applied to the bone as well as the fact that joint fluid almost always interacts with the fracture, possibly washing away hematoma critical to fracture healing.

Traditionally, scaphoid fractures are divided into three distinct categories based on anatomic fracture location: proximal pole, waist, and distal pole. One of the greatest challenges in treating scaphoid fractures lies in its tenuous and somewhat variable blood supply, leading to a relatively significant risk of nonunion.[2] The classic study performed by Gelberman in 1980 outlined the vascular supply to the scaphoid to stem from the radial artery, wherein 70%–80% of intraosseous vascularity, including the entire proximal pole, comes from branches entering through the dorsal ridge (Fig. 70.1).[3]

Pathoanatomy

The scaphoid is the most commonly fractured carpal bone, accounting for 60%–70% of all carpal fractures.[4] Acute scaphoid fractures are most commonly the result of a fall on an outstretched hand in slight pronation. In one cadaveric study, scaphoid fractures were reproduced by loading the wrist in extension.[5] The severity of pain and disability is variable after these injuries, and so any patient presenting with pain on the radial side of the wrist should be ruled out for scaphoid fracture as part of the initial workup. However, a large number of scaphoid fractures go unrecognized, or are initially diagnosed as a sprain. Any patient with radial-sided wrist pain, even with normal imaging, should be immobilized

until evaluation by an orthopedic surgeon can be arranged and repeat imaging can be obtained. Failure to follow this protocol continues to lead to missed fractures and scaphoid nonunions.

Classification

There are two popular classification systems for scaphoid fractures. These are the Herbert and Russe classifications. They vary in that the Herbert classification is based upon fracture stability, whereas the Russe classification is based upon fracture pattern.[6,7] In the Herbert classification (Fig. 70.2), type A fractures are considered stable whereas type B fractures are considered unstable.[8] Type C and D fractures are related to healing, with type C fractures indicating delayed union and type D fractures being established nonunions.[8]

In the Russe classification (Fig. 70.3), the plane of the fracture pattern is considered. There are three separate patterns, characterized by abbreviations of their pattern, with "HO" representing horizontal oblique fractures, "T" representing transverse fractures, and "VO" representing vertical oblique fractures.

In 2012, the concept of classification by displacement versus instability was evaluated with arthroscopic assessment. While

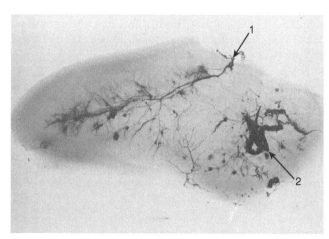

• **Fig. 70.1** Photograph of a specimen showing the internal vascularity of the scaphoid with dorsal scaphoid radial branch of the artery (1) and volar scaphoid branch (2). (From Gelberman RH, Menon J. The vascularity of the scaphoid bone. *J Hand Surg Am.* 1980;5:508-513.)

TYPE A:

STABLE ACUTE FRACTURES

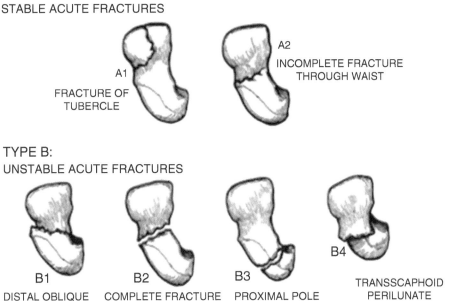

A1
FRACTURE OF
TUBERCLE

A2
INCOMPLETE FRACTURE
THROUGH WAIST

TYPE B:

UNSTABLE ACUTE FRACTURES

B1
DISTAL OBLIQUE
FRACTURE

B2
COMPLETE FRACTURE
OF WAIST

B3
PROXIMAL POLE
FRACTURE

B4
TRANSSCAPHOID
PERILUNATE
FRACTURE DISLOCATION
OF CARPUS

• **Fig. 70.2** The Herbert classification. (From Herbert TJ, Fisher WE. Management of the fractured scaphoid using a new bone screw. *J Bone Joint Surg Br.* 1984;66:114-123.)

TYPES OF FRACTURE AND RECOMMENDED TIME OF IMMOBILIZATION		
TYPES IN RELATION TO LONG AXIS OF NAVICULAR		**IMMOBILIZATION**
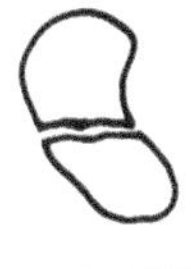	HORIZANTAL OBLIQUE 35%	DISTAL THIRD 6 WEEKS MIDDLE THIRD 6 WEEKS PROXIMAL THIRD 10–12 WEEKS
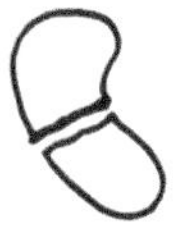	TRANSVERSE 60%	6 WEEKS (+ 4 TO 6 WEEKS)
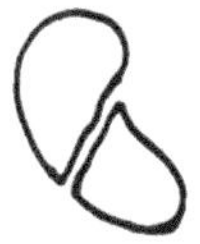	VERTICAL OBLIQUE 5%	10 – 12 WEEKS

• **Fig. 70.3** The Russe classification. (From Russe O. Fracture of the carpal navicular. Diagnosis, nonoperative treatment, and operative treatment. *J Bone Joint Surg Am.* 1960;42-A:759-768.)

not developing a traditional classification scheme, the authors challenged the equality often used for the terms "displaced" and "unstable," evaluating 58 consecutive patients with scaphoid fracture assessed arthroscopically.[9] They found that of 31 nondisplaced fractures, 11 were actually unstable upon arthroscopic evaluation, indicating a relatively high percentage of arthroscopically unstable fracture in contrast to those traditionally considered to be stable based on nondisplaced radiographs.[9]

Most commonly, scaphoid fractures are categorized based on the location of the fracture. These are broken down into distal pole, waist, or proximal pole fractures. Based on anatomical considerations discussed above and blood supply, this type of classification does have prognostic value, as proximal fractures are very prone to nonunion, while distal pole fractures have a much lower rate of nonunion. This suggestion is supported by a prospective multicenter study of 1052 patients, wherein proximal pole fractures were found in only 5% of fractures, but accounted for 23% of nonunions.[10]

Diagnosis

Any discussion of scaphoid fractures requires a careful discussion of diagnostic methodology. While fairly simple to diagnose a scaphoid fracture in some cases, these fractures are often missed

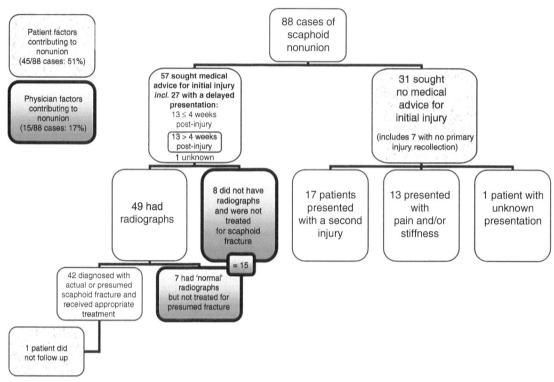

• **Fig. 70.4** Summary of presentation and initial management of 88 scaphoid fractures that became non-unions. (From Wong K, von Schroeder HP. Delays and poor management of scaphoid fractures: factors contributing to nonunion. *J Hand Surg Am.* 2011;36:1471-1474.)

upon initial presentation for a variety of reasons, so a low threshold for suspicion of a scaphoid fracture must be maintained when encountering an appropriate mechanism of injury. Any discussion of treatment decision regarding scaphoid fractures must take into account the risk of nonunion. In a study looking at 88 scaphoid nonunions, the authors found that risk factors for nonunion included delayed presentation for evaluation, as more than half of the nonunions presented late and did not receive standard initial management, with 35% not seeking medical attention at all, and 31% seeking delayed medical attention.[11] In the same study, proximal pole fractures were found to account for 23% of the nonunions encountered (Fig. 70.4).

Physical examination of the patient with a suspected scaphoid fracture based on mechanism of injury and/or location of pain must be performed carefully and can greatly add to obtaining an accurate diagnosis. The classic physical examination tests for scaphoid fractures include palpation at the anatomic snuffbox, palpation at the scaphoid tubercle, and testing for reproduction of pain with longitudinal compression of the thumb. In a study looking at the combination of physical examination maneuvers for diagnosis of scaphoid fracture, all three of the aforementioned maneuvers were 100% sensitive for detection of a scaphoid feature.[12] In the same study, anatomic snuffbox tenderness showed a specificity of 9%, whereas scaphoid tubercle tenderness and pain with longitudinal compression showed a specificity of 30% and 48%, respectively.[12] When patients were seen and examined 24 hours following injury, however, a combination of these three physical examination modalities increased total specificity to 74%, suggesting the combination of tests is more valuable and effective than each individual maneuver alone.[12]

Routine radiographic analysis should always include a posteroanterior (PA) view, oblique view, lateral view, and dedicated scaphoid view with the wrist in ulnar deviation. Placing the wrist in an ulnarly deviated position on the PA view brings the scaphoid into extension and allows the most likely view to identify a scaphoid fracture. Additional imaging modalities are also useful. The most commonly utilized advanced imaging techniques are computed tomography (CT) scan and magnetic resonance imaging (MRI). It should be noted that while CT is most useful for identifying fracture morphology and displacement, it must be performed with appropriate formating specifically for the scaphoid longitudinal axis.

According to a 2008 publication addressing the accuracy of MRI for identification of scaphoid fractures, the sensitivity was 98%, the specificity was 99%, and the accuracy was 96%.[13] While generally considered the best modality for identifying occult scaphoid fractures, the possibility exists for false-positive findings in the setting of acute injury. One of the most beneficial categories of patients for consideration of MRI would be athletes, heavy laborers, or any patient with a high impact activity who requires accurate early diagnosis to preclude return to such vocation or avocation that could potentially displace an occult fracture. In theory, use of MRI in the acute setting to rule out occult fracture could potentially limit the number of missed fractures mistakenly diagnosed as wrist sprain and allowed to return to forceful activity.

CT scan evaluation for diagnosis of scaphoid fracture shows a sensitivity of 94%, specificity of 96%, and accuracy of 98%.[13] In a meta-analysis combined with latent class analysis, CT scan was found to be imprecise due to subtlety of nondisplaced fractures having an absence of definite interpretation of small unicortical lines being a true fracture, so the authors recommended interpretation of CT scan for subtle fractures to be taken with caution.[14] In a comparison of X-ray versus CT sagittal imaging for identification of scaphoid fractures, both X-ray and CT showed a relatively high sensitivity and specificity.[15] However, it was determined that the specificities for X-ray and CT to detect displacement >1 mm are 84% and 89%, respectively, with both sensitivity and specificity increasing when studies were interpreted by fellowship-trained hand surgeons.[15]

Treatment Options

There are two general treatment options for scaphoid fractures: casting and surgical intervention. Within the surgical group are several different techniques which will be reviewed below. Indications for treatment choice depend on various factors including fracture type and location, associated injuries, medical comorbidities, and patient activity level and demands. Nonoperative treatment is indicated in stable, nondisplaced fractures or in patients unable to undergo surgery for other medical or psychosocial reasons. Surgical intervention is required for unstable injuries. Unstable injuries include displaced fractures, comminuted fractures, proximal pole fractures, and fractures associated with perilunate dislocations. As mentioned above, some nondisplaced fractures have also been shown to be unstable, and these may also require surgical stabilization.

Casting

One important consideration is that nonoperative treatment of nondisplaced, stable scaphoid fractures may require a far longer period of immobilization compared with nonoperative treatment of other types of fractures, due to the blood supply pattern and fracture location within the scaphoid. In a study using CT scan to determine union rate of nonoperatively treated scaphoid fractures, time to union for proximal pole fractures was 113 days, compared with 65 days for waist and 53 days for distal pole fractures.[16] The literature reporting the ideal type of immobilization has varied over time with controversy surrounding the length of time immobilized and type of immobilization, being long arm versus short arm casting, and whether to include the thumb in the cast. In a prospective randomized trial based on the degree of healing as observed with CT scan at 10 weeks from injury, patients had a higher percentage of healing with casts that did not include the thumb, suggesting that short arm cast without thumb spica extension is a reliable method of immobilization.[17] In a systematic review and meta-analysis of randomized controlled trials, evaluating cast techniques of above-elbow versus below-elbow, below-elbow including versus excluding the thumb, and below-elbow casting excluding the thumb with wrist in 20 degrees of flexion versus extension, there were no differences found in union rate, pain, grip strength, time to union, or osteonecrosis across all studies.[18] A study examining 51 prospective patients randomized to long arm versus short arm thumb splice casting for nondisplaced scaphoid fractures, time to union for the long arm cast group was 9.5 weeks versus 12.7 weeks for the short arm group.[19] A subsequent study evaluating 292 fractures randomized to short arm casts with or without thumb inclusion found the incidence of nonunion was independent of the type of cast.[20] In a more rigorous multicenter randomized controlled trial, 62 patients with MRI- or CT-confirmed nondisplaced fractures were treated with short arm casts including or excluding the thumb, finding a significant increase in healing at 10 weeks judged on CT scan for

the group excluding the thumb, with 85% healing compared with 70% healing for the group including the thumb.[17] Therefore it is unclear exactly which form of immobilization is superior and practitioners must use their best judgment in selecting the type of cast. The authors tend to favor below-elbow thumb spica casts for the majority of their nondisplaced fractures. In pediatric patients, the elbow is frequently included in the cast, as much to limit heavy activities as to increase fracture stability. In some office workers, the exclusion of the thumb may be appropriate to allow continued work without adding undue stress to the fracture.

Indications for Surgical Treatment

The role of surgical treatment of nondisplaced fractures is considered controversial. Multiple short-term factors, however, must be taken into account when determining the optimal choice for the patient in this setting. In an analysis of six randomized controlled trials comparing cast to operative fixation for nondisplaced fractures, the authors found that union rates were high in both treatment groups, with improved grip strength and range of motion at 8 and 16 weeks in the operative group, but advantages of surgical fixation are transient, suggesting that operative fixation would lead to a faster return to work and less time spent in a cast, with unchanged time to healing and similar union rates.[21] In order to test a suggested trend in treating nondisplaced scaphoid fractures with surgical fixation instead of casting, a review of randomized controlled trials including 419 patients found that surgical treatment was favored in improved functional outcome and less time off work; however, this led to a higher complication rate (23.7%) compared to conservative casting (9.1%).[22]

There are, therefore, situations in which even nondisplaced and stable fractures could be indicated for operative treatment, and this typically depends upon the particular patient's job or extracurricular activities, as surgical treatment of nondisplaced fractures has been shown to decrease the length of time of treatment and immobilization and may return patients to weight-bearing and sports much more quickly than nonoperative care, while maintaining equal or even better long-term outcomes.[23] There is a growing body of literature evaluating the operative treatment of stable fractures with the hope of reducing periods of disability and improving union rates. It has also been noted that surgical treatment for nondisplaced waist fractures leads to higher healing rates and more rapid time to healing.[24]

Surgical treatment for scaphoid fractures is indicated for any displaced or unstable fracture and also depends on the location of fracture. As more proximal fractures have a higher chance of nonunion when treated nonoperatively, virtually all proximal pole fractures should be fixed surgically when feasible.

Surgical Approaches

Multiple surgical approaches exist for treating scaphoid fractures. These include percutaneous screw fixation, open reduction internal fixation (ORIF), and arthroscopically assisted fracture fixation. Each of these techniques can be performed with screws placed in a dorsal antegrade or volar retrograde direction. Often the fracture pattern itself will dictate the particular screw-insertion technique, with the volar retrograde technique potentially more applicable to distal fracture patterns, while the dorsal antegrade technique may be applicable to proximal fracture patterns.

One of the greatest benefits of percutaneous technique is the limitation of soft tissue disruption around the zone of fracture, with preservation of the soft tissue envelope and, ideally, improved healing. This technique absolutely requires maintenance of reduction throughout the procedure and involves placing a cannulated headless compression screw centrally within the scaphoid, buried just below the articular surface. Percutaneous joysticks may be utilized to reduce displacement; however, any loss of reduction intraoperatively obviates the ability to perform the procedure percutaneously. It is critical to obtain the optimal starting point when performing percutaneous fixation for scaphoid fractures, and central screw placement is absolutely necessary as it leads to 39% increased load to failure compared with eccentric screw position.[25] If the ideal screw starting point cannot be obtained, it is simple to make a small incision to visualize the starting point on the scaphoid without performing a truly "open" reduction. This can sometimes simplify the procedure without adding significant soft tissue stripping.

ORIF is indicated in any setting of a displaced unstable fracture pattern, or with displacement that cannot be anatomically reduced with percutaneous techniques. Via either a dorsal or volar approach, the scaphoid fracture is reduced and most commonly stabilized with a headless compression screw placed in a similar fashion as in the percutaneous technique, with one main difference being initiation of the screw starting point under direct visualization. Additionally, the fracture itself can be visualized confirming anatomic reduction of the articular surface through direct inspection. The decision to perform ORIF using a dorsal versus a volar approach, similar to percutaneous technique, is often made based on fracture pattern and location of fracture, in that proximal fractures are more easily reduced and stabilized from a dorsal approach, while distal fractures are more readily reduced and stabilized from a volar approach. Specific surgical techniques will be discussed in detail in the following chapter.

Relevant Complications

There are many complications that must be considered in treating scaphoid fractures. The most commonly reported in the literature are delayed union, malunion, nonunion, avascular necrosis, stiffness, decreased grip strength, and arthritis.

One of the most challenging complications of scaphoid fracture treatment is nonunion, with or without avascular necrosis of the proximal pole. The most common vascular pattern of the scaphoid is a dorsal introduction of the blood supply which then travels in a retrograde direction. This blood supply may be compromised by a dorsal approach. Care must be taken, therefore, upon performing operative fixation of scaphoid fractures via a dorsal approach, to avoid surgical dissection more distal than is absolutely necessary to view the appropriate starting position for guidewire placement for the antegrade screw. It is critical to avoid stripping the soft tissue off of the dorsal ridge during surgery to avoid disruption of the dorsal blood supply insertion.

Another critical complication to avoid is the missed scaphoid fracture. It is difficult to know the incidence of missed scaphoid fractures, but there is well-documented literature supporting the increased risk of nonunion or delayed union with late presentation.[26] There is some evidence to suggest that subacute scaphoid fractures presenting between 6 weeks and 6 months from injury can be expected to heal with casting alone with a union rate of 83%, although exclusion of risk factors for healing such as diabetes, comminution, and humpback deformity within the same cohort resulted in a 96% union rate.[27]

Nonoperative treatment of scaphoid fractures is not without risk. In a meta-analysis of randomized controlled trials comparing nonoperative with operative treatment for acute scaphoid fractures, nonoperative treatment was found to have significantly decreased grip strength up to 12 months after treatment.[28] In addition, patients treated nonoperatively suffered from increased duration of absence from work and increased rate of delayed union.[28]

Complications of hardware are another potential source for failure of surgical treatment of scaphoid fractures. Screws that are too long or are placed off trajectory may impinge on the adjacent joint, leading to cartilage wear, arthritis, and pain, whereas screws not placed within the central axis of the scaphoid may not provide adequate stability and load to failure. In a postoperative comparison of antegrade versus retrograde screw placement, the antegrade screw was found to be central in 88.2% of scaphoids, compared with 51.6% of retrograde screws.[29] In a comparison between percutaneous dorsal antegrade screw fixation and mini-open dorsal antegrade screw fixation, no significant difference in complication rates was found, and the authors recommended a mini-open approach due to the ability to directly visualize the starting point and improve the accuracy of screw trajectory.[30] In another study, the scaphoid was found to be on average 4mm longer in males versus females, with a significantly wider proximal pole.[31] Such information is helpful in determining optimal screw length and size to maximize fixation strength.

Infection, as with any orthopedic surgical treatment, can lead to devastating consequences. Fortunately, the infection rate following scaphoid ORIF or percutaneous fixation is relatively low and as a result, is not reflected as a significant concern in the current literature.

Damage to the sensory branch of radial nerve or any tendon is a concern with dorsal open or percutaneous approach. A cadaveric study showed that optimal dorsal antegrade guidewire placement is 17 mm from the superficial sensory branch of the radial nerve, 5 mm from the extensor pollicis longus (EPL) tendon, and 3 mm from the extensor indicis proprius (EIP) tendon.[32] Careful attention to technique can limit these complications significantly.

Review of Treatment Outcomes

The current literature supports successful treatment of stable, nondisplaced scaphoid fractures via either operative or nonoperative approach. Treatment of unstable fractures, however, introduces a more complicated scenario with variable treatment outcomes. Proximal pole fractures, as discussed earlier, are at an increased risk of failure with conservative treatment and, therefore are most commonly treated with surgical fixation. A retrospective review of proximal pole fractures treated operatively over a 19-year period found that 43% of patients showed evidence of union at 14 weeks.[33] Union rates were 70% in nondisplaced proximal pole fractures, compared with 23% in displaced fractures, although a delay in ORIF of up to 28 days did not affect the rate of union.[33]

As sports-related scaphoid fractures are common, an understanding of return to sport becomes important in counseling athletes undergoing surgery for a scaphoid fracture. A review of current literature found that 98% of patients were able to return to their sport, with an average return to sport time of 7.3 weeks.[34]

Previously the technique of percutaneous fixation was discussed in relation to screw position within the scaphoid. Regarding outcomes of this choice of technique, in a comparison of dorsal versus volar percutaneous screw fixation in type B fractures, fracture union was achieved in 100% of patients, with no difference in either group regarding functional or clinical results.[35]

References

1. Berger RA. The anatomy of the scaphoid. *Hand Clin.* 2001;17:525–532.
2. Botte MJ, Pacelli LL, Gelberman RH. Vascularity and osteonecrosis of the wrist. *Orthop Clin North Am.* 2004;35:405–421 (xi).
3. Gelberman RH, Menon J. The vascularity of the scaphoid bone. *J Hand Surg Am.* 1980;5:508–513.
4. Green DP. *Green's Operative Hand Surgery.* 5th ed. Philadelphia, PA: Elsevier/Churchill Livingstone; 2005.
5. Weber ER, Chao EY. An experimental approach to the mechanism of scaphoid waist fractures. *J Hand Surg Am.* 1978;3:142–148.
6. Russe O. Fracture of the carpal navicular. Diagnosis, non-operative treatment, and operative treatment. *J Bone Joint Surg Am.* 1960;42-A:759–768.
7. Herbert TJ, Fisher WE. Management of the fractured scaphoid using a new bone screw. *J Bone Joint Surg Br.* 1984;66:114–123.
8. Herbert TJ. *The Fractured Scaphoid.* St. Louis, MO: Quality Medical Publishing; 1990.
9. Buijze GA, Jorgsholm P, Thomsen NO, Bjorkman A, Besjakov J, Ring D. Factors associated with arthroscopically determined scaphoid fracture displacement and instability. *J Hand Surg Am.* 2012;37:1405–1410.
10. Munk B, Frokjaer J, Larsen CF, et al. Diagnosis of scaphoid fractures. A prospective multicenter study of 1,052 patients with 160 fractures. *Acta Orthop Scand.* 1995;66:359–360.
11. Wong K, von Schroeder HP. Delays and poor management of scaphoid fractures: factors contributing to nonunion. *J Hand Surg Am.* 2011;36:1471–1474.
12. Parvizi J, Wayman J, Kelly P, Moran CG. Combining the clinical signs improves diagnosis of scaphoid fractures. A prospective study with follow-up. *J Hand Surg Br.* 1998;23:324–327.
13. Ring D, Lozano-Calderon S. Imaging for suspected scaphoid fracture. *J Hand Surg Am.* 2008;33:954–957.
14. Yin ZG, Zhang JB, Kan SL, Wang XG. Diagnostic accuracy of imaging modalities for suspected scaphoid fractures: meta-analysis combined with latent class analysis. *J Bone Joint Surg Br.* 2012;94:1077–1085.
15. Temple CL, Ross DC, Bennett JD, Garvin GJ, King GJ, Faber KJ. Comparison of sagittal computed tomography and plain film radiography in a scaphoid fracture model. *J Hand Surg Am.* 2005;30:534–542.
16. Grewal R, Suh N, MacDermid JC. Use of computed tomography to predict union and time to union in acute scaphoid fractures treated nonoperatively. *J Hand Surg Am.* 2013;38:872–877.
17. Buijze GA, Goslings JC, Rhemrev SJ, et al. Cast immobilization with and without immobilization of the thumb for nondisplaced and minimally displaced scaphoid waist fractures: a multicenter, randomized, controlled trial. *J Hand Surg Am.* 2014;39:621–627.
18. Doornberg JN, Buijze GA, Ham SJ, Ring D, Bhandari M, Poolman RW. Nonoperative treatment for acute scaphoid fractures: a systematic review and meta-analysis of randomized controlled trials. *J Trauma.* 2011;71:1073–1081.
19. Gellman H, Caputo RJ, Carter V, Aboulafia A, McKay M. Comparison of short and long thumb-spica casts for non-displaced fractures of the carpal scaphoid. *J Bone Joint Surg Am.* 1989;71:354–357.
20. Clay NR, Dias JJ, Costigan PS, Gregg PJ, Barton NJ. Need the thumb be immobilised in scaphoid fractures? A randomised prospective trial. *J Bone Joint Surg Br.* 1991;73:828–832.
21. Grewal R, King GJ. An evidence-based approach to the management of acute scaphoid fractures. *J Hand Surg Am.* 2009;34:732–734.
22. Buijze GA, Doornberg JN, Ham JS, Ring D, Bhandari M, Poolman RW. Surgical compared with conservative treatment for acute nondisplaced or minimally displaced scaphoid fractures: a systematic review and meta-analysis of randomized controlled trials. *J Bone Joint Surg Am.* 2010;92:1534–1544.
23. Al-Ajmi TA, Al-Faryan KH, Al-Kanaan NF, et al. A systematic review and meta-analysis of randomized controlled trials comparing surgical versus conservative treatments for acute undisplaced or minimally-displaced scaphoid fractures. *Clin Orthop Surg.* 2018;10:64–73.
24. McQueen MM, Gelbke MK, Wakefield A, Will EM, Gaebler C. Percutaneous screw fixation versus conservative treatment for fractures of the waist of the scaphoid: a prospective randomised study. *J Bone Joint Surg Br.* 2008;90:66–71.
25. McCallister WV, Knight J, Kaliappan R, Trumble TE. Central placement of the screw in simulated fractures of the scaphoid waist: a biomechanical study. *J Bone Joint Surg Am.* 2003;85:72–77.
26. Mack GR, Wilckens JH, McPherson SA. Subacute scaphoid fractures. A closer look at closed treatment. *Am J Sports Med.* 1998;26:56–58.
27. Grewal R, Suh N, MacDermid JC. The missed scaphoid fracture-outcomes of delayed cast treatment. *J Wrist Surg.* 2015;4:278–283.
28. Shen L, Tang J, Luo C, Xie X, An Z, Zhang C. Comparison of operative and non-operative treatment of acute undisplaced or minimally-displaced scaphoid fractures: a meta-analysis of randomized controlled trials. *PloS One.* 2015;10:e0125247.
29. Lucenti L, Lutsky KF, Jones C, Kazarian E, Fletcher D, Beredjiklian PK. Antegrade versus retrograde technique for fixation of scaphoid waist fractures: a comparison of screw placement. *J Wrist Surg.* 2020;9:34–38.
30. Dodds SD, Rush 3rd AJ, Staggers JR. A mini-open, dorsal approach for scaphoid fracture fixation with a ligament sparing arthrotomy. *Tech Hand Up Extrem Surg.* 2020;24(1):32–36.
31. Heinzelmann AD, Archer G, Bindra RR. Anthropometry of the human scaphoid. *J Hand Surg Am.* 2007;32:1005–1008.
32. Adamany DC, Mikola EA, Fraser BJ. Percutaneous fixation of the scaphoid through a dorsal approach: an anatomic study. *J Hand Surg Am.* 2008;33:327–331.
33. Brogan DM, Moran SL, Shin AY. Outcomes of open reduction and internal fixation of acute proximal pole scaphoid fractures. *Hand (N Y).* 2015;10:227–232.
34. Goffin JS, Liao Q, Robertson GA. Return to sport following scaphoid fractures: a systematic review and meta-analysis. *World J Orthop.* 2019;10:101–114.
35. Gurbuz Y, Kayalar M, Bal E, Toros T, Kucuk L, Sugun TS. Comparison of dorsal and volar percutaneous screw fixation methods in acute Type B scaphoid fractures. *Acta Orthop Traumatol Turc.* 2012;46:339–345.

71

Technique Spotlight: Scaphoid Fractures— Volar vs. Dorsal, Open vs. Percutaneous; Bone Graft Options

MICHAEL N. NAKASHIAN AND THOMAS B. HUGHES

Volar Percutaneous Technique

Indications

The indications for volar percutaneous fixation of scaphoid fractures include nondisplaced scaphoid fractures, or minimally displaced fractures that can be reduced using K-wires as joysticks. In particular, the volar approach is useful for more distal fractures which can be more challenging to manage from a dorsal approach.

Preoperative Evaluation

Standard radiographic imaging including posteroanterior (PA), oblique, lateral, and scaphoid views should be obtained. In certain cases, computed tomography (CT) scan may be obtained to evaluate fracture morphology.

Positioning and Equipment

The patient is placed in a supine position with a radiolucent hand table. Two techniques for positioning of the wrist are commonly used. In one approach, the arm is fully supinated with the volar wrist facing the ceiling. With this approach, a larger C-arm, with the image intensifier under the table, is preferred. Finger traps with 8–10 pounds of traction hang from the end of the hand table (Fig. 71.1A).

The other method for volar percutaneous scaphoid fixation is to have the elbow flexed 90 degrees with the arm strapped to the table. If an arthroscopy traction tower is used, the metal post can be a challenge to image around. Instead of a traction tower, the arm can be suspended using finger traps from an IV pole with weights hanging from the elbow. This may make imaging easier. With these techniques with the forearm positioned vertically, the mini C-arm is preferred to a standard fluoroscopy unit, as imaging occurs with the C-arm positioned horizontally. A headless compression screw of the surgeon's selection is used for fixation.

Technique Description

Fracture location, morphology, and alignment are confirmed via fluoroscopy to be sure that percutaneous fixation remains an acceptable surgical option. If necessary, one to two K-wires can be placed percutaneously to reduce a minimally displaced fracture. One to two rolled towels are placed beneath the dorsal wrist and a single finger trap is placed on the thumb. Eight to 10 pounds of weight is hung off the end of the hand table, pulling the wrist into extension and ulnar deviation. A K-wire is used to mark out the trajectory for centralized screw placement using a surgical marker, in both the anteroposterior (AP) and lateral views. This, along with palpation of the distal pole of the scaphoid, will allow for identification of the appropriate starting position. A 14-gauge needle is then placed percutaneously and advanced to the appropriate starting position on the distal pole of the scaphoid (Fig. 71.1B). The bevel should face dorsally and the needle can be used to hinge the scaphoid into flexion, levering on the trapezium to push it slightly dorsally to allow a better guidewire trajectory. The guidewire for the implant is then placed in a retrograde fashion through the needle. Positioning is confirmed in multiple views to make sure there is no violation of an articular surface. Critical views are the ulnarly deviated scaphoid view to evaluate for screw length and position, the hypersupinated PA to evaluate the scaphocapitate joint, the lateral view to check for volar penetration and volar screw trajectory, and the pronated oblique for proximal and distal penetration. Once the guidewire is determined to be in perfect position, a small incision is made along the guidewire, only large enough to allow entry of the screw. The tip is confirmed to be at the level of proximal subchondral bone and measured for length. Typically, 4 mm will be subtracted from this measurement to account for cartilage thickness. For more distal fractures, the length of the screw chosen may be even shorter and still provide adequate fixation. The guidewire is then advanced into, or through, the proximal subchondral bone to prevent its

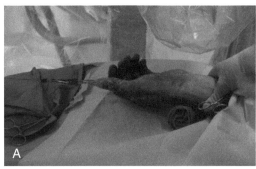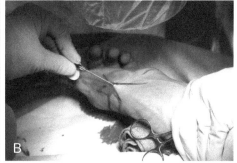

• **Fig. 71.1** Position of the hand for a volar percutaneous approach to fixation of scaphoid fractures. (A) The wrist is extended over a rolled towel while 8–10 pounds of traction is applied through a finger trap placed on the thumb. (B) A 14-gauge needle or angiocatheter is used as a cannula through which the guidewire is placed. It is placed under fluoroscopic guidance into the scaphotrapezius joint and used to lever the trapezius dorsally to improve the starting point for the guidewire.

accidental removal after drilling. The guidewire is overdrilled on power. Many systems have two diameter drills, one for the leading threads and one for the trailing threads. It is important to use the larger drill for the trailing threads to prevent hoop stresses and possible fracture around the trailing threads.

In some cases, a second, de-rotation wire may be beneficial (Fig. 71.2). This is likely more important in unstable fractures or in those that have more displacement. It tends to be used less commonly in percutaneous fixation as those fractures that may require a second wire tend not to be amenable to percutaneous reduction. However, if displaced or unstable fractures are managed percutaneously, a de-rotation wire should be strongly considered.

Traction is released and the screw is inserted. As the screw is advanced, longitudinal pressure should be placed on the screw, adding to the compression. While the variable pitch threads do lead to compression, each thread can provide only a small compressive force and the force from the screwdriver can assist in maximizing compression at the fracture site. Final imaging should confirm fracture reduction and screw positioning.

PEARLS AND PITFALLS

- It is often difficult to obtain an appropriately dorsal starting point due to interference by the trapezium. Once the scaphoid is hinged using the needle, a small mallet may be used to impact the needle and decrease the chance of losing the starting point as the wire is introduced.
- If it is too difficult to obtain a dorsal enough starting point, it is acceptable to place the guidewire through the trapezium and a transtrapezial drill and screw path is occasionally the only way to obtain adequate screw position from this approach. For this reason, dorsally placed screws tend to be more centrally placed within the scaphoid. However, for a fracture at or distal to the waist, the volar approach may be the best option despite this limitation.
- Once the screw is placed, it should be evaluated critically as far as position and length. For many of the headless compression systems that rely on the variable pitch of the screw to gain compression, taking the screw out and replacing it may not lead to the same compression obtained after the original placement. Therefore if the screw positioning is imperfect, but acceptable, it should be left in place. While it is best to make these corrections with the guidewire before drilling, it is sometimes difficult to get the same images that you can obtain after the screw is placed and the guidewire is removed.
- Screws that penetrate the articular surfaces should be repositioned. In some cases, a larger screw may be needed when repositioning in order to get adequate compression and fixation.
- It is difficult to get good fixation of very proximal fractures through the volar approach. There is far less tolerance of inaccurate screw length measurement in these cases, and a dorsal approach should be performed.

Dorsal Percutaneous Technique

Indications

The indications for dorsal percutaneous fixation of scaphoid fractures include nondisplaced scaphoid fractures, or minimally displaced fractures that can be reduced using K-wires as joysticks. Proximal pole fractures are also more indicated for dorsal percutaneous fixation compared with volar. Very distal fractures may be more challenging to address from this approach.

Preoperative Evaluation

Traditional radiographic imaging including PA, oblique, lateral, and scaphoid view X-rays should be obtained. In certain cases, a CT scan may be obtained to evaluate fracture morphology.

Positioning and Equipment

The patient is placed in a supine position with a radiolucent hand table, with the forearm in pronation. Intraoperative fluoroscopy is necessary throughout the procedure. A standard C-arm fluoroscopy unit is preferable, if available, as it is easier to place the wire without moving the fluoroscopy out of the way after imaging, as is often needed with mini C-arm fluoroscopy units. A headless compression screw of the surgeon's selection is used for fixation.

Technique Description

Fracture location, morphology, and alignment are confirmed via fluoroscopy to be sure that percutaneous fixation remains an acceptable surgical option. If necessary, one to two K-wires can be placed percutaneously to reduce a slightly displaced fracture. The wrist is flexed and radially deviated to create the signet ring sign, signifying appropriate longitudinal alignment of the scaphoid (Fig. 71.3). This positioning is best accomplished on a large stack of towels so that extreme flexion can be obtained. The guidewire for the screw is then driven in an antegrade fashion through the center point of the signet ring. The wire position is checked also on the lateral view, and then the wire is driven distally until it penetrates the volar skin. The wire is then advanced until it is just at the level of the proximal subchondral bone, so as to allow extension of the wrist for optimal fluoroscopic evaluation. However, prior to penetrating the distal cortex, a measurement for screw length is obtained. A small incision is made just large enough for the screw and blunt dissection is performed to create a path to the scaphoid cartilage. With this technique, this cartilage is not visualized, but just palpated with the scissor tip while

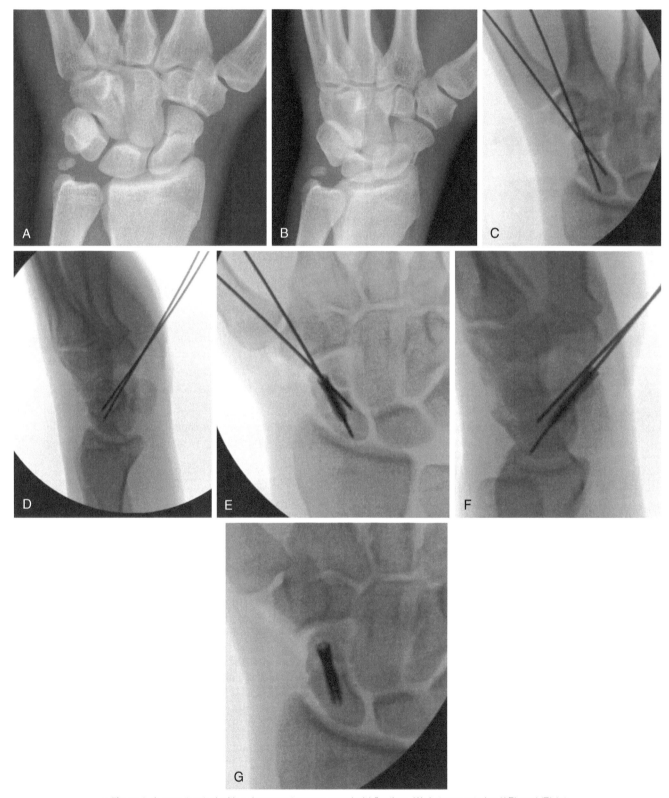

• **Fig. 71.2** A case treated with volar percutaneous scaphoid fixation. (A) Anteroposterior (AP) and (B) lateral images demonstrate a scaphoid body fracture that is distal to the midpoint of the scaphoid. For this reason, a volar approach was chosen. (C) and (D) demonstrate AP and lateral views after placement of the guidewire with a de-rotation K-wire. Note on the lateral view that the guidewire is slightly volar to the central axis as the guidewire is in contact with the volar trapezium which influences the wire's position. (E) and (F) demonstrate the screw placed over the guidewire and (G) shows the final position of the screw.

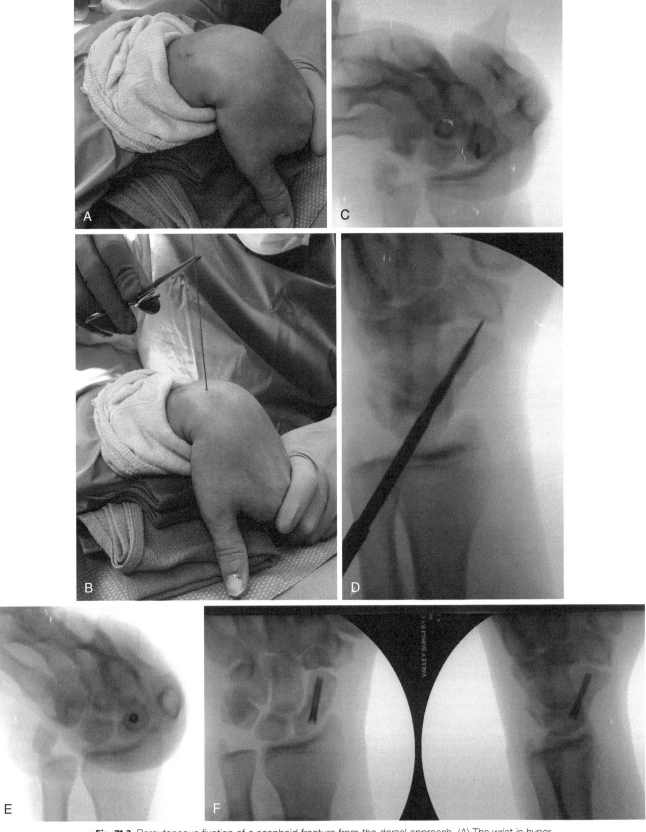

• **Fig. 71.3** Percutaneous fixation of a scaphoid fracture from the dorsal approach. (A) The wrist is hyper-flexed over a stack of towels. (B) The pin is positioned percutaneously under fluoroscopic guidance. (C) The flexed scaphoid forms a ring and the pin is placed centrally within that ring, which represents the long axis of the scaphoid. (D) The pin is measured and then advanced into the distal subchondral bone to prevent it from being accidentally removed with the cannulated drill. (E) The wrist is flexed and the perfect ring of the scaphoid can be seen at the same time that the cannulated hole in the screw is visualized, demonstrating near-perfect alignment with the long axis of the scaphoid. (F) Final positioning of the screw on anteroposterior and lateral images.

bluntly dissecting. If the measurement is not obtained then, it can be difficult to accurately gauge the distal endpoint after having penetrated the distal cortex. Typically, 4 mm will be subtracted from this measurement to account for proximal scaphoid cartilage thickness. Critical views are the ulnarly deviated scaphoid view to evaluate for screw length and position, the hypersupinated PA to evaluate the scaphocapitate joint, the lateral view to check for volar penetration, and the pronated oblique for proximal and distal penetration. Once the guidewire is determined to be in perfect position, it is then advanced back in a retrograde fashion with the wrist in extreme flexion again and brought out through the dorsal incision. The wire is left through the volar skin and distal cortex and a hemostat is placed on the wire to minimize the chance of its accidental removal with the cannulated drill. The path is drilled and the screw is inserted. As the screw is advanced, longitudinal pressure should be placed on the screw, adding to the compression. While the variable pitch threads do lead to compression, each thread can provide only a small compressive force and the force from the screwdriver can assist in maximizing compression at the fracture site. Final imaging should confirm fracture reduction and screw positioning.

PEARLS AND PITFALLS

- In order to improve accuracy of guidewire placement, it is helpful to palpate and place a finger on the distal pole of the scaphoid. This gives the surgeon a tactile feel and a target for the guidewire.
- Obtaining the appropriate starting position can be challenging. While the starting point should be just at the insertion of the scapholunate ligament, the site of skin penetration should be significantly more ulnar and proximal. By the time the pin traverses the depth of the dorsal soft tissues on the oblique course along the wrist, it will have traveled at least a centimeter radial and distal. The starting point through the skin should be chosen accordingly. For this reason, the authors prefer the mini-open technique that makes finding the starting point more reliable with minimal additional morbidity.
- It is difficult to get good fixation of very distal fractures through the dorsal approach. There is far less tolerance of inaccurate screw length measurement in these cases, and a volar approach should be considered for these distal fractures.

Dorsal Mini-Open Technique

The general technique for a mini-open dorsal approach and indications for this technique are similar to the percutaneous technique. However, some authors prefer to make a small 1- to 1.5-cm incision in order to directly visualize the starting point and improve screw trajectory. In this approach, the traditional dorsal approach as described below is not necessary. A longitudinal incision is made after first localizing the approximate starting point using fluoroscopy. A small incision is made and blunt dissection is performed to the retinaculum (Fig. 71.4). A small incision is made in the extensor retinaculum and capsule between the extensor polices longus (EPL) and the fourth compartment extensor tendons. The entire retinaculum is not released and, therefore, repair is not needed at the end of the procedure. Like with percutaneous technique, the incision should be placed sufficiently proximal and ulnar to account for the oblique path the wire will take as it crosses the wrist so that it is angled toward the proximal starting point of the wire. This allows visualization of the starting point for optimal guidewire placement. The wire should be placed into the scaphoid just at the insertion of the scapholunate ligament. The

remainder of the procedure is performed as per the percutaneous dorsal technique.

PEARLS AND PITFALLS

- The dorsal incision should be slightly proximal and ulnar to the anticipated starting point of the screw in order to select the proper path for the guidewire.

Arthroscopically Assisted ORIF

Indications

The indications for arthroscopically assisted open reduction internal fixation (ORIF) include displaced scaphoid fractures, or minimally displaced fractures. In general, arthroscopic assistance allows for percutaneous fixation techniques in the setting of unstable or comminuted fractures that would otherwise require open treatment. Arthroscopy also allows for visualization of the fracture reduction directly and permits confirmation that the articular surfaces of the scaphoid are not penetrated inadvertently during fixation.

Preoperative Evaluation

Traditional radiographic imaging including PA, oblique, lateral, and scaphoid view X-rays should be obtained. In certain cases, a CT scan may be obtained to evaluate fracture morphology.

Positioning and Equipment

The patient is placed in the supine position with a radiolucent hand table, and the initial setup mimics that for a dorsal percutaneous approach. However, the arthroscopic wrist traction tower is available, including standard wrist arthroscopic equipment such as camera, shaver, and electrocautery. A cannulated headless compression screw system is necessary for fixation.

Technique Description

Initial fracture reduction and guidewire placement are as per the dorsal percutaneous technique already described. Once the guidewire is placed, it is advanced distally through the volar skin at the point that the proximal tip is just beneath the proximal subchondral bone in order to allow wrist extension and positioning within the traction tower. Finger traps are placed, and 10–12 pounds of distraction is placed through the wrist. Diagnostic arthroscopy is then performed using the radial midcarpal portal to assess accuracy of the reduction. If the reduction is deemed to be inadequate, the guidewire can be pulled out more volarly, just distal to the fracture site, allowing mobility through the fracture zone. Percutaneous K-wire joysticks can be placed within the proximal and distal fragments to improve the reduction, and a probe can be used through the ulnar midcarpal portal to assist reduction if necessary. Once the reduction is determined to be anatomic by arthroscopic visualization, the guidewire can then be placed more proximally across the fracture site to stabilize the reduction. Fluoroscopy is used to confirm reduction. The wrist is then taken out of traction, placed in flexion, and the guidewire is advanced proximally, with the distal tip at the subchondral level of the distal pole. It is then measured, drilled, and the screw is placed per the manufacturer's technique.

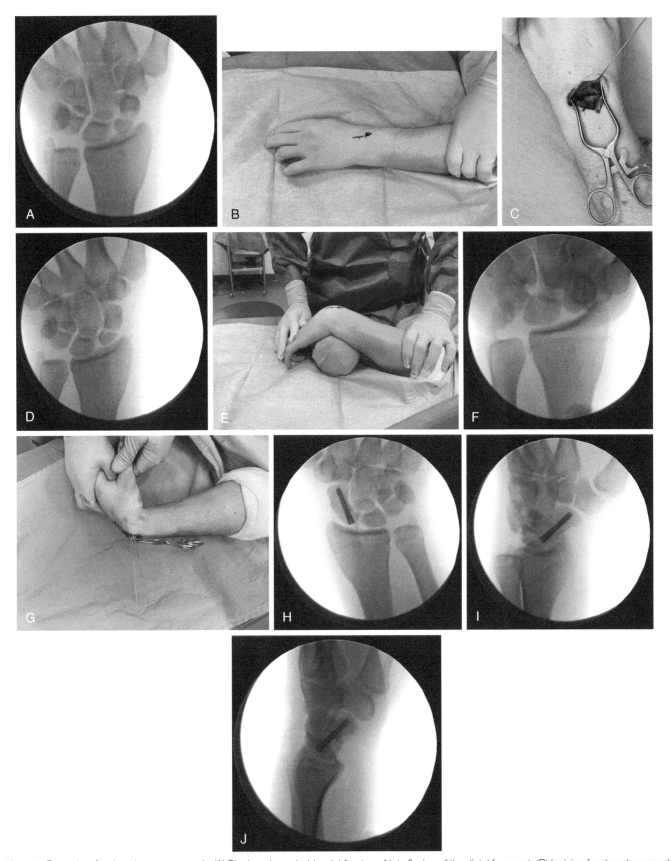

• **Fig. 71.4** Procedure for dorsal open approach. (A) Displaced scaphoid waist fracture. Note flexion of the distal fragment. (B) Incision for dorsal approach to scaphoid. The two *hash marks* would be for a "mini" open incision of approximately 1 cm. The incision can be extended past the *hash marks* for another 1 cm to provide larger exposure. The *oval circle* is Lister's tubercle. (C) Scaphoid waist fracture visualized as the dark line transversely, with a K-wire used for joystick to perform reduction. (D) Fracture reduced. Note that the distal fragment is no longer in flexion. (E) The wrist can be flexed over a bump to obtain radiographic visualization of the starting point for a dorsal guidewire. (F) Increased wrist flexion will allow visualization of the signet ring sign, to identify the appropriate starting point for guidewire position. (G) Guidewires in position. Note one guidewire in line with the thumb metacarpal, as the guidewire for the screw. An additional K-wire can be used for unstable fractures outside the trajectory of the screw guidewire. (H) Hypersupinated view to confirm the screw is not violating the scaphocapitate joint. (I) Pronated oblique view to confirm no penetration of the scaphotrapezial joint. (J) Lateral view, to confirm appropriate screw trajectory within center mass of scaphoid.

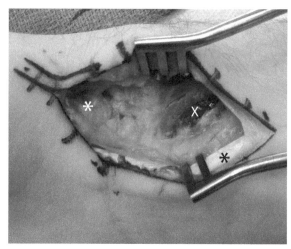

• **Fig. 71.5** The volar approach to the scaphoid. An incision is made starting proximally over the flexor carpi radialis (FCR) tendon and extended at an angle over the wrist flexion crease towards the distal pole of the scaphoid. In this image, the thumb is to the left. The FCR *(black asterisk)* can be seen retracted behind the Weitlander retractor and the distal edge of pronator is noted on the distal radius *(X)*. The scaphoid tubercle is noted distally *(white asterisk)*.

PEARLS AND PITFALLS

- Arthroscopically assisted scaphoid fracture fixation requires considerable skill with wrist arthroscopy.

Volar ORIF: Compression Screw

Indications

The indications for an open volar approach include displaced fractures of the waist or distal third that are not reducible by closed means or K-wire joystick techniques, including fractures with a humpback deformity. This approach is used most commonly for scaphoid nonunions with a humpback deformity that require volar structural bone grafting.

Preoperative Evaluation

Traditional radiographic imaging including PA, oblique, lateral, and scaphoid view X-rays should be obtained. In certain cases, a CT scan may be obtained to evaluate fracture morphology.

Positioning and Equipment

The patient is placed in a supine position with a radiolucent hand table. Intraoperative fluoroscopy is necessary throughout the procedure. A self-retainer such as a small Weitlaner retractor is helpful for visualization. A headless compression screw of the surgeon's selection is used for fixation. Bipolar cautery is useful for hemostasis and K-wires are helpful to maintain provisional fixation after reduction is obtained.

Technique Description

The incision is based on the location of the distal pole of the scaphoid which should be palpated and confirmed with fluoroscopy. The incision should be approximately 4 cm, beginning proximally along the flexor carpi radialis (FCR), and curving radially just distal to the tubercle, toward the base of the thumb metacarpal (Fig. 71.5).

Take care to avoid injury to the radial artery branch in this area, as it crosses the FCR distal to the radial wrist crease. The sheath and the subsheath of the FCR tendon are incised and the tendon is retracted. The volar capsule is encountered and incised longitudinally to allow exposure of the distal pole of the scaphoid. This portion of the capsule contains the radioscaphocapitate ligament and will be repaired after completion of the fixation. An elevator can be used between the scaphoid and trapezium to aid in visualizing the appropriate starting point. K-wires may be placed into the two fragments of the scaphoid to act as joysticks to control the reduction. Once reduction is obtained, a provisional K-wire can be placed in a retrograde fashion, outside of the expected screw pathway, to maintain reduction. Once the reduction is maintained, the guidewire for the screw can be placed without concerns over maintaining the reduction. In more stable configurations, the guidewire can be placed initially without the provisional wire. The volar lip of the trapezium may impede perfect guidewire placement. In most cases, a rongeur is used to remove a portion of the volar lip of the trapezium to aid in appropriate placement of the guidewire. An alternative to removing a portion of the trapezium is to place the guidewire directly through the trapezium. Once the position of the guidewire is confirmed with fluoroscopy, the depth gauge is used to choose a screw length. The wire is advanced into the proximal cortex to prevent accidental screw removal with the drill. The guidewire is then overdrilled after fluoroscopic confirmation of position in multiple views, and the compression screw is placed. In screw systems where there are different diameter drills for the leading and trailing threads, both drills should be used to prevent excessive hoop stresses that could lead to distal pole fracture with screw placement. In some cases, a second, de-rotation wire may be beneficial. This is likely more important in more unstable fractures or in those that have more displacement. In cases where a provisional wire is placed prior to guidewire placement, that provisional wire will act as a de-rotation wire.

As the screw is advanced, longitudinal pressure should be placed on the screw, adding to the compression. While the variable pitch threads do lead to compression, each thread can provide only a small compressive force and the force from the screwdriver can assist in maximizing compression at the fracture site. Final imaging should confirm fracture reduction and screw positioning. In the volar approach, the volar capsular tissues should be repaired as part of the closure.

PEARLS AND PITFALLS

- When freeing the soft tissue off of the distal pole of the scaphoid, care should be taken not to dissect too far radially and dorsally, as vigorous elevation in this area could strip the dorsal soft tissues and blood supply.
- It is also critical to evaluate for any volar comminution, as the compression screw could collapse the scaphoid through a zone of comminution, leading to shortening, screw penetration, and possibly accentuating a humpback deformity.

Dorsal ORIF: Compression Screw

Indications

The indications for dorsal ORIF of scaphoid fractures include displaced scaphoid fractures, or minimally displaced fractures that cannot be reduced using K-wires as joysticks. Proximal pole fractures are more easily approached in this manner compared with distal fractures which are more easily approached volarly. It is more difficult to evaluate for and correct flexion deformities from the dorsal approach. As a result of this, there are fewer indications for a full open dorsal approach (as compared with the mini-open approach), as there are limited deformity issues that can be addressed from this approach.

Preoperative Evaluation

Traditional radiographic imaging including PA, oblique, lateral, and scaphoid view X-rays should be obtained. In certain cases, a CT scan may be obtained to evaluate fracture morphology.

Positioning and Equipment

The patient is placed in a supine position with the forearm in pronation, with a radiolucent hand table. Intraoperative fluoroscopy is necessary throughout the procedure. A self-retaining retractor such as a small Weitlaner is helpful for visualization. A headless compression screw of the surgeon's selection is used for fixation. Bipolar cautery is useful for hemostasis, and K-wires are helpful to maintain provisional fixation after reduction is obtained.

Technique Description

The incision is based on the location of the proximal pole of the scaphoid which is identified based on its anatomic location in comparison to Lister's tubercle. The incision should be approximately 3 cm, beginning proximally at or just ulnar to Lister's tubercle, and extending toward the third metacarpal. The interval just ulnar to the EPL tendon is used. After skin flaps are raised, the extensor retinaculum is incised directly over the EPL. A self-retaining retractor is placed, retracting the EPL and extensor carpi radialis brevis tendons radially, and the extensor digitorum communis tendons ulnarly. This allows visualization of the dorsal capsule, which is incised longitudinally. The capsular incision length and shape will be determined based on the degree of displacement and location of the fracture. If necessary, an inverted T-shaped capsulotomy can be performed for better visualization and access

to fracture fragments. Reduction is then obtained. Once reduction is obtained, place a provisional K-wire in an antegrade fashion, outside of the expected screw pathway, to maintain reduction. The guidewire is then placed just at the membranous insertion of the scapholunate ligament and fluoroscopic confirmation of guidewire position is obtained on multiple views. Once its central position is confirmed, a depth gauge is used to select the screw size. Typically, 4 mm is subtracted to account for scaphoid cartilage depth. The wire is then advanced into the subchondral bone distally to prevent inadvertent guidewire removal with the drill. The guidewire is then overdrilled and the compression screw is placed. As the screw is advanced, longitudinal pressure should be placed on the screw, adding to the compression. While the variable pitch threads do lead to compression, each thread can provide only a small compressive force and the force from the screwdriver can assist in maximizing compression at the fracture site. Final imaging should confirm fracture reduction and screw positioning.

In screw systems where there are different diameter drills for the leading and trailing threads, both drills should be used to prevent excessive hoop stresses that could lead to distal pole fracture with screw placement. In some cases, a second, de-rotation wire may be beneficial. This is likely more important in more unstable fractures or in those that have more displacement. In cases where a provisional wire is placed prior to guidewire placement, that provisional wire will act as a de-rotation wire. In this approach, the dorsal capsular tissues should be repaired as part of the closure.

PEARLS AND PITFALLS

- Care should be taken when incising the dorsal capsule, as injury to the scapholunate ligament can occur if the incision is taken too deep on the initial approach.
- The portion of the capsule overlying the dorsal ridge should not be stripped from the scaphoid, so as to protect the blood supply.
- In reducing fractures via this approach, it may be helpful to ulnarly deviate the wrist initially while placing volar to dorsal pressure on the distal pole to bring the distal fragment into a better position.

72

Perilunate and Lunate Dislocations

JEFFREY YAO AND BRIAN CHRISTIE

Introduction

Perilunate injuries represent a challenge to the hand and wrist surgeon. Complex anatomy and kinematics, coupled with missed diagnoses and oft-delayed presentation, make the achievement of excellent outcomes difficult. It is our goal to present the essential information—anatomy, pathoanatomy, treatment options, surgical approaches, and expected outcomes—necessary for the hand and wrist surgeon to successfully identify and treat perilunate injuries.

Anatomy

Knowledge of the ligamentous and bony anatomy of the carpus is essential to properly diagnose and treat perilunate injuries. The function of the wrist is as a link between the forearm and the hand. The distal radius and distal ulna articulate with the proximal carpal row, which further articulates with the distal carpal row, which then articulates with the metacarpal bones. The distal articular surface of the radius, which consists of the scaphoid and lunate fossae, and the triangular fibrocartilage complex (TFCC) overlying the distal ulna, articulates with the proximal carpal row. The midcarpal joint can be separated into three distinct zones: radial, central, and ulnar. Radially, the scaphoid articulates with the trapezium and trapezoid, as well as with the radial capitate. Centrally, the lunate articulates with the capitate (in Type I lunates), or with both the capitate and the proximal pole of the hamate (in Type II lunates). Ulnarly, the midcarpal joint consists of the hamate-triquetral articulation.

All ligaments of the wrist are intracapsular apart from the transverse carpal ligament and the pisohamate/pisometacarpal ligaments. The remainder of the ligamentous anatomy of the wrist is separated into the extrinsic and intrinsic ligaments of the wrist. The extrinsic ligaments consist of the palmar radiocarpal ligaments, the palmar ulnocarpal ligaments, and the dorsal radiocarpal ligaments. The palmar radiocarpal ligaments consist of the radioscaphoid ligament, the radioscaphocapitate ligament, the long radiolunate ligament, and the short radiolunate ligament.[1] The space of Poirier represents a relative weak zone of the volar capsule through which the lunate may dislocate.[2] The palmar ulnocarpal ligaments consist of the ulnocapitate ligament, the ulnotriquetral ligament, and the ulnolunate ligament. The ulnocapitate ligament and the radioscaphocapitate ligament converge distally to form the arcuate ligament.[3] The ulnotriquetral and ulnolunate ligaments arise from the TFCC. The dorsal radiocarpal ligament arises from the dorsum of the radius and travels to the triquetrum (Fig. 72.1).[4,5]

The intrinsic ligaments of the wrist originate and insert within the carpus. The scapholunate ligament consists of a dorsal segment, which plays a key role in scapholunate stability; a palmar segment, which plays a lesser role; and a proximal membranous portion, which contributes minimally to stability.[6] The lunotriquetral ligaments consist of a palmar segment, which is stronger and more significant for lunotriquetral stability; a dorsal component, which is less significant; and a proximal membranous portion, which is weakest.[7] The dorsal intercarpal ligament that extends from the triquetrum across the lunate to the scaphoid, trapezium, and trapezoid functions to stabilize the lunocapitate joint, as no intrinsic ligaments link the lunate to the capitate.[8] The palmar midcarpal intrinsic ligaments extend from the triquetrum to the hamate and capitate, and function as the ulnar arm of the arcuate ligament. Other midcarpal intrinsic ligaments include the scaphocapitate and dorsal scaphotrapezio-trapezoid (STT) ligaments. Distally, strong interosseous ligaments connect the distal carpal row to the metacarpals (Fig. 72.2).[4]

Pathoanatomy of Perilunate Injuries

The pathomechanics of perilunate injuries follow progressive, predictable stages of carpal destabilization. The injury pattern is that of a forced hyperextension injury, in either ulnar or radial deviation, and is typically high energy, such as a motor vehicle collision or fall from a height.[9] The energy that is transmitted through the carpus follows a pattern that, at each stage, may pass through and disrupt either ligamentous or bony anatomy. These two pathways are termed *lesser arc injuries*, for a ligamentous pathway of disruption, or *greater arc injuries*, for pathways that contain any element of bony disruption or fracture. While trans-scaphoid greater arc injuries usually result in preserved scapholunate ligament continuity with the proximal pole of the scaphoid, perilunate injury with concomitant scaphoid fracture and scapholunate ligament disruption has been described (Fig. 72.3).[10]

First Stage: As the wrist is forced into hyperextension, the distal carpal row pulls the scaphoid into extension through the STT and scaphocapitate ligaments. The lunate, however, is constrained extrinsically by the long and short radiolunate ligaments and is unable to follow the scaphoid into extension, leading to scapholunate ligament tearing and failure. If the wrist is hyperextended in radial deviation, however, the proximal pole of the scaphoid will be constrained by the radioscaphocapitate

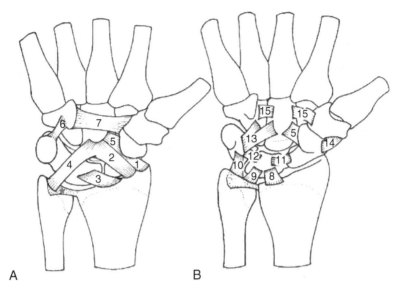

• **Fig. 72.1** Palmar ligaments. Schematic representation of the most consistently present wrist ligaments. These drawings do not aim to replicate the exact shape and dimensions of the actual ligaments, or their frequent anatomic variations. (A) Palmar superficial ligaments: radioscaphoid (1); radioscaphoid-capitate (2); long radiolunate (3); ulnar capitate (4); scaphoid capitate (5); pisohamate (6); and flexor retinaculum or transverse carpal ligament (7). (B) Palmar deep ligaments: short radiolunate (8); ulnar lunate (9); ulnar triquetrum (10); palmar scapholunate (11); palmar lunate triquetrum (12); triquetral-hamate-capitate, also known as the ulnar limb of the arcuate ligament (13); dorsolateral scaphotrapeziotrapezoid (14); and palmar transverse interosseous ligaments of the distal row (15).

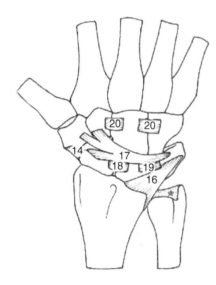

• **Fig. 72.2** Dorsal ligaments: radial triquetrum, also referred to as dorsal radiocarpal (16); triquetrum-scaphoid-trapeziotrapezoid, also known as the dorsal intercarpal ligament (17); dorsal scapholunate (18); dorsal lunate triquetrum (19); and dorsal transverse interosseous ligaments of the distal row (20). (Asterisk) Triangular fibrocartilage.

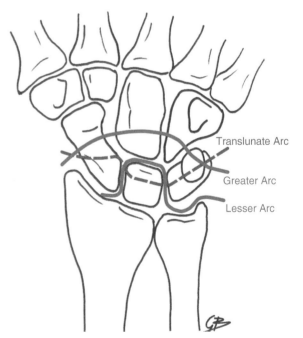

• **Fig. 72.3** Lesser versus greater arc injuries.

ligament, leading instead to scaphoid fracture as the transmission of energy. Scaphoid fracture occurs in approximately 60% of cases.[11]

Second Stage: As the distal row and scaphoid continue to extend, now unconstrained following scaphoid fracture or scapholunate dissociation, they dislocate dorsally relative to the lunate, resulting in lunocapitate dissociation. Occasionally, the capitate may instead fracture, as the distal pole of the capitate migrates with the rest of the distal row and scaphoid,

while the proximal pole of the capitate remains with the lunate. This dorsal translation may also result in tearing of the radioscaphocapitate ligament off the radial styloid with or without a fracture.

Third Stage: Dorsal translation of the capitate pulls the triquetrum dorsally through the arcuate ligament (triquetrum-hamate-capitate ligamentous complex). This tension results in tearing of the lunotriquetral ligaments, fracture of the triquetrum, or, rarely, fracture of the hamate.[12,13]

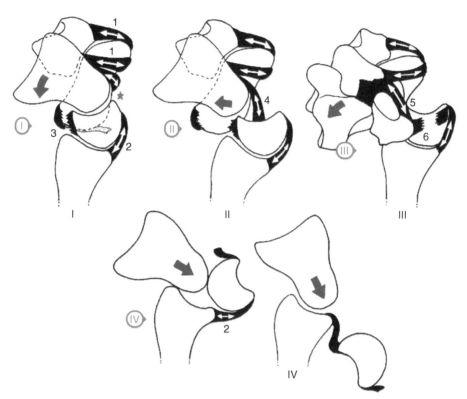

• **Fig. 72.4** Schematic representation of the four stages of perilunate instability, viewed from the ulnar side: (I) As the distal carpal row is forced into hyperextension *(red arrows)*, the scaphotrapezioid-capitate ligaments *(1)* pull the scaphoid into extension, opening the space of Poirier *(asterisk)*. The lunate cannot extend as much as the scaphoid because it is directly constrained by the short radiolunate ligament *(2)*. When the scapholunate torque reaches a certain value, the scapholunate ligaments may fail, usually from palmar to dorsal. A complete scapholunate dissociation is defined by the rupture of the dorsal scapholunate ligament *(3)*. (II) When dissociated from the lunate, the scaphoid-distal row complex may dislocate dorsally relative to the lunate *(red arrow)*. The limit of such dorsal translation is determined by the radioscaphoid-capitate ligament *(4)*. (III) If hyperextension persists, the ulnar limb of the arcuate ligament *(5)* may pull the triquetrum dorsally, causing failure of the lunate triquetrum ligaments *(6)*. (IV) Finally, the capitate may be forced by the still intact radioscaphoid-capitate ligament *(4)* to edge into the radiocarpal space and push the lunate palmar-ward until it dislocates into the carpal canal in a rotary fashion.

Fourth Stage: The lunate remains constrained now only by dorsal capsule and radiolunate ligaments. As the capitate is pulled back into the radiocarpal space, it exerts a palmarly directed force onto the lunate. This results in lunate dislocation through the space of Poirier, often rotating into the carpal tunnel (Fig. 72.4).[3]

Classification

Mayfield's cadaver studies were highly instructive in demonstrating the progressive ligamentous or osseous disruption of perilunate injuries.[14] Mayfield's classification system follows this progression in a staged fashion.

Mayfield Stages

Stage I: Scapholunate instability
Stage II: Capitolunate dissociation
Stage III: Triquetrolunate dissociation
Stage IV: Lunate dislocation

The addition of a fifth stage has been suggested for dislocation with complete enucleation of the lunate with disruption of the

short radiolunate ligament, significant for the loss of lunate vascularity and higher likelihood of avascular necrosis.[15]

Herzberg Stages

Alternately, Herzberg and colleagues broadly categorized perilunate injuries into perilunate dislocations (Stage I) and lunate dislocations (Stage II).[16] They subcategorized lunate dislocations by the degree of lunate rotation, with a subluxated and minimally rotated (<90 degrees) as Stage IIA and complete dislocation with greater rotation (>90 degrees), indicative of an intact short radiolunate ligament, as Stage IIB. Complete enucleation of the lunate with rupture of all ligamentous and vascular structures to the lunate is categorized as Stage IIC (Fig. 72.5).

Diagnosis

Determination of treatment begins with a careful clinical and radiologic examination of the patient. The mechanism of injury and chronicity of the complaint may yield helpful information driving the choice of treatment. Often the injury is open (10%), associated with other injuries of the upper extremity (11%), or associated with polytrauma (26%).[16] An estimated 16%–25%

Dorsal

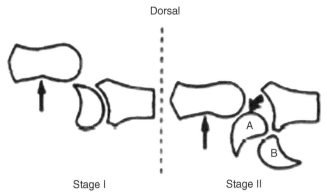

Stage I   Stage II

• **Fig. 72.5** Herzberg initial severity classification of perilunate dislocations and trans-scaphoid perilunate fracture-dislocations. The displacement is classified according to the relationships between the lunate, capitate, and radius: in Stage I, the lunate remains in place under the radius; in Stage IIA, the lunate is palmarly dislocated but rotated by <90 degrees; and in Stage IIB, the lunate is palmarly dislocated and rotated >90 degrees.

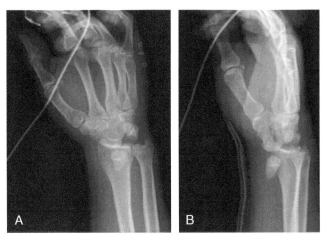

• **Fig. 72.6** Radiographs of lunate dislocation.

of perilunate injuries may be missed on initial presentation and may therefore present as their chronic sequelae.[17] Acute injuries (within 1 week of injury) may often be treated with primary repair of injured structures, while subacute (1–6 weeks) may present with an unstable, but reducible, carpus that is more difficult to repair primarily. A chronic injury (>6 weeks from injury) will often present with an irreducible carpus.[3] Physical examination of the injured extremity frequently lacks an obvious deformity and often presents with swelling only. Pain is typically diffuse, and range of motion is limited. It is critical to examine the status of the patient's median nerve, as many patients acutely will present with median neuropathy due to direct compression in the carpal tunnel by the dislocated lunate.[18] Dense, progressive median neuropathy should prompt emergent decompression via open carpal tunnel release. Other commonly associated injuries, such as carpometacarpal dislocations and distal radioulnar joint dislocations, should be ruled out (Fig. 72.6).

Imaging evaluation via standard four-view radiographs of the wrist (posteroanterior [PA], lateral, semipronated, and scaphoid views) is often sufficient to diagnose a perilunate injury. Evaluation of Gilula's lines will demonstrate step-offs indicative of carpal derangement.[19] The typical trapezoidal configuration of the lunate may be instead replaced by a wedge or triangular shape, suggestive of lunate dislocation. In Stage I perilunate injuries, addition of a clenched fist or pencil grip view can accentuate dynamic scapholunate dissociation. Measurement of standard carpal angles and relationships are also valuable in the chronic settings. The radius, lunate, capitate, and third metacarpal should be colinear on lateral radiograph, and measurement of the capitolunate angle, which normally ranges from –15 to 15 degrees, may indicate midcarpal injury. Determination of the scapholunate angle, which typically ranges from 30 to 60 degrees, may suggest scapholunate dissociation when >60 degrees. This level of angulation is termed dorsal intercalated segmental instability (DISI) deformity. Measurement of other relationships, such as the radiolunate angle, ulnar variance, carpal height, capitate/radius index, and ulnar translocation ratio, may be helpful with chronic presentations to determine the pattern of carpal instability.[3,20]

Other imaging modalities may also add valuable information driving treatment options. Computed tomography (CT) can demonstrate the amount and direction of carpal displacement. Magnetic resonance imaging (MRI) may better identify and quantify

ligamentous injury. Lastly, arthroscopy remains the gold standard for direct visualization of articular surfaces and interrogation of ligamentous integrity.

Treatment Options

Initial treatment involves acute evaluation in the emergency department with closed reduction attempted as soon as possible. The median nerve should be evaluated at the carpal tunnel, and progressive neuropathy should prompt emergent carpal tunnel release. Closed reduction of a lunate dislocation requires complete muscle relaxation, through either deep sedation, a general anesthetic, Bier block, or axillary block. Local anesthesia is typically insufficient to permit reduction. The arm should be hung from finger traps with 10–15 lbs of traction for at least 10 minutes. If the lunate is dislocated, flexion of the wrist and direct pressure onto the lunate directing it back into the lunate fossa of the radius should first be attempted. In patients with Herzberg Stage IIB (rotation >90 degrees) injuries or IIC (complete enucleation of the lunate) injuries, however, this maneuver should not be attempted, as it may disrupt the tenuous blood supply or result in further compressive injury to the median nerve.[3] Tavernier's maneuver is then performed: manual traction is maintained, and the surgeon's thumbs are placed volarly over the proximal lunate to stabilize it and prevent volar displacement. The wrist is then extended, recreating the mechanism of injury, followed by slow flexion and reduction of the capitate back onto and into the distal lunate concavity. A thumb spica splint is then applied, and definitive treatment should ideally follow within 1–2 weeks (Fig. 72.7).[11]

Various options have been described for definitive treatment of perilunate injuries. Historically, nonoperative treatment with closed reduction and casting was also the definitive treatment of choice, though this has largely fallen out of favor due to universally poor outcomes.[17,21–23] Closed reduction with percutaneous pinning may be attempted if perfect anatomic reduction of all perilunate joints is achieved.[24] Open reduction with direct ligament repair permits visualization and assessment of all bony and soft tissue injury, more accurate reduction of any displacement, and direct suturing of reparable ligaments.[3] Options include a dorsal approach, volar approach, or combined dorsal and volar approach. More recently, arthroscopically assisted direct ligament repair has been advocated to reduce disruption of uninjured structures seen with an open approach.

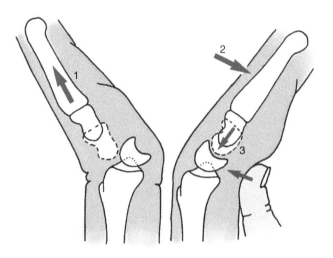

• **Fig. 72.7** Schematic representation of Tavernier's method[41] of reduction of dorsal perilunate dislocations. With the wrist slightly extended, gentle manual traction is applied *(1)*. Without releasing such traction, and while the lunate is stabilized palmarly by the surgeon's thumb, the wrist is flexed, until a snap occurs *(2)*. This indicates that the proximal pole of the capitate has overcome the dorsal horn of the lunate. At this point, traction is released, and the wrist is brought back to neutral *(3)*.

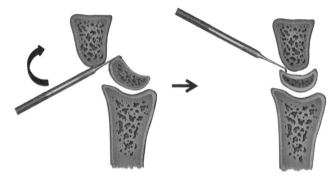

• **Fig. 72.8** "Shoehorn maneuver."

Indications for Surgical Treatment

Perilunate injuries are rarely emergent, unless the dislocation is irreducible or median neuropathy is progressive despite decompression of the carpal tunnel via reduction of the lunate. Following immediate closed reduction, operative intervention may proceed once the initial swelling has subsided. This chapter will focus on Mayfield Stage III and IV injuries, as repair of isolated scapholunate and lunotriquetral injuries involves a separate classification system, treatment algorithm, and comparison of surgical outcomes that is beyond the scope of this chapter.

Generally, owing to universally poor outcomes with closed reduction and casting alone, all patients with Stage III and IV injuries should be managed operatively. In the acute setting, arthroscopic reduction and pinning or open reduction and direct repair through a volar, dorsal, or combined volar and dorsal approach will permit the best evaluation and repair of all structures. An exception includes patients with associated comminuted distal radius fractures or extensive soft tissue injury, who may benefit instead from external fixation.[20,25]

Patients missed on initial diagnosis will often see improvement in pain but will predictably progress and collapse into a volar intercalated segment instability (VISI) or DISI deformity over time. Gradually, a reduction in mobility, loss of strength, and painful joint degeneration occur, and patients often present in the chronic settings as candidates for salvage procedures such as proximal row carpectomy (PRC) or radiocarpal fusion with scaphoid with/without triquetral excision.[3,23,26–28]

Surgical Approaches

Arthroscopic Closed Reduction and Percutaneous Pinning

As advocated by Kim et al.,[24] arthroscopic-assisted reduction and percutaneous pinning may achieve satisfactory results if restoration of normal carpal alignment is achieved and stabilized during healing. If closed reduction of the perilunate dislocation was not initially possible, this is attempted again in the operating room under regional anesthetic blockade. If reduction is still not attainable, then arthroscopic-assisted reduction of the capitolunate joint is attempted utilizing wrist tower traction. Finger traps are placed on the index and long fingers and suspended in a traction tower under 10–15 lbs of traction. Anatomic landmarks and portal site incisions are marked, and the extremity is exsanguinated with an Esmarch bandage. The tourniquet is inflated to 250 mm Hg. The three to four portal is made first. A standard technique for placement of portals is used, with insertion of an 18-gauge needle through the proposed portal site and insufflation of 5 mL of normal saline. Wet arthroscopy is our preference, but this may also be adequately performed under dry arthroscopy (no saline). With appropriate swelling of the radiocarpal joint and back-pressure return of saline into the syringe, the correct location of the portal is confirmed. A 2- to 3-mm longitudinal skin incision is made with a #11 blade. A hemostat is used to spread the tissue to the level of the dorsal capsule, which is then entered and dilated longitudinally and transversely with the hemostat. A freer elevator or arthroscopic probe is inserted and the "shoehorn maneuver" as described by Liu et al. is performed to reduce the capitolunate joint. Alternatively, the four to five portal may also be used for this maneuver (Fig. 72.8).[29]

The trochar and cannula are then inserted, and the trochar is exchanged for a 2.7-mm 30-degree arthroscope. A four to five portal is then placed in a similar fashion for introduction of an arthroscopic shaver. Clot and debris present in the radiocarpal space are removed through the three to four and four to five portals, improving visualization and permitting assessment of ligamentous disruption and cartilage and bony injury. The palmar capsular ligaments, scapholunate interosseous ligament (SLIL), lunotriquetral interosseous ligament (LTIL), TFCC, and articular surfaces of the radius, scaphoid, and lunate are inspected and interrogated with a probe. Further debridement of torn ligamentous structures is performed as needed.

Midcarpal portals (MCR and MCU) are then placed, and the SLIL, LTIL, and midcarpal joint surfaces are assessed from this perspective. Interposed soft tissue or bony fragments that may have been blocking reduction of the capitolunate joint are removed. Under fluoroscopic guidance, two parallel 0.062-inch K-wires are placed into the scaphoid, and two more K-wires are placed into the triquetrum, each aimed in the direction of the lunate without crossing the intercarpal interval (Fig. 72.9A–B).

The lunate is then reduced into the neutral position through wrist flexion under fluoroscopic guidance, and a temporary radiolunate 0.062-inch K-wire is inserted through the dorsal distal

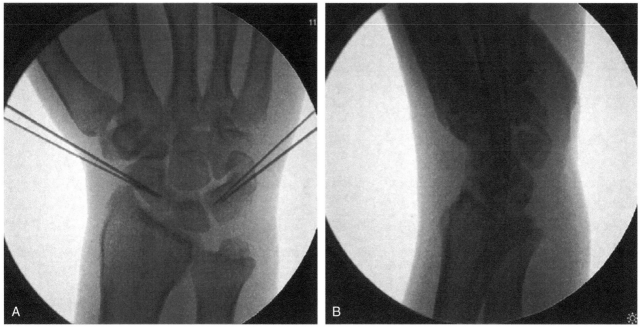

• **Fig. 72.9** (A and B) Provisional K-wire placement through Linscheid maneuver.

radius into the lunate, maintaining the lunate's neutral position (Linscheid maneuver). Under midcarpal arthroscopic visualization, the scaphoid and triquetrum are each reduced to the lunate, and the scaphoid/triquetral K-wires are then advanced across the intercarpal intervals (Figs. 72.10–72.12).

In the setting of gross instability, including disruption of both the primary and secondary stabilizers of the scapholunate or lunotriquetral intervals, the SLIL and LTIL are repaired through a mini-open incision. The three to four portal is extended to a 2-cm longitudinal incision, exposing the dorsal capsule. The dorsal capsule is incised and bone anchors are inserted and used to augment direct repair of the SLIL and/or LTIL ligaments (Figs. 72.13 and 72.14).

For trans-scaphoid injuries, two 0.045-inch K-wires are inserted into the proximal and distal fragments and manipulated as joysticks until the fracture is appropriately reduced under midcarpal arthroscopic visualization. The guidewire for a 3.0-mm cannulated screw is then advanced across the fracture site once articular congruity is obtained. One to two headless compression screws may then be placed in the scaphoid using a percutaneous technique, with one screw introduced along the central axis of the scaphoid, and another placed as an antirotation screw if needed (Figs. 72.15–72.19).

The k-wires are then cut beneath the skin in a buried fashion and the wounds are closed. The wrist is immobilized in a thumb spica cast. The k-wires are removed at 8 weeks. Hand therapy is critical in regaining hand and wrist motion, and in reducing swelling.

Open Repair

Open repair of perilunate injuries may be accomplished via an all-dorsal, all-volar, or combined dorsal and volar approach. Although most injuries may be adequately addressed with a dorsal approach alone, due to the complexity of some ligamentous disruptions and the carpal relationships, many recommend a combined two-incision approach, which will be described in the accompanying

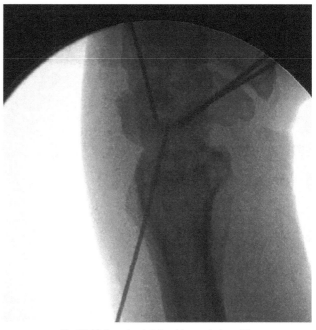

• **Fig. 72.10** Lunate stabilized in neutral position.

technique spotlight.[30–34] In this technique, the volar approach may be used for reduction of the lunate, carpal tunnel release, repair of the volar capsular tear, and repair of the volar lunotriquetral ligament. The dorsal approach may be used for repair of the SLIL and/or treatment of a scaphoid fracture in the case of trans-scaphoid injuries.

Relevant Complications

Most complications of perilunate injury and surgical treatment of perilunate injury are often related to the original trauma sustained. These include persistent median nerve dysfunction,

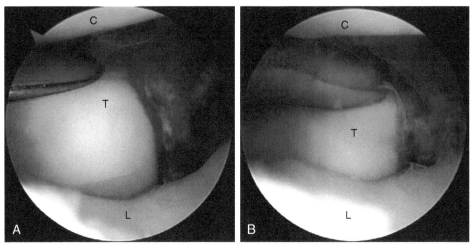

• **Fig. 72.11** (A and B) Arthroscopically reduce the scaphoid and triquetrum to the lunate through midcarpal portals. *C*, Capitate; *L*, lunate; *T*, triquetrum.

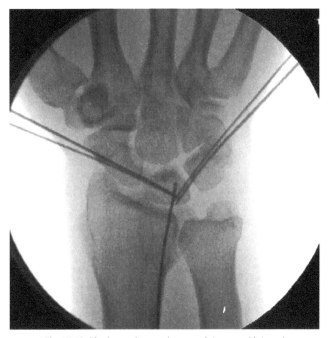

• **Fig. 72.12** K-wires advanced across intercarpal intervals.

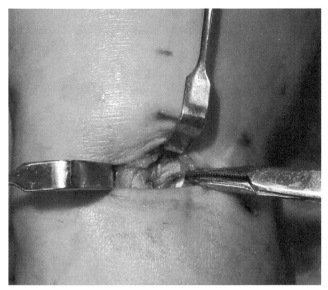

• **Fig. 72.13** Mini-open repair for gross ligamentous instability.

incomplete resolution of pain, complex regional pain syndrome, tendon rupture, residual carpal instability, and avascularity of the lunate.[11,35,36] Acute median neuropathy is found in approximately 47%–50% of patients.[18,37] Israel et al. evaluated complications in 65 patients with perilunate injury repaired through an open dorsal approach. Most patients demonstrated radiographic evidence of carpal collapse, with decreases in carpal height, increases in ulnar translation and DISI deformities common at final follow-up. Wrist arthritis was seen radiographically in 59% of cases, while osteonecrosis of the lunate was found in 8% of cases. Complex regional pain syndrome was observed in 12%, and an unplanned secondary surgery was required in 26% (Fig. 72.20).[38]

Meijer et al. evaluated 115 patients treated for perilunate injury and evaluated factors associated with unplanned reoperation.[39] Of the 16 patients (14%) who had unplanned reoperations, four were for compartment syndrome, three were for deep infections, and three were for malaligned/errant screws. Patients with unplanned operations were found to be younger and were more likely to be injured in a motor vehicle collision, perhaps indicative of higher energy injuries.

Left untreated, all perilunate injuries will progress to degenerative carpal collapse and arthrosis, resulting in pain, reduction of range of motion, and decreased grip strength.[34]

Review of Treatment Outcomes

Unfortunately, there is a lack of high-quality data reporting outcomes for perilunate injuries.[20,35] A relatively infrequent injury with a wide spectrum of severity, and outcomes that are best measured in years rather than weeks, has resulted in most studies being carried out as small retrospective case series with heterogeneous injuries and varying operative techniques. There are very few well-designed studies directly comparing different techniques. Below we present the highest quality, most up-to-date data available reviewing and comparing treatment outcomes.

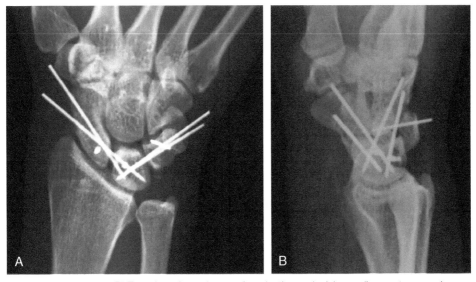

• **Fig. 72.14** (A and B) Final view after arthroscopic reduction and mini-open ligamentous repair.

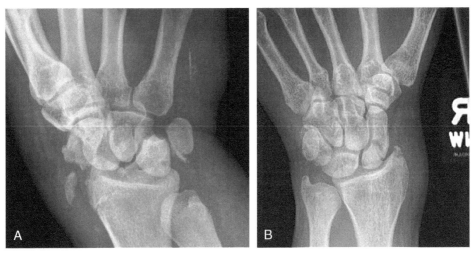

• **Fig. 72.15** (A and B) Trans-scaphoid perilunate injury.

While historically many perilunate injuries were managed with closed reduction and casting, numerous publications demonstrated the clear superiority of operative fixation.[17,40,41] Adkison reviewed 55 patients treated with a myriad of methods and demonstrated that reduction was maintained in only 31% of patients treated nonoperatively.[22] Inoue retrospectively reviewed 14 wrists: 2 were treated with casting while 12 were treated surgically. Those treated with casting alone had the only unsatisfactory results of the series.[21] Apergis followed 28 patients with perilunate injuries for an average of 6 years and found that in patients treated with closed reduction, results were fair in 3 and poor in 5, while patients treated with early open reduction had a better clinical score with 4 excellent, 9 good, 3 fair, and 4 poor results. They concluded that perilunate fracture-dislocations are too unstable to be treated with closed reduction alone.[42]

The necessity of ligament repair was studied by Minami and Kaneda, who reported on 32 patients treated with perilunate injuries, most of whom were seen >4 weeks from injury. Twelve patients underwent SL repair or reconstruction, while 20 patients did not undergo repair or reconstruction. Patients who underwent repair or reconstruction had better radiographic findings (SL diastasis, SL angle) and better modified Green-O'Brien scores compared with those who did not.[41] Comparison of closed reduction with percutaneous pinning to open reduction internal fixation (ORIF) has also demonstrated the superiority of open treatment in multiple circumstances,[35,43] although this superiority has been challenged recently by arthroscopic assistance of percutaneous pinning, in which heavy emphasis on direct visualization of restoration of carpal alignment is placed.[24]

The timing of definitive operative intervention has also been studied. Herzberg reported that acute perilunate dislocations/fracture-dislocations treated >6 weeks after injuries had significantly worse clinical outcomes than those treated within 6 weeks, a finding supported by Gupta et al.[17,44] Treatment delay of up to 18 days, however, did not affect outcomes.[45] Late treatment of unreduced injuries results in near-uniformly worse outcomes. Inoue et al. compared open reduction with or without internal fixation of the scaphoid to PRC and to partial or total lunate excision. They concluded that PRC was superior when patients present >8 weeks after injury,[46] and that internal fixation or lunate excision was less favorable.

Comparison of approaches for open reduction and direct repair also lacks strong head-to-head comparative evidence, and

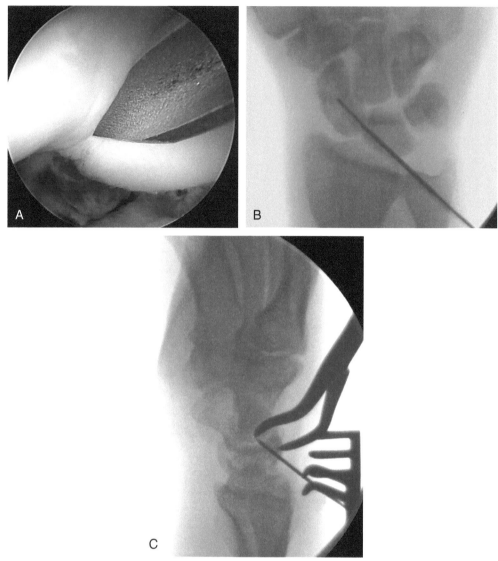

• **Fig. 72.16** (A–C) Provisional guidewire placement through scaphoid.

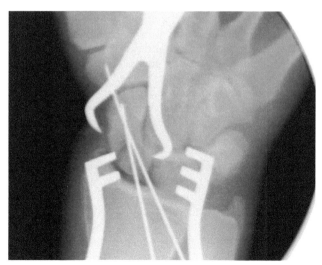

• **Fig. 72.17** Advancement of guidewires across reduced scaphoid.

the combined approach has not been definitively proven to be superior to a volar- or dorsal-only approach.[20] Minami and colleagues' report described previously did not include repair of the LT ligament in any patients, and they reported that those with LT incongruity did as well as those without LT abnormalities, suggesting that the volar approach for repair of the volar LT ligament may not be necessary.[41] Many argue that the complexity of reducing the normal intercarpal anatomy, combined with the advantages of repair of both the dorsal scapholunate ligament and volar lunotriquetral ligament, calls for a combined volar and dorsal approach.[30–34,47] Melone followed 28 patients treated with a combined approach for an average of 4.7 years and found that 86% were rated good to excellent, with 95% returning to preinjury activities.[32] Sotereanos used a combined volar and dorsal approach to treat 11 patients with perilunate injury and found that, after an average of 2.5 years following surgery, flexion-extension arc was 71% of the contralateral side and strength was 77% of the contralateral side. Seven of 11 patients had satisfactory pain control.[31] Hildebrand followed 23 perilunate injuries treated with

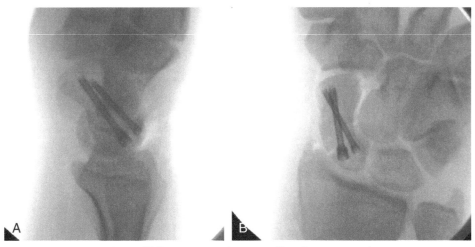

• **Fig. 72.18** (A and B) Percutaneous placement of headless compression screws.

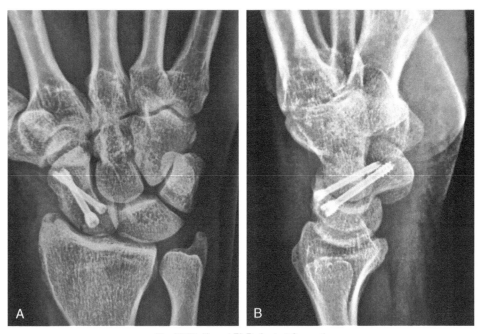

• **Fig. 72.19** (A and B) Patient at 3 months.

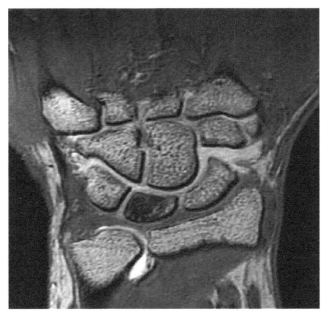

• **Fig. 72.20** Avascular necrosis of lunate.

a combined approach for an average of 3 years and found that flexion-extension arc was 57% of the contralateral side and strength was 73% of the contralateral side.[33]

Evaluation of patient-reported outcomes has been more common over the past decade. Kremer evaluated 39 patients treated through a dorsal, volar, or combined approach, at an average of 5.5 years and found an average Mayo score of 70, DASH (the Disabilities of the Arm, Shoulder and Hand) score of 23, corresponding to moderate disability after treatment.[40] Forli followed 18 patients treated with ORIF through a variety of approaches for a minimum of 10 years and found a Mayo score of 76, with evidence of arthritis in 67% and SL widening in 22% of patients, but neither correlated with poor outcomes.[48] Krief evaluated 30 patients treated with both open and closed methods with at least 15 years of follow-up and found an average Mayo score of 70, average quick DASH of 20, and average patient-rated wrist hand evaluation (PRWE) of 21.

Progression to carpal collapse and degenerative arthritis was common in all studies regardless of fixation method. Most studies, however, have found that arthritis is often asymptomatic, and that it is not correlated with functional outcomes.[16,20,31,32,36,40,48,49] In

Krief's study of patients >15 years from injury, 70% of patients developed arthritic changes in the wrist, but clinical functional impact of arthritis was felt to be low, with minimal impact on patient-reported outcomes.[49]

Expected return to work was studied by Griffin et al., who prospectively followed 16 patients treated with a combined dorsal and volar approach and found that early treatment allowed 88% of patients to return to work within 6 months and 63% of patients to return to sport within 1 year.[50]

Factors associated with poorer outcomes, regardless of method of treatment, have been studied by several authors. Delayed treatment beyond 4–6 weeks, open injuries, persistent carpal malalignment/inadequate fixation, fractures of the head of the capitate, and osteochondral defects were associated with poorer outcomes in reports by Jupiter, Weil, Herzberg, and Melone.[16,20,32,51] Kara et al. also found that Herzberg Stage II injuries (lunate dislocations), open fractures, and scapholunate dissociation >2 mm had worse functional results.[52] Dunn et al. followed 40 patients for an average of 4 years and found that injuries to the nondominant extremity resulted in better outcomes, and ligamentous-only injuries had less pain at rest and were more likely to return to sport.[37] In most cases, patients may expect decreased grip strength and limited range of motion regardless of presentation or treatment modality.[20]

External fixation may also be a reasonable treatment option in the polytrauma patient, owing to the advantages of decreased operative time in the setting of other emergent medical comorbidities/injuries. Savvidou followed 20 patients with perilunate injuries treated with external fixation and percutaneous pinning for an average of 3.3 years. Three patients required conversion to ORIF, and both radiographic and functional results were satisfactory.[25]

Arthroscopically assisted direct ligament repair has gained significant traction over the past decade as a viable method to restore articular congruity and carpal alignment while minimizing disruption of uninjured ligamentous structures.[53] Early and medium-term results have been encouraging, with outcomes similar to those for open approaches. Liu et al. reported early results of 31 patients treated with arthroscopically assisted reduction with percutaneous pinning. Twenty-four of the patients were followed for at least 15 months, and the authors found a mean flexion/extension arc of 85% of the contralateral wrist, grip strength of 83% of contralateral wrist, mean Mayo wrist score of 87, mean DASH score of 7, and PRWE score of 10. All patients returned to work.[29] Medium-term results were reported by Kim et al., who treated 20 patients with perilunate injuries with arthroscopic reduction and percutaneous pinning. They found, at an average of 2.5 years of follow-up, a mean flexion/extension arc of 79% of the contralateral wrist, grip strength of 78% of contralateral wrist, mean Mayo wrist score of 79, mean DASH score of 10, and PRWE score of 18.[24] Oh and colleagues reported a nonrandomized comparison of 20 patients with trans-scaphoid perilunate injuries, half of whom were treated with an arthroscopically assisted technique, and half treated with open reduction via a dorsal approach. Results at a minimum of 2-year follow-up demonstrated a clinically significant difference in mean DASH score (10.6 arthroscopic vs. 20.8 open); other outcome parameters were similar.[54]

Lastly, acute salvage procedures have been advocated by many for consideration in treatment of perilunate injuries.[55–58] Muller compared 8 patients treated with acute PRC with 13 patients treated with ORIF and found that outcomes at an average of 2.9 years were at least as good for PRC as ORIF. Additionally, PRC benefited from shorter operative times and shorter immobilization periods.[57]

Conclusion

Perilunate injuries represent a challenging spectrum of a progressive instability pattern and are often devastating. Unfortunately, regardless of treatment, most patients develop loss in range of motion and grip strength. Progression to radiocarpal and midcarpal arthrosis, while questionably significant, is common. Prompt identification of the injury, early treatment, and focus on open or arthroscopically assisted restoration of articular surfaces and carpal alignment results in better outcomes.

References

1. Rainbow MJ, Kamal RN, Moore DC, Akelman E, Wolfe SW, Crisco JJ. Subject-specific carpal ligament elongation in extreme positions, grip, and the Dart Thrower's Motion. *J Biomech Eng.* 2015;137(11):111006. https://doi.org/10.1115/1.4031580.
2. Mayfield JK. Patterns of injury to carpal ligaments. A spectrum. *Clin Orthop Relat Res.* 1984;187:36–42.
3. Cohen MS, Hotchkiss RN, Kozin SH, Pederson WC, Wolfe SW, Green DP. *Green's Operative Hand Surgery.* Philadelphia, PA : Elsevier; 2017. https://nls.ldls.org.uk/welcome.html?ark:/81055/vdc_1 00055965935.0x000001.
4. Berger RA. The ligaments of the wrist. A current overview of anatomy with considerations of their potential functions. *Hand Clin.* 1997;13(1):63–82.
5. Feipel V, Rooze M. The capsular ligaments of the wrist: morphology, morphometry and clinical applications. *Surg Radiol Anat.* 1999;21(3):175–180. https://doi.org/10.1007/bf01630897.
6. Berger RA. The gross and histologic anatomy of the scapholunate interosseous ligament. *J Hand Surg.* 1996;21(2):170–178. https://doi.org/10.1016/S0363-5023(96)80096-7.
7. Ritt MJ, Linscheid RL, Cooney WP, Berger RA, An KN. The lunotriquetral joint: kinematic effects of sequential ligament sectioning, ligament repair, and arthrodesis. *J Hand Surg Am.* 1998;23(3):432–445. https://doi.org/10.1016/S0363-5023(05)80461-7.
8. Mitsuyasu H, Patterson RM, Shah MA, Buford WL, Iwamoto Y, Viegas SF. The role of the dorsal intercarpal ligament in dynamic and static scapholunate instability. *J Hand Surg Am.* 2004;29(2):279–288. https://doi.org/10.1016/j.jhsa.2003.11.004.
9. Kapoor G, Heire P, Turmezei T, Chojnowski A, Toms AP. Perilunate injuries: biomechanics, imaging, and classification. *Clin Radiol.* 2020;75(2):81–87. https://doi.org/10.1016/j.crad.2019.10.016.
10. Inoue G, Miura T. Transscaphoid perilunate dislocation with a dorsal dislocated proximal scaphoid fragment. Report of 2 cases. *Acta Orthop Scand.* 1991;62(4):394–396. https://doi.org/10.3109/17453679108994481.
11. Budoff JE. Treatment of acute lunate and perilunate dislocations. *J Hand Surg.* 2008;33(8):1424–1432. https://doi.org/10.1016/j.jhsa.2008.07.016.
12. Rhind J-H, Gulihar A, Smith A. Trans-triquetral perilunate fracture dislocation. *Trauma Case Reports.* 2018;14:27–30. https://doi.org/10.1016/j.tcr.2018.01.003.
13. Alyamani AM, Alfawzan MF, Alhassan TS, Almeshal OM. Transstyloid, trans-hamate dorsal lunate dislocation: a case report. *International Journal of Surgery Case Reports.* 2019;61:96–98. https://doi.org/10.1016/j.ijscr.2019.07.011.
14. Mayfield JK, Johnson RP, Kilcoyne RK. Carpal dislocations: pathomechanics and progressive perilunar instability. *J Hand Surg Am.* 1980;5(3):226–241. https://doi.org/10.1016/s0363-5023(80)80007-4.
15. Severo AL, Lemos MB, Pereira TAP, Fajardo RDP, Maia PEC, Lech O. Trans-scaphoid perilunate fracture dislocation beyond Mayfield stage IV: a case report on a new classification proposal. *Revista*

Brasileira de Ortopedia (English Edition). 2018;53(5):643–646. https://doi.org/10.1016/j.rboe.2017.05.008.

16. Herzberg G, Forissier D. Acute dorsal trans-scaphoid perilunate fracture-dislocations: medium-term results. *J Hand Surg: British & European.* 2002;27(6):498–502.

17. Herzberg G, Comtet JJ, Linscheid RL, Amadio PC, Cooney WP, Stalder J. Perilunate dislocations and fracture-dislocations: a multicenter study. *J Hand Surg Am.* 1993;18(5):768–779. https://doi.org/10.1016/0363-5023(93)90041-Z.

18. Wickramasinghe N, Duckworth A, Clement N, Hageman M, McQueen M, Ring D. Acute median neuropathy and carpal tunnel release in perilunate injuries can we predict who gets a median neuropathy? *J Hand Microsurg.* 2016;07(02):237–240. https://doi.org/10.1007/s12593-015-0189-z.

19. Linn MR, Mann FA, Gilula LA. Imaging the symptomatic wrist. *Orthop Clin North Am.* 1990;21(3):515–543.

20. Jupiter JB, Nunez FA, Nunez F, Fernandez DL, Shin AY. Current perspectives on complex wrist fracture-dislocations. *Instr Course Lect.* 2018;67:155–174.

21. Inoue G, Kuwahata Y. Management of acute perilunate dislocations without fracture of the scaphoid. *J Hand Surg Br.* 1997;22(5):647–652. https://doi.org/10.1016/s0266-7681(97)80366-x.

22. Adkison JW, Chapman MW. Treatment of acute lunate and perilunate dislocations. *Clin Orthop Relat Res.* 1982;164:199–207.

23. Vitale MA, Seetharaman M, Ruchelsman DE. Perilunate dislocations. *J Hand Surg.* 2015;40(2):358–362. https://doi.org/10.1016/j.jhsa.2014.10.006.

24. Kim J, Lee J, Park M. Arthroscopic treatment of perilunate dislocations and fracture dislocations. *Jnl Wrist Surg.* 2015;04(02):081–087. https://doi.org/10.1055/s-0035-1550160.

25. Savvidou O, Beltsios M, Sakellariou V, Papagelopoulos P. Perilunate dislocations treated with external fixation and percutaneous pinning. *Jnl Wrist Surg.* 2015;04(02):076–080. https://doi.org/10.1055/s-0035-1550159.

26. Bhatia DN. Arthroscopic reduction and stabilization of chronic perilunate wrist dislocations. *Arthroscopy Techniques.* 2016;5(2):e281–e290. https://doi.org/10.1016/j.eats.2015.12.008.

27. Bain G, Pallapati S, Eng K. Translunate perilunate injuries—a spectrum of this uncommon injury. *J Wrist Surg.* 2013;02(01):063–068. https://doi.org/10.1055/s-0032-1333064.

28. Çolak I, Bekler HI, Bulut G, Eceviz E, Gülabi D, Çeçen GS. Lack of experience is a significant factor in the missed diagnosis of perilunate fracture dislocation or isolated dislocation. *Acta Orthop Traumatol Turcica.* 2018;52(1):32–36. https://doi.org/10.1016/j.aott.2017.04.002.

29. Liu B, Chen S, Zhu J, Tian G. Arthroscopic management of perilunate injuries. *Hand Clin.* 2017;33(4):709–715. https://doi.org/10.1016/j.hcl.2017.06.002.

30. Rettig ME, Raskin KB. Long-term assessment of proximal row carpectomy for chronic perilunate dislocations. *J Hand Surg Am.* 1999;24(6):1231–1236. https://doi.org/10.1053/jhsu.1999.1231.

31. Sotereanos DG, Mitsionis GJ, Giannakopoulos PN, Tomaino MM, Herndon JH. Perilunate dislocation and fracture dislocation: a critical analysis of the volar-dorsal approach. *J Hand Surg Am.* 1997;22(1):49–56. https://doi.org/10.1016/S0363-5023(05)80179-0.

32. Melone CP, Murphy MS, Raskin KB. Perilunate injuries. Repair by dual dorsal and volar approaches. *Hand Clin.* 2000;16(3):439–448.

33. Hildebrand KA, Ross DC, Patterson SD, Roth JH, MacDermid JC, King GJ. Dorsal perilunate dislocations and fracture-dislocations: questionnaire, clinical, and radiographic evaluation. *J Hand Surg Am.* 2000;25(6):1069–1079. https://doi.org/10.1053/jhsu.2000.17868.

34. Goodman AD, Harris AP, Gil JA, Park J, Raducha J, Got CJ. Evaluation, management, and outcomes of lunate and perilunate dislocations. *Orthopedics.* 2019;42(1):e1–e6. https://doi.org/10.3928/01477447-20181102-05.

35. Herzberg G. The treatment of perilunate injuries. *Jnl Wrist Surg.* 2015;04(02). https://doi.org/10.1055/s-0035-1550094. 075-075.

36. Meszaros T, Vögelin E, Mathys L, Leclère FM. Perilunate fracture-dislocations: clinical and radiological results of 21 cases. *Arch Orthop Trauma Surg.* 2018;138(2):287–297. https://doi.org/10.1007/s00402-017-2861-1.

37. Dunn J, Koehler L, Kusnezov N, et al. Perilunate dislocations and perilunate fracture dislocations in the U.S. Military. *J Wrist Surg.* 2018;07(01):057–065. https://doi.org/10.1055/s-0037-1603932.

38. Israel D, Delclaux S, André A, et al. Peri-lunate dislocation and fracture-dislocation of the wrist: retrospective evaluation of 65 cases. *J Orthop Traumatol: Surgery & Research.* 2016;102(3):351–355. https://doi.org/10.1016/j.otsr.2016.01.004.

39. Meijer ST, Janssen SJ, Drijkoningen T, Ring D. Factors associated with unplanned reoperation in perilunate dislocations and fracture dislocations. *Jnl Wrist Surg.* 2015;4(2):88.

40. Kremer T, Wendt M, Riedel K, Sauerbier M, Germann G, Bickert B. Open reduction for perilunate injuries—clinical outcome and patient satisfaction. *J Hand Surg Am.* 2010;35(10):1599–1606. https://doi.org/10.1016/j.jhsa.2010.06.021.

41. Minami A, Kaneda K. Repair and/or reconstruction of scapholunate interosseous ligament in lunate and perilunate dislocations. *J Hand Surg Am.* 1993;18(6):1099–1106. https://doi.org/10.1016/0363-5023(93)90410-5.

42. Apergis E, Maris J, Theodoratos G, Pavlakis D, Antoniou N. Perilunate dislocations and fracture-dislocations. Closed and early open reduction compared in 28 cases. *Acta Orthop Scand Suppl.* 1997;275:55–59.

43. Blazar PE, Murray P. Treatment of perilunate dislocations by combined dorsal and palmar approaches. *Tech Hand Up Extrem Surg.* 2001;5(1):2–7. https://doi.org/10.1097/00130911-200103000-00002.

44. Gupta RK, Kamboj K. Functional outcome after surgical treatment of perilunate injuries: a series of 12 cases. *Journal of Clinical Orthopaedics and Trauma.* 2016;7(1):7–11. https://doi.org/10.1016/j.jcot.2015.09.005.

45. Brown KV, Tsekes D, Gorgoni CG, Di Mascio L. The treatment of perilunate ligament injuries in multiply injured patients. *Eur J Trauma Emerg Surg.* 2019;45(1):73–81. https://doi.org/10.1007/s00068-017-0856-9.

46. Inoue G, Shionoya K. Late treatment of unreduced perilunate dislocations. *J Hand Surg.* 1999;24(2):221–225. https://doi.org/10.1054/JHSB.1998.0003.

47. Pappas ND, Lee DH. Perilunate injuries. *Am J Orthop.* 2015;44(9):E300–E302.

48. Forli A, Courvoisier A, Wimsey S, Corcella D, Moutet F. Perilunate dislocations and transscaphoid perilunate fracture-dislocations: a retrospective study with minimum ten-year follow-up. *J Hand Surg Am.* 2010;35(1):62–68. https://doi.org/10.1016/j.jhsa.2009.09.003.

49. Krief E, Appy-Fedida B, Rotari V, David E, Mertl P, Maes-Clavier C. Results of perilunate dislocations and perilunate fracture dislocations with a minimum 15-year follow-up. *J Hand Surg.* 2015;40(11):2191–2197. https://doi.org/10.1016/j.jhsa.2015.07.016.

50. Griffin M, Roushdi I, Osagie L, Cerovac S, Umarji S. Patient-reported outcomes following surgically managed perilunate dislocation: outcomes after perilunate dislocation. *HAND,* 2016;11(1): 22-28.

51. Weil WM, Slade JF, Trumble TE. Open and arthroscopic treatment of perilunate injuries. *Clin Orthop Relat Res.* 2006;445:120–132. https://doi.org/10.1097/01.blo.0000205889.11824.03.

52. Kara A, Celik H, Seker A, Kilinc E, Camur S, Uzun M. Surgical treatment of dorsal perilunate fracture-dislocations and prognostic factors. *Int J Surg.* 2015;24:57–63. https://doi.org/10.1016/j.ijsu.2015.10.037.

53. Herzberg G, Cievet-Bonfils M, Burnier M. Arthroscopic treatment of translunate perilunate injuries, not dislocated (PLIND). *J Wrist Surg.* 2019;08(02):143–146. https://doi.org/10.1055/s-0038-1667307.

54. Oh W-T, Choi Y-R, Kang H-J, Koh I-H, Lim K-H. Comparative outcome analysis of arthroscopic-assisted versus open reduction and fixation of trans-scaphoid perilunate fracture dislocations. *Arthrosc J Arthrosc Relat Surg*. 2017;33(1):92–100. https://doi.org/10.1016/j.arthro.2016.07.018.

55. Roberts D, Power DM. Acute scaphoidectomy and four-corner fusion for the surgical treatment of trans-scaphoid perilunate fracture dislocation with pre-existing scaphoid non-union. *BMJ Case Rep*. 2015. https://doi.org/10.1136/bcr-2015-209520. bcr2015209520. (Published Online).

56. Matthewson G, Larrivee S, Clark T. Case report of an acute complex perilunate fracture dislocation treated with a three-corner fusion. *Case Reports in Orthopedics*. 2018;2018:1–5. https://doi.org/10.1155/2018/8397638.

57. Muller T, Hidalgo Diaz JJ, Pire E, Prunières G, Facca S, Liverneaux P. Treatment of acute perilunate dislocations: ORIF versus proximal row carpectomy. *J Orthop Traumatol: Surgery & Research*. 2017;103(1):95–99. https://doi.org/10.1016/j.otsr.2016.10.014.

58. Russchen M, Kachooei A, Teunis T, Ring D. Acute proximal row carpectomy after complex carpal fracture dislocation. *J Hand Microsurg*. 2016;07(01):212–215. https://doi.org/10.1007/s12593-014-0162-2.

73

Technique Spotlight: Open Reduction and Repair of Perilunate Injuries

JEFFREY YAO AND BRIAN CHRISTIE

Treatment of perilunate injuries may be accomplished via a number of different approaches. Open repair of perilunate injuries can be accomplished via an all-dorsal, all-volar, or combined dorsal and volar approach. Due to the complexity of some ligamentous disruptions and the carpal relationships, many recommend a combined two-incision approach. In the combined volar-dorsal technique, the volar approach is used for reduction of the lunate, carpal tunnel release, repair of the volar capsular tear, and repair of the volar lunotriquetral ligament. The dorsal approach is used for repair of the scapholunate interosseous ligament and/or treatment of a scaphoid fracture in the case of trans-scaphoid injuries. Most injuries may be adequately addressed with a dorsal approach alone, images of which are included.

Indications

Indications for open management of perilunate injuries are very similar to those for perilunate injuries in general. That is, because of the poor outcomes of closed reduction and casting alone, all patients with Mayfield III/IV injuries should be managed operatively. Patients with all Herzberg stages may be treated via an open approach (Fig. 73.1).

Preoperative Evaluation

Timely diagnosis and treatment of perilunate injury is critical, as up to 25% of injuries are missed. Closed reduction of the dislocated distal row and lunate should be attempted immediately after adequate sedation and relaxation are achieved (Figs. 73.2 and 73.3). Assessment of any median neuropathy is mandatory. Dense, progressive median neuropathy that persists after reduction should prompt consideration of emergent surgical decompression of the carpal tunnel.

Standard four-view radiographs of the wrist (posteroanterior [PA], lateral, semipronated, and scaphoid views) are typically all that is required for the diagnosis of a perilunate injury. Disruption of Gilula's lines and a change in the configuration of the lunate on PA view from trapezoidal to a wedge or triangular shape indicate

carpal derangement. Computed tomography or magnetic resonance imaging may better characterize carpal displacement and ligamentous injury, although neither is necessary prior to reduction and repair.

Positioning and Equipment

Anesthesia of the wrist is achieved via regional block of the brachial plexus. The patient is positioned supine on the operating room table, with a standard hand table positioned with the shoulder at the midpoint of the table. An upper arm tourniquet is applied and the hand is prepped and draped. A standard power setup with 0.045- and 0.062-inch K-wires is required. A headless compression screw set is necessary for trans-scaphoid injuries.

Description of Technique

Dorsal Approach

A standard dorsal approach to the wrist begins with a 4- to 5-cm incision centered directly ulnar to Lister's tubercle, taking care to avoid branches of the sensory branch of the radial nerve (Fig. 73.4A). The extensor retinaculum is divided between the second and third compartments, and the extensor pollicis longus tendon is freed from its compartment and transposed radially. Dissection is carried ulnarly through the septum between the second and fourth compartments to expose the fourth compartment tendons as well. The fourth compartment tendons are retracted ulnarly and the second and third compartment tendons are retracted radially, exposing the dorsal capsule. A posterior interosseous neurectomy is then performed as a pain-relieving measure by dissecting and removing a 2-cm section at the base of the fourth compartment and cauterizing the proximal nerve (Fig. 73.4B).

The dorsal capsule/dorsal radiocarpal ligament is often found to be disrupted at its insertion onto the radius, and this tear is followed ulnarly and distally in line with the dorsal radiocarpal ligament. An incision is then made from the distal extent of the capsulotomy incision radially in line with

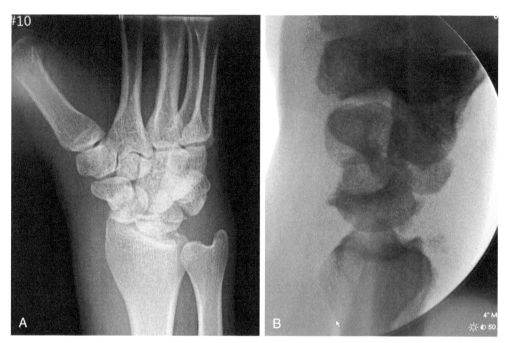

• **Fig. 73.1** Injury films: A 26-year-old male sustained a fall while skateboarding. Radiographs (A: PA and B: lateral) demonstrate a greater arc perilunate injury through the scaphoid waist, with disruption of Gilula's lines and rotation of the proximal pole of the scaphoid approximately 90 degrees. (Image courtesy Marc Richard, MD.)

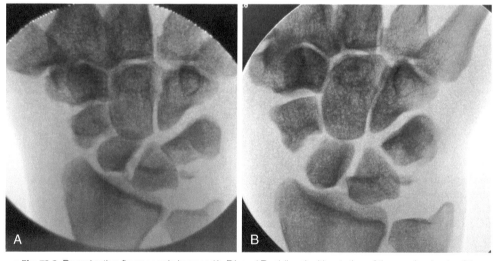

• **Fig. 73.2** Prereduction fluoroscopic images (A: PA and B: oblique) with rotation of the proximal pole of the scaphoid 90 degrees. (Image courtesy Marc Richard, MD.)

the dorsal intercarpal ligament, completing a Mayo ligament–sparing capsulotomy approach to the dorsal wrist (Figs. 73.5 and 73.6).[1] At this point, the pathology may be addressed in its entirety. If a combined dorsal/volar approach is required to address the volar pathology, the retractors are removed, moist gauze is placed in the wound, and attention is turned to the volar surface of the wrist.

Volar Approach (Optional)

The wrist is exposed volarly through an extended carpal tunnel incision, beginning 2–3 cm proximal to the distal wrist crease in line with the ulnar border of the palmaris tendon, and extending

in an angled fashion ulnarly across the wrist crease, in line with the radial aspect of the ring finger, to the level of Kaplan's cardinal line. This approach minimizes the chance of injury to the palmar cutaneous branch of the median nerve. The incision is carried through the antebrachial and palmar fascia to the level of the transverse carpal ligament. The transverse carpal ligament is divided sharply under direct visualization, exposing and decompressing the contents of the carpal tunnel. The flexor tendons and median nerve are retracted radially, exposing the rent in the volar capsule at the space of Poirier. If the lunate has remained dislocated, it is reduced directly back into the lunate facet of the distal radius using a technique identical to Tavernier's maneuver

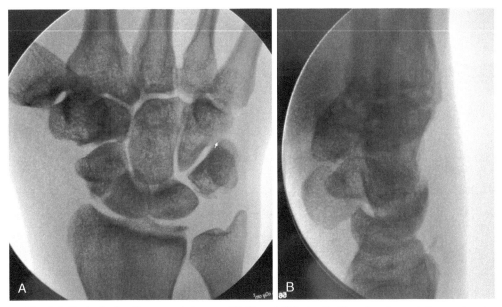

• **Fig. 73.3** Postreduction fluoroscopic images ((A) PA and (B) Lateral) with restored carpal alignment and reduction of the proximal pole of the scaphoid. (Image courtesy Marc Richard, MD.)

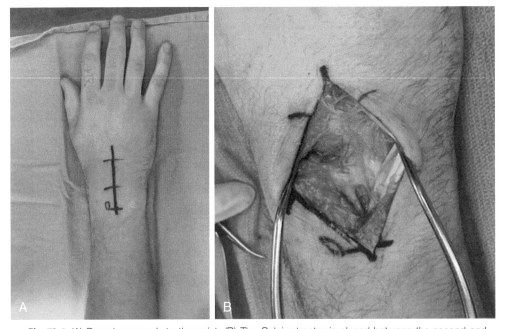

• **Fig. 73.4** (A) Dorsal approach to the wrist. (B) The Gelpi retractor is placed between the second and fourth compartments; the posterior interosseous nerve is visible on the dorsal capsule along the floor of the fourth compartment. (Image courtesy Marc Richard, MD.)

described for closed reduction. Interposed capsule prevents reduction of the lunate and should be removed, retracted, and repaired.

Fixation of Fractures

Greater arc injuries may be transulnar/radial styloid, trans-scaphoid, transcapitate, and/or transtriquetral. Scaphoid fractures may be reduced using dorsal joysticks, similar to the reduction method of the scapholunate interval, and

stabilized with a headless compression screw (Figs. 73.7 and 73.8). Reduction and fixation of capitate fractures are best approached dorsally, with care to adequately reduce the proximal pole of the capitate, which may be rotated as much as 180 degrees ("scaphocapitate syndrome"). Fixation may be accomplished via a headless compression screw, and primary bone grafting may also be indicated in cases of severe comminution. Triquetral fractures may also be stabilized using a headless compression screw.

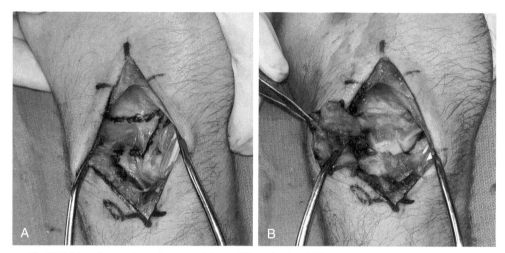

• **Fig. 73.5** Mayo ligament–sparing capsulotomy. ((A) marked and (B) capsule retracted). (Image courtesy Marc Richard, MD.)

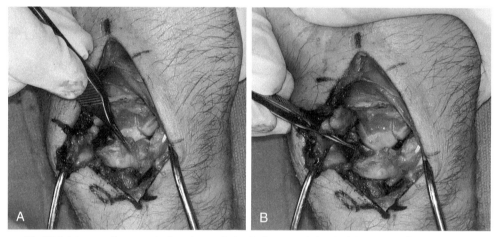

• **Fig. 73.6** Intraoperative examination demonstrates both a scapholunate interosseous ligament tear (A) and a scaphoid waist fracture (B). (Image courtesy Marc Richard, MD.)

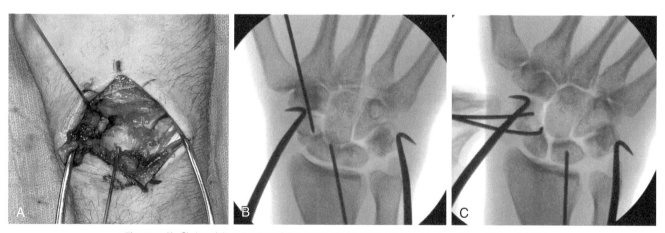

• **Fig. 73.7** (A–C) Joystick reduction of the scaphoid fracture. (Image courtesy Marc Richard, MD.)

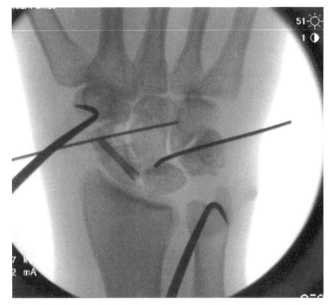

• **Fig. 73.8** Scaphoid fixation. (Image credit: Marc Richard, MD.)

Reduction of Carpus

Temporary radiolunate pinning (Linscheid maneuver) permits provisional lunate fixation in a neutral position while ligamentous repair is performed (Fig. 73.9). K-wires are then placed into the scaphoid and lunate from the dorsal exposure, to be used as joysticks to correct the intercalated segment deformity. Alternatively, a pointed reduction clamp may be used (Fig. 73.10). In particular, the scaphoid wire should be oriented at 45 degrees from distal to proximal, and the lunate wire at 45 degrees from proximal to distal, to facilitate reduction by extending the scaphoid and flexing the lunate. Once the scapholunate interval is reduced, four intercarpal 0.045-inch K-wires are placed from the (1) scaphoid to the lunate (two wires) and (2) triquetrum to the lunate (two wires). A pointed reduction clamp may be placed across the LT interval prior to K-wire fixation (Fig. 73.11). With stabilization of the proximal row, the joystick K-wires are removed and the midcarpal joint is reduced with dorsal to volar pressure on the distal carpal row, reducing the subluxated capitate back onto the distal lunate. Two additional 0.045-inch K-wires are placed from the (3) scaphoid to the

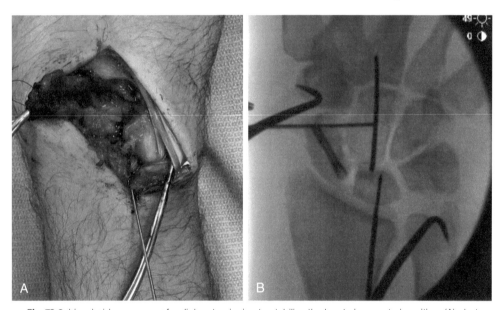

• **Fig. 73.9** Linscheid maneuver of radiolunate pinning to stabilize the lunate in a neutral position. (A) photo and (B) fluoroscopic image. (Image courtesy Marc Richard, MD.)

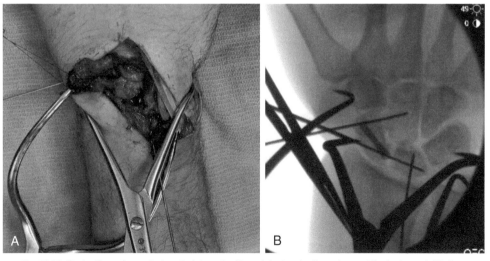

• **Fig. 73.10** Reduction of scapholunate interval with pointed reduction clamp. (A) photo and (B) fluoroscopic image. (Image courtesy Marc Richard, MD.)

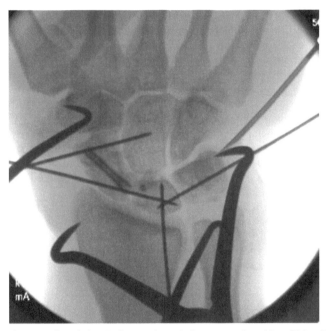

• **Fig. 73.11** Scapholunate ligament repair. (Image courtesy Marc Richard, MD.)

capitate and (4) triquetrum to the capitate. These result in a "diamond" configuration on PA fluoroscopy and stabilize the intercarpal joints in two separate planes (Fig. 73.12).

Repair of Ligaments

The strong dorsal scapholunate interosseous ligament is repaired via the dorsal incision. If the ligament is torn in its midsubstance, it is repaired using a 3-0 or 4-0 braided nonabsorbable suture (Fig. 73.13). In most circumstances, however, the ligament is avulsed directly off the dorsal lunate or scaphoid. In these circumstances, repair proceeds with one or two bone anchors onto the bone from which the ligament was avulsed. The volar lunotriquetral ligament is then repaired in a similar fashion through the volar incision.

Closure

The capsulotomy incisions and capsular rents are then reapproximated using a 4-0 braided nonabsorbable suture. The avulsed dorsal radiocarpal ligament is repaired back to the lip of the distal radius with a bone anchor. The extensor retinaculum is repaired, and the extensor pollicis longus tendon is left radially transposed. The skin is closed with nylon sutures volarly and a running 4-0

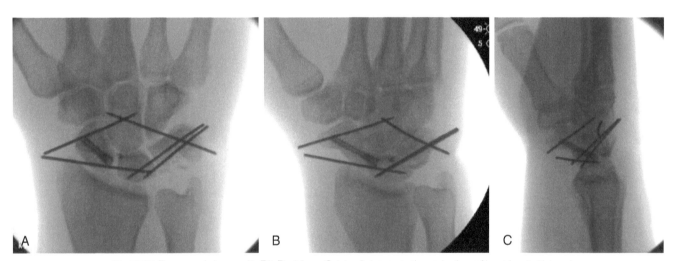

• **Fig. 73.12** Fluoroscopic images (A: PA, B: oblique, C: lateral) demonstrating reduction of lunotriquetral interval with pointed reduction clamp. (Image courtesy Marc Richard, MD.)

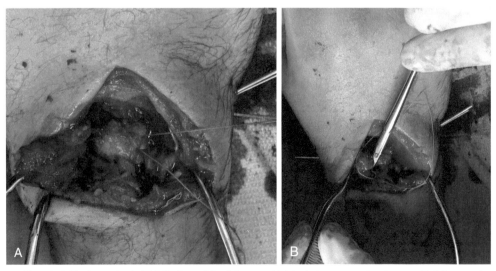

• **Fig. 73.13** Final construct: Stabilization of the intercarpal joints in two separate planes with intercarpal wires placed from the (1) scaphoid to the lunate, (2) triquetrum to the lunate (two wires), (3) scaphoid to the capitate, and (4) triquetrum to the capitate. (Image courtesy Marc Richard, MD.)

subcuticular monofilament suture dorsally. A thumb spica splint is placed with the wrist in 30 degrees of wrist extension and the patients are immobilized for 8 weeks after which the K-wires are removed and therapy is initiated.

Palmar Perilunate Injuries and Lunate Fractures

Palmar perilunate dislocations represent <3% of perilunate injuries,[2] and are often associated with fracture of the lunate.[3-5] Closed treatment is rarely effective and should be approached via combined open dorsal and palmar incisions as described above. The lunate fracture should be stabilized with a headless compression screw.

PEARLS AND PITFALLS

- Initial diagnosis is critical, as missed injuries are common and result in increased morbidity.
- Assessment should include closed reduction and determination of median nerve compression at each stage of treatment. Failure of closed reduction and/or progressive median nerve symptoms are an indication for urgent surgical management.
- Addition of the volar approach allows for carpal tunnel decompression, volar lunotriquetral ligament repair, and volar capsular repair.
- Radiolunate pinning (Linscheid maneuver) permits provisional lunate fixation in a neutral position while ligamentous repair is performed.
- Trans-scaphoid injuries may be reduced and stabilized with one to two headless compression screws prior to ligamentous repair. Scaphoid fracture with concomitant scapholunate ligament disruption, while rare, should not be missed.
- K-wire stabilization of the lunate should occur in two planes to minimize rotational instability.
- Hand therapy is critical in the postoperative setting to reduce swelling and stiffness and to maximize ultimate range of motion.

References

1. Herzberg G. The treatment of perilunate injuries. *Jnl Wrist Surg.* 2015;04(02):075. https://doi.org/10.1055/s-0035-1550094.
2. Herzberg G, Forissier D. Acute dorsal trans-scaphoid perilunate fracture-dislocations: medium-term results. *J Hand Surg: British & European.* 2002;27(6):498–502.
3. Bhatia DN. Arthroscopic reduction and stabilization of chronic perilunate wrist dislocations. *Arthroscopy Techniques.* 2016;5(2):e281–e290. https://doi.org/10.1016/j.eats.2015.12.008.
4. Meszaros T, Vögelin E, Mathys L, Leclère FM. Perilunate fracture-dislocations: clinical and radiological results of 21 cases. *Arch Orthop Trauma Surg.* 2018;138(2):287–297. https://doi.org/10.1007/s00402-017-2861-1.
5. Dunn J, Koehler L, Kusnezov N, et al. Perilunate dislocations and perilunate fracture dislocations in the U.S. Military. *J Wrist Surg.* 2018;7(1):57–65. https://doi.org/10.1055/s-0037-1603932.

74

Metacarpal Fractures

JED I. MASLOW AND R. GLENN GASTON

Introduction

The metacarpal bones make up the bony arch connecting the phalanges to the carpus and are one of the most commonly fractured bone in the hand.[1] Knowledge of the unique metacarpal anatomy, musculotendinous attachments, and surrounding neurovascular structures can allow surgeons to select the most effective and safe treatment individualized to each fracture. Several deforming forces act on the metacarpal head, neck, shaft, and base that lead to common patterns of displacement such as apex dorsal angulation and shortening. Special attention to thumb metacarpal base anatomy and common fracture patterns will lead to improved outcomes in these fractures. Nonoperative treatment is the mainstay for most metacarpal fractures, though many fixation options and approaches exist for fractures requiring surgical treatment. The ideal surgical treatment attains adequate alignment and stability while minimizing soft tissue disruption which can be accomplished with the use of percutaneous pinning, intramedullary devices, plates and screw constructs, and external fixators. When principles of metacarpal fracture management are followed, the outcomes are generally favorable with few complications. In this chapter, we will review the relevant anatomy, treatment options, surgical considerations, and outcomes of metacarpal fracture management.

Relevant Anatomy

The metacarpals are critical to the shape and function of the hand and serve as a framework to bridge the carpus to the phalanges. As the most proximal of the hand long bones, the metacarpals combine to form a concave arch in the palm. The bony anatomy can be divided into a head, neck, shaft, and base. The nonthumb metacarpals have a cam-shaped head that articulates with the proximal phalanx in a condyloid manner. This shape allows motion in flexion, extension, radial and ulnar planes. The metacarpophalangeal joint (MPJ) is stabilized by a fibrocartilaginous volar plate resisting hyperextension and a deep transverse intermetacarpal ligament connecting adjacent nonthumb metacarpals. This ligament, found approximately 2 cm proximal to the interdigital skin fold, is important in maintaining length stability in the setting of a more proximal isolated metacarpal fracture. The collateral ligaments provide varus and valgus stability to the MPJ. The proper collateral ligament travels at an angle of 30 degrees from the collateral recess dorsally on the metacarpal head to the proximal phalanx base. The accessory collateral ligament travels nearly perpendicular

to the joint inserting on the volar plate.[2–4] Testing the integrity of the proper and accessory collateral ligament can be performed at 30 degrees of MPJ flexion and full joint extension, respectively, to align with their anatomic orientation.

The nonthumb metacarpal shafts are triangular shaped with a flat dorsal surface that widens at the base.[4] The fifth metacarpal has the widest medullary canal while the second metacarpal has the longest length and largest neck width. Conversely, the ring finger has the narrowest intramedullary canal which must be considered during intramedullary fixation[5,6] The coronal plane alignment of the ring and small finger metacarpals is essentially straight while the sagittal plane apex dorsal bow is 12 and 10 degrees, respectively.[7] At their base, the metacarpals form a cuboidal shape and articulate with each other in addition to the distal carpal row. The mobility of the carpometacarpal (CMC) joints increases from radial to ulnar; the index and long finger CMC joints are more constrained with limited range of motion compared with the ring and small finger CMC joints with a much larger flexion-extension arc of motion. This allows powerful precision pinch and cupping of the hand.[3,8]

The muscular anatomy of the palm includes the interosseous muscles, the lumbricals, the thenar muscles, and the hypothenar muscles. The extrinsic extensor tendons are stabilized over the MPJ by the radial and ulnar sagittal bands originating from the lateral margins of the volar plate. The interossei muscles originate along the volar radial and volar ulnar faces of the metacarpal shaft and travel distally passing dorsal to the deep transverse intermetacarpal ligament. This ligament is continuous with the interosseous muscular fascia. Innervated by the ulnar nerve, the bipennate dorsal interossei impart a flexion and abduction moment and the unipennate palmar interossei impart a flexion and adduction moment to the MPJ. The lumbricals originate from the flexor digitorum profundus (FDP) tendons in the palm and travel volar to the deep transverse intermetacarpal ligament along with the neurovascular bundles. The four lumbrical muscles insert onto the radial extensor expansion and contribute to MPJ flexion.

Several other extrinsic muscles insert at the level of the metacarpals and can be a deforming force in the setting of a metacarpal fracture. Dorsal tendon attachments include the extensor carpi radialis longus (ECRL) and extensor carpi radialis brevis (ECRB) onto the base of the second and third metacarpals, respectively. The extensor carpi ulnaris (ECU) inserts onto the base of the fifth metacarpal. Additionally, the extensor digitorum communis (EDC) tendon to the index, long, ring, and small fingers is central over the respective metacarpal and the extensor indicis proprius

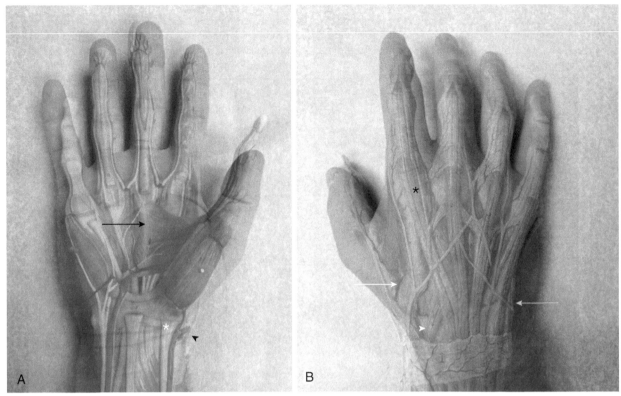

• **Fig. 74.1** Anatomy of the metacarpals with the extrinsic deforming forces highlighted. (A) The flexor carpi radialis inserts onto the base of the index metacarpal *(white asterisk)* and the adductor pollicis transverse head *(black arrow)* originates from the third metacarpal and inserts onto the ulnar thumb sesamoid and proximal phalanx. The radial artery *(black arrow head)* division into the volar and dorsal branches at the level of the radial styloid. (B) The extensor carpi radialis longus *(white arrow)* and extensor carpi radialis brevis *(white arrowhead)* insert onto the radial base of the second and third metacarpals, respectively. The extensor carpi ulnaris inserts at the ulnar base of the fifth metacarpal *(yellow arrow)* . Extensor indicis proprius tendon *(black asterisk)* is found deep and ulnar to the extensor digitorum communis tendon.

and extensor digiti minimi (EDM) are found deep and ulnar to the EDC of the index finger and small finger, respectively. On the volar aspect, the flexor carpi radialis (FCR) tendon inserts on the base of the index metacarpal and the flexor carpi ulnaris (FCU) inserts at the base of the small finger metacarpal, the pisiform, and the hook of the hamate. The adductor pollicis muscle, an important intrinsic muscle for pinch, comprises a transverse and oblique head that originates from the long finger metacarpal shaft and capitate, respectively. These two heads join to insert onto the ulnar thumb sesamoid, the base of the proximal phalanx, and the extensor apparatus (Fig. 74.1).[2–4]

The primary arterial supply to the hand originates from the radial and ulnar arteries. The radial artery branches into a dorsal branch and a volar branch at the level of the radial styloid. The dorsal branch crosses the anatomic snuffbox to then travel between the two heads of the first dorsal interosseous muscle and contribute to the deep palmar arch. Before penetrating the first dorsal interosseous muscle, this branch gives supply to the dorsal aspect of the thumb. The princeps pollicis arises from this contribution of the radial artery and supplies the palmar proper radial and ulnar digital arteries of the thumb and frequently the radial digital artery to the index finger. The volar branch contributes to the superficial arch. The ulnar artery gives a small branch to the deep palmar arch and predominantly contributes to the superficial arch. The superficial arch travels approximately 12 mm distal to the carpal tunnel with the deep palmar arch coursing more proximal. At the

mid-level of the metacarpals, the common digital arteries to the second through fourth web spaces arise from the superficial arch and subsequently bifurcate at the level of the MPJ to become the proper digital arteries. The ulnar proper digital artery is dominant in the thumb and index finger. The radial proper digital artery is dominant in the ring and small finger.[9]

The neuroanatomy of the hand comprises the median, ulnar, and radial nerves. At the level of the metacarpals, the median nerve exits the carpal tunnel to innervate the thenar musculature via the recurrent motor branch and the two most radial lumbricals via the common digital nerves. It courses dorsal to the common digital arteries to become the common digital nerves to the first, second, and third webspace. The ulnar nerve innervates the hypothenar musculature via the deep motor branch, the ulnar two lumbrical muscles, the adductor pollicis, and all of the interosseous muscles. The deep motor branch of the ulnar nerve and the deep palmar arch lie within close proximity to the volar surface of the metacarpal bones and are at risk of injury during fracture fixation, especially of the third metacarpal (Fig. 74.2). Sensory innervation to the fourth web space, the small finger, and the dorsal ulnar hand occurs via the common digital nerve, the ulnar proper digital nerve to the small finger, and the dorsal cutaneous branch from the ulnar nerve.[3,10]

The thumb is essential for normal hand function and its unique anatomy allows for prehension. The thumb metacarpal is a more cylindrical, shorter, and wider metacarpal and rests in a relative pronated position.[4,8] Distally, the MCP joint is a condyloid joint with a round, but less spherical head than the other metacarpals. The volar plate, proper collateral and accessory collateral ligaments function to stabilize this joint in a similar manner to the other digits. Proximally, the CMC joint is a biconcavoconvex joint with interlocking saddle shapes opposing one another and a notable beak at the volar metacarpal base. This anatomy allows abduction, adduction, flexion, extension, hitchhiker, circumduction, opposition, and

the ability to transition from unstable to stable. There are 16 named ligaments around the CMC joint, the most important of these for pinch is the dorsal ligament complex (comprises the dorsal radial and posterior oblique subligaments). The volar beak ligament also contributes to joint stability predominantly in a hitchhiker position.[11]

Important muscular and tendinous attachments to the thumb metacarpal act as dynamic stabilizers and potential deforming forces in trauma. The first dorsal interosseous muscle originates from the thumb metacarpal and inserts into the index finger extensor expansion to produce index finger abduction and thumb adduction.[3] The abductor pollicis longus (APL) inserts onto the dorsal radial base of the thumb metacarpal. The extensor pollicis brevis and longus cross the thumb metacarpal to insert onto the proximal and distal phalanx, respectively. Other muscles important to thumb function include the intrinsic thenar muscles, the abductor pollicis brevis (APB), flexor pollicis brevis, and opponens pollicis. Of these, the opponens pollicis inserts onto the volar radial thumb metacarpal and the flexor pollicis brevis and APB insert on the thumb MPJ capsule and radial sesamoid.[3,4,11]

Pathoanatomy

Metacarpal fractures are very common injuries affecting the hand and comprise up to 44% of all hand fractures. Fractures may be the result of a direct blow or axial loading.[2,12] An understanding of the relevant anatomy and the deforming forces is critical to effective nonoperative or operative treatment. In nonthumb metacarpal shaft fractures, the combined flexion moment on the metacarpal by the intrinsic muscles and strong extrinsic flexors typically leads to an apex dorsal angulation. The ECRL and ECRB can cause dorsal displacement of metacarpal base fractures involving the index and long finger, respectively (Fig. 74.3). The ECU causes the typical deformity seen in a reverse Bennett fracture of proximal and ulnar displacement of the metacarpal shaft.[4] Conversely, the intermetacarpal ligament imparts length stability to the nonthumb central metacarpals and prevents metacarpal shortening of >4 mm when fractured.[12]

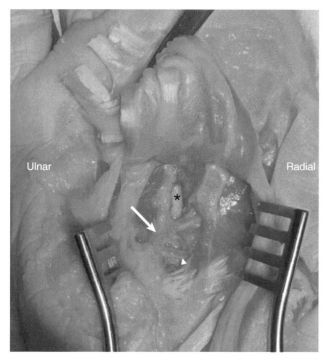

• **Fig. 74.2** Relevant neurovascular anatomy in the retroflexor space. The contents of the carpal tunnel have been cut and reflected to expose the deep palmar arch *(white arrowhead)*, the deep motor branch of the ulnar nerve *(white arrow)*, and the third metacarpal *(black asterisk)*.

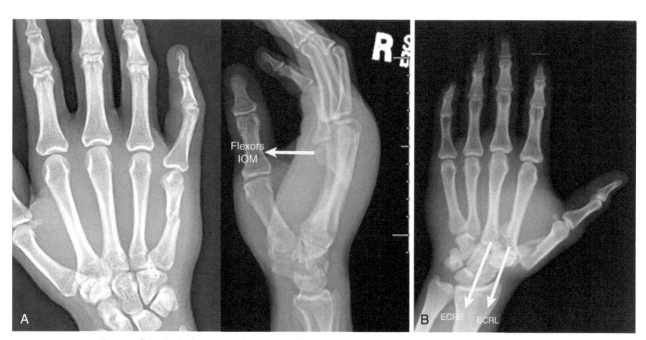

• **Fig. 74.3** Dorsal displacement of metacarpal base fractures involving the index and long finger. (A, B) Demonstrate a PA and lateral radiograph of a metacarpal shaft fracture with typical apex dorsal angulation and shortening. The shortening is limited by the transverse intermetacarpal ligament. *ECRB*, Extensor carpi radialis brevis; *ECRL*, extensor carpi radialis longus; *IOM*, interosseous muscles.

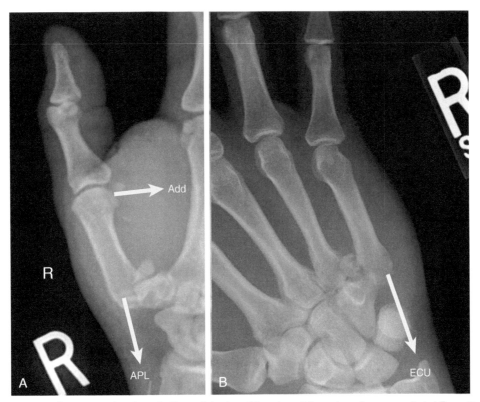

• **Fig. 74.4** Posteroanterior view of a Bennett fracture (A) and an oblique view of a reverse (baby) Bennett fracture (B) with the primary deforming forces. *Add*, Adductor pollicis; *APL*, abductor pollicis longus; *ECU*, extensor carpi ulnaris.

The deforming forces affecting the thumb are primarily the APL and the adductor pollicis. In thumb metacarpal base fractures, the Bennett or comminuted Rolando fractures, the APL pulls the metacarpal base proximal while the adductor pollicis pulls the distal fragment into flexion, adduction, and supination (Fig. 74.4).[4,13] The ligamentous attachment to the palmar beak fragment in Bennett's fractures is primarily the ulnar collateral ligament and to a lesser degree, the anterior oblique ligament.[14]

Metacarpal head fractures, although rare, often involve small fragments or articular disruption and risk osteonecrosis with operative or nonoperative treatment. Metacarpal neck fractures can result from direct axial blows, as in the common "boxer's fracture" involving the small finger. Often these injuries involve comminution of the volar metacarpal neck.[2,15] Typical apex dorsal angulation is seen just as in metacarpal shaft fractures. A "pseudoclaw" deformity may result from compensatory MPJ hyperextension and proximal interphalangeal (PIP) joint flexion due to an imbalance of extrinsic and intrinsic forces. Metacarpal shaft fractures may occur as transverse, oblique, or comminuted fractures depending on the mechanism of injury and are subject to angulation, rotation, and shortening. Metacarpal base fractures may occur as the result of a fall onto a flexed wrist with axial loading onto the metacarpal.[2,15] These fractures can present in conjunction with a CMC dislocation and may be intra-articular in nature. Injuries involving CMC fracture-dislocations are more commonly the result of a blow to a closed fist or involve high-energy mechanisms of injury such as a fall from height or motor vehicle accident. Due to the bony anatomy of the CMC articulation, the majority of fracture-dislocations displace dorsally despite the stout nature of the dorsal ligaments.[16]

Classification

Metacarpal fractures may be described as open or closed, intra- or extra-articular, or classified by fracture location, and orientation. The fracture location can be identified as the head (extra-articular or intra-articular), neck, shaft, and base (extra-articular or intra-articular). Metacarpal base fractures can be further described as those associated with CMC fracture-dislocations in the setting of CMC joint disruption. The fracture orientation can be a split, shear, or comminuted fracture in the setting of metacarpal head fractures. In metacarpal shaft fractures, the pattern may be transverse, long or short oblique, spiral, or comminuted. The displacement of each fracture pattern can be angulated, translated, rotated, or shortened.[17]

Other classification systems of metacarpal fractures have been devised and found to have good inter- and intraobserver agreement despite being used less commonly. One such classification is an extension of the AO Comprehensive Classification of long bone fractures. This system identifies the ray of the hand from radial to ulnar (1–5), the level of the hand bone (metacarpal, proximal phalanx, middle phalanx, distal phalanx), and segment of bone fractured (1–3). A letter further denotes the type of fracture pattern in extra-articular and intra-articular fractures.[18] CMC fracture-dislocations are described by the direction in which the dislocation occurs and the presence of associated fractures.[19]

The thumb metacarpal may be described in the same manner as the nonthumb metacarpals although two eponyms are frequently used. The partial articular fracture involving the volar ulnar base of the first metacarpal is termed a Bennett fracture. The term Rolando fracture was originally intended to describe a

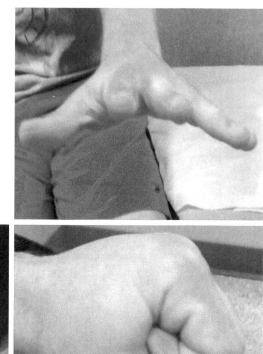

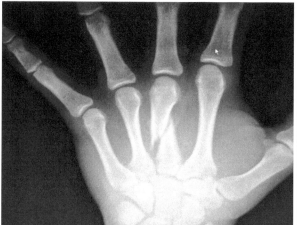

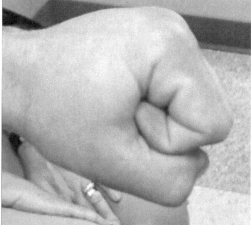

• **Fig. 74.5** Posteroanterior radiograph of a displaced midshaft long finger metacarpal fracture treated non-operatively. Clinical images show functional outcome after healing has complete range of motion without deficit.

Y-shaped base of the first metacarpal fracture with separate dorsal and volar articular fragments but is commonly used to describe any comminuted base of the first metacarpal fracture.[20]

Treatment Options

Traditionally, metacarpal fractures have been predominantly treated nonoperatively with success. The use of casts, splints, and braces protects otherwise stable fractures in amenable patients. Closed treatment can be performed with or without reduction. The necessity of immobilizing has been challenged in recent literature for some fracture patterns. For minimally displaced metacarpal shaft fractures, immediate active protected mobilization in the form of buddy taping for 4 weeks has been trialed with reliable healing and adequate return of grip strength at 2 months after injury.[21] There is a paucity of literature supporting one form of immobilization over another or that any immobilization produces superior functional outcomes to buddy taping despite more time off work (Fig. 74.5).[22–25]

If a reduction is attempted for an apex dorsal angulated metacarpal neck or shaft fracture, the classic maneuver is the Jahss maneuver. A local anesthetic hematoma block is administered into the fracture site and a dorsally directed force is applied to the proximal phalanx as the MPJ and PIPJ are both flexed to 90 degrees. After reduction, the hand was classically immobilized with the MPJ held in flexion though similar outcomes have been shown whether the MPJ is held in flexion or extension.[26]

When operative treatment is required, several options are available. The ideal treatment modality depends on both patient and fracture characteristics. Relatively simple to perform, closed reduction and percutaneous fixation has been performed successfully for metacarpal fractures of all patterns and levels. The primary advantages of percutaneous pinning are the relative ease, cost-effectiveness, and minimal soft tissue injury incurred in conjunction with either a closed reduction or a limited open reduction. Pinning may be performed antegrade, retrograde, transverse, or bouquet. Single or multiple pins may be used and these may be left exposed outside of the skin or buried.[27–29] Pinning can be combined with open reduction in CMC fracture-dislocations and provide reliably good radiographic outcomes if performed early (Fig. 74.6).[16] The primary disadvantage to percutaneous pinning is the risk of infection with exposed pins and the relatively limited rigidity that requires more conservative postoperative immobilization.[4]

Another method of osteosynthesis with minimal soft tissue damage is intramedullary fixation. Traditionally this was performed using intramedullary K-wires that acted as an internal splint. Angulation can be effectively controlled, though shortening and malrotation can still occur. More recently, retrograde screws have gained popularity and allow for fixation of metacarpal neck, shaft, or base fractures with superior biomechanical strength to crossing K-wires and minimal complications.[30–32] Some other advantages of intramedullary screw fixation include the ability to allow immediate postoperative motion without prominent hardware or the need for subsequent hardware removal.[33–35] The ideal

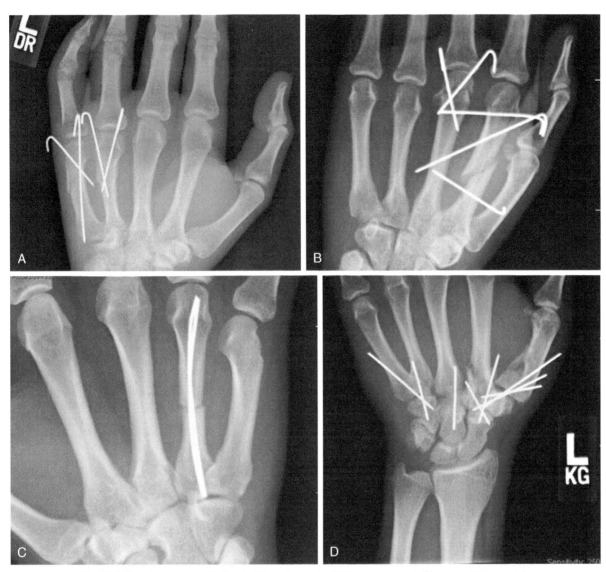

• **Fig. 74.6** Percutaneous pin fixation in (A) a retrograde, (B) transverse, and (C) bouquet intramedullary manner. (D) Pin fixation can be combined with open reduction for carpometacarpal fracture-dislocation.

fracture pattern for fixation with an intramedullary screw is transverse, although it can be effective in many oblique or comminuted fractures (Fig. 74.7). Special attention to length, alignment, and rotation in these patterns is essential to attain optimal outcomes.

Open treatment of metacarpal fractures can include osteosynthesis with K-wire pin fixation, screw fixation alone, or plate fixation. Traditionally, lag screws are indicated in spiral or oblique fractures with a fracture length equal to or greater than twice the cortical diameter of the metacarpal. When performed, two 2.0-mm interfragmentary screws have shown increased biomechanical strength compared with using three 1.5-mm screws for fixation.[36] Bicortical interfragmentary screws may offer comparable strength to a lag screw technique without as much risk for fracture propagation or displacement.[37] Plate and screw fixation offers superior biomechanical strength to the other methods of fixation at the expense of requiring a larger dissection with the risk of prominence, stiffness, or removal. When lag screw fixation is performed, a neutralization plate may be placed of similar size for additional strength. Importantly, dorsal plating should contour to the dorsal curvature of the metacarpal and can be placed in compression for

transverse fractures. Locked plating has been shown to be more stable than nonlocked plating. Modern three-dimensional plating includes double-row or multiplane plates that allow for shorter plates with staggered screw placement. These plates have even stronger biomechanical properties, specifically increased resistance to failure with less surgical dissection (Fig. 74.8).[38–40] Despite the clear increased strength advantage, plate fixation has also been associated with less postoperative motion compared with pin fixation, presumably due to increased soft tissue insult.[41]

In the setting of polytrauma, severe comminution, or severe soft tissue injury, external fixation may be appropriate as a temporizing measure or definitive fixation. Fixation from the proximal metacarpal or carpus to the phalanges can bridge significant defects or suspected infection. In comminuted or pilon-type articular fractures, the external fixator can be a useful tool to attain and maintain reduction via ligamentotaxis (Fig. 74.9).[4] Frequently when multiple metacarpals are fractured, a combination of several different techniques may be employed for optimal fixation while allowing range of motion in certain digits that may be amenable while applying increased rigidity in others. Other techniques for severe injuries with

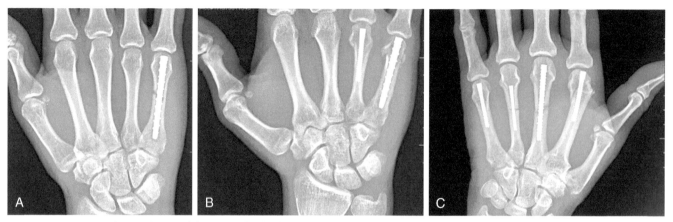

• **Fig. 74.7** Intramedullary screw fixation for variable shaft fracture location and morphology. Screw fixation for a (A) short oblique shaft fracture, (B) neck fracture, and (C) multiple adjacent metacarpal fractures of shaft and neck.

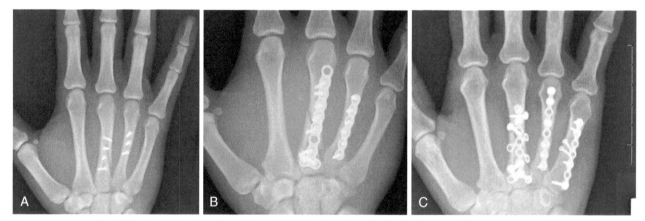

• **Fig. 74.8** Open internal fixation methods including lag screw fixation for (A) long oblique fractures or (B) plate fixation with two-dimensional or (C) three-dimensional plate options.

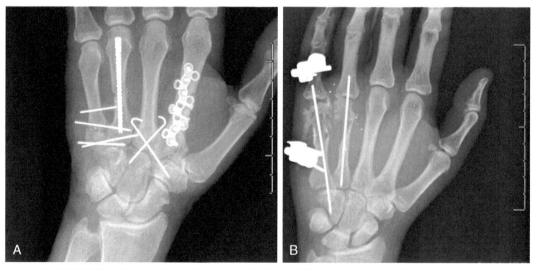

• **Fig. 74.9** (A) Combined methods of metacarpal fixation and (B) use of an external fixator and intramedullary pin fixation for temporary fixation of comminuted metacarpal head and neck fractures.

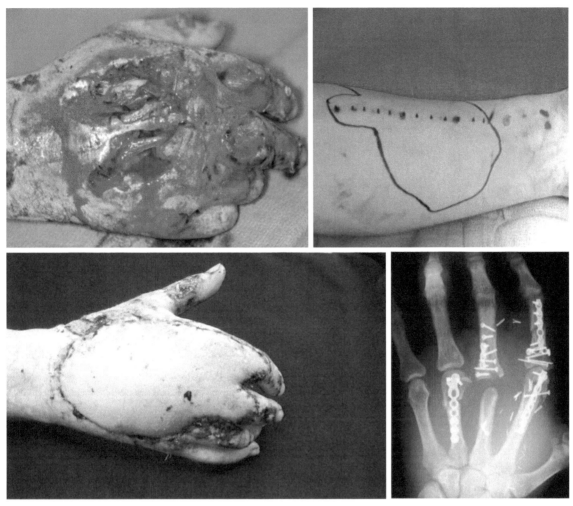

• **Fig. 74.10** Severe soft tissue injury associated with multiple metacarpal and phalangeal fractures. After debridement, coverage required a reverse radial forearm flap and several modalities of fixation including plate osteosynthesis, screw fixation, and Tupper arthroplasty.

significant comminution or bone loss include silicone arthroplasty, volar plate interposition (Tupper arthroplasty), ray resection with or without transposition, iliac crest bone grafting, Masquelet with subsequent bone grafting, and rarely arthrodesis (Fig. 74.10).[42,43] The volar plate interpositional arthroplasty is a useful salvage option for metacarpal head injuries with significant bone loss after ballistic injuries that can allow some MPJ motion. If bone loss is limited to a single metacarpal, the Masquelet induced-membrane staged technique with initial temporizing skeletal stabilization and cement spacer placement followed by cancellous autografting can effectively fill most defects in the hand. When multiple adjacent metacarpals are affected, iliac crest bone block grafting can fill the defect and offer adequate stability.

Future modalities for metacarpal fracture fixation in the United States may involve bioabsorbable implants. More frequently used in Europe, these implants have been shown to have comparable stability to traditional titanium implants without significant complications.[44] Previously, the most commonly reported complication was an aseptic inflammatory response occurring in the early postoperative period in roughly 5%–25% of patients.[45] As the material properties have evolved in newer generation implants, this rate has dropped to be as low as 2.4% when polylactic acid (PLA) or polyglycolic acid (PGA) implants are used instead of trimethylene carbonate/PLA.[46]

Indications for Surgical Treatment

The goal of treatment of metacarpal fractures is to restore anatomy to allow early range of motion and recovery of strength. Achieving this goal while preserving the aesthetic subunits of the hand will lead to functionally and cosmetically successful outcomes.[3] Several factors must be considered when deciding on surgical treatment including patient age, hand dominance, occupation, functional demands, mechanism of injury, time of injury, and prior trauma. In addition to a detailed history, physical examination and radiographic evaluation are critical to determining the stability of fractures and subsequent treatment. A detailed neurovascular examination is essential and associated soft tissue injuries should be assessed. Initial radiographic evaluation involves posteroanterior (PA), lateral, and oblique views of the hand. The hand may need to be supinated or pronated to view the true lateral of the affected ulnar or radial metacarpal, respectively.[17] Specialty views include the Roberts, Betts, and Brewerton views. The Roberts view shows an anteroposterior view of the thumb, the Betts view shows a true lateral of the thumb CMC joint, and the Brewerton view shows the metacarpal heads.[4,13]

A clear indication for operative treatment includes open fractures in the setting of significant soft tissue disruption or contamination. Multiple adjacent metacarpal fractures cause a disruption

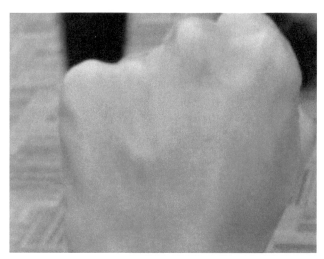

• **Fig. 74.11** The appearance of a ring finger metacarpal shaft fracture malunion that has no functional deficit but has a noticeable dorsal bony prominence and loss of knuckle contour.

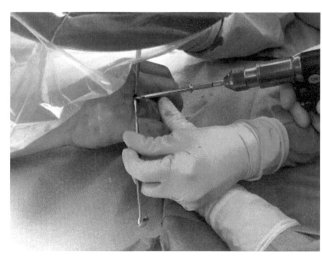

• **Fig. 74.12** Intramedullary screw fixation is performed through a dorsal incision with either a tendon splitting or sparing approach. With the digit flexed, the screw is inserted under fluoroscopic guidance.

to the inherent length stability and may be treated surgically to restore metacarpal height. Other high-energy injury fracture patterns such as segmental bone loss may also require operative intervention. Patients sustaining polytrauma may be indicated for operative treatment if they cannot tolerate immobilization or nonoperative treatment. Furthermore, open wounds overlying distal metacarpal fractures or the MPJ should raise concern for a clenched-fist "fight bite" injury. In this scenario, for early wound care, either operative or nonoperative, broad-spectrum antibiotics should be used for coverage of oral pathogens including *Streptococcus*, *Staphylococcus*, *Eikenella*, and *Corynebacterium*.[47]

The surgical indications for closed metacarpal fractures depend on which metacarpal is affected, the level of the fracture, the pattern of the fracture, and the degree of displacement. At the metacarpal head, intra-articular displacement (1 mm of step-off or greater) or comminution requires open reduction to restore congruity. If a block to motion is noted on physical examination or imaging reveals >25% joint involvement, open reduction may be required to repair osteochondral fractures.

Metacarpal neck and shaft fractures frequently displace with shortening, apex dorsal angulation, or malrotation. A small degree of shortening may be tolerated well by patients though cadaveric studies have shown that a 7-degree extensor lag results from every 2 mm of shortening.[48] In other studies, 5 mm of shortening or more may affect grip strength and displacement beyond 5 mm should be treated operatively.[49]

Angulation of the fracture can cause relative shortening of the metacarpal leading to an extensor lag. Alternatively, it can limit grip due to a prominent metacarpal head more volar in the palm. Angulation can also be aesthetically unappealing to the patient causing the loss of knuckle contour or the presence of pseudo-claw deformity (Fig. 74.11). Metacarpals with more mobile adjacent CMC joints, such as the fourth and fifth metacarpals and the thumb, can generally tolerate more angulation than the index and long finger metacarpal that have a relatively more constrained CMC joint. Additionally, the inherent ability to hyperextend roughly 20 degrees actively at the MPJ allows minor deformities to be overcome. The general indications for acceptable angulation at the metacarpal shaft and neck without leading to compensatory posturing or decreased function are: 30–40 degrees at

the thumb, 0–15 degrees at the index finger, 0–20 degrees at the long finger, 20–30 degrees at the ring finger, and 30–40 degrees at the small finger.[2,4,13] Some surgeons are more conservative in treatment indications in accepting small finger metacarpal neck angulation up to 70 degrees while others favor operative fixation for any angulated fracture >30 degrees, both reporting satisfactory outcomes.[12,50] It is important to note that measuring the angulation of metacarpal fractures, particularly neck fractures, can be inaccurate or inconsistent which can affect the type of treatment recommended.[51,52] Uniformly not well tolerated is malrotation in metacarpal fractures. Even a small degree of malrotation, 5 degrees, can lead to 1.5 cm of digital overlap and disrupt the normal cascade of composite finger flexion.[2] In general, any clinically observed malrotation is an indication for surgical intervention.

Surgical Approaches

The first discussion point in deciding on the most appropriate approach to treating metacarpal fractures is to discuss *where* to fix these fractures. With the popularization of surgical techniques with the patient wide awake under local anesthesia with no tourniquet (WALANT), these fractures may be amenable to safe, cost-effective treatment in a procedure room where the resources exist.[53,54] A recent cost evaluation of this model showed no significant differences in complications while attaining earlier fixation at a cost savings of over $2000 per encounter.[54] Several others have extended the indication from closed reduction and percutaneous pinning and have performed WALANT open reduction and internal fixation with plating or intramedullary screws with good results.[55–58]

Minimally invasive techniques of fixation such as intramedullary screw fixation can be performed through a small dorsal incision over the MCP joint for retrograde insertion. The extensor tendon can be split or retracted to one side after releasing a portion of the sagittal band to access the starting point on the dorsal third central aspect of the metacarpal head (Fig. 74.12). An arthrotomy is performed and the guidewire is inserted at a point where there is minimal contact between the proximal phalanx base and screw entry point.[59] In addition, a small dorsal approach to attain fracture reduction can be performed in addition to intramedullary screw insertion or percutaneous pinning techniques.

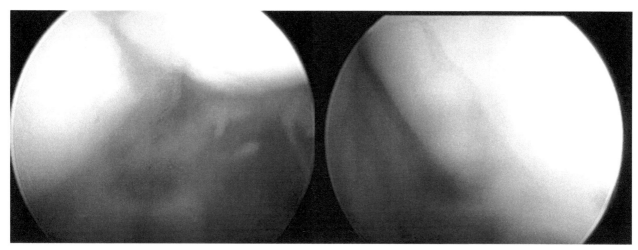

• **Fig. 74.13** Arthroscopic view of the base of the thumb metacarpal before *(left)* and after *(right)* reduction is performed and confirmed with direct visualization.

The majority of metacarpal fractures that require operative open treatment can be successfully approached dorsally. Metacarpal head fractures may be approached dorsally through an extensor tendon split or by dividing the radial or ulnar sagittal band with subsequent repair. Due to the innate ulnar pull of the extensor tendon and the reliance on the radial sagittal band to counteract this, it is recommended to divide the ulnar sagittal band if this approach is used to reduce the risk of extensor subluxation.[3] More proximally, the metacarpal shaft and base are easily approached dorsally by protecting subcutaneous dorsal cutaneous nerves and veins and subsequently mobilizing the overlying extensor tendon. The index and long finger metacarpal are found radial to the respective EDC tendon, the ring finger is directly beneath the EDC tendon, and the small finger is ulnar to the EDC tendon and directly beneath the EDM tendon. Juncturae tendinae are frequently encountered and can be incised and later repaired.[3]

A volar approach to the metacarpal can be particularly useful when treating metacarpal head volar shear fractures where the volar half of the metacarpal head needs to be accessed. The approach is performed through a standard Bruner incision centered over the MPJ with release of the A1 pulley.[60] When performing this approach in the setting of a fracture-dislocation, care must be taken to identify and protect the radial and ulnar neurovascular bundles as their superficial displacement may increase the risk of injury. The volar plate can be longitudinally incised to increase the exposure.

Displaced Bennett fractures can be approached through a dorsal approach similar to the nonthumb metacarpals, a Wagner approach, or through a direct volar approach with excellent fracture visualization.[50,61] Arthroscopy has shown promise as an adjunct to treatment of intra-articular fractures. While not frequently employed, arthroscopy has been described as a useful aid to visualize anatomic reduction of metacarpal head fractures with percutaneous pinning or internal fixation.[62] More commonly, it is used in the treatment of intra-articular base of the thumb metacarpal fractures (Fig. 74.13). Arthroscopy can be combined with traditional closed or open techniques for fixation to confirm anatomic reduction and assess the degree of cartilage injury (Fig. 74.14).[63] When comparing arthroscopically assisted percutaneous screw fixation to open surgery, arthroscopy use led to fewer complications and shorter operative times, though it may not eliminate the risk of late fracture displacement.[64,65]

Relevant Complications

Complications related to metacarpal fractures can be sequelae of the fracture itself, from the associated soft tissue injury, or from the stabilization technique. It is important to note that the risk of complications increases with open fractures and those fractures associated with significant soft tissue injury. Malunion can result from operative or nonoperative treatment and in extra- or intra-articular fractures. Malunion can occur in any of the planes of fracture displacement including angulation, rotation, and shortening. The rate of malreduction with some treatment techniques like percutaneous pinning is as high as 12%. Deforming forces acting on the metacarpal shaft fractures can lead to dorsal angulation malunion. The consequence of significant angulation can be pseudoclawing or grip weakness as a result of extensor lag.[2,66] Malrotation typically results from malunion in the setting of a spiral or oblique fracture pattern. Functionally, this becomes limiting when adjacent digital overlap occurs. Even a small degree of malrotation is not acceptable: 5 degrees of malrotation can lead to 1.5 cm of digital overlap.[66] Surgical correction of a malunion can be accomplished with a corrective osteotomy with or without bone grafting.

Infection may be superficial or deep. It is more commonly associated with open fractures and percutaneous pinning. In fact, the rate of infection associated with K-wires is relatively high if buried (4.1%–8.7%) or exposed (6.5%–17.6%), though exposed K-wires can lead to infection as much as two times more frequently.[67,68] Progression of infection to osteomyelitis is rare though the risk of amputation is increased if treatment is delayed for >6 months or requires more than three procedures.[69]

Nonunion rarely occurs at the level of the metacarpal. When it does occur, it is more commonly atrophic and associated with bone loss or infection.[70] Nonunion is typically diagnosed at 4 months but the diagnosis can be challenging because radiolucent lines may be present up to 14 months after injury and pain may be present for 1 year in healing fractures.[17] Ultimately, a combination of imaging and physical examination may lead to the diagnosis of nonunion. Treatment may involve revision osteosynthesis in the case of hypertrophic nonunion or revision fixation with bone graft in the case of atrophic nonunion (Fig. 74.15).[66]

Stiffness is most frequently observed after metacarpal fractures and can be a result of several factors. Significant soft tissue

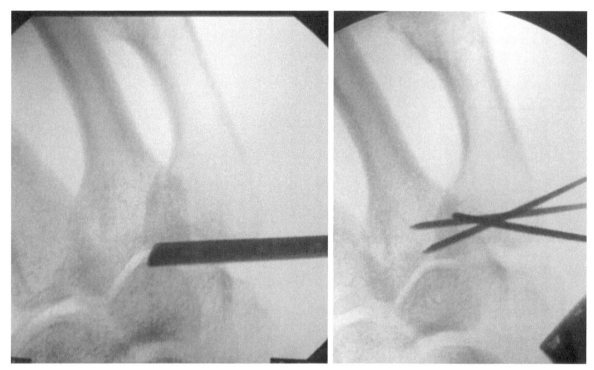

• **Fig. 74.14** Percutaneous fixation of a thumb metacarpal base fracture with the use of arthroscopy. On the *left*, the arthroscope is used to visualize the volar fragment and fixation is performed under direct visualization.

damage, intrinsic muscle dysfunction or contracture, or prolonged immobilization can negatively affect postinjury range of motion. While uncommon in isolated metacarpal fractures, tendon adhesions can occur between the extensor tendon and dorsal bony surface that may ultimately require tenolysis should therapy not succeed in attaining a functional range of motion. Metacarpal head fractures may limit the range of motion if there is an articular malunion with a block to motion or if posttraumatic arthritis develops.[15,17]

Review of Treatment Outcomes

The nonoperative treatment of metacarpal fractures is typically successful with minimal morbidity provided rotation is correct. Even a small amount of metacarpal deformity is tolerated well by patients secondary to the ability of adjacent digits to stabilize and the large arc of motion of adjacent joints to compensate. As mentioned, angulation up to 70 degrees in the ulnar digits and shortening of roughly 5 mm may be treated nonoperatively.[71,72] In fact, several reports advocate that only about 5% of metacarpal fractures require open surgical reduction and those treated nonoperatively have almost uniformly normal functional and aesthetic outcomes.[73,74]

Operative treatment, when indicated, produces good results with a low complication rate. In comparing plate fixation to percutaneous pinning, a meta-analysis of 231 fractures found 12% higher total active motion (TAM) scores for percutaneous pinning and no significant difference in functional Disabilities of the Arm, Shoulder and Hand (DASH) scores, grip

strength, time to union, or complications.[41] Total grip strength at final follow-up reached 79%–87% of the contralateral side. Intramedullary screw fixation in metacarpal head, neck, and shaft fractures has also proven to be a safe and effective form of treatment.[34,75] A meta-analysis of 169 fractures with an average 11-month follow-up found an average TAM of 251 degrees, 96% average grip strength, and no cases of nonunion or serious complications.[76]

Base of the thumb metacarpal fractures are more commonly treated operatively than nonthumb metacarpal fractures due to risk of instability, arthritis, and first webspace narrowing. Operative treatment varies from closed reduction and percutaneous fixation with or without arthroscopic assistance to open reduction and internal fixation. Historical reports show the clinical outcomes in pain, range of motion, and strength to be similar between closed pinning and open reduction in these fractures when the articular surface can be reduced to within 1–2 mm.[2,77] Long-term evaluation of 62 Bennett fractures treated by K-wire fixation at a mean 11.5 years after injury reported a patient satisfaction of 94% without any salvage procedures necessary and a mean DASH score 3.0.[78] More recent comparisons between open reduction and internal fixation and closed reduction with pinning found no significant correlation in grip or pinch strength to the specific treatment type but higher pain scores and increased reoperations (20% vs. 7%) were observed in the open reduction cohort. Furthermore, this study confirmed that an articular step-off of >2 mm correlated to posttraumatic arthritis at 10-year follow-up more than the type of fixation chosen.[79]

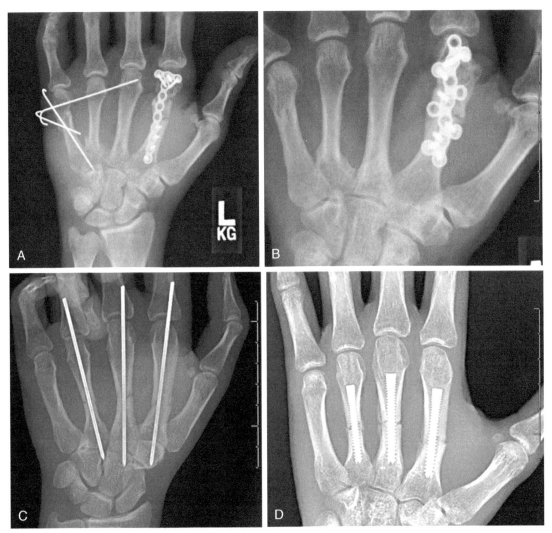

• **Fig. 74.15** (A) A patient who underwent fixation of an index finger metacarpal neck fracture with plate fixation developed a nonunion. (B) It was treated with revision three-dimensional plate fixation and bone grafting. (C) A different patient underwent closed reduction and pinning for three adjacent metacarpal shaft fractures and developed a nonunion. (D) Revision fixation was performed with intramedullary screw fixation with compression.

References

1. Nakashian MN, Pointer L, Owens BD, Wolf JM. Incidence of metacarpal fractures in the US population. *Hand (N Y)*. 2012;7(4):426–430. https://doi.org/10.1007/s11552-012-9442-0.
2. Diaz-Garcia R, Waljee JF. Current management of metacarpal fractures. *Hand Clin*. 2013;29(4):507–518. https://doi.org/10.1016/j.hcl.2013.09.004.
3. Watt AJ, Chung KC. Surgical exposures of the hand. *Hand Clin*. 2014;30(4):445–457. https://doi.org/10.1016/j.hcl.2014.07.004. vi.
4. Wong VW, Higgins JP. Evidence-based medicine: management of metacarpal fractures. *Plast Reconstr Surg*. 2017;140(1):140e–151e. https://doi.org/10.1097/PRS.0000000000003470.
5. Sephien A, Bethel CF, Doyle CM, Gulick D, Smith CJ, Schwartz-Fernandes FA. Morphometric analysis of the second through fifth metacarpal through posteroanterior X-Rays. *Clin Anat*. 2020;33(7):1014–1018. https://doi.org/10.1002/ca.23528.
6. Duarte ML, Nóbrega RR da, Prado JLM de A, Scoppetta LCD. Metacarpal stress fracture in amateur tennis player—an uncommon fracture. *Rev Bras Ortop*. 2017;52(5):608–611. https://doi.org/10.1016/j.rboe.2017.07.006.
7. Rivlin M, Kim N, Lutsky KF, Beredjiklian PK. Measurement of the radiographic anatomy of the small and ring metacarpals using computerized tomography scans. *Hand (N Y)*. 2015;10(4):756–761. https://doi.org/10.1007/s11552-015-9766-7.
8. Panchal-Kildare S, Malone K. Skeletal anatomy of the hand. *Hand Clin*. 2013;29(4):459–471. https://doi.org/10.1016/j.hcl.2013.08.001.
9. Leversedge FJ, Goldfarb CA, Boyer MI. *A Pocketbook Manual of Hand and Upper Extremity Anatomy: Primus Manus*. Philadelphia: Wolters Kluwer/Lippincott Williams & Wilkins; 2010.
10. Bertelli JA, Soldado F, Rodrígues-Baeza A, Ghizoni MF. Transferring the motor branch of the opponens pollicis to the terminal division of the deep branch of the ulnar nerve for pinch reconstruction. *J Hand Surg*. 2019;44(1):9–17. https://doi.org/10.1016/j.jhsa.2018.09.010.
11. Edmunds JO. Current concepts of the anatomy of the thumb trapeziometacarpal joint. *J Hand Surg*. 2011;36(1):170–182. https://doi.org/10.1016/j.jhsa.2010.10.029.
12. Kollitz KM, Hammert WC, Vedder NB, Huang JI. Metacarpal fractures: treatment and complications. *Hand (N Y)*. 2014;9(1):16–23. https://doi.org/10.1007/s11552-013-9562-1.
13. Bloom JMP, Hammert WC. Evidence-based medicine: metacarpal fractures. *Plast Reconstr Surg*. 2014;133(5):1252–1260. https://doi.org/10.1097/PRS.0000000000000095.

14. Kang JR, Behn AW, Messana J, Ladd AL. Bennett fractures: a biomechanical model and relevant ligamentous anatomy. *J Hand Surg.* 2019;44(2):154.e1–154.e5. https://doi.org/10.1016/j.jhsa.2018.04.024.

15. Wolfe S, Pederson W, Hotchkiss R, Kozin S, Cohen M. In: *Green's Operative Hand Surgery.* 7th ed. Philadelphia: Elsevier; 2016.

16. Steinmetz G, Corning E, Hulse T, et al. Carpometacarpal fracture-dislocations: a retrospective review of injury characteristics and radiographic outcomes. *Hand (N Y).* 2019;16(3):362–367. https://doi.org/10.1177/1558944719852743. 1558944719852743.

17. Cotterell IH, Richard MJ. Metacarpal and phalangeal fractures in athletes. *Clin Sports Med.* 2015;34(1):69–98. https://doi.org/10.1016/j.csm.2014.09.009.

18. Szwebel J-D, Ehlinger V, Pinsolle V, Bruneteau P, Pélissier P, Salmi L-R. Reliability of a classification of fractures of the hand based on the AO comprehensive classification system. *J Hand Surg Eur.* 2010;35(5):392–395. https://doi.org/10.1177/1753193409355256.

19. Pundkare G, Deshpande S. Proposal for a radiological classification system for carpo-metacarpal joint dislocations with or without fractures. *Malays Orthop J.* 2018;12(2):42–46. https://doi.org/10.5704/MOJ.1807.008.

20. Caldwell RA, Shorten PL, Morrell NT. Common upper extremity fracture eponyms: a look into what they really mean. *J Hand Surg.* 2019;44(4):331–334. https://doi.org/10.1016/j.jhsa.2018.07.012.

21. Jardin E, Pechin C, Rey P-B, Uhring J, Obert L. Functional treatment of metacarpal diaphyseal fractures by buddy taping: a prospective single-center study. *Hand Surg Rehabil.* 2016;35(1):34–39. https://doi.org/10.1016/j.hansur.2015.12.001.

22. Pellatt R, Fomin I, Pienaar C, et al. Is buddy taping as effective as plaster immobilization for adults with an uncomplicated neck of fifth metacarpal fracture? A randomized controlled trial. *Ann Emerg Med.* 2019;74(1):88–97. https://doi.org/10.1016/j.annemergmed.2019.01.032.

23. Dunn JC, Kusnezov N, Orr JD, Pallis M, Mitchell JS. The Boxer's fracture: splint immobilization is not necessary. *Orthopedics.* 2016;39(3):188–192. https://doi.org/10.3928/01477447-20160315-05.

24. van Aaken J, Fusetti C, Luchina S, et al. Fifth metacarpal neck fractures treated with soft wrap/buddy taping compared to reduction and casting: results of a prospective, multicenter, randomized trial. *Arch Orthop Trauma Surg.* 2016;136(1):135–142. https://doi.org/10.1007/s00402-015-2361-0.

25. Kaynak G, Botanlioglu H, Caliskan M, et al. Comparison of functional metacarpal splint and ulnar gutter splint in the treatment of fifth metacarpal neck fractures: a prospective comparative study. *BMC Musculoskelet Disord.* 2019;20(1):169. https://doi.org/10.1186/s12891-019-2556-6.

26. Hofmeister EP, Kim J, Shin AY. Comparison of 2 methods of immobilization of fifth metacarpal neck fractures: a prospective randomized study. *J Hand Surg.* 2008;33(8):1362–1368. https://doi.org/10.1016/j.jhsa.2008.04.010.

27. Potenza V, Caterini R, De Maio F, Bisicchia S, Farsetti P. Fractures of the neck of the fifth metacarpal bone. Medium-term results in 28 cases treated by percutaneous transverse pinning. *Injury.* 2012;43(2):242–245. https://doi.org/10.1016/j.injury.2011.10.036.

28. Foucher G. "Bouquet" osteosynthesis in metacarpal neck fractures: a series of 66 patients. *J Hand Surg.* 1995;20(3 Pt 2):S86–S90. https://doi.org/10.1016/s0363-5023(95)80176-6.

29. Yi JW, Yoo SL, Kim JK. Intramedullary pinning for displaced fifth metacarpal neck fractures: closed reduction and fixation using either an open antegrade or percutaneous retrograde technique. *JBJS Essent Surg Tech.* 2016;6(2):e21. https://doi.org/10.2106/JBJS.ST.16.00006.

30. Jones CM, Padegimas EM, Weikert N, Greulich S, Ilyas AM, Siegler S. Headless screw fixation of metacarpal neck fractures: a mechanical comparative analysis. *Hand (N Y).* 2019;14(2):187–192. https://doi.org/10.1177/1558944717731859.

31. Avery DM, Klinge S, Dyrna F, et al. Headless compression screw versus Kirschner wire fixation for metacarpal neck fractures: a biomechanical study. *J Hand Surg.* 2017;42(5):392. https://doi.org/10.1016/j.jhsa.2017.02.013. e1–392.e6.

32. Oh JR, Kim DS, Yeom JS, Kang SK, Kim YT. A comparative study of tensile strength of three operative fixation techniques for metacarpal shaft fractures in adults: a cadaver study. *Clin Orthop Surg.* 2019;11(1):120–125. https://doi.org/10.4055/cios.2019.11.1.120.

33. Warrender WJ, Ruchelsman DE, Livesey MG, Mudgal CS, Rivlin M. Low rate of complications following intramedullary headless compression screw fixation of metacarpal fractures. *Hand (N Y).* 2019;15(6):798–804. https://doi.org/10.1177/1558944719836214. 1558944719836214.

34. Ruchelsman DE, Puri S, Feinberg-Zadek N, Leibman MI, Belsky MR. Clinical outcomes of limited-open retrograde intramedullary headless screw fixation of metacarpal fractures. *J Hand Surg.* 2014;39(12):2390–2395. https://doi.org/10.1016/j.jhsa.2014.08.016.

35. Jann D, Calcagni M, Giovanoli P, Giesen T. Retrograde fixation of metacarpal fractures with intramedullary cannulated headless compression screws. *Hand Surg Rehabil.* 2018;37(2):99–103. https://doi.org/10.1016/j.hansur.2017.12.005.

36. Eu-Jin Cheah A, Behn AW, Comer G, Yao J. A biomechanical analysis of 2 constructs for metacarpal spiral fracture fixation in a cadaver model: 2 large screws versus 3 small screws. *J Hand Surg.* 2017;42(12). https://doi.org/10.1016/j.jhsa.2017.07.018. 1033.e1–1033.e6.

37. Liporace FA, Kinchelow T, Gupta S, Kubiak EN, McDonnell M. Minifragment screw fixation of oblique metacarpal fractures: a biomechanical analysis of screw types and techniques. *Hand (N Y).* 2008;3(4):311–315. https://doi.org/10.1007/s11552-008-9108-0.

38. Ochman S, Doht S, Paletta J, Langer M, Raschke MJ, Meffert RH. Comparison between locking and non-locking plates for fixation of metacarpal fractures in an animal model. *J Hand Surg.* 2010;35(4):597–603. https://doi.org/10.1016/j.jhsa.2010.01.002.

39. Tannenbaum EP, Burns GT, Oak NR, Lawton JN. Comparison of 2-dimensional and 3-dimensional metacarpal fracture plating constructs under cyclic loading. *J Hand Surg.* 2017;42(3):e159–e165. https://doi.org/10.1016/j.jhsa.2017.01.003.

40. Sohn RC, Jahng KH, Curtiss SB, Szabo RM. Comparison of metacarpal plating methods. *J Hand Surg.* 2008;33(3):316–321. https://doi.org/10.1016/j.jhsa.2007.11.001.

41. Melamed E, Joo L, Lin E, Perretta D, Capo JT. Plate fixation versus percutaneous pinning for unstable metacarpal fractures: a meta-analysis. *J Hand Surg Asian-Pac.* 2017;22(1):29–34. https://doi.org/10.1142/S0218810417500058.

42. Tupper JW. The metacarpophalangeal volar plate arthroplasty. *J Hand Surg.* 1989;14(2 Pt 2):371–375. https://doi.org/10.1016/0363-5023(89)90115-9.

43. Masquelet AC, Fitoussi F, Begue T, Muller GP. [Reconstruction of the long bones by the induced membrane and spongy autograft]. *Ann Chir Plast Esthet.* 2000;45(3):346–353.

44. Sakai A, Oshige T, Zenke Y, Menuki K, Murai T, Nakamura T. Mechanical comparison of novel bioabsorbable plates with titanium plates and small-series clinical comparisons for metacarpal fractures. *J Bone Joint Surg Am.* 2012;94(17):1597–1604. https://doi.org/10.2106/JBJS.J.01673.

45. Givissis PK, Stavridis SI, Papagelopoulos PJ, Antonarakos PD, Christodoulou AG. Delayed foreign-body reaction to absorbable implants in metacarpal fracture treatment. *Clin Orthop.* 2010;468(12):3377–3383. https://doi.org/10.1007/s11999-010-1388-3.

46. Hazan J, Azzi AJ, Thibaudeau S. Surgical fixation of metacarpal shaft fractures using absorbable implants: a systematic review of the literature. *Hand (N Y).* 2019;14(1):19–26. https://doi.org/10.1177/1558944718798856.

47. Shoji K, Cavanaugh Z, Rodner CM. Acute fight bite. *J Hand Surg.* 2013;38(8):1612–1614. https://doi.org/10.1016/j.jhsa.2013.03.002.

48. Strauch RJ, Rosenwasser MP, Lunt JG. Metacarpal shaft fractures: the effect of shortening on the extensor tendon mechanism. *J Hand Surg*. 1998;23(3):519–523. https://doi.org/10.1016/S0363-5023(05)80471-X.

49. Wills BPD, Crum JA, McCabe RP, Vanderby R, Ablove RH. The effect of metacarpal shortening on digital flexion force. *J Hand Surg Eur*. 2013;38(6):667–672. https://doi.org/10.1177/1753193412461589.

50. Xing SG, Tang JB. Surgical treatment, hardware removal, and the wide-awake approach for metacarpal fractures. *Clin Plast Surg*. 2014;41(3):463–480. https://doi.org/10.1016/j.cps.2014.03.005.

51. Leung YL, Beredjiklian PK, Monaghan BA, Bozentka DJ. Radiographic assessment of small finger metacarpal neck fractures. *J Hand Surg*. 2002;27(3):443–448. https://doi.org/10.1053/s0363-5023(06)90001-x.

52. Tosti R, Ilyas AM, Mellema JJ, Guitton TG, Ring D. Science of variation group. Interobserver variability in the treatment of little finger metacarpal neck fractures. *J Hand Surg*. 2014;39(9):1722–1727. https://doi.org/10.1016/j.jhsa.2014.05.023.

53. Gillis JA, Williams JG. Cost analysis of percutaneous fixation of hand fractures in the main operating room versus the ambulatory setting. *J Plast Reconstr Aesthetic Surg JPRAS*. 2017;70(8):1044–1050. https://doi.org/10.1016/j.bjps.2017.05.011.

54. Garon MT, Massey P, Chen A, Carroll T, Nelson BG, Hollister AM. Cost and complications of percutaneous fixation of hand fractures in a procedure room versus the operating room. *Hand (N Y)*. 2018;13(4):428–434. https://doi.org/10.1177/1558944717715105.

55. Feldman G, Orbach H, Rinat B, Rozen N, Rubin G. Internal fixation of metacarpal fractures using wide awake local anesthesia and no tourniquet. *Hand Surg Rehabil*. 2020;39(3):214–217. https://doi.org/10.1016/j.hansur.2020.01.003.

56. Nucci AM, Del Chiaro A, Addevico F, Raspanti A, Poggetti A. Percutaneous headless screws and wide-awake anesthesia to fix metacarpal and phalangeal fractures: outcomes of the first 56 cases. *J Biol Regul Homeost Agents*. 2018;32(6):1569–1572.

57. Hyatt BT, Rhee PC. Wide-awake surgical management of hand fractures: technical pearls and advanced rehabilitation. *Plast Reconstr Surg*. 2019;143(3):800–810. https://doi.org/10.1097/PRS.0000000000005379.

58. Poggetti A, Nucci AM, Giesen T, Calcagni M, Marchetti S, Lisanti M. Percutaneous intramedullary headless screw fixation and wide-awake anesthesia to treat metacarpal fractures: early results in 25 patients. *J Hand Microsurg*. 2018;10(1):16–21. https://doi.org/10.1055/s-0037-1618911.

59. ten Berg PWL, Mudgal CS, Leibman MI, Belsky MR, Ruchelsman DE. Quantitative 3-dimensional CT analyses of intramedullary headless screw fixation for metacarpal neck fractures. *J Hand Surg*. 2013;38(2):322–330. https://doi.org/10.1016/j.jhsa.2012.09.029.e2.

60. Melamed E, Calotta N, Bello R, Hinds RM, Capo JT, Lifchez S. Dorsal and volar surgical approaches to the metacarpophalangeal joint: a comparative anatomic study. *J Hand Surg Asian-Pac*. 2017;22(3):297–302. https://doi.org/10.1142/S0218810417500332.

61. Levy V, Mazzola M, Gonzalez M. Intra-articular fracture of the base of the first metacarpal bone: treatment through a volar approach. *Hand (N Y)*. 2018;13(1):90–94. https://doi.org/10.1177/1558944716685828.

62. Slade JF, Gutow AP. Arthroscopy of the metacarpophalangeal joint. *Hand Clin*. 1999;15(3):501–527.

63. Culp RW, Johnson JW. Arthroscopically assisted percutaneous fixation of Bennett fractures. *J Hand Surg*. 2010;35(1):137–140. https://doi.org/10.1016/j.jhsa.2009.10.019.

64. Pomares G, Strugarek-Lecoanet C, Dap F, Dautel G. Bennett fracture: arthroscopically assisted percutaneous screw fixation versus open surgery: functional and radiological outcomes. *Orthop Traumatol Surg Res OTSR*. 2016;102(3):357–361. https://doi.org/10.1016/j.otsr.2016.01.015.

65. Zemirline A, Lebailly F, Taleb C, Facca S, Liverneaux P. Arthroscopic assisted percutaneous screw fixation of Bennett's fracture. *Hand Surg Int J Devoted Hand Up Limb Surg Relat Res J Asia-Pac Fed Soc Surg Hand*. 2014;19(2):281–286. https://doi.org/10.1142/S0218810414970053.

66. Balaram AK, Bednar MS. Complications after the fractures of metacarpal and phalanges. *Hand Clin*. 2010;26(2):169–177. https://doi.org/10.1016/j.hcl.2010.01.005.

67. Terndrup M, Jensen T, Kring S, Lindberg-Larsen M. Should we bury K-wires after metacarpal and phalangeal fracture osteosynthesis? *Injury*. 2018;49(6):1126–1130. https://doi.org/10.1016/j.injury.2018.02.027.

68. Ridley TJ, Freking W, Erickson LO, Ward CM. Incidence of treatment for infection of buried versus exposed Kirschner wires in phalangeal, metacarpal, and distal radial fractures. *J Hand Surg*. 2017;42(7):525–531. https://doi.org/10.1016/j.jhsa.2017.03.040.

69. Reilly KE, Linz JC, Stern PJ, Giza E, Wyrick JD. Osteomyelitis of the tubular bones of the hand. *J Hand Surg*. 1997;22(4):644–649. https://doi.org/10.1016/S0363-5023(97)80122-0.

70. Ring D. Malunion and nonunion of the metacarpals and phalanges. *Instr Course Lect*. 2006;55:121–128.

71. Neumeister MW, Webb K, McKenna K. Non-surgical management of metacarpal fractures. *Clin Plast Surg*. 2014;41(3):451–461. https://doi.org/10.1016/j.cps.2014.03.008.

72. Shaftel ND, Capo JT. Fractures of the digits and metacarpals: when to splint and when to repair? *Sports Med Arthrosc Rev*. 2014;22(1):2–11. https://doi.org/10.1097/JSA.0000000000000004.

73. McKerrell J, Bowen V, Johnston G, Zondervan J. Boxer's fractures—conservative or operative management? *J Trauma*. 1987;27(5):486–490.

74. Zong S-L, Zhao G, Su L-X, et al. Treatments for the fifth metacarpal neck fractures: a network meta-analysis of randomized controlled trials. *Medicine (Baltim)*. 2016;95(11). https://doi.org/10.1097/MD.0000000000003059. e3059.

75. Eisenberg G, Clain JB, Feinberg-Zadek N, Leibman M, Belsky M, Ruchelsman DE. Clinical outcomes of limited open intramedullary headless screw fixation of metacarpal fractures in 91 consecutive patients. *Hand (N Y)*. 2020;15(6):793–797. https://doi.org/10.1177/1558944719836235. 1558944719836235.

76. Beck CM, Horesh E, Taub PJ. Intramedullary screw fixation of metacarpal fractures results in excellent functional outcomes: a literature review. *Plast Reconstr Surg*. 2019;143(4):1111–1118. https://doi.org/10.1097/PRS.0000000000005478.

77. Carter KR, Nallamothu SV. Bennett fracture. In: *StatPearls*. Treasure Island, FL: StatPearls Publishing; 2020. http://www.ncbi.nlm.nih.gov/books/NBK500035/.

78. Middleton SD, McNiven N, Griffin EJ, Anakwe RE, Oliver CW. Long-term patient-reported outcomes following Bennett's fractures. *Bone Jt J*. 2015;97-B(7):1004–1006. https://doi.org/10.1302/0301-620X.97B7.35493.

79. Kamphuis SJM, Greeven APA, Kleinveld S, Gosens T, Van Lieshout EMM, Verhofstad MHJ. Bennett's fracture: comparative study between open and closed surgical techniques. *Hand Surg Rehabil*. 2019;38(2):97–101. https://doi.org/10.1016/j.hansur.2018.11.003.

75

Metacarpal Fractures—Pins vs. Plates vs. Intramedullary Devices—When and How

CASEY SABBAG AND R. GLENN GASTON

Indications for Surgical Treatment

Metacarpal fractures can be treated nonoperatively or operatively depending on the fracture characteristics of angulation, displacement, rotation, and stability following reduction when applicable. The osseous and soft tissue anatomy of the metacarpals provides functional stability to many of the fractures that occur and contributes to the success of nonoperative treatment.[1–4] Absolute surgical indications include open fractures, open metacarpophalangeal (MP) or carpometacarpal (CMC) joints, significant malrotation resulting in digital overlap, and those fractures with associated soft tissue injuries such as tendon or nerve injuries necessitating repair. Relative indications for surgical intervention include excessive shortening (>5 mm) especially those with pseudoclawing, extensor lag, prominence of the metacarpal head in the palm, multiple fractures, and intra-articular fractures. The decision-making between three common surgical techniques will be considered: pinning, plating, and intramedullary (IM) devices.

Pinning

Closed reduction and percutaneous pinning is the most commonly used technique when a closed reduction is easily obtained. Advantages of the technique include its low cost, universal availability, being less technically demanding, and time-proven results. Disadvantages include pin tract infections, extensor tendon irritation, and the need for supplemental immobilization. This can be performed retrograde, transversely, or antegrade with a small open approach. Transverse pinning is typically reserved for border digits especially in the case of comminution, and it requires a stable adjacent metacarpal.

Plating

Dorsal plating with locking or nonlocking plates is best suited for transverse, long oblique, or spiral fractures of the metacarpal shaft and can be used in conjunction with interfragmentary compression screws if the fracture is a spiral or long oblique pattern. Typically, plating is reserved for cases where there is diaphyseal bone loss, comminution, significant soft tissue injury, or nonunion. Advantages of plating include earlier initiation of range-of-motion exercises, lessened need for immobilization, and a lack of exposed hardware. Disadvantages include higher cost, being a more technically demanding surgery, and irritation of the overlying extensor tendons.

Intramedullary Devices

IM fixation devices such as an IM compression screw, IM rods and nails, and IM K-wires are a versatile option that can be used on most length stable metacarpal fractures that do not involve the metacarpal head or base. This technique offers some unique advantages to the other options such as no exposed hardware externally, no irritation of the hardware with the extensor mechanism, a minimally invasive approach, and the ability for early range of motion with lessened need for immobilization. Disadvantages include implant cost (depending on the selected implant), technical demand, and an application limited to certain fracture locations and patterns.

Preoperative Evaluation (Imaging, Examination, etc.)

A thorough physical examination should first be performed. This includes attention to the presence of any open wounds (especially those over the dorsum of the MP joint suggestive of a "fight bite"), any clinical rotation or coronal plane malalignment, pseudoclawing, or neurovascular injury. Initial imaging studies in the evaluation of metacarpal fractures include posteroanterior (PA), lateral, and oblique views of the hand. Lateral views of each individual metacarpal can be difficult to obtain. These basic radiographic views are usually sufficient in diagnosing the majority of metacarpal head, neck, and shaft and base fractures. The Brewerton view offers an excellent anteroposterior (AP) of the MP joint and can be specified for each digit as needed. A semipronated oblique view is helpful in better visualizing the fifth CMC joint which can have subtle dorsal subluxation that is easily missed with routine imaging.

Positioning and Equipment

For all of the above methods of fixation, the patient is positioned supine on a standard operating room table with adjustable hand table attachment. The arm is prepped to the level of the elbow and a nonsterile tourniquet may be applied above the elbow. Surgeon and assistant are on either side of the extremity and mini-fluoroscopy can be introduced from either side.

Pinning

The necessary equipment for pinning includes nonthreaded K-wires which can be single or double-ended depending on the surgeon's preference as well as a wire driver and wire cutters. Typical sizes include 0.045-inch K-wires for most shaft fractures with 0.035-inch K-wires available for periarticular fractures and 0.062-inch K-wires at times for IM placement.

Plating

There are several options for metacarpal plating including 2.0-mm nonlocking and locking straight plates, H-, L-, or T-plates, and newer variable angle locking plates. The ideal plate will depend upon fracture characteristics and the surgeon's preference.

Intramedullary Devices

This fixation method utilizes IM screws (some manufactured specifically for metacarpals), IM nails, or IM K-wires. IM screw sets include a guidewire, drill, depth gauge, and variable width and length IM screws.

Detailed Technique Description

Pinning

Prior to inflating tourniquet, the reduction maneuver should be performed and checked with fluoroscopy to ensure that it can be easily performed by the surgeon and assistant and to expedite the maneuver quickly after the tourniquet is inflated. Given the apex dorsal angulation of metacarpal neck and many shaft fractures, closed reduction typically requires the Jahss maneuver where the MP joint is flexed to 90 degrees to relax the pull of the intrinsic muscles and collateral ligaments. Then a dorsally directed pressure on the metacarpal head is applied through the proximal phalanx base (Fig. 75.1).

Retrograde pinning is well suited for metacarpal neck and shaft fractures.[5] Two smooth K-wires are placed from distal to proximal starting in the collateral recess on the radial and ulnar aspect of the metacarpal head while the MP joint is held in flexion (Fig. 75.2). The trajectory is confirmed on fluoroscopic imaging, ensuring that the starting points are centered at the collateral recess of the PA view and in the dorsal one-third of the metacarpal head on the lateral view. The pins should be advanced into the distal fragment to the level of the fracture line. The fracture is then reduced as it previously was and the pins are advanced across the fracture site into the subchondral bone of the metacarpal base or bicortically into the shaft. Pin ends may either be cut external to the skin and bent to 90 degrees to aid in pin removal or cut beneath the skin. Full passive motion of the MP joint and proper rotation of the digit should be ensured. An immediate postoperative splint is placed, which is removed after 1 week and converted to a custom-made removal splint. Pins are usually removed after 3–4 weeks.

Transverse pinning is typically reserved for border digits with comminuted and length unstable fractures or metacarpal base fractures with associated fracture-dislocation (Fig. 75.3A–B). This

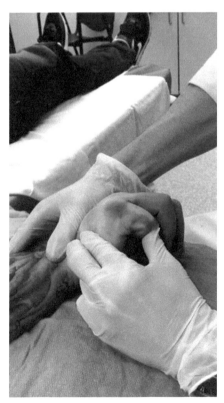

• **Fig. 75.1** Example of the Jahss maneuver used for closed reduction. The metacarpophalangeal joint is flexed to 90 degrees while dorsal pressure is transmitted to the distal segment through indirect pressure from the proximal phalanx.

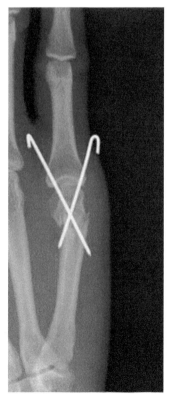

• **Fig. 75.2** Posteroanterior radiograph showing retrograde cross-pinning of the fourth and fifth metacarpal fractures.

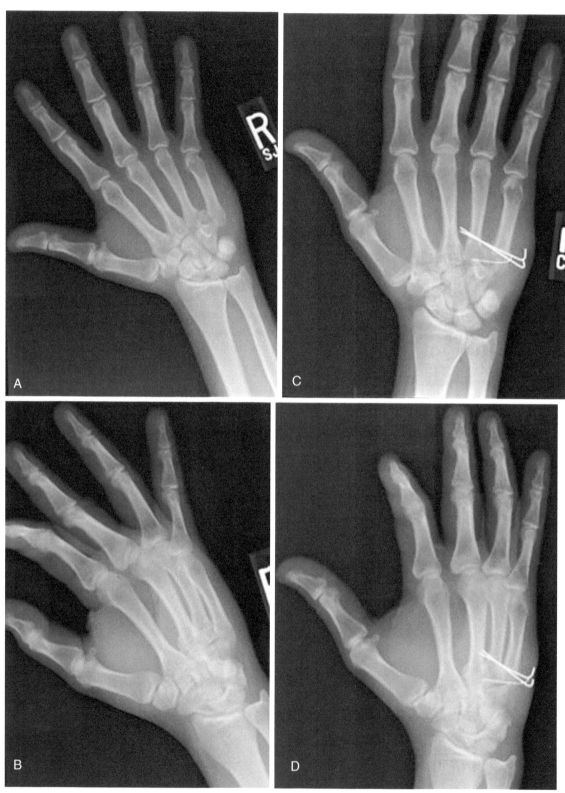

• **Fig. 75.3** Preoperative (A) posteroanterior (PA) and (B) lateral and postoperative (C) PA and (D) lateral views after transverse pinning which was utilized for this reverse Bennet's fracture. After it is reduced, it is pinned to the adjacent fourth metacarpal.

technique requires a stable adjacent metacarpal.[6,7] Longitudinal traction is applied to the digit to restore length and the distal fragment is pinned to the adjacent metacarpal to maintain length and rotation using two pins. The trajectory is typically volar to dorsal for pin placement owing to the arch-like configuration of the metacarpals (Fig. 75.3C–D). The proximal aspect of the metacarpal is then similarly pinned to the adjacent metacarpal with two K-wires. An immediate postoperative splint is placed, which is removed after 1 week and converted to a custom-made removal splint. Pins are usually removed after 3–4 weeks. In the setting of severe injuries, pins may be maintained longer depending on the clinical and radiographic healing.

Plating

If the fracture is spiral or oblique (Fig. 75.4A–B), lag screw fixation may be performed as mentioned and a neutralization plate may be added.[8] For transverse fractures, compression plating is utilized. The metacarpal fracture is approached dorsally with a longitudinal incision placed directly over or slightly radial or ulnar to the injured. If more than one metacarpal requires fixation, then an incision centered between adjacent metacarpals can allow access to both. The extensor tendons are retracted radially or ulnarly. Any juncturae that are inhibiting visualization of the fracture are divided and repaired upon closure. The periosteum is elevated and the fracture site is debrided. Care is taken to elevate a flap of periosteum that can later be used to cover the plate at the time of closure. Provisional reduction may be achieved with a combination of manual traction, reduction clamps, and K-wires. The appropriate plate is selected. In the setting of comminution, bone loss, or osteopenia, locked plating is preferred. A plate of length

allowing four to six cortices of fixation on each side of the fracture is selected.[9] If two-dimensional plating is performed, a straight plate may be cut to length and positioned onto the dorsal surface of the metacarpal ideally minimizing direct contact with the overlying extensor tendons (Fig. 75.5A–B). If three-dimensional plating is performed, a staggered plate, L-, T-, or H-plate may be selected (Fig. 75.5A–B). The plate should be bent to accommodate the dorsal curvature of the metacarpal in order to allow the plate to lay flush on the bone. Screws are placed first adjacent to the fracture in a bicortical manner. Additional screw fixation may be placed in compression mode. Adequate alignment is confirmed with fluoroscopy and the wound is thoroughly irrigated. When possible, the periosteum should be closed over the plate with absorbable suture. The skin is closed in a standard fashion and an intrinsic-plus splint with the IP joints free is applied for 3–5 days before starting therapy and gentle motion.

Intramedullary Devices

IM fixation may be achieved with antegrade K-wires (1 vs. 2 crossing), with commercially available IM rods or nails, or with IM headless compression screws.[10–13]

An antegrade IM approach can be used which has been suggested to result in increased motion and decreased shortening when compared with crossed K-wire or retrograde IM fixation.[5,14] A small longitudinal incision is made over the metacarpal base.

The dorsal sensory nerves are identified and protected and extensor tendons retracted. A curved awl or drill is then used to create a small opening in the metaphysis of the metacarpal base and ideally directed from proximal to distal. Then two or three pre-bent K-wires are passed antegrade up the metacarpal diaphysis

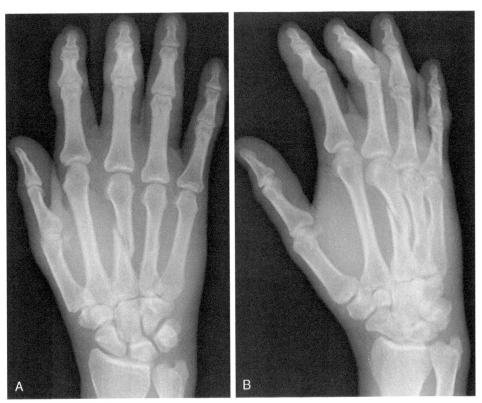

• **Fig. 75.4** PA (A) and oblique (B) radiographs demonstrate short oblique fractures of the third and fourth metacarpals could be amenable to lag screw fixation and neutralization plate or standard two-dimensional or three-dimensional plating.

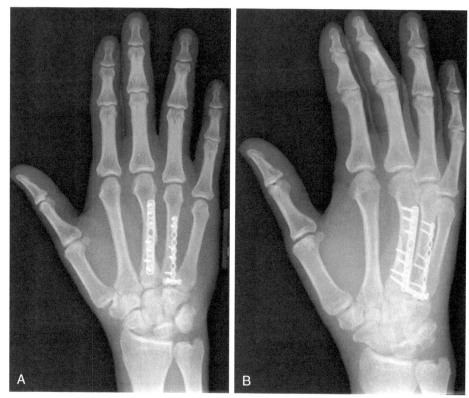

• **Fig. 75.5** (A) Posteroanterior and (B) lateral or standard two-dimensional plating of the third metacarpal and three-dimensional plating with a T-plate of the fourth metacarpal with lag screw placed through the plate.

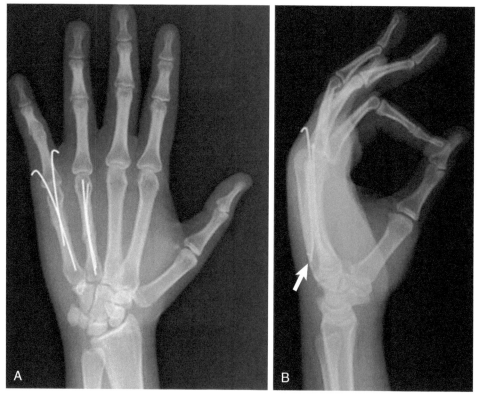

• **Fig. 75.6** The fourth metacarpal transverse fracture has been fixed using antegrade intramedullary technique as seen on the (A) posteroanterior and (B) lateral views. (B) The *arrow* shows where the antegrade wires were cut flush with the dorsal metacarpal base.

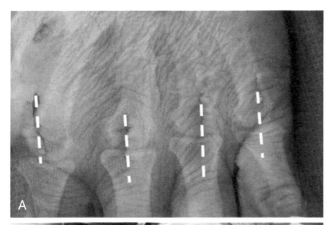

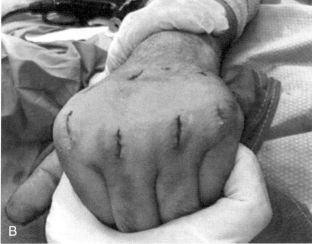

• **Fig. 75.7** (A) The dorsal incisions for the index through small finger approaches with corresponding bony architecture. (B) The 90-degree flexed position of the metacarpophalangeal joints to make the approach and for guidewire and screw placement.

up to the fracture site. The reduction maneuver is performed and then the wires are advanced across the fracture site and into the subchondral bone of the metacarpal head. Care must be taken to avoid penetrating the distal cortex. The pins may then be cut flush with the dorsal cortex and left in place permanently (Fig. 75.6A–B) or left prominent and subsequently removed. The goal is to have the tips diverge in the head to create a "flower bouquet."[14] Pins do not need to be removed, but if they are should be removed after radiographic evidence of bony union at the surgeon's discretion.

If commercial IM devices or headless compression screws are used, preoperative planning should include measurement of the medullary canal to estimate the size of the device or screw. For headless compression screws, determination of proper screw diameter and length can then be confirmed intraoperatively with a measuring guide placed over the skin which has length markings along the edge. This step is critical in order to ensure adequate purchase within the medullary canal and assurance that the screw will be able to fit within the canal. An incision is made on the dorsal metacarpal head centered over the MP joint; this should be large enough to have adequate visualization of the joint and permit screw insertion (Fig. 75.7A). There are two ways to approach the extensor mechanism: either a split of the extensor tendon over the MP joint or retraction of the tendon to one side by releasing a portion of the sagittal band. With the MP joint in 90 degrees of flexion (Fig. 75.7B), the guidewire is then placed with fluoroscopic guidance to ensure it is centered on the PA and within the dorsal third of the metacarpal head on the lateral, which is in line with the IM canal of the metacarpal shaft (Fig. 75.8A). The guidewire for the screw is then inserted through the dorsal entry point and across the fracture site. Appropriate screw length can be measured. The soft tissues surrounding the joint are protected while drilling (Fig. 75.8B). The screw is inserted over the guidewire to a depth of approximately 2 mm below the articular surface of the metacarpal head

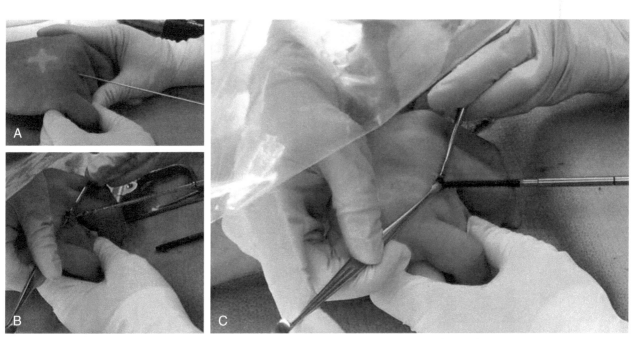

• **Fig. 75.8** (A) With the metacarpophalangeal joint flexed to 90 degrees, the guidewire is inserted under fluoroscopic guidance. (B) The length is measured using depth gauge after the guidewire has been placed into the metacarpal (MC) base. With the extensor mechanism protected, the MC is drilled to the appropriate depth and (C) the screw is inserted.

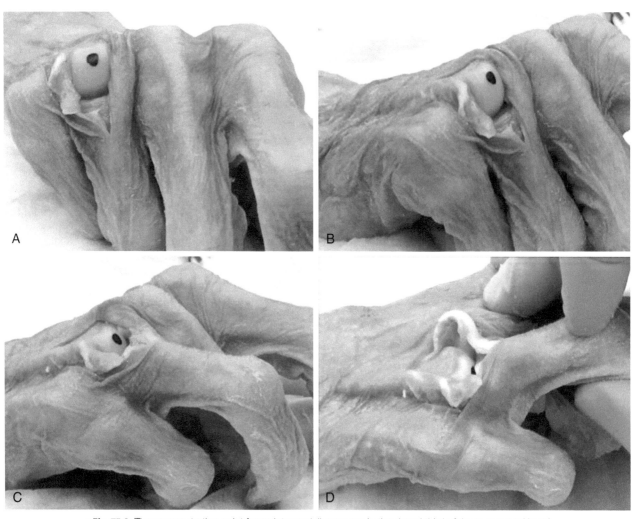

• **Fig. 75.9** The proper starting point for an intramedullary screw in the dorsal third of the metacarpal head (A) does not contact the base of the proximal phalanx in 90 degrees of flexion (B) or even 20 degrees of flexion (C) and only incompletely contacts in hyperextension (D).

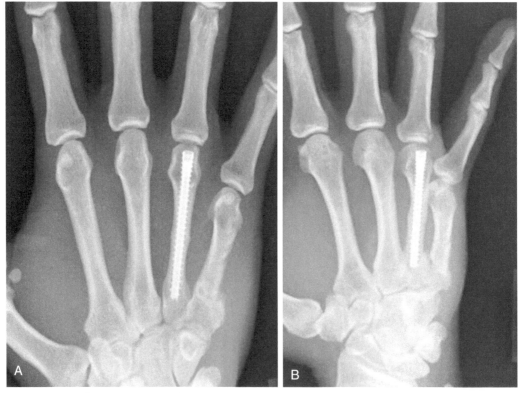

• **Fig. 75.10** The (A) posteroanterior and (B) lateral views show postoperative films follow intramedullary screw which has appropriate countersinking of the screw head, good fit within the medullary canal, and multiple threads past the fracture site.

(Fig. 75.8C). This ensures that the screw head is buried and does not impinge on the base of the proximal phalanx in flexion or extension (Fig. 75.9A–D).[15] The length should provide several threads crossing the fracture and the width should ensure good purchase within the isthmus of the metacarpal (Fig. 75.10). To maximize mechanical advantage, the screw length should be as closely matched to the length of the metacarpal as possible. The appropriate position of the screw and fracture reduction are confirmed with fluoroscopy and the guidewire is removed. If divided, the extensor tendon is repaired with an absorbable suture. The hand is placed in a soft dressing and immediate gentle range of motion is initiated.

Pearls and Pitfalls

Pinning

- Many metacarpal neck fractures amenable to pinning can be performed in the office as wide awake under local anesthesia and no tourniquet (WALANT).[7] This can be done at a significant cost saving to the patient and without risk of anesthesia-related complications in properly selected patients.
- To assist in maintaining the starting point and trajectory of K-wire insertion, a 16-gauge hypodermic needle may be inserted, positioned, and used as a guide through which a 0.045-inch K-wire may be inserted.
- Therapy should be initiated after 1 week to prevent stiffness which is a common complication of pinning.
- Multiple passes with K-wires should be avoided to decrease the risk of pin tract infection and thermal necrosis.

Plating

- If the patient has all four metacarpals fractured and all require open reduction, two longitudinal incisions can be performed between the fourth and fifth and the second and third metacarpals to access all of them.
- Care should be taken to avoid drill penetration causing damage to volar structures, especially the third metacarpal given the proximity of the ulnar nerve motor branch.
- Three-dimensional (3D) locking plates can minimize the required soft tissue dissection and provide rigid fixation over a smaller area compared with traditional plates.
- IM Devices
- The end of a freer or metal instrument of known width can be used for a quick estimation of the width of the metacarpal canal for IM devices.
- If not prepackaged, placing the proposed screw over the skin and assessing diameter and length under fluoroscopy can be very helpful in ensuring optimal screw selection.
- Typically the ring metacarpal diameter is the smallest and at times is too narrow to permit screw fixation.
- To avoid inadvertent removal during drilling, the guidewire can be temporarily advanced into the CMC joint.
- If the reduction is challenging to attain, a small incision centered over the fracture can allow open reduction without significant additional soft tissue insult.

References

1. Wong VW, Higgins JP. Evidence-based medicine: management of metacarpal fractures. *Plast Reconstr Surg.* 2017;140(1):140e–151e. https://doi.org/10.1097/PRS.0000000000003470.
2. Retrouvey H, Morzycki A, Wang AMQ, Canadian Plastic Surgery Research Collaborative, Binhammer P. Are we over treating hand fractures? Current practice of single metacarpal fractures. *Plast Surg (Oakv).* 2018;26(3):148–153. https://doi.org/10.1177/2292550318767926.
3. Neumeister MW, Webb K, McKenna K. Non-surgical management of metacarpal fractures. *Clin Plast Surg.* 2014;41(3):451–461. https://doi.org/10.1016/j.cps.2014.03.008.
4. Jardin E, Pechin C, Rey P-B, Uhring J, Obert L. Functional treatment of metacarpal diaphyseal fractures by buddy taping: a prospective single-center study. *Hand Surg Rehabil.* 2016;35(1):34–39. https://doi.org/10.1016/j.hansur.2015.12.001.
5. Kim JK, Kim DJ. Antegrade intramedullary pinning versus retrograde intramedullary pinning for displaced fifth metacarpal neck fractures. *Clin Orthop Relat Res.* 2015;473(5):1747–1754. https://doi.org/10.1007/s11999-014-4079-7.
6. Galal S, Safwat W. Transverse pinning versus intramedullary pinning in fifth metacarpal's neck fractures: a randomized controlled study with patient-reported outcome. *J Clin Orthop Trauma.* 2017;8(4):339–343. https://doi.org/10.1016/j.jcot.2017.05.015.
7. Winter M, Balaguer T, Bessière C, Carles M, Lebreton E. Surgical treatment of the boxer's fracture: transverse pinning versus intramedullary pinning. *J Hand Surg Eur Vol.* 2007;32(6):709–713. https://doi.org/10.1016/J.JHSE.2007.07.011.
8. Sohn RC, Jahng KH, Curtiss SB, Szabo RM. Comparison of metacarpal plating methods. *J Hand Surg Am.* 2008;33(3):316–321. https://doi.org/10.1016/j.jhsa.2007.11.001.
9. Tannenbaum EP, Burns GT, Oak NR, Lawton JN. Comparison of 2-dimensional and 3-dimensional metacarpal fracture plating constructs under cyclic loading. *J Hand Surg Am.* 2017;42(3):e159–e165. https://doi.org/10.1016/j.jhsa.2017.01.003.
10. Beck CM, Horesh E, Taub PJ. Intramedullary screw fixation of metacarpal fractures results in excellent functional outcomes: a literature review. *Plast Reconstr Surg.* 2019;143(4):1111–1118. https://doi.org/10.1097/PRS.0000000000005478.
11. Boulton CL, Salzler M, Mudgal CS. Intramedullary cannulated headless screw fixation of a comminuted subcapital metacarpal fracture: case report. *J Hand Surg Am.* 2010;35(8):1260–1263. https://doi.org/10.1016/j.jhsa.2010.04.032.
12. Jones CM, Padegimas EM, Weikert N, Greulich S, Ilyas AM, Siegler S. Headless screw fixation of metacarpal neck fractures: a mechanical comparative analysis. *Hand (N Y).* 2019;14(2):187–192. https://doi.org/10.1177/1558944717731859.
13. Avery DM, Klinge S, Dyrna F, et al. Headless compression screw versus Kirschner wire fixation for metacarpal neck fractures: a biomechanical study. *J Hand Surg Am.* 2017;42(5):392.e1–392.e6. https://doi.org/10.1016/j.jhsa.2017.02.013.
14. Foucher G. "Bouquet" osteosynthesis in metacarpal neck fractures: a series of 66 patients. *J Hand Surg Am.* 1995;20(3 Pt 2):S86–S90. https://doi.org/10.1016/s0363-5023(95)80176-6.
15. Gregory S, Lalonde DH, Fung Leung LT. Minimally invasive finger fracture management: wide-awake closed reduction, K-wire fixation, and early protected movement. *Hand Clin.* 2014;30(1):7–15. https://doi.org/10.1016/j.hcl.2013.08.014.

76

Technique Spotlight: Volar vs. Dorsal Approaches for Metacarpophalangeal Joint Dislocations

JED I. MASLOW AND R. GLENN GASTON

Indications

Metacarpal fractures are one of the most commonly sustained hand fractures and the overwhelming majority of these fractures may be treated nonoperatively with or without immobilization. Surgical intervention is frequently considered when the fracture leads to a functionally limiting or aesthetically displeasing deformity. In general, intra-articular displacement, malrotation, fracture shortening of ≥5 mm, and angulation that can cause compensatory posturing or extensor lag are not well tolerated (see the "Indications for Surgical Treatment" section of Chapter 74). Several methods of surgical treatment exist, each with its own advantages and disadvantages. Closed reduction with percutaneous pinning is inexpensive, readily available, and minimally invasive but carries the risk of pin site infection and stiffness due to associated immobilization. Intramedullary screw fixation is a minimally invasive option that avoids the risk associated with pin retention but is more costly and technically demanding. Other fractures are better managed with open reduction and internal fixation. In particular, intra-articular fractures with displacement, multiple metacarpal fractures, or significantly displaced fractures may require open surgical treatment through either a volar or dorsal approach highlighted in this chapter (Table 76.1).

The dorsal approach for metacarpal fracture fixation is by far most often utilized and is ideal for metacarpal neck, shaft, or base fractures. Minimal dissection is needed to reach the level of the metacarpal and the typical apex dorsal deformity can be corrected through this approach. Additionally, metacarpal head fractures that involve the dorsal half of the articular surface or a dorsal metacarpophalangeal (MCP) joint dislocation may be approached through a dorsal extensor splitting or sparing approach. The complexity of these metacarpal head fractures may require a combined volar and dorsal approach in order to attain and maintain an anatomic reduction.[1,2] Carpometacarpal (CMC) base fractures with or without dislocation may also necessitate open reduction and fixation. The typical direction of dislocation is dorsal and a dorsal approach is used in this scenario to visualize an anatomic reduction.[3]

While the majority of metacarpal fractures are adequately treated through a dorsal approach, the volar approach can be more appropriate for certain fractures and useful to be familiar with. Metacarpal head fractures that are articular shear fractures involving the volar aspect of the head can be better accessed through a volar A1 pulley approach.[4] Displaced thumb metacarpal base fractures, Bennett or Rolando fractures, may be approached through a standard dorsal approach similar to the nonthumb metacarpals, a volar Wagner approach, or a direct volar approach depending on fracture pattern and surgeon's preference.[5]

Other considerations in surgical decision-making in metacarpal fractures involve the use of arthroscopy as an aid and the use of wide-awake local anesthesia with no tourniquet (WALANT) techniques. Arthroscopy is especially helpful when performing closed or open reduction of intra-articular thumb metacarpal base fractures to confirm anatomic reduction.[6] As WALANT becomes a more commonly employed method of fracture fixation, anesthetic risk and cost can be minimized for patients. WALANT has the added advantages of allowing direct observation of active range of motion to assess rotation and less surgical waste. It can be used in the setting of closed or open treatment but has been traditionally reserved for relatively uncomplicated fracture patterns.[7,8]

Preoperative Evaluation

The preoperative evaluation of metacarpal fractures proceeds in a similar fashion as for other long bone fractures. Soft tissues are assessed for open wounds, tendon, or muscle injury, and compartment syndrome. A thorough neurovascular examination and evaluation of each tendinous unit in the hand are critical to choosing the most effective surgical approach. The initial imaging of choice when a metacarpal fracture is suspected is a three- or four-view radiographic evaluation. With radiographs alone, the fracture location, pattern, displacement, and ultimately the necessary approach for optimal fixation can be determined. It must be remembered that the metacarpals form a transverse arch and, consequently, the hand must be supinated or pronated to view the ulnar or radial metacarpals in the true lateral plane, respectively.[9] Concomitant injuries may also be diagnosed on radiographs that can affect surgical treatment. Proximal phalanx fractures or carpal fractures, specifically, may need to be addressed at the time of metacarpal fixation and can affect surgical decision-making. When a metacarpal head fracture is suspected or diagnosed on plain radiographs, computed tomography (CT) can be a helpful tool for confirming the diagnosis or planning the most appropriate surgical approach and fixation strategy (Fig. 76.1).

Positioning and Equipment

A standard operating room table and hand table attachment are used for patient positioning. A nonsterile tourniquet is placed above the elbow. The arm is prepped and draped in a standard sterile fashion and mini-fluoroscopy is utilized. When closed reduction and percutaneous pinning is performed, smooth K-wires sized 0.9–1.1 mm are utilized and a 16-gauge hypodermic needle may be utilized as a wire guide if insertion is difficult. If lag screw fixation or a plate and screw construct is to be performed, 1.1-, 1.5-, 2.0-, or 2.4-mm screws and plates are appropriately sized. If the fracture is at the proximal or distal third of the metacarpal and plating is performed, three-dimensional (3D) plates may offer multiple screw fixation points with a smaller area of dissection and should be considered.

Detailed Technique Description

Dorsal

A standard dorsal approach to the metacarpal diaphysis is performed through a longitudinal incision along the length of the fractured metacarpal. When multiple adjacent metacarpals are fractured, the incision may be positioned between two metacarpals to access both dorsal surfaces through the same incision, though this may require a slightly longer incision (Fig. 76.2). Subcutaneous veins and cutaneous branches from the radial and ulnar nerves should be identified and protected. The index and long finger metacarpals are found deep and radial to their respective extensor digitorum communis (EDC) tendon, the ring finger metacarpal is directly deep to the respective EDC tendon, and the small finger is deep and ulnar to the EDC tendon but can be found beneath the extensor digiti minimi (EDM) tendon.[10] The juncturae tendonae arise from the ring EDC and insert on the adjacent long and small finger EDC tendons. If the juncturae compromise visualization and instrumentation, they can be incised and repaired after internal fixation. Once the extensor tendon is retracted, the periosteum

TABLE 76.1	Fractures That Are Best Treated by Volar Approach or by Dorsal Approach When Open Reduction and Internal Fixation Is Required	
Volar	**Dorsal**	
Metacarpal head fracture involving volar 50%	Metacarpal head fracture involving dorsal 50%	
Metacarpal head fracture with metacarpophalangeal joint dislocation	Metacarpal neck and shaft fracture	
Base of thumb metacarpal fracture	Metacarpal base fracture with or without carpometacarpal dislocation	
	Multiple adjacent metacarpals	

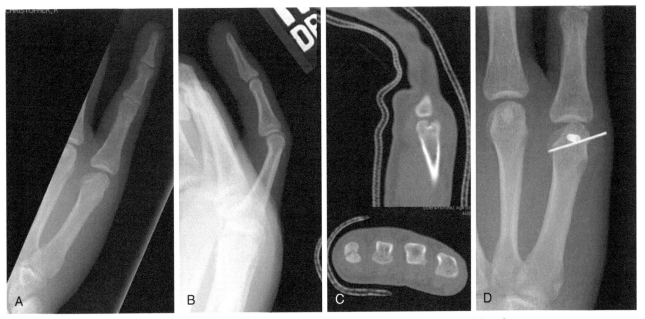

• **Fig. 76.1** (A and B) Abnormality of the metacarpal head of the small finger raises suspicion of a metacarpal head fracture. (C) Computed tomography scan reveals a displaced, depressed intra-articular fracture. (D) Open reduction and internal fixation was performed.

of the metacarpal can be incised and elevated. The fracture is then exposed long enough to perform lag screw or plate fixation. When possible, a plate can be applied to the metacarpal so that it will avoid direct extensor contact (Fig. 76.3). After fixation, if the periosteal layer is intact, it may be repaired.

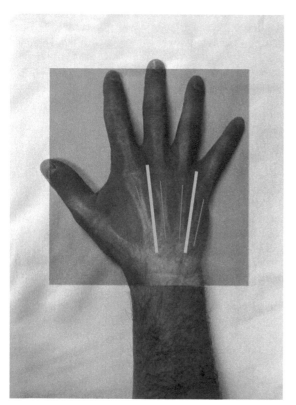

• **Fig. 76.2** Dorsal incisions used to approach one *(red lines)* or multiple metacarpals *(blue lines)*. Note the increased incision length needed to approach multiple metacarpals through one incision.

The metacarpal head and neck may be approached through a longitudinal or curvilinear dorsal incision. The dorsal cutaneous nerve and venous branches are preserved. The extrinsic extensor tendon may be split longitudinally or the sagittal band may be incised (Fig. 76.4). The digit is flexed to 90 degrees or more to avoid the proximal phalanx. When going through the sagittal band, while the radial or ulnar side may be incised, the ulnar sagittal band is preferred to prevent ulnar subluxation of the extensor tendons given the ulnar-directed force of the extrinsic extensor tendons. The capsule is incised and elevated off the metacarpal head while preserving the collateral ligament origin. After fixation of the metacarpal head and neck, the longitudinal extensor tendon split or sagittal band incision is repaired with 4-0 braided absorbable suture. When approaching the metacarpal base, a longitudinal incision may be placed over bony landmarks or with fluoroscopic localization. Similar to shaft exposure, cutaneous nerves and veins are preserved. When approaching the index or long metacarpal bases, the extensor carpi radialis longus (ECRL) and extensor carpi radialis brevis (ECRB) tendons can be identified on the most radial aspect of the base and typically do not interfere with the exposure. Similarly, the ECU inserts very proximal and ulnar on the base of the small finger metacarpal and rarely affects the exposure. The thumb metacarpal shaft is approached in a similar manner either radial to the EPL tendon or the EPB tendon. When the base is approached, the abductor pollicis longus (APL) tendon and periosteum may be elevated to visualize intraarticular fractures.

Volar

The volar approach to the metacarpal head is performed through a standard Bruner incision over the metacarpophalangeal joint (MPJ). After incising skin, identify and retract the radial and ulnar neurovascular bundles. The A1 pulley is incised longitudinally and the flexor tendons retracted radially or ulnarly to expose the volar plate. The volar plate can be longitudinally divided to expose the volar MPJ and may be repaired after fixation. The nonthumb metacarpal shaft is rarely approached from

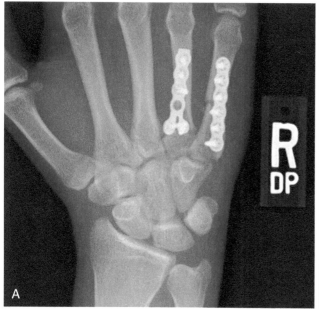

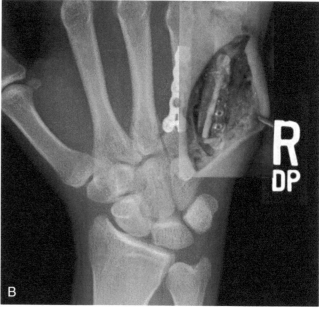

• **Fig. 76.3** (A) Dorsal approach to the ring and small finger metacarpal shaft with plate osteosynthesis. (B) The plate has been placed to avoid direct contact with the extensor tendon.

volar due to the risk of injury to neurovascular structures in close proximity (Fig. 76.5). The thumb metacarpal base may be approached through either a Wagner approach or a direct volar approach. The Wagner incision is more commonly utilized and begins at the border of the glabrous and nonglabrous skin between the APL tendon and thenar muscles. Proximally, the incision curves volar toward the flexor carpi radialis (FCR) at the wrist crease (Fig. 76.6). The thenar musculature can be elevated from the volar metacarpal and the joint capsule can be longitudinally incised. The base of the first metacarpal is visualized for reduction and fixation (Fig. 76.7). A direct volar approach is performed through a curvilinear incision at the volar base of the thumb and the thenar muscles are released from their origin. Through a volar capsulotomy, the base of the first metacarpal can be visualized.[5]

Arthroscopic-assisted surgery deserves mention in the treatment of metacarpal fractures. In particular, thumb metacarpal base and MPJ fractures are amenable to arthroscopic techniques for fracture reduction. A small joint 1.9-mm arthroscope can be inserted in the 1R or 1U portals on either side of the extrinsic extensor tendons to visualize the articular reduction and chondral injury (Fig. 76.8). A 2-mm shaver can be inserted into one of the portals for debridement and a probe can be used to attain an anatomic reduction.[6]

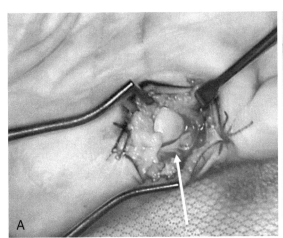

• **Fig. 76.4** The dorsal approach to the long finger metacarpal head. The digit is flexed to 90 degrees and a longitudinal incision is made through skin. The extensor tendon has been split here to expose the metacarpal head.

PEARLS AND PITFALLS

- The majority of metacarpal fractures can be effectively treated nonoperatively.
- Dorsal
  - Divide the ulnar sagittal band if preserving the extensor tendon through the dorsal approach. This can reduce the risk of extensor subluxation due to the ulnar pull of extrinsic extensor tendons.
  - Juncturae tendinae may be encountered during a dorsal approach and can be divided with later repair.
  - When performing internal fixation from the dorsal approach, care must be exercised not to plunge volar and risk injury to the deep motor branch of the ulnar nerve, especially when approaching the long finger metacarpal.
  - Aids to achieving a successful outcome with open reduction and internal fixation include WALANT surgery and arthroscopy.
- Volar
  - When a volar approach is used for metacarpal head fractures associated with MPJ dislocations, identification of the radial and ulnar neurovascular bundles is critical to avoid iatrogenic injury. In this pattern of injury, the bundles are displaced superficially and are at risk during superficial dissection.

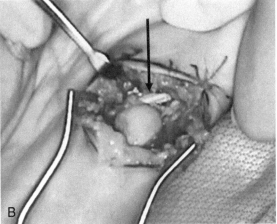

• **Fig. 76.5** Volar approach to the metacarpophalangeal joint through a Bruner incision for treatment of a metacarpophalangeal joint dislocation. (A) During the superficial dissection, the neurovascular bundle is identified and retracted (*white arrow*). (B) Deeper dissection exposes the flexor tendon and A1 pulley dorsal to the metacarpal head (*black arrow*).

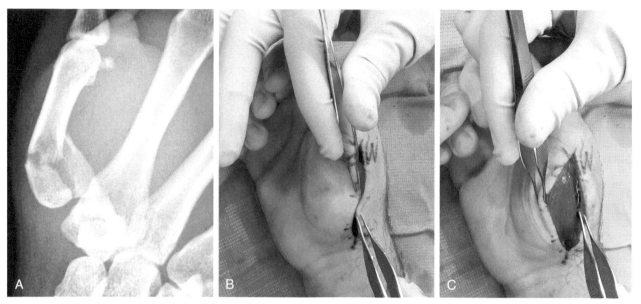

• **Fig. 76.6** A comminuted fracture of the base of the first metacarpal in a college athlete (A) treated with open reduction via a Wagner approach. (B) The incision is curvilinear along the glabrous and nonglabrous skin border. (C) Immediately after skin incision, the thenar musculature is encountered.

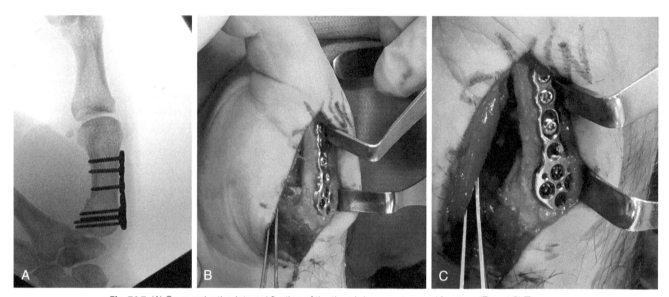

• **Fig. 76.7** (A) Open reduction internal fixation of the thumb base metacarpal fracture. (B and C) The exposure is attained with elevation of the thenar musculature origin and the joint capsule is incised to allow for plate fixation.

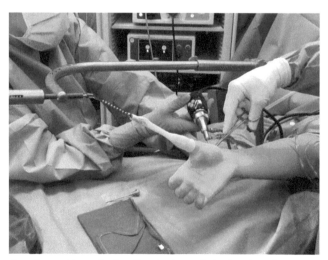

• **Fig. 76.8** Arthroscopically assisted thumb metacarpal base fixation. Traction is applied using the wrist arthroscopy tower and a 1.9-mm scope may be inserted through the 1R or 1U portal.

References

1. Hamada Y, Sairyo K, Tonogai I, Kasai T. Irreducible fracture dislocation of a finger metacarpophalangeal joint: a case report. *Hand N Y.* 2008;3(1):76–78. https://doi.org/10.1007/s11552-007-9064-0.

2. Hirata H, Tsujii M, Nakao E. Locking of the metacarpophalangeal joint of the thumb caused by a fracture fragment of the radial condyle of the metacarpal head after dorsal dislocation. *J Hand Surg Edinb Scotl.* 2006;31(6):635–636. https://doi.org/10.1016/j.jhsb.2006.07.010.

3. Steinmetz G, Corning E, Hulse T, et al. Carpometacarpal fracture-dislocations: a retrospective review of injury characteristics and radiographic outcomes. *Hand N Y.* 2019;16(3):362–367. https://doi.org/10.1177/1558944719852743. 1558944719852743.

4. Melamed E, Calotta N, Bello R, Hinds RM, Capo JT, Lifchez S. Dorsal and volar surgical approaches to the metacarpophalangeal joint: a comparative anatomic study. *J Hand Surg Asian-Pac.* 2017;22(3):297–302. https://doi.org/10.1142/S0218810417500332.

5. Levy V, Mazzola M, Gonzalez M. Intra-articular fracture of the base of the first metacarpal bone: treatment through a volar approach. *Hand N Y.* 2018;13(1):90–94. https://doi.org/10.1177/1558944716685828.

6. Culp RW, Johnson JW. Arthroscopically assisted percutaneous fixation of Bennett fractures. *J Hand Surg.* 2010;35(1):137–140. https://doi.org/10.1016/j.jhsa.2009.10.019.

7. Feldman G, Orbach H, Rinat B, Rozen N, Rubin G. Internal fixation of metacarpal fractures using wide awake local anesthesia and no tourniquet. *Hand Surg Rehabil.* 2020;39(3):214–217. https://doi.org/10.1016/j.hansur.2020.01.003.

8. Hyatt BT, Rhee PC. Wide-awake surgical management of hand fractures: technical pearls and advanced rehabilitation. *Plast Reconstr Surg.* 2019;143(3):800–810. https://doi.org/10.1097/PRS.0000000000005379.

9. Cotterell IH, Richard MJ. Metacarpal and phalangeal fractures in athletes. *Clin Sports Med.* 2015;34(1):69–98. https://doi.org/10.1016/j.csm.2014.09.009.

10. Watt AJ, Chung KC. Surgical exposures of the hand. *Hand Clin.* 2014;30(4):445–457. vi. https://doi.org/10.1016/j.hcl.2014.07.004.

77

Metacarpophalangeal Joint Dislocations

MAUREEN O'SHAUGHNESSY AND MARCO RIZZO

Introduction

Dislocations of the metacarpophalangeal (MCP) joint of the hand are caused by trauma to the hand, typically from a fall, with forced hyperextension of the joint. Athletes may more frequently sustain these injuries particularly in contact sports or ball-handling sports that require diving, setting, or catching balls at very high speeds. This chapter will focus on dislocations resulting in isolated soft tissue damage. Joint dislocations associated with fracture to the phalanx and/or metacarpal are covered in their respective chapters.

Relevant Anatomy

The MCP joint is a semiconstrained joint. The stability of the joint relies in part on the ball-in-cup design of the respective anatomy of the metacarpal head and the proximal phalanx base (Fig. 77.1). The congruency of this joint design lends a small amount of inherent stability. The ball-in-cup design allows motion in several planes including flexion and extension, abduction and adduction, and rotation.

The majority of joint stability is afforded by the soft tissue constraints around the joint. Soft tissue stability is afforded by the primary stabilizers which insert directly on the bone and joint capsule. These include the dorsal capsule, the volar plate, and the ulnar and radial collateral ligaments. Secondary stabilizers include those which do not insert directly around the joint but their presence adds to the stability. This includes the flexor tendons and associated pulley system, the extensor tendon and its mechanism, lumbricals, sagittal bands, superficial and deep intermetacarpal ligaments, and the natatory ligaments.

The metacarpal head has an eccentric, oval shape with a wider dorsal dimension that narrows palmarly in the axial plane. In the lateral plane, the MCP head is cam-shaped. The collateral ligaments arise from the concave metacarpal recess of the metacarpal head. The collateral ligaments consist of proper and accessory portions. The accessory ligaments are smaller and longitudinally oriented, lending stability in full extension. The proper collaterals are stronger ligaments, running obliquely from dorsal to palmar direction, and thus lend stability in flexion. They insert dorsally on the metacarpal and palmarly on the phalanx. Due to this anatomy, the collateral ligaments tighten as the joint flexes and are lax as the joint extends. The collaterals are lax in extension, allowing for increased side-to-side motion of the joint in full extension. With collaterals tight in flexion, this affords increased lateral stability in a clenched fist position. The proper collateral ligaments are the primary stabilizer of the MCP joint.

The dorsal capsule is relatively thin and loose, making this a weak constraint for dorsally or volarly directed forces. The volar (or palmar) plate is an extremely strong connective tissue structure that prevents joint hyperextension. The volar plates of adjacent digits are connected by the interpalmar plate ligaments (radial, central, and ulnar) that supply lateral metacarpal stability.[1]

After reduction of dorsal dislocations, the joint is ideally held at 20–50 degrees of flexion. Placing the MCP at 90 degrees of flexion places too much tension and stress on the collateral ligaments and impedes their healing potential. Placing the joint in full extension leads to improper balancing of the intrinsic and extrinsic ligaments and can lead to the intrinsic minus deformity. Placing the joint in the proper midarc of motion also prevents joint contracture and allows the MCP joint to heal in an ideal position.

Classification

Anatomic

MCP dislocations are classified anatomically by the direction of dislocation, either volar or dorsal. Dislocations are almost always dorsal, although volar dislocations have been described. The dislocation direction is classified by the position of the distal segment, that is, a dorsal dislocation notes the proximal phalanx to be dorsal (Fig. 77.2). The dorsal dislocation occurs typically from a hyperextension deformity. Volar dislocations, least commonly seen, can occur with either hyperflexion or hyperextension forces.

Complexity

MCP dislocations can be further classified as either reducible or irreducible, also referred to as simple or complex, respectively. Simple dislocations have no interposition of the volar plate, sesamoids, or other soft tissue and are typically successfully closed reduced. On clinical examination, the simple dislocation may appear more severe as the finger will typically rest in a very obvious hyperextended position (Fig. 77.3). The classic radiographic finding is the MCP joint at 90 degrees of hyperextension. An adolescent series by Maheshwari et al. noted 89% of patients with the classic 90-degree sign on radiographs were able to be successfully closed reduced.[2]

Complex or complete dislocations involve interposed soft tissue and result in complete dislocation of the joint. The volar plate and sesamoid may become entrapped within the joint. The proximal phalanx typically sits parallel to the metacarpal and clinically may, deceivingly, appear less severe (Fig. 77.4). Other methods of entrapment include the metacarpal head "button holing" in the natatory ligaments or transverse metacarpal ligament. The named "Kaplan's lesion" is rare but involves the metacarpal head button holing into the palm volarly with the volar plate interposed between the proximal phalanx and metacarpal head; it is most commonly seen in the index finger. Kaplan described dimpling of the skin over the proximal palmar crease as a pathognomonic sign for a dorsal complex dislocation.[3]

Pathoanatomy

A significant amount of force is required to dislocate the relatively stable MCP joint of the hand. If the MCP collateral ligaments, volar plate, and dorsal capsule can be thought of as the four sides of a box that support the joint, a dislocation typically indicates disruption of at least three of the four sides of the box. The thumb and index are the most commonly dislocated joints. The thumb is common in part because of its radial position on the hand without protection from adjacent digits.[1] Overall, MCP joint dislocations are relatively rare, especially when compared with proximal interphalangeal (PIP) joint dislocations. This is due, in part, to the support from adjacent digits and the strong stabilizers of the MCP joints.

With the more common dorsal dislocation, the volar plate avulses off of the metacarpal and remains attached to the dorsally displaced proximal phalanx. The volar plate with its adjoining sesamoids, if present, can entrap in the joint blocking reduction.

Palmarly, the ligamentous and tendinous structures can entrap the metacarpal head. Kaplan initially described the pathologic anatomy of the complex (irreducible) MCP joint dislocation in his classic article in 1957.[3] He believed that the palmar soft tissues around the joint create a noose which, once the metacarpal enters, cannot be removed without open reduction. The palmar soft tissues creating the noose as described by Kaplan are the natatory ligament, superficial transverse metacarpal ligament, flexor tendons, and lumbricals (Fig. 77.5). Additional blocks to reduction described are, in the index finger, the lumbrical radially and the flexor tendons ulnarly and, in the small finger, the abductor digiti quinti ulnarly and the flexor tendon radially. In the thumb, the flexor pollicis longus and adductor tendons may be involved.

Cadaveric work by Afifi et al. aimed to evaluate whether the structures as described by Kaplan were the true blocks to reduction.[4] Their anatomic modeling found that the volar plate was the structure that most often prevented successful reduction, and not the structures originally outlined by Kaplan. The authors argue

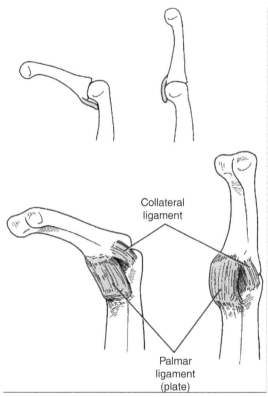

• **Fig. 77.1** Ball-in-cup design of metacarpophalangeal joint. (From Lehman T, Hildenbrand J, Rayan G. Fractures and ligament injuries of the thumb and metacarpals. In: Trumble T, Rayan G, Budoff J, Baratz M, eds. *Principles of Hand Surgery and Therapy*. Vol 2. 2nd ed. Philadelphia: Saunders Elsevier; 2010:35–50, Fig. 1–9.)

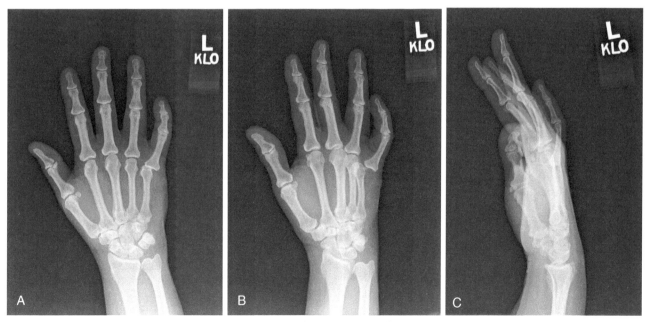

• **Fig. 77.2** Radiographs showing dorsal dislocation of small finger metacarpophalangeal joint.

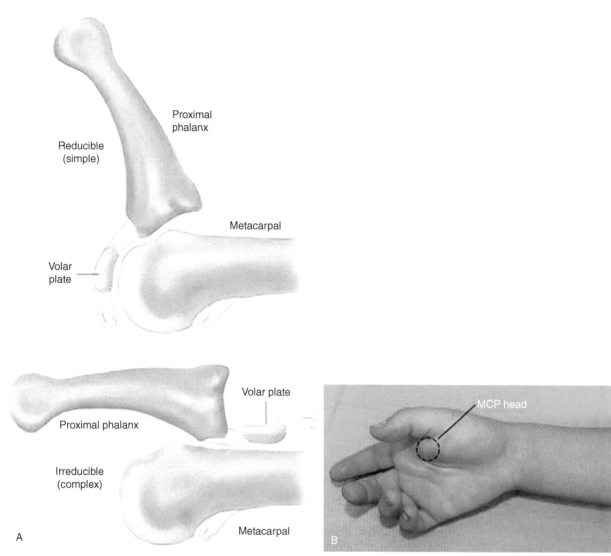

• **Fig. 77.3** Simple and complex metacarpophalangeal dislocation. (From Chung K. Open reduction for metacarpophalangeal joint dislocation. In: *Operative Techniques: Hand and Wrist Surgery.* Philadelphia: Saunders Elsevier; Figs. 15.2A–B and 15.3.)

that division of the volar plate should be the primary aim of surgery however, they note that controversy exists as to whether primary repair of the volar plate is indicated.

Treatment Options

Treatment of MCP dislocation is closed reduction unless soft tissue interposition blocks the reduction, in which case conversion to open reduction is indicated.

Appropriate assessment of the injury includes radiographs of the affected joint. At least three views (posteroanterior [PA], lateral, oblique) should be obtained. Careful scrutiny of the plain films should be undertaken looking for subtle undiagnosed fractures. Assessment of the position of the sesamoid(s) if present at the joint is important. Evidence of sesamoid(s) within the joint indicates that the volar plate is entrapped and suggests that the joint may not be reducible closed (Fig. 77.6).

Closed Reduction

Appropriate anesthesia is indicated to ensure successful closed reduction. For simple dislocations or subluxations, closed

reduction may sparingly be attempted without any sedation or analgesia, such as sideline sports, with an experienced provider such as an athletic trainer or team physician. Pediatric patients should always be provided sufficient analgesia and/or sedation and reduction should never be attempted without this. The authors prefer a 50/50 mixture of a fast-acting agent such as lidocaine for rapid anesthesia and a slower agent such as bupivacaine for lasting pain relief. Typically, 10 mL injected proximal to the MCP joint is appropriate for a successful block. Once appropriate analgesia and/or sedation is set up, reduction may be attempted.

For dorsal dislocations, the so-called McLaughlin maneuver involves hyperextension of the dorsally angulated proximal phalanx with a gentle volarly directed push of the base of the proximal phalanx up and over the metacarpal head.[5] One should avoid simple axial traction as this may lead to interposition of the volar plate and increase the likelihood of requiring open reduction. Wrist and PIP joint flexion can help relax the flexor tendons and aid in reduction. As stated by McLaughlin, if the joint is not reduced through proper technique, one can turn a simple dislocation into a complex one.[5]

For volar dislocations, the wrist and PIP are flexed to take tension off the flexors. The joint is then hyperflexed with a gentle

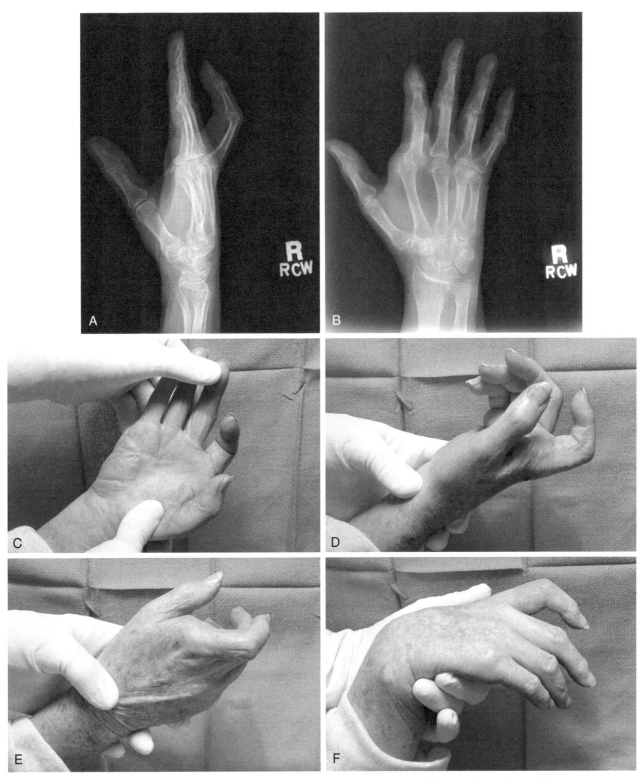

• **Fig. 77.4** Radiographic and clinical image of complex dorsal dislocation of the index finger. Note radiographic parallelism of index and metacarpal and relatively subtle clinical posturing of the digit.

dorsally directed push on the proximal phalanx base up and over the metacarpal head to reduce the dislocation.

It is crucial to avoid more than one to two attempts at closed reduction. Excessive force should be avoided as this may lead to iatrogenic fracture and may convert a simple dislocation into a complex one. The joint should be able to be reduced easily with minimal strength with the judicious use of appropriate anesthesia

and proper reduction techniques. Open reduction is imperative if the joint remains dislocated.

Postreduction Protocol

The joint should be protected in 20–50 degrees of flexion with a dorsal blocking splint for dorsal dislocations and volar blocking

Palmar view of MCP joint of index finger

Palmar view of MCP joint of 5th digit

Ulnar side
of proximal
phalanx

Radial side
of proximal
phalanx

Ulnar side
of proximal
phalanx

Radial side
of proximal
phalanx

Natatory
ligament
displaced
distally

Metacarpal
head
"button holing"

Natatory
ligament
displaced
distally

Metacarpal
head
"button holing"

Superficial
transverse
metacarpal
ligament
displaced
proximally

Superficial
transverse
metacarpal
ligament
displaced
proximally

Flexor tendon
displaced to
ulnar side

Lumbrical
displaced to
radial side

Abductor digiti
minimi muscle
displaced to
ulnar side

Flexor tendon
displaced to
radial side

A

B

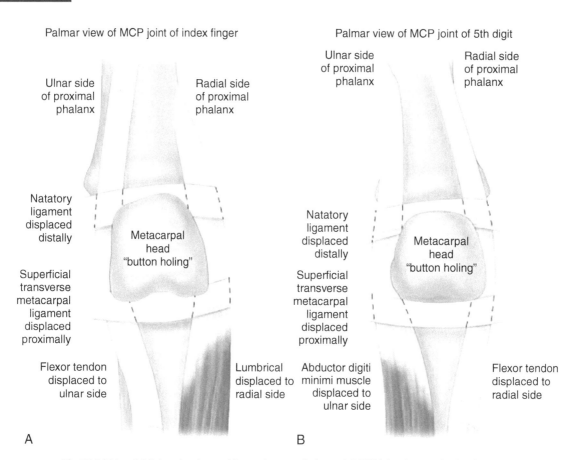

• **Fig. 77.5** Volar stabilizing structures of the metacarpophalangeal *(MCP)* joint that can lead to irreducible dislocation. (From Chung K. Open reduction for metacarpophalangeal joint dislocation. In: *Operative Techniques: Hand and Wrist Surgery*. Philadelphia, PA: Saunders Elsevier; Fig. 15.5A–B.)

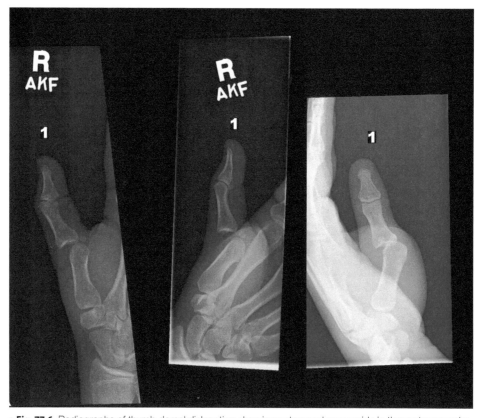

• **Fig. 77.6** Radiographs of thumb dorsal dislocation showing entrapped sesamoids in the metacarpophalangeal joint.

splint for volar dislocations. Keeping the joint blocked in flexion helps avoid redislocation. The compliant patient may begin moving the joint immediately in the protective splint. The MCP joint should be rested for 7–10 days, at which time progressive therapy and range of motion can begin.[6] After allowing time for the tissues to rest, the hand can be transitioned into a hand-based dorsal blocking splint versus a relative motion brace or yoke splint to allow range of motion at the joint while avoiding undue forces that could lead to redisplacement. The joint should be protected for 3–4 weeks while the soft tissues heal.

Return to play is considered based on sport, position, and league allowances. For example, football players who are allowed to play in a splint may return almost immediately if using a protective brace or cast.

Full return to activity without protection should be avoided until the 4- to 6-week time frame. The athlete should have 90% motion and 90% strength before return without protection.

In the athlete or other high-demand patient, one may give consideration to early advanced imaging and fixation of associated collateral injury.

Indications for Surgical Treatment

If closed reduction fails, surgical treatment is warranted for open reduction of the joint. No published guidelines exist for time to open reduction, but our preference is for joint reduction as soon as possible. Joint dislocations should typically be considered an orthopedic emergency and warrant urgent reduction to avoid further injury to the cartilage, tendons, or neurovascular structures. Prior to making surgical incisions, closed reduction should be attempted again once the patient is appropriately sedated by anesthesia and more relaxed. It is not infrequent to obtain successful closed reduction with appropriate anesthesia in an operating room setting.

Surgical Approaches

The joint can be approached from either a volar or dorsal direction, or incorporating a midaxial incision. Each approach has its own risks and benefits. The dorsal approach is typically safer as it avoids damage to critical volar structures and allows direct access to the dorsally interposed volar plate. It also allows access to the metacarpal head for fracture fixation. The volar approach affords better visualization of the typical structures that block reduction and allows anatomic repair of the volar plate if indicated. It also allows access to volar phalanx fractures or chondral lesions.

Dorsal Approach

Incision is made centered over the MCP joint. This can be straight longitudinal or curvilinear. Skin is incised and dissection is taken down by raising full-thickness skin flaps to protect the sensory nerve branches traversing the joint. The extensor tendon is identified. In the thumb, index and small fingers, the joint is approached by splitting the two tendons at the joint (i.e., extensor pollicis longus [EPL] and extensor pollicis brevis [EPB], extensor indicis proprius [EIP] and extensor digitorum communis [EDC], EDC and extensor digiti quinti [EDQ], respectively). The extensor tendons are retracted and protected. The dorsal capsule can be carefully incised but is generally thinned from trauma. Care is taken at this level to avoid iatrogenic damage to the dorsally displaced proximal phalanx. Gentle flexion of the wrist and careful mobilization allows reduction of the proximal phalanx up and over the metacarpal head. If the volar plate is noted to be entrapped

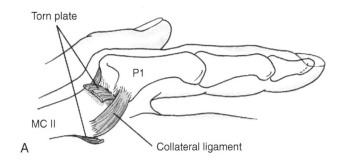

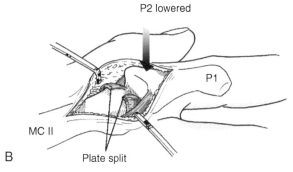

• **Fig. 77.7** Complex dorsal dislocation with the volar plate entrapped in the joint blocking reduction. (From Lehman T, Hildenbrand J, Rayan G. Fractures of the ligament injuries of the thumb and metacarpals. In: Trumble T, Rayan G, Budoff J, Baratz M, eds. *Principles of Hand Surgery and Therapy*. Philadelphia: Saunders Elsevier; 2010: 35–50, Fig. 3.47.)

and remains irreducible with direct reduction maneuvers, it may be split longitudinally along its midline to allow joint reduction (Figs. 77.7 and 77.8).

Once reduced, the joint is taken through a range of motion to ensure stability. The joint is flexed, extended, and radially and ulnarly deviated. Care is taken to look for undiagnosed fractures or cartilage lesions and these should be documented, with fractures repaired as indicated. Evaluate the status of the collateral ligaments and, if possible, the volar plate. Repair of these structures can be considered; however, studies have not shown improved outcomes with volar plate repair.[7] Postreduction stability is assessed, but is typically stable and does not require further ligamentous repair. In more chronic dislocations, residual instability can be remedied with provisional pinning for a short period. The dorsal capsule is typically thin and attenuated from the injury but should be carefully repaired whenever possible.

The thumb MCP joint may warrant increased vigilance for repair of collateral ligament injury given the additional pinch and lateral forces across the thumb. The ulnar collateral ligament (UCL) should be evaluated at the time of open reduction to assess for a Stener lesion or complete UCL avulsion, which warrants surgical fixation (Fig. 77.9). Typically, a suture anchor with 2-0 nonabsorbable suture can allow for appropriate primary repair. Thumb radial collateral ligament injury treatment is debated and is left up to the surgeon's preference.

Skin is closed and the wrist is splinted with a dorsal blocking splint keeping the MCP joint flexed to 20–50 degrees. More flexion puts undue tension on the collateral ligaments and impedes their recovery.

Volar Approach

Oblique, longitudinal, or zig-zag incisions are designed in the palm centered over the A1 pulley. Palpation of the prominent metacarpal head can help identify the correct level for incision.

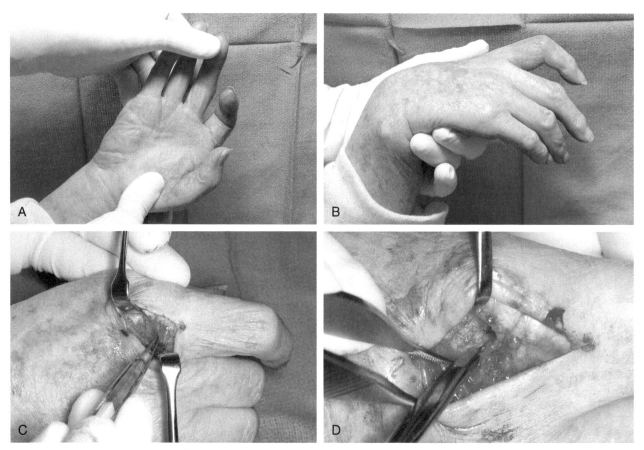

• **Fig. 77.8** Intraoperative photographs of the dorsal approach for joint reduction. Note the volar plate split required to successfully reduce the joint.

Skin is incised and careful dissection is made to the level of the flexor tendon sheath. Extreme care must be taken as the neurovascular bundles and/or flexor tendons may be displaced volarly and more superficial than their anatomic position. Care must be taken to avoid iatrogenic injury to these structures.

The metacarpal head should be readily identifiable, with the proximal phalanx and its attached volar plate dorsal to the metacarpal. The A1 pulley may be incised at this point, allowing gentle retraction on the flexor tendons. The surgeon should then be able to identify the structures trapping the metacarpal head. These may be the "noose" of the natatory ligaments, superficial transverse metacarpal ligaments, flexor tendons, and lumbricals, or the volar plate itself, as described by Kaplan. If the volar plate is tight and unable to be freed, it can be split longitudinally to allow reduction of the joint. Use of a freer below the volar plate can help prevent injury to the cartilage of the underlying metacarpal head. The wrist is flexed and the tight structures are retracted to allow gentle reduction of the proximal phalanx onto the metacarpal head. A freer elevator can be used to gently guide the reduction. The volar plate must be checked after reduction to ensure it is free from the joint and placed back into its anatomic position.

The joint is then assessed through a range of motion for stability. The joint is flexed, extended, and radially and ulnarly deviated. Careful attention is paid to rule out undiagnosed fractures or cartilage lesions, and these should be documented and, if indicated, repaired. Evaluate the status of the collateral ligaments and volar plate. Repair of these structures can be considered; however, studies have not shown improved outcomes with repair.[7] Postreduction stability is assessed, but is typically stable in the MCP joint and does not require further repair. Repair of the dorsal capsule cannot typically be addressed through the volar approach.

As described above in the dorsal approach, the volar approach of the thumb allows additional evaluation of the collateral ligaments with consideration given to repair. The volar approach should be considered in a patient with delayed presentation as it can allow easier access to offending structures.

Skin is closed and the wrist is splinted with a dorsal blocking splint keeping the MCP joint flexed to 20–50 degrees. More flexion puts undue tension on the collateral ligaments and impedes their recovery.

Postoperative Protocol

For both the dorsal and volar open approach, the operative joint is allowed to rest in a protective splint for 7–10 days after surgery with the MCP in 20–50 degrees of flexion with a dorsal blocking splint.

Keeping the joint blocked in flexion helps avoid redislocation. The compliant patient may begin moving the dislocated MCP joint almost immediately in the protective splint. The MCP joint should first be rested in an operative splint for 7–10 days, at which time more aggressive therapy and range of motion can begin.[6] After allowing time for the tissues to rest, the hand can be transitioned into a hand-based dorsal blocking splint or a relative motion splint at week 2 to allow range of motion at the MCP joint while avoiding undue forces that could lead to redisplacement. The joint should be protected for 3–4 weeks while the soft tissues heal.

Relevant Complications

The majority of complications associated with MCP dislocations are related to a failure of diagnosis and appropriate treatment. Repeated attempts at closed reduction, traumatic open reduction, or prolonged

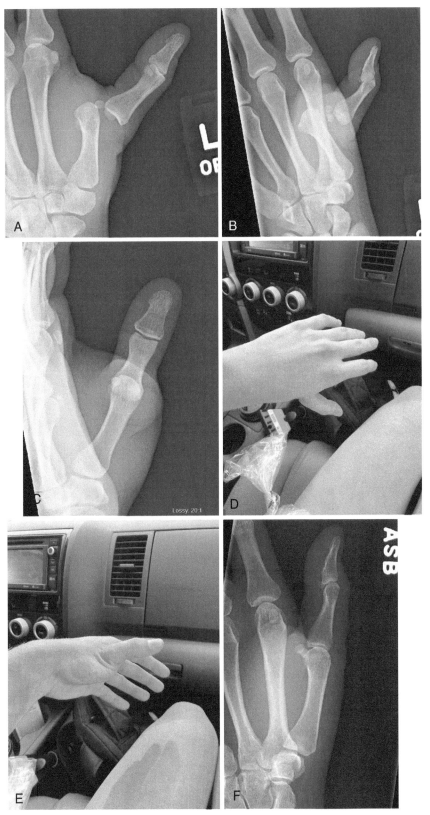

• **Fig. 77.9** Collegiate athlete with thumb dorsal dislocation. (A–D) Radiographs and injury photograph show dislocation requiring open reduction by outside surgeon (E and F), followed by operative stabilization of ulnar collateral ligament injury noted on (G and H) magnetic resonance imaging (I and J) and intraoperatively.

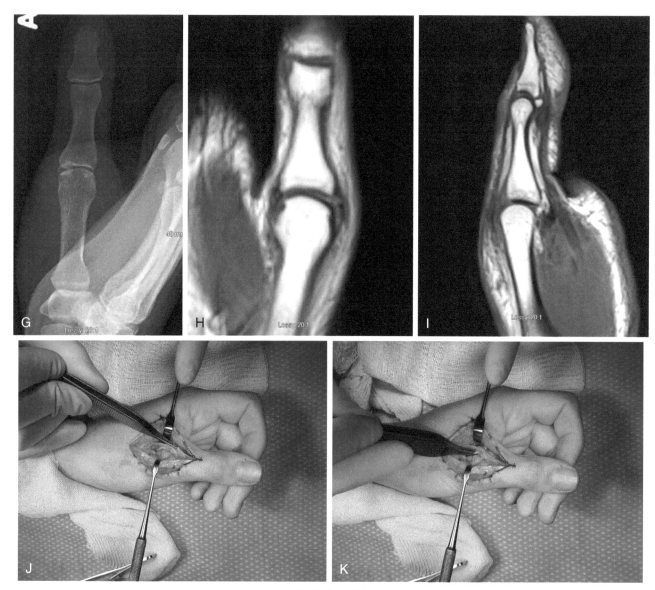

Fig. 77.9, cont'd

dislocation can lead to increased complications.[8] The complex dislocation may have a more subtle clinical examination than simple, leading to a delay in diagnosis. Patients presenting late (>2–3 weeks after injury) may require dual approach with both dorsal and volar incisions to allow reduction and potential repair of the now chronically dislocated structures. Thus radiographs and appropriate clinical examination are imperative for evaluation of hand injuries.

Joint stiffness is the primary complication associated with MCP dislocation. Ongoing stiffness and swelling are common and can often require a prolonged recovery. Persistent stiffness, swelling, and pain can be noted for up to 6–9 months. Early protected motion combined with formal therapy may help avoid this. Patients with persistent symptoms may require operative capsulotomy and/or tenolysis to improve final arc of motion.

The MCP joint of the thumb can tolerate a much higher amount of stiffness and limited motion than the MCP joint or PIP joints of the fingers. As opposed to the IP joints where stiffness and loss of motion can cause severe functional limitations, the MCP joint is a relatively forgiving joint. Ultimately, thumb MCP fusion is a salvage operation that is well tolerated.

Associated injuries are not infrequent given the amount of force required to dislocate the joint. Consideration should be given to advanced imaging in an athlete or other high-demand patient such as a surgeon or laborer in which timing of repair and return to work or sport is important. These injuries may occur with associated complete collateral ligament tears. For example, one would not want to miss a UCL complete tear with an associated Stener lesion which may prolong the postoperative course and require delayed repair or reconstruction. Additionally, up to 50% of MCP dislocations will have concurrent fracture;[8] therefore vigilance is important to identify associated fractures.

Nerve injury can occur and is typically a neurapraxic injury due to putting the nerve on stretch from the joint being dislocated. Nerve damage may also occur from reduction maneuvers. Nerve injury should be observed and will typically resolve with expectant management. Iatrogenic nerve transection has been reported in the volar approach due to the superficial displacement of the bundle by the metacarpal head and must be avoided with meticulous dissection.

Although uncommon, skeletally immature patients may experience physeal injury which can result in growth delay or arrest.

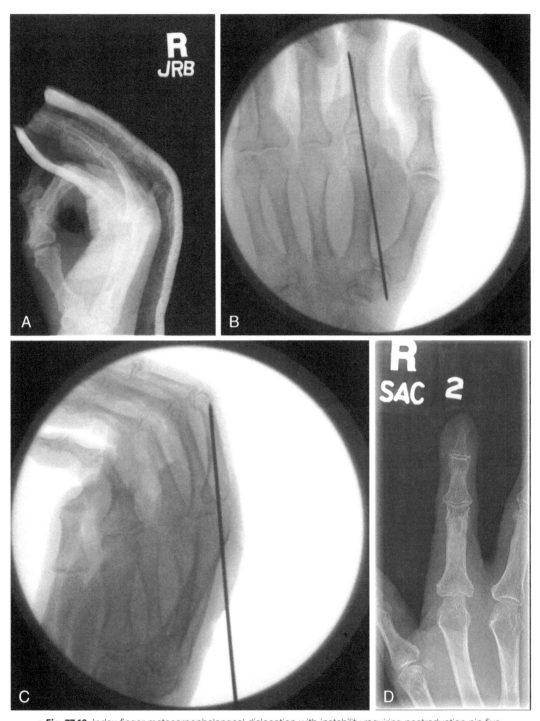

• **Fig. 77.10** Index finger metacarpophalangeal dislocation with instability requiring postreduction pin fixation. At long-term follow-up, the patient developed posttraumatic arthritis of the joint.

Multiple repeated closed reduction maneuvers should be avoided in patients with open physes to help prevent further physeal damage. Appropriate sedation and analgesia is paramount when attempting closed reduction in the pediatric patient. The surgeon should have a low threshold to take these patients to the operating room for open reduction to help avoid further physeal injury.

Avascular necrosis of the metacarpal head is an extremely uncommon complication but has been reported.[9] Posttraumatic arthritis can also occur from trauma or from prolonged dislocation,[8] although recent long-term outcomes show this is typically associated with intra-articular fractures (Fig. 77.10).[10]

Review of Treatment Outcomes

Debate persists regarding the optimal surgical approach. A recent study by Vadala and Ward sought to evaluate the two approaches.[11] They hypothesized that the dorsal approach would allow easier joint reduction, objectively defined as decreased operative time, and that a second approach would be required less frequently. They evaluated all MCP dislocations over a 10-year period at a busy trauma center and found 22 dislocations requiring open reduction. Of these, 14 underwent volar approach and 8 underwent dorsal approach. They found mean operative time was significantly shorter for dorsal approach,

70 versus 45 minutes, respectively (*P* <.05). The authors also noted that 42% of patients initially approached volarly required a second dorsal incision for successful reduction, with none of the initial dorsal approaches requiring a second incision (*P* <.05). The authors agree that a randomized controlled trial would be a superior study; however, they acknowledge this is likely not feasible given the rarity of the pathology. In summary, they found the dorsal approach to be faster and less likely to require a second approach to achieve reduction.

Outcomes are generally satisfactory, with patients achieving a functional arc of motion and grip strength. A recent series by Rubin et al. evaluated long-term outcomes of complex dislocations.[10] The authors reported on five patients with complex MCP dislocations with a median follow-up of 13 years (range: 7–36). They noted satisfactory outcomes in regard to QuickDASH and grip strength.[10] Two patients with concomitant fracture had evidence of joint changes on follow-up radiographs. The authors also reviewed the current literature, finding 12 reports of follow-up or complications, with only six containing long-term follow-up, indicating a paucity of evidence in our current body of literature regarding outcomes associated with MCP dislocations.

Summary

Although a rare injury, MCP joint dislocations require a timely and accurate diagnosis of the injury with appropriate reduction. The dorsal dislocation is far more common than volar. Keys to successful closed reduction are appropriate anesthesia and proper reduction techniques. Failure of closed reduction should be treated urgently with open reduction, with careful dissection and release of blocks to reduction. Repair of damaged structures is typically not necessary except in the UCL of the thumb. Postreduction care consists of dorsal blocking splint at 20–50 degrees of flexion to prevent redislocation combined with early active motion of the joint to help prevent adhesions and stiffness. With acute diagnosis and proper reduction, most of these injuries will have a good outcome.

References

1. Lehman T, Hildenbrand J, Rayan G. Fractures and ligament injuries of the thumb and metacarpals. In: 2nd ed. Trumble T, Rayan G, Budoff J, Baratz M, eds. *Principles of Hand Surgery and Therapy*. Vol. 2. Philadelphia, PA: Saunders Elsevier; 2010:35–50.
2. Maheshwari R, Sharma H, Duncan RDD. Metacarpophalangeal joint dislocation of the thumb in children. *J Bone Jt Surg - Ser B*. 2007;89(2):227–229.
3. Kaplan EB. Dorsal dislocation of the metacarpophalangeal joint of the index finger. *J Bone Jt Surgery*. 1957;39(5):1081–1086.
4. Afifi AM, Medoro A, Salas C, Taha MR, Cheema T. A cadaver model that investigates irreducible metacarpophalangeal joint dislocation. *J Hand Surg Am*. 2009;34(8):1506–1511.
5. McLaughlin H. Complex "locked" dislocation of the metacarpophalangeal joints. *J Trauma*. 1965;5(6):683–688.
6. Pitts G, Willoughby J, Cummings B, Uhl T. Rehabilitation of wrist and hand injuries. In: Andrews JR, Harrelson GL, Wilk KE, eds. *Physical Rehabilitation of the Injured Athlete*. 4th ed. Philadelphia, PA: Elsevier Saunders; 2012:259–280.
7. Sodha S, Breslow GD, Chang B, Disa JJ. Percutaneous technique for reduction of complex metacarpophalangeal dislocations. *Ann Plast Surg*. 2004;52(6):562–566.
8. Dinh P, Franklin A, Hutchinson B, Schnall SB, Fassola I. Metacarpophalangeal joint dislocation. *J Am Acad Orthop Surg*. 2009;17(5):318–324.
9. Gilsanz V, Cleveland RH, Wilkinson RH. Aseptic necrosis: a complication of dislocation of the metacarpophalangeal joint. *Am J Roentgenol*. 1977;129(4):737–738.
10. Rubin G, Orbach H, Rinott M, Rozen N. Complex dorsal metacarpophalangeal dislocation: long-term follow-up. *J Hand Surg Am*. 2016;41(8):e229–e233.
11. Vadala CJ, Ward CM. Dorsal approach decreases operative time for complex metacarpophalangeal dislocations. *J Hand Surg Am*. 2016;41(9):e259–e262.

78

Phalanx Fractures

FRANK A. RUSSO AND LOUIS W. CATALANO III

Introduction

Fractures of the phalanges are common injuries, with reported rates of 340,000 per year.[1] The majority occur following an accidental fall followed closely by injuries sustained after being struck by an object or person.[1] While these are common injuries across all ages and demographics, there is a higher incidence in children and adolescents.[1] They are commonly managed nonoperatively however, surgery plays an important role in the treatment algorithm.

Relevant Anatomy

Proximal Phalanx

The proximal phalanx is a tubular bone that consists of a base, a diaphysis, and a head. It tapers from proximal to distal and exhibits a slight convexity on the dorsum and a slight concavity on its volar surface. This shallow concavity palmarly supports the floor of the flexor sheath. Distally, the head consists of two condyles covered with hyaline cartilage for the proximal interphalangeal (PIP) joint. The radial and ulnar collateral ligaments of the metacarpophalangeal (MCP) joint insert at the base of the proximal phalanx. Distally, tubercles on the corresponding condyles serve as the origins of the radial and ulnar collateral ligaments of the PIP joint. The only tendinous insertion is a portion of the intrinsic muscles. With the exception of the third proximal phalanx, the superficial belly of the dorsal interossei inserts onto the lateral tubercle at the base of the proximal phalanx via the medial tendon.[2]

Middle Phalanx

The osteology of the middle phalanx is very similar to that of the proximal phalanx. It too is a tubular bone, although it demonstrates an hourglass shape in cross section.[3] Distally, the condyles are covered with articular cartilage to form the base of the distal interphalangeal (DIP) joint. Radial and ulnar collateral ligaments arise from a tubercle just proximal to the articular surface on either condyle. The central slip of the extensor mechanism inserts proximally on the dorsum of the middle phalanx; palmarly, the flexor digitorum superficialis (FDS) inserts just distal to the insertion of the volar plate.

Distal Phalanx

The distal phalanx can be divided into a base, a shaft, and the tuft distally. Dorsally, the terminal extensor tendon inserts onto a tubercle. The radial and ulnar collateral ligaments of the DIP joint insert on either side of this tubercle. Palmarly, there is another tubercle where the volar plate of the DIP inserts. The flexor digitorum profundus (FDP) inserts just distal to the insertion of the volar plate. Multiple fibrous septae anchor the palmar skin to the tuft of the distal phalanx, providing support to the pulp of the digit and minimizing displacement of underlying fractures. The germinal matrix of the nail originates just distal to the insertion of the terminal tendon; the sterile matrix supports and adheres to the overlying nail plate.

Pathoanatomy/Classification

Fractures of the Proximal Phalanx

Proximal phalanx fractures typically present with apex volar angulation, commonly with comminution of the dorsal cortex. The primary deforming force is the central slip, which extends the distal fragment, and the intrinsic muscles, which flex the proximal fragment. The reduction maneuver for these fractures primarily involves flexion at the MCP joint, which decreases tension on the intrinsic muscles and corrects the apex volar angulation by flexing the distal fragment. Malunion of these fractures results in pseudoclawing, where shortening of the proximal phalanx leads to an extensor lag at the PIP joint.[4]

Condylar Fractures of the Proximal Phalanx

Condylar fractures of the proximal phalanx are relatively common injuries. Though the exact mechanism of injury can vary, they can occur following a combination of axial loading with a shear stress through the PIP joint. Given the typical oblique pattern of these fractures, they are inherently unstable which could lead to articular incongruity. London first classified these injuries: type 1 fractures are stable unicondylar injuries without displacement, type 2 fractures are unicondylar and unstable with any degree of displacement, and type 3 are bicondylar injuries (Fig. 78.1).[5] Weiss and Hastings recommend that unicondylar fractures undergo open reduction for any degree of displacement, owing to the inherent instability of this fracture pattern.[6] They also commented that coronal plane injuries portend a poor prognosis, given disruption to the blood supply at the time of injury.

Fractures of the Middle Phalanx

Fractures of the middle phalanx can present as transverse, spiral, or oblique, with variable angulation. Treatment of displaced unstable

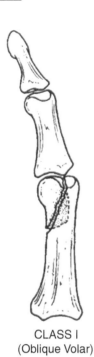 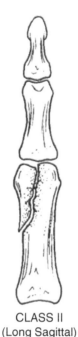 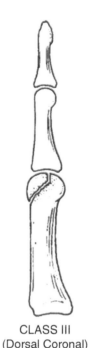 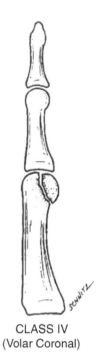

CLASS I
(Oblique Volar)

CLASS II
(Long Sagittal)

CLASS III
(Dorsal Coronal)

CLASS IV
(Volar Coronal)

• **Fig. 78.1** Diagram demonstrating unicondylar fracture patterns of the proximal phalanx as classified by Weiss and Hastings. (From Weiss AP, Hastings 2nd H. Distal unicondylar fractures of the proximal phalanx. *J Hand Surg Am*. 1993;18:594-599.)

fractures is determined by their location with respect to the insertion of the extrinsic flexor and extensor tendons. Fractures that occur proximal to the insertion of the FDS tendon assume an apex dorsal angulation, as the FDS tendon flexes the distal fragment and the dorsal insertion of the central slip extends the proximal fragment. Those fractures that occur distal to the insertion of the FDS present with apex volar angulation (Fig. 78.2).

Fractures of the Distal Phalanx

Fractures of the distal phalanx typically occur secondary to a crush injury or an axial load. Other mechanisms include lacerations, hyperextension/hyperflexion injuries, or shearing forces. Tuft fractures are commonly associated with an injury to the nail matrix, which should be directly inspected and repaired at the time of injury.

Treatment Options and Operative Indications

Extra-Articular Fractures of the Base of the Proximal Phalanx

Nonoperative management typically is achieved by immobilizing the MCP joint in 70–90 degrees of flexion and extending the PIP joint. This degree of flexion is critical in order to bring the distal portion of the proximal phalanx in line with the flexed proximal fragment. This position is maintained for a duration of 3–4 weeks with an extension block splint. Coonrad and Pohlman reported on 27 adults, 7 required corrective osteotomy following closed reduction and splinting.[7] If postreduction radiographs demonstrate recurrent displacement with apex volar angulation >25 degrees, closed reduction with percutaneous fixation versus open reduction with internal fixation may be required.[8]

A

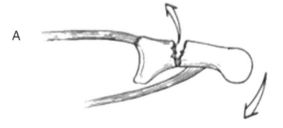

B

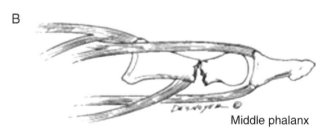

Middle phalanx

• **Fig. 78.2** (A) Fracture proximal to flexor digitorum superficialis insertion, dorsal angulation. (B) Fracture distal to flexor digitorum superficialis insertion, volar angulation. (From Hastings H, Rettig A, Strickland J. *Management of Extra-Articular Fractures of the Phalanges and Metacarpals*. Philadelphia, PA: Elsevier; 1992.)

Diaphyseal Fractures of the Proximal and Middle Phalanx

Nonoperative management follows that of extra-articular base fractures, with immobilization in 70–90 degrees of flexion at the MCP joint and extending the PIP and DIP joints. This reduction should be maintained for 3–4 weeks, with range of motion initiating at that time to prevent stiffness.[9–11] If nonoperative measures fail, several methods of stabilization are available. Closed reduction percutaneous fixation provides immediate stability and therefore some surgeons elect to start with early motion protocol. The senior author's preference is to immobilize the joint immediately proximal and distal to the pins for 3–4 weeks; however, whenever possible, the DIP should be left free for range of motion to permit FDP tendon gliding. If the fracture cannot be closed reduced, open reduction and percutaneous fixation versus internal fixation with screws or plates is indicated.

Condylar Fractures of the Proximal Phalanx

Indications for treating condylar fractures nonoperatively are limited. In the rare circumstance of a nondisplaced unicondylar fracture, splint immobilization in the position of safety can be elected. Vigilance is required to treat these fractures nonoperatively. The patients must be followed up with serial X-rays every 5–7 days for 3–4 weeks to ensure that the condylar fragment does not displace, as it often can. In the setting of nondisplaced fractures, the authors recommend to fix these fractures with percutaneous pins, rather than observe the predictable progression of fracture displacement over 3–4 weeks. At that point, an osteotomy would be required to achieve an anatomic joint surface. If the fracture involves >25% of the articular surface with a step-off of >1 mm, then operative intervention is indicated.[12]

Bicondylar fractures are inherently unstable injuries, which require operative management. Given their periarticular nature, open reduction is typically warranted. Multiple fixation options can be considered in treating these injuries including percutaneous pinning, lag screws, and plating.

Tuft Fractures of the Distal Phalanx

As these injuries tend to occur following a crush mechanism, they commonly present with soft tissue compromise. A subungual hematoma can form in closed fractures, for which decompression can be considered for pain relief. This can be performed using a trephine or electrocautery to perforate the nail plate and permit egress of the hematoma.[13] This decompression theoretically converts a closed injury to an open fracture, and therefore the treating physician should consider antibiotic prophylaxis.[14]

With respect to open injuries, the disruption of the soft tissue envelope secondarily destabilizes the fracture fragments. However, careful reapproximation of the volar pulp, removal of the nail plate, and suture repair of the nail matrix will commonly realign the injured phalanx. Following suture repair, the nail plate should be used to splint the eponychial fold open; postprocedure radiographs should then be obtained to confirm realignment of the fracture.[15] Both the distal and middle phalanges should be immobilized with a splint spanning the DIP for a duration of 2 weeks; the PIP should be left free to permit range of motion and promote tendon gliding. In rare circumstances, operative intervention may be indicated.

Shaft Fractures of the Distal Phalanx

These injuries tend to be stable, given the stout insertions of the fibrous septae that anchor the pulp to the underlying bone. Fractures through the midshaft of the phalanx can also be associated with injuries to the nail matrix, for which the nail plate should be removed to inspect and reapproximate the underlying sterile matrix. Only in exceptional circumstances, such as considerable injury to the surrounding soft tissues, is operative fixation indicated. Angulated shaft fractures can result in an obvious cosmetic

fingertip deformity, and in the author's opinion, these injuries should be closed reduced with or without pinning to restore length and alignment.[16]

Operative Techniques

Extra-Articular Fractures of the Base of the Proximal Phalanx

Several methods have been described for stabilizing extra-articular fractures at the base of the proximal phalanx. Belsky et al. describe an effective closed reduction and percutaneous fixation technique; following the reduction maneuver as described above, a K-wire is drilled anterograde through the metacarpal head into the reduced proximal phalanx (Fig. 78.3).[17] A cross-pinning technique can also be used, in which two K-wires are inserted percutaneously at the level of proximal fragment and drilled into the contralateral cortex of the distal fragment. Faruqui et al. compared transarticular pinning with extra-articular pinning and found a higher rate of complications than previously published. They reported an average loss of 27 degrees of flexion at the PIP joint in over half the patients in each group.[18] Despite the transarticular group requiring more secondary procedures than the extra-articular group, this was not found to be statistically significant; they concluded that neither technique demonstrated superiority with respect to their measured outcomes.[18]

Diaphyseal Fractures of the Proximal and Middle Phalanges

If closed reduction fails, percutaneous fixation with K-wires provides the advantage of immediate stabilization and permits early active range of motion (Fig. 78.4).[16] Reduction is obtained with longitudinal traction and 60–80 degrees of flexion at the MCP joint. After restoring length, alignment, and rotation, pins can be drilled perpendicular to the fracture site. In the setting of significant comminution or poor bone stock, the Belsky technique as described above can be utilized.[17] It should be noted, K-wire fixation primarily yields a biomechanical environment that results in indirect fracture healing. This can manifest as radiographic healing of the fracture lagging considerably behind clinical healing, with fracture gaps visible for 4 months following surgery.[19]

Another option is extra-articular cross-pin configuration. This can be achieved by placing the pins radial and ulnar to the extensor mechanism at the base of the phalanx (Fig. 78.5). A cadaveric study showed that K-wires placed away from the extensor mechanism permitted more excursion at the PIP joint than pins that were abutting or placed through it.[20] Al-Qattan compared transmetacarpal head pinning and cross-pin configuration and found less residual extensor lag with the cross-pin configuration.[21]

Lag screw fixation is an excellent technique and is indicated in the setting of spiral or oblique fracture configurations. The length of the fracture should be two to three times the width of the diaphysis to permit lag screw fixation. Screws are placed perpendicular to the fracture site and countersunk to avoid irritation of the extensor mechanism; as they compress across the fracture site, they provide absolute stability with direct fracture healing. Two screws have been found to provide adequate stability.[22] This method permits an early motion protocol to prevent adhesion formation. A randomized controlled trial comparing K-wires and screw fixation for oblique and spiral fractures of the proximal phalanx demonstrated no difference in the rate of malunion, grip strength, or active range of motion.[23]

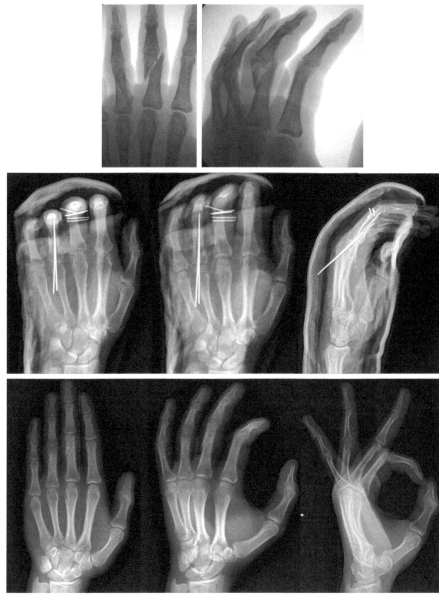

• **Fig. 78.3** A 24-year-old male who sustained ring and middle finger proximal phalanx fractures treated with closed reduction and percutaneous fixation, placed transarticular for the ring and perpendicular to the fracture for the middle.

Intramedullary fixation of proximal phalanx fractures has been used for a considerable length of time.[24] In the setting of transverse and short oblique diaphyseal fractures of the proximal phalanx, intramedullary screw fixation can provide an effective and relative minimally invasive construct. This technique avoids periosteal stripping and permits an early range-of-motion protocol. In a recent article reviewing 69 metacarpal and phalangeal shaft fractures treated with intramedullary screw fixation, all fractures healed with an average return to work in 76 days.[25] However, they noted that increased comminution or significant obliquity at the fracture site can raise the level of technical difficulty and may require a different method of fixation.[25]

Plate fixation provides increased rigidity as compared to other forms of fixation. However, they require extensive soft tissue mobilization which could lead to adhesion formation secondary to a foreign body reaction. Basar et al. compared screw fixation with plating in phalangeal fractures. They found range of motion and Q-DASH

scores were significantly better in those treated with screws alone.[26] They discouraged the use of mini-plate and screw fixation in treating spiral and oblique phalangeal fractures when possible.

External fixation is another option for stabilization, which can be particularly useful in the setting of open fractures, permitting access for wound care and avoiding disruption of tenuous blood supply to small fracture fragments. If external fixation is elected, the frame should be left in place for 4 weeks. During this time, range of motion of the surrounding joints is encouraged to minimize the formation of adhesions. The time frame with the fixator in place could be extended in the setting of significant comminution, bone loss, or soft tissue compromise.

Condylar Fractures of the Proximal Phalanx

K-wire fixation of unicondylar fractures is an excellent option and is minimally invasive. With regard to fixation, Weiss and Hastings noted the wire should be placed first into the fractured fragment then into the intact condyle to mitigate multiple passes.[6] They also noted that a single wire was susceptible to displacement, and that at least two wires should be employed for adequate fixation.[6]

Screws are another option in treating these injuries, particularly those in the setting of simple fracture patterns. Ford et al. described using 1.5- and 2.0-mm lag screws, for which they noted the most common deformity being a loss of 10–30 degrees of extension at the PIP joint.[27] The stability afforded with lag screw fixation permits an early motion protocol, which could lessen the degree of adhesion formation. Care should be taken to preserve the collateral ligament attachments, as stripping these from their

origin or insertion devascularizes the fragment and could lead to avascular necrosis.[28]

Mini-plates have a significant role in treating condylar fractures of the proximal phalanx. They are anatomically contoured and work to engage the diaphysis while buttressing the articular fragments. However, they require significant soft tissue mobilization in their application, thus inevitability leading to a higher likelihood of scarring. Their utility would be most advantageous in the setting of open fractures, where the wound already provides access for plate positioning. In their seminal article, Page and Sern found a 57% overall complication rate in plating of metacarpal and phalangeal fractures.[29] Within the phalangeal fracture cohort, 28.2% were found to have MCP or PIP flexion contracture of >35 degrees with total range of motion <180 degrees.[29] They concluded that treating these injuries with plate and screw constructs leads to a high incidence of unsatisfactory results.

Distal Phalanx Fractures

If indicated, K-wire fixation of the distal phalanx provides adequate stability. The tip of the distal phalanx lies just deep to the hyponychium. Using the fluoroscopy, a 0.028- or 0.035-inch K-wire should be inserted in a retrograde fashion. In the setting of open injuries, the wire can be inserted anterograde through the fracture site, followed by reduction of the fracture and retrograde drilling into the proximal fragment. A single wire can be used; however, a second wire adds further stiffness and stability to the construct.

Surgical Approaches

Proximal Phalanx

Several approaches have been described, with the traditional approach to the proximal phalanx being dorsal; however, there are advocates for lateral and volar approaches.[30] Swanson described the dorsal extensor splitting approach, in which the extensor mechanism is split in line with the tendon to expose the dorsum of the proximal phalanx.[31] This is the authors' preferred approach. Additionally, a Chamay approach has been described, in which a distally based triangular flap is created in the extensor tendon, permitting the lateral bands to fall volarly.[32] A midaxial approach can also be utilized, in which the proximal phalanx is exposed through

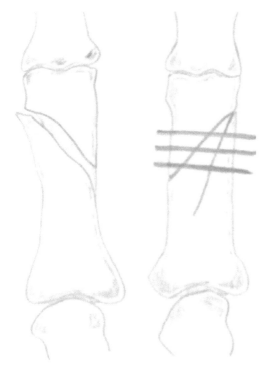

• **Fig. 78.4** Transverse K-wire fixation of long oblique fracture of proximal phalanx. (From Gregory S, Lalonde DH, Leung LTF. Minimally invasive finger fracture management: wide-awake closed reduction, K-wire fixation, and early protected movement. *Hand Clin*. 2014;30:7-15.)

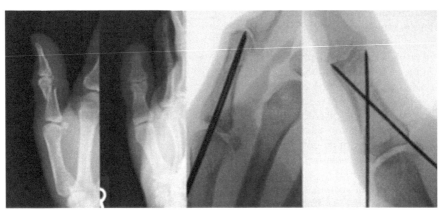

• **Fig. 78.5** K-wires are inserted in a crossed fashion, aiming to achieve multidirectional stability and maintain reduction. (From Carpenter S, Rohde RS. Treatment of phalangeal fractures. *Hand Clin*. 2013; 29[4]:519-534.)

the interval between the central slip and the lateral band. With a volar approach, a Bruner incision or hybrid Bruner-midaxial is marked out, and dissection is carried down to the flexor sheath. Lin et al. described incising the entire flexor sheath and raising it as a laterally based flap.[33] The flexor tendons are then retracted to one side to expose the proximal phalanx. After exposing and reducing the fracture, internal fixation can be achieved with K-wires, lag screws, or low-profile contoured plates.

Middle Phalanx

The dorsal approach is easily utilized for exposing fractures of the middle phalanx. Full-thickness skin flaps are elevated. Instead of splitting the extensor tendon as in the case of the proximal phalanx, the transverse retinacular ligament on each side can be divided to permit mobilization of the extensor mechanism. This allows excellent visualization of the fracture from both the radial and ulnar aspects.

A midaxial approach also permits access for fracture reduction and stabilization. Incision is marked out by flexing the digit and connecting the dorsal aspect of the skin creases that correspond with the center axis of rotation of the PIP and DIP joints. Full-thickness flaps are raised, with the neurovascular bundle protected with the volar tissues. The transverse retinacular ligament is exposed and divided, reflecting the lateral band dorsally. Subperiosteal exposure at the fracture site is performed to permit reduction and internal fixation.

Relevant Complications

The majority of these fractures are healed enough to permit return to work by 6 weeks but continue to remodel up to 5 months post injury.[34] However, independent of the method of treatment, phalanx fractures are susceptible to multiple adverse events such as stiffness, malunion, and infection among others.

Stiffness is the most common adverse outcome following these injuries. Risk factors for developing a contracture include multiply injured digits, periarticular fractures, crush mechanism, and significant soft tissue stripping.[4] To mitigate this, mobilization should begin no longer than 3–4 weeks following the injury. Treating stiffness involves a dedicated hand therapy program emphasizing active and passive range of motion. If needed, dynamic splinting can be custom-made for the patient. If edema has been controlled and the patient's progress has plateaued (typically around 6 months post injury), surgical intervention could be considered.

Malunion is a relatively common complication following non-operative management of a phalanx fracture, with different fracture patterns exhibiting a predilection for particular deformities. Malrotation can be seen following a spiral fracture, whereas shortening can be seen following a comminuted midshaft fracture. If an issue is identified in the acute to subacute setting, takedown of the nascent malunion may permit the surgeon to use the existing fracture lines to recreate the injury. In the chronic setting, prior to considering surgical intervention, attention should be focused on mobilizing the hand to optimize range of motion. In the event that surgery is indicated, various techniques in osteotomy can be utilized, though this is beyond the scope of this chapter.

Infection is rare, even in the setting of open fractures, with the incidence ranging from 2% to 11.1% in the literature.[35,36] The use of antibiotics in the treatment of open fractures is widely acknowledged as the standard of care, with multiple randomized prospective trials demonstrating their effectiveness.[37–39] However, the use of antibiotics in treating open fractures of the hand is controversial. A recent review demonstrated patients undergoing surgery for phalangeal fractures are not at increased risk of infection based on the diagnosis of open fracture alone.[40] Another study comparing two groups of patients with open fractures, with one receiving antibiotic therapy and the other not receiving any, failed to find a difference in infection rates between the two groups.[41] Botte et al. echoed these conclusions, finding no correlation between open injuries and infections in a review of patients treated with internal fixation for fractures or dislocations of the hand or wrist.[42]

References

1. Chung KC, Spilson SV. The frequency and epidemiology of hand and forearm fractures in the United States. *J Hand Surg Am.* 2001;26:908–915.
2. Smith RJ. Intrinsic muscles of the fingers: function, dysfunction, and surgical reconstruction. *AAOS Instr Course Lect.* 1975;24:200–220.
3. Panchal-Kildare S, Malone K. Skeletal anatomy of the hand. *Hand Clin.* 2013;29:459–471.
4. Wolfe S, Hotchkiss R, Pederson W, Kozin SH, Cohen M. *Green's Operative Hand Surgery.* Philadelphia, PA: Elsevier; 2017:231–275.
5. London PS. Sprains and fractures involving the interphalangeal joints. *Hand.* 1971;3:155–158.
6. Weiss AP, Hastings 2nd H. Distal unicondylar fractures of the proximal phalanx. *J Hand Surg Am.* 1993;18:594–599.
7. Coonrad RW, Pohlman MH. Impacted fractures in the proximal portion of the proximal phalanx of the finger. *J Bone Joint Surg.* 1969;51(A):1291–1296.
8. Green DP. Complications of phalangeal and metacarpal fractures. *Hand Clin.* 1986;2:307–328.
9. Wright TA. Early mobilization in fractures of the metacarpals and phalanges. *Can J Surg.* 1968;11:491–498.
10. Barton NJ. Fractures of the shafts of the phalanges of the hand. *Hand.* 1979;11:119–133.
11. James JI. Fractures of the proximal and middle phalanges of the fingers. *Acta Orthop Scand.* 1962;32:401–412.
12. Freeland AE, Sud V. Unicondylar and bicondylar proximal phalangeal fractures. *J Am Soc Surg Hand.* 2001;1:14–24.
13. Carpenter S, Rohde RS. Treatment of phalangeal fractures. *Hand Clin.* 2013;29(4):519–534.
14. Sloan J, Dove A, Maheson M, Cope AN, Welsh KR. Antibiotics in open fractures of the distal phalanx? *J Hand Surg Br.* 1987;12(1):123–124.
15. Zook EG, Guy RJ, Russel RC. A study of nail bed injuries: causes, treatment, and prognosis. *J Hand Surg Am.* 1984;9A:246–252.
16. Gregory S, Lalonde DH, Leung LTF. Minimally invasive finger fracture management: wide-awake closed reduction, K-wire fixation, and early protected movement. *Hand Clin.* 2014;30:7–15.
17. Belsky MR, Eaton RG, Lane LB. Closed reduction and internal fixation of proximal phalangeal fractures. *J Hand Surg Am.* 1984;9:725–729.
18. Faruqui S, Stern PJ, Kiefhaber TR. Percutaneous pinning of fractures in the proximal third of the proximal phalanx: complications and outcomes. *J Hand Surg Am.* 2012;37(7):1342–1348.
19. Logters TT, Lee HH, Gehrmann S, Windolf J, Kaufmann RA. Proximal phalanx fracture management. *Hand (N Y).* 2018;13(4):376–383.
20. Sela Y, Peterson C, Baratz ME. Tethering the extensor apparatus limits PIP flexion following K-wire placement for pinning extra-articular fractures at the base of the proximal phalanx. *Hand (N Y).* 2016;11(4):433–437.
21. Al-Qattan MM. Displaced unstable transverse fractures of the shaft of the proximal phalanx of the fingers in industrial workers: reduction and K-wire fixation leaving the metacarpophalangeal and proximal interphalangeal joints free. *J Hand Surg Eur.* 2011;36(7):577–583.

22. Zelken JA, Hayes AG, Parks BG, Al Muhit A, Means Jr KR. Two versus 3 lag screws for fixation of long oblique proximal phalanx fractures of the fingers: a cadaver study. *J Hand Surg Am*. 2015;40(6):1124–1129.

23. Horton TC, Hatton M, Davis TR. A prospective randomized controlled study of fixation of long oblique and spiral shaft fractures of the proximal phalanx: closed reduction and percutaneous Kirschner wiring versus open reduction and lag screw fixation. *J Hand Surg Br*. 2003;28(1):5–9.

24. Gonzalez MH, Igram CM, Hall RF. Intramedullary nailing of proximal phalanx fractures. *J Hand Surg Am*. 1995;20(5):808–812.

25. Del Pinal F, Moraleda E, Ruas J, De Piero GH, Cerezal L. Minimally invasive fixation of fractures of phalanges and metacarpals with intramedullary headless compression screws. *J Hand Surg Am*. 2015;40(4):692–700.

26. Basar H, Basar B, Basci O, Topkar OM, Erol B, Tetik C. Comparison of treatment of oblique and spiral metacarpal and phalangeal fractures with mini plate plus screw or screw only. *Arch Orthop Trauma Surg*. 2015;135(4):499–504.

27. Ford DJ, El-Hadidi S, Lunn PG, Burke FD. Fractures of the phalanges: results of internal fixation using 1.5mm and 2mm A. O. screws. *J Hand Surg Br*. 1987;12:28–33.

28. Yousif NJ, Cunningham MW, Sanger JR, Gingrass RP, Matloub HS. The vascular supply to the proximal interphalangeal joint. *J Hand Surg*. 1985;10A:852–861.

29. Page SM, Sern PJ. Complications and range of motion following plate fixation of metacarpal and phalangeal fractures. *J Hand Surg Am*. 1998;23(5):827–832.

30. Cheah AEJ, Yao J. Surgical approaches to the proximal interphalangeal joint. *J Hand Surg Am*. 2016;41(2):294–305.

31. Swanson AB, Maupin BK, Gajjar NV, Swanson GD. Flexible implant arthroplasty in the proximal interphalangeal joint of the hand. *J Hand Surg Am*. 1985;10(6):796–805.

32. Chamay A. A distally based dorsal and triangular tendinous flap for direct access to the proximal interphalangeal joint. *Ann Chir Main*. 1988;7(2):179–183.

33. Lin HH, Wyrick JD, Stern PJ. Proximal interphalangeal joint silicone replacement arthroplasty: clinical results using an anterior approach. *J Hand Surg Am*. 1995;20(1):123–132.

34. Smith FL, Rider DL. A study of the healing of one hundred consecutive phalangeal fractures. *J Bone Joint Surg Am*. 1935;17:91–109.

35. Swanson TV, Szabo RM, Anderson DD. Open hand fractures: prognosis and classification. *J Hand Surg Am*. 1991;16:101–107.

36. McLain RF, Steyers C, Stoddard M. Infections in open fractures of the hand. *J Hand Surg Am*. 1991;16(1):108–112.

37. Dunn JC, Means KR, Desale S, Giladi AM. Antibiotic use in hand surgery: surgeon decision making and adherence to available evidence. *Hand (NY)*. 2018;22:1–8.

38. Boyd RJ, Burke JF, Colton T. A double-blind clinical trial of prophylactic antibiotics in hip fractures. *J Bone Joint Surg Am*. 1973;55(6):1251–1258.

39. Burnett JW, Gustilo RB, Williams DN, Kind AC. Prophylactic antibiotics in hip fractures. A double-blind, prospective study. *J Bone Joint Surg Am*. 1980;62(3):457–462.

40. Minhas SV, Catalano 3rd LW. Comparison of open and closed hand fractures and the effect of urgent operative intervention. *J Hand Surg Am*. 2019;44:65. E1-65.E7.

41. Suprock MD, Hood JM, Lubahn JD. Role of antibiotics in open fractures of the finger. *J Hand Surg Am*. 1990;15: 761-674.

42. Botte MJ, Davis JL, Rose BA, et al. Complications of smooth pin fixation of fractures and dislocations in the hand and wrist. *Clin Orthop Relat Res*. 1992;276:194–201.

79

Technique Spotlight: Phalanx Fractures—Pins vs. Screws vs. Plates—When and How

FRANK A. RUSSO AND LOUIS W. CATALANO III

Diaphyseal Fractures of the Proximal and Middle Phalanx

Closed Reduction Percutaneous Pinning

The majority of proximal phalanx fractures displace with apex volar angulation. Therefore closed reduction involves traction with simultaneous flexion at the metacarpophalangeal (MP) joint to 70–90 degrees and extension at the proximal interphalangeal (PIP) joint. This maneuver relaxes the intrinsic muscles, which flex the proximal fragment, and permits the extensor hood to aid the reduction by serving as a tension band dorsally. Several percutaneous fixation constructs have been described. Our preference is to perform a closed reduction and place pins perpendicular to the plane of the fracture. The senior author uses one to two fracture-reduction clamps applied percutaneously to anatomically reduce and maintain the reduction while the pins are inserted. Using intraoperative fluoroscopy, a single 0.035- or 0.045-inch K-wire can be inserted into the near cortex perpendicular to the fracture site. We prefer multiple pins, at least three, to increase the stiffness of the construct. The pins can then be cut and bent above the skin or cut short and buried beneath the skin to be removed in the operative theater at 3–4 weeks.

In the setting of significant comminution, very proximal extra-articular base fractures, or if placing a perpendicular pin could tether the flexor or extensor tendons from a volar or dorsal starting point, we prefer the Belsky technique of anterograde transarticular pinning through the metacarpal head. Following closed reduction as described above, a single 0.045-inch K-wire is drilled anterograde through the metacarpal head across the MP joint and into the medullary canal of the proximal phalanx, stopping short of the articular surface of the condyles. It should be noted that the exact angle of insertion is determined under fluoroscopy. An additional wire can be added for increased stability; however, we feel a single wire is adequate for most fracture patterns (Fig. 79.1).

Fractures of the middle phalanx can present with variable angulation depending on where they occur with respect to the insertion of the flexor digitorum superficialis (FDS). The method of closed reduction is variable based on the location of the fracture in relation to the insertion of the FDS; fractures proximal to the insertion require flexion proximally and extension of the distal fragment. Conversely, those fractures distal to the insertion require extension of the proximal fragment and flexion of the distal fragment. Percutaneous fixation with K-wires can be achieved via a variety of techniques; however, the senior author's preferred method is placing multiple 0.035- or 0.045-inch K-wires perpendicular to the plane of the fracture, similar to that described for the proximal phalanx (Fig. 79.2).

Postoperatively, the digit should be immobilized in an intrinsic plus position, with the distal interphalangeal (DIP) joint left free to permit active range of motion and promote flexor digitorum profundus (FDP) tendon gliding. It is critical that the patient be instructed to work on active DIP joint flexion. This helps eliminate FDP tendon adhesions within the zone of injury. Also, the PIP and/or MP joints should be immobilized for no more than 4 weeks, at which point the pins should be removed and active range of motion should be initiated.

Open Reduction Internal Fixation With Lag Screws

The authors, preferred approach to both the proximal and middle phalanx is dorsal. The proximal phalanx is exposed via an extensor tendon splint, which provides excellent visualization and can be extended if need be. The tendon is retracted radially and ulnarly, which permits the lateral bands to fall volarly. The dorsal approach to the middle phalanx is slightly variable, where the transverse retinacular ligament is divided to allow the lateral band to be mobilized dorsally exposing the underlying cortex (Figs. 79.3 and 79.4).

Lag screw fixation is amenable for specific fracture orientations, such as long oblique and spiral patterns. We recommend close radiographic and clinical examination to ensure the length

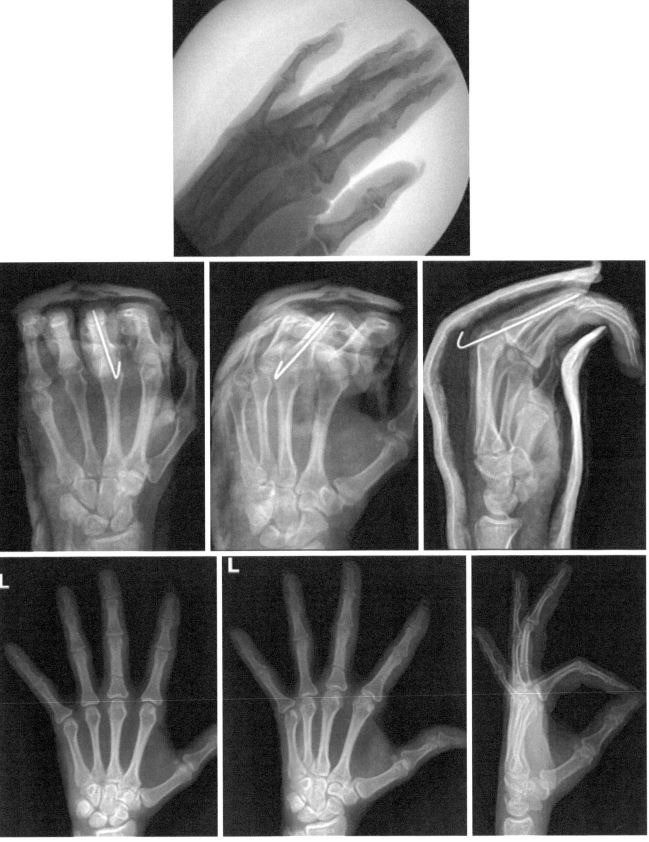

• **Fig. 79.1** A 48-year-old woman who sustained an extra-articular base fracture of her middle finger proximal phalanx, treated with closed reduction and transarticular pinning (Belsky technique).

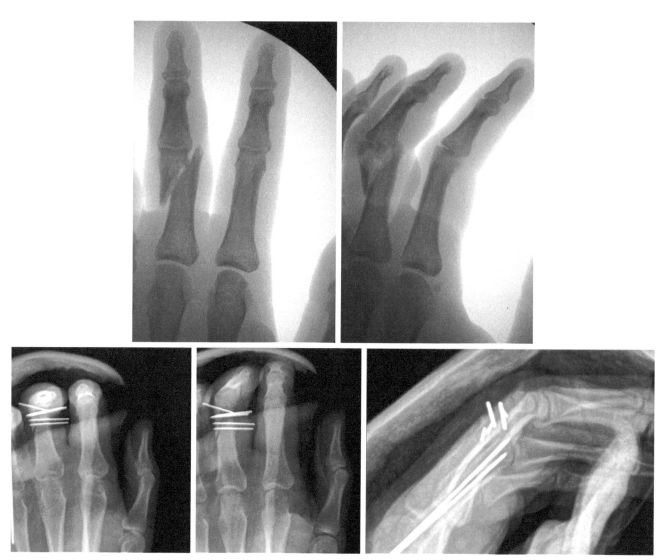

• **Fig. 79.2** A 24-year-old male who sustained ring and middle finger proximal phalanx fractures treated with closed reduction and percutaneous fixation. The posteroanterior and oblique views best demonstrate multiple K-wires placed perpendicular to the middle finger proximal phalanx. The lateral radiograph demonstrates the ring proximal phalanx fixed with a Belsky pinning technique.

of the fracture to be at least twice the width of the diaphysis to accommodate lag screws. After the reduction is obtained, two to three lag screws 1.5–2.0 mm in diameter should be placed orthogonal to the plane of the fracture. It is advisable to always have at least two points of fixation on the fracture fragments at all times. Small pointed bone tenaculums can be placed perpendicular to the fracture and in an unobstructed position to permit placement of the first lag screw.

The near cortex should be overdrilled to the outer diameter of the screw to allow for compression across the fracture site. The near cortex should be countersunk to limit the prominence of the screw head and prevent soft tissue irritation, thus decreasing the likelihood of adhesion formation. After the first lag screw is placed, one bone tenaculum can be removed and exchanged for a second lag screw. Once two lag screws are placed, the remaining tenaculum is removed, and if space permits, a third lag screw is placed.

If provisional fixation is achieved with K-wires, consider using a K-wire of the same diameter as the drill bit required for the screws that you are using. For example, if a 1.5-mm screw uses a drill bit of 1.1 mm, this is equivalent to a 0.045-inch K-wire. Often, the tract of the provisional fixation is also a potential trajectory for a

lag screw. In this case, the K-wire can be removed, the near cortex overdrilled, and a lag screw can be placed (Fig. 79.5).

This construct permits early motion protocols to help prevent significant adhesion formation. Therefore postoperatively we prefer a short period of immobilization to allow the incision to heal for 5–7 days, after which they are transitioned into a removable custom orthosis to allow for immediate active range of motion under the guidance of a hand therapist.

Open Reduction Internal Fixation With Plate and Screws

The dorsal extensor splitting approach provides an extensile exposure of the proximal phalanx. Mobilizing the tendon permits access proximally to the MP joint and distally to the articular surface at the PIP joint. The middle phalanx is approached as described above, with release of either the radial or ulnar transverse retinacular ligament for exposure. Following reduction, provisional fixation is obtained with reduction clamps and/or K-wires. For proximal phalanx fractures, a transarticular pin placed anterograde through the metacarpal head, as described by Belsky, is an excellent

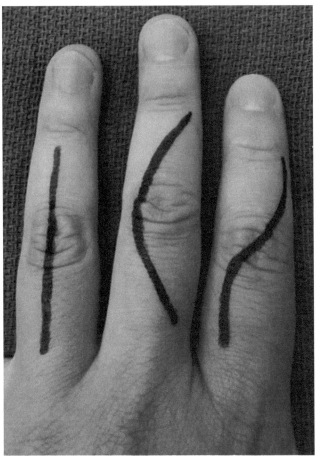

• **Fig. 79.3** Skin markings for the choice of dorsal skin incisions. From left to right, midline longitudinal incision, curvilinear incision, and a lazy S incision.

option for provisional fixation. As an alternative, a pointed reduction clamp or two can also be used for provisional fixation. After reestablishing length, alignment, and rotation, a dorsal plate can be fixed in place with an assortment of locking and nonlocking screws. Alternatively, if the fracture pattern prevents placement or adequate fixation with a dorsal plate, a lateral plate should be utilized. We prefer a dorsal approach as described above. If there is concern for tendon adhesions to the plate, the lateral band and oblique fibers can be excised. The extensor apparatus should then be reapproximated using 4-0 PDS and the skin closed (Fig. 79.6).

Condylar Fractures of the Proximal Phalanx

Closed Reduction Percutaneous Fixation

These injuries are invariably unstable; however, in simple fracture patterns we believe closed reduction and percutaneous fixation is an excellent option. A single 0.028- or 0.035-inch K-wire can be placed into the free condylar fragment, which can then be used as a joystick to perform a closed reduction. Once length, alignment, and rotation at the articular surface are confirmed under fluoroscopy, a fracture-reduction clamp is used to compress and maintain reduction. The K-wires should be advanced perpendicular to the fracture site. An additional two to three wires should be inserted to provide increased stiffness to the construct. The wires should then be cut short and buried beneath the skin, with planned removal after union is achieved (Fig. 79.7).

Open Reduction Internal Fixation With Plate and Screws

Lag screw and plate fixation for condylar fractures are ideal options to provide absolute stability and permit early motion. The approach varies slightly as compared with the approach for

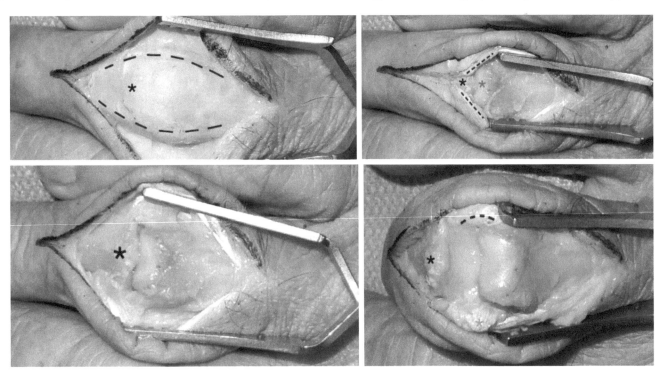

• **Fig. 79.4** Exposed extensor apparatus after elevation of skin flaps. *Asterisk* shows insertion of the central slip; *dashed lines* indicate the course of the lateral bands. Central slip splitting approach to expose the proximal interphalangeal (PIP) joint. *Black* and *red asterisks* show the central slip insertion and P1 head, respectively. Detachment of the central slip *(asterisk)* to afford greater exposure of the PIP joint. An increase in exposure gained to the PIP joint by proximal release of one collateral ligament *(blue asterisk)*. *Black asterisk* shows the central slip insertion; *dashed line* shows the intact collateral ligament.

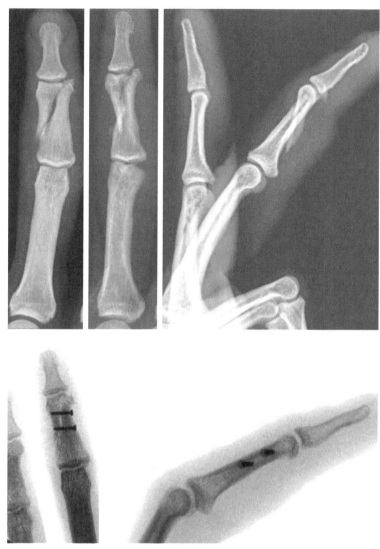

• **Fig. 79.5** A 32-year-old male who sustained a middle finger middle phalanx fracture treated with open reduction and lag screw fixation.

diaphyseal fractures described above. A portion of the radial or ulnar lateral band can be excised or released and reflected dorsally. This permits excellent exposure of the condyle and diaphysis proximally to position the plate. Because the vascular supply to the condyles is through the collateral ligaments, care is taken to avoid excessive stripping of the condylar fragment. These fractures are prone to osteonecrosis, often through iatrogenic injury to the blood supply via collateral ligament release in order to visualize and reduce the fracture. Every attempt is made to preserve the collateral ligament attachment to these fragments. The congruency of the articular surface should be reestablished before fixing the joint to the diaphysis. Fracture reduction can be obtained with a combination of reduction clamps and/or K-wires. These K-wires are placed as far dorsal or volar as possible to avoid preventing placement of the plate centrally on the condyle and in line with the shaft. Following provisional fixation of the articular segment, it should be approximated to the diaphysis with a precontoured low-profile plate. Intraoperative fluoroscopy should then be used to confirm restoration of length, alignment, and rotation of the fracture and ensure the plate is not malpositioned or oversized, especially on the lateral view. The majority of plates available provide locking and nonlocking screw options. We prefer to place a

single K-wire in the most proximal portion of the plate to ensure the entire plate is well positioned on bone. The first screw should be placed immediately proximal to the fracture to buttress the fragment. Following this, a screw should be placed into the fracture fragment distally. Next, the most proximal screw hole is filled to seat the plate onto bone proximally. The remaining holes are filled with a combination of locking and nonlocking screws.

Postoperative Protocol

Aside from when used as a bridge construct, plate and screws provide absolute stability and promote direct fracture healing; therefore they allow for an early motion protocol. We prefer a brief period of immobilization allowing the incision to heal over 5–7 days, during which the digit is placed in an intrinsic plus position with the DIP joint left free. They are then transitioned to a removable custom orthosis for protection and to initiate immediate active range of motion.

Fractures of the Distal Phalanx

For significantly displaced fractures of the distal phalanx recalcitrant to closed treatment, or open injuries, percutaneous fixation is

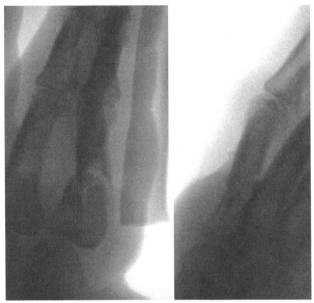

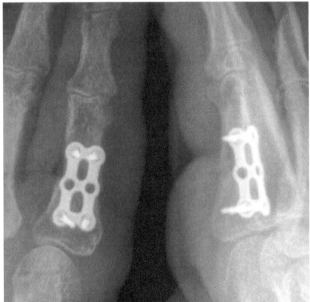

• **Fig. 79.6** A 48-year-old male with a 4-week-old proximal phalanx fracture of the index finger treated with open reduction and internal fixation with a plate and screw construct.

an excellent option. The starting point for the K-wire is just below the hyponychium; a 0.028- or 0.035-inch wire is then placed into the distal fragment and used as a joystick to help approximate the reduction. The wire is then drilled retrograde into the proximal fragment across the DIP and into the middle phalanx. In the setting of open injuries, a K-wire can be placed anterograde through the fracture site into the distal fragment out through the pulp just below the hyponychium. The fracture is then reduced, and the wire drilled retrograde back across the fracture site into the proximal fragment crossing the DIP, if need be, for further stability. Postoperatively, the DIP should be splinted in extension and the PIP should be left free to permit range of motion. The wire should be removed at 4 weeks, and immediate active range of motion with emphasis on tendon gliding should be initiated under the guidance of a hand therapist.

PEARLS AND PITFALLS

- Percutaneous reduction with clamps and fixation using pins is the preferred treatment option for the majority of these fractures.
- Intraoperatively, the surgeon must confirm restoration of length, alignment, and joint congruity using multiple fluoroscopic views (e.g., posteroanterior [PA], lateral, and multiple obliques) before and after fixation.
- Prior to leaving the operating room, passive range of motion and rotational alignment of the digits must be assessed, as malrotation cannot be appreciated on fluoroscopy alone.
- Pins that limit motion should be removed no later than 4 weeks and range of motion should be initiated immediately afterwards.
- Constructs that require extensive soft tissue dissection should be used judiciously given the increased likelihood of adhesions.
- A certified hand therapist is crucial for fabricating custom-made splints, guiding the patient through range of motion, and using modalities to decrease edema and formation of postoperative adhesions.

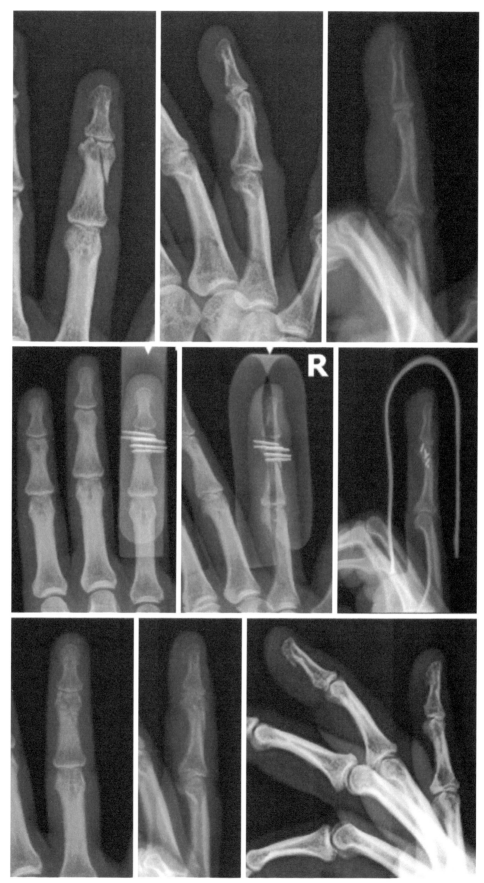

• **Fig. 79.7** A 42-year-old woman with a unicondylar fracture treated with closed reduction and percutaneous fixation with five 0.028-inch K-wires.

80

Proximal Interphalangeal Joint Dislocations

MARC J. O'DONNELL AND WARREN C. HAMMERT

Introduction

Proximal interphalangeal (PIP) joint injuries are common and in spite of seemingly minor injuries, these can affect the overall hand function. Stiffness is common with these injuries and there is often permanent residual swelling, changing the size of the digit. Patients often present in a delayed manner as it was assumed to be a "jammed finger" that would get better. When it does not improve as anticipated, they present with pain, stiffness, or residual deformity. Basic management principles are similar to other musculoskeletal injuries and include examination and imaging. The digit is evaluated for edema and the cascade for alignment of the finger in relation to adjacent digits. With flexion, the digits should point to the scaphoid tubercle and any scissoring or malalignment should be noted. While hand radiographs are appropriate for screening, radiographs of the injured digit are needed, and orthogonal views should be obtained to avoid missing subtle injuries. For finger injuries, three views of the digit are preferred.

Relevant Anatomy

The PIP joint is a complex ginglymus joint formed by the convex head of the proximal phalanx, concave base of the middle phalanx, volar plate, and collateral ligaments. There are associated bony attachments of the extensor apparatus (central slip) as well as the flexor digitorum superficialis (FDS). The osseous anatomy and relationship between the two bones impart stability to the joint.

The head of the proximal phalanx is in the shape of a trapezoid, with an intercondylar groove that allows it to articulate with the two facets of the base of the middle phalanx, with an intervening ridge.[1] There is palmar tilt to the head of the proximal phalanx, which results in an average arc of motion of 0 to 100 degrees. In a recent paper by Dumont et al., they demonstrated that the PIP joint is nonconforming, with the base of the middle phalanx having a lesser curvature than the condyles of the proximal phalanx.[2] This difference in curvature results in incongruity of the joint with range of motion. Furthermore, there is slight asymmetry between the condyles of the proximal phalanx, with the width of the radial condyles narrower in the index and long fingers, and wider in the ring and small fingers when compared to the ulnar condyles, allowing the digit to point toward the scaphoid tubercle with flexion.[3]

The radial and ulnar collateral ligaments originate from the collateral recess of the head of the proximal phalanx and are essential for stability of the PIP joint against lateral force. The proper collateral ligament is a stout structure that has a broad insertion on the lateral base of the middle phalanx, while the accessory collateral ligament is a more diminutive structure that inserts on the volar plate and can be thought of as an extension of the joint capsule rather than a discrete ligament.[4]

The volar plate of the PIP joint is a thickening of the capsule that prevents hyperextension of the joint. It is a fibrocartilaginous structure that has a robust insertion on the base of the middle phalanx through Sharpey's fibers and proximally has radial and ulnar extensions known as checkrein ligaments that loosely blend into the periosteum of the proximal phalanx.[5] The loose proximal insertion allows the volar plate to slide proximally with finger flexion.

The FDS and flexor digitorum profundus (FDP) traverse the palmar aspect of the joint. While the FDP continues to insert onto the base of the distal phalanx, the FDS has two slips that allow the FDP to pass through it at Camper's chiasma, then coalesce and insert broadly onto the proximal half of the middle phalanx. The extensor apparatus over the dorsal aspect of the joint is a complex structure, with its most important components relative to the joint being the central slip and lateral bands, which are formed from both the extrinsic and intrinsic muscles of the hand. The central slip inserts on the dorsal base of the middle phalanx, while the radial and ulnar lateral bands pass dorsal/lateral to the joint to then insert on the base of the distal phalanx.

Pathoanatomy and Classifications

Dislocations and fracture-dislocations are described by the direction of the distal structure, in this case, the middle phalanx, such as dorsal, volar, and lateral. A special category of middle phalanx base articular fractures is the pilon fracture, where the central portion of the joint is injured, but the dorsal and volar aspects are intact.

Dorsal Dislocation

The most common PIP dislocations are dorsal, typically occurring from an axial load on a hyperextended finger (Fig. 80.1). This injury pattern necessitates complete rupture of the volar plate, and variable degree of injury to the collateral ligaments, sparing the central slip. It is common to have small fracture fragments at the

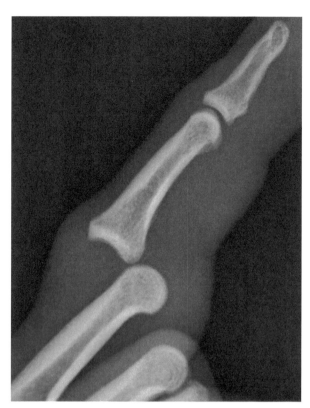

• **Fig. 80.1** Type II dorsal proximal interphalangeal joint dislocation.

TABLE 80.1	Descriptive Classification for Dorsal Proximal Interphalangeal Joint Dislocations	
Type	Description
I	Hyperextension deformity, joint surfaces still touch
II	Bayonet apposition of joint surfaces
III	Fracture-dislocation

base of the middle phalanx reflecting a volar plate avulsion injury. In some instances, the avulsed volar plate can become interposed in the joint upon attempt at closed reduction, necessitating open reduction of the injury.[6]

A simple descriptive classification system has been developed to detail three types of dorsal PIP joint dislocations (Table 80.1).

Volar Dislocation

Volar dislocation is much less common than dorsal. These include volar dislocation with or without a rotatory component (Fig. 80.2). This is the most common type of dislocation to result in an open injury. A volar-rotatory dislocation occurs when one collateral ligament remains intact. The typical mechanism of injury is torque on the finger, such as when the finger gets caught in something and the arm pulls away. This may result in a condyle of the proximal phalanx being button-holed between the central slip and the lateral band.[7] The standard reduction maneuver, which includes traction, may tighten the "noose" that the extensor apparatus (central extensor tendon and lateral band) creates around the entrapped condyle, making the injury irreducible by closed means. The favored reduction maneuver includes flexion at the

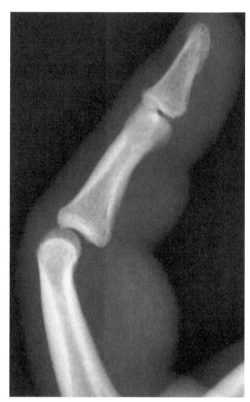

• **Fig. 80.2** Joint incongruency from volar-rotatory proximal interphalangeal joint dislocation. Note the condyles of the proximal phalanx are aligned while those of the middle phalanx are not.

metacarpophalangeal (MP) joint as well as the PIP joint to relax the flexor apparatus.

If there is no rotatory component, then closed reduction is easier to obtain, but there should be a high suspicion for a central slip injury. The integrity of the central slip must be tested after closed reduction with active extension as well as the Elson test (Fig. 80.3), which is performed by flexing the PIP joint and maintaining the MP and distal interphalangeal (DIP) joint in extension. If the central slip is intact, attempted extension of the digit at the PIP joint will leave the DIP joint supple due to the pull of the central slip on the middle phalanx. If the central slip is disrupted, the pull will be at the DIP joint through the terminal tendon and the joint will be rigid. Central slip injury necessitates immobilization of the joint after closed reduction. Missed or inadequate management of a central slip injury could result in future boutonnière deformity to the finger.

Lateral Dislocation

Lateral dislocations of the PIP joint necessitate rupture of at least one of the collateral ligaments (Fig. 80.4). The typical mechanism of injury is axial load and varus or valgus stress on the finger. These can often be reduced by closed means, and stable, stiff joints frequently result.

Dorsal Fracture-Dislocation

When considering dorsal fracture-dislocations, the size of the fracture fragment directly correlates to the postreduction stability of the joint. The small volar plate avulsion fracture can be thought of more as a ligamentous injury than a fracture

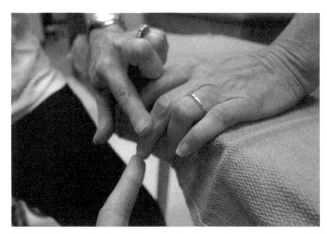

• **Fig. 80.3** Demonstration of Elson test—the metacarpophalangeal joint is extended, and the proximal interphalangeal joint is flexed over the edge of the table. The middle phalanx is extended against resistance. While resisting the middle phalanx extension, the distal phalanx is evaluated and should be easily flexible, indicating intact central slip. If the distal interphalangeal joint is firm/rigid, this indicates the central slip is not in continuity and the pull of the extensor mechanism is directed solely to the terminal tendon.

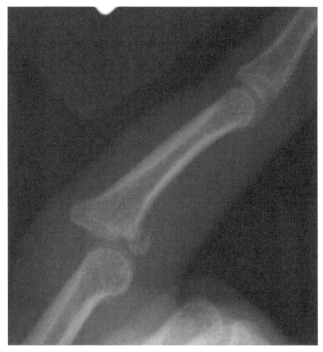

• **Fig. 80.5** Unstable proximal interphalangeal joint dorsal fracture-dislocation. Note the "V" sign.

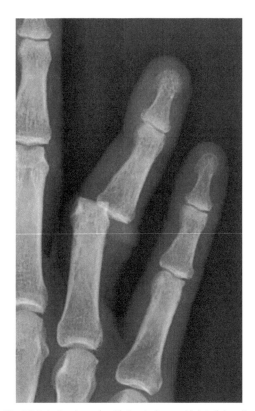

• **Fig. 80.4** Lateral proximal interphalangeal joint dislocation.

and this fracture can often be ignored, treating the injury as a simple dislocation instead if the middle phalanx base is largely intact.

It is important to look for subtle joint instability after reduction by assessing for congruency of the joint on the lateral view. The so-called "V" sign should be assessed, evaluating for dorsal subluxation of the middle phalanx (Fig. 80.5). The Hastings classification has been developed to help predict postreduction

stability of these injuries. The stability of the joint is based on the size of the fracture of the volar-lip of the middle phalanx: <30% is stable, 30%–50% tenuous, and >50% unstable.[8]

Volar Fracture-Dislocation

Volar fracture-dislocations are much less common. With this type of injury, the size of the dorsal-lip fracture fragment should be assessed, similar to dorsal fracture-dislocations. The larger the fragment, the higher the chance of joint instability. Importantly, the central slip of the extensor apparatus inserts on this fragment. These may be "missed" injuries that present to the office weeks out from the injury.

Pilon Fracture

This injury occurs from axial load when the joint is colinear, often resulting in a comminuted, impacted fracture of the base of the middle phalanx, similar to axial load injuries to the lower extremity. The joint itself may appear relatively congruent. Plain radiographs may appear rather benign, and computed tomography (CT) scan is needed to evaluate the articular surface. These injuries often require operative intervention, which may be quite challenging, as will be discussed later.

Treatment Options

Treatment of PIP joint dislocations is based upon examination and radiographic findings. Standard treatments for most injuries include closed reduction, which can often be done with digital block anesthesia. It is important to classify the injury to apply the appropriate reduction maneuver. Following reduction, joint stability should be assessed with active and passive range of motion of the finger.

For dislocations and fracture-dislocations that are reduced and stable, buddy taping to an adjacent digit and early motion is the

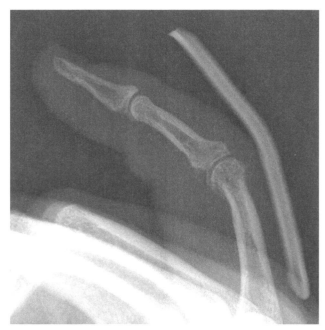

• **Fig. 80.6** Dorsal extension block splint limiting terminal 30 degrees of proximal interphalangeal extension, taped to proximal phalanx, with middle phalanx free.

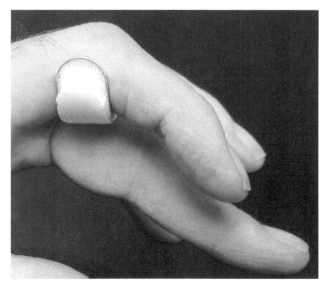

• **Fig. 80.7** Relative motion flexion orthosis.

preferred treatment. Buddy taping imparts stability by using the uninjured finger as a dynamic splint, limiting recurrent episodes of instability, while allowing motion. Buddy taping may cause skin breakdown and is known to have low patient compliance, which may allow for recurrent joint injury as well as stiffness.[9] These injuries are often protected with a splint after closed reduction by emergency department or urgent care providers, potentially resulting in substantial stiffness.

Dorsal fracture-dislocations with a volar fracture fragment larger than 30% of the joint surface should be carefully assessed for stability after reduction, as these may or may not be stable. If stable, buddy taping is the preferred treatment. If the joint is found to be unstable, then an extension block splint should be applied to block terminal extension, which is the direction of instability. The point of subluxation/dislocation should be measured, and the splint should be applied with 10 degrees of additional flexion (Fig. 80.6). There are a multitude of splint designs, including aluminum-foam, figure-eight, dynamic extension block splints, and custom fabricated splints typically molded and managed by a certified hand therapist.[10] The patient should be seen on a weekly basis by a provider or hand therapist, and the splint should be extended 10 degrees at each visit. The splint should allow finger flexion to minimize finger stiffness. If the joint is found to be unstable, or if flexion of >30 degrees is required to hold reduction, then surgery should be considered. While there is no high-quality literature that supports the 30-degree flexion rule, increased joint flexion can cause joint flexion contracture.[11]

When dealing with a volar dislocation or fracture-dislocation, there should be high suspicion for central slip injury. Following closed reduction of the injury, integrity of the central slip should be assessed. This can be done with the Elson test, as previously described. It is generally thought that the central slip must be injured for a volar dislocation event to occur (with the exception of a volar-rotatory injury). Therefore it is recommended that the PIP joint is splinted in full extension, similar to treatment for a boutonnière deformity. The DIP joint should be kept free and

motion through this joint should be encouraged to mobilize the lateral bands. Full extension should be maintained for 3–4 weeks, as further immobilization has a high probability of irreversible joint stiffness in a nonfunctional position. After the extension splint is removed, hand therapy referral may be beneficial for fabrication of a relative motion flexion orthosis, to decrease the force on the healing central slip[12] (Fig. 80.7). If the joint is incongruent after closed reduction or there is a large displaced fracture fragment, then surgery should be considered.

Indications for Surgery

Surgery is often indicated when closed reduction cannot be achieved under digital block anesthesia. This would apply to any of the aforementioned dislocations or fracture-dislocations.

Other common indications for surgery include:
- Open injuries: on a case-by-case basis depending on level of contamination and associated soft tissue injuries.
- Persistent joint incongruence, such as the "V" sign after closed reduction.
- Dorsal fracture-dislocations that require >30 degrees of flexion to maintain reduction.
- Volar-rotatory dislocations, which are commonly irreducible by closed means.
- Volar fracture-dislocations with a large displaced bony fragment.
- Pilon injury: on a case-by-case basis, depending on articular incongruity.
- Chronic injuries (6 weeks out from time of injury) on a case-by-case basis.

There are many surgical treatment options. The Technique Spotlight chapter (Chapter 81) will review extension block pinning, ORIF (open reduction internal fixation) with hemihamate arthroplasty, and dynamic external fixation.

Surgical Approaches

For PIP joint dislocations and fracture-dislocations that are found to be irreducible in the emergency department or office, an attempt at closed reduction in the operating room should be done. If closed reduction can be obtained, and the joint is found

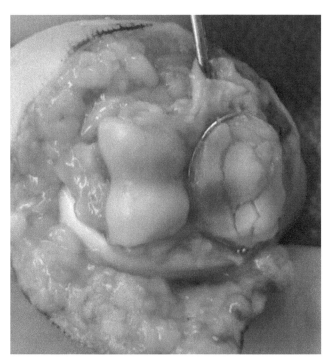

• **Fig. 80.8** Proximal interphalangeal joint exposure from "shotgun" approach. Note cerclage wire around base of middle phalanx.

to be stable, then buddy taping can be commenced. If the joint is unstable, then extension block splinting or extension block pinning can be done.

If reduction cannot be achieved closed, then open reduction should be performed. There are three approaches to the PIP joint: volar, lateral, and dorsal. Frequently, the type of injury will dictate the surgical approach. Anesthesia may be done with local-only anesthesia, monitored anesthesia care, regional anesthesia, or general anesthesia. Local-only anesthesia is beneficial when active motion needs to be assessed.

The volar approach to the PIP joint is most often utilized for dorsal irreducible dislocations and fracture-dislocations. This approach begins with a standard Bruner incision over the proximal and middle phalanges. Caution should be exercised as the trauma may displace the digital neurovascular bundles. Soft tissue dissection should come down directly on top of the flexor sheath. The sheath should be opened between the A2 and A4 pulleys; if required, 50% of the A2 and A4 pulleys may be vented. There is evidence that judicious venting of the pulleys is safe and does not result in enough tendon bowstringing to cause a clinically functional disturbance.[13] The volar plate will commonly be avulsed from the base of the middle phalanx, but often scarred back down. This is released with a transverse incision along the base of the middle phalanx and the fragments are removed from the volar plate, allowing proximal retraction to visualize the joint surface.

If the articular surface of the joint needs to be further assessed, then the joint can be "shot-gunned" open (Fig. 80.8). This requires excision of the collateral ligaments from the base of the middle phalanx to facilitate exposure. Failure to do so could result in further articular injury when the joint is forcefully hyperextended. This allows for excellent exposure for surgical fixation of the articular surface.

It is vital to restore the cup-shaped morphology of the volar-lip of the base of the middle phalanx, as failure to do so may cause recurrent instability. After reduction has been achieved, reduction

may be held with extension block pinning, small screws (1.0–1.5 mm), cerclage wires, or small volar buttress plates. If there is articular comminution that is found to be irreducible, then hemihamate arthroplasty may be employed to reconstruct the volar base of the middle phalanx. This is often performed for chronic injuries, and when >50% of the articular surface is involved.[14] Volar plate arthroplasty is a technique that was historically used when the joint surface could not be reconstructed, but this has fallen out of favor as it is technically demanding, and results were not consistently reproducible. The techniques for ORIF and hemihamate arthroplasty will be discussed in Chapter 81. The dorsal cortex needs to remain intact for the hemihamate graft. The lateral approach to the PIP joint is not frequently applied for dislocations or fracture-dislocations.

The dorsal approach to the PIP joint is performed when repair of a dorsal fracture fragment is required and to obtain open reduction of an irreducible volar-rotatory injury. The skin incision can be direct posterior, or curvilinear, preserving the dorsal veins when possible. If the injury is volar-rotatory, one condyle of the proximal phalanx will often be button-holed between the central slip and lateral band. Once reduced, the joint will often be stable. The integrity of the central slip should be assessed, although it is often intact with volar-rotatory injuries, negating the need for immobilization.

If there is a dorsal fracture fragment that requires reduction and fixation, this may require incision of the extensor apparatus. Multiple options exist for this, including extensor tendon sparing, extensor tendon splitting, and extensor tendon reflecting (Chamay) approaches. The amount of exposed PIP joint per approach has been found to be 16%, 41%, and 52%, respectively.[15] There is no consensus on the best form of internal fixation for these injuries. Techniques described include K-wires, lag screws, cerclage wires, suture anchors, and plates.[16,17] After bony fixation has been achieved, the extensor apparatus repair should be protected. Often, the dorsal fragment will contain the central slip insertion. It can be challenging to hold the reduction and some malalignment of the joint often occurs.

Pilon fractures can be challenging to treat. Depending on the fracture pattern, they may be treated with closed or open techniques. An open approach is dictated by the location of the major fracture fragments, whether volar or dorsal. Fixation techniques are similar to those above. Often, the injury is comminuted, and fracture stabilization with open reduction may not be achievable. In these situations, closed reduction and dynamic external fixation is the preferred treatment.[18] This technique will be highlighted in Chapter 81.

Salvage techniques for failed acute treatment and missed chronic injuries may be required to treat pain and improve the posture of the finger and include arthrodesis in a functional position and arthroplasty.[19]

Relevant Complications

Common complications from PIP joint dislocations and fracture-dislocations include PIP and DIP stiffness, tendon imbalance (swan-neck or boutonnière deformity), and recurrent instability. DIP stiffness is often the result of immobilization of the DIP joint, which can often be seen when these injuries are treated by emergency department and urgent care staff. It is important to leave the DIP joint free and encourage motion of this joint to keep the lateral bands mobilized. Swan-neck deformity occurs with dorsal injuries secondary to incompetence of the volar plate.

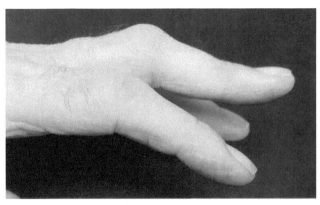

• **Fig. 80.9** Boutonnière deformity from central slip injury.

Boutonnière deformity is less common and occurs with a central slip injury from volar dislocations or fracture-dislocations (Fig. 80.9). These deformities can often be mitigated by timely referral to a certified hand therapist for splint fabrication, modalities, and motion exercises.

The vascular supply to the volar aspect of the base of the middle phalanx, at the attachment site of the volar plate, is sparse, and nonunion is a possibility, although this is infrequently encountered.[20] Nonunion is more likely to present in patients who have chronic missed PIP joint fracture-dislocations, rather than from the treatment of the injury.[21]

Each fixation technique has associated complications. Anytime a percutaneous wire is left in place, infection is possible, as is wire breakage.[22] Volar plate arthroplasty has a high risk of recurrent instability,[23] while ORIF has the risk of malunion, especially if the volar or dorsal-lip alignment of the base of the middle phalanx is not restored, sometimes necessitating corrective osteotomy.[24] Hemihamate arthroplasty has a complication rate of 35%, including minor complications such as tenderness and radiographic signs of arthritis in up to 50% of cases.[25]

Review of Treatment Outcomes

PIP joint injuries include simple dislocations that are easily reducible and complex fracture patterns that require open treatment, and the outcomes are often correlated to the chronicity of the injury and the treatment required. PIP joint motion exists on a spectrum with instability on one end, and stiffness on the other. By far, stiffness and flexion contracture are the most common outcomes when the joint is injured. The average PIP joint range of motion (ROM) after operative management is 65 to 90 degrees, with diminished motion caused by joint incongruity, hemarthrosis, and joint adhesions, lack of extension power from central slip injury, edema, prolonged immobilization, and poor compliance with therapy.[26] Chronic swelling is normal, which may also limit joint motion during recovery. This can improve over 9–12 months and typically does not completely resolve.

In a paper reviewing 12 patients treated with extension block pinning for unstable PIP joint injuries with a mean follow-up of 35.5 months, average PIP joint ROM was 84 degrees, with 11 of 12 patients maintaining radiographic reduction, and average QuickDASH score 5.7.[27]

At average follow-up of 29 months in 21 patients who underwent ORIF with a shotgun approach for PIP joint dorsal fracture-dislocations, mean ROM was 80 degrees (78% of the contralateral joint), with mean DASH (The Disabilities of the Arm, Shoulder

and Hand) score of 5.5, and only two patients demonstrating radiographic findings of arthritis.[28]

Meyer et al. reported on eight patients with central slip avulsion fractures with PIP joint volar instability, with an average follow-up of 43 months, average passive and active PIP joint ROM was 62 and 54 degrees, respectively, with six of eight patients developing radiographic signs of arthritis, and four of eight requiring additional interventions.[16] Volar fracture-dislocations are less common than dorsal fracture-dislocations and often portend a worse long-term prognosis.

Ruland et al. treated 34 patients with dynamic external fixation, with a final arc of PIP motion of 88 degrees at 16 months; 8 patients required oral antibiotics for superficial pin site infection, with no patients having loss of reduction.[29]

Summary

PIP joint dislocations and fracture-dislocations present treatment challenges. Simple dislocations that are immediately reduced and then appropriately mobilized often have excellent clinical outcomes, whereas complex articular injuries, such as pilon fractures, are often treated in a delayed fashion with a high risk of stiffness and posttraumatic arthrosis. Depending on the injury classification, various treatment options may be employed. Overall, the goal of treatment is to obtain a congruent articulation, minimize soft tissue trauma, and maximize joint ROM. Stiffness is a much more common occurrence than recurrent instability. Chapter 81 will highlight a few of the many techniques available for the surgical treatment of these injuries.

References

1. Leibovic SJ, Bowers WM. Anatomy of the proximal interphalangeal joint. *Hand Clin.* 1994;10(2):169–178.
2. Dumont C, Albus G, Kubein-Meesenburg D, Fanghänel J, Stürmer KM, Nägerl H. Morphology of the interphalangeal joint surface and its functional relevance. *J Hand Surg.* 2008;33(1):9–18.
3. Lawrence T, Trail IA, Noble J. Morphological measurements of the proximal interphalangeal joint. *J Hand Surg.* 2004;29(3):242–247.
4. Allison DM. Anatomy of the collateral ligaments of the proximal interphalangeal joint. *J Hand Surg.* 2005;30(5):1026–1031.
5. Williams EH, McCarthy E, Bickel KD. The histologic anatomy of the volar plate. *J Hand Surg.* 1998;23(5):805–810.
6. Green SM, Posner MA. Irreducible dorsal dislocations of the proximal interphalangeal joint. *J Hand Surg.* 1985;10(1):85–87.
7. Deshmukh NV. Irreducible volar dislocations of the proximal interphalangeal joint. *Emergency Med J.* 2005;22(3):221–223.
8. Kang R, Stern PJ. Fracture dislocations of the proximal interphalangeal joint. *J Am Society Surg Hand.* 2002;2:47–59.
9. Won SH, Lee S, Chung CY, et al. Buddy taping: is it a safe method for treatment of finger and toe injuries? *Clin Orthopedic Surg.* 2014;6(1):26.
10. Abboudi J, Jones CM. Proximal interphalangeal joint extension block splint. *Hand.* 2016;11(2):152–160.
11. Green DP, Wolfe SW. *Greens Operative Hand Surgery.* Philadelphia: Elsevier; 2017.
12. Merritt WH. Relative motion splint: active motion after extensor tendon injury and repair. *J Hand Surg.* 2014;39(6):1187–1194.
13. Tang JB. Recent evolutions in flexor tendon repairs and rehabilitation. *J Hand Surg.* 2018;43(5):469–473.
14. Gonzalez RM, Hammert WC. Dorsal fracture-dislocations of the proximal interphalangeal joint. *J Hand Surg.* 2015;40(12):2453–2455.
15. Wei DH, Strauch RJ. Dorsal surgical approaches to the proximal interphalangeal joint: a comparative anatomic study. *J Hand Surg.* 2014;39(6):1082–1087.

16. Meyer ZI, Goldfarb CA, Calfee RP, Wall LB. The central slip fracture: results of operative treatment of volar fracture subluxations/dislocations of the proximal interphalangeal joint. *J Hand Surg.* 2017;42(7)572.e1-572.e6.

17. Kang GC-W, Yam A, Phoon ES, Lee JY-L, Teoh L-C. The hook plate technique for fixation of phalangeal avulsion fractures. *J Bone Joint Surg Am.* 2012 Jun 6;94(11):e72. doi: 10.2106/JBJS.K.00601.

18. Henn CM, Lee SK, Wolfe SW. Dynamic external fixation for proximal interphalangeal fracture-dislocations. *Operative Techniques Orthopaed.* 2012;22(3):142–150.

19. Kamnerdnakta S, Huetteman HE, Chung KC. Complications of proximal interphalangeal joint injuries. *Hand Clin.* 2018;34(2):267–288.

20. Freiberg A, Pollard BA, Macdonald MR, Duncan MJ. Management of proximal interphalangeal joint injuries. *Hand Clin.* 2006;22(3):235–242.

21. Lu J, Xu L, Xu J, Gu Y. Individualized reconstruction of chronic fractures affecting the PIP joint. *J Hand Surg.* 2015;40(9):e23.

22. Pichler W, Mazzurana P, Clement H, Grechenig S, Mauschitz R, Grechenig W. Frequency of instrument breakage during orthopaedic procedures and its effects on patients. *J Bone Joint Surg-Am.* 2008;90(12):2652–2654.

23. Deitch MA, Kiefhaber TR, Comisar B, Stern PJ. Dorsal fracture dislocations of the proximal interphalangeal joint: surgical complications and long-term results. *J Hand Surg.* 1999;24(5):914–923.

24. Piñal FD, García-Bernal FJ, Delgado J, Sanmartín M, Regalado J. Results of osteotomy, open reduction, and internal fixation for late-presenting malunited intra-articular fractures of the base of the middle phalanx. *J Hand Surg Am.* 2005;30(5)1039.e1-1039.e14.

25. Frueh FS, Calcagni M, Lindenblatt N. The hemi-hamate autograft arthroplasty in proximal interphalangeal joint reconstruction: a systematic review. *J Hand Surg.* 2014;40(1):24–32.

26. Mangelson JJ, Stern P, Abzug JM, Chang J, Osterman AL. Complications following dislocations of the proximal interphalangeal joint. *J Bone Joint Surg-Am.* 2013;95(14):1326–1332.

27. Bear DM, Weichbrodt MT, Huang C, Hagberg WC, Balk ML. Unstable dorsal proximal interphalangeal joint fracture-dislocations treated with extension-block pinning. *Am J Orthop.* 2015;44(3):122–126.

28. Mazhar FN, Jafari D, Taraz H, Mirzaei A. Treatment of dorsal fracture-dislocations of the proximal interphalangeal joint using the shotgun approach. *J Hand Surg.* 2018;43(5):499–505.

29. Ruland RT, Hogan CJ, Cannon DL, Slade JF. Use of dynamic distraction external fixation for unstable fracture-dislocations of the proximal interphalangeal joint. *J Hand Surg.* 2008;33(1):19–25.

81

Technique Spotlight: ORIF vs. Extension Block Pinning vs. Dynamic External Fixation for Proximal Interphalangeal Joint Dislocations

MARC J. O'DONNELL AND WARREN C. HAMMERT

Introduction

This chapter will highlight three available techniques to achieve a stable proximal interphalangeal (PIP) joint after dislocation and fracture-dislocations: extension block pinning, open reduction internal fixation (ORIF) including hemihamate arthroplasty, and dynamic external fixation. Many other treatment options exist. Treatment should be tailored to the injury pattern and patient demographics.

Extension Block Pinning

Indications

Extension block pinning may be done when a PIP joint dorsal dislocation or fracture-dislocation can be reduced but is still unstable. It has the benefit of minimizing soft tissue trauma, which reduces the likelihood of stiffness. This technique may also be used to supplement ORIF, depending on the stability of fixation and the joint.

Preoperative Evaluation

A thorough history should be performed, including the date and mechanism of injury. Chronic injuries, defined as injuries >6 weeks old, have worse outcomes when treated surgically including diminished range of motion by 14 degrees, and increased risk of recurrent instability by 43%, when compared with comparable injuries treated within 2 weeks.[1]

As with all hand injuries with suspicion for PIP joint pathology, physical examination should be performed to assess for deformity, skin integrity, swelling, pain, sensation, and range of motion. Occasionally the PIP joint will have gross deformity to it, such as with lateral dislocations, but frequently the joint is simply swollen and painful, with diminished range of motion.

Three plain radiographic views of the finger should be obtained, including a true lateral view, to assess for joint congruency. Subtle joint incongruity may demonstrate the dorsal "V" sign. Computed tomography (CT) scan may be obtained when there is extensive comminution but is not generally needed. Magnetic resonance imaging (MRI) scan is rarely of any utility in the acute setting.

Positioning and Equipment

The patient is often positioned in the supine position on the operative table with an arm board. The procedure can be done with straight local anesthesia, monitored anesthesia care, regional block, or general anesthesia. Local anesthesia is helpful as active motion can be assessed, and the patient can witness intraoperative motion.

Imaging intensification, with mini C-arm fluoroscopy, is used whenever possible as it has lower radiation dose for the patient and staff, can be operated by the surgeon, and often has improved resolution for the small bones of the hand through beam collimation, when compared with standard C-arm fluoroscopy.[2,3] K-wires of various sizes should be available.

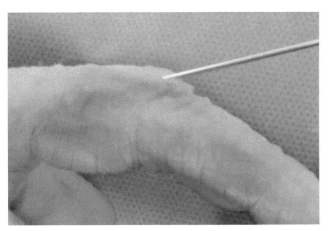

• **Fig. 81.1** Clinical picture demonstrating trajectory of extension block K-wire on a cadaver.

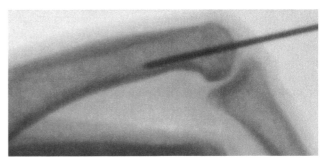

• **Fig. 81.2** Fluoroscopic image of extension block K-wire on a cadaver.

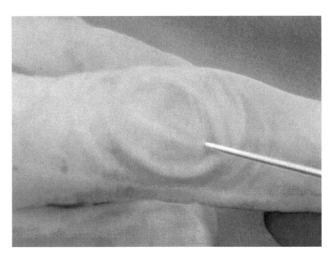

• **Fig. 81.3** Clinical picture demonstrating oblique position of K-wire between the central slip and lateral band on a cadaver.

Technique Description

Closed reduction of the joint should be done with axial traction and dorsal to volar pressure applied to the base of the middle phalanx. Flexion of the PIP joint will help hold the reduction. With the PIP joint held in flexion, one or two K-wires may be placed retrograde, through the dorsal aspect of the joint (Fig. 81.1). Commonly used wire diameters include 1.1 mm (0.045 inch) and 1.4 mm (0.054 inch), depending on the size of the patient and digit. The wire should enter the dorsal aspect of the proximal phalanx at an acute angle, 0 to 31 degrees from the coronal plane, and an attempt should be made to place the wire bicortically to prevent migration (Fig. 81.2).[4] The wire should be placed obliquely, between the central slip and lateral band (Fig. 81.3), sparing the middle phalanx. Static and dynamic imaging should be obtained to ensure the joint maintains reduction after wire placement with active or passive motion. The wire may be bent and cut short, to avoid pressure on the skin, or a rubber or plastic pin cap may be applied; these techniques will help avoid wire migration. After the procedure, the patient is encouraged to perform active finger flexion at the metacarpophalangeal and distal interphalangeal joints, and passive flexion of the PIP joint, to minimize stiffness. The patient may be seen weekly or every 2 weeks for radiographs, motion assessment, and reiteration of motion instructions. The wire is typically removed in the office 3–4 weeks later.

PEARLS AND PITFALLS

- Closed reduction must be obtained prior to placing the wire.
- Appropriate wire size should be used (1.1 or 1.4 mm); small wires may break in the joint.
- Wire migration can occur, bicortical placement minimizes this risk.
- Dynamic fluoroscopy is helpful after wire placement to ensure joint reduction is maintained.
- Finger motion is encouraged after the procedure to minimize stiffness.

ORIF and Hemihamate Arthroplasty

Indications

PIP joint fracture-dislocation ORIF is performed when closed reduction does not achieve a stable, congruent joint. Frequently

an attempt at closed reduction will be done first, and if fracture alignment is satisfactory, with restoration of the volar lip of the base of the middle phalanx, then transarticular or extension block pinning can be performed. If closed reduction does not restore articular alignment, then ORIF should be done.

Preoperative Evaluation

As for extension block pinning.

Positioning and Equipment

As for extension block pinning. K-wires and 1.3- and 1.5-mm cortical screws should be available. The size is dependent on the size of the finger and size of the graft.

Technique Description

A dorsal PIP joint fracture-dislocation is most often addressed with a volar approach to the joint to shotgun it open. The volar incision is outlined from the palmar digital crease to the distal interphalangeal crease. Skin flaps are elevated, protecting and mobilizing the neurovascular bundles as these can be stretched when the joint is "shotgunned" open. A flap of the flexor sheath is created between the distal aspect of the A2 pulley and the proximal aspect of the A4 pulley, exposing the flexor tendons. The flexor digitorum superficialis (FDS) slips can be separated proximally allowing each slip to be reflected. The volar plate is released from the middle phalanx and the collateral ligaments must be released from the proximal phalanx to achieve full exposure of the articular surface of the middle phalanx. The collateral ligaments are left attached to the base of the middle phalanx for future repair of the volar plate. The joint can now be clearly visualized allowing disimpaction and reduction of the fracture. A dental pick is useful to obtain reduction of the fracture fragments. Depending on the size of the fragments, various forms of fixation or replacement can be utilized. Larger fragments are often amenable to small screw fixation. More comminuted fragments are typically stabilized with a cerclage wire around the base of the middle phalanx, volar buttress plate with subchondral screws, or replaced with a graft from the dorsal distal hamate. When screws are used, they are frequently 1.0–1.5 mm in diameter, and care should be exercised to avoid dorsal prominence as these can be easily palpated and can tether the extensor apparatus. A minimum of two screws should be used, or 24- to 26-gauge stainless steel wire for cerclage wiring (Figs. 81.4 and 81.5).

When the volar 50% of the articular surface is involved and comminuted, hemihamate arthroplasty should be considered. The dorsal cortex must be in continuity to create a buttress for the graft (Fig. 81.6). The volar approach is utilized, and the joint is exposed as previously described. The fracture site is then prepared to receive the autograft. A box-shaped portion of bone is removed, using an oscillating saw (Fig. 81.7). Care must be taken not to cut too closely to the dorsal cortex to minimize the risk of fracturing this fragment. The size of the defect of the volar base of the middle phalanx should be carefully measured and recorded, including width, height, and depth.

To harvest the graft, a dorsal approach over the ulnar aspect of the hand is made centered over the fourth and fifth carpometacarpal joints. Imaging may help localize the incision. The dorsal cutaneous branches of the ulnar nerve may be encountered and should be protected. The carpometacarpal joint capsule is opened with a transverse incision. The distal hamate is now exposed. The distal ridge of the hamate, which lies between the fourth and fifth metacarpal bases, will be the center of the graft (Fig. 81.8). The graft size should now be outlined on the dorsal hamate. When performing the osteotomy, adequate and equal depth of the graft should be achieved. This is very important as the depth of the graft is vital to restore the volar lip of the base of middle phalanx. A frequent mistake is to create a thin or obliquely oriented graft. A trough in the proximal portion of the hamate can be made to facilitate graft extraction and avoid these complications.[5] Furthermore, the

dorsal base of the fourth and fifth metacarpals can be partially removed to improve ease of graft extraction without additional

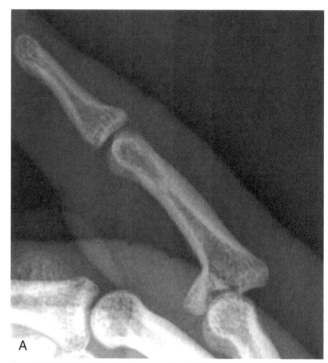

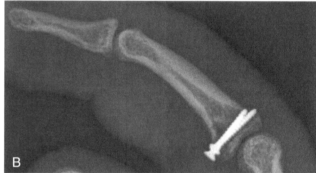

• **Fig. 81.4** A 17-year-old male who underwent open reduction internal fixation of an unstable proximal interphalangeal joint dorsal fracture-dislocation using 1.3-mm screws. (A) Pre-op X-ray. (B) Post-op X-ray.

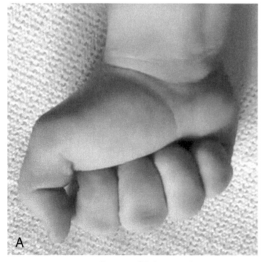
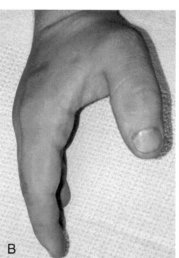
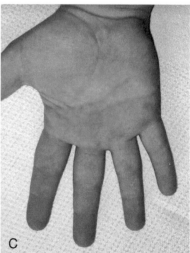

• **Fig. 81.5** Clinical motion 1 year later. (A-C) Clinical photographs of patient's motion whose radiographs are shown in Fig 81.4.

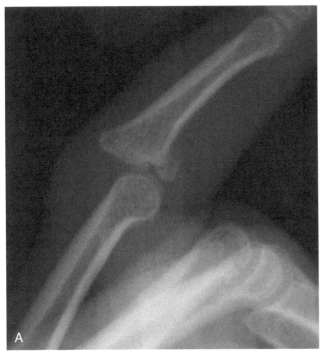

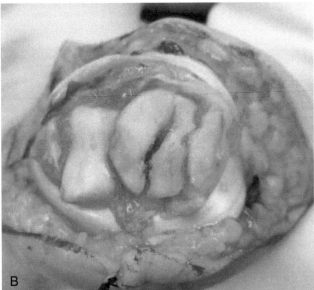

• **Fig. 81.6** Lateral radiograph (A) and clinical photograph (B) demonstrating base of middle phalanx fracture with >50% articular involvement.

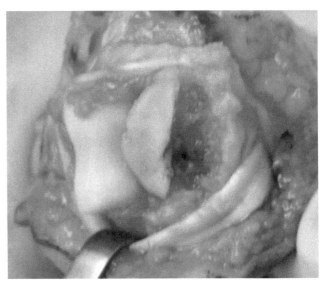

• **Fig. 81.7** Hemihamate fracture-site preparation.

seen about 5 days following the procedure and radiographs of the finger are obtained to confirm appropriate reduction of the joint and fixation of the graft. The patient is referred to a hand therapist for a wrist orthosis and figure-eight finger orthosis to block the final 20 degrees of extension. A therapy and home exercise program begins with edema control using an elastic bandage and active flexion and extension of all joints in the finger.

PEARLS AND PITFALLS

- ORIF can be performed when the fracture pattern is simple with minimal comminution.
- Devascularized fracture fragments can go on the avascular necrosis; maintain soft tissue attachments when possible.
- Be prepared to convert ORIF to hemihamate arthroplasty if extensive comminution precludes ORIF.
- Extensive comminution, involvement of >50% of the articular surface, and chronic injuries are often amenable to hemihamate arthroplasty.
- For hemihamate arthroplasty, the graft must have appropriate dimensions to adequately recreate the volar lip of the middle phalanx, and a trough in the proximal hamate, as well as removing the dorsal base of the fourth and fifth metacarpals, may help facilitate this.
- The cartilage of the hamate is thicker than that of the base of the middle phalanx, giving the appearance of articular step-off on radiographs.
- With stable fixation, early active motion should be encouraged to prevent finger stiffness.

---

graft site morbidity.[6] A small oscillating saw is used to harvest the graft, and a curved osteotome may be used to make the final coronal cut to the graft. The graft should be measured to be just larger than required and then trimmed to fit the fracture site (Fig. 81.9).

Once the graft is obtained, it should be inset in the correct orientation to recreate the volar lip of the base of the middle phalanx. Fixation can be obtained with two small screws (Figs. 81.10 and 81.11). The cartilage of the distal hamate is thicker than the cartilage of the base of middle phalanx (0.73 vs. 0.40 mm, respectively), and while the graft may look congruent on clinical examination, it may have an apparent step-off on radiographs due to this mismatch.[7] Closure is completed with reattachment of the volar plate to the remnant cuff of collateral ligaments, and by placing the flap of flexor sheath deep to the flexor tendons. The skin is closed, and a postoperative splint is applied. The patient is

Dynamic External Fixation

Indications

PIP joint dynamic external fixation is reserved for injuries not amenable to other techniques. This often includes pilon fractures, where extensive articular comminution makes internal fixation challenging, if not impossible. It is also commonly used when both the dorsal and volar cortex are fractured and is our preferred treatment in patients with early arthritis where stiffness is already a concern.

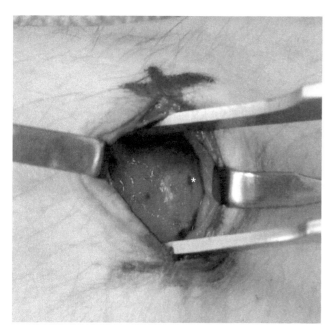

• **Fig. 81.8** Hemihamate graft harvest site. Note the distal ridge of the hamate graft *(star)*.

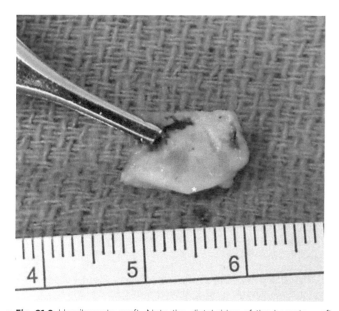

• **Fig. 81.9** Hemihamate graft. Note the distal ridge of the hamate graft *(star)*.

Preoperative Evaluation

As for extension block pinning. These injury patterns often benefit from preoperative CT scan.

Positioning and Equipment

As for extension block pinning. K-wires and orthodontic elastics (dental rubber bands) should be available. While there are some implant systems specifically designed for this, it is most common to make a "homemade" dynamic external fixation with K-wires, possibly augmented with dental rubber bands.

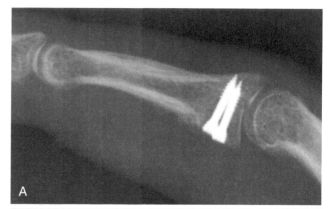

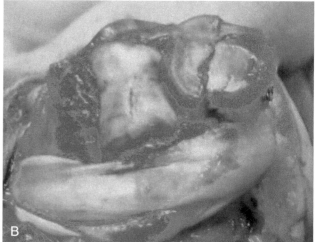

• **Fig. 81.10** Proximal interphalangeal joint hemihamate arthroplasty with graft inset. Note appearance of step-off in the joint—this is due to the difference in thickness of cartilage on hamate and middle phalanx. (A) Post-op radiograph. (B) Intraoperative picture of graft in place.

Technique Description

There are two common designs for PIP joint dynamic external fixation: with or without dental rubber bands. The following technique, first described by Hynes and Giddins in 2001,[8] and subsequently by Badia and colleagues,[9] does not require the addition of rubber bands and is thought to be a simpler design with higher reproducibility. This technique is best for pilon fractures with minimal to no dorsal subluxation. When subluxation is present, a third wire can be used to provide a volar-directed force to the middle phalanx and distraction provided with rubber bands as popularized by Joe Slade.[10]

Under image intensification, a 1.1- or 1.4 mm K-wire is placed through the center of rotation of the head of the proximal phalanx. The wire must be perpendicular to the shaft of the proximal phalanx (Fig. 81.12). A second K-wire is placed through the distal third of the middle phalanx, also perpendicular to the shaft (Fig. 82.13). The proximal wire is then bent at 90 degrees on each side, leaving space between the wire and skin to accommodate swelling. Too much space will cause the fixator to impinge on adjacent digits. With traction on the finger to distract the joint, the proximal wire is bent dorsally and then volarly to create a dorsal hook for the distal wire, maintaining distraction of the joint (Figs. 81.14 and 81.15). Imaging should be performed to demonstrate a reduced joint. If needed, a percutaneous or open approach can be done to improve the alignment of major fracture fragments.

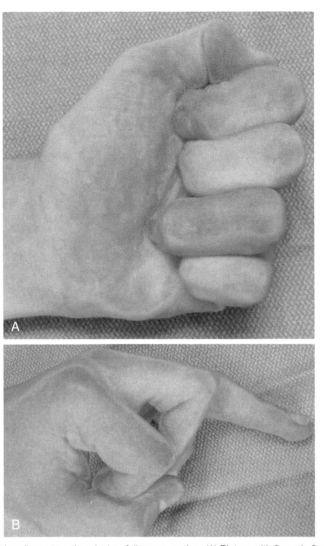

• **Fig. 81.11** Proximal interphalangeal joint hemihamate arthroplasty—follow-up motion. (A) Picture with finger in flexion. (B) Picture with finger in extension.

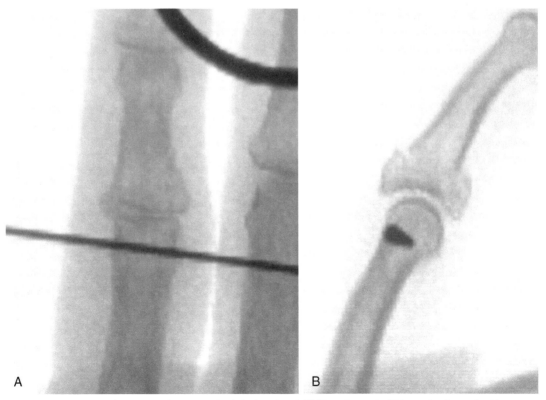

• **Fig. 81.12** K-wire centered in the proximal phalanx head. (A) PA radiograph. (B) Lateral radiograph with K-wire in place.

In the event that there is dorsal or volar subluxation, a third wire is placed in the proximal third of the middle phalanx, perpendicular to the middle phalanx shaft. This third wire is placed dorsal (for dorsal fracture-dislocations) to create a volar-directed force to maintain reduction of the joint. In this situation, the proximal wire is bent similarly and the dental rubber bands are used between the proximal and distal wires to maintain the distraction of the joint. The patient may, thereafter, move the joint actively. This technique requires close follow-up to monitor the construct. The fixator is typically left in place for 4–6 weeks.

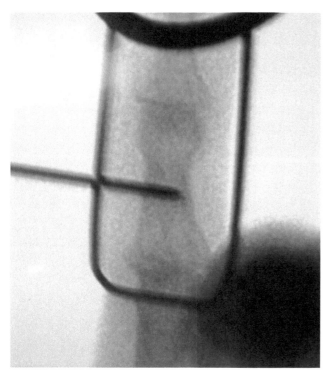

• **Fig. 81.13** Second K-wire placed in the middle phalanx. Note 90-degree bend on the proximal wire.

PEARLS AND PITFALLS

- K-wires should be long enough to create the construct, and sharp on both ends.
- Nine-inch wires are generally used for the proximal wire, and 6-inch wires for the distal and middle phalanx.
- K-wire placement must be perfect (center of rotation of the proximal phalanx head) to realign the joint anatomically and allow motion.
- The distal K-wire may be placed slightly dorsal to the axis of the middle phalanx to create a volar fulcrum to align the joint (similar to third "fulcrum" wire if rubber bands are used).
- Fixators should only be placed on patients who will be compliant and able to tolerate them.
- The fixator can easily be caught on clothes and other objects leading to failure, and close follow-up is needed.
- Infection is possible and diligent pin care is required.

Conclusion

These are just a few of the many techniques that can be used to operatively treat a PIP joint dislocation or fracture-dislocation. Whenever the patient is brought to the operative room, a "bailout" procedure should be anticipated should primary intervention be unsuccessful. The procedures are technically demanding and while joint reduction is essential, it is even more important to have close follow-up and hand therapy referral to optimize motion and hand function.

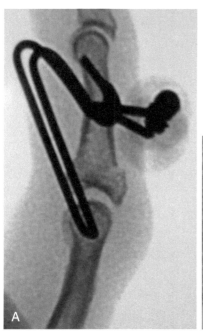
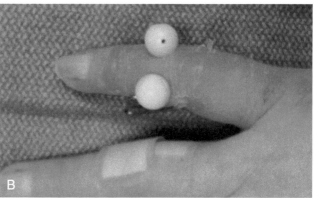

• **Fig. 81.14** Final dynamic external fixator construct. (A) Radiograph with external fixator in position demonstrating congruent joint. (B) Clinical picture with external fixator in place.

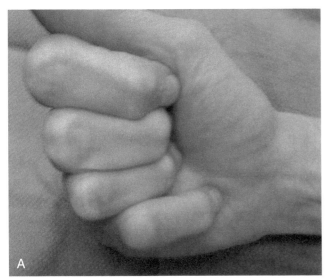

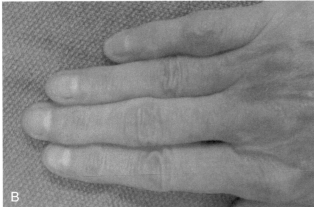

• **Fig. 81.15** Proximal interphalangeal joint dynamic external fixator—long-term follow-up motion. (A) A. Clinical picture of finger in flexion and (B) finger in extension.

References

1. Grant I, Berger AC, Tham SKY. Internal fixation of unstable fracture dislocations of the proximal interphalangeal joint. *J Hand Surg.* 2005;30(5):492–498.
2. Giordano BD, Baumhauer JF, Morgan TL, Rechtine GR. Patient and surgeon radiation exposure: comparison of standard and mini-C-arm fluoroscopy. *J Bone Joint Surg-Am Vol.* 2009;91(2):297–304.
3. Rappard JRMV, Hummel WA, Jong TD, Mouës CM. A comparison of image quality and radiation exposure between the mini C-arm and the standard C-arm. *Hand.* 2018;14(6):765–769.
4. Waris E, Mattila S, Sillat T, Karjalainen T. Extension block pinning for unstable proximal interphalangeal joint dorsal fracture dislocations. *J Hand Surg.* 2016;41(2):196–202.
5. Calfee R, Kiefhaber T, Sommerkamp T, Stern P. Hemi-hamate arthroplasty provides functional reconstruction of acute and chronic proximal interphalangeal fracture-dislocations. *J Hand Surg.* 2009;34(7):1232–1241.
6. Denoble PH, Record NC. A modification to simplify the harvest of a hemi-hamate autograft. *J Hand Surg.* 2016;41(5):e99–e102.
7. Podolsky DJ, Mainprize J, McMillan C, Binhammer P. Suitability of using the hamate for reconstruction of the finger middle phalanx base: an assessment of cartilage thickness. *Plast Surg.* 2019;27(3):211–216.
8. Hynes MC, Giddins GEB. Dynamic external fixation for pilon fractures of the interphalangeal joints. *J Hand Surg.* 2001;26(2):122–124.
9. Badia A, Riano F, Ravikoff J, Khouri R, Gonzalez-Hernandez E, Orbay JL. Dynamic intradigital external fixation for proximal interphalangeal joint fracture dislocations. *J Hand Surg.* 2005;30(1):154–160.
10. Ruland RT, Hogan CJ, Cannon DL, Slade JF. Use of dynamic distraction external fixation for unstable fracture-dislocations of the proximal interphalangeal joint. *J Hand Surg.* 2008;33(1):19–25.

Page numbers followed by "f" indicate figures, "t" indicate tables, and "b" indicate boxes.